D1345930

Cardiac Nuclear Medicine

NOTICE

Medicine is an ever-changing science. As new research and clinical experience broaden our knowledge, changes in treatment and drug therapy are required. The editor and the publisher of this work have checked with sources believed to be reliable in their efforts to provide information that is complete and generally in accord with the standards accepted at the time of publication. However, in view of the possibility of human error or changes in medical sciences, neither the editor nor the publisher nor any other party who has been involved in the preparation or publication of this work warrants that the information contained herein is in every respect accurate or complete. Readers are encouraged to confirm the information contained herein with other sources. For example and in particular, readers are advised to check the product information sheet included in the package of each drug they plan to administer to be certain that the information contained in this book is accurate and that changes have not been made in the recommended dose or in the contraindications for administration. This recommendation is of particular importance in connection with new or infrequently used drugs.

Cardiac Nuclear Medicine

THIRD EDITION

Editor

Myron C. Gerson, M.D.
Professor of Medicine
Associate Professor of Radiology
Division of Cardiology
University of Cincinnati Medical Center
Cincinnati, Ohio

McGraw-Hill
Health Professions Division

New York St. Louis San Francisco Auckland
Bogotá Caracas Lisbon London Madrid
Mexico City Milan Montreal New Delhi San Juan
Singapore Sydney Tokyo Toronto

McGraw-Hill

A Division of The **McGraw·Hill** *Companies*

Cardiac Nuclear Medicine, 3/e

1234567890 KGPKGP 9876

ISBN 0-07-032848-X

This book was set in Sabon Roman by Bi-Comp, Inc.
The editors were James T. Morgan and Peter J. Boyle;
the production supervisor was Richard Ruzycka;
the cover designer was Matthew Dvorozniak;
the indexer was Tony Greenberg, M.D.
Quebecor Printing/Kingsport was printer and binder.

This book is printed on acid-free paper.

Cataloging-in-publication data is on file for this book at the Library of Congress.

To Joanne
    with thanks for your support and understanding

CONTENTS

CONTRIBUTORS*

James A. Arrighi, M.D. [5]
Assistant Professor of Medicine and Diagnostic
  Radiology
Yale University School of Medicine
New Haven, Connecticut

Thomas M. Bashore, M.D. [15]
Professor of Medicine
Director, Cardiac Catheterization Laboratory
Duke University Medical Center
Durham, North Carolina

Steven R. Bergmann, M.D., Ph.D. [9]
Professor of Medicine and Radiology
Cardiovascular Division
College of Physicians and Surgeons
Columbia University
New York, New York

Ajit R. Bhagwat, M.D. [17]
Fellow in Cardiovascular Diseases
Division of Cardiology
University of Cincinnati
Cincinnati, Ohio

Danuta Biniakiewicz, Ph.D. [1]
Research Assistant Professor of Radiology
E. L. Saenger Radioisotope Laboratory
University of Cincinnati
Cincinnati, Ohio

Elias H. Botvinick, M.D. [13]
Professor of Medicine and Radiology
Cardiovascular Division
University of California, San Francisco Medical Center
San Francisco, California

Kenneth A. Brown, M.D. [23]
Professor of Medicine
Director, Nuclear Cardiology
Division of Cardiology
University of Vermont
College of Medicine
Burlington, Vermont

Robert W. Burt, M.D. [8]
Professor of Radiology
Director, Nuclear Medicine
Indiana University School of Medicine
Indianapolis, Indiana

Michael W. Dae, M.D. [13,29]
Professor of Radiology and Medicine
Department of Nuclear Medicine
University of California School of Medicine
San Francisco, California

E. Gordon DePuey, M.D. [4]
Professor of Radiology
Columbia University
College of Physicians and Surgeons
Director, Division of Nuclear Medicine
Dept. of Radiology, St. Luke's-Roosevelt Hospital
New York, New York

Vasken Dilsizian, M.D. [5]
Senior Investigator and Director of Nuclear
  Cardiology
National Heart, Lung and Blood Institute
Bethesda, Maryland

Claire S. Duvernoy [24]
Cardiology Trainee
Division of Cardiology
University of Michigan Medical Center
Ann Arbor, Michigan

*The numbers in brackets following the contributor name refer to chapter(s) authored or co-authored by the contributor.

Daniel Edmundowicz, M.D.   [25]
Assistant Professor of Medicine
Division of Cardiology
University of Pittsburgh Medical Center
Pittsburgh, Pennsylvania

Tracy L. Faber, Ph.D.   [3]
Assistant Professor of Radiology
Emory University School of Medicine
Atlanta, Georgia

Michael W. Farrar, M.D.   [17]
Assistant Professor of Clinical Medicine
University of Missouri-Kansas City
Kansas City, Missouri

William P. Follansbee, M.D.   [6,25]
Professor of Medicine & Radiology
Director, Nuclear Cardiology
University of Pittsburgh
Pittsburgh, Pennsylvania

Michael J. Gelfand, M.D.   [27]
Professor of Radiology and Pediatrics
Director, Pediatric Nuclear Medicine
Children's Hospital Medical Center
Cincinnati, Ohio

Myron C. Gerson, M.D.   [1,2,12,18,20,21]
Professor of Medicine and Radiology
Director, Nuclear Cardiology and Exercise Laboratory
University of Cincinnati
Cincinnati, Ohio

David W. Hannon, M.D.   [27]
Associate Professor of Pediatrics
Director, Pediatric Cardiology
East Carolina University School of Medicine
Greenville, North Carolina

Christopher L. Hansen, M.D.   [7]
Associate Professor of Medicine
Section of Cardiology
Temple University Health Science Center
Philadelphia, Pennsylvania

Brian D. Hoit, M.D.   [21]
Professor of Medicine
Director, Echocardiographic Laboratory
Division of Cardiology
University of Cincinnati
Cincinnati, Ohio

James M. Hurst, M.D.   [26]
Professor of Surgery
Vice Chairman/Clinical Department of Surgery
University of Cincinnati
Cincinnati, Ohio

Diwakar Jain, M.D.   [16]
Assistant Professor of Medicine
Section of Cardiovascular Medicine
Yale University School of Medicine
New Haven, Connecticut

Jay A. Johanigman, M.D.   [26]
Assistant Professor
Department of Surgery
University of Cincinnati
Cincinnati, Ohio

Daniel J. Lenihan, M.D.   [15,18]
Assistant Professor
Uniformed Services University for the Health Sciences
Director, Coronary Care Unit
Wright-Patterson AFB, Ohio

Anthony McGoron, Ph.D.   [1]
Assistant Professor of Radiology
University of Cincinnati
Cincinnati, Ohio

Ronald W. Millard, Ph.D.   [1]
Professor of Pharmacology and Cell Biophysics
Professor of Radiology
University of Cincinnati
Cincinnati, Ohio

D. Douglas Miller, M.D.   [22]
Associate Professor of Medicine
Director, Nuclear Cardiology
Division of Cardiology
St. Louis University Medical Center
St. Louis, Missouri

Anthony P. Morise, M.D.   [19]
Professor of Medicine
Division of Cardiology, West Virginia University
Morgantown, West Virginia

J. William O'Connell, B.S.   [13]
Director, Nuclear Medicine Computer Facility
University of California Medical Center
San Francisco, California

Ronald Rohe, Ph.D.   [12]
Assistant Professor of Radiology
E. L. Saenger Radioisotope Laboratory
University of Cincinnati
Cincinnati, Ohio

Nancy Roszell, M.S.   [1]
Doctoral Candidate
Department of Pharmacology and Cell Biophysics
University of Cincinnati
Cincinnati, Ohio

Mark R. Starling, M.D.   [24]
Professor of Medicine
Chief, Cardiology Section
Veterans Affairs Medical Center
Ann Arbor, Michigan

John R. Stratton, M.D.   [28]
Professor of Medicine
Cadiovascular Disease Section
University of Washington School of Medicine
Seattle, Washington

Frans J. Th. Wackers, M.D.   [10,11,14]
Professor of Radiology and Medicine
Director, Cardiovascular Nuclear Imaging and
    Exercise Laboratories
Yale University School of Medicine
New Haven, Connecticut

Barry L. Zaret, M.D.   [14,16]
Robert W. Berliner Professor of Medicine
Professor of Diagnostic Radiology
Chief, Section of Cardiovascular Medicine
Yale University School of Medicine
New Haven, Connecticut

PREFACE

Cardiac nuclear medicine procedures provide a practical approach to the diagnostic and prognostic assessment of patients with suspected coronary artery disease. Furthermore, recent data suggest that in some patient subsets, noninvasive stress radionuclide testing is a more cost-effective approach to the diagnosis of patients with chest pain compared to initial invasive strategies. Progress in the noninvasive detection of coronary artery disease has not, however, been limited to the scintigraphic approach—particular progress has been made with stress echocardiography. To maintain a dominant role of nuclear imaging in the noninvasive detection of coronary disease, continuing advances in the radionuclide approach are essential. Recent advances have come in the areas of 1) new radiotracer development, 2) improved nuclear medicine instrumentation, 3) documentation of the prognostic implications of scintigraphic assessment of myocardial ischemia, and 4) accurate prediction of myocardial viability. Future advances will also be essential in further documenting the cost-effectiveness of nuclear cardiology. Progress is needed in the use of radioisotopes to characterize systolic and diastolic ventricular function, atherosclerotic plaque, intravascular thrombus, and autonomic influences on the heart.

The third edition of *Cardiac Nuclear Medicine* provides extensive new information concerning advances in the field. It also provides a renewed emphasis on the interpretation of myocardial perfusion images and radionuclide studies of ventricular function. The fundamental mission of the book remains unchanged—to provide information to clinicians to allow knowledgeable cardiac test selection and test result interpretation so that patient care will be benefitted.

The first six chapters provide a detailed examination of methods used for myocardial perfusion imaging. A new chapter on radiopharmaceuticals reviews the properties of clinically available and emerging ^{99m}Tc myocardial perfusion imaging agents and compares these tracers to one another and to ^{201}Tl. Following a detailed chapter on interpretation of planar myocardial perfusion images, there follows a review of instrumentation for SPECT (single-photon emission computed tomography) including principles of attenuation and scatter correction.

Chapter 4 provides a step-by-step approach to the interpretation of myocardial perfusion tomograms. Identification of SPECT artifacts, use of functional images (e.g. bull's-eye displays), and interpretation of gated ^{99m}Tc tomograms are emphasized.

This is followed by a detailed review of myocardial imaging in the assessment of tissue viability and a discussion of methods alternative to dynamic leg exercise for identification of myocardial ischemia. Chapters 7 through 9 focus on the assessment of myocardial metabolism through the use of fatty acid tracers, SPECT imaging of ^{18}F fluorodeoxyglucose, and positron emission tomography.

The following eight chapters deal with methods for radionuclide assessment of ventricular function by blood-pool imaging. A new chapter on equilibrium gated blood-pool imaging is provided, including illustration of scintigraphic findings in coronary artery disease, valvular heart disease, cardiomyopathy, pericardial disease, hypertensive heart disease, and aortic disease. This is followed by chapters reviewing radionuclide assessment of left ventricular volumes, phase imaging, assessment of right ventricular function, diastolic left ventricular function, ambulatory monitoring of left ventricular function, and assessment of left ventricular response to pharmacologic therapy.

The remaining chapters focus on clinical applications of nuclear cardiology in specific diseases or pathophysiologic states. The basis for radioisotope test selection is examined in patients with coronary artery disease, with separate chapters considering patients presenting to the emergency department or the coronary care unit, evaluation of patients following acute myocardial infarction, the work-up in the exercise laboratory of patients with symptoms of chronic coronary artery disease, and assessment following coronary artery revascularization. Chapter 21 compares directly the diagnostic strengths and weaknesses of stress nuclear imaging to stress echocardiography. Assessment of patient prognosis by radionuclide imaging and by stress echocardiography is considered in Chapter 23. Chapters 24 through 29 review the use of radionuclide testing in valvular heart disease, cardiomyopathy, cardiac trauma, congenital heart disease, detection of intra-cardiac thrombi, and assessment of autonomic innervation.

Nineteen of the 29 chapters in the third edition of *Cardiac Nuclear Medicine* are either new chapters or have been extensively re-written. The remaining chap-ters, most of which deal with specialized areas of gated blood-pool imaging, have been updated. This textbook is designed for cardiologists, radiologists, and nuclear medicine physicians in training, but should be of substan-tial interest to practicing physicians in these fields.

Cardiac Nuclear Medicine

MYOCARDIAL PERFUSION IMAGING

Myocardial Perfusion Imaging: Radiopharmaceuticals and Tracer Kinetics

Myron C. Gerson
Anthony McGoron
Nancy Roszell
Danuta Biniakiewicz
Ronald W. Millard

Myocardial perfusion scintigraphy is widely used in the evaluation of patients with known or suspected coronary artery disease (CAD). The extensive clinical use of stress myocardial perfusion imaging has resulted largely from its demonstrated improved diagnostic sensitivity and specificity for detection of CAD compared to the exercise electrocardiogram.[1] The myocardial perfusion scintigram can also reveal the functional consequence of an anatomic coronary artery stenosis demonstrated by coronary arteriography and can differentiate viable myocardium from myocardial scar. However, unlike the coronary arteriogram, the myocardial scintigram is used to examine the heart at the myocardial level and may also demonstrate abnormal myocardial blood flow related to myocardial processes such as cardiac metastases or granulomas.

Thallium 201 (^{201}Tl) has been the principal tracer used for myocardial perfusion imaging over the last two decades. Recently, numerous myocardial perfusion tracers have been developed that use to advantage the favorable physical imaging properties of technetium 99m (^{99m}Tc). When comparing the strengths and weaknesses of different myocardial radiotracers, it is helpful to consider the biological and physical properties that would characterize an ideal myocardial imaging agent (Table 1-1). A brief review of some of the information derived from animal models used to evaluate new tracers is also instructive.

WHOLE ANIMAL MODELS

The relationship between initial myocardial distribution of a myocardial perfusion tracer and corresponding regional myocardial blood flow has been assessed in anesthetized canine and porcine models. A wide range of blood flows can be induced in an individual heart by occluding a coronary artery to produce a central zone of profound ischemia surrounded by zones of progressively less severe ischemia. Substantially increased blood flow can be produced in nonischemic areas in the same heart by intravenous infusion of a potent coronary artery vasodilator, usually dipyridamole or adenosine.[2] Myocardial blood flow at the time of injection of the myocardial perfusion tracer may be quantitated by injection of radiolabeled microspheres into the left atrium. The microspheres mix in the blood in the left ventricular cavity, and on ventricular ejection, enter the coronary arteries. The microspheres become trapped in a small fraction (less than 0.1 percent) of myocardial precapillary arterioles in direct relationship to regional myocardial blood flow. A reference sample of arterial blood must be withdrawn into a syringe (which serves as a surrogate organ) at a fixed withdrawal rate concurrent with microsphere injection followed by measurement of the concentration of microspheres (activity) in the syringe. Following euthanasia of the animal, the heart is sectioned, and both

Table 1-1   Properties of an Ideal Myocardial Perfusion Tracer

1. Uptake like a chemical microsphere (i.e., uptake closely related to myocardial blood flow over a wide range of normal, ischemic, and augmented flows)
2. Prompt uptake under temporary hemodynamic conditions, including peak exercise (i.e., high extraction fraction)
3. Negligible interference with myocardial visualization from adjacent organs and tissues (i.e., Compton scatter)
4. No significant attenuation of myocardial tracer activity by tissues between the heart and the activity detector
5. Constant location and concentration of tracer in the myocardium during image acquisition
6. Lack of interference with tracer uptake into the myocardium by pharmacologic agents or impaired myocardial metabolism
7. High photon flux detectable on standard imaging equipment
8. Low tracer cost
9. High tracer safety
10. Rapid tracer availability for imaging patients with acute chest pain syndromes

microsphere concentration (activity) and myocardial perfusion tracer activity per gram of myocardium are counted in a well counter. The ratio of the rate of blood flow into the syringe to the number of microspheres (activity) in the syringe is equal to the ratio of blood flow to the myocardium divided by the number of microspheres (activity) in the myocardial sample. Therefore, myocardial blood flow per gram of myocardium may be calculated from the measured concentrations (activity) of microspheres in the myocardium and in the syringe, together with the reference syringe (surrogate organ) arterial blood withdrawal rate.[3] This approach allows comparison of the myocardial perfusion tracer activity per gram of myocardium to the corresponding myocardial blood flow per gram of myocardium for each myocardial sample (Fig. 1-1A).

After initial uptake of a myocardial perfusion radiotracer, the subsequent kinetic properties of the tracer over time can be characterized using an open-chest anesthetized animal. Transient or a constant reduction in coronary blood flow can be produced by coronary artery occlusion. Flow through an unobstructed coronary artery can be maximized by pharmacologic coronary artery vasodilation at the time of injection of the myocardial perfusion agent. Flow may then be allowed to gradually return to baseline levels. With this type of model, tracer activity in the myocardium can be monitored continuously with either external or directly implanted scintillation counters.[2] Alternatively, radioactivity may be counted from biopsy samples removed directly from the myocardium at various times following tracer injection.[4] A perfusion tracer that "washes out" of the myocardium would be expected to decrease in myocardial concentration over time (beyond the decrease in activity resulting from physical decay of the tracer). Perfusion tracers that do not wash out of the myocardium over time will have a constant myocardial concentration. In the myocardial region supplied by a stenotic coronary artery, tracer activity may increase over time relative to myocardial regions supplied by normal coronary arteries, indicating differential tracer washout or actual tracer redistribution. Activity in all regions may also remain unchanged if no washout or redistribution of tracer occurs.

Clearance of a myocardial perfusion imaging agent from the blood by target and nontarget organs alike can also be assessed in an intact animal model. For such assessment, disappearance of a tracer from the circulation may be quantitated from serial blood samples withdrawn following tracer injection. Specific organ instantaneous extraction fraction of tracer may also be evaluated by securing time-matched blood samples from inflow artery and outflow vein.

Data from Whole Animal Models

An example of a relationship in a canine model between (absolute) myocardial blood flow on the x-axis and ^{99m}Tc counts per gram of myocardium (normalized) on the y-axis is shown in Fig. 1-1A. The correlation of tracer activity and myocardial blood flow is high ($r = 0.94$) and statistically significant ($p < 0.01$). However, for each increment in myocardial blood flow, the increment in tracer activity is modest, yielding a slope of the relationship of 0.46. The graph is based on 27 myocardial samples from a single animal and ^{99m}Tc counts per gram have been normalized to the mean number of counts per gram for the entire ventricular myocardium.

In Fig. 1-1B, data from 7 animals studied with the same tracer as in Fig. 1-1A have been combined to provide data from 315 postmortem tissue samples. The resultant data provide greater statistical certainty in characterizing the relationship of tracer activity and myocardial blood flow. The relationship is characterized over a range of myocardial blood flow from 0 to 8 ml/min/g of myocardium. A high correlation ($r = 0.88$) of tracer activity to myocardial blood flow is again demonstrated when data from 0 to 2 ml/min/g blood flow are analyzed. However, normalized ^{99m}Tc counts per gram reach a plateau as a myocardial blood flow of 2 ml/min/g is reached. This is referred to as a "roll-off" phenomenon. It is also noted that in myocardial regions with very low levels of myocardial blood flow from microsphere measurements that normalized ^{99m}Tc counts per gram are higher than expected for the tracer under evaluation, resulting in a y-intercept of 0.35. This commonly observed phenomenon may reflect overextraction of perfusion tracer by myocardial regions served by very low levels of blood flow.

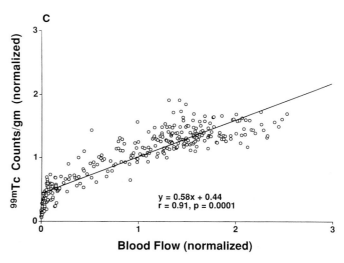

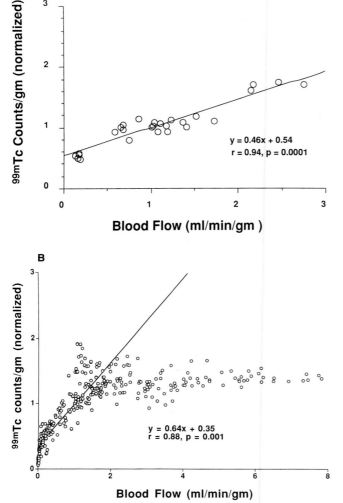

Figure 1-1 **A:** Plot of [99mTc] counts per gram of myocardium, normalized to the mean number of counts per gram in the entire left ventricle, versus myocardial blood flow in ml/min/g in each tissue sample. Samples are from a single animal. **B:** Plot of [99mTc] counts per gram of myocardium versus myocardial blood flow in ml/min/g. The [99mTc] counts have been normalized to the mean number of counts per gram in the entire left ventricle facilitating combination of data from seven different animals. **C:** Plot of [99mTc] counts per gram (normalized) versus myocardial blood flow, which has now also been normalized for each animal to the mean myocardial blood flow to the left ventricle. (Adapted from Gerson et al,[4] by permission of the American Heart Association, Inc.)

Figure 1-1C presents data from the same 7 animals shown in Fig. 1-1B. Myocardial blood flow (x-axis) has now been normalized within each heart sample to the mean myocardial blood flow for the heart samples from a given animal by the method of Bassingthwaighte et al.[5] Displayed in this manner, a linear relationship of normalized [99mTc] tracer counts per gram to normalized myocardial blood flow is suggested over a broad range of flows. However, it is also apparent that different methods of data normalization can also modify the slopes, intercepts, and correlation coefficients that characterize these data plots. The importance of comparing tracer activity versus myocardial blood flow plots using the same methods of data normalization is illustrated by these examples. Such analysis is necessary when attempts are made to contrast properties of different tracers.

Results of myocardial tracer kinetic studies are illus-

trated by Figs. 1-2 and 1-3. As effects of pharmacologic coronary artery vasodilation dissipate in the distribution of the left anterior descending (LAD) coronary artery, coronary blood flow decreases significantly over 4 h (see Fig. 1-2). Myocardial blood flow in the ischemic left circumflex artery distribution is severely reduced initially and remains reduced over time due to a sustained induced stenosis. Figure 1-3 shows that endocardial activity of a [99mTc] tracer measured by serial direct subendocardial tissue biopsies did not change over 4 h following tracer injection. This demonstrates lack of statistically significant washout for this [99mTc] tracer from myocardium with high (vasodilated) or low (ischemic) blood flow.

Figure 1-4 illustrates clearance of a [99mTc] myocardial perfusion tracer from the central circulation after intravenous injection. In this example, clearance of the [99mTc] perfusion tracer from the circulating blood volume was

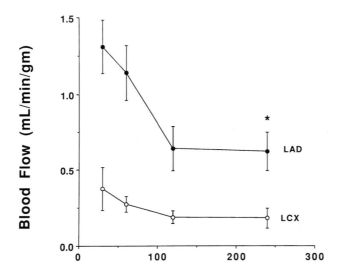

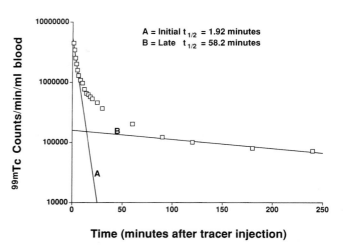

Figure 1-4 Clearance of a 99mTc myocardial tracer from the blood following intravenous injection. Blood clearance in this canine model was biexponential with initial half-time of 1.92 min and late half-time of 58.2 min.

Figure 1-2 Plot of transmural myocardial blood flow measured by radiolabeled microspheres in nine animals from 30 to 240 minutes following injection of a 99mTc myocardial tracer. Myocardial blood flow in the territory of the left anterior descending (LAD) coronary artery decreased significantly from 30 to 240 min following tracer injection (*p < 0.05) as dipyridamole-induced vasodilation dissipated. Myocardial blood flow in the distribution of the left circumflex (LCX) artery was reduced by a hydraulic occluder and remained unchanged over time. (Adapted from Gerson et al,[6] Myocardial uptake and kinetic properties of technetum-99m-Q3 in dogs, reprinted with permission from the *Journal of Nuclear Medicine* 35:1968, 1994.)

rapid and biexponential with an initial clearance half-time of 1.9 min.

ISOLATED PERFUSED HEART MODELS

Uptake of a perfusion tracer into the myocardium is determined by coronary blood flow and the extraction fraction of the tracer by the myocardium. The extraction fraction can be accurately assessed in the isolated perfused rodent or rabbit heart.[7] With the Langendorff preparation, the isolated heart is suspended on a stand (Fig. 1-5) and perfused retrograde through the aorta at constant pressure or flow.[7] The heart may be perfused with a buffered electrolyte solution but high Po_2 and high coronary flow are required to provide neccessary myocardial tissue oxygen delivery. Myocardial oxygen demand can be obtained at more physiologic coronary blood flows and near normal Po_2 if the perfusate is an erythrocyte-containing solution. Heart rate may be regulated by electrical pacing. The isolated perfused heart provides a number of advantages for measurement of tracer kinetics compared to whole animal models. Physiologic parameters including coronary flow, cardiac work, substrate availability, and drug delivery can be controlled independently under baseline conditions and in response to pharmacologic or physiologic intervention. In some cases, baseline measurements and serial responses to interventions may be compared in the same heart. In addition, the coronary venous effluent can be collected for assessment of tracer extraction or transit through the heart. Alternatively, tracer "residue" in the

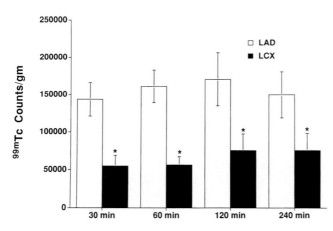

Figure 1-3 Counts of 99mTc per gram of myocardium from Cope needle myocardial biopsies taken from the left anterior descending (LAD) and left circumflex (LCX) coronary artery territories at 30, 60, 120, and 240 min following tracer injection. Although myocardial blood flow decreased in the LAD territory and remained constant in the LCX territory over this time interval (see Fig. 1-2), there was no change in 99mTc counts per gram over time in either coronary artery distribution for the six animals studied. The findings are consistent with absence of tracer redistribution over 3½ h. (Adapted from Gerson et al,[6] Myocardial uptake and kinetic properties of technetrium-99m-Q3 in dogs, reprinted with permission from the *Journal of Nuclear Medicine* 35:1968, 1994).

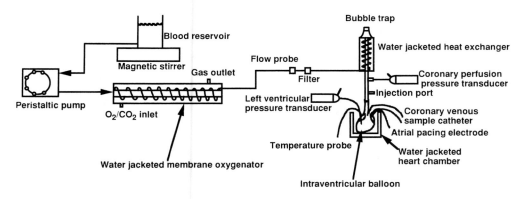

Figure 1-5 Constant flow Langendorff isolated heart perfusion apparatus.

myocardium may be directly monitored with radiation detectors placed externally over the heart.[8]

When a diffusible tracer is added to the coronary artery inflow of the isolated heart, a fraction of the tracer is extracted by the myocardium, and a fraction of the tracer is present in the coronary venous effluent. Extraction of tracer from the coronary vascular space can be determined by a multiple tracer indicator-dilution technique.[7,8] This method uses an intravascular reference tracer, such as indium 111 (^{111}In)-labeled albumin, which passes through the coronary circulation without leaving the vascular space, that is, none enters cardiac myocytes or the interstitial space. One or more diffusible myocardial perfusion tracers can be injected simultaneously with the intravascular reference tracer. The diffusible tracers pass from the coronary intravascular space into the interstitial space and into the myocytes.

Following a rapid injection containing reference and diffusible tracers into the coronary artery inflow, timed samples of cardiac effluent are collected in serial fashion. The amount of each tracer is determined in the effluent. Tracers with widely divergent physical energy levels can be counted simultaneously using energy gated spectrometry and correction for downscatter of high energy nuclides. For tracers with overlapping energy levels, those with a short physical half-life are measured first, then allowed to decay to low levels before counting tracers with a longer half-life.

Data from Isolated Perfused Hearts

The transport function, $h(t)$, describes the fraction of injected tracer transported through the coronary circulation and recovered in the effluent per second.[7] A plot of $h(t)$ versus time after tracer injection is illustrated in Fig. 1-6. Instantaneous extraction of tracer by the myocardium is characterized at each point in time by the difference between the transport function of the reference tracer, in this case ^{111}In-labeled albumin, and the trans-

port function of the diffusible tracers ^{201}Tl and the ^{99m}Tc-labeled agent. The maximum instantaneous extraction fraction, E_{max}, describes the largest fraction of tracer extracted from the blood by the myocardium during a given increment of time. The net extraction, E_{net}, for a diffusible tracer represents the cumulative fraction of injected tracer retained by the tissue (i.e., heart) (Fig. 1-7). Measurement of E_{max} and E_{net} by the indicator–dilution method provides an analysis of tracer extraction from the coronary circulation and can provide a basis for comparison of different diffusible tracers. Alternatively, serial measurements of E_{max} and E_{net} can provide a basis for analyzing changes in extraction of a single tracer in response to a physiologic or pharmacologic intervention.

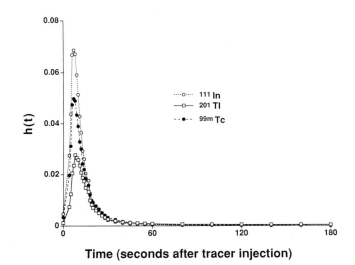

Time (seconds after tracer injection)

Figure 1-6 Plot of the transport function, $h(t)$, which is the fraction of injected tracer transported through the coronary circulation and recovered in the effluent per second, versus time after tracer injection in seconds. The reference tracer, ^{111}In-labeled albumin, remains in the intravascular compartment of the coronary circulation and provides a reference marker of coronary flow transit time. The maximum extraction fraction, E_{max}, for a diffusible tracer is the maximum measured difference between the diffusible tracer curve and the reference tracer curve.

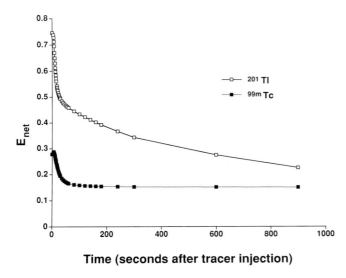

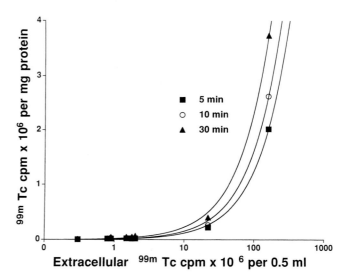

Figure 1-7 The net extraction, E_{net}, is the cumulative fraction of injected tracer retained by the heart. Early extraction of ^{201}Tl is greater than for the ^{99m}Tc tracer. However, ^{201}Tl washes out of the myocardium more rapidly than the ^{99m}Tc tracer so that E_{net} becomes similar for both tracers late (1000 s) after injection.

Figure 1-9 Plot of myocyte tracer content versus time for varying tracer concentration in the extracellular medium.

Isolated Myocyte Models

Suspension or cultures of freshly isolated cardiac myocytes (Fig. 1-8) provide convenient models for study of the effects of physiologic and pharmacologic interventions on net uptake and retention of a diffusible myocardial tracer. Unlike whole animal and isolated heart models, net uptake of tracer can be studied independently of myocardial blood flow in isolated cardiac myocytes. These cardiac myocyte preparations also remove other cardiac anatomic components (endothelial cells, vascular smooth muscle cells, fibroblasts, and neural elements) from the study preparation. One popular cardiac myocyte preparation derives ventricular cells from 10-day-

old chick embryos. The atria and connective tissue are trimmed away, and the ventricles are cut into several pieces. These pieces are then exposed to trypsin, which disaggregates the tissue into individual cells. Following standard cell culture techniques, the myocytes are grown in monolayers on coverslips, which can be immersed into buffers containing radiopharmaceuticals and any other pharmaceuticals of interest.[9]

Another isolated myocyte preparation consists of adult rat ventricular cardiocytes in suspension medium. These cells are obtained by a 30-min coronary artery perfusion of the isolated heart with a physiologic salt solution containing collagenase. The initial digestion is followed by removal of the atria, gentle mincing of the softened ventricles, and filtration and washing to obtain suspensions of mostly rod-shaped cells.[10] Agents of interest can then be added to cell suspensions to study cellular handling.

Cell suspension preparations provide a practical model for screening potential perfusion tracers for favorable net tracer uptake and retention properties as a function of cell exposure time and concentrations presented to the cell. Tracer in the extracellular space can enter the myocyte directly, for example, according to a unidirectional rate constant (passive diffusion), or in accord with its lipophilicity, or by an energy-dependent uptake mechanism. The observed retention of tracer in the myocyte depends on the size and physicochemical characteristics of the intracellular compartment available to contain the tracer and the rate constant at which the tracer diffuses out of the cell. Additionally, the response of tracer kinetics to interventions designed to alter specific components of myocyte metabolism and function permit investigation of the mechanisms of tracer accumulation.

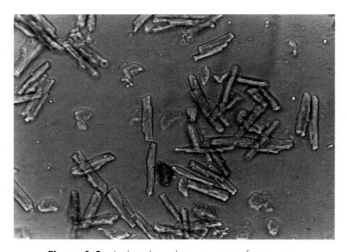

Figure 1-8 Isolated cardiac myocytes from a rat.

Data from Isolated Cardiac Myocyte Models

Flow-independent myocardial net tracer uptake may be plotted for multiple tracer concentrations (Fig. 1-9) at a constant exposure time. For a specific extracellular tracer concentration, the effects of interventions that alter metabolic rates (e.g., administration of cyanide-containing compounds to uncouple oxidative phosphorylation) can be determined. Interventions that alter electrochemical gradients or interfere with cellular structure (e.g., plasma membrane disruption by digitonin to produce chemically "skinned" myocytes) can also be used to evaluate the role of the sarcolemma in tracer uptake and retention.

Animal models of radiotracer uptake and retention can provide valuable insight into tracer mechanisms and potential clinical utility. However, tracer function in humans has been observed, on occasion, to be significantly less optimal than predicted for the same tracer from studies in animal models.[11] Therefore, use of myocardial perfusion imaging tracers in humans requires that results for tracer performance in animal models be confirmed in human clinical trials.

MYOCARDIAL PERFUSION TRACERS—THALLIUM 201

Much of the clinical acceptance of myocardial perfusion imaging has resulted from the early development of ^{201}Tl as a clinical imaging agent. Early interest in thallium as a myocardial tracer stemmed from its biological similarities to potassium, the principal cation in the human myocyte. Potassium is concentrated in the myocyte by the adenosine triphosphate (ATP)-dependent sodium–potassium exchange pump. Gehring and Hammond observed that the ATP-dependent sodium–potassium pump does not differentiate between potassium and thallium.[12] Subsequently, several investigators have provided indirect evidence for a role of the ATP-dependent sodium–potassium pump in the myocardial handling of thallium by demonstrating suppression of thallium accumulation in the myocardium when the pump mechanism is inhibited by administration of a digitalis glycoside.[13–16] McCall et al[13] found that 60 percent of radiolabeled thallium uptake occurred by an active process that could be inhibited by the digitalis glycoside, ouabain. Others have found little effect of digitalis glycosides on initial thallium accumulation in myocytes, suggesting the importance of an alternative mechanism for initial thallium uptake.[17–21] This alternative mechanism for entry of thallium into the myocardium may relate to the size of the hydrated thallium ion radius, which is intermediate between

Table 1-2   Radiation Dose Estimates for ^{201}Tl and ^{99m}Tc Sestamibi in Humans at Rest

	^{201}Tl (rad/3 mCi)	^{99m}Tc Sestamibi (rad/30 mCi)
Gallbladder	0.93	2.44
Heart	1.02	0.53
Kidneys	4.40	2.01
Liver	1.86	0.59
Lower large intestine	3.60	3.33
Lungs	0.51	0.28
Ovaries	1.70	1.33
Red marrow	1.02	0.77
Small intestine	1.94	2.89
Testes	1.62	0.31
Thyroid	2.24	0.63
Upper large intestine	3.60	4.77
Urinary bladder wall	0.57	1.89
Total body	0.72	0.49

Effective dose equivalent, see Table 1-4.
From New England Nuclear,[23] Atkins et al,[24] and Wackers et al,[74] adapted with permission.

those of K$^+$ and Rb$^+$ and favorable for passive diffusion through the myocyte cell membrane.[22] It is currently believed that thallium enters into the myocardium by a combination of active (energy-dependent) and passive (chemical gradient) mechanisms.

Physical Properties

Thallium 201 is cyclotron generated. It decays by electron capture to mercury 201, emitting mercury x-rays of 69 to 83 keV (94.4 percent abundant) and thallium gamma rays of 167 keV (10 percent abundant) and 135 keV (3 percent abundant). The physical half-life of ^{201}Tl is 73 h. For ^{201}Tl, the usual intravenously administered activity for clinical imaging in adults is approximately 2.0 to 3.0 mCi (74 to 111 MBq). Radiation dose estimates for a 3.0-mCi ^{201}Tl dose at rest are given in Table 1-2.[23–25]

Kinetics

INITIAL MYOCARDIAL UPTAKE

Initial regional distribution of ^{201}Tl in the myocardium is a function of regional myocardial blood flow and extraction of the tracer from the blood supply by the myocardium. In the in situ canine heart, regional myocardial uptake of ^{201}Tl is linearly related to regional myocardial blood flow at normal resting levels and at reduced levels of myocardial blood flow.[26] The linear relationship between ^{201}Tl myocardial uptake and myocardial blood flow is maintained during conditions of increased myocardial oxygen demand.[27] When coronary blood flow is increased without a corresponding increase in myocardial oxygen demand (e.g., during pharmacologic coronary artery vasodilation with intravenous dipyridamole) myocardial uptake of ^{201}Tl increases substantially less than myocardial blood flow.[28] The mechanism for this phenomenon requires further investigation.

In patients with normal coronary arteries, ^{201}Tl is homogeneously distributed to the left ventricle. In patients with a flow-limiting coronary artery stenosis, the relative spatial distribution of ^{201}Tl activity on an exercise perfusion scintigram reflects the maldistribution of regional myocardial blood flow.[29] Nichols et al[29] studied 14 patients with a 70 percent or greater stenosis in a branch of the left coronary artery.[29] Ratios of regional ^{201}Tl activity in the LAD and left circumflex distributions on exercise ^{201}Tl scintigrams correlated well ($r = 0.84$) with ratios of regional myocardial blood flow during exercise measured by the xenon 133 (^{133}Xe) myocardial clearance method. In patients with single-vessel CAD and absent collateral vessels, a somewhat weaker relationship has been observed between myocardial ^{201}Tl concentration ratios in ischemic and normal segments relative to minimal coronary artery luminal diameter ($r = 0.73$) and minimal luminal area ($r = 0.72$) by quantitative coronary arteriography.[30] In these same patients, only a weak correlation was observed between myocardial ^{201}Tl concentration ratios in ischemic and normal segments in comparison to the percent diameter stenosis by coronary arteriography.[30] Thus, initial myocardial distribution of ^{201}Tl is closely related to myocardial blood flow but less closely related to standard coronary arteriographic measurements.

In addition to myocardial blood flow, initial uptake of ^{201}Tl by the myocardium depends on the proportion of ^{201}Tl in coronary artery blood that is extracted by the heart muscle (e.g., the extraction fraction). The extraction fraction of ^{201}Tl was reported to be 88 ± 2 percent for the canine myocardium and was not significantly changed when the heart rate was raised from 105 to 195 beats/min by atrial pacing.[17] In isolated perfused rabbit hearts, Leppo and Meerdink[31] observed a similar extraction fraction (E_{max}) for ^{201}Tl at normal levels of myocardial blood flow. However, over a broad range of flows from 0.52 to 3.19 ml/min/g, the mean extraction fraction was 0.73 ± 0.04 and extraction fraction was found to decrease steadily with increasing levels of coronary blood flow from a high of 0.9 at 0.5 ml/min/g to a low of 0.6 at 3.0 ml/min/g.

Effects of metabolic and pharmacologic interventions on the extraction of ^{201}Tl by the myocardium have also been investigated. The effect of hypoxia on myocardial extraction of ^{201}Tl has been the subject of controversy, but there is probably minimal[17,20,32-34] effect on ^{201}Tl uptake. Grunwald et al[35] studied the effects of progressive coronary artery narrowing to induce regional ischemia on the myocardial extraction fraction of ^{201}Tl in anesthetized dogs.[35] A reduction in coronary artery distal perfusion pressure from 110 ± 20 mmHg to levels in the range of 25 to 63 mmHg produced no change in the extraction fraction of [201]Tl. The authors concluded that in normal or low flow conditions, the myocardial extraction fraction for ^{201}Tl was independent of coronary flow provided that myocardial necrosis was not induced. In other studies, acetylstrophanthidin, propranolol, and insulin did not alter the extraction fraction for ^{201}Tl by canine myocardium.[17]

Myocardial ^{201}Tl activity reaches 80 percent of peak activity within 1 min following intravenous injection, and peak ^{201}Tl activity occurs 23.7 min following intravenous injection in anesthetized dogs.[36] As myocardial blood flow is progressively reduced, the percentage of peak activity reached in 1 min is reduced and the time to peak myocardial ^{201}Tl activity is prolonged.[37] This delay in peak myocardial ^{201}Tl activity was not observed under conditions of extreme flow restriction, probably because of cell death, with a resultant decreased ability to accumulate [201]Tl.[38] A similar pattern of delay in the peak myocardial accumulation of ^{201}Tl in the distribution of coronary artery stenoses has also been observed in clinical studies.[39]

THALLIUM REDISTRIBUTION

Following initial extraction of ^{201}Tl by the myocardium, the subsequent myocardial concentration of ^{201}Tl at any point in time is determined by an equilibration process of ^{201}Tl between the myocardium and the blood pool. This equilibration process has two components—washout of ^{201}Tl from the myocardium and new myocardial uptake of ^{201}Tl from the blood pool.

Thallium 201 leaves (diffuses out of) normal myocardium at a fixed rate, referred to as the *intrinsic washout rate*. The intrinsic washout rate for ^{201}Tl has been determined in anesthetized canine models by directly injecting ^{201}Tl into a coronary artery and then monitoring the concentration of tracer remaining in the myocardium over time.[35,36] Reuptake of tracer via systemic recirculation is minimized in this model. Tracer washout from the heart is monoexponential with a myocardial half-time of approximately 84 min.[36]

In the intact circulation, the tracer equilibration process is also influenced by continuous new uptake of tracer delivered to the myocardium. Initially, following intravenous injection, ^{201}Tl is extracted from the blood into body tissues including the heart. In the same way that ^{201}Tl washes out of the heart, ^{201}Tl taken up in other organs and body tissues then slowly washes out of those tissues, replenishing the systemic blood pool. This persistent washout of ^{201}Tl from systemic organs and tissues provides a low residual concentration of tracer in the

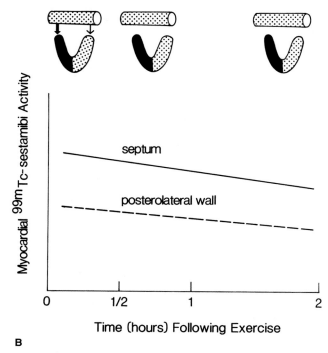

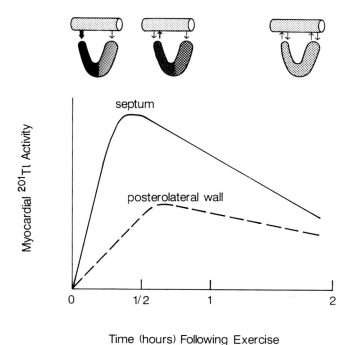

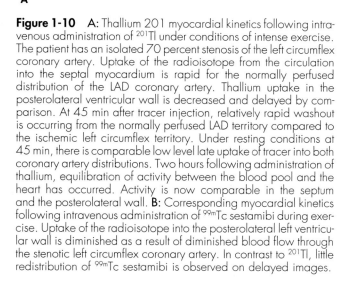

A

B

Figure 1-10   A: Thallium 201 myocardial kinetics following intravenous administration of ²⁰¹Tl under conditions of intense exercise. The patient has an isolated 70 percent stenosis of the left circumflex coronary artery. Uptake of the radioisotope from the circulation into the septal myocardium is rapid for the normally perfused distribution of the LAD coronary artery. Thallium uptake in the posterolateral ventricular wall is decreased and delayed by comparison. At 45 min after tracer injection, relatively rapid washout is occurring from the normally perfused LAD territory compared to the ischemic left circumflex territory. Under resting conditions at 45 min, there is comparable low level late uptake of tracer into both coronary artery distributions. Two hours following administration of thallium, equilibration of activity between the blood pool and the heart has occurred. Activity is now comparable in the septum and the posterolateral wall. B: Corresponding myocardial kinetics following intravenous administration of ⁹⁹ᵐTc sestamibi during exercise. Uptake of the radioisotope into the posterolateral left ventricular wall is diminished as a result of diminished blood flow through the stenotic left circumflex coronary artery. In contrast to ²⁰¹Tl, little redistribution of ⁹⁹ᵐTc sestamibi is observed on delayed images.

Figure 1-10   *(Continued)*

blood and permits a sustained low level ²⁰¹Tl uptake into the myocardium.

The difference between the amount of tracer leaving the heart at the intrinsic washout rate and the amount of new tracer uptake from the circulation is the net myocardial washout. It is this net washout that can be detected by external counting over the heart in an intact circulation. Following intravenous ²⁰¹Tl injection in animal models, one-half of myocardial thallium washes out of normally perfused myocardium over 5 to 8 h.[40,41]

Effect of ischemia on redistribution   Under conditions of myocardial ischemia resulting from reduced myocardial

blood flow, the intrinsic myocardial washout rate for ²⁰¹Tl is reduced substantially.[35] In one study in a canine model, the intrinsic washout rate from the myocardium was prolonged from a half-time of 52 min in the absence of coronary artery obstruction to a half-time of 311 min following coronary occlusion.[35] Delayed uptake of ²⁰¹Tl from the blood pool into the myocardium continues in the presence of myocardial ischemia as late blood pool ²⁰¹Tl activity is primarily contributed by tracer washout from noncardiac organs. Therefore, with intrinsic myocardial washout diminished and late tracer uptake from the circulation continued, the net myocardial ²⁰¹Tl washout rate is reduced in the presence of myocardial ischemia. This contributes to equalization of late tracer activity between initially ischemic and initially normally perfused myocardial segments, and is referred to as *tracer redistribution.*

Effects of exercise and other interventions on ²⁰¹**Tl washout**   When ²⁰¹Tl enters the myocardium initially under conditions of hyperemia (supranormal blood flow), as occurs during exercise, the concentration of ²⁰¹Tl in normally perfused myocardium becomes substantially greater than the systemic blood pool concentration following recovery from exercise. This results in a steep washout gradient between normal myocardium and the blood pool, producing a high net myocardial ²⁰¹Tl washout rate. Hypoperfused myocardial segments that do not receive fully increased myocardial blood flow with exercise will not accumulate as high a concentration of

[201]Tl. The ^{201}Tl gradient between hypoperfused myocardium and the blood pool will be smaller than for normal segments, and the net myocardial ^{201}Tl washout from hypoperfused segments will be less. This observation has been confirmed in humans by Sklar et al,[42] who noted that ^{201}Tl washed out more rapidly from normal myocardial segments than from the systemic blood pool and that ^{201}Tl washed out less rapidly from underperfused myocardium than from the blood pool. Principles of postexercise ^{201}Tl kinetics are illustrated diagrammatically in Fig. 1-10A.

Numerous additional factors appear to influence the rate of ^{201}Tl washout from the myocardium. Higher peak exercise heart rates result in greater initial ^{201}Tl myocardial uptake and more rapid thallium washout rates.[43–45] Lower peak heart rates relate to slower ^{201}Tl myocardial washout. Increased initial ^{201}Tl lung uptake with subsequent replenishment of blood ^{201}Tl levels by tracer washout from the lungs provides a source of late tracer uptake into the heart, reducing net myocardial tracer washout.[44] More rapid myocardial ^{201}Tl washout following exercise has been reported in women compared to men.[46] Accelerated ^{201}Tl washout, from both normal and ischemic myocardial segments, may be produced by a high carbohydrate meal consumed between poststress and delayed images.[47,48] Increasing severity of a coronary artery stenosis and increasing severity of exercise-induced ischemia can produce increasing delay in thallium washout.[30,49] It appears that other cardiac disorders (e.g., hypertensive heart disease, hypertrophic cardiomyopathy) that can limit the hyperemic coronary blood flow response to exercise can limit myocardial thallium uptake and produce slow washout of thallium from the myocardium.[50,51]

Reverse redistribution and diffuse slow washout   Reverse redistribution (Fig. 1-11) is defined as the new appearance or worsening of a perfusion defect during the redistribution phase of ^{201}Tl myocardial imaging.[52–56] It has been observed in 5 to 15 percent of patients with chronic stable CAD who undergo exercise and rest ^{201}Tl imaging,[53,54,57] but it may also be detected in up to 75 percent of patients with a recent myocardial infarction treated with a thrombolytic drug.[58] In the latter setting, Weiss et al[58] studied 67 patients 10 days after streptokinase therapy. Patients with reverse redistribution following injection of ^{201}Tl at rest were characterized by the presence of a nontransmural myocardial infarction pattern, a patent infarct-related artery, and normal or nearly normal regional wall motion in the infarct segment. The authors postulated that higher than normal blood flow to the noninfarcted tissue within the reperfused zone could explain the absence of an initial perfusion defect in that area. Because ^{201}Tl washout rate is related to initial tracer concentration in the myocardium, the washout rate of the noninfarcted tissue in the reperfusion

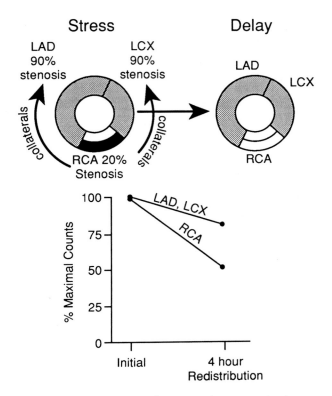

Figure 1-11   Diagrammatic illustration of reverse redistribution in a zone of previous nontransmural inferior myocardial infarction in the territory of the right coronary artery (RCA). With exercise, myocardial blood flow and tracer delivery increase greatly to the noninfarcted epicardial territory supplied by the patent RCA. There is minimal tracer activity in the adjacent infarcted subendocardial tissue. Because the gamma camera lacks sufficient resolution to separate subendocardium from subepicardium, the inferior wall is represented by an average of the number of counts per pixel across the entire inferior wall. Therefore, the inferior wall has a similar count density to the anterior and lateral walls, which are supplied by the severely stenotic LAD and left circumflex arteries. This gives the appearance of similar myocardial tracer activity in all three coronary artery distributions (i.e., uniform myocardial activity on exercise images). On delayed imaging 4 h later, washout of ^{201}Tl from the severely hypoperfused LAD and left circumflex territories is reduced, resulting in substantial residual tracer activity in these areas. Tracer washout from the normally perfused epicardial portion of the RCA distribution is rapidly leaving relatively reduced ^{201}Tl activity across the transmural inferior wall territory of the RCA and a pattern of reverse redistribution.

zone might exceed that of the contralateral myocardial segments resulting in accelerated tracer washout and a reverse redistribution pattern. Alternatively, ^{201}Tl may have been taken up initially into the interstitial compartment associated with the nontransmural infarct with subsequent accelerated tracer washout.

Patients who develop reverse redistribution in a setting of acute infarction and thrombolysis usually have persistence of the reverse redistribution pattern at follow-up 8 weeks later.[58] Thus, these patients provide an example in which reverse redistribution persists into a setting of more chronic CAD. In this instance, apparent worsening of tracer distribution occurs in a myocardial segment containing viable myocardium (i.e., the salvaged myocardium surrounding a nontransmural infarct) and a relatively mild or no regional coronary artery stenosis (see Fig. 1-11). The presence of viable myocardium in most segments with reverse redistribution is consistent with observations of investigators who have documented retained fluorodeoxyglucose extraction on positron emission tomography or active ^{201}Tl accumulation on thallium reinjection in segments showing the reverse redistribution phenomenon.[57,59–61] In other cases, reverse redistribution has been observed in the myocardium supplied by a severely stenotic coronary artery,[46,47,53] but the mechanism by which reverse redistribution occurs in these cases remains incompletely defined.

A possibly related phenomenon has been described as "diffuse slow washout."[62] This phenomenon, which was observed with quantitative planar ^{201}Tl imaging, consists of uniform initial thallium myocardial distribution followed by delayed tracer washout from all regions and was described in patients with multivessel CAD.

Artifactual patterns suggesting reverse redistribution have also been described.[63–65] Brown et al[63] showed that reverse redistribution on a stress–rest imaging sequence was simulated by oversubtraction of background activity from planar ^{201}Tl images acquired at rest. When the images were reviewed without background subtraction, apparent worsening of defects on the resting images was no longer observed. Reverse redistribution may also be simulated on ^{201}Tl tomograms. In a patient with patent coronary arteries, initial ^{201}Tl distribution is uniform. However, as thallium clears from the body, prominent ^{201}Tl activity may be present at rest in the large bowel or liver resulting in overlap of noncardiac tracer activity with the inferior myocardial segment, falsely suggesting the presence of heterogeneous myocardial activity. Reverse redistribution may also be simulated by nonconcordant defects on stress and redistribution ^{201}Tl images resulting from inconsistent location of soft-tissue attenuation. For example, in women, if position of the left breast is different on stress and redistribution images, a new defect may appear on the rest images, falsely suggesting reverse redistribution. In the presence of uniform initial tracer distribution, careful attention must be given to the exclusion of artifactual causes for new defects on redistribution images before identifying reverse redistribution.

Implications of Thallium 201 Uptake and Redistribution

Extraction of ^{201}Tl by the myocardium implies the presence of structurally intact myocytes and viable myocardial tissue.[38] With irreversible myocardial injury, ^{201}Tl may be present in the intramyocardial vascular space but may not be extracted into injured myocardial cells. An imaging correlate of this observation is that irreversibly damaged myocardium will contain severely diminished levels of ^{201}Tl activity.[66–68] If the maximum ^{201}Tl count rate on a myocardial tomographic image slice is assigned a value of 100 percent, then the relative tracer distribution in myocardial segments supplied by a diseased coronary artery can be assigned a relative count rate. Under resting conditions, myocardial perfusion defects having less than 50 percent of the ^{201}Tl count rate of normal segments usually correspond to the presence of irreversibly damaged myocardium. Myocardial segments that demonstrate ^{201}Tl redistribution or that, at rest, contain 50 percent or more of the ^{201}Tl distribution of normal myocardial segments generally contain viable myocardium.

Advantages and Disadvantages of Thallium 201

Advantages and disadvantages of ^{201}Tl for myocardial perfusion imaging are listed in Table 1-3. Despite these limitations of ^{201}Tl as an imaging agent, it remains the most widely used myocardial tracer at this time.

TECHNETIUM 99m MYOCARDIAL PERFUSION IMAGING AGENTS

In the past decade, myocardial perfusion agents have been developed that use the favorable physical properties of [99m]Tc. Potential advantages of a ^{99m}Tc myocardial perfusion agent in comparison to ^{201}Tl include:

1. The 140-keV gamma ray emission of ^{99m}Tc is ideally suited for imaging on a standard gamma camera.
2. The 140-keV energy of ^{99m}Tc is less attenuated by soft tissue compared to the 69- to 83-keV lower energy emissions of [201]Tl.
3. The shorter (6 h) half-life of ^{99m}Tc compared to the 73-h half-life of ^{201}Tl permits greater administered ^{99m}Tc activity and improved counting statistics.
4. Because ^{99m}Tc is produced by the molybdenum-99m generator at the medical use site, it is more readily available for urgent use.

Technetium-99m Sestamibi

A ^{99m}Tc myocardial perfusion agent that has been studied extensively[73–76] and has entered into general clinical use

Table 1-3   Advantages and Disadvantages of Thallium 201 for Myocardial Perfusion Imaging

Advantages	Disadvantages
1. Rapid myocardial extraction (i.e., facilitating imaging with conditions of temporary stress)	1. Low energy emissions attenuated by overlying soft tissue, particularly diaphragm[70,71] and left breast[72]
2. Minimal uptake by abdominal organs during exercise	2. Long physical half-life
3. Delayed ^{201}Tl washout, late ^{201}Tl uptake, and resultant redistribution permit differentiation of myocardial ischemia from scar[69]	a. Unfavorable dosimetry resulting in limited counting statistics
4. Not significantly affected by cardiac drugs	b. Limited use for serial studies
5. Diagnostic and prognostic implications of ^{201}Tl lung uptake (see Chap. 2)	3. Cyclotron-generated
	a. Difficult to maintain on hand for acute dosing in patients with chest pain
	b. Costly
	4. Slow course of ^{201}Tl redistribution results in long imaging sequences

is ^{99m}Tc hexakis-2-methoxyisobutyl isonitrile (i.e., ^{99m}Tc sestamibi). Technetium-99m sestamibi is a monovalent cation consisting of a central Tc(I) core surrounded in an octahedral configuration by six identical methoxyisobutyl isonitrile ligands coordinated through the isonitrile carbon atoms. This structure is associated with sufficient lipophilicity to enable it to partition across biological membranes. However, the entry of ^{99m}Tc sestamibi into myocardial cells cannot be explained by passive diffusion across the myocyte cell membrane alone.[77] Piwnica-Worms et al[78,79] demonstrated that the distribution of ^{99m}Tc sestamibi in myocytes is strongly dependent on plasma membrane and mitochondrial membrane potentials. In cultured chick myocytes, depolarization of plasma membrane potentials by raising extracellular potassium concentrations to 130 mM, the same level as intracellular potassium, resulted in a severely reduced net accumulation of intracellular ^{99m}Tc sestamibi (Fig. 1-12). Addition of the potassium ionophore valinomycin to cells incubated in buffer containing 130 mM potassium further reduced net uptake of ^{99m}Tc sestamibi to levels observed in nonviable cells apparently by depolarizing mitochondrial membrane potentials. In chick myocytes placed in physiologic buffer, the protonophore carbonyl cyanide-m-chlorophenylhydrazone (CCCP), which rapidly uncouples mitochondria by depolarizing the inner mitochondrial membrane potential, inhibited 90 percent of net ^{99m}Tc sestamibi uptake.[78] Conversely, ^{99m}Tc sestamibi uptake was augmented in studies in which mitochondrial membrane potentials were hyperpolarized with oligomycin, an inhibitor of mitochondrial ATP synthase.[78] These findings were corroborated in subcellular distribution studies following administration of ^{99m}Tc sestamibi in isolated perfused rat hearts.[80] Nevertheless, Maublant et al[21] found no effect on ^{99m}Tc sestamibi uptake after 15 min incubation of isolated rat cardiac myocytes in either sodium cyanide (5 mM), an inhibitor of the respiratory chain, sodium iodoacetate (0.1 mM), an inhibitor of glycolysis, or ouabain (10 M), an inhibitor of the ATP-dependent sodium–potassium pump. Piwnica-Worms et al[14] also found no effect of iodoacetate (1 mM)

on ^{99m}Tc sestamibi uptake in cultured chick myocytes. The authors postulated that interventions that slowly deplete myocyte substrate, enzymes, or ATP stores do not interfere with ^{99m}Tc sestamibi uptake until sufficient metabolic inhibition has occurred to neutralize cellular or mitochondrial membrane potentials, thereby inducing irreversible myocyte injury.[14] The latter conclusion is supported by the studies of Beanlands et al.[81] These authors induced irreversible injury in isolated rat hearts by infusing Krebs–Henseleit buffer containing either sodium cyanide (10

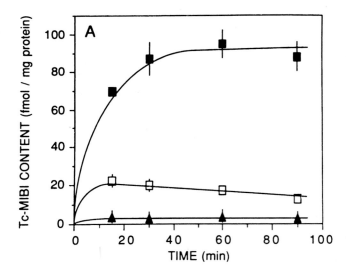

Figure 1-12   Plot of effects of high potassium buffer and valinomycin on ^{99m}Tc sestamibi (MIBI) net uptake by cultured chick cardiac myocytes. Control net uptake of ^{99m}Tc sestamibi in buffer containing a normal (5.4 mM) concentration of potassium is shown with black squares. Net uptake of tracer in the presence of plasma membrane depolarizing buffer concentrations (130 mM) of potassium is shown with white squares. Net uptake of tracer in the presence of both a 130 mM potassium concentration and the potassium ionophore valinomycin (1 μg/ml) is shown with black triangles. Depolarization of the plasma membrane with 130 mM potassium concentration in the buffer reduced tracer net uptake substantially. Addition of valinomycin resulted in a further reduction in tracer net uptake with the postulated mechanism consisting of depolarization of mitochondrial membrane potentials. (From Piwnica-Worms et al,[78] by permission of the American Heart Association, Inc.)

mM/l) for 30 min or by chemically skinning sarcolemmal membrane with the detergent triton X-100 (0.5%) for 5 min. Irreversible cell injury was documented by cardiac enzyme release, triphenyl tetrazolium chloride staining, and electron microscopy. Both cyanide and triton X-100 infusion significantly reduced ^{99m}Tc sestamibi accumulation. These studies demonstrate that myocardial accumulation of ^{99m}Tc sestamibi depends on maintenance of myocyte viability, including intact plasma membrane and mitochondrial membrane potentials.

PHYSICAL PROPERTIES

Technetium 99m is a metastable radionuclide produced from a molybdenum-99m generator. It is a gamma ray emitter with a physical half-life of 6.0 h. Radiation dose esimates for 30 mCi of ^{99m}Tc sestamibi administered at rest are given in Table 1-2.[74] At 60 min after injection, approximately 1 percent of the administered activity is localized in the heart, 5.6 percent is localized in the liver, and 0.9 percent is localized in the lung.[74]

INITIAL MYOCARDIAL DISTRIBUTION

In an anesthetized canine model of left circumflex coronary artery occlusion, Okada et al[75] demonstrated a linear relationship ($r = 0.92$) of myocardial ^{99m}Tc sestamibi activity and myocardial blood flow by microsphere measurement over a range of flows from approximately 0.1 to 0.9 ml/min/g. In a similar model[2] in which myocardial blood flow was increased to levels up to 5 ml/min/g by intravenous administration of dipyridamole, the relationship between ^{99m}Tc sestamibi and myocardial blood flow was linear up to flows of 2 ml/min/g. However, at higher myocardial blood flows, there was little further increase in ^{99m}Tc sestamibi activity. This plateau in ^{99m}Tc sestamibi uptake with pharmacologically induced increases in myocardial blood flow above 2 ml/min/g in the absence of a corresponding increase in myocardial oxygen consumption is similar to that observed with ^{201}Tl.[2]

Following a complete coronary artery occlusion for 1 min in an anesthetized canine model, Li et al[82] observed a consistent excess of ^{99m}Tc sestamibi myocardial activity for myocardial blood flows less than 40 percent of that in normal myocardial regions. This excess of tracer activity at very low myocardial blood flows was apparent both with direct tissue counting and with scintigraphic imaging. This finding has been postulated to result from increased myocardial extraction of ^{99m}Tc sestamibi by viable myocardium at very low myocardial blood flows.[82–84] Studies in guinea pigs suggest that myocardial extraction of ^{99m}Tc sestamibi is not significantly altered by commonly used cardiac pharmaceutical agents, including propranolol, digoxin, and verapamil.[85]

COMPARISON OF INITIAL UPTAKE OF THALLIUM 201 AND TECHNETIUM-99M SESTAMIBI

Because the mechanisms of tracer uptake into the myocardium differ for ^{201}Tl and for ^{99m}Tc sestamibi, it is not surprising that the rates of myocardial tracer uptake are also different. Leppo and Meerdink[15,83] used a paired indicator–dilution method in isolated, blood-perfused, contracting rabbit hearts to quantitate myocardial extraction of these radiotracers. They observed substantially higher capillary transport of ^{201}Tl compared to ^{99m}Tc sestamibi resulting in a peak value of the instantaneous extraction fraction (E_{max}) of 0.31 to 0.39 for ^{99m}Tc sestamibi versus 0.59 to 0.73 for ^{201}Tl ($p < 0.001$). Although ^{201}Tl left the intramyocardial capillaries and entered the extravascular myocardial space more rapidly compared to sestamibi, the net extraction of ^{99m}Tc sestamibi over time approached that of ^{201}Tl by approximately 5 to 10 min after injection. This occurred because ^{99m}Tc sestamibi enters the parenchymal cell more rapidly than ^{201}Tl, the volume of distribution of ^{99m}Tc sestamibi is greater than that for ^{201}Tl in the myocyte, and because ^{201}Tl washes back out of myocardial cells more rapidly than does ^{99m}Tc sestamibi.[83] Therefore, at the time of clinical imaging following tracer injection, net myocardial tracer content is similar for ^{201}Tl and ^{99m}Tc sestamibi, even though earliest tracer extraction is more rapid for ^{201}Tl.

In the absence of myocardial infarction, partial coronary artery obstruction has been associated with less severe stress ^{99m}Tc sestamibi defects compared to ^{201}Tl defects.[86–89] This observation has been reported in canine models of coronary artery occlusion during pharmacologic coronary artery vasodilation.[86,87] Here, tomographic myocardial imaging with ^{99m}Tc sestamibi during moderately severe partial coronary artery occlusion underestimated the area of perfusion defect relative to ^{201}Tl defect size and relative to the defect size on pathology specimens.[86] The ^{99m}Tc sestamibi defect size also underestimated the magnitude of the flow disparity between stenotic and normal coronary perfusion beds, with the degree of flow underestimation greater for ^{99m}Tc sestamibi than for ^{201}Tl for both mild and severe coronary stenoses.[87] It has also been noted on exercise imaging studies in patients with angiographic CAD disease that ^{99m}Tc sestamibi images yield smaller perfusion defects compared to ^{201}Tl images obtained in the same patients.[88,89]

In addition to greater underestimation of regional differences in myocardial blood flow, ^{99m}Tc sestamibi also differs from ^{201}Tl in its uptake characteristics under conditions of myocellular injury (Fig. 1-13). Piwnica-Worms et al[90] examined the effects on cultured chick ventricular myocytes of metabolic inhibition with iodoacetate (1 mM) and rotenone (10 μM). Initial myocyte uptake of ^{99m}Tc sestamibi increased by 42 percent with mild cell injury resulting from 10 min of metabolic inhi-

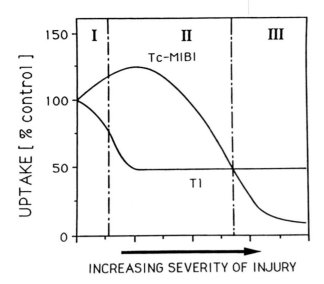

Figure 1-13 Diagram of the effect of severity of injury on initial uptake rates of ^{99m}Tc sestamibi and ^{201}Tl into chick cardiac myocytes. Zones I, II, and III represent mild, moderate, and severe myocellular injury respectively. (From Piwnica-Worms et al,[90] by permission of the American Heart Association, Inc.)

bition, whereas ^{201}Tl uptake did not change substantially. With moderate myocyte injury produced by 60 min of metabolic inhibition, ^{201}Tl uptake decreased by 42 percent, whereas ^{99m}Tc sestamibi uptake had essentially returned to control levels. However, after 90 min of metabolic inhibition resulting in severe myocyte injury, ^{201}Tl uptake remained decreased by approximately 50 percent, but ^{99m}Tc sestamibi uptake was decreased to approximately 25 percent of control values. Thus, mild myocyte injury appears to produce augmented ^{99m}Tc sestamibi uptake, whereas profound metabolic dysfunction produces profound depression of ^{99m}Tc sestamibi accumulation.[90] These observations of augmented ^{99m}Tc sestamibi uptake in the presence of mild metabolic inhibition may provide an additional mechanism responsible for the smaller ischemic defects detected with ^{99m}Tc sestamibi compared to [201]Tl.

TECHNETIUM-99m SESTAMIBI MYOCARDIAL CLEARANCE

Studies of ^{99m}Tc sestamibi myocardial clearance have focused on the presence or absence of tracer washout, assessment of relative washout from ischemic compared to normal myocardium, and attempts to detect tracer redistribution from myocardial images. Although initial studies by Okada et al[2,75] and by Mousa et al[73] did not document significant myocardial clearance of ^{99m}Tc sestamibi over 4 h, several recent studies in canine models have documented a limited amount of ^{99m}Tc sestamibi washout from the heart.[82,91-93] Li et al[82] used direct myocardial biopsies in anesthetized dogs to demonstrate an increase in absolute ^{99m}Tc sestamibi activity in previously

ischemic myocardial zones as well as reduction of tracer activity in normal myocardium. After 3 h of reperfusion, there was 15 percent redistribution of ^{99m}Tc sestamibi compared to a 96 percent redistribution of [201]Tl. This resulted in a small but visible reduction in ischemic defect size on tomographic imaging of ^{99m}Tc sestamibi activity. In other studies, the amount of ^{99m}Tc sestamibi redistribution has been too small to produce a visible reduction in the ischemic zone size as assessed by planar imaging methods.[2,93] Others have been able to document limited ^{99m}Tc sestamibi redistribution from tomographic images when a quantitative approach was used.[82]

In summary, ^{99m}Tc sestamibi does wash out of the myocardium, but the rate of washout is slow relative to washout of [201]Tl. Differential washout, in which ^{99m}Tc sestamibi clears more rapidly from normal than from ischemic myocardium, has been documented in several but not all animal models in which it has been evaluated. Redistribution of ^{99m}Tc sestamibi in ischemic defects has been described in animal studies using quantitative approaches with tomographic gamma camera images, but the changes are subtle and may be of limited utility for detection of viable myocardium.

ADVANTAGES AND DISADVANTAGES OF TECHNETIUM-99M SESTAMIBI FOR MYOCARDIAL IMAGING

Technetium-99m sestamibi provides superior physical imaging properties compared to ^{201}Tl for myocardial imaging. It can be used to provide higher myocardial image quality with reduced soft-tissue attenuation effect. It can also provide sufficient counting statistics to permit gating of perfusion images or acquisition of high quality first-pass angiocardiograms. It has several disadvantageous biological properties compared to ^{201}Tl, including prominent distribution in the liver, which may interfere with myocardial visualization. Distribution of ^{99m}Tc sestamibi in the lungs is not related to the number of diseased coronary arteries or to the level of left ventricular function and, therefore, provides less prognostic information than pulmonary ^{201}Tl activity.[94-98] Importantly, limited redistribution of ^{99m}Tc sestamibi has resulted in more limited prediction of viable myocardial tissue compared to [201]Tl.

Technetium-99m Teboroxime

A second class of ^{99m}Tc myocardial imaging agents is the boronic acid adducts of technetium dioxime or bato compounds.[99] Of these compounds, teboroxime is approved by the Food and Drug Administration for clinical use in the United States. Like ^{99m}Tc sestamibi, ^{99m}Tc teboroxime is highly lipophilic. Unlike ^{201}Tl and ^{99m}Tc sestamibi, teboroxime has a neutral valence that permits it to diffuse rapidly back out of the myocardium after initial uptake.

In comparison to ^{201}Tl and ^{99m}Tc sestamibi, ^{99m}Tc teboroxime functions as a nearly pure myocardial blood flow tracer. In cultured rat myocardial cells, Maublant et al[100] observed little effect over 1 h on teboroxime uptake in the presence of sodium cyanide (5 mM) to inhibit mitochondrial respiration. Inhibition of glycolysis with sodium iodoacetate (0.1 mM) and of the ATP-dependent sodium–potassium pump with ouabain (0.1 mM) had little or no effect on teboroxime uptake into the myocardium. Thus, myocardial uptake of ^{99m}Tc teboroxime shows less sensitivity to metabolic impairment compared with ^{201}Tl or ^{99m}Tc sestamibi.[100]

Radiation dosimetry of ^{99m}Tc teboroxime has been reported by Narra et al.[101] The gallbladder and upper large intestine are the target organs and receive, respectively, 98 and 123 mrad per mCi ^{99m}Tc teboroxime.

INITIAL MYOCARDIAL UPTAKE

Di Rocco and associates[102] studied the relationship of ^{99m}Tc teboroxime, ^{99m}Tc sestamibi, and ^{201}Tl myocardial uptake to myocardial blood flow measured by radiolabeled microspheres in a single-pass model in rats and in a multiple-pass model in dogs. In both models, ^{99m}Tc teboroxime and ^{201}Tl better approximated myocardial blood flow than did ^{99m}Tc sestamibi, which underestimated flows over a wide range. Variable results have been reported in the evaluation of initial myocardial ^{99m}Tc teboroxime activity versus myocardial blood flow. This variability appears to result from the superimposed effects of very rapid myocardial washout of the tracer.[103] In addition, although initial extraction of ^{99m}Tc teboroxime from the circulation is high, continued extraction of ^{99m}Tc teboroxime is limited by binding to red blood cells.[104,105]

Stewart et al[106] reported 90 ± 4 percent myocardial retention following intracoronary injection of ^{99m}Tc teboroxime in open-chest dogs. No significant relationship was found between retention fraction of teboroxime and myocardial blood flow over a wide range of flows from 0.3 to 7.7 ml/min/g, suggesting high tracer extraction over a wide range of flows. Localization of retained tracer to the myocardium versus the intramyocardial vascular space was examined by Leppo and Meerdink[99] using the paired-indicator dilution technique in isolated, blood-perfused rabbit hearts. Peak myocardial extraction (E_{max}) of ^{99m}Tc teboroxime exceeded that for ^{201}Tl over a wide range of myocardial blood flows from approximately 0.3 to 2.4 ml/min/g. The mean value for E_{max} was 0.72 ± 0.09 for ^{99m}Tc teboroxime versus 0.57 ± 0.10 for ^{201}Tl ($p < 0.01$). The mean value for net myocardial extraction (E_{net}) was 0.55 ± 0.18 for ^{99m}Tc teboroxime compared to 0.46 ± 0.17 for ^{201}Tl ($p < 0.05$).

Separation of ischemic from normally perfused myocardium was evaluated for ^{99m}Tc teboroxime, ^{99m}Tc sestamibi, and ^{201}Tl in rabbit hearts studied by dual-isotope autoradiography by Weinstein et al.[107] In this study, ^{99m}Tc teboroxime and ^{99m}Tc sestamibi produced greater normal-to-defect contrast than ^{201}Tl in each heart. Tomography with ^{99m}Tc teboroxime generated larger ischemic defect images than did ^{201}Tl-generated images in the same hearts.

TECHNETIUM-99m TEBOROXIME MYOCARDIAL WASHOUT

In the clinical setting ^{99m}Tc teboroxime clears rapidly from the myocardium—substantially more rapidly than does ^{201}Tl. Furthermore, myocardial washout is flow related in the clinical setting. In normal volunteers injected with ^{99m}Tc teboroxime at rest, myocardial activity washed out with a half-time of 9.1 min, whereas with higher myocardial blood flows associated with exercise, the half-time for myocardial washout shortened to 6.6 min.[108] Studies of washout from isolated perfused rabbit hearts have not demonstrated accelerated clearance of ^{99m}Tc teboroxime relative to ^{201}Tl.[99,105,109] The difference in ^{99m}Tc teboroxime washout in these settings appears to be a result of binding of teboroxime to red blood cells.[104,105] In isolated rabbit hearts perfused with blood-free buffer, Dahlberg et al[105] found that only 18 percent of injected ^{99m}Tc teboroxime washed out from the myocardium with a rapid half-time of 31 s, whereas 82 percent cleared with a long half-time of 22 min. In isolated rabbit hearts perfused with a solution containing human red blood cells, 61 percent of injected ^{99m}Tc teboroxime washed out of the myocardium rapidly with a half-time of 23 sec. This suggests that a significant amount of ^{99m}Tc teboroxime remains bound to blood components and may be imaged in the intramyocardial vascular space. Red blood cell-bound ^{99m}Tc teboroxime has minimal myocardial extraction and may rapidly leave the intravascular compartment of the myocardium, giving the appearance of rapid myocardial washout. Technetium-99m teboroxime that is in a blood-free perfusate is more highly extracted into the myocardium and may also have a lesser gradient for washout because red blood cells and plasma protein are not present in the perfusate.[105] These factors appear to explain the lower myocardial washout rate for ^{99m}Tc teboroxime from isolated buffer-perfused hearts compared to washout in human studies. These observations also suggest that ^{99m}Tc teboroxime reaching the human heart may include a significant component that cannot be extracted into myocytes.

In a canine model, Stewart et al[110] observed washout of 67 percent of initially extracted ^{99m}Tc teboroxime with a rapid half-time of 2.3 ± 0.6 min and clearance of 18 percent of tracer with a slow half-time of 20 min.[110] Beanlands et al[111] injected ^{99m}Tc teboroxime in dogs with a wide range of coronary blood flows induced by LAD artery occlusion and dipyridamole infusion. The animals were killed 1, 2, or 5 min later. In comparison to myocardial blood flow by microsphere determination, tracer retention significantly underestimated flow changes at moderate and high flow rates by 5 min after ^{99m}Tc teboroxime injection. Noting rapid tracer washout from the myocardium, the authors concluded that rapid acquisition protocols are needed to fully exploit the potential of ^{99m}Tc teboroxime for imaging myocardial perfusion.

Technetium-99m teboroxime clears more rapidly from myocardium supplied by an unobstructed coronary artery than it does from myocardium supplied by a stenotic artery.[110,112] Stewart et al[106] studied this phenomenon in a canine model in which blood flow through one coronary artery was reduced with an occluder and blood flow through the remaining coronary arteries was increased by pharmacologic means. Initial ^{99m}Tc teboroxime perfusion defects distal to the coronary occluder resolved in 71 percent of the animals by 8.8 ± 2.5 min postinjection of tracer. Gray and Gewirtz[113] also found evidence of differential washout of ^{99m}Tc teboroxime from ischemic and nonischemic myocardium in a swine model of coronary artery stenosis. Unlike ^{201}Tl redistribution, which is related to the gradient between myocardial and blood ^{201}Tl concentration and less influenced by myocardial blood flow,[114,115] differential washout of ^{99m}Tc teboroxime from ischemic and normally perfused myocardium is related to myocardial blood flow during the tracer clearance phase. Therefore, serial ^{99m}Tc teboroxime scans would be expected to show resolution of perfusion defects only if regional flow differences present at the time of tracer injection persisted during tracer washout, producing reduced washout from the ischemic zone. Conversely, equalization of myocardial blood flows to normal and previously ischemic regions, soon following tracer injection, would result in similar tracer washout rates from both zones producing persistent defects and falsely suggesting the presence of myocardial scar. As is the case for ^{201}Tl, evaluation of defect severity, evaluation of tracer distribution at rest, and evaluation for reversible tracer defects may all be necessary to detect fully the presence of viable myocardium with ^{99m}Tc teboroxime imaging.

IMPLICATIONS OF TECHNETIUM-99m TEBOROXIME KINETICS FOR CLINICAL IMAGING

The kinetic properties of teboroxime translate into a requirement for rapid clinical imaging. A brief blood pool phase of approximately 0.5 to 1.5 min follows intravenous ^{99m}Tc teboroxime injection. Myocardial uptake is apparent within 1 min after tracer injection. Although initially low, hepatic activity becomes prominent by 5 to 10 min after teboroxime injection and can interfere with visualization of the inferior wall of the left ventricle. Myocardial washout is rapid, with a half-time of approximately 6 to 12 min following intravenous injection.[108,116] Consequently, imaging should be started within 2 min following tracer injection and completed over approximately 10 min. As a result of high myocardial count rates, a series of three planar ^{99m}Tc teboroxime views may be acquired with an average total imaging time of 4 to 5 min. Planar imaging may be performed in an upright position to improve separation of myocardial activity from background activity in the liver.[116,117]

Because of the requirement for rapid image acquisition, tomographic imaging of ^{99m}Tc teboroxime activity in the heart is best accomplished with a multidetector camera.[118] Li et al[119] studied ischemic myocardial defects in dogs using single-detector tomographic images after ^{99m}Tc teboroxime administration. The authors concluded that ischemia was underestimated in the inferior wall, apparently due to photon scatter from the liver. In the Canadian multicenter ^{99m}Tc teboroxime study reported by Burns et al,[120] there was no significant difference in detection of angiographic coronary artery stenoses using ^{99m}Tc teboroxime versus ^{201}Tl with a single-detector gamma camera. Nevertheless, the sensitivity for detection of individual right coronary artery and left circumflex artery stenoses tended to be higher with [201]Tl (40 of 53 stenoses, 78 percent) compared to ^{99m}Tc teboroxime (34 of 53 stenoses, 64 percent).

In cardiac phantom studies designed to evaluate the effects of changes in myocardial tracer concentration during tomographic image acquisition, Bok et al[121] found no significant image distortion provided that acquisition time was less than twice the myocardial half-time of the tracer. However, if differential washout from myocardial regions occurs, as can occur with ^{99m}Tc teboroxime, then to keep resultant quantitative errors in the ratio of septal-to-lateral wall activity under 5 percent, the acquisition time must be shorter than half of the tracer's half-time in the myocardium[122] or less than 3 min.[123,124] This can then be followed by a second brief acquisition for evaluation of differential tracer washout as an indication of reversible myocardial ischemia.[125,126] A separate injection of ^{99m}Tc teboroxime at rest is typically used 1 to 4 h following stress injection for evaluation of myocardial viability.[108,116,127]

SECOND-GENERATION TECHNETIUM 99m MYOCARDIAL PERFUSION IMAGING AGENTS

The continued widespread use of ^{201}Tl for myocardial perfusion imaging illustrates not only the favorable biological properties of ^{201}Tl, but also the need for further innovation in the development of new ^{99m}Tc perfusion tracers. Technetium 99m myocardial imaging tracers are needed that permit convenient, brief imaging sessions and define accurately myocardial viability as well as perfusion. Second-generation ^{99m}Tc myocardial imaging agents, including tetrofosmin, furifosmin, and N-NOET, were developed as an attempt to combine the favorable physical imaging properties of a ^{99m}Tc complex with improved target-to-nontarget tracer distribution to enable myocardial imaging early after tracer injection. These second-generation tracers may also provide valuable insights into the synthesis of future tracers which, in addition to providing accurate assessment of myocardial perfusion, can measure accurately myocardial metabolism and viability.

Radiochemical Correlates of Clinical Imaging Properties

The design of new ^{99m}Tc-containing tracers has been guided by observation of the relationships between basic biological and chemical properties and corresponding myocardial images. Technetium-99m-1,2-bis(dimethyl-phosphino)ethane (DMPE)$_2$ Cl$_2$, the first ^{99m}Tc-containing myocardial imaging agent to be investigated in humans,[128,129] yielded excellent myocardial visualization in dogs, cats, rats, and baboons but virtually no detectable myocardial activity in pigs and highly variable myocardial activity in humans.[11,129] The Tc(III) complex, (DMPE)$_2$ Cl$_2$, undergoes reduction in vivo to a neutral Tc(II) complex, allowing it to wash out of the heart rapidly and to be taken up into the liver.[130] Changes in oxidation state of ^{99m}Tc to the Tc(I) complexes, (DMPE)$_3$ or hexakis t-butylisonitrile (TBI) largely eliminated myocardial washout but resulted in prolonged blood pool activity in the former and excessive tracer activity in the lungs for the latter.[131,132] A more successful approach to reducing excessive myocardial washout and hepatic uptake of tracer has involved the addition of ether functionalities. Addition of symmetric ether groups to the diphosphine backbone of (DMPE)$_2$ Cl$_2$ led to the synthesis of ^{99m}Tc tetrofosmin.[133,134] Replacement of the diphosphine backbone of (DMPE)$_2$ Cl$_2$ with a Schiff base N$_2$O$_2$ ligand and moving the phosphorus atoms and ether functionalities to a separate pair of pendant ligands led to the mixed ligand complex, furifosmin.[135,136]

Technetium-99m Tetrofosmin

Similarly to ^{99m}Tc sestamibi, ^{99m}Tc tetrofosmin is concentrated in myocardial mitochondria. In isolated rat mitochondria, accumulation of ^{99m}Tc tetrofosmin requires the presence of substrates for cell respiration and is inhibited by the presence of 5 μM 2,4-dinitrophenol, an uncoupler of oxidative phosphorylation.[137,138] Dependence of ^{99m}Tc tetrofosmin uptake on cellular viability has also been inferred from observations in rat[139] and canine[140,141] mod-

els of myocardial reperfusion in which tetrofosmin uptake underestimated myocardial blood flow in irreversibly injured myocardium.

Myocardial uptake of ^{99m}Tc is linearly related to myocardial blood flow for regions of normal flow, mild-to-moderate ischemia, and moderate hyperemia. In an open-chest, anesthetized canine model, Sinusas et al[142] found a good relation of tracer activity to myocardial blood flow for flows from 0.2 to 2.0 ml/min/g, but there was a plateau of the relationship with underestimation of flows above 2.0 ml/min/g. In addition, low myocardial blood flows of less than 0.2 ml/min/g were accompanied by excess tracer uptake, apparently related to prolonged transit time with improved tissue extraction.[142] In isolated perfused rabbit hearts, Dahlberg et al[143] observed a linear relationship of ^{99m}Tc tetrofosmin myocardial activity to coronary blood flow for flows up to 2.5 ml/min/g, however, myocardial uptake of tetrofosmin increased less than myocardial uptake of ^{201}Tl with increasing coronary blood flow.[143]

Following intravenous injection, ^{99m}Tc tetrofosmin clears rapidly from the blood. Blood activities at 5 and 15 min after injection in the canine model were 2.8 $\pm$ 0.9 percent and 0.8 $\pm$ 0.3 percent of peak activity, respectively.[142] Extraction of ^{99m}Tc tetrofosmin from the blood into the myocardium is less efficient than for ^{201}Tl. At a mean coronary blood flow of 2.7 ml/min/g, Dahlberg et al,[144] using blood-perfused isolated rat hearts, found maximum extraction (E$_{max}$) of 0.24 $\pm$ 0.09 for tetrofosmin compared to an E$_{max}$ of 0.69 $\pm$ 0.08 for ^{201}Tl ($p < 0.0001$). Between 5 and 15 min after tracer injection, net extraction (E$_{net}$) for tetrofosmin (0.16 $\pm$ 0.10) remained unchanged, whereas E$_{net}$ for ^{201}Tl fell significantly from 0.44 $\pm$ 0.12 to 0.35 $\pm$ 0.12, reflecting moderate ^{201}Tl washout. Therefore, although ^{201}Tl is more avidly extracted into the myocardium compared to tetrofosmin initially, tetrofosmin myocardial content approaches that of thallium because of progressive loss of ^{201}Tl through washout.

Technetium-99m tetrofosmin also shows minimal washout from the myocardium in a canine model[142] and in humans.[145] Because its clearance from the blood is rapid and its myocardial and lung washout are minimal, it would be anticipated that ^{99m}Tc tetrofosmin does not show clinically significant tracer redistribution. Lack of ^{99m}Tc tetrofosmin redistribution has been confirmed in a number of clinical reports.[146–148]

The human biodistribution of ^{99m}Tc tetrofosmin has been the subject of recent reports. At 5 min after resting injection, 1.2 to 1.8 percent of the ^{99m}Tc tetrofosmin dose is localized in the myocardium,[134,149] compared to 1.2 percent of the injected dose for ^{99m}Tc sestamibi.[74] With resting injection, heart-to-liver ^{99m}Tc tetrofosmin activity ratios increase from 0.8 $\pm$ 0.2 at 5 min to 1.3 $\pm$ 0.4 at 60 min and 2.1 $\pm$ 0.4 at 180 min[145] whereas the corresponding ratios for ^{99m}Tc sestamibi are 0.5 $\pm$ 0.1,

0.6 ± 1, and 1.4 ± 0.2, respectively.[74] When ^{99m}Tc tetrofosmin is injected at exercise, heart-to-liver ratios increase from 1.3 ± 0.4 at 5 min to 1.6 ± 0.4 at 60 min and 2.0 ± 0.4 at 180 min, with similar corresponding ^{99m}Tc sestamibi heart-to-liver ratios of 1.3 ± 0.1, 1.8 ± 0.3, and 2.4 ± 0.3, respectively.[74] As is the case for ^{99m}Tc sestamibi,[74] heart-to-lung ratios of both rest and exercise distributions of ^{99m}Tc tetrofosmin activity are favorable by 5 min after tracer injection and remain so over the ensuing 3 h.[145] Human absorbed radiation doses have been reported by Higley et al[134] and are similar for ^{99m}Tc tetrofosmin compared to ^{99m}Tc sestamibi. In comparison to available ^{99m}Tc myocardial perfusion tracers, potential advantages of ^{99m}Tc tetrofosmin include relatively rapid hepatic clearance, which may permit earlier imaging following injection at rest,[150] and room temperature tracer preparation.

Technetium-99m Furifosmin (Q12)

From the mixed ligand series of "Q complexes," ^{99m}Tc furifosmin or Q12 has completed phase three clinical studies. Similar to ^{99m}Tc sestamibi, and in contrast to ^{201}Tl, ^{99m}Tc furifosmin does not appear to be actively transported into the myocyte by the ATP-dependent sodium–potassium exchange pump.[151] In isolated rat myocyte preparations, Roszell et al[152] observed a linear relationship between ^{99m}Tc furifosmin uptake over 30 min and furifosmin concentration of the suspension medium for tracer concentrations between 1 and 200 μCi/ml. Using suspensions of rat myocytes and rat myocardial mitochondria, furifosmin concentration was 5 to 10 times greater on a per gram basis in mitochondria compared to intact myocardial cells. Thus, as is the case for ^{99m}Tc sestamibi and ^{99m}Tc tetrofosmin, mitochondrial mechanisms appear to account for further ^{99m}Tc furifosmin concentrating potential within myocytes.

Blood clearance of ^{99m}Tc furifosmin is biexponential in an open-chest canine model, with initial half-time of 1.8 ± 0.01 min and late half-time of 69.0 ± 8.2 min.[4] The relationship of ^{99m}Tc furifosmin activity per gram of myocardium to myocardial blood flow measured by microsphere methods in an open-chest canine model is shown in Fig. 1-1**A**, **B**, and **C**. For myocardial blood flows up to 2 ml/min/g, there was a significant ($p < 0.001$) linear relationship between myocardial tracer activity and myocardial blood flow ($r = 0.88$). In isolated rabbit hearts[152] perfused at rates from 0.56 to 2.92 ml/min/g of tissue, maximal fractional extraction (E_{max}) of ^{99m}Tc furifosmin (0.26 ± 0.05) was significantly less than that for ^{201}Tl (0.71 ± 0.05, $p < 0.01$). Net extraction (E_{net}) of furifosmin (0.12 ± 0.05) was also less than for ^{201}Tl (0.57 ± 0.11, $p < 0.001$). In human studies,[153,154] 1.2 to 2.2 percent of an injected ^{99m}Tc furifosmin dose localized in the heart.

Uptake and clearance of ^{99m}Tc furifosmin from the heart does not appear to be substantially influenced by the metabolic state of the myocardium. Thus, McGoron et al[155] found that acidemia (pH = 6.7), which reduced left ventricular pressures by 50 percent and ^{201}Tl E_{net} by 11.2 percent, had no significant effect on the uptake or clearance of ^{99m}Tc furifosmin in isolated, blood-perfused rat hearts. In contrast to ^{99m}Tc furifosmin, ^{201}Tl clearance was accelerated by acidemia.[155] Similarly, Johnson et al[156,157] found no effect of hypoxia or severely reduced buffer flow rate (ischemia) on ^{99m}Tc furifosmin clearance in isolated perfused rat hearts.

Once ^{99m}Tc furifosmin is extracted into the myocardium, there is no significant tracer clearance over 4 h.[4] Therefore, separate stress and rest tracer injections are required to detect myocardial viability. The principal clinical advantage of ^{99m}Tc furifosmin relates to its rapid hepatic clearance following both exercise and rest injection. Rapid hepatic clearance of tracer may facilitate the use of rapid imaging protocols.[153,154]

Technetium-99m N-NOET

Bis(N-ethoxy,N-ethyl dithiocarbamato)nitrido ^{99m}Tc(V) is a neutral lipophilic myocardial imaging agent referred to as TcN-NOET.[158] From a series of ^{99m}Tc nitrido complexes, the lateral groups attached to the dithiocarbamate ligand were varied to optimize myocardial uptake and washout. Consequently, as much as 5.2 percent of the injected dose of TcN-NOET has been reported to localize in the heart at 30 min following tracer injection in humans.[159] The mechanism of TcN-NOET uptake into the myocardium has not been established clearly. The tracer appears to be associated with various membranes of the myocardial cell and is absent from the cytosol. A neutral compound, TcN-NOET differs from cationic ^{99m}Tc myocardial imaging agents because selective binding to mitochondria is not observed.[160]

High myocardial uptake of TcN-NOET has been documented in a variety of animal species.[158] In anesthetized, open-chest canines, Ghezzi et al[161] observed a linear relationship of normalized TcN-NOET activity to normalized myocardial blood flow over a broad range of ischemic, normal, and hyperemic flows. At very low myocardial blood flows (mean = 0.28 ± 0.14 ml/min/g), TcN-NOET activity overestimated myocardial blood flow, whereas at very high flows (mean = 3.22 ± 1.64 ml/min/g) TcN-NOET activity underestimated myocardial blood flow. The first-pass extraction fraction of TcN-NOET was 76 ± 4 percent with basal myocardial blood flow and 85 ± 2 percent with pharmacologically induced hyperemic conditions as measured from arterial-coronary sinus differences relative to a nondiffusible intravascular tracer.[161]

Table 1-4 Properties of Thallium 201 and Five Technetium 99m Myocardial Tracers

	^{201}Tl	Sestamibi	Teboroxime	Tetrofosmin	Furifosmin (Q12)	NOET
Classification	Element	Isonitrile	Boronic acid adduct	Diphosphine	Mixed ligand	Nitrido
Charge	Cation	Cation	Neutral	Cation	Cation	Neutral
Uptake	Active	Passive	Passive	Passive	Passive	Passive
Preparation	Cyclotron	Kit	Kit	Kit	Kit	Kit
E_{max}	0.69–0.73	0.39	0.72	0.24	0.26	—
Myocardial clearance	T½ approx. 6 h	Minimal at 5 h	T½ approx. 10 min	Minimal at 3 h	Minimal at 4 h	—
Injection to imaging time	1–15 min	15 min (stress) 60 min (rest)	1–2 min	Approx. 15 min	Approx. 15 min	30 min
Differential washout	Yes	Negligible	Yes	Negligible	Negligible	Yes
SPECT studies	Yes	Yes	Possible	Yes	Yes	Yes
Gated SPECT	No	Yes	No	Yes	Yes	—
%ID in heart (at 60 min at rest)	1–2.7	1.0	Minimal, due to washout	1.2	1.2–2.3	5.2
Heart/liver (at 60 min at rest)	2.6	0.3–0.6	Minimal, due to washout	1.4	1.0–1.6	—
Blood pool, initial T½	5 min	2.2 min	<2 min	<5 min	1.8 min	4.7 min
Effective dose equivalent	2.6 rem/2 mCi	1.1 rem/30 mCi	1.8 rem/30 mCi	0.8 rem/30 mCi	0.9 rem/30 mCi	—
Clearance	Renal	Hepatic	Hepatic	Hepatic	Hepatic and renal	—

E_{max}, maximum extraction fraction (values not directly comparable as coronary flows vary); ID, injected dose;—insufficient or no data

Blood clearance of TcN-NOET is slower than for ^{99m}Tc sestamibi. Blood TcN-NOET activity at 30 min following intravenous injection was 20 percent of that observed at 2 min and the blood tracer level remained relatively constant until 90 min after injection.[161] Myocardial clearance of TcN-NOET is prominent in isolated rat hearts perfused with Krebs–Henseleit buffer enriched with red blood cells but negligible in the absence of red blood cells.[162,163] In the presence of an experimental coronary artery stenosis and pharmacologic coronary artery vasodilation, the relationship between myocardial blood flow and TcN-NOET myocardial retention is maintained for up to 90 min after tracer injection. However, with coronary reflow following tracer injection nearly complete tracer redistribution was observed.[161] In humans, reversibility of perfusion defects with TcN-NOET has correlated well with ^{201}Tl redistribution.[164]

In animals and in humans, TcN-NOET activity is initially prominent in the lungs, but lung activity then clears more rapidly than myocardial activity.[161,164] For this reason, in the European multicenter study,[164] tomographic myocardial imaging was delayed for 30 min following TcN-NOET injection. Nevertheless, imaging with TcN-NOET offers substantial promise of combining the favorable physical imaging properties of ^{99m}Tc

with potentially advantageous biological properties resembling ^{201}Tl.

Comparison of Current Myocardial Perfusion Imaging Agents

Properties of six myocardial perfusion imaging agents are summarized in Table 1-4. Direct comparison between tracers has been hampered by methodologic differences among experimental studies. For example, normalization of data in plots of myocardial tracer activity versus myocardial blood flow has varied substantially from study to study. Additionally, methods for calculation of heart-to-organ tracer activity ratios have not been fully standardized.

TRACER ACCUMULATION IN ISCHEMIC MYOCARDIUM

A novel approach to the detection of reversibly ischemic myocardium involves the development of nitroimidazole tracers that are selectively trapped in hypoxic myocardial tissue.[165] The "hypoxic sensitizer" misonidazole has been shown to accumulate in hypoxic tissue related to tumors, stroke, or myocardial ischemia. F-18 misonidazole has been imaged with positron emission tomography,[166-169] and iodinated[170] and ^{99m}Tc-labeled nitroimidazole tracers have been developed.[171-175] In animal models, ^{99m}Tc nitroimidazole has shown selective retention in ischemic but viable myocardium in animal models.[171-174] This approach appears to show substantial clinical potential. However, low target-to-nontarget activity ratios of hypoxic myocardium to background liver activity may limit the effectiveness of currently available agents.[171]

CONCLUSIONS

Thallium 201 continues to be used widely for noninvasive detection of CAD and identification of viable myocardium. The physical imaging properties of ^{99m}Tc are clearly superior to those of ^{201}Tl, so that the challenge remains to develop a ^{99m}Tc myocardial tracer with biological properties that compare favorably to those of [201]Tl. Thus, ^{99m}Tc myocardial tracers are needed with (1) improved tracer localization in the myocardium, (2) better tracer contrast between ischemic and normal myocardium, (3) improved detection of myocardial viability, and (4) reduced interference from tracer activity in nontarget organs, particularly the liver and lungs. Progress has been made in developing ^{99m}Tc myocardial imaging agents that represent advances in these areas but substantial further improvements in tracer development are needed.

REFERENCES

1. Ritchie JL, Zaret BL, Strauss HW, et al: Myocardial imaging with thallium-201: A multicenter study in patients with angina pectoris or acute myocardial infarction. *Am J Cardiol* 42:345, 1978.
2. Glover DK, Okada RD: Myocardial kinetics of Tc-MIBI in canine myocardium after dipyridamole. *Circulation* 81:628, 1990.
3. Heymann MA, Payne BD, Hoffman JIE, Rudolph AM: Blood flow measurements with radionuclide-labeled particles. *Prog Cardiovasc Dis* 20:55, 1977.
4. Gerson MC, Millard RW, Roszell NJ, et al: Kinetic properties of ^{99m}Tc-Q12 in canine myocardium. *Circulation* 89:1291, 1994.
5. Bassingthwaighte JB, Malone MA, Moffett TC, et al: Validity of microsphere depositions for regional myocardial flows. *Am J Physiol* 253:H184, 1987.
6. Gerson MC, Millard RW, McGoron AJ, et al: Myocardial uptake and kinetic properties of technetium-99m-Q3 in dogs. *J Nucl Med* 35:1968, 1994.
7. Meerdink DJ, Leppo JA: Experimental studies of the physiologic properties of technetium-99m agents: Myocardial transport of perfusion imaging agents. *Am J Cardiol* 66:9E, 1990.
8. Bassingthwaighte JB, Holloway GA Jr: Estimation of blood flow with radioactive tracers. *Semin Nucl Med* 6:141, 1976.
9. Horres CR, Lieberman M, Purdy JE: Growth orientation of heart cells on nylon monofilament. *J Membr Biol* 34:313, 1977.
10. Powell T, Twist VW: A rapid technique for the isolation and purification of adult cardiac muscle cells having respiratory control and a tolerance to calcium. *Biochem Biophys Res Comm* 72:327, 1976.
11. Deutsch E, Ketring AR, Libson K, et al: The Noah's Ark experiment: Species dependent biodistributions of cationic Tc-99m complexes. *Int J Radiat Appl Instrum* 16:191, 1989.
12. Gehring PJ, Hammond PB: The interrelationship between thallium and potassium in animals. *J Pharm Exp Ther* 155:187, 1967.
13. McCall D, Zimmer LJ, Katz AM: Kinetics of thallium exchange in cultured rat myocardial cells. *Circ Res* 56:370, 1985.
14. Piwnica-Worms D, Kronauge JF, Delmon L, et al: Effect of metabolic inhibition on technetium-99m-MIBI kinetics in cultured chick myocardial cells. *J Nucl Med* 31:464, 1990.
15. Meerdink DJ, Leppo JA: Comparison of hypoxia and ouabain effects on the myocardial uptake kinetics of technetium-99m hexakis 2-methoxyisobutyl isonitrile and thallium-201. *J Nucl Med* 30:1500, 1989.
16. McGoron AJ, Millard RW, Biniakiewicz DS, et al: Effects of ouabain on technetium-99m-Q12 and thallium-201 extraction and retention by isolated heart. *J Nucl Med* 37:752, 1996.
17. Weich HF, Strauss HW, Pitt B: The extraction of thallium-201 by the myocardium. *Circulation* 56:188, 1977.
18. Hamilton GW, Narahara KA, Yee H, et al: Myocardial imaging with thallium-201: Effect of cardiac drugs on myocardial images and absolute tissue distribution. *J Nucl Med* 19:10, 1978.
19. Krivokapich J, Shine KI: Effects of hyperkalemia and glycoside on thallium exchange in rabbit ventricle. *Am J Physiol* 240:H612, 1981.
20. Melin JA, Becker LC: Quantitative relationship between global left ventricular thallium uptake and blood flow: Effects of propranolol, ouabain, dipyridamole, and coronary artery occlusion. *J Nucl Med* 27:641, 1986.
21. Maublant JC, Gachon P, Moins N: Hexakis (2-methoxy isobutylisonitrile) technetium-99m and thallium-201 chloride: Uptake and release in cultured myocardial cells. *J Nucl Med* 29:48, 1988.
22. Lebowitz E, Greene MW, Fairchild R, et al: Thallium-201 for medical use. *J Nucl Med* 16:151, 1975.
23. New England Nuclear: Thallous chloride Tl-201. North Billerica, MA, November 1977 (package insert).
24. Atkins HL, Budinger TF, Lebowitz E, et al: Thallium-201 for medical use. Part 3: Human distribution and physical imaging properties. *J Nucl Med* 18:133, 1977.

25. Krahwinkel W, Herzog H, Feinendegen LE: Pharmacokinetics of thallium-201 in normal individuals after routine myocardial scintigraphy. *J Nucl Med* 29:1582, 1988.
26. Mueller TM, Marcus ML, Ehrhardt JC, et al: Limitations of thallium-201 myocardial perfusion scintigrams. *Circulation* 54:640, 1976.
27. Nielsen AP, Morris KG, Murdock R, et al: Linear relationship between the distribution of thallium-201 and blood flow in ischemic and nonischemic myocardium during exercise. *Circulation* 61:797, 1980.
28. Gould KL: Noninvasive assessment of coronary stenoses by myocardial perfusion imaging during pharmacologic coronary vasodilatation. *Am J Cardiol* 41:279, 1978.
29. Nichols AB, Weiss MB, Sciacca RR, et al: Relationship between segmental thallium-201 uptake and regional myocardial blood flow in patients with coronary artery disease. *Circulation* 68:310, 1983.
30. Hadjimiltiades S, Watson R, Hakki A-H, et al: Relation between myocardial thallium-201 kinetics during exercise and quantitative coronary angiography in patients with one vessel coronary artery disease. *J Am Coll Cardiol* 13:1301, 1989.
31. Leppo JA, Meerdink DJ: Comparison of the myocardial uptake of technetium-labelled isonitrile analogue and thallium. *Circ Res* 65:632, 1989.
32. Leppo JA: Myocardial uptake of thallium and rubidium during alterations in perfusion and oxygenation in isolated rabbit hearts. *J Nucl Med* 28:878, 1987.
33. Friedman BJ, Beihn R, Friedman JP: The effect of hypoxia on thallium kinetics in cultured chick myocardial cells. *J Nucl Med* 28:1453, 1987.
34. Leppo JA, Macneil PB, Moring AF, et al: Separate effects of ischemia, hypoxia, and contractility on thallium-201 kinetics in rabbit myocardium. *J Nucl Med* 27:66, 1986.
35. Grunwald AM, Watson DD, Holzgrefe HH Jr, et al: Myocardial thallium-201 kinetics in normal and ischemic myocardium. *Circulation* 64:610, 1981.
36. Okada RD, Jacobs ML, Daggett WM, et al: Thallium-201 kinetics in nonischemic canine myocardium. *Circulation* 65:70, 1982.
37. Okada RD, Leppo JA, Strauss HW, et al: Mechanisms and time course for the disappearance of thallium-201 defects at rest in dogs. *Am J Cardiol* 49:699, 1982.
38. Goldhaber SZ, Newell JB, Alpert NM, et al: Effects of ischemic-like insult on myocardial thallium-201 accumulation. *Circulation* 67:778, 1983.
39. Berger BC, Watson DD, Taylor GJ, et al: Quantitative thallium-201 exercise scintigraphy for detection of coronary artery disease. *J Nucl Med* 22:585, 1981.
40. Nishiyama H, Adolph RJ, Gabel M, et al: Effect of coronary blood flow on thallium-201 uptake and washout. *Circulation* 65:534, 1982.
41. Bradley-Moore PR, Lebowitz E, Greene MW, et al: Thallium-201 for medical use. II: Biologic behavior. *J Nucl Med* 16:156, 1975.
42. Sklar J, Kirch D, Johnson T, et al: Slow late myocardial clearance of thallium: A characteristic phenomenon in coronary artery disease. *Circulation* 65:1504, 1982.
43. Kaul S, Chesler DA, Pohost GM, et al: Influence of peak exercise heart rate on normal thallium-201 myocardial clearance. *J Nucl Med* 27:26, 1986.
44. Nishimura T, Uehara T, Hayashida K, et al: Quantitative assessment of thallium myocardial washout rate: Importance of peak heart rate and lung thallium uptake in defining normal values. *Eur J Nucl Med* 13:67, 1987.
45. Nordrehaug JE, Danielsen R, Vik-Mo H: Effects of heart rate on myocardial thallium-201 uptake and clearance. *J Nucl Med* 30:1972, 1989.
46. Rabinovitch M, Suissa S, Elstein J, et al: Sex-specific criteria for interpretation of thallium-201 myocardial uptake and washout studies. *J Nucl Med* 27:1837, 1986.
47. Wilson RA, Sullivan PJ, Okada RD, et al: The effect of eating on thallium myocardial imaging. *Chest* 89:195, 1986.
48. Angello DA, Wilson RA, Palac RT: Effect of eating on thallium-201 myocardial redistribution after myocardial ischemia. *Am J Cardiol* 60:528, 1987.
49. Gutman J, Berman DS, Freeman M, et al: Time to completed redistribution of thallium-201 in exercise myocardial scintigraphy: Relationship to the degree of coronary artery stenosis. *Am Heart J* 106:989, 1983.
50. Kimball BP, Shurvell BL, Mildenberger RR, et al: Abnormal thallium kinetics in postoperative coarctation of the aorta: Evidence for diffuse hypertension-induced vascular pathology. *J Am Coll Cardiol* 7:538, 1986.
51. Takata J, Counihan PJ, Gane JN, et al: Regional thallium-201 washout and myocardial hypertrophy in hypertrophic cardiomyopathy and its relation to exertional chest pain. *Am J Cardiol* 72:211, 1993.
52. Tanasescu D, Berman D, Staniloff H, et al: Apparent worsening of thallium-201 myocardial defects during redistribution—What does it mean? *J Nucl Med* 20:688, 1979 (abstr).
53. Hecht HS, Hopkins JM, Rose JG, et al: Reverse redistribution: Worsening of thallium-201 myocardial images from exercise to redistribution. *Radiology* 140:177, 1981.
54. Silberstein EB, DeVries DF: Reverse redistribution phenomenon in thallium-201 stress tests: Angiographic correlation and clinical significance. *J Nucl Med* 26:707, 1985.
55. Popma JJ, Smitherman TC, Walker BS, et al: Reverse redistribution of thallium-201 detected by SPECT imaging after dipyridamole in angina pectoris. *Am J Cardiol* 65:1176, 1990.
56. Pace L, Cuocolo A, Maurea S, et al: Reverse redistribution in resting thallium-201 myocardial scintigraphy in patients with coronary artery disease: Relation to coronary anatomy and ventricular function. *J Nucl Med* 34:1688, 1993.
57. Marin-Neto JA, Dilsizian V, Arrighi JA, et al: Thallium reinjection demonstrates viable myocardium in regions with reverse redistribution. *Circulation* 88:1736, 1993.
58. Weiss AT, Maddahi J, Lew AS, et al: Reverse redistribution of thallium-201: A sign of nontransmural myocardial infarction with patency of the infarct-related coronary artery. *J Am Coll Cardiol* 7:61, 1986.
59. Soufer R, Dey HM, Lawson AJ, et al: Relationship between reverse redistribution on planar thallium scintigraphy and regional myocardial viability: A correlative PET study. *J Nucl Med* 36:180, 1995.

60. Ohte N, Hashimoto T, Banno T, et al: Clinical significance of reverse redistribution on 24-hour delayed imaging of exercise thallium-201 myocardial SPECT: Comparison with myocardial fluorine-18-FDG-PET imaging and left ventricular wall motion. *J Nucl Med* 36:86, 1995.

61. Pace L, Cuocolo A, Nicolai E, et al: Reverse redistribution in Tl-201 stress-redistribution myocardial scintigraphy. Effect of rest reinjection. *Clin Nucl Med* 19:956, 1994.

62. Bateman TM, Maddahi J, Gray RJ, et al: Diffuse slow washout of myocardial thallium-201: A new scintigraphic indicator of extensive coronary artery disease. *J Am Coll Cardiol* 4:55, 1984.

63. Brown KA, Benoit L, Clements JP, et al: Fast washout of thallium-201 from area of myocardial infarction: Possible artifact of background subtraction. *J Nucl Med* 28:945, 1987.

64. Lear JL, Raff U, Jain R: Reverse and pseudo redistribution of thallium-201 in healed myocardial infarction and normal and negative thallium-201 washout in ischemia due to background oversubtraction. *Am J Cardiol* 62:543, 1988.

65. Leppo J: Thallium washout analysis: Fact or fiction? *J Nucl Med* 28:1058, 1987.

66. Bonow RO, Dilsizian V, Cuocolo A, et al: Identification of viable myocardium in patients with chronic coronary artery disease and left ventricular dysfunction. Comparison of thallium scintigraphy with reinjection and PET imaging with ^{18}F-fluorodeoxyglucose. *Circulation* 83:26, 1991.

67. Ragosta M, Beller GA, Watson DD, et al: Quantitative planar rest-redistribution ^{201}Tl imaging in detection of myocardial viability and prediction of improvement in left ventricular function after coronary bypass surgery in patients with severely depressed left ventricular function. *Circulation* 87:1630, 1993.

68. Zimmermann R, Mall G, Rauch B, et al: Residual ^{201}Tl activity in irreversible defects as a marker of myocardial viability. Clinicopathological study. *Circulation* 91:1016, 1995.

69. Pohost GH, Alpert NM, Ingwall JS, et al: Thallium redistribution: Mechanism and clinical utility. *Semin Nucl Med* 10:70, 1980.

70. Gordon DG, Pfisterer M, Williams R, et al: The effect of diaphragmatic attenuation on ^{201}Tl images. *Clin Nucl Med* 4:150, 1979.

71. Johnstone DE, Wackers FJTh, Berger HJ, et al: Effect of patient positioning on left lateral thallium-201 myocardial images. *J Nucl Med* 20:183, 1979.

72. Stolzenberg J, Kaminsky J: Overlying breast as cause of false-positive thallium scans. *Clin Nucl Med* 3:229, 1978.

73. Mousa SA, Williams SJ, Sands H: Characterization of in vivo chemistry of cations in the heart. *J Nucl Med* 28:1351, 1987.

74. Wackers FJTh, Berman DS, Maddahi J, et al: Technetium-99m hexakis 2-methoxyisobutyl isonitrile: Human biodistribution, dosimetry, safety, and preliminary comparison to thallium-201 for myocardial perfusion imaging. *J Nucl Med* 30:301, 1989.

75. Okada RD, Glover D, Gaffney T, et al: Myocardial kinetics of technetium-99m-hexakis-2-methoxy-2-methylpropyl-isonitrile. *Circulation* 77:491, 1988.

76. Kahn JK, McGhie I, Akers MS, et al: Quantitative rotational tomography with ^{201}Tl and 99mTc 2-methoxy-isobutyl-isonitrile. A direct comparison in normal individuals and patients with coronary artery disease. *Circulation* 79:1282, 1989.

77. Piwnica-Worms D, Kronauge JF, Holman BL, et al: Comparative myocardial uptake characteristics of hexakis (alkylisonitrile) technetium(I) complexes: Effect of lipophilicity. *Invest Radiol* 24:25, 1989.

78. Piwnica-Worms D, Kronauge JF, Chiu ML: Uptake and retention of hexakis (2-methoxyisobutyl isonitrile) technetium(I) in cultured chick myocardial cells. Mitochondrial and plasma membrane potential dependence. *Circulation* 82:1826, 1990.

79. Backus M, Piwnica-Worms D, Hockett D, et al: Microprobe analysis of Tc-MIBI in heart cells: Calculation of mitochondrial membrane potential. *Am J Physiol* 265:C178, 1993.

80. Carvalho PA, Chiu ML, Kronauge JF, et al: Subcellular distribution and analysis of technetium-99m-MIBI in isolated perfused rat hearts. *J Nucl Med* 33:1516, 1992.

81. Beanlands RSB, Dawood F, Wen W-H, et al: Are the kinetics of technetium-99m methoxyisobutyl isonitrile affected by cell metabolism and viability? *Circulation* 82:1802, 1990.

82. Li Q-S, Frank TL, Franceschi D, et al: Technetium-99m methoxyisobutyl isonitrile (RP30) for quantification of myocardial ischemia and reperfusion in dogs. *J Nucl Med* 29:1539, 1988.

83. Leppo JA, Meerdink DJ: Comparison of the myocardial uptake of a technetium-labeled isonitrile analogue and thallium. *Circ Res* 65:632, 1989.

84. Canby RC, Silber S, Pohost GM: Relations of the myocardial imaging agents ^{99m}Tc-MIBI and ^{201}Tl to myocardial blood flow in a canine model of myocardial ischemic insult. *Circulation* 81:289, 1990.

85. Mousa SA, Carroll TR, Morgan RA: Acute effects of commonly used drugs in the cardiac care unit on the myocardial extraction kinetics of ^{99m}Tc-sestamibi. *Int J Clin Pharmacol Ther Toxicol* 29:14, 1991.

86. Leon AR, Eisner RL, Martin SE, et al: Comparison of single-photon emission computed tomographic (SPECT) myocardial perfusion imaging with thallium-201 and technetium-99m sestamibi in dogs. *J Am Coll Cardiol* 20:1612, 1992.

87. Glover DK, Ruiz M, Edwards NC, et al: Comparison between ^{201}Tl and ^{99m}Tc sestamibi uptake during adenosine-induced vasodilation as a function of coronary stenosis severity. *Circulation* 91:813, 1995.

88. Narahara KA, Villanueva-Meyer J, Thompson CJ, et al: Comparison of thallium-201 and technetium-99m hexakis 2-methoxyisobutyl isonitrile single-photon emission computed tomography for estimating the extent of myocardial ischemia and infarction in coronary artery disease. *Am J Cardiol* 66;1438, 1990.

89. Maublant JC, Marcaggi X, Lusson J-R, et al: Comparison between thallium-201 and technetium-99m methoxyiso-

butyl isonitrile defect size in single-photon emission computed tomography at rest, exercise and redistribution in coronary artery disease. *Am J Cardiol* 69:183, 1992.

90. Piwnica-Worms D, Chiu ML, Kronauge JF: Divergent kinetics of ^{201}Tl and ^{99m}Tc-sestamibi in cultured chick ventricular myocytes during ATP depletion. *Circulation* 85:1531, 1992.

91. Mousa SA, Cooney JM, Stevens S: Kinetics of technetium-99m- sestamibi and thallium-201 in a transient ischemic myocardium animal model: Insight into the 'redistribution' phenomenon. *Cardiology* 81:157, 1992.

92. Sinusas AJ, Bergin JD, Edwards NC, et al: Redistribution of ^{99m}Tc-sestamibi and ^{201}Tl in the presence of a severe coronary artery stenosis. *Circulation* 89:2332, 1994.

93. Glover DK, Okada RD: Myocardial technetium 99m sestamibi kinetics after reperfusion in a canine model. *Am Heart J* 125:657, 1993.

94. Giubbini R, Campini R, Milan E, et al: Evaluation of technetium-99m-sestamibi lung uptake: Correlation with left ventricular function. *J Nucl Med* 36:58, 1995.

95. Saha M, Farrand TF, Brown KA: Lung uptake of technetium 99m sestamibi: Relation to clinical, exercise, hemodynamic, and left ventricular function variables. *J Nucl Cardiol* 1:52, 1994.

96. Hurwitz GA, Fox SP, Driedger AA, et al: Pulmonary uptake of sestamibi on early post-stress images: Angiographic relationships, incidence and kinetics. *Nucl Med Commun* 14:15, 1993.

97. Gill JB, Ruddy TD, Newell JB, et al: Prognostic importance of thallium uptake by the lungs during exercise in coronary artery disease. *N Engl J Med* 317:1485, 1987.

98. Boucher CA, Zir LM, Beller GA, et al: Increased lung uptake of thallium-201 during exercise myocardial imaging: Clinical, hemodynamic and angiographic implications in patients with coronary artery disease. *Am J Cardiol* 46:189, 1980.

99. Leppo JA, Meerdink DJ: Comparative myocardial extraction of two technetium-labeled BATO derivatives (SQ30217, SQ32014) and thallium. *J Nucl Med* 31:67, 1990.

100. Maublant JC, Moins N, Gachon P, et al: Uptake of technetium-99m-teboroxime in cultured myocardial cells: Comparison with thallium-201 and technetium-99m-sestamibi. *J Nucl Med* 34:255, 1993.

101. Narra RK, Feld T, Nunn AD: Absorbed radiation dose to humans from technetium-99m-teboroxime. *J Nucl Med* 33:88, 1992.

102. Di Rocco RJ, Rumsey WL, Kuczynski BL, et al: Measurement of myocardial blood flow using a co-injection technique for technetium-99m-teboroxime, technetium-96-sestamibi and thallium-201. *J Nucl Med* 33:1152, 1992.

103. Glover DK, Ruiz M, Bergmann EE, et al: Myocardial technetium-99m-teboroxime uptake during adenosine-induced hyperemia in dogs with either a critical or mild coronary stenosis: Comparison to thallium-201 and regional blood flow. *J Nucl Med* 36:476, 1995.

104. Rumsey WL, Rosenspire KC, Nunn AD: Myocardial extraction of teboroxime: Effects of teboroxime interaction with blood. *J Nucl Med* 33:94, 1992.

105. Dahlberg ST, Gilmore MP, Leppo JA: Interaction of technetium 99m-labeled teboroxime with red blood cells reduces the compound's extraction and increases apparent cardiac washout. *J Nucl Cardiol* 1:270, 1994.

106. Stewart RE, Schwaiger M, Hutchins GD, et al: Myocardial clearance kinetics of technetium-99m-SQ30217: A marker of regional myocardial blood flow. *J Nucl Med* 31:1183, 1990.

107. Weinstein H, Reinhardt CP, Leppo JA: Teboroxime, sestamibi and thallium-201 as markers of myocardial hypoperfusion: Comparison by quantitative dual-isotope autoradiography in rabbits. *J Nucl Med* 34:1510, 1993.

108. Seldin DW, Johnson LL, Blood DK, et al: Myocardial perfusion imaging with technetium-99m SQ30217: Comparison with thallium-201 and coronary anatomy. *J Nucl Med* 30:312, 1989.

109. Marshall RC, Leidholdt EM Jr, Zhang D-Y, et al: The effect of flow on technetium-99m-teboroxime (SQ30217) and thallium-201 extraction and retention in rabbit heart. *J Nucl Med* 32:1979, 1991.

110. Stewart RE, Heyl B, O'Rourke RA, et al: Demonstration of differential post-stenotic myocardial technetium-99m-teboroxime clearance kinetics after experimental ischemia and hyperemic stress. *J Nucl Med* 32:2000, 1991.

111. Beanlands R, Muzik O, Nguyen N, et al: The relationship between myocardial retention of technetium-99m teboroxime and myocardial blood flow. *J Am Coll Cardiol* 20:712, 1992.

112. Johnson G III, Glover DK, Hebert CB, et al: Myocardial clearance kinetics of technetium-99m-teboroxime following dipyridamole: Differentiation of stenosis severity in canine myocardium. *J Nucl Med* 36:111, 1995.

113. Gray WA, Gewirtz H: Comparison of ^{99m}Tc-teboroxime with thallium for myocardial imaging in the presence of a coronary artery stenosis. *Circulation* 84:1796, 1991.

114. Okada RD, Leppo JA, Boucher CA, et al: Myocardial kinetics of thallium-201 after dipyridamole infusion in normal canine myocardium and in myocardium distal to a stenosis. *J Clin Invest* 69:199, 1982.

115. Leppo JA, Okada RD, Strauss HW, et al: Effect of hyperaemia on thallium-201 redistribution in normal canine myocardium. *Cardiovasc Res* 19:679, 1985.

116. Hendel RC, McSherry B, Karimeddini M, et al: Diagnostic value of a new myocardial perfusion agent, teboroxime (SQ 30,217), utilizing a rapid planar imaging protocol: Preliminary results. *J Am Coll Cardiol* 16:855, 1990.

117. Dahlberg ST, Weinstein H, Hendel RC, et al: Planar myocardial perfusion imaging with technetium-99m-teboroxime: Comparison by vascular territory with thallium-201 and coronary angiography. *J Nucl Med* 33:1783, 1992.

118. Nakajima K, Taki J, Bunko H, et al: Dynamic acquisition with a three-headed SPECT system: Application to technetium 99m-SQ30217 myocardial imaging. *J Nucl Med* 32:1273, 1991.

119. Li Q-S, Solot G, Frank TL, et al: Tomographic myocardial perfusion imaging with technetium-99m-teboroxime

at rest and after dipyridamole. *J Nucl Med* 32:1968, 1991.

120. Burns RJ, Iles S, Fung AY, et al: The Canadian exercise technetium 99m-labeled teboroxime single-photon emission computed tomographic study. *J Nucl Cardiol* 2:117, 1995.

121. Bok BD, Bice AN, Clausen M, et al: Artifacts in camera based single photon emission tomography due to time activity variation. *Eur J Nucl Med* 13:439, 1987.

122. Nakajima K, Shuke N, Taki J, et al: A simulation of dynamic SPECT using radiopharmaceuticals with rapid clearance. *J Nucl Med* 33:1200, 1992.

123. O'Connor MK, Cho DS: Rapid radiotracer washout from the heart: Effect on image quality in SPECT performed with a single-headed gamma camera system. *J Nucl Med* 33:1146, 1992.

124. Links JM, Frank TL, Becker LC: Effect of differential tracer washout during SPECT acquisition. *J Nucl Med* 32:2253, 1991.

125. Henzlova MJ, Machac J: Clinical utility of technetium-99m-teboroxime myocardial washout imaging. *J Nucl Med* 35:575, 1994.

126. Chua T, Kiat H, Germano G, et al: Technetium-99m teboroxime regional myocardial washout in subjects with and without coronary artery disease. *Am J Cardiol* 72:728, 1993.

127. Labonte C, Taillefer R, Lambert R, et al: Comparison between technetium-99m-teboroxime and thallium-201 dipyridamole planar myocardial perfusion imaging in detection of coronary artery disease. *Am J Cardiol* 69:90, 1992.

128. Deutsch E, Bushong W, Glavan KA, et al: Heart imaging with cationic complexes of technetium. *Science* 214:85, 1981.

129. Gerson MC, Deutsch EA, Nishiyama H, et al: Myocardial perfusion imaging with ^{99m}Tc-DMPE in man. *Eur J Nucl Med* 8:371, 1983.

130. Vanderheyden J-L, Heeg MJ, Deutsch E: Comparison of the chemical and biological properties of trans-$(Tc(DMPE)_2Cl_2)^+$ and 1,2-bis(dimethylphosphino) ethane. Single-crystal structural analysis of trans-$(Re(DMPE)_2Cl_2)PF_6$. *Inorg Chem* 24:1666, 1985.

131. Gerson MC, Deutsch EA, Libson KF, et al: Myocardial scintigraphy with technetium-^{99m}Tc-Tris-DMPE in man. *Eur J Nucl Med* 9:403, 1984.

132. Holman BL, Jones AG, Lister-James J, et al: A new Tc-99m- labeled myocardial imaging agent, hexakis (t-butyl-isonitrile)-technetium(I) [Tc-99m TBI]: Initial experience in the human. *J Nucl Med* 25:1350, 1984.

133. Kelly JD, Forster AM, Higley B, et al: Technetium-99m-tetrofosmin as a new radiopharmaceutical for myocardial perfusion imaging. *J Nucl Med* 34:222, 1993.

134. Higley B, Smith FW, Smith T, et al: Technetium-99m-1,2- bis[bis(2-ethoxyethyl)phosphino]ethane: Human biodistribution, dosimetry and safety of a new myocardial perfusion imaging agent. *J Nucl Med* 34:30, 1993.

135. Deutsch E, Vanderheyden J-L, Gerundini P, et al: Development of nonreducible technetium-99m(III) cations as myocardial perfusion imaging agents: Initial experience in humans. *J Nucl Med* 28:1870, 1987.

136. Gerundini P, Savi A, Gilardi MC, et al: Evaluation in dogs and humans of three potential technetium-99m myocardial perfusion agents. *J Nucl Med* 27:409, 1986.

137. Younes A, Songadele JA, Maublant J, et al: Mechanism of uptake of technetium-tetrofosmin. II: Uptake into isolated adult rat heart mitochondria. *J Nucl Cardiol* 2:327, 1995.

138. Platts EA, North TL, Pickett RD, et al: Mechanism of uptake of technetium-tetrofosmin. I: Uptake into isolated adult rat ventricular myocytes and subcellular localization. *J Nucl Cardiol* 2:317, 1995.

139. Takahashi N, Reinhardt CP, Marcel R, et al: Comparative analysis of Tc-99m tetrofosmin and thallium uptake in a rat model of acute coronary reperfusion. *J Nucl Med* 36:101P, 1995 (abstr).

140. Glover DK, Ruiz M, Sansoy V, et al: Myocardial uptake of Tc-99m tetrofosmin in canine models of coronary occlusion and reperfusion. *Circulation* 88:I-441, 1993 (abstr).

141. Glover DK, Ruiz M, Allen TR, et al: Assessment of myocardial viability by Tc-99m tetrofosmin in a canine model of coronary occlusion and reperfusion. *J Am Coll Cardiol* 23:475A, 1994 (abstr).

142. Sinusas AJ, Shi Q-X, Saltzberg MT, et al: Technetium-99m-tetrofosmin to assess myocardial blood flow: Experimental validation in an intact canine model of ischemia. *J Nucl Med* 35:664, 1994.

143. Dahlberg ST, Gilmore MP, Leppo JA: Effect of coronary blood flow on the "uptake" of tetrofosmin in the isolated rabbit heart. *J Nucl Med* 33:846, 1992 (abstr).

144. Dahlberg ST, Gilmore MP, Flood M, et al: Extraction and washout of Tc-99m tetrofosmin in the isolated rat heart. *J Nucl Med* 35:47P, 1994 (abstract).

145. Jain D, Wackers FJTh, Mattera J, et al: Biokinetics of technetium-99m-tetrofosmin: Myocardial perfusion imaging agent: Implications for a one-day imaging protocol. *J Nucl Med* 34:1254, 1993.

146. Jain D, Wackers FJTh, McMahon M, et al: Is there any redistribution with ^{99m}Tc-tetrofosmin imaging? A quantitative study using serial planar imaging. *Circulation* 86(suppl I):I-46, 1992 (abstr).

147. Lahiri A, Higley B, Crawley JCW, et al: Novel functionalised diphosphine complexes of Tc-99m for myocardial imaging in man. *J Nucl Med* 30:818, 1989 (abstr).

148. Sridhara BS, Braat S, Rigo P, et al: Comparison of myocardial perfusion imaging with technetium-99m tetrofosmin versus thallium-201 in coronary artery disease. *Am J Cardiol* 72:1015, 1993.

149. Sasaki Y, Nishikawa J, Ohtake T, et al: Clinical evaluation of myocardial SPECT using a new technetium-99m diphosphine agent (PPN.1011). *J Nucl Med* 33:875, 1992 (abstr).

150. Flamen P, Bossuyt A, Franken PR: Technetium-99m-tetrofosmin in dipyridamole-stress myocardial SPECT imaging: Intraindividual comparison with technetium-99m-sestamibi. *J Nucl Med* 36:2009, 1995.

151. Roszell NJ, McGoron AJ, Biniakiewicz DS, et al: ^{99m}Tc Q12 handling by isolated rat cardiac myocytes and mitochondria. *Circulation* 92(suppl I):I-181, 1995 (abstr).

152. Meerdink DJ, Dahlberg ST, Gilmore M, et al: Transcapillary exchange of Q12 and thallium-201 in isolated rabbit hearts. *Circulation* 88:I-249, 1993 (abstr).

153. Gerson MC, Lukes J, Deutsch E, et al: Comparison of technetium 99m Q12 and thallium 201 for detection of angiographically documented coronary artery disease in humans. *J Nucl Cardiol* 1:499, 1994.

154. Rossetti C, Vanoli G, Paganelli G, et al: Human biodistribution, dosimetry and clinical use of technetium(III)-99m-Q12. *J Nucl Med* 35:1571, 1994.

155. McGoron AJ, Biniakiewicz DS, Roszell NJ, et al: Extraction and retention of ^{99m}Tc Q12, ^{99m}Tc sestamibi and ^{201}Tl imaging agents in isolated rat head during acidemia. *Circulation* 92(suppl I):I-180, 1995 (abstr).

156. Johnson G III, Nguyen KN, Okada RD: Myocardial Tc-99m Q-12 (TechneCardTM) clearance is not affected by hypoxia or low flow in an isolated perfused rat heart model. *Circulation* 88:I-249, 1993 (abstr).

157. Johnson G III, Nguyen KN, Alton IL, et al: Myocardial Tc-99m Q-12 (TechneCardTM) clearance is not affected by ischemia and reperfusion in an isolated perfused rat heart model. *J Am Coll Cardiol* 23:422A, 1994 (abstr).

158. Pasqualini R, Duatti A, Bellande E, et al: Bis(dithiocarbamato) nitrido technetium-99m radiopharmaceuticals: A class of neutral myocardial imaging agents. *J Nucl Med* 35:334, 1994.

159. Giganti M, Duatti A, Uccelli L, et al: Biodistribution and preliminary clinical evaluation of 99mTc-NOET as myocardial perfusion tracer. *J Nucl Cardiol* 2:S44, 1995 (abstract).

160. Uccelli L, Bolzati C, Comazzi V, et al: Subcellular distribution of bis(dithiocarbamato) nitrido Tc(V) radiopharmaceuticals in myocardium cells of male rats. *J Nucl Med* 33:850, 1992 (abstr).

161. Ghezzi C, Fagret D, Arvieux CC, et al: Myocardial kinetics of TcN-NOET: A neutral lipophilic complex tracer of regional myocardial blood flow. *J Nucl Med* 36:1069, 1995.

162. Johnson G III, Nguyen KN, Duatti A, et al: Interaction of 99mTcN-NOET with blood components in isolated, perfused rat myocardium: A potential mechanism of radiotracer redistribution. *J Nucl Cardiol* 2:S44, 1995 (abstr).

163. Johnson G III, Allton IL, Nguyen KN, et al: Clearance of technetium 99m N-NOET in normal, ischemic-reperfused, and membrane-disrupted myocardium. *J Nucl Cardiol* 3:42, 1996.

164. Fagret D, Marie P-Y, Brunotte F, et al: Myocardial perfusion imaging with technetium-99m-Tc NOET: Comparison with thallium-201 and coronary angiography. *J Nucl Med* 36:936, 1995.

165. Nunn A, Linder K, Strauss HW: Nitroimidazoles and imaging hypoxia. *Eur J Nucl Med* 22:265, 1995.

166. Grierson JR, Link JM, Mathis CA, et al: A radiosynthesis of fluorine-18 fluoromisonidazole. *J Nucl Med* 30:343, 1989.

167. Martin GV, Caldwell JH, Graham MM, et al: Noninvasive detection of hypoxic myocardium using fluorine-18-fluoromisonidazole and positron emission tomography. *J Nucl Med* 33:2202, 1992.

168. Shelton ME, Dence CS, Hwang D-R, et al: Myocardial kinetics of fluorine-18 misonidazole: A marker of hypoxic myocardium. *J Nucl Med* 30:351, 1989.

169. Martin GV, Caldwell JH, Rasey JS, et al: Enhanced binding of the hypoxic cell marker [^{3}H]fluoromisonidazole in ischemic myocardium. *J Nucl Med* 30:194, 1989.

170. Martin GV, Biskupiak JE, Caldwell JH, et al: Characterization of iodovinylmisonidazole as a marker for myocardial hypoxia. *J Nucl Med* 34:918, 1993.

171. Shi CQ-X, Sinusas AJ, Dione DP, et al: Technetium-99m-nitroimidazole (BMS181321): A positive imaging agent for detecting myocardial ischemia. *J Nucl Med* 36:1078, 1995.

172. Rumsey WL, Patel B, Linder KE: Effect of graded hypoxia on retention of technetium-99m-nitroheterocycle in perfused rat heart. *J Nucl Med* 36:632, 1995.

173. Kusuoka H, Hashimoto K, Fukuchi K, et al: Kinetics of a putative hypoxic tissue marker, technetium-99m-nitroimidazole (BMS181321), in normoxic, hypoxic, ischemic and stunned myocardium. *J Nucl Med* 35:1371, 1994.

174. Dahlberg ST, Gilmore MP, Flood M, et al: Effect of hypoxia and low-flow ischemia on the myocardial extraction of technetium-99m-nitroimidazole. *Circulation* 88:I-250, 1993 (abstr).

175. Strauss HW, Nunn A, Linder K: Nitroimidazoles for imaging hypoxic myocardium. *J Nucl Cardiol* 2:437, 1995.

Myocardial Perfusion Imaging: Planar Methods

Myron C. Gerson

Following administration of a myocardial perfusion tracer, the heart may be visualized by planar or tomographic imaging methods. With planar imaging, the gamma-camera face is placed over the thorax, and all tracer activity in the field of view is collected into a two-dimensional image. Activity from opposing cardiac walls, soft tissue activity, and non-target-organ activity, both in front of and behind the heart, are all superimposed. Superimposition of opposing left ventricular segments limits localization of perfusion defects and detection of defects in separate myocardial regions. Regardless of these limitations, planar imaging of myocardial perfusion has much to offer in the diagnosis of coronary artery disease, both as a stand-alone diagnostic method and as a supplement to tomographic imaging. The relative simplicity of the planar method avoids many of the potential technical pitfalls that may be encountered with tomography. For patients who are unable to remain motionless and hold their arm or arms elevated during image acquisition, the planar approach may be preferred. In addition, valuable information from planar images, including quantification of lung thallium activity, can provide important supplementary information to myocardial tomograms.

IMAGING PROCEDURE

Imaging Equipment: Gamma Camera

Clinical imaging is best performed using an Anger camera equipped with at least 37 photomultiplier tubes. For imaging thallium 201 (^{201}Tl), a 20 percent window is centered on the 69- to 83-keV mercury x-ray photopeak.[1] This energy level of the mercury x-rays is below the optimal 100- to 200-keV range for conventional NaI crystal scintillation cameras, but the 94.4 percent abundance makes this photopeak preferable to the higher-energy gamma photons of ^{201}Tl for clinical imaging. Use of a ¼-inch-thick crystal results in improved ^{201}Tl image resolution, with a negligible effect on image acquisition time.[2,3] A parallel-hole collimator is usually employed.[4] Although the optimal collimator selection has not been determined, a high-resolution collimator reduces background activity from scattered counts. A general-purpose collimator permits a faster count rate from the myocardium, enabling the collection of a large number of counts from the myocardium in multiple projections before substantial thallium redistribution occurs. For imaging technetium-99m (^{99m}Tc) hexakis-2-methoxyisobutyl isonitrile (sestamibi), the equipment requirements are similar, and the energy window is centered on the 140-keV photopeak of ^{99m}Tc. Anger-camera quality control should be performed daily by flood-field assessment, by maintaining a stable energy window, as well as by periodic evaluation of camera resolution.

Patient Preparation

Patients should fast for at least 4 h prior to imaging in order to minimize tracer activity in digestive organs. The patient is interviewed and examined to ensure that no contraindication to exercise testing is present. Exclusion of the presence of clinically important coronary artery disease with a high level of certainty by exercise myocardial scintigraphy requires a high level of exercise heart rate[5] (usually 85 percent or more of predicted maximum). This is usually not possible in the presence of beta-adrenergic blockade.[6,7] Therefore, when the purpose of the exercise myocardial scintigram is to exclude the presence of clinically important coronary disease, it is desirable that beta blockers be stopped for at least 48 h prior to testing. In patients with a stable pattern of chest pain who require chest-pain diagnosis, long-acting nitrates and calcium channel blockers are withheld for 24 h prior to testing in our laboratory in order to prevent masking of exercise-induced ischemia. In some patients, withholding antianginal drugs may not be acceptable clinically. In these individuals, withholding antianginal drugs (particularly beta-adrenergic blocking drugs) may unmask severe hypertension or induce unstable angina pectoris. In these patients or in patients who are physically or emotionally unable to exercise vigorously, pharmacologic stress testing with intravenous dipyridamole or adenosine should be substituted for exercise testing. Pharmacologic stress testing is reviewed in detail in Chap. 6.

Test Procedure: Thallium 201

An intravenous line is placed prior to exercise. Graded treadmill[8] or bicycle exercise is performed. The patient exercises to at least 85 percent of predicted maximum heart rate for age or to limiting symptoms, falling systolic blood pressure, or serious arrhythmia. With careful monitoring of the patient's blood pressure, heart rhythm, and general response to exercise, it will be possible for some patients to exercise maximally. This may improve the ability to detect ischemia and may be particularly helpful in patients having a history of symptoms that occur only with strenuous exercise. In clinically stable patients with a recent myocardial infarction, the peak exercise level is commonly limited to a heart rate of 120 to 130 beats/min. The prognostic implications of exercise ^{201}Tl testing following a recent myocardial infarction may relate in part to the presence of myocardial ischemia that can be produced by low levels of exercise.[9]

As the patient reaches the target level of exercise, 2.0 to 3.0 mCi of ^{201}Tl is injected through a previously established intravenous line. The patient continues to exercise for 45 to 90 s to permit a high level of myocardial extraction of ^{201}Tl under exercise conditions. Imaging is started within 5 or 10 min after cessation of exercise, before substantial redistribution of myocardial ^{201}Tl can occur. In female patients, a breast binder can be used to flatten the breast against the chest wall, resulting in more uniform attenuation of tracer activity from the different myocardial segments and thereby minimizing breast attenuation artifacts.[10]

No study has clearly defined the optimal imaging projections. It is apparent that cardiac rotation can substantially alter the configuration of ^{201}Tl myocardial images if the same imaging angles (e.g., a 40° left anterior oblique view) are used in all patients. In particular, when quantitative approaches are applied that compare the configuration of ^{201}Tl activity in the patient's heart to the distribution of ^{201}Tl in the myocardium of a reference population, imaging projections must be selected to minimize variation related to cardiac rotation. This can be accomplished by locating a *best septal* image as soon as the patient's heart rhythm, blood pressure, and symptoms have stabilized (usually within 2 to 3 min) following exercise. A left anterior oblique view is selected (commonly at 30° to 45°) in which the inferoapical segment is directed inferiorly and both the septum and posterolateral wall are vertically oriented. Selection of this angle is guided by brief acquisition of counts from the heart onto the computer display terminal. The angle should be determined rapidly so that imaging can begin promptly after cessation of exercise. Imaging in *standardized* projections is ordinarily started by rotating the detector 45° from the best septal view toward the patient's right side. This results in the first image being a standardized *anterior* view. The first view is used to assess pulmonary as well as myocardial ^{201}Tl activity. If quantitative methods are to be applied, images must be acquired for the same preset time (typically 10 min per view, with at least 300,000 counts per image). The third view is a standardized decubitus *lateral* view, rotated 40° to the patient's left from the best septal left anterior oblique view and with the patient lying with the right side down on the imaging table. The decubitus view minimizes diaphragmatic attenuation of the inferior and posterior walls.[11,12] This imaging sequence is completed within 30 or 40 min after cessation of exercise so as to minimize the effects of ^{201}Tl redistribution. If quantitation of ^{201}Tl washout rates is performed, it is advisable to image briefly over the injection site to ensure that no infiltration of the ^{201}Tl dose has occurred, as this will substantially alter ^{201}Tl myocardial uptake and washout rates. The use of additional views of the heart may be of help in individual cases. However, substantial ^{201}Tl redistribution may have already occurred within 30 min following ^{201}Tl injection.

Separation of Myocardial Ischemia from Myocardial Scar by Thallium Imaging

Imaging is ordinarily repeated 3 to 4 h following exercise ^{201}Tl injection in order to identify regions of thallium redistribution. In most cases, exercise-induced ischemia will result in a region of decreased ^{201}Tl myocardial activity immediately following exercise with subsequent redistribution of ^{201}Tl, resulting in uniform ^{201}Tl activity 3 to 4 h after exercise-induced ischemia has resolved.[13] Thallium redistribution is enhanced by the presence of high residual blood thallium levels during the redistribution process. Eating reduces blood thallium levels and diminishes thallium redistribution into reversibly ischemic myocardium. Therefore, intake of food between the time of initial and delayed thallium images should be minimized to facilitate detection of reversible myocardial ischemia.[14-16]

In some patients, an exercise-induced or pharmacologically induced defect on initial ^{201}Tl distribution images may not improve on delayed images acquired 4 h later. Approximately 40 to 50 percent of these perfusion defects that are unimproved on 4-h delayed images will be comprised of reversibly ischemic myocardium. Persistent or fixed myocardial defects that are only mild or moderate in severity (i.e., diminished by less than 50 percent compared with normal myocardial zones on a 4-h delayed image) usually correspond to viable myocardium and may show improved perfusion and contractile function following successful coronary artery revascularization.[17,18] Severe persistent defects may also contain reversibly ischemic myocardium, and this can be demonstrated by reinjection of 1 mCi of ^{201}Tl following the 4-h delayed images. Reinjection images are then acquired approximately 30 min after ^{201}Tl reinjection.

Reversibly ischemic myocardial segments are characterized by stress-induced myocardial perfusion defects that show improvement on thallium redistribution or reinjection imaging. Viable myocardium, which may or may not be ischemic, may be represented by a mild to moderate (less than 50 percent decreased compared with normal areas) irreversible defect on thallium redistribution or reinjection images. In contrast, severe (greater than 50 percent decreased compared with normal areas) irreversible perfusion defects on redistribution images, which are unimproved on thallium reinjection, will generally correspond to metabolically inactive myocardium[18] or myocardial scar. An in-depth discussion of radionuclide assessment of myocardial viability is presented in Chap. 5.

A second function of comparing immediate postexercise and 4-h redistribution images is in analyzing the rate of ^{201}Tl washout from myocardial segments. In the presence of multivessel coronary disease, initial exercise ^{201}Tl myocardial distribution may be uniformly decreased in all myocardial segments, making disease detection difficult or impossible from initial images alone. However, the clearance rate of ^{201}Tl from these segments may be decreased compared with the myocardial ^{201}Tl clearance from normal segments in other subjects. This phenomenon is referred to as *diffuse slow washout.*[19]

Test Procedure: Technetium-99m Sestamibi, Technetium-99m Tetrofosmin, and Technetium-99m Furifosmin (Q12)

The clinical utility of postexercise ^{99m}Tc-sestamibi imaging with comparison resting images obtained on a separate day has been documented.[20,21] However, the inconvenience for the patient and diagnostic delay of serial ^{99m}Tc-sestamibi imaging sequences on separate days make a single-day protocol desirable.

Taillefer and associates have described an imaging protocol for ^{99m}Tc sestamibi that permits stress and rest imaging on the same day.[22] At rest, 7 to 10 mCi of ^{99m}Tc sestamibi is injected intravenously. One hour later, planar images are acquired in three or more projections for 10 min per view. On completion of the resting images, exercise testing is performed with injection of 25 to 30 mCi of ^{99m}Tc sestamibi during the last minute of stress. Stress images are acquired 15 to 60 min later. No loss of diagnostic accuracy was observed with the single-day compared with the multiple-day imaging protocol.[22,23] With the newer ^{99m}Tc myocardial perfusion imaging agents, tetrofosmin and furifosmin, the principal difference in the imaging protocol is that rest imaging may be started earlier following tracer injection at rest (i.e., approximately 15 min).[24,25]

A very useful property shared by ^{99m}Tc sestamibi, ^{99m}Tc tetrofosmin, and ^{99m}Tc furifosmin is the potential for assessment of both myocardial perfusion and function from a single tracer dose (see Fig. 10-3). First-pass radionuclide angiography can be used to measure right and left ventricular ejection fraction and to visualize ventricular regional wall motion during the initial transit of ^{99m}Tc tracer through the heart.[26-29] Baillet and colleagues validated measurement of right and left ventricular ejection fraction from the initial cardiac transit of 20 mCi of ^{99m}Tc sestamibi in comparison with first-pass radionuclide angiography using ^{99m}Tc diethylenetriamine penta-acetic acid (DTPA). The authors also observed an excellent correlation of left ventricular regional wall motion from the ^{99m}Tc-sestamibi first-pass radionuclide angiogram and contrast ventriculography.[27] Therefore, the same dose of ^{99m}Tc sestamibi can be used to measure ventricular function and left ventricular myocardial perfusion. However, combination of the 7- to 10-mCi rest ^{99m}Tc-sestamibi injection from the single-day imaging protocol of Taillefer et al with first-pass radionuclide angiography will likely produce inadequate counting statistics on the first-pass radionuclide angiographic study if imaging is performed on most conventional single-crystal gamma cameras.

A second approach to the combined study of left ventricular myocardial perfusion and function involves gating the ^{99m}Tc- myocardial perfusion images with the R wave of the patient's electrocardiogram (ECG).[30-33] This enables the generation of a series of myocardial images spanning the cardiac cycle and allows the assessment of systolic myocardial regional wall motion and systolic thickening. Although exercise injection of a non-redistributing ^{99m}Tc perfusion tracer yields perfusion images of the distribution of myocardial blood flow during exercise, ECG-gated images of wall motion from the same tracer injection demonstrate regional ventricular function at the time of imaging and, hence, provide a resting wall-motion study. Assessment of regional left ventricular function from planar gated ^{99m}Tc- sestamibi studies has been found to be reproducible and correlates well with echocardiographic assessment of left ventricular regional wall motion (Kappa 0.93 to 1.00).[32] An alternative method to assess regional left ventricular function from planar gated ^{99m}Tc-sestamibi images is by assessment of regional wall thickening. The limited spatial resolution of a conventional gamma camera may make detection of small increments in the size of an object impossible (i.e., in this case, the thickness of the left ventricular regional wall). However, an increment in left ventricular wall thickness will increase the intensity recorded per picture element (pixel) over the left ventricular wall. Because of this partial volume effect, left ventricular wall thickening will be assessed more accurately by measuring the change in count density over the left ventricular segment rather than by directly assessing apparent changes in wall thickness from the images.[31] The principal limitation of these methods is that perfusion defects demonstrated by severely reduced regional ^{99m}Tc-tracer activity make observation of left ventricular wall motion or thickening in the same area difficult. In addition to assessment of regional left ventricular function, it is possible to estimate left ventricular global ejection fraction from planar gated ^{99m}Tc-myocardial perfusion images.[33]

Test Procedure: Technetium-99m Teboroxime

Following intravenous injection of ^{99m}Tc teboroxime at peak exercise, a 1- to 2-min blood-pool phase is followed by intense myocardial uptake and then by rapid myocardial tracer washout and hepatic accumulation over 5 to 10 min.[34] These kinetic properties of ^{99m}Tc teboroxime dictate a rapid myocardial imaging sequence. Because myocardial washout is rapid, a same-day stress–rest (or rest–stress) imaging sequence is possible. Image acquisition parameters are set up before exercise is started. In a typical stress–rest imaging protocol, the patient is injected with 15 to 20 mCi of ^{99m}Tc teboroxime during peak treadmill exercise. Imaging is started within 1 min after cessation of exercise. The patient is imaged in an upright position to improve separation of the heart from the liver. In one protocol, to facilitate rapid patient positioning, the patient is imaged while sitting on a swivel

chair in front of the gamma camera.[34-36] Images are acquired for approximately 60 to 90 s in each of three views.[34-37] The left lateral view may be acquired first to minimize overlap by hepatic activity that is typically prominent by the end of a three-image sequence. Images are also acquired in an anterior and 45° left anterior oblique projection. Immediately following acquisition of the initial three images, the imaging sequence can be repeated in order to detect rapid resolution of initial perfusion defects as a result of differential washout of ^{99m}Tc teboroxime from normal and ischemic myocardium.[38] After a delay of 1 to 3 h, a second dose of ^{99m}Tc teboroxime is injected at rest and the images are again acquired.

COMPUTER QUANTITATIVE METHODS

A trend toward improved overall diagnostic accuracy for detection of coronary artery disease has been observed using computer quantitation of planar ^{201}Tl images compared with subjective interpretation. Other important benefits from the routine application of computer methods to planar ^{201}Tl scintigrams include improved reproducibility of image interpretation, improved quantitation of the extent of coronary disease, quantitation of tracer washout kinetics, and a more objective basis for separating normal from abnormal perfusion patterns. In the following sections, representative methods are presented for background correction and analysis of myocardial ^{201}Tl activity using horizontal or circumferential profiles. These same methods may be modified to facilitate quantitation of planar ^{99m}Tc-sestamibi myocardial images.[39,39a] Difficulties involved in comparing various computer approaches in the quantitation of planar myocardial scintigrams are noted.

Background Subtraction

Noncardiac activity in the region of the heart is best described as *tissue cross talk*,[40] which includes activity related to Compton scatter from structures on each side of the heart as well as posteriorly, attenuated by the heart. Since ^{201}Tl (or ^{99m}Tc sestamibi) activity in structures adjacent to the heart is not uniform, tissue cross talk in the region of the heart is also not uniform. For this reason, the use of a simple uniform background subtraction (in which a fixed percentage of activity is removed from all image pixels) may produce inhomogeneity of activity in the region of the heart in the absence of nonuniform myocardial perfusion. A method of background subtraction is needed for which the amount of back-

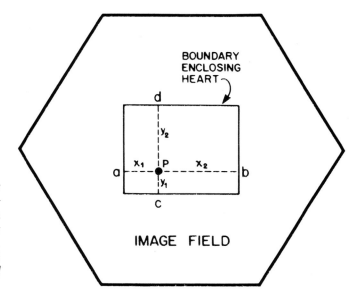

Figure 2-1 Bilinear interpolative background subtraction by the method of Watson et al. The heart is enclosed by a rectangular boundary. The contribution of activity from tissue cross talk at pixel *P* in the region of the heart is estimated from the activity observed at points *a*, *b*, *c*, and *d* outside the myocardium. Details are given in the text. (From Watson et al,[42] Spatial and temporal quantitation of plane thallium myocardial images, *J Nucl Med* 22:577, 1981, reproduced with permission.)

ground activity removed from each pixel in the region of the heart accurately reflects the activity due to tissue cross talk for that particular point on the myocardial contour. This is commonly estimated by a modification of the bilinear interpolated background subtraction described by Goris and associates.[41] A boundary is created surrounding the heart. Each point on the myocardial contour is related to points on the boundary outline by a horizontal line and a vertical line (see Fig. 2-1). The influence of activity at points *a*, *b*, *c*, and *d* on the contribution of tissue cross talk to the activity observed at point *P* over the myocardium is estimated by a weighting function. A widely used weighting function devised by Watson and associates[42] relates the importance of the contribution to tissue cross talk at point *P* to the proximity of point *P* to the four corresponding boundary points:

$$\text{background} = \frac{W_a a + W_b b + W_c c + W_d d}{W_a + W_b + W_c + W_d}$$

where $W_a = \dfrac{x_2}{x_1} + k$ $W_b = \dfrac{x_1}{x_2} + k$

$W_c = \dfrac{y_2}{y_1} + k$ $W_d = \dfrac{y_1}{y_2} + k$

and $k = 2$.

Introduction of the constant k produces rapid falloff of the calculated contribution of tissue cross talk when moving to the heart from a region of intense extracardiac activity such as the liver.[42]

The removal of tissue cross-talk activity overlying the heart is a necessary precursor to any attempt to quantitate myocardial activity. The subjective assessment of myocardial perfusion should also be simpler and

more reproducible if activity from tissue cross talk is removed, although this hypothesis has not been proven.

Figure 2-2 illustrates diagrammatically the effect of prominent pulmonary ^{201}Tl activity on the appearance of activity in the myocardium. Following interpolative background subtraction, myocardial ^{201}Tl activity is uniform.

Rationale for the Quantitative Approach

Quantitation of planar exercise myocardial perfusion scintigrams improves reproducibility of test interpretation, diagnostic accuracy, definition of the extent of coronary artery disease, and localization of individual coronary artery lesions. In a study of interobserver variability in the subjective interpretation of ^{201}Tl scintigrams, four experienced observers disagreed as to whether a scan was normal or abnormal in 13 percent of cases.[43] Scans

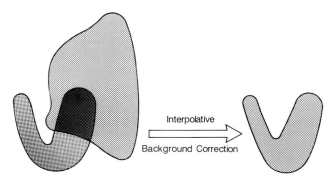

Figure 2-2 Diagrammatic illustration of the effect of prominent pulmonary thallium activity on regional myocardial activity. Following an idealized interpolative background subtraction, only net myocardial counts remain.

were considered to be borderline abnormal in 23 percent of cases. Exact agreement among all four observers as to whether a scan was normal, borderline, or abnormal occurred in 44 percent of cases.[43] Although the level of reproducibility is no worse than for other subjectively interpreted diagnostic procedures, such as coronary arteriography,[44] multiple readers would be required in order to establish which individual patient has a reproducible result. This is not feasible in most clinical settings. In one study[45] using quantitative analysis of myocardial perfusion scintigrams, concordant results were obtained by two observers in the evaluation of 115 of 126 myocardial segments (93 percent agreement), suggesting improved reproducibility of test interpretation compared with subjective methods. The presence or absence of angiographically important coronary artery disease was also concordantly predicted in 14 patients by quantitative thallium imaging methods.[45]

Does quantitation improve the diagnostic accuracy of postexercise planar myocardial perfusion scintigraphy? In a study by Berger and associates,[46] 60 of 70 patients with a 50 percent or greater coronary artery luminal diameter stenosis had a subjectively abnormal exercise ^{201}Tl scintigram, whereas 66 of 70 patients had abnormal findings by quantitative criteria ($p < 0.08$). Of 30 patients without angiographic coronary artery disease, 22 had a normal subjective exercise ^{201}Tl scintigram, compared with 27 of 30 patients by quantitative criteria ($p < 0.08$).[46] This trend toward improved diagnostic accuracy for determining the overall presence or absence of coronary disease by using quantitative criteria was less pronounced in the series reported by Maddahi and associates.[45]

In the series published by Berger et al,[46] extensive coronary artery disease was detected in 40 of 51 patients with multivessel disease by using quantitative exercise ^{201}Tl scintigraphy, compared with the detection of multivessel disease in only 20 of 51 patients by subjective criteria ($p < 0.002$). A 50 percent or greater stenosis in an individual coronary artery was detected with higher sensitivity and comparable specificity by computer quantitation versus subjective criteria in the study by Maddahi et al.[45] A large comparison study of subjective versus quantitative interpretation of planar ^{99m}Tc-sestamibi scintigrams is not available.[39]

Quantitative Computer Methods: Horizontal Profiles

Following the protocol of Watson and associates,[42,46,47] data are acquired beginning 10 min after ^{201}Tl injection at peak exercise (optionally again at 1 h) and 2 to 3 h following exercise. Images are identically positioned and image alignment is accomplished by a two-dimensional least squares fit. Data are collected in the anterior and

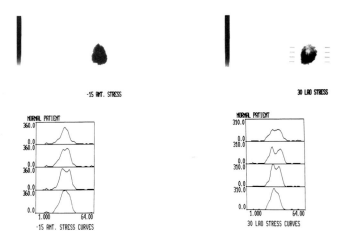

Figure 2-3 A normal postexercise thallium scintigram processed by the method of horizontal profiles. Following an interpolative bilinear background subtraction, the anterior (ANT) image (*top left*) and 30° left anterior oblique (LAO) image (*top right*) are seen. The myocardium is transected by four horizontal profiles producing the count profiles shown below each image.

45° and 70° left anterior oblique projections in a 64 × 64 matrix for 10 min per view. Following an interpolated background subtraction,[42] a 9-point spatial smoothing operation is performed. Four horizontal profiles are then generated across each myocardial image (Fig. 2-3). The slices are one picture element (pixel) in height, but each pixel samples a 9-pixel region because of the smoothing operation. Myocardial activity is determined from peak profile counts from regions in the anterolateral and inferior walls on the anterior images; from septal, inferoapical, and posterolateral segments on the 45° left anterior oblique images; and from anterior and posterior segments on the 70° left anterior oblique views. Time—activity curves are constructed by plotting peak profile counts from the same myocardial region for the initial and delayed images.

The ^{201}Tl study is interpreted from the unprocessed raw data along with the quantitative results. Three criteria for abnormality are used: (1) A focal area of decreased uptake is considered abnormal if the uptake is decreased by more than 25 percent compared with an adjacent or contralateral myocardial region. The 25 percent criterion represents more than 1.6 standard deviations (SD) from the mean for a population of normal subjects. The inferior wall on the anterior image is considered abnormal if there is a 35 percent decrease in peak activity compared with the anterolateral wall. This criterion compensates for attenuation of the inferior wall of the left ventricle by the overlying right ventricle. (2) Abnormal segmental ^{201}Tl washout is indicated by constant or increasing activity from a myocardial segment on delayed images compared with postexercise images. This pattern of abnormal ^{201}Tl washout following exercise is more than 2 SD

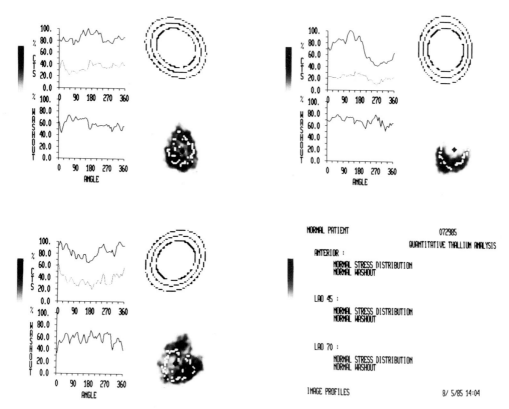

Figure 2-4 Quantitation of myocardial thallium activity by circumferential profiles by using the Cedars-Sinai method. Data are illustrated for the same normal patient shown in Fig. 2-3. *Top left panel:* The *lower figure* illustrates background-subtracted myocardial activity in the anterior projection, with *white blocks* identifying the points of maximal net myocardial counts along each radius. The *upper line graph* is a plot of the percentage of the maximal counts along the circumference of the left ventricle in this projection on the ventricle axis versus the circumferential angle on the horizontal axis. The left ventricular apex is located at 90°, and maximal count profiles are plotted in a clockwise direction from 0° to 360°. Initial (*black line*) and delayed (*gray line*) circumferential counts are displayed. The *lower line graph* is a plot of the percentage washout versus the circumferential angle. Comparison of the patient's data with a reference normal population is shown in the concentric circular (*upper*) figure. The *inner circle* corresponds to the position of the left ventricle in the anterior projection. The *middle circle* illustrates portions of the left ventricular circumference for which the percentage of maximal initial counts falls within the normal reference range. A break in this circumference would denote abnormal myocardial perfusion. The *outer circle* represents areas of the myocardial circumference for which the percentage of myocardial washout is within the normal range. *Top right panel:* Best septal left anterior oblique projection. *Bottom left panel:* 70° left anterior oblique projection. The format is the same for each projection. *Bottom right panel:* Quantitative test results by projection.

from the mean ^{201}Tl washout rate in a normal population. (3) Relative redistribution on the delayed images is represented by a change in the ratio of activity from two different myocardial segments between initial and delayed images.

This horizontal profiles method has been altered and validated for quantitation of myocardial perfusion scintigrams acquired following administration of ^{99m}Tc sestamibi. Changes include modification of the weighted background subtraction protocol to reflect the different distribution of ^{99m}Tc sestamibi in background tissues, quantitative comparison with a normal database, and

a *flashback method* for enhanced visual detection of myocardial viability.[39]

Quantitative Computer Methods: Circumferential Profiles

By following the protocol of Garcia and associates,[45,48] data are acquired beginning 6 min after ^{201}Tl injection at peak exercise (optionally again at 40 min) and 3 to 5 h following ^{201}Tl injection. Images are collected in a best septal left anterior oblique view, selected so that the septum and posterolateral walls are vertically oriented; in a standardized anterior view with the detector rotated 45° toward the patient's right side from the left anterior oblique view; and in a decubitus lateral view selected 40° lateral to the best septal left anterior oblique view. Each view is collected for 10 min using a gamma camera equipped with a high-resolution collimator. Following a bilinear interpolated background subtraction,[42] a 9-point smoothing operation is performed. The operator locates the centroid of the left ventricular myocardium, the left ventricular apex, and a circle enclosing the outer edge of the left ventricular myocardium for each projection. The myocardial contour is then divided by 60 radii extending from the centroid of the left ventricle to the outer edge of the left ventricular myocardium. The point of maximal activity along each of the radii is located and confirmed by the operator. With the left ventricular apex oriented at 90° for each projection, a profile of maximal counts at each successive clockwise 6° radius is plotted. The maximal number of counts along each radius is then normalized as a percentage of the maximum counts over all cardiac profiles in that projection, which is set at 100 percent.

Data are analyzed in terms of initial ^{201}Tl distribution and ^{201}Tl washout rate from each myocardial segment. The normal range for ^{201}Tl distribution and washout from each myocardial segment is based on a range of 2.5 SD from the mean determination derived from a population of 31 subjects having a less than 1 percent probability of coronary artery disease by Bayesian analysis.[49] Three myocardial segments are analyzed in each of three projections (see Fig. 2-4). The distribution of the left anterior descending coronary artery is represented by the anterior wall on the anterior and decubitus lateral views and by the septum on the left anterior oblique view. The distribution of the circumflex coronary artery is represented by the posterolateral wall on the left anterior oblique view. The distribution of the right coronary artery is represented by the inferior wall on the anterior and lateral decubitus views. Apical and inferoapical abnormalities do not localize to a specific coronary artery distribution. Data observed between 210° and 330° are localized to the left ventricular outflow tract and are not evaluated quantitatively for abnormality.

With the use of these methods, normal subjects were best separated from patients with coronary artery disease by the following criteria: (1) initial postexercise distribution of ^{201}Tl activity falling below normal limits for any contiguous 18° segment or (2) slower than normal washout of ^{201}Tl activity between the postexercise and 4-h delayed image for any contiguous 18° segment. To be considered abnormal, a patient must have abnormal initial distribution or washout of ^{201}Tl activity on at least two 18° segments taken from the three views. When this combination of initial ^{201}Tl distribution and washout criteria was used, no further diagnostic information resulted from analysis of the delay in the time of peak initial ^{201}Tl uptake.

Several other methods for quantitative analysis of planar ^{201}Tl activity from circumferential profiles have been described.[50-53] In addition, methods for quantitative analysis of planar [99mTc]- sestamibi myocardial perfusion images by circumferential profiles have been developed.[54] These methods require modification of the background subtraction methods developed for use with ^{201}Tl, to take into account the different distribution of sestamibi into tissues adjacent to the heart. Also, these methods require a new normal database to account for differences in the normal myocardial distribution of activity associated with [99mTc] sestamibi, compared with that associated with [201]Tl.

INTERPRETATION OF MYOCARDIAL PERFUSION STUDIES

Normal Myocardial Perfusion Images

In general, the principles of interpretation of ^{201}Tl images and [99mTc] myocardial perfusion images are very similar.[54a,54b] An example of a normal postexercise ^{201}Tl myocardial scintigram is shown in Fig. 2-5**A**. A normal postexercise [99mTc]-sestamibi study is shown in Fig. 2-5**B**. Myocardial activity is normally reduced at the left ventricular base, resulting from the presence of the aortic and mitral valves in this area.[55] A narrow, often linear region of diminished myocardial activity may be present in one or more views extending from the endocardial to epicardial surface of the left ventricular apex.[55] This finding reflects the decreased myocardial thickness of the left ventricular apex compared with the myocardial thickness at the remaining subvalvular regions of the left ventricle.[56] If the left anterior oblique image is carefully selected so that the myocardium appears to be vertically oriented, the height and intensity of tracer activity in the septal and posterolateral walls will be nearly symmetric. If the image is rotated toward an anterior view, the aortic valve plane will be moved into the position normally occupied by the base of the septum on a best septal left anterior oblique view. A region of hypoperfusion limited to the septum at the cardiac base commonly corresponds to the presence of the aortic valve apparatus in that area[57] or to attenuation of tracer activity by breast tissue. In a similar manner, myocardial perfusion images that are laterally rotated from a true vertically oriented modified left anterior oblique view may result in the suggestion of a perfusion abnormality high on the posterolateral left ventricular wall. This may correspond to the location of the mitral valve apparatus rather than posterolateral wall hypoperfusion if the left ventricle is not properly oriented.

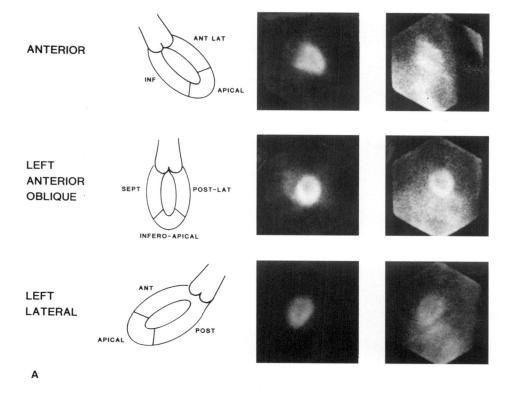

ANTERIOR

LEFT
ANTERIOR
OBLIQUE

LEFT
LATERAL

A

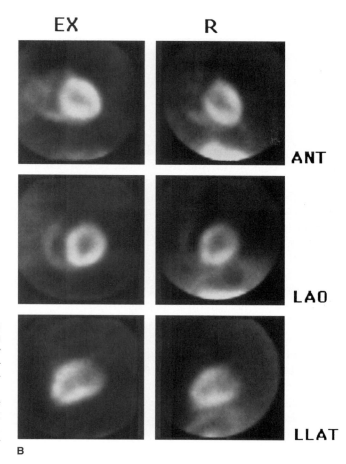

Figure 2-5   A: Normal thallium scintigrams immediately following treadmill exercise (*left images*) and 3 h later (*right images*) from a patient with a less than 1 percent probability of coronary artery disease. A high myocardial-to-background activity ratio is observed following stress with uniform myocardial distribution of activity. ANT LAT, anterolateral; INF, inferior; SEPT, septal; POST-LAT, posterolateral; ANT, anterior; POST, posterior. **B:** Postexercise (EX) and rest (R) myocardial images following injection of ^{99m}Tc sestamibi in a patient with no evidence of coronary artery disease. ANT, anterior; LAO, left anterior oblique; L LAT, left lateral. (Courtesy of Frans J. Th. Wackers, M.D.)

ANT   45° LAO

ANT   45° LAO

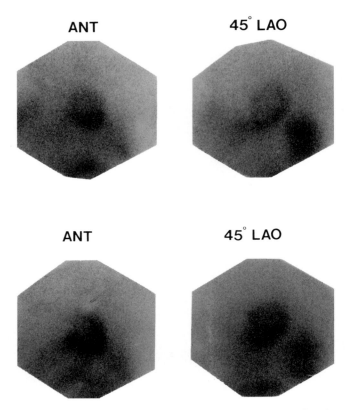

Figure 2-6 *Top:* Postexercise thallium scintigrams in a female patient with a less than 1 percent probability of coronary artery disease. Diminished activity in the anterolateral myocardium on the anterior (ANT) view and in the ventricular septum on the 45° left anterior oblique (LAO) view is observed when breast tissue overlies the myocardium. *Bottom:* Repeat study in the same patient. The breasts have been shifted away from a position overlying the heart, resulting in normal postexercise thallium scintigram findings.

Other normal variant myocardial perfusion patterns may result from soft tissue attenuation. Diaphragm attenuation of the inferior and posterior left ventricular myocardium as visualized on an anterior or a supine lateral view appears to be particularly common with ^{201}Tl imaging in obese subjects. Attenuation of myocardial activity by overlying breast tissue is a common problem with ^{201}Tl imaging in female patients and may involve the anterior wall on the anterior view, the septum on the left anterior oblique view, and the anterior or posterior wall on the left lateral view (Fig. 2-6).

Abnormal Tracer Distribution Suggestive of Coronary Artery Disease: Exercise-Induced Abnormalities

The presence of segmental hypoperfusion in response to exercise with uniform myocardial perfusion on the corresponding rest or redistribution images is suggestive of exercise-induced ischemia due to coronary artery disease.[13] The likelihood of exercise-induced myocardial

hypoperfusion is further increased when multiple regions of decreased myocardial tracer activity are present immediately following exercise or when concordant regions of hypoperfusion are present on multiple views.[58] A 25 percent or greater difference between adjacent myocardial segments is commonly observed when ischemia related to a hemodynamically important coronary artery stenosis is present.[42] Exercise-induced hypoperfusion related to coronary artery disease most commonly involves the distal distribution of the coronary arteries so that the left ventricular apex is more commonly hypoperfused as compared with the left ventricular base. An exception is the posterobasal or posterolateral wall, which may involve the distal distribution of the right or left circumflex coronary artery. Exercise-induced perfusion abnormalities limited to the septum at the base of the left

STRESS   REST

ANT

45° LAO

70° LAO

LT LAT

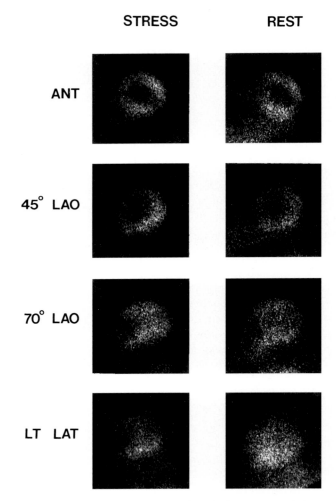

Figure 2-7 Postexercise (stress) and rest thallium myocardial scintigrams from a patient with occlusion of the left anterior descending coronary artery resulting in an anteroseptal myocardial infarction. Diminished myocardial activity is present at the left ventricular apex on the anterior (ANT) view, in the ventricular septum on the 45° left anterior oblique (LAO) view, and in the anteroapical regions in the 70° LAO and left lateral (LT LAT) views.

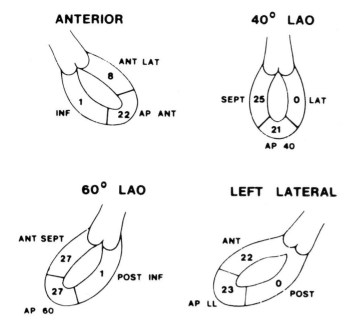

Figure 2-8 Distribution of postexercise thallium defects in 32 patients with a 70 percent or greater stenosis of the left anterior descending coronary artery and no 50 percent or greater stenosis of the luminal diameter in any other coronary artery. Numbers refer to the frequency of defects for each segment. LAO, left anterior oblique; ANT LAT, anterolateral; AP ANT, left ventricular apex as viewed on the anterior projection; INF, inferior; SEPT, septal; AP 40, apex as viewed in the 40° LAO projection; LAT, lateral; ANT SEPT, anteroseptal; AP 60, apex on the 60° LAO view; POST INF, posteroinferior; ANT, anterior; AP LL, apex as viewed in the left lateral projection; POST, posterior. (From Dunn et al,[59] Exercise thallium imaging: Location of perfusion abnormalities in single-vessel coronary disease, *J Nucl Med* 21:717, 1980, reproduced with permission.)

ventricle or to the anterior wall near the cardiac base represent an unlikely pattern of exercise-induced ischemia related to coronary artery disease.

Segmental abnormalities in the washout of ^{201}Tl from the myocardium following exercise also suggest a segmental disease process. Following exercise, a myocardial segment that fails to decrease in net thallium concentration on the 2- to 3-h delayed images is considered to be abnormal.[42] Alternatively, the rate of ^{201}Tl washout in a myocardial segment may be compared with a reference range of washout rates derived from a population of normal subjects.[45]

Findings Suggestive of Disease in the Distribution of a Specific Coronary Artery

The septum, anterior wall, and apex of the left ventricle (see Figs. 2-7 and 2-8) are commonly perfused by the left anterior descending coronary artery.[59] Rotation of the left anterior oblique projection toward the right will

increase overlap of the septum with the posterobasal and posteroseptal myocardium. If the image projection is not selected so that the left ventricle appears to be vertically oriented, an abnormal distribution of activity may be seen in which a posterior wall perfusion abnormality may mimic septal hypoperfusion (Fig. 2-9) related to the left anterior descending coronary artery.[59] Depending on the length of each coronary artery, the apex of the left ventricle may be variously supplied by any combination of one or more coronary arteries.

The distribution of myocardial perfusion related to the left circumflex coronary artery is illustrated in Figs. 2-10 and 2-11. Dunn and associates,[60] using ^{201}Tl myocardial scintigraphy, studied 32 patients with angiographic evidence of a 70 percent luminal diameter reduction in the left circumflex artery and no stenosis greater than 50 percent in the right coronary or left anterior descending coronary artery as well as no stenosis producing a greater than 30 percent luminal

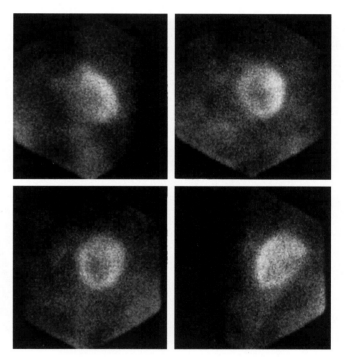

Figure 2-9 Postexercise thallium scintigrams in the anterior (*top left*), 30° left anterior oblique (*top right*), 50° left anterior oblique (*bottom left*), and decubitus left lateral (*bottom right*) projections from a patient with persistent angina pectoris following myocardial infarction. At coronary arteriography, there was total occlusion of the proximal right coronary artery. The left main, left anterior descending, and left circumflex coronary arteries were free of obstruction. A prominent thallium defect involving the inferior and posterior left ventricular walls is seen on the anterior and left lateral projections. In the 30° left anterior oblique projection, the septum appears to contain diminished thallium activity. This is a result of overlap of the septum and the posterior left ventricular wall. When the myocardium is imaged in the 50° left anterior oblique projection, the septum is more vertically oriented and is observed to be normally perfused.

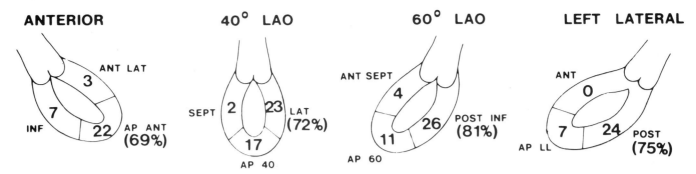

Figure 2-10 Diagrammatic representation of four postexercise thallium views from 32 patients with significant isolated left circumflex coronary artery disease, defined as a 70 percent or greater luminal reduction with no 50 percent or greater stenosis of any other coronary artery (abbreviations as in Fig. 2-8). (From Dunn et al,[60] reproduced with permission of the American Heart Association, Inc.)

diameter reduction in the left main coronary artery. The posterolateral wall on a 40° left anterior oblique view was more commonly hypoperfused in patients having a proximal left circumflex artery lesion compared with patients having disease limited to the distal left circumflex coronary artery.[60] The left circumflex artery most commonly contributed to the perfusion of the left ventricular posterior wall as assessed on a steep left anterior oblique or left lateral view. Abnormal perfusion of the left ventricular apex as assessed on the anterior view was also observed in the majority

of patients with single-vessel left circumflex coronary artery disease. Evidence of exercise-induced anteroseptal ^{201}Tl myocardial hypoperfusion was highly uncommon in these patients with single-vessel left circumflex artery disease but was observed in patients having a stenotic lesion in an intermediate artery arising directly from the left main coronary artery.[60]

The right coronary artery provides perfusion to the inferior left ventricular wall as visualized on the anterior view. The inferoposterior wall, as visualized on a steep left anterior oblique or a left lateral projection, may be

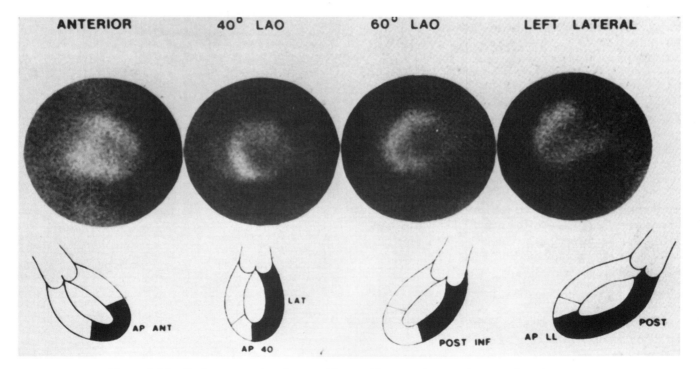

Figure 2-11 Thallium scintigram from a 49-year-old man with a single circumflex obstruction proximal to the first marginal branch. Defects illustrated diagrammatically in *black* are located in the apical, lateral, posteroinferior, and posterior left ventricular segments (abbreviations as in Fig. 2-8). (From Dunn et al,[60] reproduced with permission of the American Heart Association, Inc.)

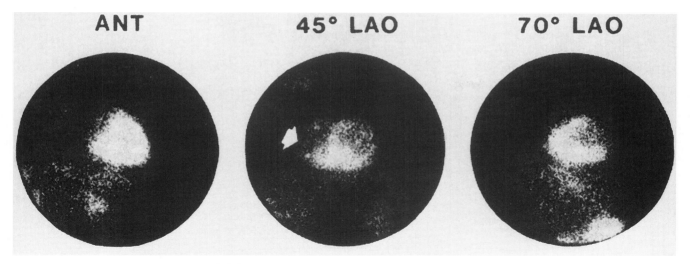

Figure 2-12 Proximal defect (*arrow*) on the right ventricular postexercise thallium scintigram in the 45° left anterior oblique (LAO) view of a patient with proximal right coronary artery stenosis. Diminished activity is also noted in the posterolateral left ventricular wall but not in the inferior wall. ANT, anterior. (From Gutman et al,[62] reproduced with permission of the American Heart Association, Inc.)

perfused by either the right or the left circumflex artery (Fig. 2-10). Decreased perfusion of the inferior wall on the anterior projection may be difficult to assess as a result of attenuation by the overlying right ventricle or by the diaphragm. Reversible hypoperfusion or nonvisu-

alization of the free wall of the right ventricle with exercise on the left anterior oblique view has also been described as a sign of stenosis (Fig. 2-12) in the proximal right coronary artery.[61–63] Enhanced hepatic uptake of ^{201}Tl after treadmill exercise has also been described as

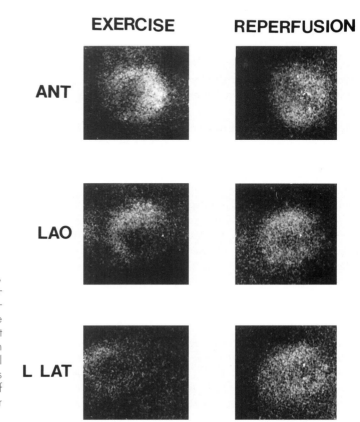

Figure 2-13 Exercise-induced ischemia of the anterior, septal, and posterolateral left ventricular segments, suggesting the presence of left main coronary artery disease. At coronary arteriography, greater than 70 percent stenoses were present in the left main, left anterior descending, left circumflex, and right coronary arteries. Severely diminished postexercise thallium activity at the body and apex of the left ventricle, with residual activity at the base of the left ventricle (as observed in this scintigram), has been described by Dash et al,[68] as a sign of triple-vessel coronary disease. ANT, anterior; LAO, left anterior oblique; L LAT, left lateral.

DIPYRIDAMOLE

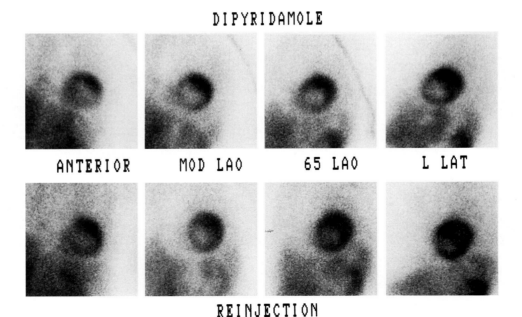

ANTERIOR   MOD LAO   65 LAO   L LAT

REINJECTION

Figure 2-14 ^{201}Tl myocardial perfusion images acquired following dipyridamole infusion and again after reinjection in a 79-year-old woman with typical angina pectoris. There is prominent tracer activity at the cardiac base, with extensive hypoperfusion of the apical two-thirds of the heart. Coronary arteriography confirmed the presence of severe triple-vessel coronary disease.

a sign of severe narrowing of the right coronary artery.[63a] This finding may be a result of exercise-induced right ventricular ischemia with consequent right heart failure.

Myocardial Tracer Distribution Suggestive of Multivessel or Left Main Coronary Artery Disease

The presence of a 50 percent or greater stenosis in either the left main coronary artery or each of the three major epicardial coronary arteries identifies a patient group with improved survival with surgical compared with medical treatment.[64–67] Consequently, an important function of the myocardial scintigram is to identify specifically those patients with high-risk coronary anatomy who might benefit most from coronary angiography and aggressive therapeutic intervention. A number of scintigraphic patterns have been described that suggest the presence of left main or triple-vessel coronary disease. The scintigraphic appearance and basic pathophysiology associated with these patterns is described here, whereas the diagnostic correlates are detailed in Chap. 20.

A *left main pattern* has been described when perfusion defects are present in the anterior, septal, and posterolateral walls (Fig. 2-13).[68] This pattern of hypoperfusion implies that blood flow during exercise or pharmacologic stress is restricted in the entire distribution of both the left anterior descending and left circum-

flex coronary arteries. By subjective interpretation, the left main pattern is present in only 13 to 24 percent of patients with a 50 percent or greater stenosis of the left main coronary artery.[69,70] This is probably a consequence of more critical coexistent coronary lesions compared with the left main lesion.[70,71] In addition, the left main scintigraphic pattern is more readily detected in patients with a patent rather than an occluded right coronary artery.[69] This likely is a result of a greater contrast between the normally perfused distribution of the right coronary artery and an underperfused left main distribution. Use of a quantitative approach to the detection of the left main coronary artery stenosis pattern improved diagnostic sensitivity for left main disease from 15 percent (two of 15 patients) to 77 percent (10 of 15 patients) in one study,[72] but others have observed a sensitivity of just 14 percent with quantitative planar methods.[71]

The presence of triple-vessel coronary artery disease is strongly suggested by the presence of perfusion defects in the distributions of all three coronary vessels. Myocardial perfusion defects involving more than 40 percent of the left ventricular perimeter have proven helpful in the identification of multivessel compared with single-vessel coronary disease. Perfusion defect size alone has been less helpful in separating double-vessel from triple-vessel disease.[73] An additional sign of triple-vessel coronary disease is the presence of prominent tracer activity at the base of the left ventricle with severely reduced tracer activity in the midventricular and apical segments (Fig. 2-14).[68]

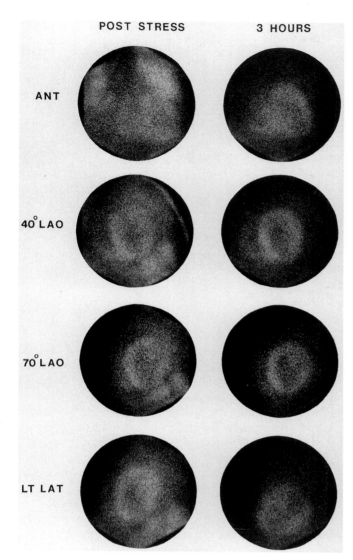

POST STRESS   **3 HOURS**

ANT

40° LAO

70° LAO

LT LAT

Figure 2-15 Extensive pulmonary thallium activity following exercise in a patient with coronary artery disease: 3 h later, pulmonary thallium activity has returned to normal levels. ANT, anterior; LAO, left anterior oblique; LT LAT, left lateral.

TRANSIENT LEFT VENTRICULAR CAVITY DILATION

Dilation of the left ventricular cavity with exercise[74-76] or with pharmacologic coronary artery vasodilation[77-79] in comparison with resting cavity size is a useful sign of severe myocardial ischemia. In patients evaluated for diagnosis of chest pain, it is usually a marker for multivessel coronary disease.[74-78] In addition to an actual increase in left ventricular cavity size, an apparent enlargement in left ventricular cavity size results from extensive stress-induced subendocardial ischemia. Transient dilation has been identified either by subjective observation of left ventricular cavity size or by measurements from hand-drawn regions of interest.

PULMONARY ACTIVITY RELATED TO MYOCARDIAL PERFUSION TRACERS

Prominent pulmonary ^{201}Tl activity (Fig. 2-15) in response to exercise has been described as a sign of multivessel coronary artery disease.[80] In a canine model, Bingham et al[81] showed that pulmonary thallium accumulation increases in the presence of a prolonged transit time through the lungs or with increased left atrial pressure. Similarly, increased pulmonary ^{99m}Tc-sestamibi activity is related to elevated left ventricular end-diastolic pressure and pulmonary transit times in dogs.[82] These findings suggest that increased pulmonary ^{201}Tl or ^{99m}Tc-sestamibi activity is a nonspecific indicator of impaired left ventricular function rather than a specific sign of coronary artery disease.

The hemodynamic correlates of pulmonary thallium activity in humans were studied by Boucher et al.[83] Five patients with increased postexercise lung activity on thallium scanning had an increase in pulmonary capillary wedge pressure from 12 ± 1 mmHg (mean $\pm$ 1 SD) at rest to 24 ± 3 mmHg with supine bicycle exercise ($p < 0.05$) without an increase in cardiac index. In contrast, seven patients without increased pulmonary thallium activity demonstrated an increase in mean cardiac index with exercise without a rise in pulmonary capillary wedge pressure. Exercise pulmonary thallium activity is inversely related to exercise peak heart rate and is also related to propranolol use.[84]

Increased pulmonary thallium activity can often be detected visually. However, Levy et al[85] have illustrated that the degree of photographic exposure may substantially alter the appearance of thallium activity in the lungs. Kushner et al[80] proposed a method of pulmonary thallium quantitation employing a ratio of pulmonary to myocardial activity. These authors found that a ratio of left lung counts to maximal myocardial counts at exercise greater than 0.545 was more than 2 SD above the mean for a normal population and was associated with multivessel coronary disease. Levy et al[85] quantitated pulmonary thallium activity following exercise and on a redistribution anterior image (Fig. 2-16). The difference between mean postexercise and mean redistribution pulmonary counts was divided by the mean postexercise pulmonary counts, yielding a pulmonary thallium washout value. A pulmonary thallium washout value of 41 percent or greater (Fig. 2-17) was considered abnormal (more than 2 SD above the mean value observed in patients with a less than 1 percent likelihood of coronary artery disease). Although not specific for the presence of coronary disease, abnormal postexercise pulmonary thallium activity does appear to be more common in patients with multivessel compared with single-vessel coronary artery disease.[80,85,86] In patients with single-vessel left anterior descending coronary artery disease (50 percent or more luminal diameter narrowing), the presence of abnormal pulmonary thallium activity following

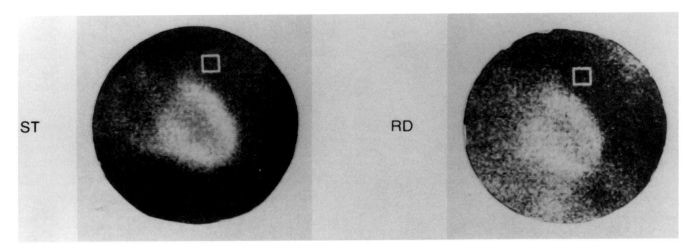

Figure 2-16   For determination of pulmonary thallium washout, a 10 × 10 pixel region of interest was placed over the medial aspect of the left upper lung field on the anterior view from the poststress (ST) and redistribution (RD) images. (From Levy et al,[85] *J Am Coll Cardiol* 2:719, 1983, reproduced with permission of the American College of Cardiology.)

exercise correlates with a larger number of abnormal thallium scintigraphic segments and with a more severe reduction in coronary luminal diameter.[87] With quantitative approaches to the analysis of ^{201}Tl myocardial activity distribution and washout that permit detection of coronary artery disease with approximately 90 percent sensitivity, the additional diagnostic role of pulmonary thallium activity is debatable. The added use of pulmonary thallium criteria for detecting an abnormal exercise

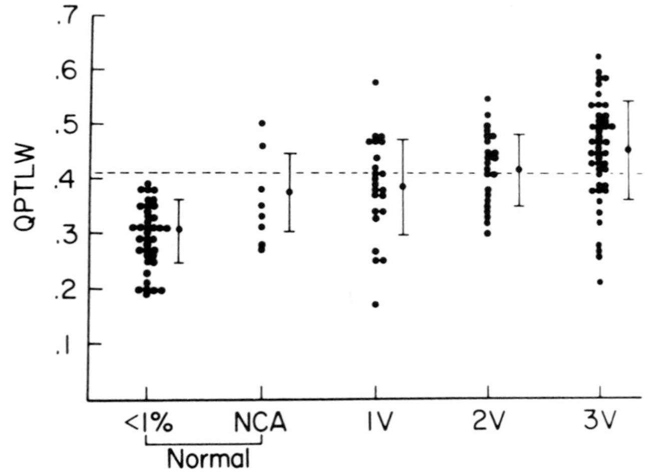

Figure 2-17   Comparison of the quantitative pulmonary thallium washout (QPTLW) values in 139 patients subgrouped by disease category. *Bars*, mean value ± SD; *dashed horizontal line*, pulmonary thallium washout value of 0.41 (mean ± 2 SD); <1%, patients with less than 1 percent probability of coronary artery disease; NCA, patients with normal coronary arteriograms; 1V, 2V, and 3V, patients with single-, double-, and triple-vessel coronary artery disease, respectively. (From Levy et al,[85] *J Am Coll Cardiol* 2:719, 1983, reproduced with permission of the American College of Cardiology.)

thallium scintigraphic result might be expected to yield a substantial percentage of *false-positive* scans when applied to patient populations with a high prevalence of noncoronary heart disease.[88] Therefore, the presence of abnormal pulmonary thallium activity with exercise would appear most helpful in confirming the presence of abnormality detected by myocardial segment analysis, in suggesting the presence of multivessel disease, and in providing indirect information concerning the functional consequence of detected heart disease.

An increased ratio of pulmonary to myocardial ^{201}Tl activity (e.g., greater than 0.50) with infusion of dipyridamole or adenosine is more frequently observed in patients with coronary artery disease than in controls.[89–92] In the larger available studies, prominent pulmonary thallium activity has correlated with a greater number of critical coronary stenoses,[91] a larger number of perfusion defects,[90,92] multivessel compared with single-vessel disease,[92] and evidence of left ventricular dysfunction[91] and previous myocardial infarction.[90] Increased pulmonary thallium activity also correlates with the presence of redistributing thallium defects and transient left ventricular cavity dilation.[90] The mechanism by which pharmacologic coronary artery vasodilation increases pulmonary thallium uptake is unclear. It has been suggested that a dipyridamole-induced increase in pulmonary thallium activity may result from ischemic left ventricular dysfunction induced by a pharmacologically provoked coronary artery steal.[90]

A weak relation between a pulmonary-to-myocardial ^{99m}Tc-sestamibi activity ratio and the presence of coronary artery disease has been reported (r = 0.33), but sestamibi lung images were acquired 4 min following tracer injection.[93] At 1 to 2 h after sestamibi injection, pulmonary activity had largely cleared and no relation

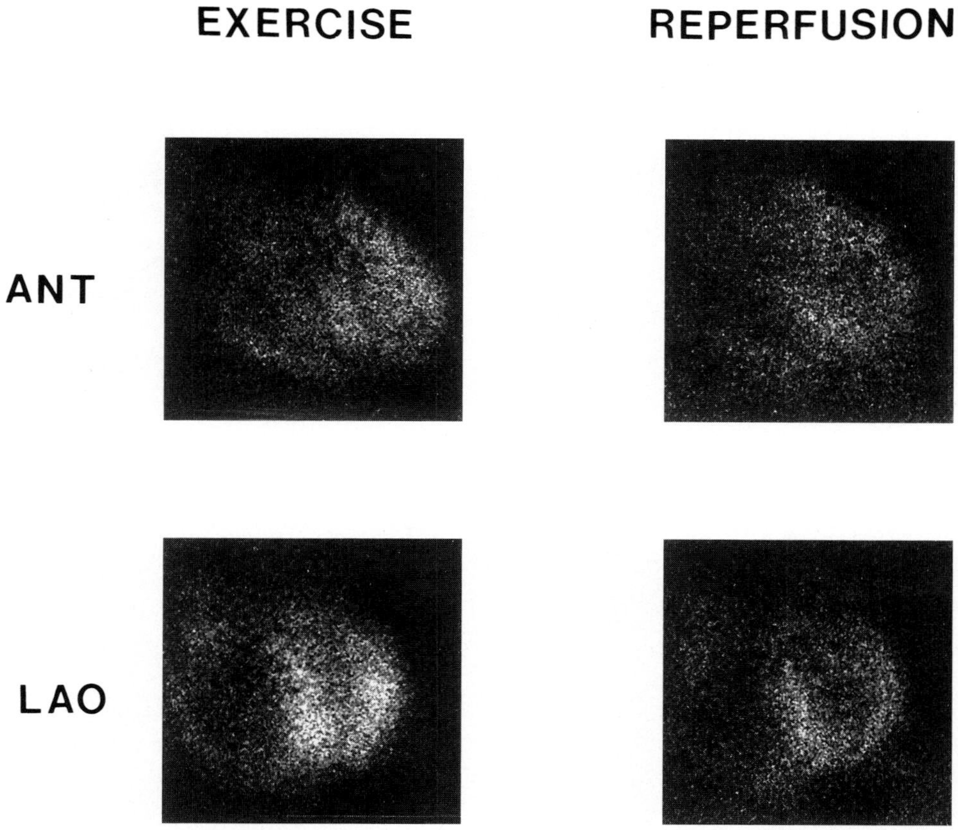

EXERCISE   REPERFUSION

ANT

LAO

Figure 2-18 Thallium scintigram demonstrating a dilated right ventricular cavity with hypertrophied right ventricular myocardium in a patient with cor pulmonale. There is a reversal of the normal convexity of the ventricular septum. ANT, anterior; LAO, left anterior oblique.

of ^{99m}Tc-sestamibi pulmonary-to-myocardial activity and the presence or absence of coronary artery disease was detectable.[93] A preliminary report[94] has suggested that a pulmonary-to-myocardial ratio of ^{99m}Tc-tetrofosmin activity (acquired at 26 ± 16 min after injection during exercise) is related to the corresponding ratio for ^{201}Tl, but further confirmation is needed. Technetium-99m—furifosmin (Q12) pulmonary-to-myocardial activity ratios do not appear to relate to the number of angiographic coronary artery stenoses present.[24] Currently, it appears that evaluation of pulmonary-to-myocardial activity ratios for ^{99m}Tc myocardial tracers does not yield predictive information for the presence and extent of coronary disease in the manner that the information is provided by ^{201}Tl imaging.

Right Ventricular Myocardial Tracer Activity

The thin-walled right ventricle normally receives less myocardial blood flow than the left ventricle, and uptake of ^{201}Tl is minimal in the right ventricle (Fig. 2-5A) com-pared with the left. Under conditions of right ventricular pressure or volume overload, the relative coronary blood flow to the right ventricular myocardium increases and ^{201}Tl activity is observed at rest in the right ventricular myocardium.[95-100] Thallium-201 scintigraphic signs to aid in the differentiation of right ventricular pressure and volume overload have been described. In isolated right ventricular pressure overload, the thickness of the right ventricular free wall increases, and there is straightening of the interventricular septum with loss of the normal convexity of the septum (Fig. 2-18) into the right ventricle.[98] In isolated right ventricular volume overload, the right ventricle is dilated, resulting in a cavity size greater than the left ventricle, and convex curvature of the interventricular septum into the right ventricle remains. Visualization of right ventricular ^{201}Tl activity greater than background activity at rest has been correlated with a right ventricular systolic pressure greater than 30 mmHg. It is also correlated with higher values of right ventricular diastolic pressure, mean pulmonary artery pressure, pulmonary vascular resistance, and right ventricular stroke–work index.[96,98] Right ventricular ^{201}Tl activity greater than background activity is found

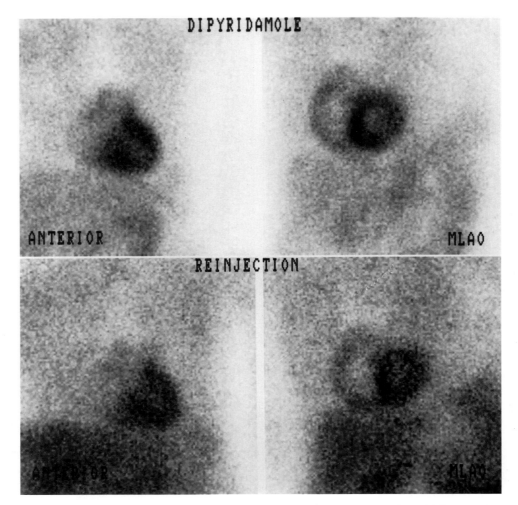

Figure 2-19 Demonstrates apparent reduction in inferoapical and posterolateral left ventricular ^{201}Tl activity. In this woman with mitral stenosis, right ventricular hypertrophy, and a normal coronary arteriogram, inhomogeneity of left ventricular tracer activity is a result of hypertrophy of the interventricular septum. LAO, left anterior oblique.

infrequently in nontachycardic patients with a right ventricular systolic pressure less than 30 mmHg and without a right ventricular volume overload.[96] Interobserver and intraobserver variability in the detection of right ventricular ^{201}Tl activity has not been clearly established, and quantitative criteria for the detection of abnormal right ventricular ^{201}Tl activity are needed.[101] The favorable physical imaging properties of ^{99m}Tc sestamibi can be expected to facilitate visualization of right ventricular myocardium, quantitation of right ventricular tracer activity, and identification of right ventricular perfusion defects.[102]

A potential pitfall in the interpretation of myocardial perfusion images may occur in the presence of right ventricular hypertrophy and associated hypertrophy of the interventricular septum. Figure 2-19 illustrates ^{201}Tl images from a woman with mitral stenosis and right ventricular hypertrophy. Septal hypertrophy is accompanied by prominent ^{201}Tl activity in the septum, giving rise to a false impression of hypoperfusion of the posterolateral and inferoapical segments. Coronary arteriography was normal.

Extracardiac Uptake of Myocardial Perfusion Tracers

During the acquisition or interpretation of myocardial perfusion studies, localized tracer activity may be noted in noncardiac tissues. Localized extracardiac ^{201}Tl activity has been identified in bronchogenic carcinoma,[103-110] adenocarcinoma of the lung,[103,111-113] carcinoma of the breast,[113-115] head and neck cancer,[116] gliomas,[117,118] sarcoma,[119] bronchopneumonia,[103] pulmonary tuberculosis,[103] goiters,[120] thyroid cancer,[120] meningiomas,[121] epidermoid inclusion cysts,[122] pulmonary actinomycosis,[123] collapsed lung,[124] and pectoralis muscle.[125] Similarly, localized uptake of [99mTc] isonitriles by a variety of benign and malignant tumors has been noted.[126–135]

REFERENCES

1. Hines HH, Glass EC, DeNardo GL: Spatial resolution for Tl-201 as a function of window width. *J Nucl Med* 21:P92, 1980 (abstr).
2. Muehllehner G: Effect of crystal thickness on scintillation camera performance. *J Nucl Med* 20:992, 1979.
3. Chapman D, Newcomer K, Berman D, et al: Half-inch vs quarter-inch Anger camera technology: Resolution and sensitivity differences at low photopeak energies. *J Nucl Med* 20:610, 1980 (abstr).
4. Nishiyama H, Romhilt DW, Williams CC, et al: Collimator evaluation for Tl-201 myocardial imaging. *J Nucl Med* 19:1067, 1978.
5. McLaughlin PR, Martin RP, Doherty P, et al: Reproducibility of thallium-201 myocardial imaging. *Circulation* 55:497, 1977.
6. Hockings B, Saltissi S, Croft DN, et al: Effect of beta adrenergic blockade on thallium-201 myocardial perfusion imaging. *Br Heart J* 49:83, 1983.
7. Pohost GM, Boucher CA, Zir LM, et al: The thallium stress test: The qualitative approach revisited. *Circulation* 60(part II):II-149, 1979 (abstr).
8. Bruce RA, Kusumi F, Hosmer D: Maximal oxygen intake and nomographic assessment of functional aerobic impairment in cardiovascular disease. *Am Heart J* 85:546, 1973.
9. Weld FM, Chu KL, Bigger JT Jr, et al: Risk stratification with low-level exercise testing 2 weeks after acute myocardial infarction. *Circulation* 64:306, 1981.
10. Stolzenberg J, Kaminsky J: Overlying breast as cause of false-positive thallium scans. *Clin Nucl Med* 3:229, 1978.
11. Gordon DG, Pfisterer M, Williams R, et al: The effect of diaphragmatic attenuation on [201Tl] images. *Clin Nucl Med* 4:150, 1979.
12. Johnstone DE, Wackers FJTh, Berger HJ, et al: Effect of patient positioning on left lateral thallium-201 myocardial images. *J Nucl Med* 20:183, 1979.
13. Pohost GM, Zir LM, Moore RH, et al: Differentiation of transiently ischemic from infarcted myocardium by serial imaging after a single dose of thallium-201. *Circulation* 55:294, 1977.
14. Angello DA, Wilson RA, Palac RT: Effect of eating on thallium-201 myocardial redistribution after myocardial ischemia. *Am J Cardiol* 60:528, 1987.
15. Nelson CW, Wilson RA, Angello DA, et al: Effect of thallium-201 blood levels on reversible myocardial defects. *J Nucl Med* 30:1172, 1989.
16. Angello DA, Wilson RA, Gee D: Effect of ribose on thallium-201 myocardial redistribution. *J Nucl Med* 29:1943, 1988.
17. Gibson RS, Watson DD, Taylor GJ, et al: Prospective assessment of regional myocardial perfusion before and after coronary revascularization surgery by quantitative thallium-201 scintigraphy. *J Am Coll Cardiol* 1:804, 1983.
18. Bonow RO, Dilsizian V, Cuocolo A, Bacharach SL: Identification of viable myocardium in patients with chronic coronary artery disease and left ventricular dysfunction: Comparison of thallium scintigraphy with reinjection and PET imaging with [18F]–fluorodeoxyglucose. *Circulation* 83:26, 1991.
19. Bateman TM, Maddahi J, Gray RJ, et al: Diffuse slow washout of myocardial thallium-201: A new scintigraphic indicator of extensive coronary artery disease. *J Am Coll Cardiol* 4:55, 1984.
20. Wackers FJTh, Berman DS, Maddahi J, et al: Technetium-99m hexakis 2-methoxyisobutyl isonitrile: Human biodistribution, dosimetry, safety, and preliminary comparison to thallium-201 for myocardial perfusion imaging. *J Nucl Med* 30:301, 1989.
21. Kahn JK, McGhie I, Akers MS, et al: Quantitative rotational tomography with [201Tl] and [99mTc] 2-methoxy-isobutyl-isonitrile: A direct comparison in normal individuals and patients with coronary artery disease. *Circulation* 79:1282, 1989.
22. Taillefer R, Laflamme L, Dupras G, et al: Myocardial perfusion imaging with Tc-99m methoxy-isobutyl isonitrile (MIBI): Comparison of short and long time intervals between rest and stress injections. *Eur J Nucl Med* 13:515, 1988.
23. Borges-Neto S, Coleman RE, Jones RH: Perfusion and function at rest and treadmill exercise using technetium-99m–sestamibi: Comparison of one- and two-day protocols in normal volunteers. *J Nucl Med* 31:1128, 1990.
24. Gerson MC, Lukes J, Deutsch E, et al: Comparison of technetium 99m Q12 and thallium 201 for detection of angiographically documented coronary artery disease in humans. *J Nucl Cardiol* 1:499, 1994.
25. Heo J, Cave V, Wasserleben V, et al: Planar and tomographic imaging with technetium 99m-labeled tetrofosmin: Correlation with thallium 201 and coronary angiography. *J Nucl Cardiol* 1:317, 1994.
26. Sporn V, Balino NP, Holman BL, et al: Simultaneous measurement of ventricular function and myocardial perfusion using the technetium-99m isonitriles. *Clin Nucl Med* 13:77, 1988.
27. Baillet GYU, Mena IG, Kuperus JH, et al: Simultaneous technetium-99m MIBI angiography and myocardial perfusion imaging. *J Nucl Med* 30:38, 1989.
28. Villanueva-Meyer J, Mena I, Narahara KA: Simultaneous assessment of left ventricular wall motion and myocardial perfusion with technetium-99m–methoxy isobutyl isonitrile at stress and rest in patients with angina: Comparison with thallium-201 SPECT. *J Nucl Med* 31:457, 1990.
29. DePuey EG, Salensky H, Melancon S, et al: Simultaneous biplane first-pass radionuclide angiocardiography using a scintillation camera with two perpendicular detectors. *J Nucl Med* 35:1593, 1994.
30. Marcassa C, Marzullo P, Parodi O, et al: A new method for noninvasive quantitation of segmental myocardial wall thickening using technetium-99m 2-methoxy-isobu-

tyl-isonitrile scintigraphy results in normal subjects. *J Nucl Med* 31:173, 1990.

31. Marzullo P, Marcassa C, Parodi O, et al: Noninvasive quantitative assessment of segmental myocardial wall motion using technetium-99m 2-methoxy-isobutyl-isonitrile scintigraphy. *Am J Noninvas Cardiol* 4:22, 1990.

32. Tischler MD, Niggel JB, Battle RW, et al: Validation of global and segmental left ventricular contractile function using gated planar technetium-99m sestamibi myocardial perfusion imaging. *J Am Coll Cardiol* 23:141, 1994.

33. Williams KA, Taillon LA: Gated planar technetium 99m–labeled sestamibi myocardial perfusion image inversion for quantitative scintigraphic assessment of left ventricular function. *J Nucl Cardiol* 2:285, 1995.

34. Leppo JA, DePuey EG, Johnson LL: A review of cardiac imaging with sestamibi and teboroxime. *J Nucl Med* 32:2012, 1991.

35. Seldin DW, Johnson LL, Blood DK, et al: Myocardial perfusion imaging with technetium-99m SQ30217: Comparison with thallium-201 and coronary anatomy. *J Nucl Med* 30:312, 1989.

36. Hendel RC, McSherry B, Karimeddini M, et al: Diagnostic value of a new myocardial perfusion agent, teboroxime (SQ30,217), utilizing a rapid planar imaging protocol: Preliminary results. *J Am Coll Cardiol* 16:855, 1990.

37. Taillefer R, Lambert R, Essiambre R, et al: Comparison between thallium-201, technetium-99m–sestamibi and technetium-99m–teboroxime planar myocardial perfusion imaging in detection of coronary artery disease. *J Nucl Med* 33:1091, 1992.

38. Weinstein H, Dahlberg ST, McSherry BA, et al: Rapid redistribution of teboroxime. *Am J Cardiol* 71:848, 1993.

39. Smith WH, Watson DD: Technical aspects of myocardial planar imaging with technetium 99m sestamibi. *Am J Cardiol* 66:16E, 1990.

39a. Sinusas AJ, Beller GA, Smith WH, et al: Quantitative planar imaging with technetium-99m methoxyisobutyl isonitrile: Comparison of uptake patterns with thallium-201. *J Nucl Med* 30:1456, 1989.

40. Goris ML: Nontarget activities: Can we correct for them? *J Nucl Med* 20:1312, 1980.

41. Goris ML, Daspit SG, McLaughlin P, et al: Interpolative background subtraction. *J Nucl Med* 17:744, 1976.

42. Watson DD, Campbell NP, Read EK, et al: Spatial and temporal quantitation of plane thallium myocardial images. *J Nucl Med* 22:577, 1981.

43. Trobaugh GB, Wackers FJTh, Sokole EB, et al: Thallium-201 myocardial imaging: An interinstitutional study of observer variability. *J Nucl Med* 19:359, 1978.

44. DeRouen TA, Murray JA, Owen W: Variability in the analysis of coronary arteriograms. *Circulation* 55:324, 1977.

45. Maddahi J, Garcia EV, Berman DS, et al: Improved noninvasive assessment of coronary artery disease by quantitative analysis of regional stress myocardial distribution and washout of thallium-201. *Circulation* 64:924, 1981.

46. Berger BC, Watson DD, Taylor GJ, et al: Quantitative thallium-201 exercise scintigraphy for detection of coronary artery disease. *J Nucl Med* 22:585, 1981.

47. Watson DD, Teates CD, Gibson RS: Myocardial perfusion imaging, in *Critical Problems in Diagnostic Radiology.* Philadelphia, JB Lippincott, 1983, p 241.

48. Garcia E, Maddahi J, Berman D, et al: Space/time quantitation of thallium-201 myocardial scintigraphy. *J Nucl Med* 22:309, 1981.

49. Diamond GA, Forrester JS: Analysis of probability in the diagnosis of coronary-artery disease. *N Engl J Med* 300:1350, 1979.

50. Burow RD, Pond M, Schafer AW, et al: "Circumferential profiles": A new method for computer analysis of thallium-201 myocardial perfusion images. *J Nucl Med* 20:771, 1979.

51. Goris ML, Gordon E, Kim D: A stochastic interpretation of thallium myocardial perfusion scintigraphy. *Invest Radiol* 20:253, 1985.

52. Brown KA, Weiss RM, Clements JP, et al: Usefulness of residual ischemic myocardium within prior infarct zone for identifying patients at high risk late after acute myocardial infarction. *Am J Cardiol* 60:15, 1987.

53. Wackers FJT, Fetterman RC, Mattera JA, et al: Quantitative planar thallium-201 stress scintigraphy: A critical evaluation of the method. *Semin Nucl Med* 15:46, 1985.

54. Koster K, Wackers FJTh, Mattera JA, et al: Quantitative analysis of planar technetium-99m–sestamibi myocardial perfusion images using modified background subtraction. *J Nucl Med* 31:1400, 1990.

54a. Kiat H, Maddahi J, Roy LT, et al: Comparison of technetium 99m methoxy isobutyl isonitrile and thallium 201 for evaluation of coronary artery disease by planar and tomographic methods. *Am Heart J* 117:1, 1989.

54b. Taillefer R, Lambert R, Dupras G, et al: Clinical comparison between thallium-201 and Tc-99m–methoxy isobutyl isonitrile (hexamibi) myocardial perfusion imaging for detection of coronary artery disease. *Eur J Nucl Med* 15:280, 1989.

55. Cook DJ, Bailey I, Strauss HW, et al: Thallium-201 for myocardial imaging: Appearance of the normal heart. *J Nucl Med* 17:583, 1976.

56. Gray H: *Anatomy of the Human Body,* Clemente CD (ed), 30th ed. Philadelphia, Lea and Febiger, 1985, p 637.

57. Wackers FJTh, Sokole EB, Samson G, et al: Atlas of ²⁰¹Tl myocardial scintigraphy. *Clin Nucl Med* 2:64, 1977.

58. Dunn RF, Wolff L, Wagner S, et al: The inconsistent pattern of thallium defects: A clue to the false positive perfusion scintigram. *Am J Cardiol* 48:224, 1981.

59. Dunn RF, Freedman B, Bailey IK, et al: Exercise thallium imaging: Location of perfusion abnormalities in single-vessel coronary disease. *J Nucl Med* 21:717, 1980.

60. Dunn RF, Newman HN, Bernstein L, et al: The clinical features of isolated left circumflex coronary artery disease. *Circulation* 69:477, 1984.

61. Brown KA, Boucher CA, Okada RD, et al: Serial right ventricular thallium-201 imaging after exercise: Relation to anatomy of the right coronary artery. *Am J Cardiol* 50:1217, 1982.

62. Gutman J, Brachman M, Rozanski A, et al: Enhanced detection of proximal right coronary artery stenosis with the additional analysis of right ventricular thallium-201

uptake in stress scintigrams. *Am J Cardiol* 51:1256, 1983.

63. Brown KA, Boucher CA, Okada RD, et al: Initial and delayed right ventricular thallium-201 rest-imaging following dipyridamole-induced coronary vasodilation: Relationship to right coronary artery pathoanatomy. *Am Heart J* 103:1019, 1982.

63a. Chuttani K, Metherall J, Griffith J, et al: Enhanced hepatic uptake of thallium-201 in patients with severe narrowing of the right coronary artery. *Am J Cardiol* 76:1020, 1995.

64. Takaro T, Hultgren HN, Lipton MJ, et al: The VA cooperative randomized study of surgery for coronary arterial occlusive disease. II. Subgroup with significant left main lesions. *Circulation* 54(suppl III):III-107, 1976.

65. Detre K, Peduzzi P, Murphy M, et al: Effect of bypass surgery on survival in patients in low- and high-risk subgroups delineated by the use of simple clinical variables. *Circulation* 63:1329, 1981.

66. European Coronary Surgery Study Group: Long-term results of prospective, randomized study of coronary-artery bypass surgery in stable angina pectoris. *Lancet* 2:1173, 1982.

67. Passamani E, Davis KB, Gillespie MJ, et al: A randomized trial of coronary artery bypass surgery: Survival of patients with a low ejection fraction. *N Engl J Med* 312:1665, 1985.

68. Dash H, Massie BM, Botvinick EH, et al: The noninvasive identification of left main and three-vessel coronary artery disease by myocardial stress perfusion scintigraphy and treadmill exercise electrocardiography. *Circulation* 60:276, 1979.

69. Chikamori T, Doi YL, Yonezawa Y, et al: Noninvasive identification of significant narrowing of the left main coronary artery by dipyridamole thallium scintigraphy. *Am J Cardiol* 68:472, 1991.

70. Rehn T, Griffith LSC, Achuff SC, et al: Exercise thallium-201 myocardial imaging in left main coronary artery disease: Sensitive but not specific. *Am J Cardiol* 48:217, 1981.

71. Nygaard TW, Gibson RS, Ryan JM, et al: Prevalence of high-risk thallium-201 scintigraphic findings in left main coronary artery stenosis: Comparison with patients with multiple- and single-vessel coronary artery disease. *Am J Cardiol* 53:462, 1984.

72. Maddahi J, Abdulla A, Garcia EV, et al: Noninvasive identification of left main and triple vessel coronary artery disease: Improved accuracy using quantitative analysis of regional myocardial stress distribution and washout of thallium-201. *J Am Coll Cardiol* 7:53, 1986.

73. Iskandrian AS, Hakki A-H, Segal BL, et al: Assessment of the myocardial perfusion pattern in patients with multivessel coronary artery disease. *Am Heart J* 106:1089, 1983.

74. Stolzenberg J: Dilatation of left ventricular cavity on stress thallium scan as an indicator of ischemic disease. *Clin Nucl Med* 5:289, 1980.

75. Weiss AT, Berman DS, Lew, AS, et al: Transient ischemic dilatation of the left ventricle on stress Tl-201 scintigrams: A marker of severe and extensive coronary artery disease. *J Am Coll Cardiol* 9:752, 1987.

76. Canhasi B, Dae M, Botvinick E, et al: Interaction of "supplementary" scintigraphic indicators of ischemia and stress electrocardiography in the diagnosis of multivessel coronary disease. *J Am Coll Cardiol* 6:581, 1985.

77. Chouraqui P, Rodrigues EA, Berman DS, et al: Significance of dipyridamole-induced transient dilation of the left ventricle during thallium-201 scintigraphy in suspected coronary artery disease. *Am J Cardiol* 66:689, 1990.

78. Lette J, Lapointe J, Waters D, et al: Transient left ventricular cavitary dilation during dipyridamole–thallium imaging as an indicator of severe coronary artery disease. *Am J Cardiol* 66:1163, 1990.

79. Iskandrian AS, Heo J, Nguyen T, et al: Left ventricular dilatation and pulmonary thallium uptake after single-photon emission computer tomography using thallium-201 during adenosine-induced coronary hyperemia. *Am J Cardiol* 66:807, 1990.

80. Kushner FG, Okada RD, Kirshenbaum HD, et al: Lung thallium-201 uptake after stress testing in patients with coronary artery disease. *Circulation* 63:341, 1981.

81. Bingham JB, McKusick KA, Strauss HW, et al: Influence of coronary artery disease on pulmonary uptake of thallium-201. *Am J Cardiol* 46:821, 1980.

82. Miller DD, Heyl BL, Walsh RA: Lung uptake of technetium-99m hexamibi isonitrile during acute reversible ischemic left ventricular dysfunction in conscious dogs. *Circulation* 78(suppl II):II-387, 1988 (abstr).

83. Boucher CA, Zir LM, Beller GA, et al: Increased lung uptake of thallium-201 during exercise myocardial imaging: Clinical, hemodynamic and angiographic implications in patients with coronary artery disease. *Am J Cardiol* 46:189, 1980.

84. Brown KA, Boucher CA, Okada RD, et al: Quantification of pulmonary thallium-201 activity after upright exercise in normal persons: Importance of peak heart rate and propranolol usage in defining normal values. *Am J Cardiol* 53:1678, 1984.

85. Levy R, Rozanski A, Berman DS, et al: Analysis of the degree of pulmonary thallium washout after exercise in patients with coronary artery disease. *J Am Coll Cardiol* 2:719, 1983.

86. Homma S, Kaul S, Boucher CA: Correlates of lung/heart ratio of thallium-201 in coronary artery disease. *J Nucl Med* 28:1531, 1987.

87. Liu P, Kiess M, Okada RD, et al: Increased thallium lung uptake after exercise in isolated left anterior descending coronary artery disease. *Am J Cardiol* 55:1469, 1985.

88. Martinez EE, Horowitz SF, Castello HJ, et al: Lung and myocardial thallium-201 kinetics in resting patients with congestive heart failure: Correlation with pulmonary capillary wedge pressure. *Am Heart J* 123:427, 1992.

89. Okada RD, Dai Y-H, Boucher CA, et al: Significance of increased lung thallium-201 activity on serial cardiac images after dipyridamole treatment in coronary heart disease. *Am J Cardiol* 53:470, 1984.

90. Villanueva FS, Kaul S, Smith WH, et al: Prevalence and correlates of increased lung/heart ratio of thallium-

201 during dipyridamole stress imaging for suspected coronary artery disease. *Am J Cardiol* 66:1324, 1990.

91. Hurwitz GA, O'Donoghue JP, Powe JE, et al: Pulmonary thallium-201 uptake following dipyridamole–exercise combination compared with single modality stress testing. *Am J Cardiol* 69:320, 1992.

92. Nishimura S, Mahmarian JJ, Verani MS: Significance of increased lung thallium uptake during adenosine thallium-201 scintigraphy. *J Nucl Med* 33:1600, 1992.

93. Hurwitz GA, Fox SP, Driedger AA, et al: Pulmonary uptake of sestamibi on early post-stress images: angiographic relationships, incidence and kinetics. *Nucl Med Commun* 14:15, 1993.

94. Barr SA, Jain D, Wackers FJTh, et al: Are there correlates of increased thallium lung uptake on planar tetrofosmin perfusion imaging? *Circulation* 88:I-582, 1993 (abstr).

95. Cohen HA, Baird MG, Rouleau JR, et al: Thallium 201 myocardial imaging in patients with pulmonary hypertension. *Circulation* 54:790, 1976.

96. Kondo M, Kubo A, Yamazaki H, et al: Thallium-201 myocardial imaging for evaluation of right-ventricular overloading. *J Nucl Med* 19:1197, 1978.

97. Khaja F, Alam M, Goldstein S, et al: Diagnostic value of visualization of the right ventricle using thallium-201 myocardial imaging. *Circulation* 59:182, 1979.

98. Ohsuzu F, Handa S, Kondo M, et al: Thallium-201 myocardial imaging to evaluate right ventricular overloading. *Circulation* 61:620, 1980.

99. Yasuno M, Kawamura O, Watanabe T, et al: Diagnostic value of thallium-201 myocardial imaging in pulmonary embolism. *Angiology* 34:293, 1983.

100. Schulman DS, Lazar JM, Ziady G, et al: Right ventricular thallium-201 kinetics in pulmonary hypertension: Relation to right ventricular size and function. *J Nucl Med* 34:1695, 1993.

101. Nakajima K, Taki J, Ohno T, et al: Assessment of right ventricular overload by a thallium-201 SPECT study in children with congenital heart disease. *J Nucl Med* 32:2215, 1991.

102. DePuey EG, Jones ME, Garcia EV: Evaluation of right ventricular regional perfusion with technetium-99m–sestamibi SPECT. *J Nucl Med* 32:1199, 1991.

103. Tonami N, Shuke N, Yokoyama K, et al: Thallium-201 single photon emission computed tomography in the evaluation of suspected lung cancer. *J Nucl Med* 30:997, 1989.

104. Basara BE, Wallner RJ, Hakki A-H, et al: Extracardiac accumulation of thallium-201 in pulmonary carcinoma. *Am J Cardiol* 53:358, 1984.

105. Eisenberg B, Velchik MG, DeVries DFL: Thallium-201 chloride uptake in a lung tumor during a routine stress thallium examination. *Clin Nucl Med* 13:214, 1988.

106. Fakier DR, Strauss EB: Thallium-201 accumulation in an unsuspected bronchogenic carcinoma. *Clin Nucl Med* 14:460, 1989.

107. Salvatore M, Carratu L, Porta E: Thallium-201 as a positive indicator for lung neoplasms: Preliminary experiments. *Radiology* 121:487, 1976.

108. Cox PH, Belfer AJ, van der Pompe WB: Thallium-201 chloride uptake in tumors: A possible complication in heart scintigraphy. *Br J Radiol* 49:767, 1976.

109. Tonami N, Yokoyama K, Shuke N, et al: Evaluation of suspected malignant pulmonary lesions with ^{201}Tl single photon emission computed tomography. *Nucl Med Commun* 14:602, 1993.

110. Tonami N, Yokoyama K, Taki J, et al: Thallium-201 SPECT depicts radiologically occult lung cancer. *J Nucl Med* 32:2284, 1991.

111. Togawa T, Yui N, Koakutsu M, et al: Two cases of adenocarcinoma of the lung in which thallium-201 gave a better delineation of metastatic lesions than gallium-67. *Clin Nucl Med* 14:197, 1989.

112. Tonami N, Yokoyama K, Michigishi T, et al: Thallium-201 single photon emission computed tomograms of double cancers: Lung and breast. *Clin Nucl Med* 14:594, 1989.

113. Tonami N, Yokoyama K, Taki J, et al: [201]Tl SPECT in the detection of mediastinal lymph node metastases from lung cancer. *Nucl Med Commun* 12:779, 1991.

114. Waxman AD, Ramanna L, Memsic LD, et al: Thallium scintigraphy in the evaluation of mass abnormalities of the breast. *J Nucl Med* 34:18, 1993.

115. Lee VW, Sax EJ, McAneny DB, et al: A complementary role for thallium-201 scintigraphy with mammography in the diagnosis of breast cancer. *J Nucl Med* 34:2095, 1993.

116. El-Gazzar AH, Sahweil A, Abdel-Dayem HM, et al: Experience with thallium-201 imaging in head and neck cancer. *Clin Nucl Med* 13:286, 1988.

117. Black KL, Hawkins RA, Kim KT, et al: Use of thallium-201 SPECT to quantitate malignancy grade of gliomas. *J Neurosurg* 71:342, 1989.

118. Oriuchi N, Tamura M, Shibazaki T, et al: Clinical evaluation of thallium-201 SPECT in supratentorial gliomas: Relationship to histologic grade, prognosis and proliferative activities. *J Nucl Med* 34:2085, 1993.

119. Ramanna L, Waxman A, Binney G, et al: Thallium-201 scintigraphy in bone sarcoma: Comparison with gallium-67 and technetium–MDP in the evaluation of chemotherapeutic response. *J Nucl Med* 31:567, 1990.

120. Fukuchi M, Kido A, Hyodo K, et al: Uptake of thallium-201 in enlarged thyroid glands: Concise communication. *J Nucl Med* 20:827, 1979.

121. Jinnouchi S, Hoshi H, Ohnishi T, et al: Thallium-201 SPECT for predicting histological types of meningiomas. *J Nucl Med* 34:2091, 1993.

122. Bordlee RP, Ware RW: Thallium-201 accumulation by epidermoid inclusion cyst. *J Nucl Med* 33:1857, 1992.

123. Aktolun C, Demirel D, Kir M, et al: Technetium-99m–MIBI and thallium-201 uptake in pulmonary actinomycosis. *J Nucl Med* 32:1429, 1991.

124. Lee JD, Lee BH, Kim SK, et al: Increased thallium-201 uptake in collapsed lung: A pitfall in scintigraphic evaluation of central bronchogenic carcinoma. *J Nucl Med* 35:1125, 1994.

125. Campeau RJ, Garcia OM, Correa OA, et al: Pectoralis muscle uptake of thallium-201 after arm exercise ergome-

try: Possible confusion with lung thallium-201 activity. *Clin Nucl Med* 15:303, 1990.

126. Piwnica-Worms D, Holman BL: Noncardiac applications of hexakis(alkylisonitrile) technetium-99m complexes. *J Nucl Med* 31:1166, 1990 (editorial).

127. O'Doherty MJ, Kettle AG, Wells P, et al: Parathyroid imaging with technetium 99m–sestamibi: Preoperative localization and tissue uptake studies. *J Nucl Med* 33:313, 1992.

128. Geatti O, Shapiro B, Orsolon PG, et al: Localization of parathyroid enlargement: Experience with technetium-99m methoxyisobutylisonitrile and thallium-201 scintigraphy, ultrasonography and computed tomography. *Eur J Nucl Med* 21:17, 1994.

129. Benard F, Lefebvre B, Beuvon F, et al: Rapid washout of technetium-99m–MIBI from a large parathyroid adenoma. *J Nucl Med* 36:241, 1995.

130. Caner B, Kitapcl M, Unlu M, et al: Technetium-99m–MIBI uptake in benign and malignant bone lesions: A comparative study with technetium-99m–MDP. *J Nucl Med* 33:319, 1992.

131. Hassan IM, Sahweil A, Constantinides C, et al: Uptake and kinetics of Tc-99m hexakis 2-methoxy isobutyl isonitrile in benign and malignant lesions in the lungs. *Clin Nucl Med* 14:333, 1989.

132. Balon HR, Fink-Bennett D, Stoffer SS: Technetium-99m–sestamibi uptake by recurrent Hürthle cell carcinoma of the thyroid. *J Nucl Med* 33:1393, 1992.

133. Pietrzyk U, Scheidhauer K, Scharl A, et al: Presurgical visualization of primary breast carcinoma with PET emission and transmission imaging. *J Nucl Med* 36:1882, 1995.

134. Khalkhali I, Cutrone J, Mena I, et al: Technetium-99m–sestamibi scintimammography of breast lesions: Clinical and pathological follow-up. *J Nucl Med* 36:1784, 1995.

135. Taillefer R, Robidoux A, Lambert R, et al: Technetium-99m–sestamibi prone scintimammography to detect primary breast cancer and axillary lymph node involvement. *J Nucl Med* 36:1758, 1995.

Tomographic Imaging: Methods

Tracy L. Faber

The utility of nuclear medicine for evaluating cardiac perfusion and left ventricular function was originally demonstrated by planar imaging, yet planar studies are suboptimal in a number of ways. They are created using a projection technique in which counts throughout the depth of the torso are combined in a single image. Therefore, the portion of the image containing the heart also will contain counts from structures in front of and behind it. This superimposition property implies that the heart cannot be isolated from other regions of the chest, nor can one area of the heart be truly isolated from another. In addition, the two-dimensional aspect of projection images means that structures perpendicular to the imaging plane are viewed in a foreshortened manner, if they are viewed at all. Single photon emission computed tomography (SPECT) eliminates these shortcomings and is now the preferred technique for myocardial perfusion imaging.

SPECT combines planar views acquired over multiple angles around the axis of the body to provide transaxial slices that show the relative amounts of radioactivity detected at each point in the imaged three-dimensional volume. This is demonstrated in Fig. 3-1. Unlike planar projections, SPECT does not suffer from occlusion or superimposition of other structures in front of or behind the organ of interest, thus improving image contrast and allowing smaller defects to be accurately diagnosed. SPECT gives a fully three-dimensional view of radiotracer distribution in a slice-by-slice manner, thus enabling better localization of abnormalities and improved analysis of their extent. These properties of

SPECT make it a superior technique for cardiac imaging. It has in fact been demonstrated that the sensitivity and specificity of SPECT for the extent of coronary artery disease are higher compared with qualitative planar techniques.[1-3]

However, SPECT is very technically demanding; it requires complex equipment, dedicated quality control, and a multitude of careful, informed acquisition and processing protocol decisions to ensure high image quality. In turn, the accuracy of the diagnosis often depends on image quality. Therefore, knowledge of how the many factors in SPECT affect cardiac images, positively or negatively, is essential for patient care. This chapter describes the basic issues in SPECT acquisition and processing, and discusses aspects of new techniques that are just now being used clinically.

SPECT IMAGE PROPERTIES

Three common parameters that contribute importantly to the technical adequacy of cardiac radionuclide images are contrast, noise, and spatial resolution. These three properties are somewhat different from each other in character. All three can be altered through image processing. However, spatial resolution more often depends on equipment choices; in particular, there is an upper limit placed on spatial resolution by the detector hardware. Conversely, noise and contrast are more com-

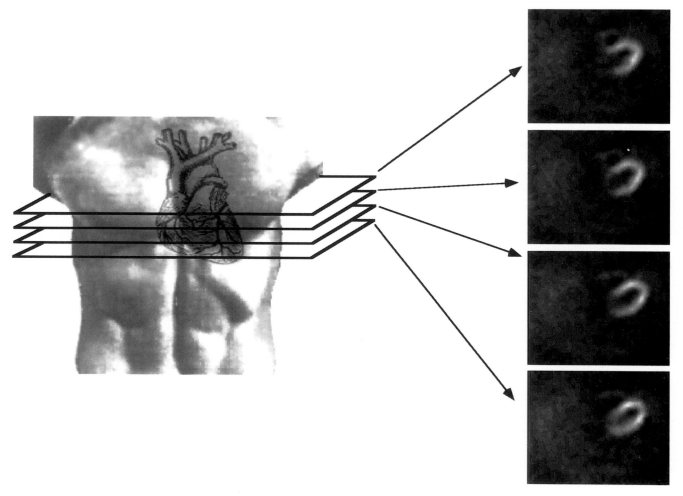

Figure 3-1 Tomography creates a stack of slices through the axis of the body; the slices show the distribution of radionuclide at each point. Here, myocardial perfusion images that slice through the chest are displayed.

monly affected by a combination of many image acquisition and processing factors, including, for example, radionuclide properties. Because spatial resolution is limited by hardware, it is the only one of these three parameters measured on a common basis, as a quality-control technique. However, because all three are indicators of image quality and because all can be affected by image acquisition and processing choices, they are important to understand.

Contrast is a measure of intensity or counts in a target organ compared with the intensity in a background region. It is often measured as $(C_o - C_b)/C_b$, where C_o are the organ counts and C_b are the background counts. The higher the contrast, the more visible is the organ of interest. In an extreme case, low contrast can make the target organ undetectable against a high-count background. Contrast is most easily measured by graphing the counts encountered along a line drawn through a region of interest in the image; such a line is called a

profile. The peak counts in the graph are taken to be C_o, and the minimum count level is taken to be C_b. Figure 3-2 shows profiles taken through the left ventricular myocardium in both a planar and a tomographic image. The decreased background count level in the tomographic image causes increased contrast compared with the planar image.

Spatial resolution is a measure of how close two point sources can get and still be distinguished as separate. Because no medical imaging modality is perfect, a point source never appears as a single point but instead as a blurred distribution. Two blurry points eventually smear btogether into a single spot when they are moved close enough to each other. Resolution is measured by taking a profile though a point source and analyzing the resulting curve. A profile through a perfect point source would look like a sharp single spike rising above the flat background. A profile through a real point source appears as a Gaussian-shaped curve.

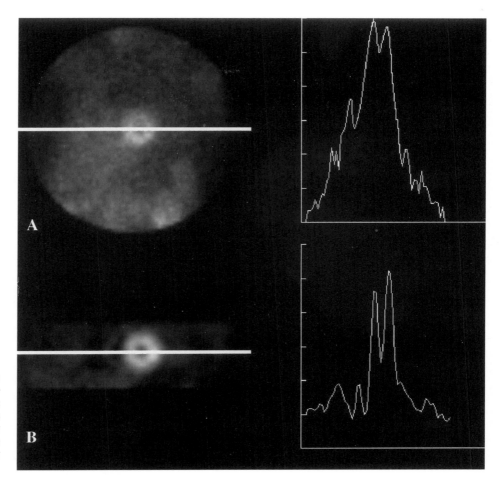

Figure 3-2 Profiles taken through the myocardium in a planar perfusion image **(A)** and a tomographic perfusion image **(B)** show properties related to image quality. The higher background count level seen in the planar image profile causes lower contrast.

Resolution is the width of the Gaussian curve at a level of one-half of its maximum, or the full-width half-maximum (FWHM).

Noise can be thought of as a measure of irrelevant information or a disturbance of the useful data in the image. Noise appears as a speckle in nuclear medicine images and is particularly noticeable in background or otherwise constant regions. Noise is measured relative to the useful image information, called the *signal*. In nuclear medicine, the signal is proportional to the counts, N, while the noise is proportional to $\sqrt{N}$. Thus, the relative amount of noise—the signal/noise ratio—is $N/\sqrt{N}$, or $\sqrt{N}$. Note that the signal, N, increases faster than the noise, $\sqrt{N}$. The implication of this fact is that noise is a more serious problem in low-count studies. As image counts increase, noise becomes less evident. Therefore, image *noise quality* can be improved by a factor of 2 by increasing the acquired counts by a factor of 4. Thus, the absolute number of increased counts required to improve the noise quality of a low-count image will be substantially less that the number of additional counts needed to improve substantially the noise quality of a high-count image.

SPECT EQUIPMENT

Camera Heads

The main components of a SPECT system are the camera heads, the frame supporting the head(s) known as the gantry, the computer hardware, and the computer software. The properties of each of these components interact to determine the quality of the final image and the speed at which it can be acquired.

Each head of a system is a separate scintillation detector, comprised of a collimator, a NaI crystal, photomultiplier tubes (PMTs), pulse height analyzers (PHAs), and spatial positioning circuitry. A gamma ray travels through the collimator and strikes the crystal, causing a scintillation; this glow is converted into an electrical signal by the PMTs. The intensity of this signal is related to the energy of the gamma ray, and this is measured by the PHAs. The location of the scintillation in the crystal is determined by the spatial positioning hardware, which compares relative signals from adjacent PMTs. Traditionally, output signals from the PHA and positioning circuitry were analog; they were then converted to digital signals for input into the nuclear medicine computer. New *digital* cameras convert the output from each PMT to a digital signal, which then can be analyzed for energy and position by using digital electronics. The primary advantage of this early digitizing is greater processing flexibility and spatial resolution, since programming can be used to change or improve energy and/or spatial analysis.

Circular camera heads were the norm for many years; today, rectangular heads dominate the market for general-purpose SPECT, since they increase the acquisition speed of whole-body bone scans. For cardiac imaging, there is little advantage to rectangular heads, and in fact the patient's arms may interfere with the corners of the rectangular camera during SPECT. Related to the shape of the head is its field of view, or the size of the usable imaging area of the camera when a parallel-hole collimator is used. Small-field-of-view cameras which "cut off" the outer portion of the torso can produce image artifacts, but these artifacts generally only affect the periphery of the image and not the cardiac region. Such field-of-view artifacts are more problematic when performing transmission studies with a SPECT system as a precursor to attenuation correction. This is discussed more fully later in the chapter.

MULTIHEADED SYSTEMS

SPECT systems with a single head were the only option up until the late 1980s; multiheaded cameras now make up a large proportion of all new systems sold. The addition of more heads to a SPECT system increases its overall sensitivity; that is, the number of counts that can be detected per unit time. There are currently three configurations for multiheaded SPECT systems. There are triple-headed cameras with detectors positioned 120° apart, and there are dual-headed systems with detectors positioned 90° or 180° apart. Some manufacturers offer dual-headed systems in which the detectors can be positioned at either 90° or 180° apart.

The ability to acquire two or even three times the counts detected from a single-headed system in the same time period has many implications. A study requiring 20 min on a single-headed camera can be finished in 10 min on a dual-headed camera whose heads are oriented at 90° apart. The reconstructions from the corresponding single- and dual-headed acquisitions will be essentially identical if the imaged radiopharmaceutical does not wash in or out of the myocardium significantly over the course of the acquisition. This is true for both sestamibi (hexakis-2-methoxyisobutyl isonitrile) and ^{201}Tl; therefore, patient throughput can be increased with multiheaded systems with no loss of image quality, assuming all other acquisition parameters are identical.

For radiopharmaceuticals that do wash out of the myocardium rapidly over the course of the acquisition, speed is of the utmost importance to assure that the radionuclide distribution seen in the reconstruction is accurate. For example, one-half of the original concentration of ^{99m}Tc teboroxime in the myocardium will wash out 4 min following its point of maximum uptake. To ensure a high-quality, artifact-free reconstruction that accurately represents the maximum teboroxime uptake, the acquisition should be finished in less than 4 min.[4,5] This restriction is obviously easier to meet with a multiheaded system. In fact, *dynamic* tomographic images of teboroxime, consisting of multiple sequential high-speed acquisitions, have been performed with multiheaded cameras.[6,7]

Decreased acquisition time should also lead to less patient motion. More importantly, there is some preliminary evidence that if a patient does move during an acquisition with a multiheaded system, the reconstruction is affected less than if similar motion occurred during a single-headed acquisition.[8]

The increased sensitivity gained from multiheaded systems may be used to improve image quality. High-resolution collimators and cardiac gating both decrease the collected counts (the details are provided later in this chapter), and this decrease will degrade image quality by increasing the amount of noise. With a single-headed camera, this degradation can be lessened by increasing imaging time to restore the missing counts lost to collimation or the division of the study into multiple time bins. By switching from a single- to a dual-headed system, a loss of half the original counts can be restored with no increase in original imaging time.

Finally, one of the heads of a multiheaded system can be used to acquire a transmission image while the other heads are acquiring the emission data, in order to apply attenuation correction algorithms. The topic of attenuation correction is discussed more fully later in the chapter.

COLLIMATORS

The collimator is positioned between the detector and the patient. It is used to ensure that photons detected at each projection angle have traveled perpendicularly to the camera face or detector crystal from their original emission point. Collimators are rated as to their sensitivity and resolution. Sensitivity describes how many counts are collected in a given time. Resolution describes how close two point sources can get and still be distinguished as separate when imaged with that collimator. In general, the sensitivity and resolution of a collimator are inversely related; a very highly sensitive collimator will have a low resolution, and a very high-resolution collimator will have a low sensitivity. Collimators affect these properties by the area, shape, and length of their holes.

General all-purpose (GAP) collimators have relatively short, wide holes; they can acquire many more counts than those with long, narrow holes. This is explained geometrically. If a hole is wide and short, more photons at oblique angles will be able to travel through them to reach the detector. This increases the number of collected counts, i.e., sensitivity, but the overlapping of oblique counts causes a blur that decreases image resolution. High-resolution collimators with relatively long, narrow holes will create higher-resolution images than a GAP collimator. This is because only those nuclei directly in line with a collimator hole will be able to emit photons that can get through the hole and strike the detector. Unfortunately, the improved resolution comes at the cost of decreased sensitivity, since fewer photons are detected overall. This is illustrated in Fig. 3-3**A** and **B**. Finally, there is an inherent relationship between the resolution of a collimator and the distance of the source being imaged. The closer to the collimator that a nucleus is, the less likely that photons traveling obliquely will get through any of the collimator holes. Oblique photons emitted farther away from the collimator are more likely to travel through adjacent collimator holes, causing a blur. This can also be seen in Fig. 3-3**A** and **B**. The collimator–source distance relationship is called the *detector response* or *geometric response* of the camera system. Its effect on tomographic images is that areas in the center of the body are usually blurred more than those near its surface.

Parallel-hole collimators are the most common in SPECT. However, higher sensitivity can be obtained with converging collimators, i.e., fan-beam or cone-beam collimators. The improved sensitivity arises because the converging collimator "views" a source through a larger solid angle than a parallel-hole collimator and thus enables more of the photons to be detected. This can be visualized in Fig. 3-3**C**.

For cardiac SPECT, the problem with converging collimators is that their field of view does not necessarily cover the entire thorax in every view. If the cardiac region is truncated, artifacts may badly degrade the reconstruction. Currently, the best compromises have been either to use fan-beam collimators with a very slight angle in order to improve resolution slightly with no truncation, or to create a collimator with holes that change the pitch of their angles depending on their location in the field

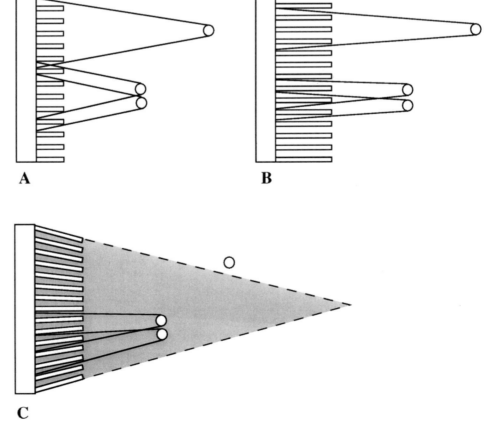

Figure 3-3 Collimators affect system sensitivity and image resolution. **A:** A general all-purpose collimator. The *lines drawn* indicate the angular range of directions that photons may travel and still proceed through the collimator. In a parallel-hole collimator, a wide angle indicates that many counts are collected (high sensitivity), but close points will overlap (low resolution). Note that counts from the source farthest from the collimator spread out farther than those from the closer sources—this is the detector response function. **B:** A high-resolution collimator. The sources shown here are at the same distance from this collimator as those shown in A. Note that the counts from these sources do not spread as far when imaged with the high-resolution collimator as they do when imaged with the all-purpose collimator. This indicates that the resolution is higher but sensitivity is lower with collimator B. **C:** A fan-beam collimator. Note how the spread of counts from the two close sources is larger than those in the high-resolution collimator, indicating higher sensitivity. Also note that the field of view of this collimator excludes imaging of the farthest point source.

of view. This type of collimator has holes that get closer to parallel toward their sides; this means objects in the center of the field of view will be imaged with higher sensitivity than those at the edges, but there will be no truncation.

Gantry

The frame that supports the camera head(s) contains the machinery to rotate and position them. The primary concerns with the gantry are its size and stability. Size is mostly a practical issue; since the gantry is the largest part of a SPECT system, its size will determine the amount of room space needed. Likewise, since the gantry supports the heads that may have heavy lead collimators, it is often the heaviest part of a SPECT system. Thus, its weight may determine the amount of floor support needed prior to installation. Finally, the heavy camera heads are difficult to move swiftly and surely from point to point; there is usually some amount of settling time for the heads to become completely stationary after a rotation. This manifests itself as part of the system *dead time*, which can greatly increase the length of an acquisition. Dead time and camera rotation acquisition modes are discussed later in the acquisition section.

Computers

The task of a nuclear medicine computer is to acquire the projections, reconstruct them into a tomographic image, analyze and process the reconstructions if necessary, display all images and graphic results, and store all of this information. Computer hardware determines the upper limit of how fast each step can be completed, how much data can be stored and processed, and how many and how well images can be displayed. Software can also play a role in speed, but its more obvious quality is a nebulous trait called *usability*. Software provides the link between the operator and the hardware, and it can either help or hinder the speed and quality of each operation.

HARDWARE

There are four main hardware components of a nuclear medicine computer system: the processor, memory, storage, and display. The processor (also called the *CPU* or central processing unit) is the electronic circuitry that actually performs mathematical operations. Often, the speed of the CPU determines how fast the computer is, overall. Both memory and storage are places that hold data for the short and long term, respectively. In order for the CPU to access data, it must be stored in the computer's memory. Data are stored for longer periods of time on hard disks, optical disks, floppy disks, or magnetic tape. Finally, text, images, and other graphics are output to the computer's display hardware. The faster each of these four components is, the "better" the computer will perform.

Memory and disk space requirements can be determined by considering a typical SPECT data set. Note that a basic cardiac SPECT acquisition of 64 × 64 pixel projections from 64 angles requires a half-million bytes of disk space to be stored on a disk or tape, and 32 reconstructed slices created from this projection set will require another quarter-million bytes of disk space. In order to perform the reconstruction process, the original projections, the intermediate reconstructed slices, and numerous temporary storage areas should be able to fit in memory. Therefore, a computer will need at least 4 million bytes of memory to perform this very basic, low-end process. To reconstruct projections having 128 pixels per side, both the amounts of disk space and memory needed are increased by 16 times. Gated acquisitions increase disk storage requirements by a factor equal to the number of frames acquired; i.e., an 8-frame gated projection set will require about 4 million bytes of disk space to store. Memory requirements for reconstructing gated studies are not necessarily increased, since frames are usually reconstructed one at a time. Instead, the amount of time needed for reconstruction of the entire set increases as the number of frames increase, and thus processor speed becomes more important for gated SPECT.

Because nuclear medicine is a visual discipline, the computer display is very important. Display hardware is described by its spatial resolution; that is, the size of the screen in discrete elements, called *pixels* or dots. This determines how many images can be displayed on the screen at the same time. An additional concern in selecting a display is how fast an image can be displayed on the screen; this becomes an issue when attempting to view gated cardiac images. If the transfer from memory to display is slow, then "beating" slices must be displayed in a very small format in order to move at a reasonable speed. The number of colors that can be displayed at one time on a computer screen is generally described as graphics *bits*; that is, a 256-color screen has 8-bit graphics, since $2^8 = 256$. Most workstation displays are about 1000 × 1000 pixels in size with 8-bit graphics that allow 256 different colors or shades of gray to be displayed on the screen at one time. This is adequate for most basic clinical displays. Older and cheaper stations may be only 512 × 512 pixels; this may be enough for many uses, but realize that only sixty-four 64 × 64 images can be displayed on such a screen. Often it is useful to view various slices of rest and stress cardiac studies together, and 512 × 512 pixels may be barely adequate for this. In addition, more than 8 bits of graphics are useful in order to create high-quality three-dimensional graphics; *true-color* displays offer 24-bit graphics. Note that programs generally must be written to take advantage of high-resolution and true-color displays; not all software can support all hardware.

Three types of computer systems are available from various manufacturers. Originally, each vendor designed (or at least customized) its own hardware and software, since over-the-counter systems were incapable of performing the demanding reconstruction and processing tasks in SPECT. Today, the trend is toward using either workstations or personal computers (PCs) as the main components in SPECT system hardware.

IN-HOUSE SYSTEMS

Even today, hardware specifically designed to perform the computations for SPECT can offer some advantages over less specialized electronics. Such hardware can be faster than off-the-shelf systems for both processing and display. Often, companies use specially designed hardware dedicated to controlling the camera and handling the acquisition, since these tasks are very time dependent. However, an in-house-designed system used as a basic processing and display station has some serious disadvantages. Users are completely dependent on the nuclear medicine company for upgrades and maintenance; similarly, upgrades and maintenance may be far more expensive for in-house systems because of the economics of scale.

PERSONAL COMPUTERS

The biggest advantage of PC-based hardware, that is, either IBM-compatible or Macintosh-based systems, is the relatively low cost of the basic hardware, and the availability of many software packages that can be used with them. Many useful programs can be purchased or even obtained free to perform SPECT-related tasks, such as image processing and display, report generation, and patient scheduling and billing. PC-based systems are ideal low-cost viewing stations, and ever-improving hardware has made most new systems capable of basic SPECT acquisition, reconstruction, and processing at reasonable speeds.

WORKSTATIONS

Workstations are the most common type of hardware sold by nuclear medicine companies. They combine off-the-shelf availability and price with speed and capacity of in-house systems. Most workstations are standardized with the UNIX operating system and X-windows graphical user interfaces. Workstations are generally faster with more memory (and higher prices) than PCs, although these differences in capacity, performance, and price are becoming less well defined.

SOFTWARE

Software can be categorized in a number of ways. There are menu-driven systems where options are listed at each step and selecting one menu option brings up a more specific menu or starts a process. They usually limit the user to doing one thing at a time. Window-based systems are more flexible, as they generally provide more choices and allow many things to proceed simultaneously. However, they can be more confusing to use and are harder to design well. The most important aspect to software is its availability and its usability. The necessary programs to perform every task needed in the clinic must be on the system (and run correctly), and they should be simple to use. Availability of software is easily determined; usability is generally only found to be lacking after the system is delivered. Some factors which improve user friendliness are

Use of familiar terms

Provision of *default* answers to questions, and the ability to change them to new defaults

Ability to perform basic functions (such as displaying an image) with a minimal amount of user interaction

Availability of macros to perform related functions or protocols with few interactions, and the ability to create new ones

Speed

Useful error messages that advise you how to fix a problem

Inclusion of hints and *help* functions that can offer instructions specific to whatever you are doing (context-sensitive help)

Well-written manuals with extensive cross-referenced indexes.

TOMOGRAPHIC ACQUISITIONS

Cross-sectional tomographic images are created by mathematically combining multiple planar views, called *projections*, that have been collected at many angles around the body. There are numerous variables that define exactly how the rotating gamma camera travels around the patient and how and when each projection is obtained. These acquisition parameters help to determine the quality of the final tomographic image.

General

For cardiac SPECT, three important variables are the size of the planar projection image in pixels, the average number of counts collected for each pixel, and the number of views obtained. For typical cardiac SPECT system resolution on the order of 1 cm, an acquisition projection matrix size of 64 × 64 is adequate. Generally, the number of counts acquired should be maximized, without exceeding radiation dosage limits or the patient's ability to remain immobile; 100 counts/pixel in the myocardium is typical for a stress sestamibi image. Finally, 64 projections over 180° are sufficient for most cardiac studies.

In SPECT, the appearance of the final reconstruction depends on numerous physical factors besides the radiotracer distribution within the body. Many things can happen to a photon after it is emitted and before it strikes the crystal. First, it can be absorbed by another nucleus; the likelihood of absorption depends on a parameter termed the *attenuation coefficient*. The attenuation coefficient, in turn, depends on the photon energy of the radiotracer and the electron density of the tissue through which the photon is passing. The relationship is described mathematically by $N = N_o\, e^{-\mu l}$, where N_o is the number of photons emitted, N is the number which escape attenuation, l is the length of the path that the photon travels through the tissue, and μ is the attenuation coefficient of the tissue. For instance, a photon emitted near a bone is more likely to be absorbed than one emitted near the surface of the body. Generally, a high-energy photon is less likely to be absorbed by another nucleus than a low-energy photon.

A gamma ray may also "bounce off" of another atom and be redirected in a new path. This effect, called *Compton scatter*, also depends on photon energy and tissue electron density. Scatter causes higher background count levels and thus reduces contrast.

Finally, the likelihood of a photon traveling through a collimator hole and striking the detector depends on the properties of the collimator, along with the direction the photon is traveling and its point of emission. This property, termed *detector response*, was discussed previously in the equipment section. These three things—absorption, scatter, and detector response—mean that the projection depends on a combination of the physical properties of the collimator, the energy of the emitted gamma ray, the detector distance from each emission point, and the shape and composition of the body. This will be different for every patient, radioisotope, collimator, and exact position of the detector, so the path of the gamma camera as it rotates, i.e., its orbit, becomes an important variable for SPECT image quality.

Orbits

180° VERSUS 360° ORBITS

Historically, 180° acquisitions have been preferred for cardiac SPECT. The angles chosen for the 180° arc are those closest to the heart, from 45° right anterior oblique (RAO) to 45° left posterior oblique (LPO). These projections are those that suffer least from attenuation, scatter, and detector response, because they are the ones that get the camera head as close as possible to the heart. Reconstructions from 180° acquisitions are felt to have higher resolution and contrast than those from 360°; this is particularly true for ^{201}Tl images.[9,10] However, because 180° reconstructions are not truly complete—that is, new information is available from the other 180° of projections—there are occasional artifacts seen with 180° reconstructions that can be avoided with 360° reconstructions.[11–13]

Perhaps the greatest advantage to 180° orbits is that, historically, they could be completed in half of the time as a 360° acquisition. This is no longer true with some of the new multiple-headed cameras. Relative speed of an acquisition depends on the number of heads, the configuration of the heads, and whether the acquisition covers 180° or 360°. For example, a three-headed camera (with heads spaced at 120°) will acquire an entire 360° set of projections even if only 180° of the data is to be reconstructed. Since the costs of the two acquisitions are equal, 360° reconstructions may be preferred for ^{99m}Tc-based radionuclides in order to avoid the possible artifacts generated in 180° reconstructions.

CIRCULAR VERSUS NONCIRCULAR ORBITS

Initially, SPECT rotating gamma cameras were limited to rotating in a circle; that is, the position of the detectors with respect to the center of rotation was fixed to a given radius for a given acquisition. The radius chosen was that which would allow the head to just clear the patient's body at every angle. Circular orbits are still used; however, forcing the camera to stay at a fixed radius in order to clear the patient at one angle may cause the camera to be very far from the body surface at another angle. New cameras are able to change their radius angle by angle in order to travel in elliptical or even body-contoured orbits. Elliptical orbits are presumed to be better than circular for getting the camera close to an average person, and contoured orbits get the camera as close as possible to every patient at every angle, using either sophisticated hardware or preacquisition setup by the user. By keeping the detector as close as possible to the patient, detector response is minimized and resolution is made as high as possible.[14] However, because the resolution will vary from angle to angle, the resulting reconstruction may be different from one created with a circular orbit. In cardiac SPECT, the heart is often put at or near the center of rotation when a circular orbit is used; this ensures that the heart will be imaged with approximately the same resolution for all angles. The use of a noncircular orbit will change the distance of the detector to the center of rotation, or the heart, at each angle. This may cause the base and septum of the heart to appear as having slightly decreased counts, because these regions are relatively farther away from the detector during a body-contoured orbit.[15] These "artifacts" may be related to exactly how the noncircular orbit is effected; that is, how the gantry, camera heads, and patient table are moved during the acquisition. At least one recent study has in fact found no significant difference in perfusion quantification applied to acquisitions performed with circular and noncircular orbits.[16]

Acquisition Modes

The most common method of acquiring projections is called *step-and-shoot*, in which the camera is turned off while it rotates, and in which data collection occurs only while the camera is stopped at a given projection angle. The time during which the camera is moving and turned off is termed *dead time*, and it is typically 3 to 5 s per projection, but may be as high as 8 s/projection. This increases acquisition time without benefit to image quality and reduces patient comfort.

A second acquisition mode for gathering projection data is termed *continuous rotation* acquisition. In this mode, the camera acquires data constantly while it slowly rotates about the patient. Counts over contiguous arcs are combined into discrete projection sets. The elimination of dead time with continuous rotation acquisition can allow an image to be acquired in less time, without loss of counts. However, continuous rotation acquisition can add image blur because data over a range of projection angles are averaged prior to reconstruction, but those data are used in the backprojection algorithm as though they originated from a single discrete angle. In general though, this blur is not very significant compared with the benefits of a faster scan with no count loss, particularly when the radionuclide concentration is rapidly redistributing.

A final acquisition mode combines step-and-shoot with continuous acquisition; thus, it is termed *continuous step-and-shoot*. The camera is stopped at discrete projection angles, but is not turned off during rotation. This minimizes the blur seen with continuous rotation acquisition but maximizes the number of collected counts in a given time.

Gated Acquisitions

Standard cardiac SPECT images suffer from motion blur, since the heart is always in motion. These images can only show a picture of the average position of the heart. It is well known that, because the heart is moving and contracting and relaxing, perfusion defects can be missed or underestimated, since they are in a sense "averaged" with normal myocardium that may move into the location previously occupied by the defect earlier in the cardiac cycle. In addition, it is well understood that the intensity of the myocardium in nuclear medicine images is related not only to radiotracer uptake, but also to relative myocardial thickness.[17] As the heart contracts, the myocardium appears brighter in the reconstructed image. This effect also gets "averaged" in a standard static (ungated) acquisition and may result in impaired diagnostic accuracy.[18]

Cardiac gating allows heart motion and contraction to be resolved by dividing the projections into discrete time parts, or frames, coupled to the cardiac cycle. The electrocardiogram (ECG) is used to determine the heart rate as well as the onset of contraction at the QRS complex. The cardiac cycle is divided into a set number of predetermined time intervals, called *frames*, and counts collected during each different frame are directed to a different projection set. Counts are directed into the first frame during the initial T/N seconds after the QRS complex is detected, where N is the number of frames and T is the length in seconds of the cardiac cycle. Then, counts are directed into the second frame for the second T/N seconds, and so on. This is repeated for each heartbeat during the acquisition, at every angle. At the end of the acquisition, there are N sets of complete projection images. When these are reconstructed, the result is N three-dimensional sets of slices showing the heart at N points during the cardiac cycle. These four-dimensional data enable three-dimensional analysis of motion and myocardial thickening,[19–22] as well as perhaps enabling better discrimination of the extent and location of perfusion abnormalities.[23] It has even been proposed that exercise ejection fraction can be measured using gated tomographic perfusion imaging by acquiring gated projections rapidly—in about 6 min—during stress. While the resulting images are of poor quality and probably not useful for perfusion analysis, the endocardial surfaces may be detected with enough accuracy to compute end-diastolic and end-systolic volumes for ejection fraction calculation.[24]

There are a number of practical considerations for cardiac gating. First, each projection set and reconstruction will be reduced in counts by a factor equal to the number of collected frames. This precludes gating studies, which are normally low count, as image quality becomes too poor. Also, gating software should be able to deal with abnormal heartbeats and "reject" or ignore counts from these contractions. Similarly, the acquisition should be able to adjust to changing heart rates and direct counts to the projection frames accordingly. One commonly seen result of changing heart rate is late frame drop-off. If the heart rate speeds up but the software fails to adjust, the heartbeat will end before counts have been directed into the last few frames. When the next contraction begins, counts will be directed back into the first frames. Therefore, relatively fewer counts will be seen in the late end-diastolic frame. In addition, motion blur is also reintroduced, since for some early projection angles the cardiac cycle is divided into 8 frames, but for late projection angles, it is divided into fewer frames. Finally, the size of a gated data set increases proportionally to the number of frames collected. This raises both processing time and storage space for gated studies.

Patient Positioning

For 180° acquisitions, the patient should be supine so that his or her left side is as close as possible to the edge of the table. This enables the camera to get as close as possible to the body and not be restricted by the table edge. As noted previously, maintaining a minimal distance between the patient and camera maximizes image resolution. For 360° acquisitions, the patient should be centered on the table, and the camera positioned so that it passes as close as possible to the anterior chest wall. For all acquisitions, attenuation can be minimized by having patients position their arms over their head; specialized arm rests are available to make this position as comfortable as possible. A pillow or other support should be placed under a patient's knees to help ease back strain. Patient comfort is of utmost importance for the quality of the scan, since it minimizes the chance of patient motion. Again the camera should come as close to the patient as possible, and it can even touch the patient at some angles, as long as the contact does not cause alarm, movement, or discomfort. Warning the patient of possible contact should minimize such reactions.

Quality Control

High-quality reconstructions depend on high-quality projections. Tomographic cameras require quality-control procedures similar to those performed for planar cameras, but these procedures are even more important with SPECT imaging. Improper performance can introduce unexpected errors into the reconstruction; in a clinical setting, these errors could be mistaken for perfusion abnormalities. Additional quality-control procedures specific to rotating systems are also necessary to ensure accurate reconstructions.

Tomographic systems must be tested as soon as they are installed to verify that their performance matches the manufacturer's specifications. These acceptance tests can then be used as a standard to which daily quality-control results can be compared. Deviations from the standard can indicate equipment problems that will compromise image quality.

Numerous reports have detailed proper procedures for both acceptance testing and quality control of gamma cameras in general and SPECT systems in specific. Comprehensive publications have been provided by manufacturers' and scientists' associations.[25,26] This discussion focuses on the most common procedures and the effects of typical quality-control problems on reconstructed images.

UNIFORMITY

Modern gamma cameras are not designed to be uniform; that is, the output of the electronics to the same source will vary over the field of view. The input–output relationship is modified by internal correction circuitry, but it must be further corrected weekly or at least monthly with high-count flood-correction images, and then checked on a daily basis to ensure that the image from a gamma camera of a uniform source is truly uniform. These tests should be performed with each isotope to be used that day. Detailed information can be found in references 27 and 28.

Daily uniformity tests may be done intrinsically (without a collimator) by placing a point source at a distance from the detector at least five times the crystal field of view. Alternatively, daily extrinsic uniformity tests may be performed by placing a sheet source on the collimator. In either case, the count rate of the source should be kept low enough so that the camera's electronics and correction circuitry can respond rapidly enough; 20,000 counts per second is generally acceptable. Daily flood images should be acquired for 5 million counts (for a 64×64 matrix with "1–2–1" smoothing). Integral uniformity is calculated by computing the difference of the maximum (max) and minimum (min) count rates over the field of view: Integral uniformity = 100% * (max − min)/(max + min). Differential uniformity is computed similarly but defined for smaller areas. Uniformity values should not exceed 4 percent for corrected flood fields. In some systems, it is impossible to acquire intrinsic flood images; in this case, the manufacturer's instructions for daily uniformity tests should be followed.

High-count extrinsic flood images should be acquired weekly; these are used to incorporate the effects of collimation on the flood field for correction of clinical images. A separate flood correction image should be collected for each collimator, as differences in hole and septum geometry change the flood field. The most commonly used flood source for cardiac imaging is a ^{57}Co sheet source; however, a refillable liquid sheet source can be used if necessary. The main precaution with refillable sources is to ensure that the center does not bulge; that is, that the source is truly uniform. Weekly flood-correction fields are acquired with a large number of counts in order to compute uniformity with an accuracy of 1 percent.

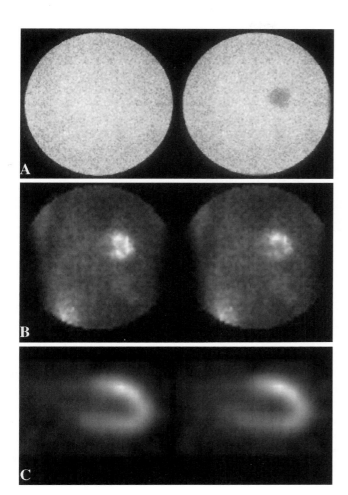

Figure 3-4 Quality-control problems with nonuniformity. **A:** Flood images from a system working correctly (*left*) and from a system with a faulty photomultiplier tube (*right*). **B:** Effect of the nonuniformity on planar images. *Left:* Image acquired with uniform flood field. *Right:* Image acquired using nonuniform field. Note the decreased intensity in the inferior wall of the left ventricle, entirely attributable to the faulty PMT. **C:** Effect of the nonuniformity in reconstructed images. *Left:* Vertical long-axis slice through the left ventricle acquired with the uniform flood field. *Right:* Vertical long-axis slice through the left ventricle acquired with the nonuniform system. Note the decreased counts in the inferior wall of the ventricle resulting from the uniformity problem; this could be easily mistaken for a perfusion abnormality. (Courtesy of James R. Galt, PhD, Emory University.)

For 64 × 64 matrices, 30 M count floods should be acquired; for 128 × 128 matrices, 120 M will provide better results.

Nonuniformities in a rotating gamma camera cause cold spots or cold-ring *bull's-eye* artifacts in the reconstructed image. This can be seen in Fig. 3-4. While such an artifact is often visibly obvious in a flood image, it is less obvious in a planar clinical image, since only portions of the ring artifact may be visible. For SPECT cameras, flood nonuniformity must be analyzed by computer. Nonuniformities (e.g., in integral or differential uniformity) from 3 to 8 percent are often impossible to

detect visually but can lead to substantial visible artifacts after reconstruction.

CENTER OF ROTATION

Center of rotation (COR) is the x, y position in the projection of the gamma camera's axis of rotation. The center of rotation is used during reconstruction in order to backproject counts from the planar view into the "correct" pixel of the reconstruction. During backprojection, projections are placed so that the center of rotation backprojects into a single point. If the COR is not correct, the reconstruction of a point source will be blurred and, in extreme cases, may even become a ring. Reconstructions with center-of-rotation error are displayed in Fig. 3-5.

COR is measured by placing a point source off-center and extended over the edge of the imaging table. The point source is imaged in as many projections as practical, and software provided by the manufacturer is used to determine the proper COR. Note that an off-center point source imaged in two opposing views will project to opposite sides of the projection matrix; the COR is the mean of those x–y positions.

CAMERA/TABLE ALIGNMENT

The camera face must be parallel to the axis of rotation throughout the SPECT orbit in order to ensure that each slice of the reconstruction contains data from only one transaxial plane. Errors in camera head orientation are difficult to detect in the reconstruction but can seriously compromise image resolution. This problem is most easily avoided by using a bubble level to ensure the camera head is level at four angles, 90° apart.

SENSITIVITY

Sensitivity is a measure of how many counts are acquired per unit time by a SPECT system. Because of the count–noise relationship described in the beginning of the chapter, sensitivity affects image quality. The limiting piece of equipment affecting sensitivity is the collimator. To measure sensitivity, a source of known activity is placed on the collimator. The source should be thin but distributed; usually a Petri dish is used. Sensitivity is reported in terms of counts/(minute * microCurie).

PATIENT MOTION

If the patient moves during the tomographic acquisition, image quality may suffer. Various reports have suggested that motion of as little as one-half pixel may induce "abnormalities" in a truly normal image.[29,30] Patient motion should ideally either be eliminated by reimaging

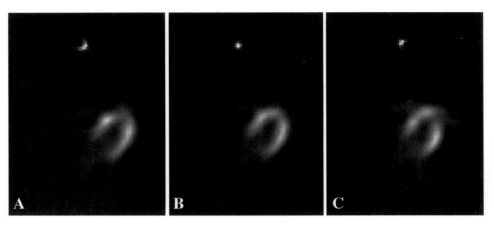

Figure 3-5 Quality-control problems with center of rotation. **A:** Transaxial slices of a point source (*top*) and a clinical study (*bottom*) reconstructed with a negative center-of-rotation error. **B:** Transaxial slices of a point source (*top*) and a clinical study (*bottom*) reconstructed using the correct center of rotation. **C:** Transaxial slices of a point source (*top*) and a clinical study (*bottom*) reconstructed with a positive center-of-rotation error. (Courtesy of James R. Galt, PhD, Emory University.)

those who move during the scan or by using corrective software.

Motion can be identified best by viewing a cine loop of the projections. A recent study has reported that visual analysis is accurate for motion of more than one 3.2-mm pixel of axial displacement and for motion of more than two 3.2-mm pixels for lateral displacement.[31]

It is always easier to prevent than to correct for patient motion. Ensuring that the patient is comfortable before the scan is important; see the patient-positioning section in this chapter for details. In addition, various types of straps may be used to immobilize the torso relative to the table and prevent most types of movement.

When motion does occur, it may be possible to "correct" the data and remove artifacts. Abrupt motion can be corrected easily if a point source is placed on the outside of the body prior to imaging. Body motion is then reflected in motion of the point source. Unfortunately, a major source of motion artifact in cardiac tomography is the *upward creep* of the heart seen after exercise; this movement is attributable to diaphragmatic relaxation.[32] Obviously, an external point source will not reflect this slow upward movement of the heart. Upward creep can be minimized by allowing 15 min between injection and start of imaging, but is difficult to eliminate entirely in every case.

Software has been developed to correct for abrupt patient movements; the most popular is a cross-correlation technique. The method finds the displacement that must be applied to each successive projection frame so that it "matches" the previous one in an optimal mathematical sense.[33] Unfortunately, this method may be less appropriate for gradual or rotational patient motion.

In cases of severe motion, some correction must be used. If necessary, the projection frames can always be manually corrected for motion. Following the correction, the projection images should again be evaluated for motion. If the projection data as well as the motion-corrected reconstruction indicate that the perfusion is normal, then it is unlikely that there are motion artifacts remaining in the study. An abnormality in a motion-corrected reconstruction, particularly when the user is unsure of the success of the correction, indicates that the study should be repeated.

Examples of Clinical Acquisition Protocols

THALLIUM-201 ACQUISITION PROTOCOLS

The physical and biological properties of ^{201}Tl result in relatively few photons being emitted and fewer being detected during the acquisition. The low-energy 80-keV photons are highly attenuated and scattered, particularly in the posterior views. These considerations affect the acquisition protocol.

The most common protocols for ^{201}Tl SPECT acquisition advocate use of a large field-of-view camera equipped with a low-energy all-purpose parallel-hole collimator. The all-purpose collimator with its high sensitivity helps maximize the number of collected counts and minimize the effects of noise in what is normally a relatively low-count study.

A 3- to 4-mCi dose of ^{201}Tl is injected into the patient 1 min prior to the termination of stress testing. The start of acquisition is delayed for 10 min after injection to minimize upward creep of the heart. A total of 32 projections are acquired over a 180° arc from 45° RAO to 45° LPO. This acquisition arc eliminates the highly attenuated posterior projections and improves contrast in the reconstruction. A circular orbit may be used with the left ventricle at the approximate center of the circle in order to avoid artifacts related to the varying detector response effects associated with noncircular orbits. Imaging time at each projection stop is generally 40 s; images are usually acquired into a 64 × 64 matrix.

Historically, the stress acquisition has been followed by a delayed ^{201}Tl redistribution, or washout, acquisition 4 h later. Washout imaging has been largely superseded or at least complemented by a reinjection protocol, however, as it has been demonstrated that a significant number of nonreversible defects seen in redistribution images demonstrate viability when imaged using reinjection.[34,35]

TECHNETIUM-99m—SESTAMIBI ACQUISITION PROTOCOLS

The higher energy of ^{99m}Tc and the higher allowable dosage of sestamibi compared with ^{201}Tl result in more emitted photons and less attenuation and scatter during an acquisition. Therefore, sestamibi studies are generally high-count, low-noise studies. Protocols for same-day rest–stress imaging, 2-day stress–rest imaging, and dual-isotope rest ^{201}Tl–stress ^{99m}Tc-sestamibi imaging have been developed. A comparative analysis of these three protocols can be found in the analysis by Berman et al.[36] A same-day stress–rest imaging protocol is also possible; however, most evidence indicates that this approach underestimates perfusion defect reversibility.[37,38]

For same-day rest–stress imaging, an average-sized patient is injected with 8 to 10 mCi ^{99m}Tc sestamibi for the initial rest study, which should begin 1 h after injection. Stress injections must be delayed for 3 to 4 h after the rest injection to allow the initial radioactivity to decay; the stress dosage ranges from 25 to 30 mCi, depending on the patient's weight. Stress imaging should not begin until 15 min after this injection in order to minimize the upward creep of the heart. The 2-day protocol is similar, except that the stress study is performed on the first day; therefore, the resting study may be eliminated when stress perfusion is determined to be normal. Also, the second-day resting dose should be higher—20 to 30 mCi—because there will be no later studies with which this radioactivity could interfere.

The acquisition protocols are similar for both same-day and 2-day injections. The following protocol was optimized for same-day imaging.[39] A total of 64 projections over 180° from 45° RAO to 45° LPO are acquired; however, 360° acquisitions with 64 or 128 projection stops may also be used since attenuation in posterior projections is less of a problem with ^{99m}Tc compared with ^{201}Tl; 360° acquisitions are adopted primarily by those with multiheaded cameras that can provide a full 360° of data in the same time as 180°. High-resolution collimators are advocated because the improved detector response of these collimators maximizes image quality while the loss of counts is usually inconsequential. Frequently, a circular orbit is used with the left ventricle in the approximate center of rotation.

Acquisition time is 20 to 25 s per projection for a 180° stress study and for the second-day resting study. A same-day resting study requires a longer acquisition time—at least 25 s and perhaps as long as 40 s per projection because of its lower count rate. Images are acquired into a 64 × 64 matrix.

The high count rates of stress ^{99m}Tc-sestamibi studies allow gated acquisitions. Gated reconstructions will enable the evaluation of both endocardial motion and myocardial thickening. Usually, 8 to 16 frames are collected.

DUAL-ISOTOPE THALLIUM-201 AND TECHNETIUM-99m—SESTAMIBI ACQUISITION PROTOCOLS

Because most SPECT systems are capable of acquiring data in more than one energy window simultaneously, ^{201}Tl and ^{99m}Tc-sestamibi images can be acquired at the same time or sequentially. This allows a relatively rapid acquisition protocol, as there does not have to be a delay for radioactive decay or radionuclide washout between rest and stress studies.

Although simultaneous acquisition of the two isotopes is possible, there is a problem with scattered ^{99m}Tc photons contaminating the ^{201}Tl energy window when both radionuclides are present.[40] For this reason, a sequential injection–acquisition protocol is recommended. The ^{201}Tl resting study is performed first, with acquisition beginning at least 10 min after injection of a 3.0-mCi dose. Immediately afterward, stress testing is begun. A 25-mCi injection of ^{99m}Tc sestamibi is administered at near-maximal exercise, and imaging is started 15 min later. Because no ^{99m}Tc is present during the ^{201}Tl acquisition, downscatter of the ^{99m}Tc into the ^{201}Tl window is not a problem, and scatter of the higher-energy ^{201}Tl emission (167 keV) into the ^{99m}Tc window during the later stress acquisition has been shown to be negligible.[41]

Both rest and stress acquisitions are performed with a high-resolution collimator, in order to compare better the resulting reconstructions. A total of 64 projections over 180° from 45° RAO to 45° LPO are acquired with a circular orbit, with an acquisition time of 25 s per projection stop for the resting ^{201}Tl and 20 s per projection for the stress sestamibi. For ^{201}Tl imaging, two energy windows are employed, with a 15 percent window centered on the 80-keV peak and a 10 percent window centered on the 167-keV peak. This helps maximize the number of collected counts for the relatively small injected dose. Then a relatively narrow 15 percent window centered on the 140-keV peak of ^{99m}Tc is used during the second acquisition; this smaller window reduces the possibility of contamination from scattered ^{201}Tl photons.

TECHNETIUM-99m—TEBOROXIME ACQUISITION PROTOCOLS

The outstanding characteristic of ^{99m}Tc teboroxime is its extremely high rate of myocardial clearance. An obvious advantage of this property is that both stress and rest SPECT acquisitions can be performed rapidly, usually within 60 to 90 min. An obvious disadvantage is that such rapid washout mandates a similarly rapid tomographic acquisition in order to prevent image artifacts.[4,5] An undesirable property of teboroxime is its high hepatic uptake; this frequently causes difficulties in the analysis of inferior wall perfusion.

Both rest and stress acquisitions of ^{99m}Tc teboroxime should be started within 3 min after injection of a 15- to 20-mCi dose. Continuous-mode acquisition is recommended in order to eliminate the dead time associated with step-and-shoot, and to shorten acquisition time while maintaining acceptable count rates. An acquisition arc of 180° is used; imaging starts at 45° LPO and ends at 45° RAO; this helps to minimize the effect of liver activity, which peaks toward the end of the acquisition. A high-resolution collimator is generally preferred, and images are collected into a 64 × 64 matrix. Images should be acquired as rapidly as possible; multiheaded cameras can be used to their best advantage with this radiopharmaceutical. With all cameras, however, a ^{99m}Tc-teboroxime acquisition should be completed in 5 min or less.

TOMOGRAPHIC RECONSTRUCTION

Following acquisition, projection images are combined mathematically to create cross-sectional pictures of the radionuclide distribution through the chest. A number of methods can be used; the most common is the filtered backprojection technique.[42] Complicated corrections for attenuation and other degradations require more complex iterative reconstruction techniques.

Filtered Backprojection

Filtered backprojection is, as its name implies, a combination of filtering and backprojection. Backprojection involves smearing the counts in each projection back out over the transverse slice from which they were acquired.

This is illustrated in Fig. 3-6. The counts from each angle are summed together. The resulting image is very blurred; this blur is removed through a filtering operation. The projection is first smoothed with a low-pass filter to reduce noise and prevent it from being magnified in the later processes. The backprojection operation is then combined with a sharpening filter to remove the blur. Following such a filtering, backprojection creates a much sharper image, as seen in Fig. 3-6.

Filtering

In SPECT, filters are used either to enhance or to remove the high-frequency components of the image.[43] High-frequency components are sharp changes in image intensity, such as those seen at edges between the heart and the background, or in noise points. Low frequencies contain information about slowly changing or constant intensities of the image, such as uniform regions of perfusion. Filters that remove high frequencies are called *low-pass filters* because they preserve (pass) only the low frequencies. This reduces noise but blurs edges. Filters that enhance high frequencies are called *high-pass filters*. They operate in the opposite manner from low-pass filters; they pass only the high frequencies while attenuating low frequencies. This sharpens organ boundaries but increases noise.

Filters are usually specified by a cutoff value (sometimes called a *critical frequency*) in units of frequency. In a low-pass filter, low frequencies are retained (passed), but higher and higher frequencies are more and more diminished. The cutoff parameter specifies the properties of this decrease; that is, which frequencies get passed and which get reduced. The lower the cutoff is, the more high frequencies are removed. Some filters have an additional parameter called the *order* or *roll-off*. This parameter relates to whether the decrease in high frequencies happens slowly, over a large range of frequencies, or very quickly, through a smaller range of frequencies. The lower the order, the more slowly the higher frequencies are attenuated. Practically, the order affects image quality less than the cutoff.

In some nuclear medicine systems, the order parameter is defined differently as the *power*; power is related to the order as power = 2 * order. Additionally, different manufacturers specify cutoff values by using different units, including cycles/centimeter, cycles/pixel, and Nyquist, which is equivalent to cycles/2 pixels. Table 3-1 may help you convert one to another.

In tomography, the first filter applied to the projections is called a *prefilter*. It is a low-pass filter used to remove noise from the projections. Two commonly used filters in tomography are the Hanning and Butterworth filters. The Hanning filter is specified using a cutoff value; the Butterworth filter is specified using both a cutoff frequency and an order.

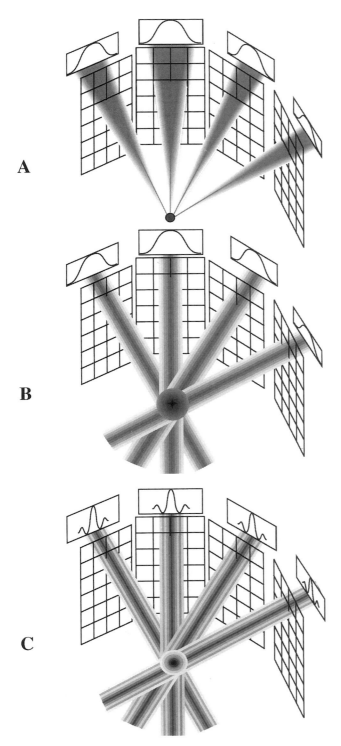

Figure 3-6 Filtered backprojection. **A:** A point source projects as a blurry spot in all planar views collected. Profiles through the source in the projections are shown above and behind the projection matrices. **B:** Backprojection involves smearing the projection data back out over the plane from which they were collected. The result is a very blurred point in the reconstruction. **C:** A high-pass filter applied to the projection data sharpens the point, as seen in the profiles shown *over* and *behind* the planar views. Backprojection then results in a much sharper, although never ideal, reconstruction of the original point source.

The second filter used during filtered backprojection is a ramp filter. This is a high-pass filter used to remove the blur that is inherent in backprojection. A ramp filter has no parameters. The two filters—the prefilter and the ramp filter—work together to achieve a balance between noise and blur removal. Results of applying the ramp filter after prefilters of various cutoff values to both ^{201}Tl and ^{99m}Tc-sestamibi images are demonstrated in Figs. 3-7 and 3-8.

Some SPECT systems combine the prefilter and ramp filter into a single filter applied during backprojection. This option alone is less desirable because it smooths only within the transaxial plane. In contrast, prefilters applied prior to backprojection smooth the two-dimensional projection both within and *across* planes. Nevertheless, a single reconstruction filter is generally specified exactly the same as a prefilter would be; the ramp filter is usually not mentioned but is "understood."

Iterative Reconstruction

It is difficult to correct for attenuation or detector response effects with much accuracy when using filtered backprojection. However, more complex iterative reconstruction techniques allow these complicated degradations to be modeled and theoretically corrected. Iterative techniques use the original projections and models of the attenuation and detector response to predict a reconstruction. The predicted reconstruction is then used again with the attenuation and detector response models to recreate new predicted projections. If the predicted projections are different from the actual projections, these differences are used to modify the reconstruction. This process is continued until the reconstruction is such that the predicted projections match the actual projections. The primary differences between various iterative methods are how the predicted reconstructions and projections are created, and how they are modified at each step. Practically speaking, the more theoretically accurate the iterative technique, the more time-consuming is the process. Maximum likelihood methods enable the noise to be modeled, while least squares techniques, such as the conjugate gradient method, generally ignore noise.[44–46] Iterative filtered backprojection methods create the new reconstruction at every iteration by using filtered backprojection.[47,48] Correction for detector response requires modeling the collimator and takes much more time for each iteration than simply modeling the attenuation process. For this reason, commercially available iterative reconstruction methods generally only contain models of attenuation and do not correct for detector response.

Corrections

As discussed in the acquisition section, the effects of scatter, attenuation, and detector response imply that

TABLE 3-1 Conversions: multiply column to get row

	From Nyquist	From cycles/cm	From cycles/pixel
To get Nyquist	1	2 * pixel size	2
To get cycles/cm	1/(2 * pixel size)	1	1/pixel size
To get cycles/pixel	1/2	pixel size	1

Pixel sizes are assumed to be in centimeters.

the normal tomographic appearance of myocardial perfusion depends not only on radiotracer uptake, but also on body shape and composition, photon energy, collimator choice, and orbit of the gamma camera. For example, the anterior left ventricular wall often appears to have abnormally low perfusion in women with large breasts. This artifact is entirely due to attenuation of emitted photons by breast tissue in the anterior projection views. Such effects make it difficult to determine whether the findings of a study are normal; the physician must be aware of all possible contributing factors affecting the final image. New software methods that can eliminate or at least mitigate all three degradations—attenuation, scatter, and detector response—may help create tomograms that accurately depict the true distribution of myocardial perfusion. This would theoretically reduce normal variations and make diagnosis of any defects more straightforward and accurate.

SCATTER CORRECTION

Many of the emitted photons interact with atoms in the body and are scattered in a new direction. Most scattered photons are incorrectly detected as arising from the direction in which they scattered instead of from the direction in which they were emitted, leading to decreased contrast in SPECT images. However, in the process of the collision they lose energy; therefore, analysis of the energy of detected photons enables a type of correction for scatter. A simple scatter-reduction technique is to narrow the energy window used during acquisition. This is most effective for high-count studies, as it will effectively eliminate some unscattered photons from the acquisition. More complicated scatter-correction algorithms use the ability of modern SPECT systems to acquire photons in more than one energy window at once.

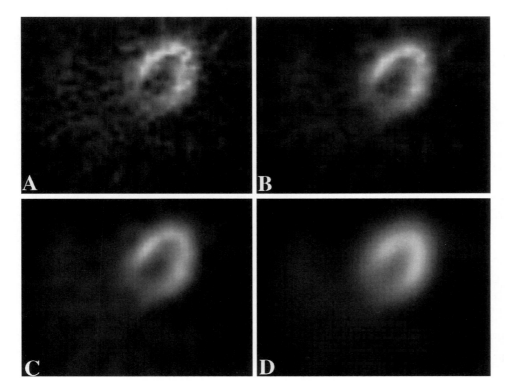

Figure 3-7 Results of applying a Hanning filter of various cutoff values to a thallium-201 acquisition. **A:** Ramp filter only. **B:** Hanning filter with cutoff of 1.2 cyc/cm (followed by a ramp filter). **C:** Hanning filter with cutoff of 0.8 cyc/cm. **D:** Hanning filter with cutoff of 0.4 cyc/cm.

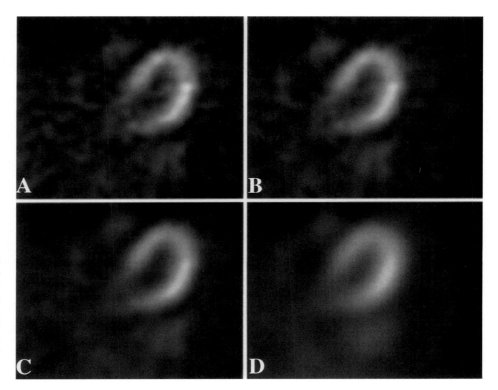

Figure 3-8 Results of applying a Butterworth filter of various cutoff values to a technetium-99m–sestamibi acquisition. The order of the filter in each case was 5. **A:** Ramp filter only. **B:** Butterworth filter with a cutoff of 0.75 cyc/cm. **C:** Butterworth filter with cutoff of 0.5 cyc/cm. **D:** Butterworth filter with cutoff of 0.25 cyc/cm.

Multienergy window scatter-correction methods use one window centered on the photopeak of the radionuclide's energy spectrum and a second centered on a lower-energy region associated with scattered photons, generally termed the *Compton region*.[49] Reconstructed images from the two acquisition windows can be mathematically combined; some fraction of the scatter image is subtracted from the primary one. The resulting scatter-corrected image has higher contrast but, owing to decreased counts, increased noise. A variation on this approach places the two windows so that they "split" the photopeak; again the scatter component is calculated as a function of the counts in the two windows and subtracted from the total image.[50] A related technique that uses three windows has also been described.[51] An example of this method applied to cardiac perfusion images is shown in Fig. 3-9. Scatter may also be corrected at the data acquisition stage of SPECT imaging.[52,53] The energy-weighted acquisition method uses a preprocessor between the input and output of the gamma-camera circuitry to analyze both energy and position signals from each event. This information is used to determine the likelihood that a photon is scattered, and to weight each one accordingly.

ATTENUATION CORRECTION

Most software packages available in SPECT computers offer an attenuation correction package that can be used with filtered backprojection. A commonly used technique is the Chang algorithm.[54] In this method, a map of the attenuation coefficients in the thorax is used to determine the average amount of attenuation seen at each pixel of the image over the directions of the acquired projections. The reconstruction is multiplied by correction factors based on these average attenuation values. This method is not a particularly accurate one; in fact, its original description included iterative corrections that are generally ignored by most manufacturers. The noniterative first step, or *multiplicative Chang*, that is commonly provided is known to overcorrect the center of the image and may introduce new errors and artifacts in cardiac images. More accurate methods of attenuation correction require iterative reconstruction techniques, as just described.

A critical issue for all attenuation correction methods is the creation of the attenuation map; that is, an image that shows the attenuation coefficient of each pixel in the thorax region. Many commercially available attenuation correction programs make the simplifying assumption that attenuation is constant throughout the area being imaged. Thus, creation of the attenuation map requires only the definition of the body surface, which can be done automatically or with minimal operator intervention. This assumption of constant attenuation is so poor for the chest region, however, that corrections based on such a map are not worthwhile. Recently, a number of researchers have described using transmission scans acquired with a SPECT camera to create the attenuation map.[55,56] An example of such a transmission image is

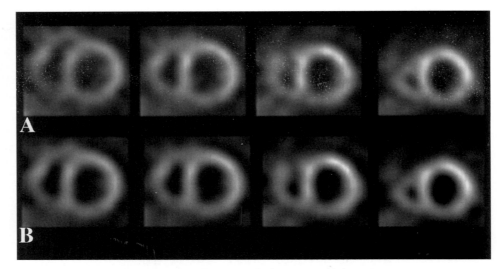

Figure 3-9   Technetium-99m–sestamibi images before **(A)** and after **(B)** scatter correction. Note the higher contrast and the better separation of the inferior myocardium from the adjacent liver in the scatter-corrected images. (Courtesy of S. James Cullom, PhD, Emory University, and Toshiba America Medical Systems.)

shown in Fig. 3-10. It has also been suggested that scatter images or ^{99m}Tc macroaggregated albumin emission images may be used to segment the chest into lung and soft tissue as a basis for creation of attenuation maps.[57,58]

Transmission scans are most frequently acquired by using multiheaded SPECT cameras with special hardware, so the emission images can be acquired in one or two heads while the remaining head acquires the transmission scan. Two main different approaches are used. One method uses a line source positioned opposite to the third head of a triple-headed camera.[56] The detector acquiring the transmission data is equipped with a focusing collimator, while those acquiring the emission data are equipped with parallel-hole or focusing collimators. One commercially available program uses this approach to create the attenuation map and then applies maximum likelihood iterative reconstruction to correct the emission data for attenuation. An example of this technique is displayed in Fig. 3-11.

A second approach uses a *scanning* line source, mounted opposite one of the detectors in a dual-headed, 90° system. The line source is slowly moved across the field of view of the camera at each projection stop; this enables the use of standard parallel-hole collimators for

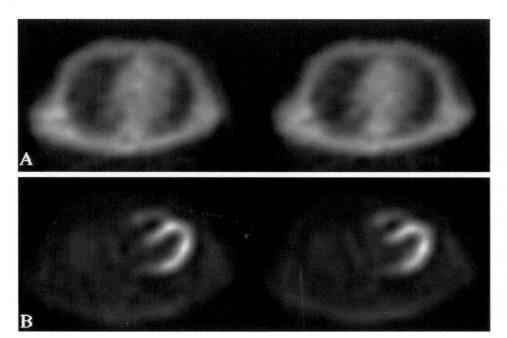

Figure 3-10   **A:** Serial transaxial transmission images of a patient's thorax created using a gadolinium-153 scanning line source. Image intensity is proportional to tissue electron density; therefore, bright areas of this image indicate regions that will attenuate photons more heavily during the emission acquisition. **B:** Corresponding technetium-99m–sestamibi emission images provided for reference. These emission studies have *not* been corrected for attenuation. (Courtesy of S. James Cullom, PhD, Emory University.)

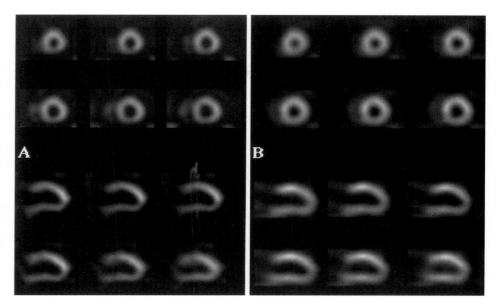

Figure 3-11 Results of applying the attenuation methods of Tung et al.[56] to a technetium-99m–sestamibi image. **A:** Original short-axis (*top*) and vertical long-axis (*bottom*) sections from a 49-year-old male patient with end-stage renal disease. The inferior wall demonstrates decreased activity. **B:** Corresponding sections after attenuation correction using a maximum likelihood reconstruction with an attenuation map created from a transmission scan. The inferior wall was read as normal after attenuation correction; catheterization results confirmed normal coronary arteries. (Courtesy of Karl Kellar, Picker Nuclear Medicine Division.)

transmission image acquisition and eliminates the possibility of truncation sometimes seen with focusing collimators.[55]

Transmission acquisitions may be performed either simultaneously with or separately from emission scans. If the two scans are done separately, there are two issues of concern. The total time required for acquisition will increase, and the patient may move between the emission and transmission scans. Mismatches between transmission and emission images are highly likely to result in image artifacts.

If the two scans are performed simultaneously, then correction for Compton scatter is the most important issue. Current setups use a ^{99m}Tc or ^{241}Am transmission source in conjunction with ^{201}Tl. Because the photopeak of ^{99m}Tc is above the primary photopeak of ^{201}Tl, some photons emitted from the higher energies will be scattered, lose energy, and then be detected in the ^{201}Tl window. Therefore, the ^{201}Tl emission data require careful correction for contamination by scattered photons from a ^{99m}Tc transmission source when the two acquisitions are done concurrently.[55,56] Transmission sources for use during ^{99m}Tc *emission* studies include ^{153}Gd or ^{241}Am. Both of these radionuclides have primary photopeaks below the energy of ^{99m}Tc, so contamination is less of a problem. In all cases, however, additional scatter correction of the emission data itself, as just discussed, may be a necessity in order to get an accurate picture of the radionuclide distribution in the inferior wall of the heart,[59,60] as this area is most vulnerable to interference by scattered photons originating in the liver.

DETECTOR RESPONSE CORRECTION

The position dependence of resolution in SPECT results in deep objects having a lower resolution than those closer to the surface of the body. If this difference is accounted for and corrected, then image resolution is homogenized, and improved, overall. Three main techniques are used to achieve this result. First, complex filters can be designed to *restore* the original resolution.[61] These filters are very dependent on the choices of input parameters, however.[62] With an iterative reconstruction method, the effects of collimation and photon path can be modeled in the projection and backprojection steps.[48,63,64] The models can be quite sophisticated, including size and shape of collimator holes and septa. A simpler technique relies on the theory that detector response effects are visible as frequency variations of the sinogram and can be filtered out.[65] The iterative reconstruction approach is computationally demanding and can slow the reconstruction process down by a factor of 2 or 3. The sinogram approach is much faster and is more likely to be used in the near future as a clinical method, although it may be less accurate than the iterative technique.

Examples of Clinical Reconstruction Protocols

THALLIUM-201 RECONSTRUCTION PROTOCOLS

All SPECT acquisitions must be corrected for uniformity, center of rotation, and radioactive decay prior to reconstruction. Filtered backprojection is the most common reconstruction technique; the primary variable is which filter(s) to use. Due to the lower counts in ^{201}Tl images, filter cutoffs are generally low compared with those used with ^{99m}Tc. This helps reduce the noise associated with count-poor images. A typical selection is a Hanning prefilter with a cutoff of 0.82 cyc/s and a ramp reconstruction filter. Thallium-201 images are usually reconstructed into enough 64 × 64 pixel slices to span the left ventricle. Pixel sizes in these reconstructions are on the order of 5 to 7 mm, and the slices are generally 1 pixel thick.

TECHNETIUM-99m—SESTAMIBI RECONSTRUCTION PROTOCOLS

Filtered backprojection is used to create transaxial reconstructions following correction for uniformity, center of rotation, and radioactive decay. The relatively high count rates in sestamibi images enable the use of a less restrictive filter, since noise is less of an issue. A typical prefilter choice is a Butterworth filter of cutoff frequency of 0.52 cyc/cm and an order of 2.5 for the stress study. The lower-count rest study is filtered more heavily to reduce noise with a cutoff of 0.4 cyc/cm and an order of 5. As with ^{201}Tl, the reconstruction filter is a ramp. Transaxial slices spanning the left ventricle are created; each slice is 64 × 64 pixels. Again, pixel sizes are generally 5 to 7 mm, and each slice is one pixel thick.

DUAL-ISOTOPE THALLIUM-201 AND TECHNETIUM-99m—SESTAMIBI RECONSTRUCTION PROTOCOLS

To compare the ^{201}Tl and ^{99m}Tc-sestamibi images for clinical evaluation, they must be processed similarly. Following corrections for radioactive decay, uniformity, and center of rotation, projections are prefiltered with a Butterworth filter using a cutoff of 0.52 cyc/cm and order of 2.5 for the stress ^{99m}Tc images and a cutoff of 0.4 cyc/cm and an order of 5 for the ^{201}Tl rest images. They are reconstructed using filtered backprojection with a ramp filter. Each reconstructed slice is 64 × 64 pixels in size, with each pixel being 5 to 7 mm long on each side, and slices are again one pixel thick.

TECHNETIUM-99m—TEBOROXIME RECONSTRUCTION PROTOCOLS

Technetium-99m—teboroxime projections must be corrected as always for uniformity and center of rotation. Because of the extremely short acquisition time, radioactive decay correction can probably be omitted with no noticeable effect. Projections are prefiltered with a Butterworth filter with a cutoff of 0.3 cyc/cm and an order of 5, and then reconstructed with a ramp filter. Reconstruction limits should be placed as close as possible to the inferior wall of the left ventricle in order to reduce the effects of liver activity. Images are reconstructed into a 64 × 64 matrix with pixel sizes on the order of 5 to 7 mm; each slice is one pixel thick.

PROCESSING

Oblique Reorientation and Reslicing

Once the projections have been reconstructed, a three-dimensional block of data indicating the distribution of radionuclide throughout the chest is available. This block of data is in the reference frame, or coordinate system, of the body. Therefore, each slice of the three-dimensional block is perpendicular to the body axis. These slices are known as either transverse or transaxial; such slices are shown in Fig. 3-12**A**. However, because the location and orientation of the heart within the chest can vary greatly from person to person, standardized slices that use the left ventricle itself as a frame of reference have been created.[66,67] Some published methods for automatic reorientation and reslicing of cardiac data have been published;[68,69] however, most commercial systems offer only interactive approaches. Next, a typical interactive algorithm is presented, along with descriptions of the three standard oblique sections that it creates.

VERTICAL LONG-AXIS SLICES

Oblique axis slices are created in a standard manner. Using a display of a transaxial slice through the middle of the left ventricle, the position of the long axis is denoted with a line drawn by the user. Slices created parallel to the drawn line and perpendicular to the stack of transaxial images are then created. The user again identifies the long axis on these images. This completely specifies the three-dimensional orientation of the long axis, which is used as a basis for standardized oblique cardiac images. Slices created parallel to the long axis and approximately perpendicular to the transverse slices are called *vertical long-axis slices,* as shown in Fig. 3-12**B**. The long axis in the left ventricle is horizontal in these slices. They are displayed with the base of the left ventricle toward the left side of the image and the apex toward the right. Serial slices are displayed from medial to lateral, left to right.

HORIZONTAL LONG-AXIS SLICES

Oblique slices taken parallel to the long axis and approximately parallel to the original transverse images are called *horizontal long-axis slices,* presented in Fig. 3-12**C**. The long axis of the left ventricle is vertical in these images. They contain the left ventricle with the base toward the bottom of the image and the apex toward the top. The right ventricle appears on the left side of the image. Serial horizontal long-axis slices are displayed from inferior to anterior, from left to right.

SHORT-AXIS SLICES

Slices perpendicular to the denoted long axis and perpendicular to the vertical long-axis slices are also cut from the stack. These are termed *short-axis slices;* they contain the left ventricle with its anterior wall toward the top, its inferior wall toward the bottom, and its septal wall toward the left. Serial short-axis slices are displayed from apex to base, from left to right. Short-axis slices are shown in Fig. 3-12**D**.

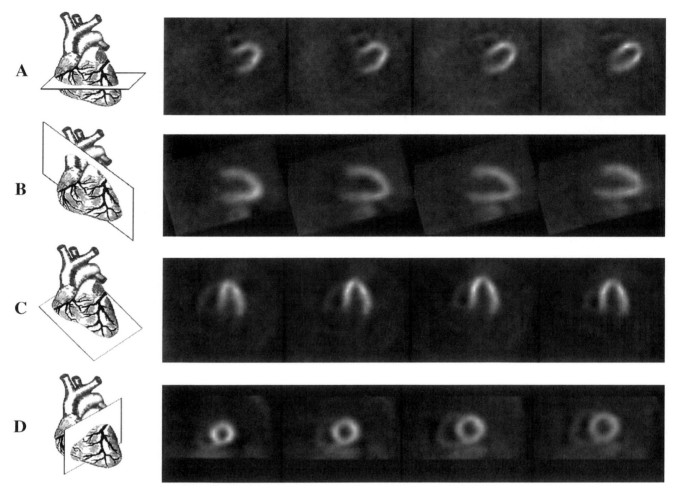

Figure 3-12 Standard image sections for viewing cardiac data. **A:** Original transaxial slices. The left side of the body is to the *right* in each slice, with the anterior side at the *top*. Slices are displayed from inferior to superior, left to right. **B:** Vertical long-axis slices. The base of the left ventricle is toward the *left* side of the image and the apex is toward the *right*. Slices are displayed from medial to lateral, left to right. **C:** Horizontal long-axis slices. The base of the left ventricle is toward the *bottom* of the image and its apex is toward the *top*. The right ventricle appears on the *left* side of the image. Serial slices are displayed from inferior to anterior, from left to right. **B:** Short-axis slices. The anterior wall of the left ventricle is toward the *top*, the inferior wall is toward the *bottom*, and the septal wall is toward the *left*. Slices are displayed from apex to base, from left to right.

Quantitation

PERFUSION QUANTITATION AND CIRCUMFERENTIAL PROFILES

Left ventricular counts can be investigated with computer software to calculate relative myocardial perfusion and localize both reversible and irreversible defects. Such automated quantification methods can be used as teaching tools or as independent second opinions, but, most importantly, they provide an objective and standardized analysis of perfusion tomograms. It has been shown that automated perfusion quantitation techniques improve the sensitivity of perfusion SPECT for detecting disease.[70,71]

Most commercially available quantification methods for myocardial perfusion in SPECT are based on the idea that sampled counts in the myocardium of a patient's image can be compared with similar counts sampled from a set of normal subjects. In its basic form, the quantitation algorithm samples the left ventricular myocardium in short-axis slices to determine the maximal count values within the myocardium at evenly spaced angles about the left ventricular long axis. For each short-axis slice, the resulting maximal count values are graphed against the angle at which they were encountered; such a graph is called a *circumferential profile*. Figure 3-13 demonstrates the creation of circumferential profiles.

Circumferential profiles are amassed for a large number of normal subjects. The profiles are generally normalized for each person so that the maximum count value

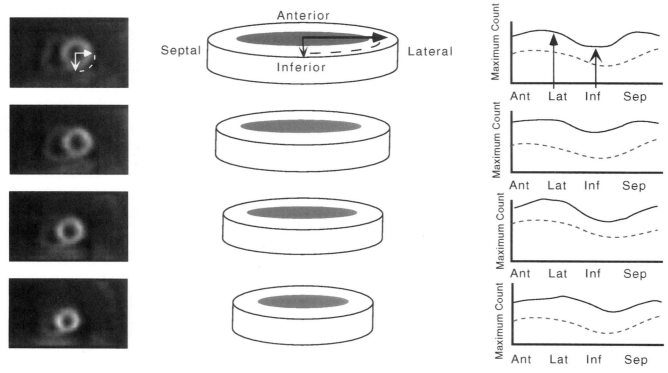

Figure 3-13 Creation of circumferential profiles. Short-axis slices are sampled at numerous angles about the center of the left ventricle; the maximal count in the myocardium at each angle is graphed against the angle. The result is a circumferential profile for each short-axis slice, seen as the *solid line* in the graphs at the *right*. Normal limits are created for each profile by studying normal subjects; these normal limits are shown as *dotted lines* in the graphs. Whenever a part of the circumferential profile falls below the normal limit, that portion of the patient's myocardium is considered to have a perfusion defect. The subject shown here is normal.

in each study is rescaled to a standard value such as 100. This accounts for variations in uptake, dose, and overall perfusion rates. For each angle on each slice, both a mean normal value and its standard deviation are computed over the set of normal subjects. Normal boundaries or normal limits for each point in each profile are created based on these statistical values; for example, they may be set at 2 or 2.5 standard deviations below the mean normal value. By comparing a patient's circumferential profile angle by angle and slice by slice to the normal limits, perfusion defects can be pointed out automatically.

Generally, analysis is performed and normal limits are created for the stress study and for a normalized difference between the stress and rest studies. (If ^{201}Tl washout images are being quantitated, the percent change between the stress and washout image is analyzed instead of the normalized difference between the two.) Separate normal limits must be created for males and females because normal differences in body shape cause different normal attenuation and scatter artifacts in the reconstructions. Abnormal areas or defects seen in the stress images that persist on the rest study are considered fixed. Abnormal regions in the stress that improve or normalize in the rest study are considered reversible.

There are many variations on this basic technique. The exact manner in which the myocardium is sampled varies. The method used to determine the lower limit of *normal* may be very simple or very complex. Also, the way in which studies are normalized differs among approaches. All the methods are similar, however, in that they sample the counts at discrete points in the myocardium and compare those values to some known normal values to localize perfusion defects.

For example, the original quantitative approach to ^{201}Tl SPECT perfusion quantification, developed at Cedars–Sinai Hospital, analyzes short-axis slices extending from the subendocardial limit of the apex to about 1.5 cm below the base of the left ventricle.[72] Vertical long-axis sections, which extend from the subendocardial portion of the septum to the subendocardial limits of the lateral wall, are also analyzed. Midventricular perfusion is quantitated by circumferential sampling of the short-axis slices, while apical perfusion is analyzed from the vertical long-axis sections. The stress and rest profiles are normalized so that the maximum count in each is set to 100. Finally, the lower limit to normal perfusion was taken to be the lowest observed value for each myocardial sample in the resulting set of circumferential profiles from the normal patient group. This method was extensively validated (see reference 73).

A more recent approach to quantification of ^{201}Tl SPECT studies, developed at Emory University (Atlanta, GA), creates circumferential profiles for each short-axis slice extending from apex to base.[74] Profiles from a particular study are interpolated in order to produce a total of 15 profiles independent of the left ventricular size or the number of short-axis slices actually analyzed. The ratio of the average raw counts per pixel to the counts in the normal profiles is computed for four midventricular sections around the left ventricle, and the section with the highest ratio is considered to be normal. The profiles are normalized by dividing each of them by this ratio. Normal limits were determined by computing both the mean and the standard deviation for each sample of the 15 profiles created from the normal subjects. For each sample in each profile, 2.5 standard deviations below the mean was used for the lower limit of normal. This approach was validated in a multicenter trial.[75]

A third method expands on the Emory technique with additional automation and analysis features.[76,77] Most circumferential sampling is performed using base-to-apex short-axis slices, but apical perfusion analysis samples long-axis slices by using spherical coordinates to create five additional circumferential profiles. The resulting collection of profiles is interpolated to create a final set of 15. The lower limit of normal for each sample is set to a fixed multiple of standard deviations below the mean of the normal subjects' profiles; this level can be set by the user.

Circumferential profile-based techniques have also been applied to ^{99m}Tc-sestamibi perfusion images.[39,78] In one approach, the myocardium is sampled in a three-dimensional manner. Midventricular and apical short-axis slices are sampled circumferentially, while the apical hemispherical cap is sampled using a spherical coordinate system. Normalization is performed by computing the ratio between mean count values in eight midventricular sectors and their corresponding means from the normal database. The sector with the highest ratio is considered the most normal, and all sectors are normalized by dividing each by this ratio. Normal limits were computed by finding the number of standard deviations below the mean for each of four left ventricular sectors (anterior, septal, inferior, and lateral) that best separated normal from abnormal in a prospective patient group, where normal and abnormal were defined by expert visual readings, and the "best" separation was determined by receiver–operator curves. A multicenter trial was performed for extensive validation of these methods.[79]

There have been few studies comparing these various approaches to perfusion quantification with one another. Therefore, it is not a simple matter to choose one based on its comparative accuracy. Instead, more practical issues may be the best guide to choosing which of the methods may be best for your clinical use. Certainly it is important that the approach has been validated and the results published. The manufacturer should have FDA approval to market it for clinical use. It is also important that the methodologies be kept up to date. New normal files are often required for new protocols, and a program that is no longer in active development will not be applicable to the latest technologies. For instance, some programs may not have normal files for dual-isotope perfusion analysis. Others that were developed for use with all-purpose collimators may never provide normal limits for use with high-resolution collimators. Certainly, a new normal database will be necessary for use with attenuation-corrected images. In any case, the most important thing to keep in mind when using quantitative programs is to follow the acquisition and processing protocols developed for the technique exactly. Even small changes in reconstruction filtering or acquisition time can compromise the accuracy of the quantitation.

DISPLAY

Polar maps   Polar maps, or bull's-eye displays, are another way to view circumferential profiles. They give a quick and comprehensive overview of the circumferential samples from all slices by combining these into a color-coded image. The points of each circumferential profile are assigned a color based on normalized count values, and the colored profiles are shaped into concentric rings. The most apical slice processed with circumferential profiles forms the center of the polar map, and each successive profile from each successive short-axis slice is displayed as a new ring surrounding the previous. The most basal slice of the left ventricle makes up the outermost ring of the polar map. Plate **1A** shows polar maps created from applying a perfusion quantification method to a ^{99m}Tc-sestamibi study. This kind of display enables immediate and comprehensive viewing of the quantitative results of the entire myocardium.

The use of color can help identify abnormal areas at a glance, as well. Abnormal regions from the stress study are often assigned black, thus creating a blackout map. Blacked-out areas that normalize at rest are color coded white, thus creating a whiteout reversibility map.[80] This can also be seen in Plate **1A**. Additional maps, such as a standard deviation map that shows the number of standard deviations below normal of each point in each circumferential profile, can aid in evaluation of the study by indicating the severity of any abnormality.

Polar maps, while offering a comprehensive view of the quantitation results, distort the size and shape of the myocardium and any defects. There have been numerous improvements in the basic polar map display to help overcome some of these problems.[39] For instance, *distance-weighted maps* are created so that each ring is the same thickness. These maps have been shown to be useful for accurate localization of abnormalities. *Volume-weighted maps* are constructed such that the area of each ring is proportional to the volume of the corresponding slice. This type of map has been shown to be best for estimating defect size. However, more realistic displays have been introduced that do not suffer from the distortions of polar maps.

Three-dimensional displays Three-dimensional graphics techniques can be used to overlay results of perfusion quantification onto a representation of a specific patient's left ventricle.[81,82] In its most basic form, the pixel locations of the maximal-count myocardial points sampled during quantitation are used to estimate the myocardial surface. These points can be connected into triangles, which are then color coded similarly to the polar map. Plate 1**B** displays the same information seen in the polar maps of Plate 1**A** using a three-dimensional representation. Such displays can routinely be rotated in real time and viewed from any angle with current computer power. They have the advantage of showing the actual size and shape of the left ventricle, and the extent and location of any defect in a very realistic manner. Preliminary studies have demonstrated that such three-dimensional displays are better for estimating the size and location of defects than either polar maps or the original slice-by-slice displays.[83,84]

The biggest disadvantage of three-dimensional displays is that they require more computer screen space (and therefore more film or paper for hard copies) than do polar maps. The entire left ventricle can be visualized in a single circular polar map, but only one side of the left ventricle can be seen when it is displayed using three-dimensional graphics.

QUANTITATION OF GATED PERFUSION TOMOGRAMS

Quantitative function information can be obtained from gated perfusion SPECT images. Global variables such as left ventricular volumes, mass, and ejection fraction can be calculated. Local properties of wall motion and myocardial thickening are also obtainable; these can then be displayed using either polar maps or three-dimensional graphics. Some of the software to compute these variables is available clinically; some of it is still in the domain of research. A number of methods are likely to cross from research to clinical application shortly; therefore, an overview of these methods is provided.

Global variables Probably the most accurate way to obtain volume, mass, and ejection fraction measure-

ments from SPECT perfusion tomograms is to detect the left ventricular endocardial and epicardial boundaries in the actual images. The number of pixels within the chamber or left ventricular wall can then be determined. Because the pixel sizes are known, the total volume in the chamber or myocardium can be computed. Myocardial mass is calculated by multiplying the myocardial volume by an assumed density, usually 1 gm/cc. The end-diastolic volume is determined to be the largest chamber volume found in the gated set of images; the end-systolic volume is the smallest. Ejection fraction is computed using these values.

Detection of left ventricular boundaries is very complicated, but most methods use as a basis the fact that image count levels rise across the edge of the chamber to the endocardial edge of the left ventricular myocardium, and then fall again across the edge of the epicardium to the outside of the left ventricle.[19,20] These points where image intensity changes quickly can be located and serve as at least a first estimate of endocardial and epicardial surfaces. Some kind of constraint is used to ensure a smooth, "reasonable" surface, and some kind of interpolation is used to fill in the surface when a severe perfusion defect would otherwise create a "hole" in the boundary. An example of the results of applying the endocardial surface detection methods described in reference 85 to a gated perfusion SPECT image can be seen in Plate 2**C**; slices from the original images are shown in Plate 2**A** and **B**.

Endocardial wall motion If the endocardial surface is detected at each point in the cardiac cycle, then regional endocardial wall motion can be assessed by computing how each surface point moves. Wall motion is difficult to compute with much accuracy because it is impossible to say with certainty that a particular point in one time frame moves to a particular location in the next. In addition, there is a global translational component to left ventricular motion which is difficult to assess and/ or remove. In fact, most analyses of left ventricular wall motion rely heavily on simplified models of motion originally developed for two-dimensional contrast ventriculograms or radionuclide ventriculograms. They may assume, for example, that every point moves radially toward the left ventricular center of mass; regional motion is therefore forced to be *radial*. Two approaches[19,20] use a three-dimensional extension of the centerline method originally developed for contrast ventriculograms.[86] In this method, each left ventricular surface point is assumed to move in a direction perpendicular to the surface at that point. Results of this approach applied to the patient of Plate 2**A** and **B** are shown in Plate 2**D**. Note that no method for modeling endocardial motion is completely accurate in every case; therefore, quantitated left ventricular wall motion should be considered in conjunction with perfusion information.

Myocardial thickening Myocardial thickening is known to be a better indicator of myocardial viability than endocardial wall motion; therefore, the ability to quantify this variable accurately from perfusion tomograms would be very valuable. The most promising methods use the fact that, due to detector response, myocardial thickness is linearly related to image intensity in perfusion images when the myocardial thickness is less than two times the resolution of the reconstructed images.[17] Since current SPECT systems provide resolution on the order of 1 cm, this thickness–intensity relationship should hold true for the vast majority of cases where the range of myocardial thickness is 0.5 to 2 cm. Note that there is no way to tell absolute thickness with this method; instead, only the change in thickness over the cardiac cycle can be assessed. For example, if the peak counts at one point of the myocardium double from end diastole to end systole, it can be postulated that the wall has doubled in thickness during contraction at that point.

One approach to quantification of wall thickening by using this theory samples the myocardial counts at numerous locations (>4000) for every gated frame.[21] Then a time/intensity curve is created for each of the myocardial points. The curve is *smoothed* by fitting a cosine function to its values. The amplitude of the fitted cosine wave is used as a measure of the change in thickness from end diastole to end systole at the point in question. Thickening polar plots or three-dimensional displays can be created to show the resulting *percent thickening* computed around the left ventricle. The results of applying this wall-thickening method to the patient in Plate 2A and B are shown in Plate 2E. This method has shown to be very robust with respect to noise in simulation studies. However, quantification of myocardial thickening from perfusion SPECT images has not at this writing been truly tested in the clinic. It remains an intriguing possibility for the future.

CONCLUSION

Cardiac SPECT provides superior contrast resolution compared with planar imaging and offers a fully three-dimensional view of the heart. Its high technological demands require careful decisions about equipment selection, as image quality is affected by the hardware and software used. In particular, throughput and image quality is affected most by the number of camera heads and the collimator choice, respectively. Software usability is the major factor that determines whether the technology can be used to its best ability.

Acquisition of the studies is very flexible and can be tailored to fit different needs of each clinic or even each patient. New acquisition modes such as continuous rotation can improve throughput, whereas noncircular orbits may improve image resolution. Cardiac gating enables left ventricular motion to be resolved and enables evaluation of endocardial motion and myocardial thickening. Quality control is extremely important in order to maintain study accuracy no matter which type of acquisition is performed.

Filtered backprojection is the standard algorithm used for creating transaxial reconstructions from the acquired projections; selection of the reconstruction filter is the most important part of filtered backprojection. Iterative reconstruction methods provide better correction for attenuation or detector response degradations. Accurate attenuation correction methods require knowledge of patient-specific thoracic attenuation coefficients. This information can be obtained by using multiheaded cameras to acquire simultaneous emission and transmission studies of the thorax. Correction for photon scatter is performed by acquiring data in multiple energy windows and removing from the primary window a fraction from the other windows. This correction is especially important when performing attenuation correction, but is compatible with standard filtered backprojection.

Reconstructed image datasets are resliced into standard views for display and analysis. This enables comparisons between the perfusion tomograms of a particular patient and a set of normal subjects. Quantitative analysis samples the myocardium around its circumference (circumferential sampling) to find maximal counts; these numbers are compared with known values created by performing similar analyses on normal subjects. Results are commonly displayed by color-coding relative count values in polar maps, but three-dimensional representations enable improved evaluation of the size and shape of the myocardium and any perfusion defect. Gated perfusion tomograms can be analyzed to evaluate left ventricular volume, mass, and ejection fraction; regional values of endocardial motion and thickening may also be obtained. The circumferential sampling quantitation techniques objectify and standardize analysis of perfusion; the gated analyses provide important functional knowledge of the left ventricle.

Basic SPECT and cardiac perfusion examinations provide essential diagnostic information. Significant new technical advances promise improved and more accurate studies and additional important functional data.

ACKNOWLEDGMENTS

The assistance of the following people is greatly appreciated: James R. Galt, Ph.D., S. James Cullom, Ph.D., Johnathan P. Vansant, M.D., Ernest V. Garcia, Ph.D.,

Russell D. Folks, CNMT, all from Emory University; and Karl Kellar, from Picker Nuclear Medicine Division.

REFERENCES

1. Kiat H, Berman DS, Maddahi J: Comparison of planar and tomographic exercise thallium-201 imaging methods for the evaluation of coronary artery disease. *J Am Coll Cardiol* 13:613, 1989.
2. Tamaki S, Nakajima H, Murakami T, et al: Estimation of infarct size by myocardial emission computed tomography with thallium-201 and its relation to creatine kinase-MB release after myocardial infarction in man. *Circulation* 66:994, 1982.
3. Fintel DJ, Links JM, Brinker JA, et al: Improved diagnostic performance of exercise thallium-201 single photon emission computed tomography over planar imaging in the diagnosis of coronary artery disease: A receiver–operator characteristic analysis. *J Am Coll Cardiol* 13:600, 1989.
4. Bok BD, Bice AN, Clausen M, et al: Artifacts in camera-based single photon emission tomography due to time–activity variation. *Eur J Nucl Med* 13:439, 1987.
5. O'Connor MK, Cho DS: Rapid radiotracer washout from the heart: Effect on image quality in SPECT performed with a single-headed gamma camera system. *J Nucl Med* 33:1146, 1992.
6. Chua T, Kiat H, Germano G, et al: Rapid back-to-back adenosine stress/rest technetium-99m teboroxime myocardial perfusion SPECT using a triple-detector camera. *J Nucl Med* 34:1485, 1994.
7. Nakajima K, Taki J, Bunko H, et al: Dynamic acquisition with a 3-headed SPECT system: Application to Tc-99m SQ30217 myocardial imaging. *J Nucl Med* 32:1273, 1991.
8. Cullom SJ, Folks RD, Vansant JP, Nowak DJ: The differences in motion artifacts for single and dual 90° detector cardiac SPECT. *J Nucl Med* 36;168P, 1995 (abstr).
9. Maublant JC, Peycelon P, Kwiatkowski F, et al: Comparison between 180° and 360° data collection in technetium-99m MIBI SPECT of the myocardium. *J Nucl Med* 30:295, 1989.
10. Hoffman EJ: 180° compared to 360° sampling in SPECT. *J Nucl Med* 23:745, 1982.
11. Eisner RL, Nowak DJ, Pettigrew RI, Fajman W: Fundamentals of 180° reconstruction in SPECT imaging. *J Nucl Med* 27:1717, 1986.
12. Go RT, MacIntyre WJ, Houser TS, et al: Clinical evaluation of 360° and 180° data sampling techniques for transaxial SPECT thallium-201 myocardial perfusion imaging. *J Nucl Med* 26:695, 1985.
13. Knesaurek K, King MA, Glick SJ, Penney BC: Investigation of causes of geometric distortion in 180° and 360° angular sampling in SPECT. *J Nucl Med* 30:1666, 1989.
14. Gottschalk SC, Salem D, Lim CB, Wake RH: SPECT resolution and uniformity improvements by noncircular orbit. *J Nucl Med* 24:822, 1983.
15. Maniawski PJ, Morgan HT, Wackers FJT: Orbit-related variation in spatial resolution as a source of artifactual defects in thallium-201 SPECT. *J Nucl Med* 32:871, 1991.
16. Van Train KF, Silagan G, Germano G, et al: Non-circular vs. circular orbits in quantitative analysis of myocardial perfusion SPECT. *J Nucl Med* 36:46P, 1995 (abstr).
17. Galt JR, Garcia EV, Robbins WL: Effects of myocardial wall thickness on SPECT quantification. *IEEE Trans Med Imaging* 9:144, 1990.
18. Eisner RL, Schmarkey S, Martin SE, et al: Defects on SPECT "perfusion" images can occur due to abnormal segmental contraction. *J Nucl Med* 35:638, 1994.
19. Faber TL, Akers MS, Peshock RM, Corbett JR: Three dimensional motion and perfusion quantification in gated single photon emission computed tomograms. *J Nucl Med* 32:2311, 1990.
20. Germano G, Kavanagh PB, Kiat H, et al: Automatic analysis of gated myocardial SPECT: Development and initial validation of a method. *J Nucl Med* 35:116P, 1994 (abstr).
21. Cooke CD, Garcia EV, Cullom SJ, et al: Determining the accuracy of calculating systolic wall thickening using a fast Fourier transform approximation: A simulation study based on canine and patient data. *J Nucl Med* 35:1185, 1994.
22. Buvat I, Bacharach SL, Bartlett ML, et al: Wall thickening from gated SPECT/PET: Evaluation of four methods. *J Nucl Med* 36:8P, 1995 (abstr).
23. Corbett JR, McGhie AI, Faber TL: Perfusion defect size and severity using gated SPECT sestamibi: Comparison to ungated imaging. *J Nucl Med* 35:115P, 1994 (abstr).
24. Germano G, Kiat H, Mazzant M, et al: Stress perfusion/stress wall motion with fast (6.7 min) Tc sestamibi myocardial SPECT. *J Nucl Med* 35:81P, 1994 (abstr.)
25. National Electrical Manufacturer's Association: *Performance Measurement of Scintillation Cameras*. Standards publication NU1-1986. Washington, DC, National Electrical Manufacturer's Association, 1986.
26. AAPM SPECT Task Group: Rotating scintillation camera SPECT acceptance testing and quality control. AAPM Report 22. Woodbury, NY, American Institute of Physics, 1987.
27. Rogers WL, Clinthorne MH, Harness BA, et al: Field-flood requirements for emission computed tomography with an Anger camera. *J Nucl Med* 23:162, 1982.
28. O'Connor MK, Vermeersch C: Critical examination of the uniformity requirements for single-photon emission computed tomography. *Med Phys* 18:190, 1991.
29. Botvinick EH, Zhu YY, O'Connell WJ, Dae MW: A quantitative assessment of patient motion and its effect on myocardial perfusion SPECT images. *J Nucl Med* 34:303, 1993.
30. Eisner R, Churchwell A, Noever T, et al: Quantitative analysis of the thallium-201 myocardial bullseye display: Critical role of correcting for patient motion. *J Nucl Med* 29:91, 1988.
31. Cooper JA, Neumann PH: Visual detection of patient motion during tomographic myocardial perfusion imaging. *Radiology* 185:284, 1992.
32. Friedman J, Van Train K, Maddahi J, et al: "Upward creep" of the heart: A frequent source of false positive reversible defects during thallium-201 stress-redistribution SPECT. *J Nucl Med* 30:1718, 1989.
33. Eisner RL, Noever T, Nowak D, et al: Use of cross-correla-

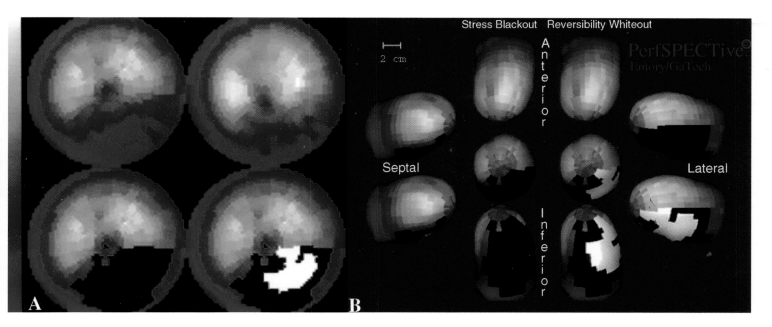

Plate 1 Polar (bull's-eye) plots and three-dimensional displays from a technetium-99m–sestamibi image.

A: Polar plots of stress perfusion (*top left*), rest perfusion (*top right*), stress blackout (*bottom left*) and reversibility whiteout (*bottom right*). In polar plots, the anterior wall is toward the *top*, the septal side is toward the *left*, the lateral wall is toward the *right*, and the inferior wall is toward the *bottom*. For each plot, colors are scaled from 0 to 100 percent of the maximum myocardial counts. The blackout plot shows in *black* all abnormal regions in the stress image, determined from comparison to normal limits. Those regions that normalize at rest are shown in *white* in the whiteout map.

B: Three-dimensional displays of the same data as in A. Here, only stress blackout and reversibility whiteout data are shown. Five different views of the left ventricle are provided; *clockwise from top*, they are anterior, lateral, inferior, and septal. An apical view is in the *center*. Note how the size and shape of the left ventricle can be better appreciated in this three-dimensional display; also, the size, shape, and location of the defects are immediately obvious.

Plate 2 Functional variables determined from a gated technetium-99m—sestamibi image.

A: Slices from the end-diastolic frame of the gated set. From *left* to *right* are the vertical long axis, horizontal long axis, and apical, midventricular, and basal short-axis slices. This patient has a large apical perfusion defect resulting from an infarction.

B: Corresponding sections from the end-systolic frame.

C: Posterolateral (~45° LPO) view of the left ventricular endocardial surface at near end-systole detected using methods described by Quaife et al (*J Nucl Med* 36:12P, 1995). The surface is color coded for left ventricular perfusion, quantified using methods of Garcia et al.[39] Colors range from 0 to 100 percent of maximal counts in this end-systolic frame.

D: Same end-systolic, LPO view of the left ventricular endocardial surface. Surface is color coded for endocardial motion from end diastole to end-systole, quantified using methods of Faber et al.[19] Colors range from –2 mm to 8 mm of motion.

E: Same end-systolic, LPO view of the left ventricle at near end systole. Surface is color coded for myocardial thickening, quantified using the approach of Cooke et al (*J Nucl Med* 35:1185, 1994). Colors range from 0 to 100 percent thickening as compared with end diastole. For all three-dimensional displays, note the obvious apical aneurysm and the corresponding defects in perfusion, motion, and thickening.

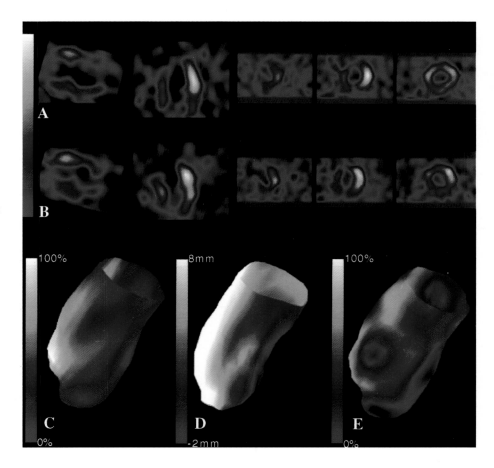

Breast Attenuation

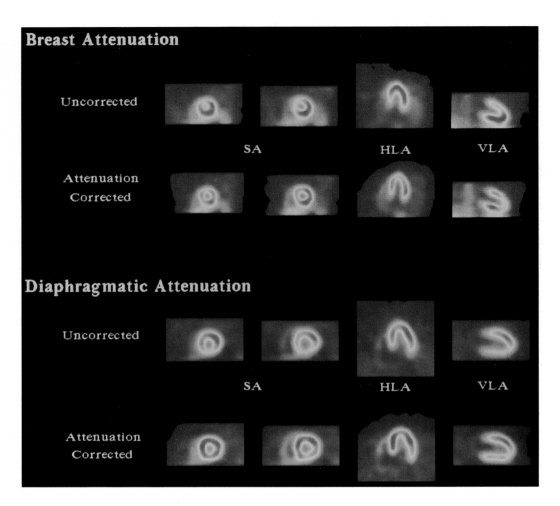

Plate 3 Comparison of uncorrected and attenuation-corrected ^{99m}Tc sestamibi images. Breast attenuation and diaphragmatic attenuation artifacts apparent in the uncorrected images are properly corrected in the attenuation-corrected images. The breast artifact is most evident in the anterior wall of the short-axis (SA) and vertical long-axis (VLA) slices. The diaphragmatic attenuation artifact is seen in the inferior wall of the SA and VLA slices. HLA indicates horizontal long axis. (From Ficaro et al, *Circulation* 93:463, 1996, reproduced by permission of the American Heart Association, Inc.)

Diaphragmatic Attenuation

Plate 4 Mid-ventricular vertical long axis Tc-99m sestamibi tomogram obtained with this male patient supine *(left)* demonstrates a moderate decrease in inferior wall count density. In repeat SPECT performed with the patient prone *(right)* inferior count density is normal. Normalization of inferior count density with the patient prone favors diaphragmatic attenuation rather than scar as a cause of the inferior wall defect.

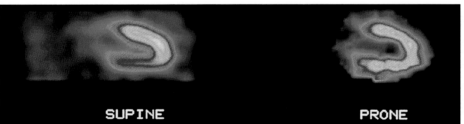

Plate 5 Stress *(left)*, and rest *(right)* raw *(top)* and severity *(bottom)* polar plots from a ^{201}Tl SPECT scan. Liver uptake of ^{201}Tl was included in the stress polar plot radius of search, resulting in an intense "hot spot" over the apex and inferior wall. The stress polar plot is normalized to this "hot spot," resulting in an artifactual severe reversible defect involving the remainder of the left ventricle.

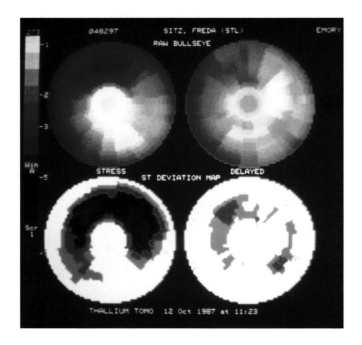

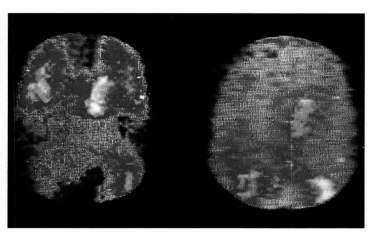

Plate 6 Immediate postexercise *(left)* and 4-h delayed *(right)* anterior planar ^{201}Tl projection images demonstrating markedly increased lung uptake in the stress images. This finding has been associated with deterioration of ventricular function during exercise and severe, multivessel coronary disease.

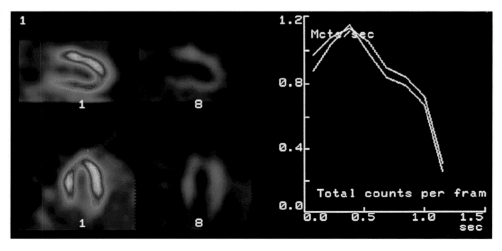

Plate 7 Stress and 4-h delay ^{201}Tl polar maps *(top row)* demonstrate only mild, partially reversible inferior and anteroseptal perfusion defects. However, in this patient, subsequently demonstrated angiographically to have severe multivessel coronary disease, the washout polar map *(lower left)* demonstrates markedly and diffusely delayed washout.

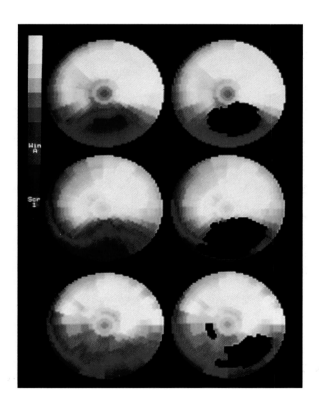

Plate 8 Three sequential stress ^{201}Tl perfusion scans in a patient with right coronary artery stenosis. The stress polar plots are shown in the column on the left, and the corresponding quantitative extent maps on the right. In the initial study *(top row)* there is a marked inferior perfusion defect in the right coronary artery territory (extent score = 485). The second study *(middle row)* was performed seven months later following medical therapy. The inferior perfusion defect is very slightly more marked (extent score = 510). Shortly thereafter a right coronary artery PTCA was performed. A follow-up scan with the patient asymptomatic was performed three months thereafter and is shown in the bottom row. Incomplete resolution of the inferior perfusion defect is apparent (extent score = 370) . All three resting perfusion scans were normal. The extent score is calculated as the sum of the number of standard deviations below mean normal limits of all pixels identified as abnormal ($\geq$2.5 standard deviations below mean normal limits and blackened on the extent map).

Plate 9 In a patient with marked arrhythmia there is considerable data dropout at end-diastole in this eight frame per cardiac cycle gated ^{99m}Tc-sestamibi SPECT scan. A time-activity curve of mean myocardial count density *(right)* demonstrates an initial increase in count density during ventricular systole, associated with myocardial wall thickening. However, there is a marked decrease in count density subsequently at end-diastole due to arrhythmic beats. Comparing frame #1 (end diastole triggered by the R wave) and frame #8 *(middle)* in vertical long axis *(top)* and horizontal long axis *(bottom)* tomograms, there is a marked decrease in count density in frame #8 due to arrhythmia (Provided courtesy of Kenneth Nichols, PhD.)

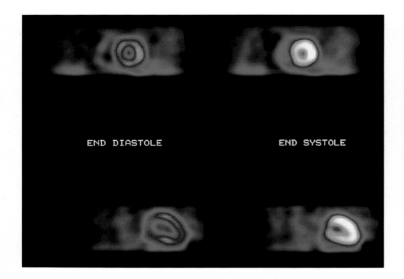

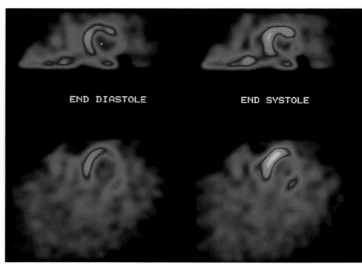

Plate 10 **A:** Normal ⁹⁹ᵐTc sestamibi gated SPECT images in short axis *(top)* and vertical long axis projections *(bottom)*. **B:** Patient with marked and extensive inferoposterior and lateral wall scar. The color images demonstrated absent inferoposterior and lateral wall thickening (i.e., lack of inferoposterior and lateral wall intensification from end diastole to end systole).

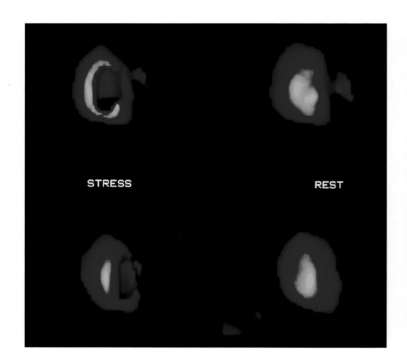

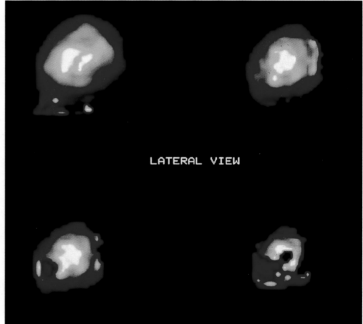

Plate 11 Three-dimensional surface map displays of stress *(left)* and rest *(right)* ⁹⁹ᵐTc sestamibi SPECT in a patient with a large, reversible posterolateral perfusion defect. Images in the top row view the postero-lateral wall (apex at top, valve plane at bottom). Images in the bottom row "look down" on the anterior wall (septum to the left, posterolateral wall to the right).

Plate 12 Effect of thresholding on three-dimensional surface map displays. In this normal ⁹⁹ᵐTc sestamibi SPECT scan three-dimensional images viewed from the posterolateral wall are displayed. The image in the upper right corner is thresholded correctly: normal perfusion is apparent with a very slight amount of the right ventricular myocardium displayed. In the image in the upper left corner the threshold is too low: background activity from abdominal viscera merges with the left ventricle, and nearly the entire right ventricle is displayed. In images in the lower left and right corners increasingly high thresholds were selected, creating increasingly severe artifactual perfusion defects involving the apex and lateral wall.

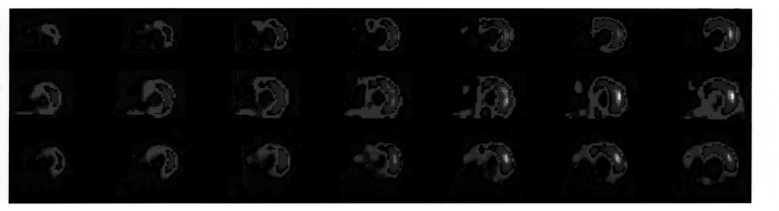

Plate 13   Top row: Fifteen-minute postinjection rest thallium short axis sections. **Middle row:** Three-hour delay thallium short axis section. **Bottom row:** One-hour postinjection short axis FDG SPECT. There are no significant differences between the examinations. Viability in the septum and inferior wall is unlikely in this patient with multivessel coronary artery disease and infarction.

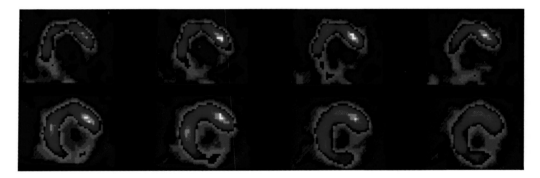

Plate 14   Top row: Short axis rest (3-h delay) ^{201}Tl images. No uptake is present in the inferior septum, inferior and lateral segments. **Bottom row:** Short axis FDG SPECT shows uptake (probable viability) in the inferior septum and inferior segments. The lateral wall is probably not viable.

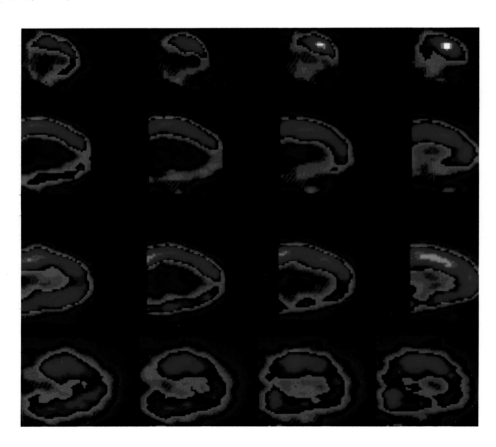

Plate 15   Top row: Rest thallium (SPECT). **Second row:** Rest ^{13}N NH$_3$ (PET). **Third row:** ^{18}F FDG (PET). **Fourth row:** ^{18}F FDG (SPECT). Patient with severe right coronary artery and left circumflex artery stenoses with evidence of akinesis in the inferior and posterior basal segments. Thallium 201 and NH$_3$ images show reduced perfusion. FDG images show uptake with both PET and SPECT. Delayed SPECT images show more uptake than PET.

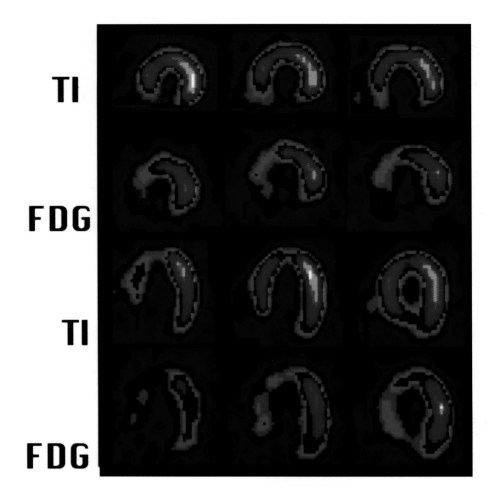

Plate 16 Representative short (**top**) and horizontal long axis (**bottom**) sections (SPECT) of rest thallium and FDG images showing a nonviable inferior wall. There is ^{201}Tl uptake in the septum, anterior wall, and lateral wall.
There is FDG uptake primarily in the lateral wall indicating hypermetabolism (ischemia).

Plate 17 A single midventricular tomographic reconstruction obtained in a healthy human volunteer after the intravenous administration of $H_2^{15}O$ (**top left**), after inhalation of ^{15}O-labeled carbon monoxide to label the vascular pool (**top right**), and after the $H_2^{15}O$ data have been corrected for radioactivity in the vasculature (**bottom left**). The same corrected image displaying myocardial regions of interest in the lateral (LAT), anterior (ANT), and septal (SEP) walls is shown at the **bottom right**. The mitral valve plane is posterior. Although $H_2^{15}O$ is the flow tracer least effected by myocardial metabolism, because of the necessity to correct activity for tracer in the vasculature in order to "image" myocardium and because of the high count rates achieved after administration of $H_2^{15}O$, it is the most technically demanding tracer for quantitation of flow. [From Herrero and Bergmann, in Schwaiger M (ed): *Cardiac PET*, with permission of Kluwer Academic Publishers, Inc., 1996 (in press).]

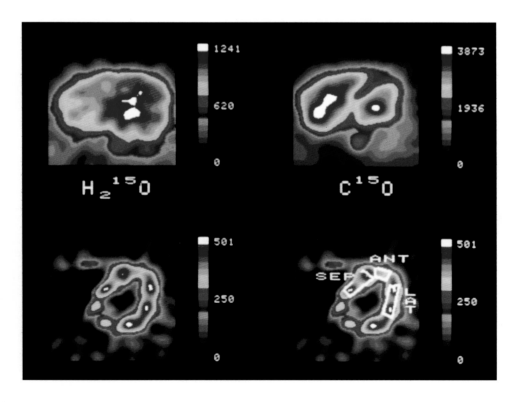

Plate 18 Sequential tomograms obtained on days 1, 2, and 7 in a patient with acute myocardial infarction treated with thrombolytic therapy. As depicted in the midventricular tomograms on the **top**, myocardial perfusion at rest is initially diminished in the anterior myocardium but recovers by day 2 and is then maintained. The accumulation of ^{11}C acetate (**bottom**) is delayed compared with the recovery of perfusion and indicative of delayed recovery of myocardial oxygen consumption compared with perfusion. By day 7, both perfusion and metabolism have recovered to near normal levels indicative of substantial myocardial salvage. Recovery of oxidative metabolism presages recovery of mechanical function. PET enables delineation of the efficacy of therapeutic interventions designed to improve myocardial perfusion and metabolism.

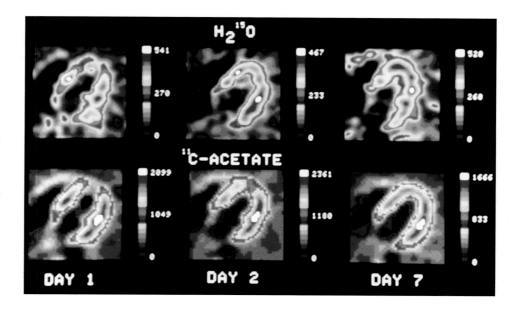

Plate 19 Four transverse midventricular tomographic reconstructions from data acquired 45 to 75 min after intravenous infusion of ^{18}F FDG and 3 to 8 min after intravenous infusion of ^{11}C acetate in the same subject under fasting conditions (**left**) and after glucose loading (**right**). The top of each image represents anterior, and the left of each image represents the patient's right. Under fasting conditions, there was a large deficit in the anteroseptal uptake of ^{18}F FDG, whereas uptake of ^{11}C acetate was homogeneous. The deficit became less after glucose loading. This suggests that there are regional differences in the utilization of glucose that must be taken into account in interpreting images obtained with ^{18}F FDG, especially under fasting conditions. (From Gropler et al, J Nucl Med 31:1749, 1990, reproduced with permission.)

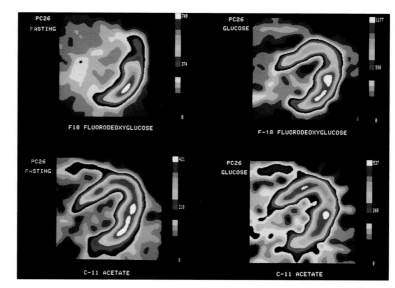

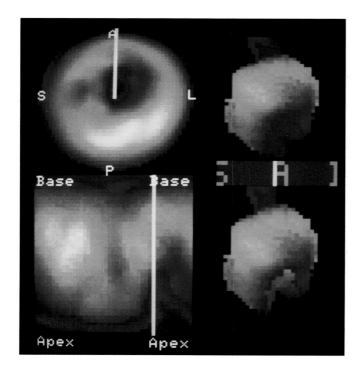

Plate 20 Parametric images of myocardial oxidative metabolism (i.e., in micromoles of oxygen per gram per minute) obtained from a patient with anterior infarction in the bull's-eye and Mercator projections (*left, top,* and *bottom,* respectively) as well as in two three- dimensional surface-shaded projections (*right*). These images represent the state of the art in tomographic reconstructions, since they represent delineation of actual metabolic utilization in absolute terms and in three dimensions using a physiologically based tracer and a mathematical model correlating the kinetic data with a metabolic process. (Computer reconstructions performed by Dr. Tom Miller.)

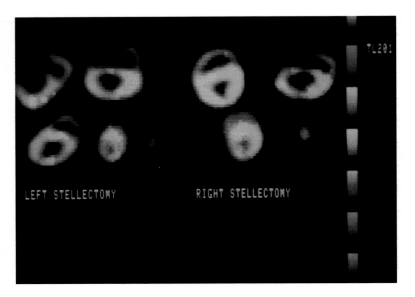

Plate 21 Dual-isotope color functional maps of myocardial slices from dogs with left and right stellectomy. The *area of yellow to green* represents denervated myocardium (reduced MIBG uptake relative to thallium 201), while the *red* represents normally innervated myocardium. The posterior left ventricle is denervated in left stellectomy, while the anterior left ventricle is denervated in right stellectomy. (From Dae et al, *Circulation* 79:634, 1989, reproduced with permission of the American Heart Association, Inc.)

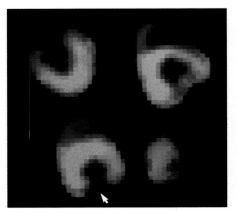

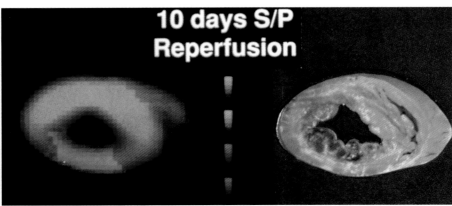

Plate 22 Color functional maps of myocardial slices from a dog with transmural myocardial infarction. Note the area of absent activity in the slice proximal to the apex (*arrow*). This represents a region of transmural scar. Adjacent and distal to this region of scar is an area of denervated myocardium, represented by the *yellow to green*. The *red* regions represent normally innervated myocardium. (From Dae et al, *J Am Coll Cardiol* 17:1416, 1991, reproduced with permission of the American College of Cardiology.)

Plate 23 Myocardial slice from a dog studied 10 days following intracoronary occlusion and reperfusion (*right*), and the corresponding dual-isotope functional map (*left*). There is an area of subendocardial necrosis, with morphologically normal-appearing myocardium at the middle-to-epicardial territory. This area is denervated on the functional map. (From Dae et al, *Cardiovasc Res* 30:270, 1995, reproduced with permission.)

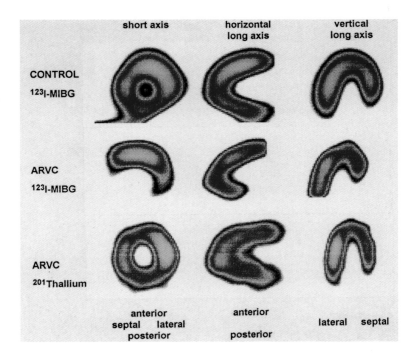

Plate 24 Iodine-123 MIBG images in the basal short axis (*left*), vertical long axis (*middle*), and horizontal long axis (*right*) in a patient of the control group and in a patient with arrhythmogenic right ventricular cardiomyopathy (ARVC) and right ventricular outflow tract tachycardia. There is a normal distribution of MIBG in the control subject (*top*), whereas, in the patient with ARVC, MIBG imaging demonstrates a reduced tracer uptake in the basal posteroseptal area of the left ventricle (*middle*). The corresponding thallium-201 images of the ARVC patient (*bottom*) show normal perfusion in the areas of demonstrated sympathetic dysinnervation. (From Wichter et al, *Circulation* 89:667, 1994, reproduced with permission of the American Heart Association, Inc.)

tion function to detect patient motion during SPECT imaging. *J Nucl Med* 28:97, 1987.

34. Dilsizian V, Rocco TP, Freedman NM, et al: Enhanced detection of ischemic but viable myocardium by the reinjection of thallium after stress-redistribution imaging. *N Engl J Med* 323:141, 1990.

35. Cloninger KG, DePuey EG, Garcia EV, et al: Incomplete redistribution in delayed thallium-201 single photon emission computed tomographic (SPECT) images: An overestimation of myocardial scarring. *J Am Coll Cardiol* 12:955, 1988.

36. Berman DS, Kiat HS, Van Train KF, et al: Myocardial perfusion imaging with technetium-99m sestamibi: Comparative analysis of available imaging protocols. *J Nucl Med* 35:683, 1994.

37. Taillefer R, Laflamme L, Dupras G, et al: Same day injections of Tc-99m methoxy isobutyl isonitrile (hexamibi) for myocardial tomographic imaging: Comparison between rest–stress and stress–rest injection sequences. *Eur J Nucl Med* 15:113, 1989.

38. Heo J, Kegel J, Iskandrian AS, et al:. Comparison of same-day protocols using technetium-99m sestamibi myocardial imaging. *J Nucl Med* 33:186, 1992.

39. Garcia EV, Cooke CD, Van Train KF, et al: Technical aspects of myocardial perfusion SPECT imaging with Tc-99m sestamibi. *Am J Cardiol* 66:23E, 1990;

40. Watson DD, Smith WE, Glover DK, et al: Dual isotope SPECT imaging of Tc-99m sestamibi and Tl-201: Comparing myocardial defect magnitudes. *Circulation* 84(Suppl II):314, 1991.

41. Kiat H, Germano G, Friedman J, et al: Comparative feasibility of separate or simultaneous rest thallium stress technetium-99m sestamibi dual isotope myocardial perfusion SPECT. *J Nucl Med* 35:542, 1994.

42. Brooks RA, DiChiro G: Principles of computer assisted tomography (CAT) in radiographic and radioisotopic imaging. *Phys Med Biol* 21:689, 1976.

43. Galt JR, Hise LH, Garcia EF, Nowak DJ: Filtering in frequency space. *J Nucl Med Technol* 14:152, 1986.

44. Shepp LA, Vardi Y: Maximum likelihood reconstruction for emission tomography. *IEEE Trans Med Imaging* 1:113, 1982.

45. Budinger TF, Gullberg GT: Three-dimensional reconstruction in nuclear medicine emission imaging. *IEEE Trans Nucl Sci* 21:2, 1974.

46. Tsui BMW, Zhao X, Frey E, Gullberg GT: Comparison between ML-EM and WLS-CG algorithms for SPECT image reconstruction. *IEEE Trans Med Imaging* 38:1766, 1991.

47. Galt JR, Cullom SJ, Garcia EV: SPECT quantification: A simplified method for attenuation correction for cardiac imaging. *J Nucl Med* 33:2232, 1992.

48. Ye J, Cullom SJ, Kearfott KK, et al: Simultaneous attenuation and depth-dependent resolution compensation for 180° myocardial perfusion SPECT. *IEEE Trans Nucl Sci* 39:1056, 1992.

49. Floyd CE, Jaszczak RJ, Greer KL, Coleman RE: Deconvolution of Compton scatter in SPECT. *J Nucl Med* 26:403, 1985.

50. King MA, Hadamenos GJ, Glick SJ: A dual-photopeak window methods for scatter correction. *J Nucl Med* 33:605, 1992.

51. Ogawa K, Harata Y, Ichihara T, et al: A practical method for position-dependent compton scatter correction in single photon emission CT. *IEEE Trans Med Imaging* 10:408, 1991.

52. Hamill JJ, DeVito RP: Scatter reduction with energy-weighted acquisition. *IEEE Trans Nucl Sci* 36:1334, 1989.

53. DeVito RP, Hamill JJ: Determination of weighting functions for energy-weighted acquisition. *J Nucl Med* 32:343, 1992.

54. Chang LT: A method for attenuation correction in radionuclide computed tomography. *IEEE Trans Nucl Sci* 25:638, 1978.

55. Frey EC, Tsui BMW, Perry JR: Simultaneous acquisition of emission and transmission data for improved thallium-201 cardiac SPECT imaging using a technetium-99m transmission source. *J Nucl Med* 33:2238, 1992.

56. Tung CH, Gullberg GT, Zeng GL, et al: Non-uniform attenuation correction using simultaneous transmission and emission converging tomography. *IEEE Trans Nucl Sci* 39:1134, 1992.

57. Pan TS, King MA, Penney BD, Rajeevan N: Segmentation of the body, lungs, and patient table from scatter and primary window images in SPECT. *J Nucl Med* 34:195P, 1993 (abstr).

58. Wallis JW, Miller TR, Koppel P: Attenuation correction in cardiac SPECT without a transmission measurement. *J Nucl Med* 36:506, 1995.

59. Frey EC, Li J, Tsui BMW: The importance of combined scatter and attenuation compensation in Tl-201 SPECT. *J Nucl Med* 36:60P, 1995 (abstr).

60. King MA, Xia W, de Vries DJ, et al: A Monte Carlo investigation of artifacts caused by the liver in perfusion imaging. *J Nucl Med* 36:29P, 1995 (abstr).

61. King MA, Schwinger RB, Doherty PW, Penney BC: Two-dimensional filtering of SPECT images using the Metz and Wiener filters. *J Nucl Med* 25:1234, 1984.

62. Penney BC, Glick SJ, King MA: Relative importance of the error sources in Wiener restoration of scintigrams. *IEEE Trans Med Imaging* 9:60, 1990;

63. Zeng GL, Gullberg GT, Tsui BMW, Terry JA: Three-dimensional algorithms with attenuation and geometric point response correction. *IEEE Trans Nucl Sci* 38:693, 1991.

64. Liang Z, Turkington TG, Gilland DR, et al: Simultaneous compensation for attenuation, scatter, and detector response for SPECT reconstruction in three dimensions. *Phys Med Biol* 37:587, 1992.

65. Xia W, Lewitt RM, Edholm PR: Fourier correction for a spatially variant collimator blurring in SPECT. *IEEE Trans Med Imaging* 14:100, 1995.

66. Borello JA, Clinthorne NH, Rogers WL, et al: Oblique-angle tomography: A restructuring algorithm for transaxial tomographic data. *J Nucl Med* 22:471, 1981.

67. O'Brien A, Gemmell H: Effectiveness of oblique section display in thallium-201 myocardial tomography. *Nucl Med Commun* 7:609, 1986.

68. Mullick R, Ezquerra NF: Automatic determination of left ventricular orientation from SPECT data. *IEEE Trans Med Imaging* 14:88, 1995.

69. Germano G, Kavanagh PB, Su HT, et al: Automatic reorientation of 3-dimensional transaxial myocardial perfusion SPECT images. *J Nucl Med* 36:1107, 1995.

70. DePasquale EE, Nody AC, DePuey EG, et al: Quantitative rotational thallium-201 tomography for identifying and localizing coronary artery disease. *Circulation* 77:316, 1988.

71. Maddahi J, Garcia EV, Berman DS, et al: Improved noninvasive assessment of coronary artery disease by quantitative analysis of regional stress myocardial distribution and washout of thallium-201. *Circulation* 64:924, 1981.

72. Garcia EV, Van Train K, Maddahi J, et al: Quantification of rotational thallium-201 myocardial tomography. *J Nucl Med* 26:17, 1985.

73. Van Train KF, Maddahi J, Berman DS, et al: Quantitative analysis of tomographic stress thallium-201 myocardial scintigrams: A multicenter trial. *J Nucl Med* 31:1168, 1990.

74. DePasquale E, Nody A, DePuey EG, et al: Quantitative rotational thallium-201 tomography for identifying and localizing coronary artery disease. Circulation 77:316, 1988.

75. Garcia EV, DePuey EG, Sonnemaker RE, et al: Quantification of the reversibility of stress induced SPECT thallium-201 myocardial perfusion defects: A multicenter trial using bull's-eye polar maps and standard normal limits. *J Nucl Med* 31:1761, 1990.

76. Eisner RL, Tamas MJ, Cloninger KG, et al: The normal SPECT thallium-201 bullseye display: Gender differences. *J Nucl Med* 29:1901, 1989.

77. Schonkoff D, Eisner RL, Gober A, et al: What quantitative criteria should be used to read defects on the SPECT Tl-201 bullseye display in men? ROC analysis. *J Nucl Med* 28:674, 1987 (abstr).

78. Van Train KF, Areeda J, Garcia EV, et al: Quantitative same-day rest-stress technetium-99m sestamibi SPECT: Definition and validation of stress normal limits and criteria for abnormality. *J Nucl Med* 34:1494, 1993.

79. Van Train KF, Garcia EV, Maddahi J, et al: Multicenter trial validation for quantitative analysis of same-day rest-stress technetium-99m sestamibi myocardial tomograms. *J Nucl Med* 35:609, 1994.

80. Klein JL, Garcia EV, DePuey EG, et al: Reversibility bulls eye: A new polar bull's-eye map to quantify reversibility of stress-induced SPECT Tl-201 myocardial perfusion defects. *J Nucl Med* 31:1240, 1990.

81. Faber TL, Cooke CD, Pettigrew RI, et al: Three-dimensional displays of left ventricular epicardial surface from standard cardiac SPECT perfusion quantification techniques. *J Nucl Med* 36:697, 1995.

82. Cooke CD, Garcia EV, Folks RD: Three-dimensional visualization of cardiac single photon emission computed tomography studies, in Robb RA (ed): *Visualization in Biomedical Computing 1992: Proc SPIE 1808-671-675.* Chapel Hill, NC.

83. Quaife RA, Faber TL, Corbett JR: Visual assessment of quantitative three-dimensional displays of stress thallium-201 tomograms: Comparison with visual multislice analysis. *J Nucl Med* 32:1006P, 1991 (abstr).

84. Cooke CD, Vansant JP, Krawczynska E, Garcia EV: Clinical validation of 3-d color-modulated displays of myocardial perfusion. *J Nucl Med* 36:12P, 1995 (abstr).

85. Faber TL, Cooke CD, Pettigrew RI, Garcia EV: Left ventricular volumes, and mass from gated perfusion tomograms using a standard processing program. *J Nucl Med* 36:12P, 1995.

86. Sheehan FH, Bolson EL, Dodge HT, et al: Advantages and applications of the centerline method for characterizing region ventricular function. *Circulation* 74:293, 1986.

A Stepwise Approach to Myocardial Perfusion SPECT Interpretation

E. Gordon Depuey

Single photon emission computed tomography (SPECT) is used in the majority of myocardial perfusion scintigraphic studies acquired in the United States. SPECT imaging provides clear advantages compared to planar imaging in the noninvasive localization of coronary artery disease and in determining disease extent. However, every step of SPECT myocardial perfusion image acquisition and processing is fraught with potential errors that can result in false-positive scans. For this reason, it is essential that patient studies be interpreted in a systematic, stepwise fashion.[1] A critical aspect of the interpretation of each patient study is careful review of the image data at each step of image acquisition and processing. Although image interpretation can be accomplished either from the computer console or from film or paper hard copy, review of quality control measures and any associated reprocessing of images are facilitated by study review at the computer. Thus, the reviewing physician must become thoroughly familiar with the processing algorithms and image review formats available on the particular computer that is used.

There are many possible approaches to the interpretation of SPECT myocardial perfusion images. This chapter presents one systematic approach that has proven effective in the detection of coronary artery disease and determination of disease extent, while avoiding many sources of false-positive tomogram interpretations. It should be emphasized that before this systematic approach to image interpretation can succeed, each of the instrumentation quality assurance measures described in Chap. 3 must be carried out.

PREPARATION FOR INTERPRETATION OF MYOCARDIAL PERFUSION SPECT

Preparation for SPECT interpretation should proceed in a stepwise sequence: 1) Information regarding the patient's body habitus should be available; 2) the planar projections should be reviewed to assess overall image quality and detect evidence of artifacts related to patient motion, soft tissue attenuation, and high tracer activity in organs adjacent to the heart; 3) accurate selection of the left ventricular long axis for tomogram orientation should be confirmed; 4) the tomographic slices should be examined closely to verify that the data have been correctly normalized to maximal myocardial counts; 5) the planar projections and tomographic slices should be reviewed to assess for the presence of artifact patterns; and 6) myocardial polar maps and electrocardiographically gated perfusion tomograms should be reviewed for the possible presence of technical or attenuation artifacts.

Patient Body Habitus

Before image interpretation, it is essential to obtain specific relevant information concerning the patient's body habitus. This information includes height, weight, chest circumference, bra cup size in female patients, history of mastectomy or breast implantation, the presence of

Table 4-1   Body Habitus Profile

Patient _____ X-ray # _____ Date _____
Height _____ Weight _____

FEMALES

Chest circumference	____inches
Bra cup size	____(A–D)
Left mastectomy	____no ____yes
Breast prosthesis	____no ____yes
Breast implant	____no ____yes
Breast position	____anterior ____anterolateral
	____lateral ____inferolateral
Breast density (chest x-ray)	____low ____modt ____marked
Lateral chest wall fat	____mild ____modt ____high
Abdominal protuberance	____mild ____modt ____marked
Immediate images	____bra off ____bra on
Delayed images	____bra off ____bra on
Additional delayed images	____bra off ____bra on

MALES

Chest circumference	____inches
Gynecomastia	____no ____yes
Pectoral development	____mild ____modt ____marked
Lateral chest fat	____mild ____modt ____marked
Abdominal protuberance	____mild ____modt ____marked

COMMENTS:

chest wall deformity or previous lung resection, and abdominal girth (Table 4-1). Attenuation artifacts are much more likely to occur in an obese woman with large, dense breasts than in a tall, thin man. Knowledge of body habitus alerts the interpreting physician to such potential artifacts.

Review of Planar Projection Images

Planar projection images should be reviewed at the computer console in endless-loop cinematic format (Fig. 4-1). This format provides a highly effective means to detect subtle degrees of motion, which can both degrade spatial resolution and introduce motion artifacts. At the time that these projection images are inspected, the physician can assess overall image quality in terms of cardiac count density, target-to-background ratio, and evidence of dose infiltration. The position and relative density of attenuators, including the left breast and left hemidiaphragm, can also be determined. In addition, the presence of increased lung tracer concentration can be assessed from the anterior planar projection image.

LEFT VENTRICULAR AXIS SELECTION

Accurate interpretation of myocardial tomograms is fundamentally dependent on display of myocardial activity in a format that allows correct localization of left ventricular myocardial segments. A joint committee of the American College of Cardiology, the American Heart Association, and the Society of Nuclear Medicine has issued a policy statement standardizing the format and orientation of myocardial perfusion tomograms.[2] These standardized projections are each oriented orthogonal to the long axis of the left ventricle. Therefore, standardized image orientation requires precise localization of the long axis of the left ventricle. In addition to correct identification of myocardial segments, precise localization of the left ventricular long axis is critically important in identifying the boundaries of the left ventricle. To determine if a defect in the circumference of a myocardial slice is a result of impaired perfusion within the myocardial wall or a result of inclusion of a region outside the border of the left ventricle, myocardial activity must be accurately oriented orthogonal to the ventricular long axis.

In general, following filtered backprojection, the long axis of the left ventricle is first determined from the transaxial mid-ventricular slice. After a mid-ventricular vertical long axis slice is thereby reconstructed, the long axis of the left ventricle is again selected from that mid-ventricular vertical long axis slice. Both the transaxial and vertical long axis slices should precisely bisect the left ventricular cavity, from the midpoint of the valve plane to the apex (Fig. 4-2). Moreover, in order that both stress and rest tomograms encompass identical myocardial regions or segments, the angulation of these axes should be identical.

On most nuclear medicine computers it is possible to review the apical and basal limits set for short axis slice selection, the ventricular axis of the transaxial tomogram used for reconstruction of the vertical long axis slices, and the ventricular axis of the mid-ventricular vertical long axis tomogram used for reconstruction of short axis and horizontal long axis slices (Fig. 4-3). Review of these limits and axes is required to ensure congruency of the stress and rest tomograms.

Tomographic Slice Inspection

Once correct axis selection has been assured, the tomographic slices themselves should be systematically inspected. Most commonly, the corresponding stress and rest slices are viewed together in the short axis, horizontal long axis (Fig. 4-4), and vertical long axis projections. An advantage of this combined method of interpreting stress and rest perfusion tomograms is that studies can be interpreted on x-ray film or paper printout. However, two potentially serious pitfalls of the "offline" method of interpretation are that 1) if stress and rest tomographic slices are not congruently aligned with

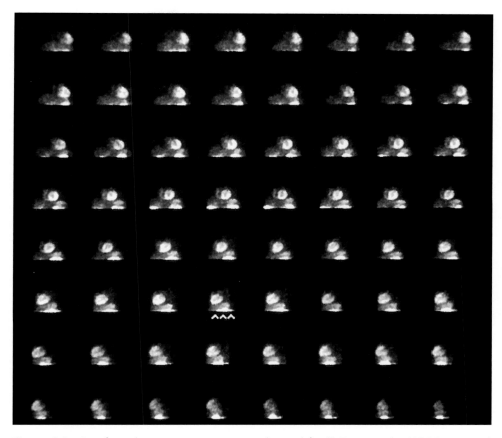

Figure 4-1 Sixty-four planar projection images obtained for ^{99m}Tc sestamibi SPECT, acquired over 180°, from the 45° right anterior oblique to the 45° left posterior oblique view. Transient, abrupt, upward motion is present (arrows).

one another, corresponding segments will not be compared, and 2) if both stress and rest images are not correctly normalized to the myocardium, comparison of relative segmental count density is very difficult, if not impossible. If stress and rest tomographic slices are not correctly aligned with one another, then they must be realigned before interpretation can proceed. This process is facilitated if the physician who is interpreting the study can quickly reconstruct the tomographic images. An alternate method of inspecting tomographic slices, which requires viewing at the computer console, is to first inspect the stress tomographic slice images in all projections and then inspect the rest images. Each tomographic projection can be viewed slowly in dynamic format (e.g., one can "page-through" the short axis slices from the base to the apex), first for stress, then for rest. Alternately, this dynamic method can be applied to the stress and rest images simultaneously. This approach may provide the observer with a more three-dimensional appreciation of the extent and vascular distribution of perfusion defects. The choice of a static versus "dynamic" approach is a matter of reader preference.

Normalization of Tomographic Slices

Tomographic slices are usually normalized to the hottest region of the entire left ventricular myocardium. This is done separately for the stress and rest images. Thereby defect intensity can be readily compared to that of normal myocardium. An alternative method is to normalize each tomographic slice to the hottest region in that particular slice alone. The latter approach allows the reader to determine relative tracer distribution within regions of severely decreased perfusion (which can also be done easily on the computer console using the "whole heart-normalized" method, merely by increasing the image intensity). However, a serious drawback of the slice-normalized approach is to severely underestimate the severity of perfusion defects involving an entire tomographic slice, a situation not uncommonly encountered in apical short axis slices in patients with disease of a "wraparound" left anterior descending coronary artery, supplying the entire apex and distal left ventricle. Therefore, it appears preferable to normalize the tomographic slices to the hottest region of the entire left ventricle (Fig. 4-5).

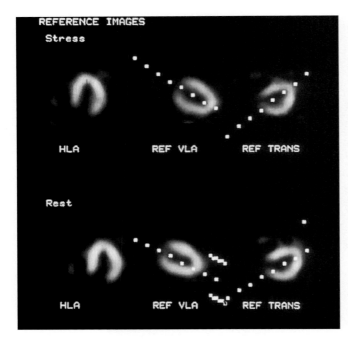

Figure 4-2 Correct selection of the long axes of the left ventricle from stress and rest vertical long axis (VLA) and transaxial (TRANS) tomograms. (HLA is horizontal long axis. Ref is reformatted.)

Display Method

Controversy exists among experts regarding the best display format for perfusion tomograms—color, monochrome, or black and white. A wide variety of color scales are available on nuclear medicine computer systems. If gradations between colors are too abrupt (e.g., a 10 percent change in count density resulting in a change from white to red) normal, physiologic variations in count density may be misinterpreted as perfusion defects. A limitation of many color scales is that at the lower end of the scale, with count densities below approximately 35 percent of maximum, there is very little color variation. Consequently, changes in count density of severe perfusion defects, often indicative of slight defect reversibility and myocardial viability, can be easily overlooked. Although subtle perfusion defects may be difficult to detect with some black-and-white displays, a linear black-and-white scale will show gray-scale gradations in areas of severely decreased count density, allowing subtle degrees of defect reversibility to be discerned. It should be noted, however, that many computers offer the options of "logarithmic" or "exponential" black-and-white scales, both of which may decrease or eliminate gray scale gradations in the low count density range. Thus, both color and

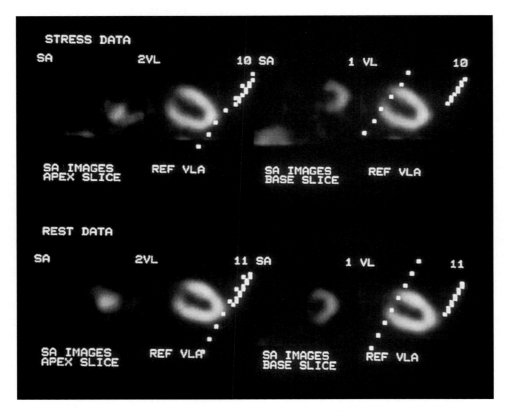

Figure 4-3 Correct selection of apical and basal limits of the left ventricle at stress and rest from mid-ventricular vertical long axis (VLA) tomograms. (SA is short axis.)

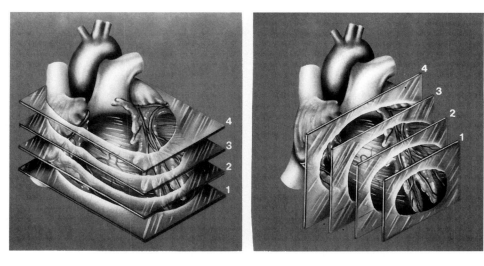

HORIZONTAL LONG AXIS   SHORT AXIS

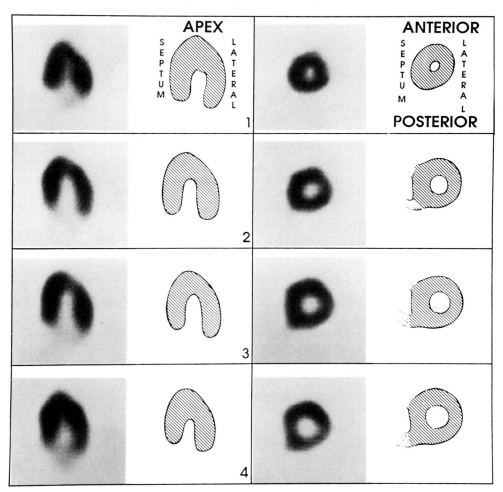

Figure 4-4   Normal myocardial perfusion tomograms. (Courtesy of General Electric Medical Systems.)

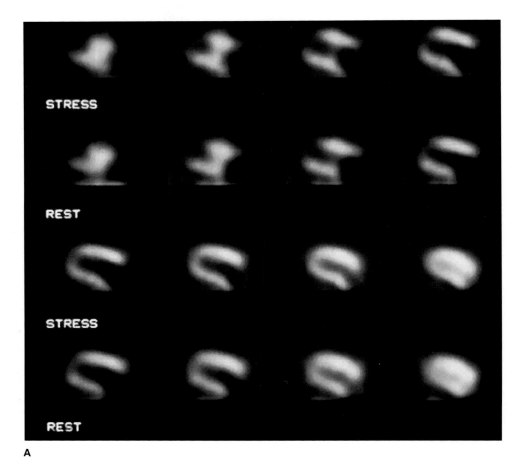

A

Figure 4-5 A severe, fixed apical perfusion defect is present in stress and rest vertical long axis tomograms **(A)**. When short axis tomograms are displayed normalized to activity within the entire left ventricle **(B)**, absent apical activity is portrayed correctly. However, when the short axis tomograms are slice-normalized **(C)**, the fixed apical defect is underestimated.

black-and-white displays have distinct advantages and disadvantages for interpretation of perfusion tomograms. To gain the potential advantages of both display methods it may be helpful to display the SPECT images side by side on both black-and-white and color monitors.

An alternate display format that many experts have found useful is a monochromatic red or green color scale. It has been suggested that a monochromatic scale allows subtle perfusion defects to be detected more readily and that it also provides a dynamic range in regions of low count density to allow for detection of reversibility of severe perfusion defects. Although it provides a good single display format, the monochromatic scale is nevertheless somewhat of a compromise between the color and black-and-white displays. The optimal display method for interpretation of perfusion tomographic slices has not been established in a large-scale, blinded study.

AVOIDANCE AND DETECTION OF ARTIFACTS

Patient Motion

The most sensitive means to detect patient motion is to inspect the planar projection images in an endless-loop rotating cinematic format. The eye is quite sensitive in detecting subtle degrees of motion in either the vertical (axial) or rotational (lateral) direction (Fig. 4-1).

Patient motion most often occurs because the patient is uncomfortable or anxious during image acquisition.[3,4,5,6,7] Therefore, every effort should be made by the technologist and physician to reassure the patient and make him or her as comfortable as possible. The neck and lumbar vertebral region should be supported, and the knees should be slightly flexed and supported to minimize low back strain during imaging. For the camera head to closely approximate the chest wall and to minimize the SPECT radius of rotation, it is essential that

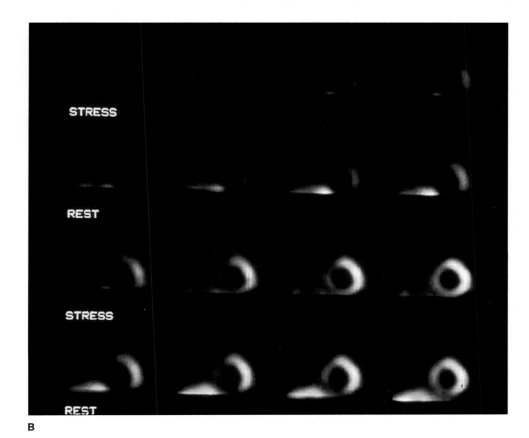

Figure 4-5 (*Continued*)

the patient's arms be extended above the head. A support for the shoulder and arms is extremely helpful in decreasing shoulder discomfort. Moreover, the hands can be restrained lightly or strapped together to further decrease arm and shoulder strain. It has been reported that such measures decrease motion artifacts by approximately two-thirds.[8] Owing to arthritis, some patients are unable to elevate both arms above the head. If a 180° image arc [45° right anterior oblique (RAO) to 45° left posterior oblique (LPO)] is used, it is possible to perform SPECT with only the left arm elevated. If for some reason the patient must move his or her arm during SPECT acquisition, the arm should be moved by the technologist, taking care to minimize associated motion of the chest. However, left arm motion may also result in a shift in position of the left breast, creating a variable attenuation artifact (see the following). In some patients it is not possible to perform SPECT without significant motion. These patients include individuals with arthritis or pain of the shoulders or low back, those who are uncooperative, and those who may be dyspneic owing to congestive heart failure. In such individuals, planar imaging may be preferable to SPECT.

Motion detected on planar projection images viewed in endless loop cinematic format may be characterized as follows:

a) bounce: often due to coughing, sighing, or snoring. The patient should be instructed to breathe normally. It is inadvisable to allow the patient to fall asleep since respirations may be unusually deep or irregular.

b) abrupt vertical motion: usually due to a shift in the position of the patient on the imaging table.

c) gradual motion/creep: often due to the patient sliding up or down on the imaging table through movement of the back or legs. Another source of gradual motion is "upward creep" encountered in stress thallium-201 images in which acquisition is begun soon after the termination of exercise when the patient's respirations are still deep.[9] With deep respiration the diaphragm is pushed down, and the heart lies lower in the thorax. During SPECT acquisition, the depth of respiration decreases, and consequently the heart gradually rises or "creeps up" in the thorax. Such an "upward creep" artifact can be avoided by postponing image acquisition for 15 min after the termination of exercise or until the respiratory rate has returned to normal.

d) horizontal/rotational motion: usually due to rotation of the thorax consequent to arm motion. Occasionally small patients may actually move horizontally on the imaging pallet.

Although inspection of planar projection data in cinematic format is the best way to detect any of these types of motion, these cinematic data cannot be captured in hard-copy format for the patient record. Alternate meth-

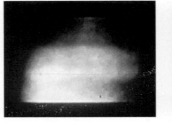 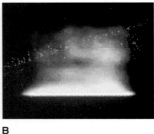

Figure 4-6 A: Summed planar projection images from a 180° acquisition. No patient motion is present. B: Summed projection images from a patient who moved approximately two pixels in the cephalad direction (arrows) at the midpoint of the 180° SPECT acquisition.

ods of detecting motion are less sensitive, but provide a permanent record. Image acquisition data can be summed as a "summed projection image" (Fig. 4-6). Since the heart is not at the center of the camera radius of rotation, it "moves" across the planar projection image as the camera rotates around the thorax, from right to left using a 45° RAO to 45° LPO 180° arc. The superior and inferior borders of the left ventricular "stripe" should be horizontal. Gradual motion, or "creep," is easily detected. Abrupt motion can be detected if the patient remains in the altered position for the remainder of the acquisition (Fig. 4-6B). However, if the patient returns to his or her original position, abrupt motion is much less apparent. Patient bounce and lateral or rotational motion are difficult or impossible to detect by this means.

An image sinogram can be generated to assist in detecting motion (Fig. 4-7A). In this format each projection image is "flattened," or compressed, with maintenance of the count density distribution in the X-axis but minimization of the count density distribution in the

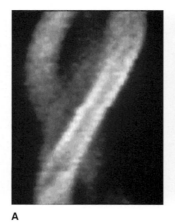 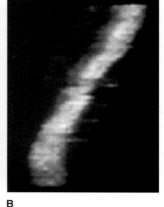

Figure 4-7 A: Sinogram from a 180° SPECT acquisition. No patient motion is present. B: Sinogram from a 180° SPECT acquisition during which multiple episodes of patient motion occurred as indicated by discontinuities in the sinogram.

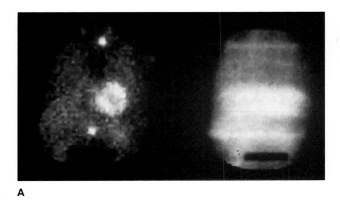

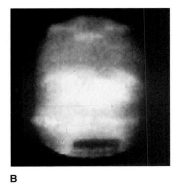

Figure 4-8 **A:** Thallium-201 point source markers placed on the anterior chest wall above and below the level of the heart (**left**). Summed planar projection images (**right**) demonstrate smooth horizontal lines produced by the point sources, indicating no patient motion. **B:** In a patient with transient downward motion during the mid third of SPECT acquisition, there is discontinuity of the horizontal lines (**arrows**) formed by the point sources.

Y-axis. Projection image frames are then progressively "stacked." Since the heart is not at the center of the camera radius of rotation, the position of the left ventricle in the stacked frames varies sinusoidally. Sinograms are most helpful in detecting abrupt patient motion and lateral motion, which are manifest as a discontinuity of the smooth ventricular borders of the sinogram (Fig. 4-7B). Patient bounce is usually too subtle to detect. Gradual motion can seldom if ever be detected.

Another method of monitoring patient motion is to affix small ^{201}Tl or ^{99m}Tc point sources to the patient's chest wall above and below the heart. With no patient motion, the summed projection image demonstrates two horizontal lines created as the stationary point sources are imaged (Fig. 4-8A). With abrupt or gradual patient motion, the lines are broken or tilted (Fig. 4-8B). However, cardiac motion, particularly "upward creep" or motion due to periodic deep respiration, can occur without associated chest wall motion. Therefore, the point source method is insensitive to these types of motion.

Multidetector systems for myocardial perfusion SPECT are now in widespread use. By maintaining a count density identical to those of single detector systems

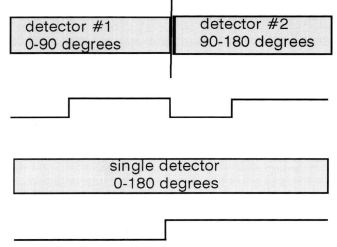

Figure 4-9 Effect of abrupt patient motion imaged over 180° with dual 90°-opposed detectors compared to a single detector.

while shortening the 180° image acquisition time (by 50 percent for two 90°-angled detectors and by 33 percent for three 120°-detectors), these new instruments offer a significant advantage in decreasing the potential for patient motion. However, when motion does occur, the effect is compounded with the multidetector configuration. For instance, using a 90°-angled, two-detector system, if a patient moves abruptly, the motion is "seen" by both detectors (Fig. 4-9). In addition, at the "seam" between the two detectors a third change in cardiac posi-

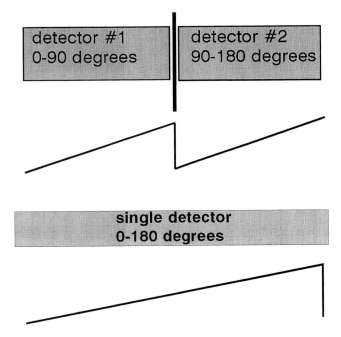

Figure 4-10 Effect of gradual patient motion ("creep") imaged over 180° with dual 90°-opposed detectors compared to a single detector.

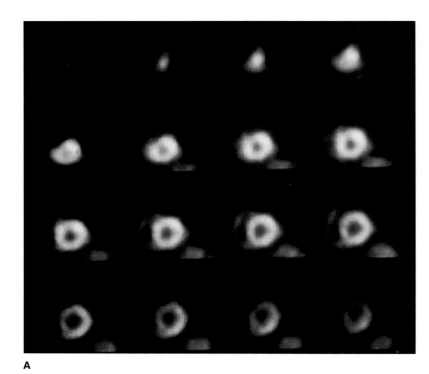

A

Figure 4-11 Characteristic artifacts in short axis (**A**), horizontal long axis (**B**), and transaxial (**C**) tomograms and raw (**left**) and severity (**right**) polar plots (**D**) in a patient who moved approximately two pixels in the cephalad (vertical) direction midway through a 180° SPECT acquisition. For images in this chapter, short axis tomograms proceed from apex to base, vertical long axis tomograms from septum to lateral wall, and horizontal long axis tomograms from inferior to anterior wall.

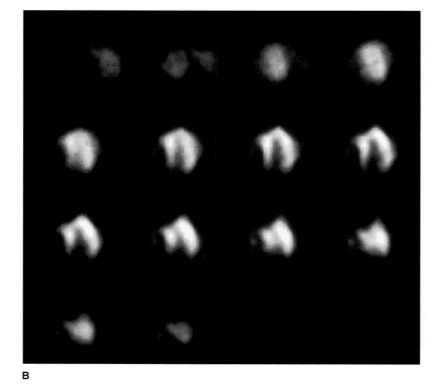

B

tion occurs as the heart shifts from its final position back to its original position. With upward creep, gradual motion is detected by both detectors, and, in addition, an abrupt shift of cardiac position is present at the "seam" (Fig. 4-10).

A SPECT acquisition method has been described whereby multiple rapid tomographic acquisitions are performed and then summed.[10] If patient motion occurs during one of the acquisitions, those data are discarded. In this way, a single episode of patient motion will not confound the entire study. This method is of greatest benefit when there is one episode of vertical or horizontal

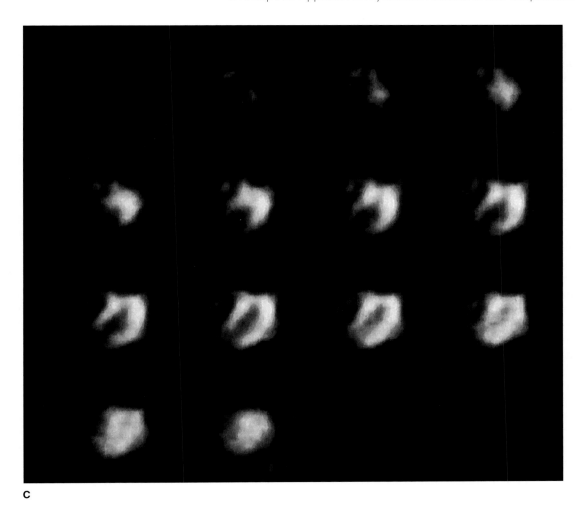

C

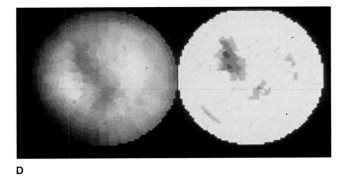

D

Figure 4-11   (Continued)

motion and the patient returns to his or her original position. If the original position is not resumed, the heart is in different positions before and after the discarded single rapid acquisition. This method is also useful for eliminating the effects of motion at the very beginning or end of SPECT acquisition.

Artifacts caused by patient motion are a very significant source of false-positive myocardial perfusion tomograms. Motion resulting in an image defect misinterpretable as a true perfusion abnormality is estimated to

occur in as many as 10 to 15 percent of patient studies.[11] Unfortunately, associated artifact characteristics are variable and not always predictable from the planar projection image quality control images. However, vertical (and particularly rotational) motion that occurs at the midpoint (45° LAO) of the acquisition is most problematical.

The most characteristic artifact created by patient motion can be observed in the short axis tomograms as opposed anterior and inferior, somewhat linear defects (Fig. 4-11). This artifact is caused by filtered backprojection of data onto different points in the volume matrix when the heart is in different positions at different times during the acquisition. These "opposed" defects can be observed with greater difficulty in the orthogonal horizontal long axis and vertical long axis tomograms. More commonly, in these views the apex will appear skewed, with its anteroseptal and posterolateral margins misaligned. Inspection of transaxial tomograms is often helpful to better delineate the motion artifact. This type of artifact can be observed with either abrupt patient motion in the horizontal or vertical directions or gradual motion.

It is often possible to fully, or at least partially, computer-correct for patient motion and thereby salvage myocardial perfusion scans. Software is available to correct motion in ^{201}Tl SPECT.[12,13,14,15] However, visceral uptake in the bowel and liver, sometimes present in ^{201}Tl studies and frequently in studies using ^{99m}Tc labeled tracers, may confound this automated technique. Therefore, many laboratories have found it more reliable to correct for patient motion by manually shifting individual projection image frames in the vertical direction to compensate for vertical motion of the heart. After all appropriate frames have been shifted, the planar projection images displayed in cinematic format and the summed projection image should demonstrate a smooth horizontal path of the heart throughout the acquisition, although the frames themselves will appear to "jump" since they have been shifted during the correction process. Although this method is somewhat labor-intensive and tedious, it can often avoid the discarding and reacquisition of a study. It is important to note, however, that this method cannot correct for horizontal or rotational patient motion.

Soft Tissue Attenuation Artifacts

BREAST ATTENUATION ARTIFACTS

Breast attenuation artifacts are encountered very frequently with ^{201}Tl SPECT and less commonly with myocardial perfusion SPECT performed with the ^{99m}Tc labeled tracers such as sestamibi. Although breast attenuation usually produces a diffuse, fixed anterior defect, the location and severity of the artifact depend on the size, density, and position of the breasts. Infrequently, the breast can vary in position between the stress and rest images, creating a "shifting" breast attenuation artifact, simulating a reversible perfusion defect, i.e., ischemia. Knowledge of these parameters can aid the interpreting physician considerably in anticipating a breast artifact. The following serve as valuable means to assess parameters relating to breast attenuation:

1. The patient's height, weight, chest circumference, and bra cup size should be recorded. Also, as the technolo-

gist or physician observes the patient lying supine on the imaging table, the approximate position of the breast should be recorded (i.e., anterior, anterolateral, lateral).

2. The patient should be imaged in such a manner as to minimize the effect of breast attenuation. The patient should not wear a bra and should wear loose-fitting clothing or a hospital gown so the breasts are pendulous or lie flat against the chest wall. A bra will position the breasts anteriorly and thicken them, considerably increasing photon attenuation. Other laboratories elevate the breasts above the level of the heart by taping them. Although taping may be effective, it is objectionable to some women. Moreover, if the breast is not fully elevated, it can overlie the superiormost aspect of the left ventricle and create a severe attenuation artifact. Another approach is to bind the chest with an elastic bandage to flatten the breasts. However, the breasts may vary in position under the binder from stress to rest and create an artifact that mimics ischemia.

3. The position of the left breast will vary depending on the degree of elevation of the left arm. Therefore, if the left arm moves during image acquisition, not only may a motion artifact result, but there may also be a second artifact created by the varying position of the breast attenuator. Similarly, if the position of the left arm is different in the stress and rest SPECT acquisitions, a shifting breast attenuation artifact, simulating ischemia, may be encountered. Therefore, precise repositioning, support, and gentle restraint of the left arm are important measures to avoid a shifting breast artifact.

4. It is important that the planar projection images should be viewed in endless-loop cinematic format. Large, dense breasts will create a discrete "shadow" when silhouetted against the background tracer concentration in the thorax and chest wall. Thereby, the density of the breast, its position, and the portion of the left ventricular myocardium that is "eclipsed," or most markedly attenuated, can be determined. In general, if the breast shadow markedly and abruptly eclipses just a portion of the left ventricle (e.g., the anterolateral wall), an attenuation artifact should be anticipated (Fig. 4-12). However, if the breast is large and pendulous and overshadows the entire left ventricle, the attenuation effect is more diffuse, so the location of the attenuation artifact is more difficult to predict (Fig. 4-13). Finally, the position and density of the breast shadow in the stress and rest planar projection images should be compared to determine the possibility of a shift in breast position. Moreover, when the "rotating" planar projection images are viewed, motion of the left arm should alert the interpreting physician to the possibilities of patient motion and a shifting breast attenuation artifact.

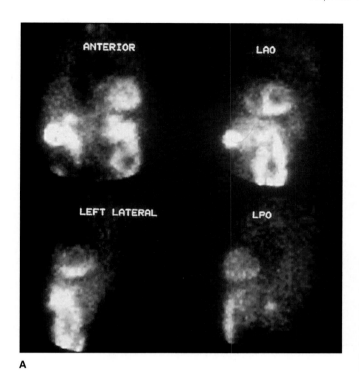

A

Figure 4-12 Marked breast attenuation is noted in projection images **(A)** in this woman with a large chest (44D bra cup) imaged with ^{99m}Tc sestamibi. Anterior and anterolateral fixed defects are apparent in short axis **(B)**, vertical long axis **(C)**, and horizontal long axis **(D)** tomograms and quantitative polar plots **(E)**. Gated vertical long axis **(top)** and short axis **(bottom)** tomograms **(F)** demonstrate normal wall motion and thickening, indicating an attenuation artifact rather than scar. (LAO is left anterior oblique, LPO is left posterior oblique.)

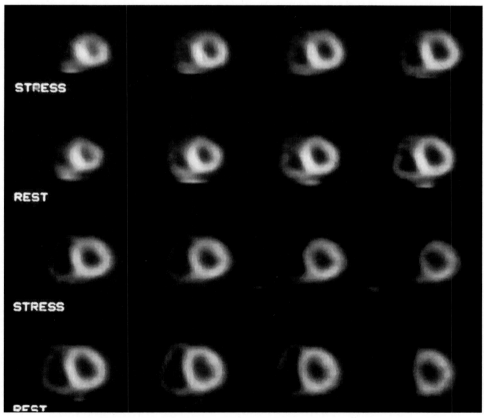

B

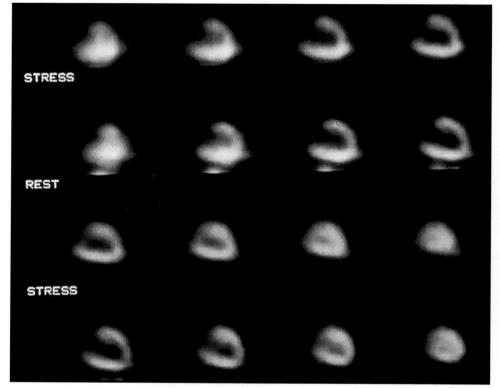

C

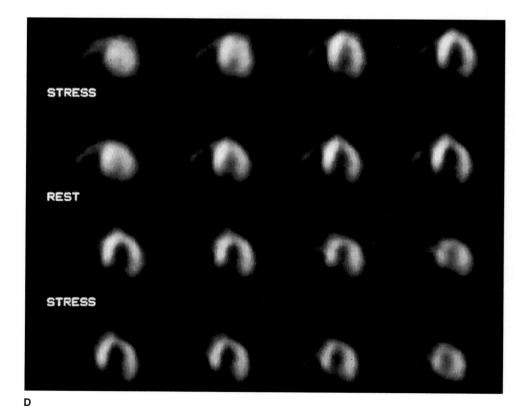

D

Figure 4-12   (*Continued*)

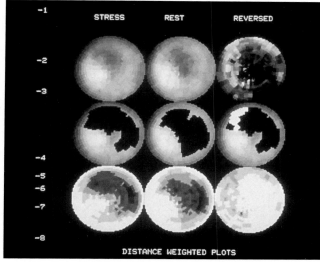

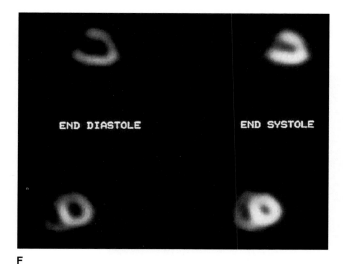

Figure 4-12   (Continued)

The effect of breast attenuation on tomograms depends on the size, density, and position of the breast. In Figs. 4-12 and 4-13 the attenuation effects in women with various breast sizes imaged with ^{99m}Tc sestamibi are illustrated. The attenuation effect is best observed in the planar projection images. The resulting impact on perfusion tomograms and quantitative polar plots is illustrated.

Gated SPECT with ^{99m}Tc sestamibi has been shown to be very useful in differentiating fixed scan defects due to breast attenuation from those due to myocardial scarring. Areas of myocardial scarring will demonstrate decreased wall thickening and, usually, abnormal wall motion, whereas attenuation artifacts will demonstrate totally normal wall thickening and motion.[16] The normal pattern of wall motion and thickening in a woman with

large breasts is illustrated in Fig. 4-12. Taillefer et al have reported an increase in test specificity in women with gated ^{99m}Tc sestamibi SPECT as compared with nongated sestamibi or ^{201}Tl SPECT.[17]

LATERAL CHEST WALL ATTENUATION ARTIFACTS

In obese patients, both men and women, adipose tissue may be prominent in the lateral chest wall, resulting in photon attenuation. The thickness of soft tissue in the lateral chest wall is accentuated when a patient lies supine.

The technologist should note if marked lateral wall soft tissue is present. In the planar projection images displayed in endless-loop cinematic format, the entire heart will exhibit a marked decrease in count density in the left lateral and left posterior oblique views (Fig. 4-14). In tomograms and polar plots a diffuse decrease in count density is frequently observed throughout the entire lateral wall of the left ventricle, mimicking scarring in the circumflex coronary artery territory.

The most reliable method of recognizing a lateral wall attenuation artifact is to anticipate it from knowledge of the patient's body habitus. Also, gated SPECT is of value, because, like other attenuation artifacts, the lateral wall attenuation artifact will be accompanied by normal wall motion and thickening.

DIAPHRAGMATIC ATTENUATION ARTIFACTS

Photon attenuation by the left hemidiaphragm has proved to be one of the most problematical sources of myocardial perfusion SPECT artifacts. In most instances diaphragmatic attenuation artifacts are found in men. The reason for this preponderance in men is unclear, but it has been observed that the diaphragm is more muscular and thicker in men, creating more marked attenuation than in women. Alternately, others believe that, unlike women, who primarily use the chest musculature to breathe, men use their abdominal musculature, elevating the diaphragm during expiration. In obese patients and those with protuberant abdomens, the diaphragm is often elevated, resulting in decreased lung volume. Therefore, before scan interpretation, the interpreting physician, in order to anticipate artifacts from diaphragmatic attenuation, should be cognizant of the patient's gender, height, weight, and body habitus, especially with regard to abdominal protuberance.

The first clue to diaphragmatic attenuation of the inferior wall of the left ventricle is revealed, again, by inspection of the planar projection images displayed in cinematic format. With diaphragmatic elevation, the right lobe of the liver, which invariably has some trace uptake, may be noted to extend into the right hemithorax, often to the level of the anterior wall of the left ventricle (Fig. 4-15). Although the left hemidiaphragm

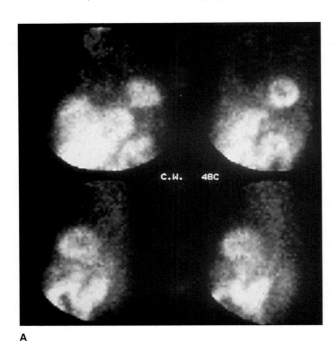

A

Figure 4-13 Marked breast attenuation is less apparent in this ^{99m}Tc sestamibi SPECT scan than in Fig. 4-12 because the large, laterally positioned left breast (48C bra cup) eclipses the entire left ventricle in the lateral views **(A)**. A fixed anterior and lateral defect is apparent in short axis **(B)**, and vertical long axis **(C)**.

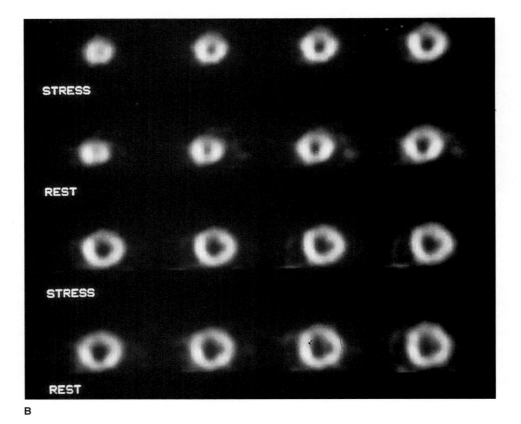

B

itself is seldom visualized, a "stomach bubble" due to air or fluid within the stomach can be visualized in the left lateral projection images. Similarly, tracer concentration within the splenic flexure of the colon, the stomach, and occasionally the small bowel frequently defines the location of the left hemidiaphragm (Fig. 4-16). If any of these structures is noted to overlie or "indent" the inferior wall of the left ventricle in the left lateral view, diaphragmatic attenuation should be anticipated. Some laboratories have found the left lateral projection image so useful in estimating the position of the left hemidiaphragm that they routinely obtain a separate three to

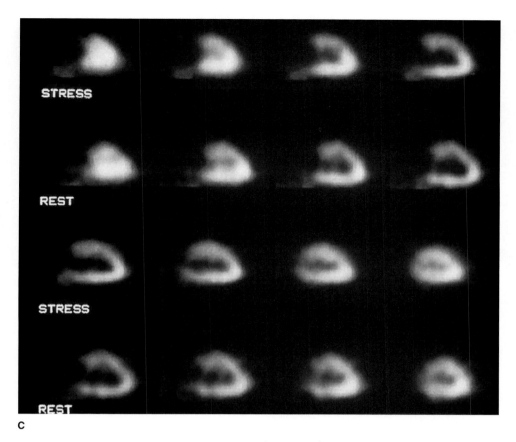

Figure 4-13   (Continued)

five minute left lateral planar image either before or after SPECT acquisition.

From myocardial perfusion tomograms alone it is very difficult, if not impossible, to differentiate diaphragmatic attenuation from a true inferior myocardial perfusion defect. Diaphragmatic attenuation artifacts are most frequently inferior, at the 6 o'clock position in the short axis projection, and more marked in the basal half of the heart. However, inferolateral, inferoseptal, and even inferoapical attenuation artifacts are not uncommon. As for the planar projection images, if the "stomach bubble" or abdominal visceral tracer concentration is located immediately adjacent to the inferior defect, attenuation by an interposed left hemidiaphragm should be suspected.

Fortunately, in most instances of diaphragmatic attenuation artifacts are fixed in both stress and rest images and mimic scars rather than ischemia. However, there is one potential scenario wherein diaphragmatic height could change from stress to rest, mimicking ischemia. If during exercise or pharmacologic stress the patient swallows air, distending the stomach and elevating the left hemidiaphragm, attenuation of the inferior wall will be present in subsequent stress images. If in resting images the air is expelled, diaphragmatic

height will decrease, and the artifacts will be less marked or absent.

Polar maps and quantitative analysis are virtually useless in differentiating a diaphragmatic attenuation artifact from a true inferior perfusion defect. In fact, they have the disadvantage compared with both the planar projection images and tomograms that there are no extracardiac "clues" to suggest diaphragmatic elevation.

Attenuation and scatter correction of myocardial perfusion SPECT images is now commercially available. Simultaneously with the emission scan, a transmission scan is performed, usually using a ^{99m}Tc or ^{153}Gd line source.[18,19,20,21,22,23] Such attenuation correction methodology has been demonstrated to decrease artifacts created by breast and diaphragmatic soft tissue attenuation (Plate 3, Fig. 4-17). As the methodology was being developed, it was noted that when the transmission scan does not encompass the entire thorax, truncation artifacts may be introduced. More recently, commercially available approaches have been developed that appear to have resolved this problem.

An effective means of differentiating diaphragmatic attenuation from an inferior scar is to perform an additional SPECT acquisition with the patient prone.[24,25] In

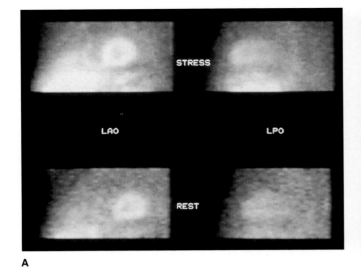

A

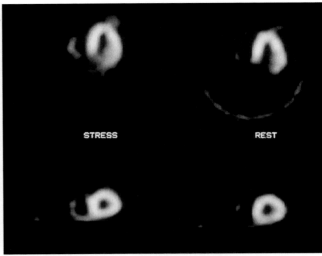

B

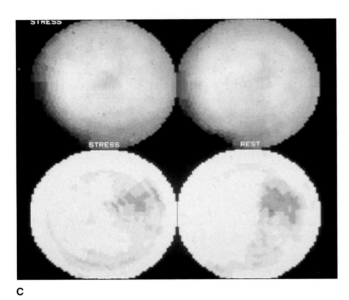

C

Figure 4-14 In this obese man (47-inch chest circumference) imaged with ^{99m}Tc sestamibi, stress and rest planar projection images **(A)** demonstrate decreased myocardial count density in the lateral view, indicating attenuation by lateral chest wall fat. Tomograms **(B)** and raw and severity polar plots **(C)** demonstrate a mild-to-moderate fixed lateral wall defect.

this position, the diaphragm is pushed down as the abdomen is flattened on the imaging table, and the heart moves slightly cephalad, increasing the distance between the inferior wall of the left ventricle and the diaphragm (Plate 4). Prone imaging is well tolerated by patients and, in fact, patient motion is less likely in the prone position. However, there are several limitations to this approach. First, an additional SPECT acquisition is required. Second, unless additional prone imaging is to be performed in all patients, SPECT images must be processed and the interpreting physician or a very experienced technologist must view them and decide if additional prone SPECT is necessary. Otherwise, the patient must be recalled to the laboratory, and a repeat tracer injection is often required. Third, prone images cannot be compared to supine SPECT normal limits for purposes of quantitation. Although some laboratories perform prone rather than supine SPECT routinely, a "cut-out" table is required to eliminate anterior/septal attenuation by the imaging table, and quantification is again not possible owing to lack of commercially available prone SPECT normal limits.[26]

A much simpler means of differentiating fixed diaphragmatic attenuation artifacts from inferior myocardial scarring is to perform gated SPECT using ^{99m}Tc sestamibi (or tetrofosmin). As stated earlier for breast attenuation artifacts, a myocardial segment containing a diaphragmatic attenuation artifact will move and thicken normally, whereas a scar will demonstrate decreased thickening and abnormal wall motion (Figs. 4-15 and 4-18). DePuey et al demonstrated a decrease in the rate of false-positive sestamibi SPECT from 14 to 3 percent, due in part to the ability of gating to exclude an inferior scar as a cause of a fixed defect.[16]

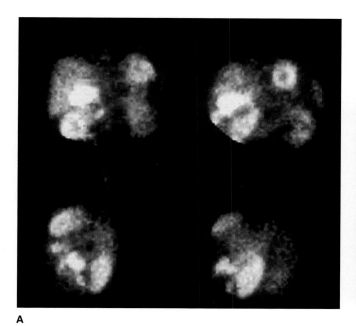

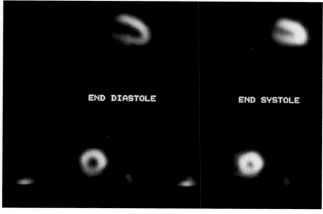

END DIASTOLE END SYSTOLE

A **B**

Figure 4-15 Diaphragmatic elevation is manifested in this obese man by the cephalad position of the liver in the anterior view (upper left) and attenuation of the inferior wall of the left ventricle in the left posterior oblique view (lower right) in planar projection images **(A)**. A moderate decrease in inferior wall count density is present on the vertical long axis and short axis gated tomograms at end diastole **(B)**. The gated tomograms demonstrate normal wall motion and thickening in systole, indicating an attenuation artifact rather than scar.

ABDOMINAL VISCERAL TRACER CONCENTRATION ARTIFACTS

When planar projection images are viewed in endless loop rotating cinematic format, it is useful to observe the presence, location, and intensity of abdominal visceral activity and its proximity to the heart. Adjacent abdominal visceral activity frequently results in problems with

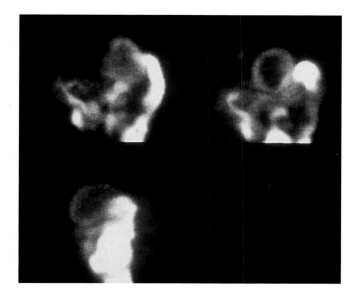

Figure 4-16 Technetium-99m-sestamibi concentration in the splenic flexure of the colon in a patient with marked left hemidiaphragmatic elevation. Marked left ventricular dilatation is also apparent in these planar projection images.

myocardial perfusion image display and SPECT artifacts. The distribution and degree of visceral uptake will vary with the radiopharmaceutical employed.

With ^{201}Tl SPECT, abdominal visceral uptake of tracer is usually confined to the liver, although activity may be observed occasionally in the spleen, stomach, bowel, or muscular diaphragm. In contrast, with the ^{99m}Tc labeled perfusion agents, which are excreted via the hepatobiliary system, activity is much more frequently present in the small and large bowel and the stomach, the latter due to duodenogastric reflux. The clinical applicability of ^{99m}Tc teboroxime has been substantially limited by very rapid tracer clearance by the myocardium and intense accumulation in the liver. Uptake of ^{99m}Tc sestamibi in the liver is much less, but nevertheless somewhat limits laboratory efficiency because of the delay from tracer injection to imaging necessary for hepatic clearance. The newer ^{99m}Tc labeled tracers, tetrofosmin and furifosmin (Q12), demonstrate more rapid hepatic clearance but minimal myocardial washout, partially circumventing these problems. However, unlike with ^{201}Tl marked gastrointestinal uptake of ^{99m}Tc labeled radiopharmaceuticals often creates an even greater problem with abdominal visceral artifacts.

In patients with diaphragmatic elevation, abdominal visceral activity may occasionally overlie the inferior or inferoposterior wall of the left ventricle, confounding interpretation of those myocardial segments. This is particularly problematic with ^{99m}Tc activity in the splenic flexure

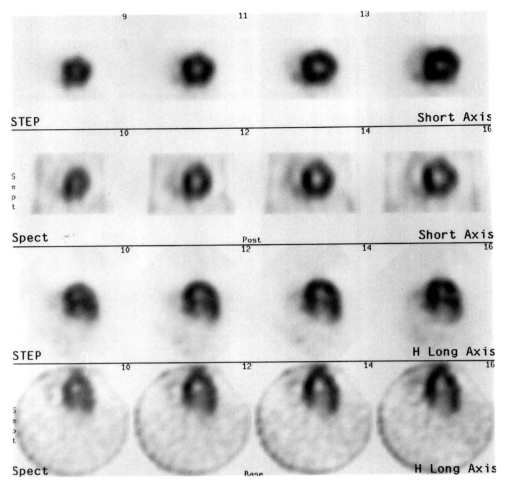

Figure 4-17 Short axis **(top)** and horizontal long axis **(bottom)** ^{201}Tl tomograms from a markedly obese woman (320 lbs) acquired without (2nd and 4th rows) and with (1st and 3rd rows, labeled "STEP") attenuation compensation. In the uncorrected SPECT images an artifactual decrease in count density is apparent throughout the anterior and lateral walls. With attenuation compensation count density distribution is much more uniform throughout the myocardium. (Provided courtesy of Myron Gerson, MD.)

of the colon (Fig. 4-19) and in the stomach. In patients with hiatal hernias (Fig. 4-20), scans are occasionally uninterpretable. Also, for either ^{201}Tl or ^{99m}Tc agents, hepatic tracer concentration is markedly increased with the pharmacologic stress agents dipyridamole and adenosine. The regions of abdominal visceral/myocardial overlap may appear "hot" and, obviously, uninterpretable. More frequently, however, tomographic slices are normalized to the spuriously intense region of the myocardium, giving the false impression of decreased tracer uptake in the remainder of the myocardium.

Abdominal visceral activity not necessarily overlapping the myocardium but just adjacent to the inferior wall frequently creates artifacts in polar maps. For polar map reconstruction, a region of interest is positioned around the left ventricle in the short axis projection, which defines the limits of the radius of search used for polar map reconstruction. If this limiting region of interest encompasses adjacent abdominal visceral activity, it will be projected onto the polar plot (Fig. 4-21). Since polar maps, either "slice-normalized" or "heart-normalized" plots, are normalized to the most intense region, the overlapping abdominal visceral activity will appear normal (100 percent intensity), whereas the remainder of the myocardium will appear to exhibit abnormally decreased activity (Plate 5). Regions that are normally decreased in intensity (the inferior wall in men and the anterior wall in women) will appear particularly abnormal. Computer software programs that provide a mid-ventricular short axis slice for the technologist to draw a limiting region of interest are particularly subject to this type of artifact since, although abdominal visceral activity may be completely excluded from this mid-ventricular region, in more basal or apical slices that same region may encompass significant extra-cardiac activity.

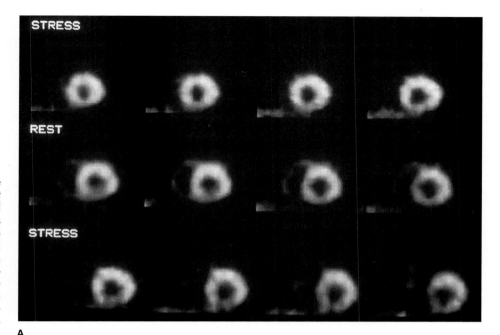

Figure 4-18 In this markedly obese man (320 lbs), ⁹⁹ᵐTc sestamibi short axis (**A**), vertical long axis (**B**), and horizontal long axis (**C**) tomograms and raw polar plots (**D**) demonstrate a moderate decrease in inferior wall count density. Gated vertical long axis (**top**) and short axis (**bottom**) tomograms (**E**) demonstrate normal inferior wall motion and thickening, consistent with diaphragmatic attenuation rather than scar as a cause of the fixed interior wall defect.

A

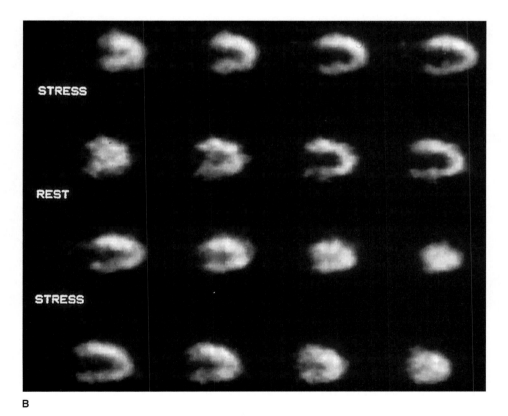

B

A more common problem results from inappropriate formatting or display of tomographic myocardial perfusion images. Images are usually "frame-normalized," ie, the region of maximal tracer activity in the entire frame is set to 100 percent. Depending on the field of view of the scintillation camera used and the horizontal boundaries set by the technologist, considerable, often intense, extra-cardiac activity may be included in the frame. If images are normalized to such extra-cardiac activity, the entire heart will appear to demonstrate decreased tracer concentration. For this reason also, when the intensity of extra-cardiac activity differs in stress and rest images (i.e., more intense liver uptake in resting images), myocardial intensity will vary inversely, ren-

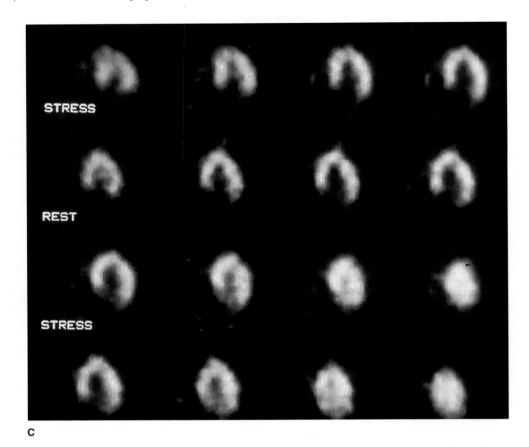

C

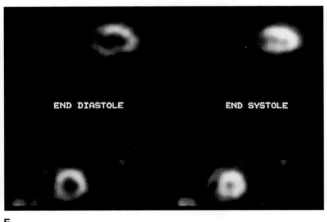

D

E

Figure 4-18 *(Continued)*

dering comparison of stress and rest tomograms difficult, if not impossible.

It has also been observed that when significant hepatic tracer localization is present, inconsistencies in the projections inherent to SPECT imaging will result in an apparent decrease in inferior wall myocardial counts.[27] The effect on the inferior wall is most marked with 180° imaging, most likely because the acquisition arc used to acquire cardiac data is not ideal for the hepatic activity distribution (Fig. 4-22). Utilization of a 360° acquisition

and attenuation/scatter correction minimizes such artifacts.

How can these abdominal visceral artifacts be minimized or eliminated?

1. Minimize hepatic trace uptake.
   a) During dynamic exercise, blood flow to the liver decreases relative to the myocardium and working musculature. Therefore, by assuring maximal

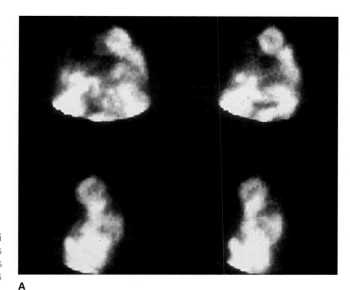

A

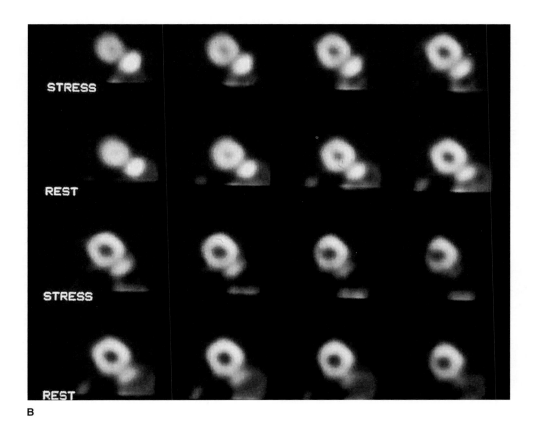

Figure 4-19   A loop of bowel containing excreted ^{99m}Tc sestamibi adjacent to the heart is noted on stress planar projection images (A) and both stress and rest short axis (B), and vertical long axis (C) tomograms. With good spatial resolution bowel activity is separated from the left ventricle.

B

treadmill or bicycle exercise, hepatic uptake in stress images will be minimized.

b) Food in the gut increases abdominal visceral blood flow. Therefore, by withholding food before resting tracer injection and during the stress-to-rest interval, liver tracer uptake may be minimized.

c) When combined with dipyridamole pharmacologic stress, dynamic exercise decreases hepatic blood flow, decreases tracer uptake by the liver, and improves myocardial perfusion image quality.

d) With ^{99m}Tc sestamibi, furifosmin (Q12), or tetrofosmin, hepatic tracer concentration decreases over time. Therefore, particularly for resting images, an injection-to-imaging interval shorter than that recommended in the radiopharmaceutical package insert should not be used. Moreover,

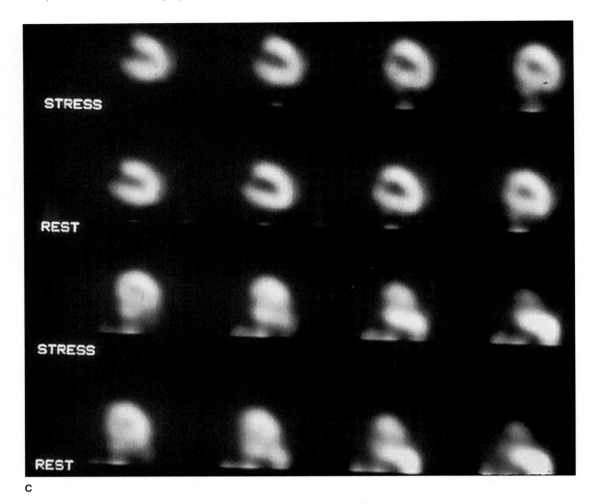

c

Figure 4-19   (Continued)

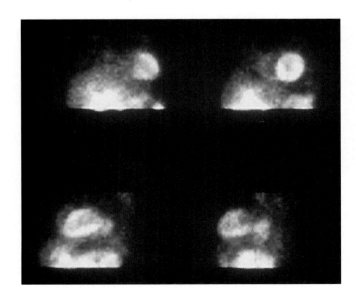

Figure 4-20   Planar projection images demonstrate ^{99m}Tc sestamibi concentration in the stomach in a patient with a hiatal hernia and duodeno-gastric reflux. The fundus of the stomach lies posterior to the heart.

when a patient is positioned under the scintillation camera, the technologist should observe the degree of hepatic uptake before initiating SPECT acquisition and delay imaging for at least 30 min if it is excessive.

2. Minimize bowel and stomach activity
   a) Although milk or a fatty meal was initially prescribed between ^{99m}Tc sestamibi injection and SPECT acquisition, it is now felt to be inadvisable since fat in the bowel promotes gallbladder contraction, subsequently increasing tracer concentration in the bowel and stomach (the latter if duodenogastric reflux is present).
   b) If the technologist observes excessive bowel or stomach activity, particularly activity overlapping the heart, before SPECT acquisition, he or she should offer the patient one or two glasses of water to drink to promote tracer clearance from the gut and delay image acquisition for 30 min. In some laboratories water is given routinely 30 min before imaging. Alternatively, in patients with marked stomach or bowel activity, metoclopramide (10 mg IV) may be administered by the nurse

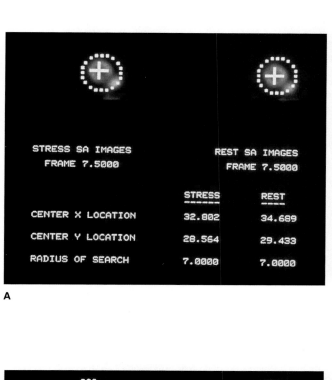

A

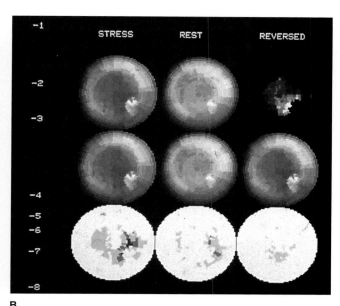

B

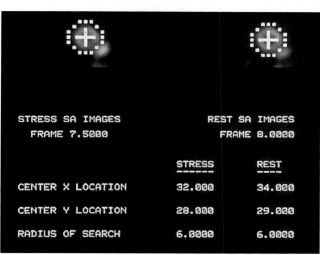

C

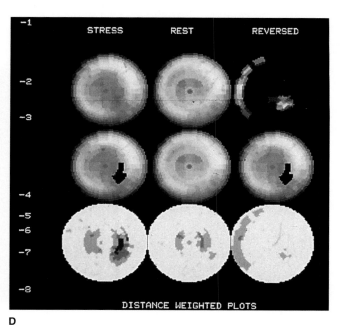

D

Figure 4-21 For the patient example shown in Fig. 4-19, a limiting ROI used for polar map reconstruction was positioned incorrectly, encompassing adjacent bowel activity (**A**). The resulting polar plots (**B**) demonstrate a "hot spot" corresponding to bowel activity included in the bull's-eye radius of search. Correct placement of the limiting ROI to exclude adjacent bowel activity (**C**) eliminates the artifactual "hot spot" in the polar plots (**D**).

or physician to produce visceral contraction and bowel clearance of tracer.

c) High-resolution collimation is useful for improving image resolution, thereby better separating myocardial and abdominal visceral activity. Also, by decreasing Compton scatter, high-resolution collimation improves overall image quality, particularly for ^{99m}Tc labeled tracers, and limits scatter

of abdominal visceral activity into the inferior wall of the left ventricle.

3. Process and display studies to exclude bowel activity
   a) When polar maps are reconstructed, care should be taken to exclude abdominal visceral activity from the limiting region of interest placed around the left ventricle. Once a limiting region of interest has been selected, the short axis tomograms

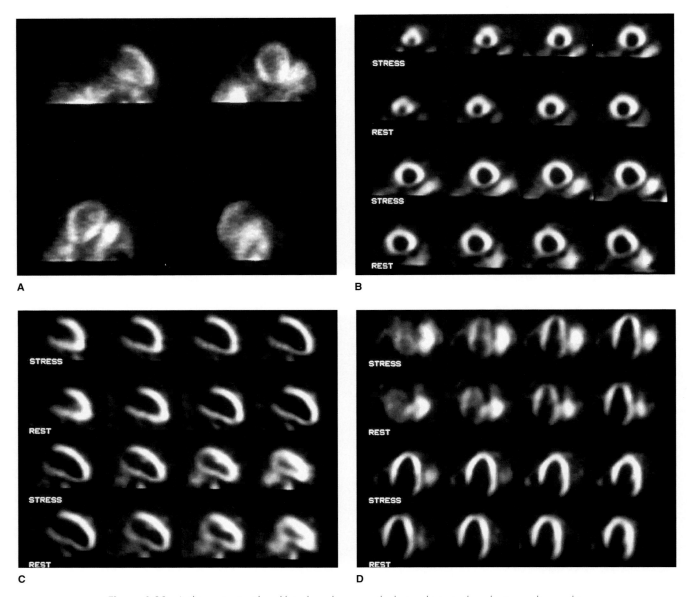

Figure 4-22   In this patient with a dilated cardiomyopathy but no historical or electrocardiographic evidence of myocardial infarction, ^{99m}Tc sestamibi activity is present in the stomach, which lies considerably cephalad due to left hemidiaphragmatic elevation (**A**). In short axis (**B**) vertical long axis (**C**), and horizontal long axis (**D**) tomograms a moderate to marked fixed inferior defect is apparent. This is also demonstrated on the polar map display (**E**). Gated horizontal long axis (**top**) and short axis (**bottom**) tomograms (**F**) demonstrate moderate-to-marked, diffuse hypokinesis, consistent with cardiomyopathy. However, inferior wall motion is no worse than that of the remainder of the ventricle, suggesting that the fixed inferior defect is not due to scar. The defect is more likely due to either diaphragmatic attenuation or the negative component of the ramp filter subtracting inferior wall myocardial activity because of the intense adjacent stomach activity.

should be visualized sequentially ("snaked") to ensure that, if possible, abdominal visceral activity has been excluded from all short axis slices. Note that, if the limiting region of interest is too small, portions of the myocardium may be excluded from the short axis slices and hence from the polar plot radius of search, creating photopenic defects

in the polar map, particularly at the base, where the left ventricular dimensions are the greatest (Fig. 4-21).

b) Some laboratories have found computer "masking" to be useful in simplifying this normalization process. A mask surrounding the entire heart or one manually drawn to exclude only abdominal

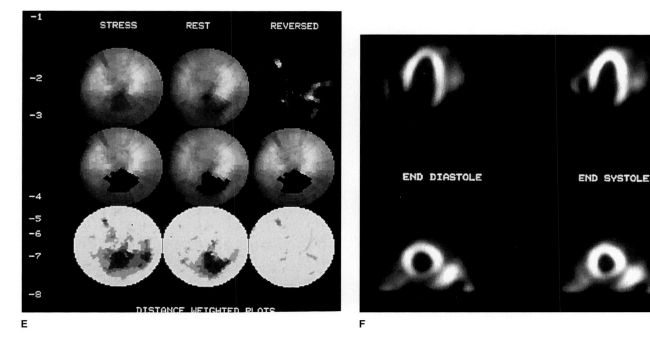

Figure 4-22 (*Continued*)

visceral activity (Fig. 4-23) may be useful. However, great care must be taken not to mask out portions of the left ventricular myocardium. Another "masking" method frequently employed is to drape a lead apron over the patient during SPECT acquisition to exclude abdominal visceral activity. Apart from being uncomfortable for the patient, this method risks attenuating myocardial counts and has no advantage over post-acquisition computer masking since SPECT acquisition intervals, or "stops," are prescribed for a specified time, not total counts per image.

INTERPRETATION OF MYOCARDIAL PERFUSION TOMOGRAMS

Once all of the critical quality control checks described earlier have been performed, the physician is ready to interpret the study.

Characterization of Perfusion Defects

Tomograms should be evaluated systematically (e.g., from base to apex or from apex to base) in the short axis projection, from septum to lateral wall in the vertical long axis projection, and from inferior to superior segments in the horizontal long axis projection). Defects should be subjectively evaluated for *extent* (large, moderate, or small), *severity* (marked, moderate, or mild), and *reversibility* (completely reversible, partially reversible, or fixed), since each of these parameters is an important determinant of patient prognosis. Also, defects should be ascribed to one or more vascular territories.

A left ventricular myocardial segmentation scheme is commonly used for purposes of tomogram analysis for research studies (Fig. 4-24). Vascular territories can be assigned to these various segments. However, for clinical purposes, such a segmental description of perfusion defects is probably too detailed and may result in awkward reports to referring physicians. In contrast, polar maps (even without quantitative analysis) are extremely helpful in determining defect extent, severity, and reversibility, and determining the vascular territory involved and will be discussed in a later section.

Description of defect extent and severity is subjective and therefore varies among interpreting physicians. However, if several physicians interpret myocardial perfusion SPECT studies at a particular laboratory or institution, it is preferable that all of these physicians reach a consensus regarding the terminology used to describe defects. Once this terminology has been standardized, it should be communicated to referring physicians so that scan reports can be meaningfully applied to patient management. Although such terminology will undoubtedly vary from institution to institution, the following may serve as a useful example:

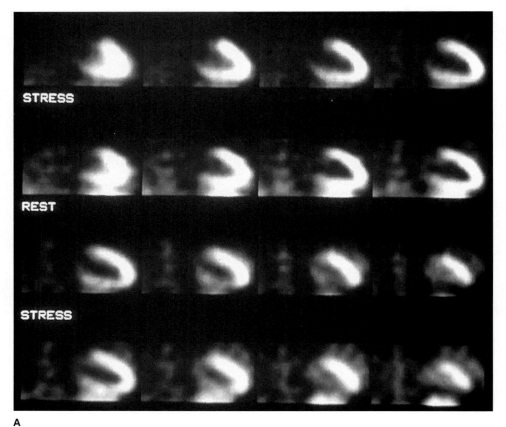

A

Figure 4-23 Technetium-99m sestamibi SPECT vertical long axis slices **(A)** in a patient with a large inferoposterior myocardial infarction. In **B** the tomograms are displayed using a mask around the left ventricle to exclude background activity.

DEFECT EXTENT

large: >⅓ left anterior descending (LAD) territory, or >½ right coronary artery (RCA) or left circumflex artery (LCX) territory

moderate: ⅙ to ⅓ LAD territory, or ¼ to ½ RCA or LCX territory

small: <⅙ LAD territory, or <¼ RCA or LCX territory

DEFECT SEVERITY

marked: <40% maximal myocardial count density

moderate: 40% to 59% maximal count density

mild: 60% to 80% maximal count density

DEFECT REVERSIBILITY

complete: >90% reversible

partial: 30% to 90% reversible

primarily fixed: 10% to 30% reversible

fixed: <10% reversible

With regard to assigning defects to vascular territories, the interpreting physician should be aware of the considerable variability in coronary anatomy. In general, if a large perfusion defect in a single vascular territory extends slightly into an adjacent territory, it is most likely that a single large coronary vessel is involved.

Examples of perfusion abnormalities in tomograms and polar maps are presented in Figs. 4-25, 4-26, and 4-27.

Indirect Indicators of Severe Coronary Artery Disease

Although sensitivities of approximately 98 percent are reported in the literature in detecting perfusion defects in patients with triple vessel coronary artery disease, very occasionally in such patients the perfusion scan will be falsely negative, demonstrating normal, homogeneous perfusion. Moreover, frequently the stress perfusion scan may underestimate the extent and severity of disease in such patients. Abnormalities other than discrete perfusion defects in SPECT myocardial perfusion scans may indicate multivessel coronary disease.

ABNORMAL LUNG UPTAKE

For ^{201}Tl scintigraphy, increased lung uptake with stress has been associated with decreased left ventricular func-

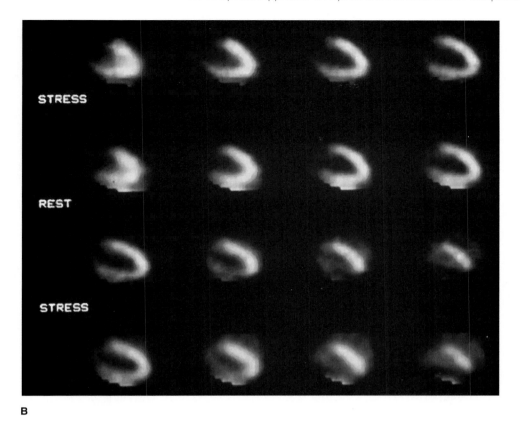

B

Figure 4-23   (Continued)

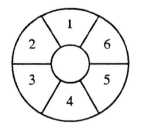

DISTAL SHORT AXIS

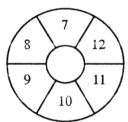

MID SHORT AXIS

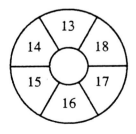

BASAL SHORT AXIS

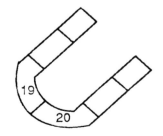

VERTICAL LONG AXIS

Figure 4-24   Segmentation scheme for left ventricular tomography (1) anterior; (2) anteroseptal; (3) inferoseptal; (4) inferior; (5) inferolateral; (6) high lateral; (7) anterior; (8) anteroseptal; (9) inferoseptal; (10) inferior; (11) inferolateral; (12) high lateral; (13) anterior; (14) anteroseptal; (15) inferoseptal; (16) inferior; (17) inferolateral; (18) high lateral; (19) anteroapical; (20) inferoapical.

tion, multivessel or severe coronary disease, and poor patient prognosis.[28,29,30,31,32,33] Increased pulmonary ^{201}Tl activity can often be detected by subjective review of the planar projections viewed in cinematic format (Plate 6). Because of the important clinical implications of increased ^{201}Tl pulmonary activity, routine quantitation of the ratio of pulmonary-to-myocardial activity with stress is highly advisable. Many laboratories perform a separate anterior planar image of the chest before SPECT acquisition to assess pulmonary ^{201}Tl activity. In the anterior view a maximal lung/maximal myocardial uptake ratio greater than 0.55 is considered abnormal. More recently, increased lung uptake of ^{99m}Tc sestamibi in images acquired 30–40 min following a stress injection has also been associated with severe coronary disease and poor left ventricular function.[34] For sestamibi an abnormal lung/maximal myocardial ratio is greater than 0.40. Since the threshold value for abnormal pulmonary sestamibi activity is considerably lower (40 percent) than for ^{201}Tl, and is in a range in which there is little variability in image contrast, increased sestamibi lung uptake is more difficult to detect visually than is increased pulmonary ^{201}Tl activity. For this reason, and to document and quantify the degree of increased lung uptake, many laboratories routinely determine the maximal lung/maximal myocardial count density ratio using a simple region-of-interest analysis (Fig. 4-28). Of note, sestamibi lung uptake progressively decreases following tracer injec-

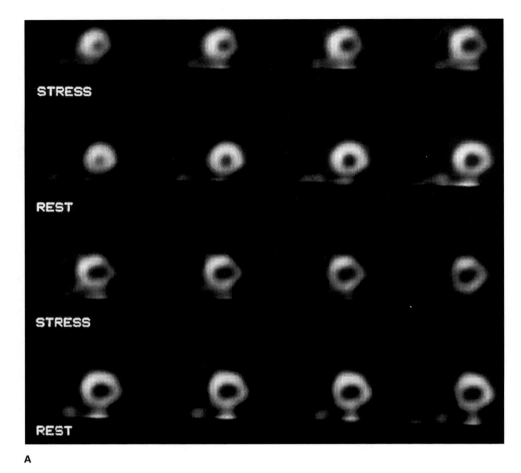

A

Figure 4-25   Stress/rest ^{99m}Tc sestamibi SPECT **(A–D)** in a male patient with a marked, extensive, primarily reversible posterolateral and inferolateral perfusion defect. Angiography demonstrated a critical proximal left circumflex coronary artery stenosis.

tion, so this abnormal threshold value probably cannot be applied to images obtained at different times.[35,36] Technetium 99m sestamibi imaging appears to be less sensitive compared to ^{201}Tl imaging for detecting high-risk pulmonary tracer activity. It should also be noted that patients with impaired left ventricular function due to other etiologies (e.g., cardiomyopathy, valvular heart disease) may demonstrate abnormally increased pulmonary tracer activity with stress, in the absence of coronary artery disease.

TRANSIENT LEFT VENTRICULAR DILATATION

For ^{201}Tl SPECT, "transient ischemic dilatation" of the left ventricle has been described in patients with severe or multivessel coronary disease and is related to a decrease in ventricular function during stress and a consequent increase in left ventricular chamber volume.[37,38,39] The ventricular dilatation persists while the stress ^{201}Tl SPECT images are acquired. Therefore, in stress images the left ventricular cavity will appear larger than in corresponding resting tomograms. Misalignment of stress and

rest images may mimic transient ischemic dilatation if a more basal short axis stress slice is compared to a more apical resting slice. With ^{99m}Tc sestamibi SPECT "transient ischemic dilatation" has also been described in patients with severe or multivessel coronary disease and is related to a decrease in ventricular function during stress and a consequent increase in left ventricular chamber volume. Since sestamibi stress tomographic acquisition is usually not begun until 30 min following the termination of stress, left ventricular dilatation associated with stress in patients with coronary disease may no longer be present unless the deterioration of function during stress is severe. However, if patients develop subendocardial ischemia during stress, with the high spatial resolution of ^{99m}Tc sestamibi SPECT, the stress subendocardial defect adjacent to the left ventricular cavity may make the cavity appear larger and sometimes eccentric in stress images (Fig. 4-29). Poor patient prognosis and the association with multivessel disease has been less well established for transient, stress-induced left ventricular cavity dilatation with sestamibi SPECT than for thallium planar or SPECT imaging.

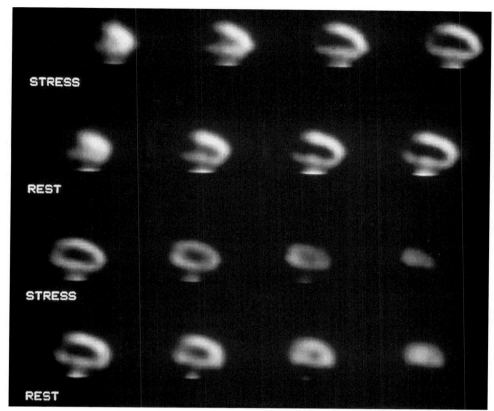

B

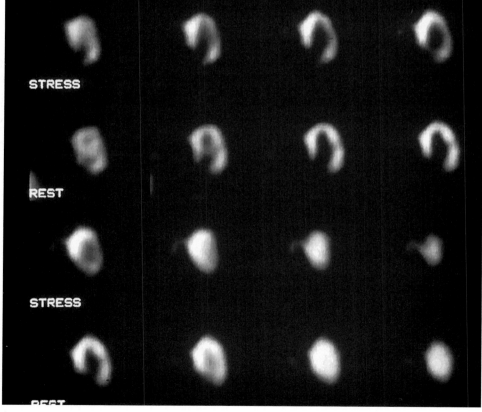

C

Figure 4-25   (Continued)

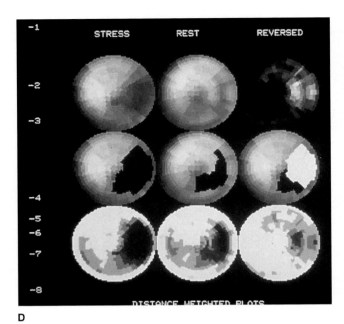

D

Figure 4-25 (Continued)

In patients with severe transmural myocardial infarction a left ventricular aneurysm may form. Such aneurysms have a characteristic appearance on myocardial perfusion tomography.[40] Instead of the walls of the left ventricle being parallel and eventually converging toward the apex in vertical long axis and horizontal long axis tomograms, in the presence of a left ventricular aneurysm they may diverge (Fig. 4-30). Thus, diverging ventricular walls adjacent to a severe, fixed perfusion defect are highly suggestive of an aneurysm. With gated perfusion SPECT, although the myocardium may not be visualized in the aneurysm itself, akinesis or dyskinesis can often be observed in perfused myocardium immediately adjacent to the defects.

"REVERSE REDISTRIBUTION"

Practically since ^{201}Tl myocardial perfusion SPECT was first introduced, a pattern of "reverse redistribution" has been observed in some patients.[41] Since the introduction of ^{99m}Tc labeled agents a similar pattern has been observed. Because ^{99m}Tc sestamibi and tetrofosmin do not redistribute, the term "reverse perfusion" has often been applied. Over the years considerable debate has ensued regarding the etiology of this "reverse redistribution" pattern. Currently the consensus opinion among experts is that it is due to subendocardial scarring distal to a patent proximal coronary artery.[42,43,44,45,46,47] At rest, decreased tracer concentration is present regionally owing to the subendocardial scar. With coronary hyperemia and increased tracer uptake by myocardium overlying the subendocardial scar, the defect is much less evident. Therefore, whereas the stress images may appear normal or nearly normal, a regional perfusion defect is evident in resting images (Fig. 4-31). Clinical circumstances that may result in a subendocardial scar with a patent proximal vessel include myocardial infarction with subsequent successful thrombolysis, infarction with subsequent successful percutaneous transluminal coronary angioplasty, transient coronary artery spasm resulting in infarction, and small vessel occlusive disease resulting in infarction.

However, technical artifacts may mimic "reverse redistribution."[48,49] Owing to tracer washout, the count density of ^{201}Tl images is approximately 50 percent of that in immediate images. Since the same filter is usually applied to both data sets, images often appear more impixelated and attenuation defects appear more marked in the lower count density resting images. This "pseudo-reverse redistribution" pattern is also frequently observed in single-day, low-dose rest/high-dose stress ^{99m}Tc sestamibi SPECT, particularly in obese patients with low count density resting studies where attenuation artifacts are pronounced. Although an image reconstruction filter with a lower cutoff frequency (and sometimes higher power) is often prescribed for such low-dose resting studies, the filter alteration is sometimes inadequate to compensate for very low count density resting studies. Therefore, when a pattern of "reverse redistribution" is observed with myocardial perfusion SPECT, a compatible history should be documented before reporting such a scan finding.

Right Ventricular Perfusion Abnormalities

With the high count density and improved spatial resolution afforded with ^{99m}Tc labeled myocardial perfusion tracers it is usually possible to visualize the right ventricular myocardium.[50] In patients with right coronary artery disease right ventricular ischemia and infarction occur frequently. In approximately 40 percent of patients with infarction of the inferior wall of the left ventricle there is extension to the diaphragmatic wall of the right ventricle.[51,52,53] Right ventricular infarct extension has been associated with increased patient morbidity.[54] Therefore, it is worthwhile to evaluate the right ventricle routinely when myocardial perfusion SPECT is performed with ^{99m}Tc labeled tracers. The right ventricle is not well visualized in perfusion tomograms at the optimal image intensity used to display left ventricular tracer distribution on the computer or on conventional x-ray film, since right ventricular tracer concentration is considerably less. Similarly, right ventricular activity is poorly visualized using color scale displays. However, if short axis tomograms are viewed at the computer console in black and white, the intensity of the monitor can be increased to optimally visualize the right ventricle (Fig. 4-32). In patients with moderate to marked liver tracer concentra-

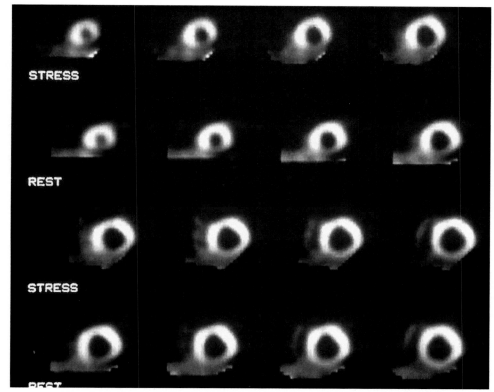

A

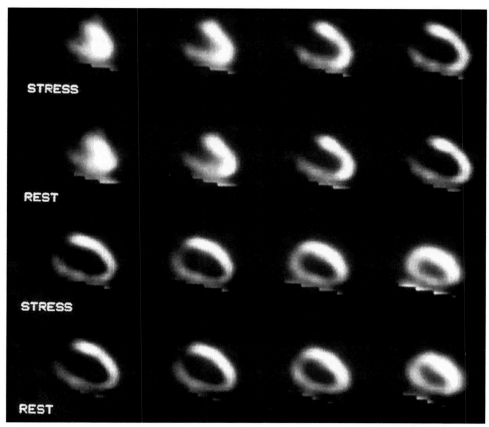

B

Figure 4-26 Stress/rest ^{99m}Tc sestamibi SPECT (A–D) in a male patient with a moderate, extensive, fixed inferior perfusion defect. Left ventricular dilatation is also present. Angiography demonstrated a 100 percent proximal right coronary artery occlusion.

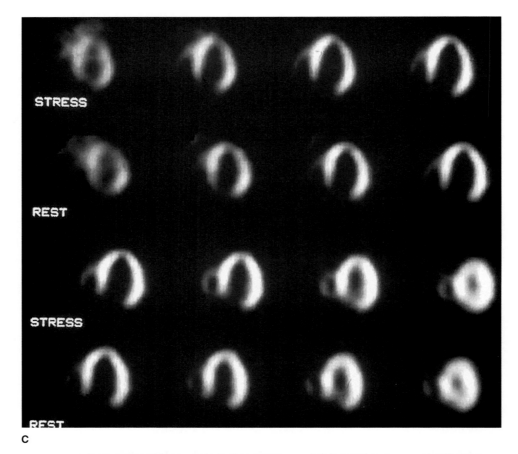

C

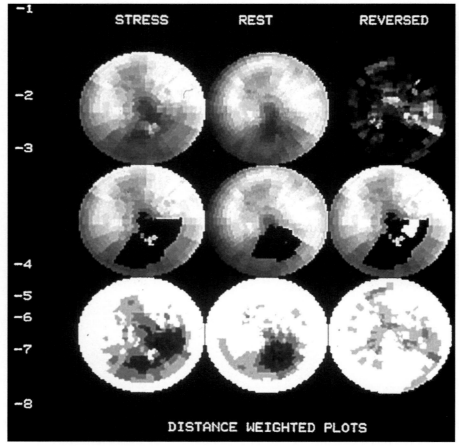

D

Figure 4-26 (*Continued*)

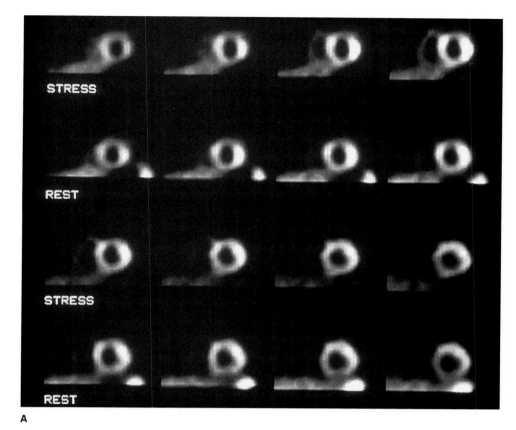

A

B

Figure 4-27 Stress/rest ^{99m}Tc sestamibi SPECT **(A–D)** in a male patient with a moderately severe, moderately extensive, minimally reversible anterior and apical perfusion defect. Angiography demonstrated a 100 percent mid–left anterior descending coronary artery occlusion.

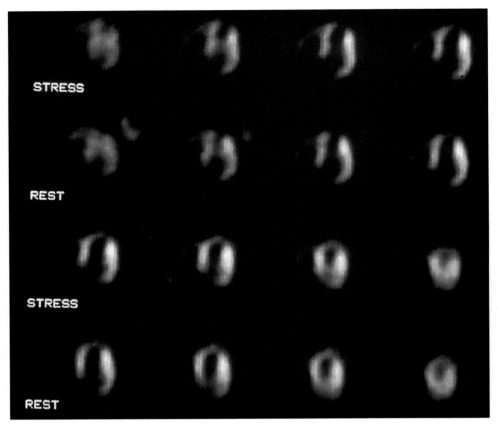

C

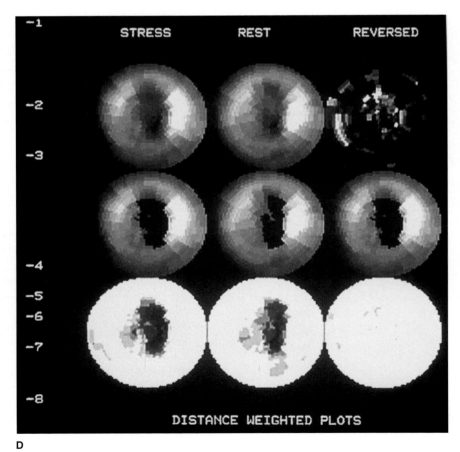

D

Figure 4-27 (*Continued*)

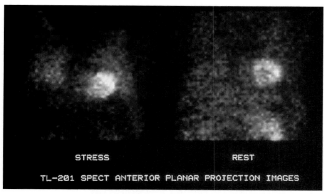

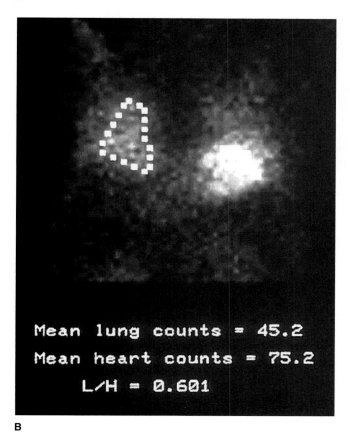

Figure 4-28 **A:** Stress and 4-h delayed ^{201}Tl anterior planar projection images from a SPECT acquisition demonstrating moderately and diffusely increased lung uptake in the stress image. **B:** Regions of interest are placed over the mid right lung and the most intense myocardial region. The calculated lung/heart ratio is 0.601.

of the right ventricle are interpreted with greater confidence than defects at the base near the valve plane. At the base of the right ventricle the pulmonary outflow tract is visualized, and short axis tomograms demonstrate decreased uptake in the region of the right atrium and tricuspid valve plane. Proceeding apically, the anterior free wall and diaphragmatic wall of the right ventricle are visualized. More distally, the right ventricular apex appears to blend with the distal septum. Because of difficulties in differentiating decreased uptake at the base of the right ventricle from a physiologic decrease at the tricuspid valve plane, it is difficult to evaluate the basal third of the right ventricle. However, fixed and reversible perfusion defects involving the distal half of the right ventricle can be discerned with confidence (Fig. 4-32).

Alterations of Tracer Distribution in Patients with Noncoronary Disease

Conditions other than coronary artery disease may result in alterations in tracer distribution within the left ventricular myocardium. Since perfusion scans should be first interpreted without the knowledge of the patient's history (other than gender and body habitus), electrocardiogram, or stress test results, recognition of noncoronary causes of scan abnormalities has been reserved for discussion toward the end of this chapter.

LEFT BUNDLE BRANCH BLOCK (LBBB)

As first described by Hirzel et al for planar ^{201}Tl perfusion imaging, tracer concentration in the septum may be decreased in patients with LBBB.[55] This is postulated to be secondary to contraction and relaxation of the septum out of synchrony with that of the remainder of the left ventricle. Since coronary flow occurs primarily during ventricular diastole, asynchronous septal relaxation results in an actual decrease in septal perfusion. This decrease is more marked at higher heart rates when the period of septal relaxation occupies a greater proportion of the cardiac cycle. Therefore, septal perfusion defects are more marked in stress studies wherein tracer is injected at high heart rates. These defects are partially or entirely reversible in delayed or resting studies where thallium has redistributed in a pattern reflecting resting coronary blood flow or where the ^{99m}Tc labeled tracers have been injected with the patient at rest. By visual scan inspection approximately 50 percent of patients with LBBB but no coronary artery disease undergoing exercise SPECT perfusion imaging demonstrate reversible septal perfusion defects.[56-59]

To avoid such reversible septal perfusion defects, in patients with LBBB pharmacologic coronary vasodila-

tion, visualization of the diaphragmatic wall of the right ventricle with resting ^{99m}Tc sestamibi SPECT is sometimes suboptimal. A more elaborate display and evaluation of the right ventricle can be accomplished by means of a polar map display wherein activity from the adjacent left ventricle is first masked.[50]

Perfusion abnormalities involving the distal portion

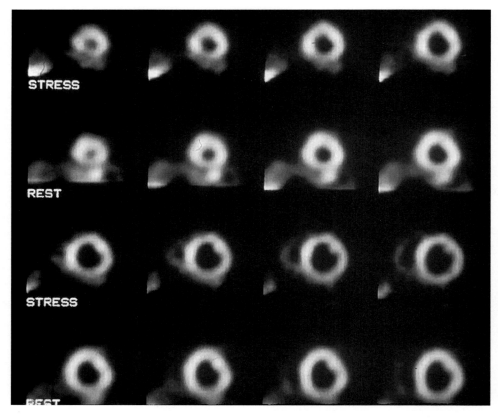

Figure 4-29 Stress/rest ^{99m}Tc sestamibi SPECT in a patient with severe, multivessel coronary disease. Although only minor perfusion abnormalities in the inferior and posterolateral walls are apparent, the left ventricular cavity is more dilated in the stress tomograms compared with the resting tomograms.

tion should be substituted for treadmill exercise since it increases the heart rate only slightly (approximately ten beats/min on average) (Fig. 4-33). Only a minimal incidence of false positive reversible septal perfusion defects have been reported when dipyridamole stress is used in LBBB patients.[60,61] However, occasionally pharmacologic stress results in an unexpected, dramatic increase in heart rate. In such patients decreased septal perfusion may occur owing to the physiologic mechanisms described previously for patients undergoing exercise.

HYPERTENSION AND MYOCARDIAL HYPERTROPHY

Since hypertension is a risk factor for coronary artery disease, hypertensive patients are frequently referred for stress myocardial perfusion imaging. With long-standing hypertension, myocardial hypertrophy frequently occurs, which may alter relative tracer distribution within the myocardium. Similarly, other diseases that result in myocardial hypertrophy such as valvular heart disease may alter tracer distribution.

In patients with myocardial hypertrophy a relative increase in tracer concentration in the septum has been described.[62] This phenomenon has been observed for both ^{201}Tl and ^{99m}Tc sestamibi. This septal increase in tracer concentration is not necessarily attributable to isolated or asymmetric septal hypertrophy, but may possibly be due to blood flow alterations in the septum. The relative increase in septal uptake may be more marked in stress images, with either exercise or pharmacologic agents.

When tomograms and polar maps are displayed, they are normalized to the region of greatest count density. In hypertensive patients with increased septal uptake, images are normalized to the septum, making the remainder of the left ventricular myocardium, particularly the lateral wall, appear to have decreased tracer concentration. When quantitative analysis is performed, these regions are often incorrectly identified as abnormal. Since increased septal uptake is sometimes more marked with stress, these lateral wall defects may appear slightly reversible, mimicking left circumflex coronary ischemia (Fig. 4-34).

HOT SPOTS

In hypertensive patients and in those with myocardial hypertrophy, the papillary muscles may also become hy-

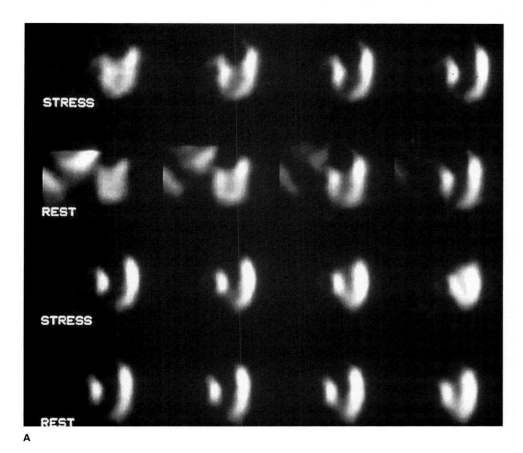

A

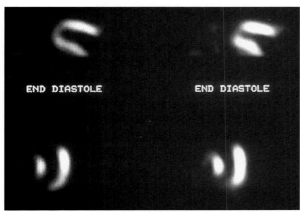

B

Figure 4-30 In this patient with a large apical aneurysm, divergence of the walls of the left ventricle is apparent in ^{99m}Tc sestamibi vertical long axis (shown as Fig. 4-5A) and horizontal long axis **(A)** tomograms. In vertical long axis **(top)** and horizontal long axis **(bottom)** gated tomograms **(B)** there is essentially no activity in the aneurysm, rendering direct assessment of regional function impossible. However, at end-systole divergence of the distal walls of the ventricle is accentuated.

pertrophied. Since the spatial resolution of myocardial perfusion SPECT is usually inadequate to differentiate the papillary muscles from the remainder of the myocardium, particularly with ^{201}Tl, the hypertrophied papillary muscles may appear as localized "hot spots" within the myocardium. With high-resolution images obtainable with the ^{99m}Tc labeled tracers, it is often possible to resolve the anterior and posterior papillary muscles to reveal the cause of the "hot spot" (Fig. 4-35).

"Hot spots" may also occur in the lateral wall and other regions of the myocardium, unrelated to the loca-

tion of the papillary muscles. These seem to occur more frequently with ^{201}Tl than with ^{99m}Tc sestamibi. A frequent location for "hot spots" is the left ventricular apex. These may be due to isolated apical hypertrophy (a variation of asymmetrical septal hypertrophy), the insertion of the right ventricular myocardium into the distal (apical) septum, and, occasionally, attenuation effects in obese women. The last may be due to attenuation of the anterior and lateral walls by the left breast, the inferior wall by the diaphragm, and the septum by the right breast, leaving only the apex relatively unattenuated.

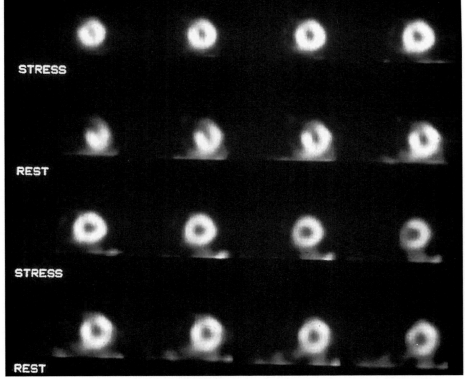

A

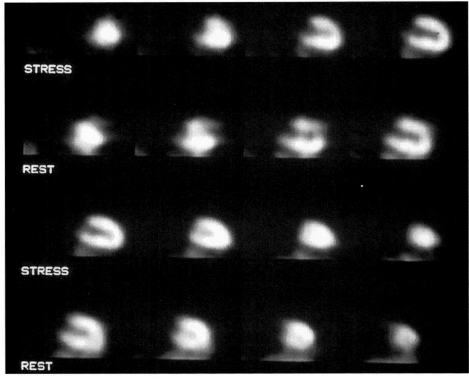

B

Figure 4-31 In this patient with an anterior myocardial infarction who underwent successful thrombolysis, stress/rest ^{99m}Tc sestamibi, short axis **(A)** and vertical long axis **(B)** tomograms and quantitative polar plots **(C)** demonstrate a mild anterior stress perfusion abnormality, which appears more marked in resting images. This "reverse perfusion" pattern has been observed in patients with subendocardial infarction and a patent coronary artery supplying that region of myocardium. Gated SPECT **(D)** demonstrates normal wall motion and thickening.

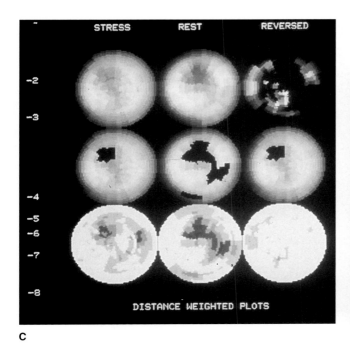

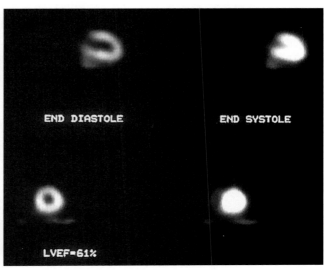

C   D

Figure 4-31 **(Continued)**

As with septal increased count density in hypertensive patients, in patients with "hot spots" as described previously, interpretation of tomograms and polar plots may be confounded because images are normalized to the hot spots, making other myocardial regions appear to have decreased count density. Quantitative analysis can be particularly misleading in such cases. Therefore, it is recommended to "read around" the "hot spot," normalizing image intensity to unaffected regions.

POLAR MAPS

Polar maps are merely a two-dimensional representation of three-dimensional tomographic data. The distribution of tracer can be conveniently evaluated with this display, and perfusion defects can be readily assigned to specific vascular territories.[63] (Fig. 4-36). The polar maps may be used as a hard-copy record of the patient's study and may also serve as a useful means to communicate information to referring physicians. Even without quantitative analysis, i.e., comparison of patient data to gender-matched normal limits, the extent and severity of perfusion defects can be assessed comparatively easily. By direct, side-by-side comparison of stress and rest polar map displays, the extent and degree of defect reversibility can be determined readily.

All of the information contained in tomographic slices is also contained in polar map displays—no less and no more. Therefore, all of the artifacts that affect tomograms will also create defects in the polar map. However, as described previously, whereas inspection of tomograms often suggests the presence of artifacts, there are few if any "clues" to artifacts in the polar maps themselves. For example, whereas apparent misalignment of the contralateral walls of the left ventricle and curvilinear "tails" of activity extending from the edges of opposed anterior and inferior defects ("hurricane sign") suggest patient motion,[64] the polar map will contain only anterior or inferior defects, indistinguishable from perfusion abnormalities involving the left anterior descending and right coronary arteries, respectively (Fig. 4-11). Likewise, whereas differences in left ventricular cavity configuration in corresponding stress and rest tomograms suggest an error in left ventricular axis selection as a cause of a localized basal perfusion defect, only the perfusion defect is observed in the polar map, with no "clues" that it is a technical artifact (Fig. 4-37). Therefore, in order to best recognize artifacts and maintain high diagnostic specificity, inspection of polar map displays should *never* substitute for a careful systematic inspection of planar projection images, quality control images including left ventricular axis, base and apex selection, and tomograms displayed in multiple projections. Instead, the polar map should be used to reinforce and refine the diagnostic impression gained by careful inspection of the tomographic slice inspection.

There are, however, a few artifacts that are unique to polar map reconstruction and display. When apical and basal limits of the left ventricle are selected appropriately, a thin "rim" of decreased activity is usually observed at the periphery (base) of the polar map, always

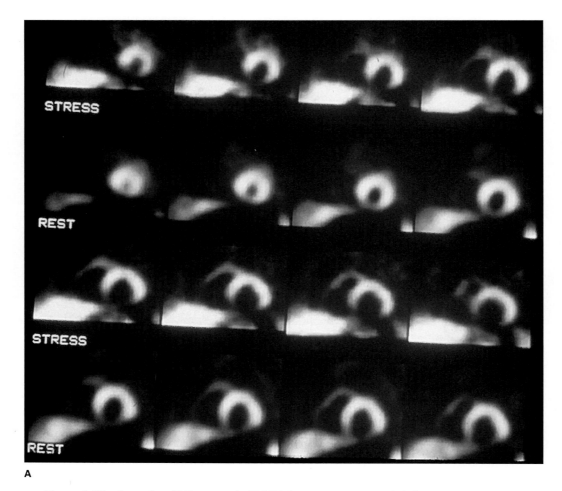

Figure 4-32   Stress/rest ^{99m}Tc sestamibi SPECT short axis tomograms **(A)** demonstrate a marked, extensive, fixed inferior left ventricular perfusion defect. By increasing image intensity **(B)**, an extensive partially reversible defect involving the right ventricle is also apparent.

thickest between the 7-o'clock and 11-o'clock positions because of absent uptake in the membranous septum. However, if the basal limit of the left ventricle is too generous (i.e., positioned in the left atrium), the photopenic rim will be accentuated (Fig. 4-38). In contrast, if the basal limit is too tight, ie, distal to the base, no rim will appear and true basal perfusion defects might be eliminated. Likewise, selection of apical limits too distally will create apparent apical perfusion defects in the polar map (Fig. 4-39), whereas limits that are too tight may eliminate true apical perfusion abnormalities.

Polar Maps: Quantitative Analysis

Quantitative analysis of myocardial perfusion SPECT is most commonly performed by comparison of patient data mapped in polar coordinates (Fig. 3-13, Plate 1A) to gender-matched normal limits. Normal databases are acquired from patients with a very low likelihood of coronary artery disease. In the normalized patient polar maps, pixels more than a specified number of standard deviations below gender-matched mean normal limits are identified. In the "extent" quantitative display all pixels below the specified standard deviation (usually 2.5) are blackened.[63] In one vendor's updated quantitative software for ^{99m}Tc sestamibi SPECT a variable standard deviation threshold is used for different myocardial regions because of greater variability in count density in those regions in the normal population. In the "severity" quantitative display, normal pixels are coded in white and abnormal pixels are color-coded according to the number of standard deviations below normal limits (Plate 5). By these means the quantitative polar map display identifies perfusion defects, potentially increasing test sensitivity for detection of coronary artery disease, but is more likely to identify physiologic variations in count density (e.g., breast attenuation in women, excessive diaphragmatic attenuation in obese patients) as abnormal, potentially increasing test specificity. Moreover, the extent and severity of perfusion defects are quanti-

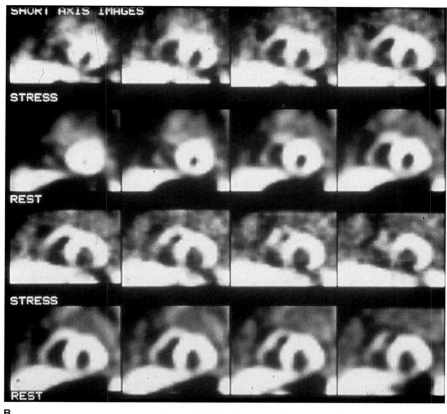

B

Figure 4-32   (Continued)

fied, potentially improving inter- and intraobserver reproducibility.

All of these potential advantages of polar maps are based on the naive assumption that all normal patients free of coronary disease have an actual or apparent distribution of tracer within the left ventricle very similar to the gender-matched normal file. Unfortunately, there is considerable variability in body habitus, cardiac position within the thorax, and so on among the general patient population. Moreover, the patient-to-normal limits comparison assumes the absence of all technical artifacts, no patient motion, etc. Therefore, in patients with a body habitus significantly different from the "normal" population, quantitative analysis will incorrectly identify perfusion defects. Women with very large breasts will be identified incorrectly as having anterior perfusion defects. Men with excessive lateral wall fat will be incorrectly identified as having lateral perfusion defects. Patients who move during SPECT acquisition will be identified as having defects, which may vary in location and severity depending on the time, severity, and direction of motion. Therefore, the interpreting physician must be extremely cautious when interpreting quantitative polar maps. As stated previously for visual analysis of "raw" polar maps, the quantitative polar plots should be inspected only after careful interpretation of tomographic slices. Quantitative data should only be used to

refine interpretations already determined from inspection of tomograms and the raw polar plot.

The reversibility of tomographic ^{201}Tl myocardial perfusion defects can be displayed through the use of a "reversibility" polar plot. By subtracting the normalized stress and rest polar plots, a "reversibility" polar plot is generated, whereby pixels with relatively greater count density at rest compared to stress are identified. These "reversible" pixels are then compared to pixel "reversibility" encountered in normal individuals, and the extent and severity of abnormal reversibility can be identified.

For planar ^{201}Tl imaging delayed tracer washout from the myocardium observed in 3- to 4-h postexercise images has been associated with multivessel coronary artery disease.[29] Similarly, for exercise ^{201}Tl SPECT, delayed tracer washout at 3–4 h following injection can be determined using quantitative polar plot analysis and has been used to demonstrate multivessel disease (Plate 7). However, to evaluate ^{201}Tl washout, several criteria must be met:

1. The patient must achieve ≥ 85 percent of the maximal predicted heart rate since lower levels of exercise will result in less delivery of tracer to the myocardium and consequently less washout.
2. The tracer dose must not be infiltrated, since thallium

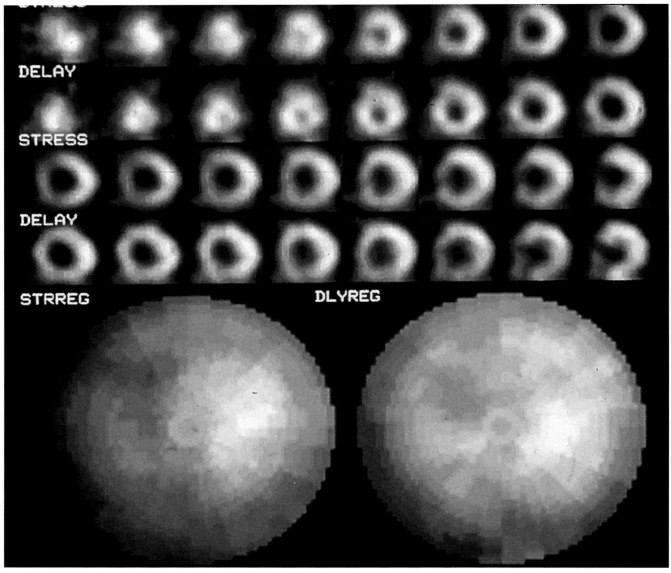

Figure 4-33 Exercise and resting ⁹⁹ᵐTc sestamibi short axis tomograms and polar plots **(A)** in a patient with left bundle branch block and normal coronary arteries. A moderate, reversible septal perfusion defect is present. When the study was repeated with a dipyridamole pharmacologic stress **(B)**, stress images were normal. (Provided courtesy of Alan Rozanski, MD.)

infiltrated into the soft tissues may gradually enter the blood pool and be delivered to the myocardium while myocardial activity extracted previously is washing out.

3. Normal limits for postexercise ²⁰¹Tl washout are not applicable to ²⁰¹Tl washout studies using pharmacologic stress.

4. Many laboratories have adopted a thallium reinjection method to assess myocardial viability whereby a 3- to 4-h delayed image is not obtained, but instead, following stress image acquisition, the patient is reinjected with a "booster" dose of ²⁰¹Tl at rest and rest-

ing/delayed images are obtained subsequently. This stress/reinjection protocol negates the value of ²⁰¹Tl washout analysis.

5. Finally, with ⁹⁹ᵐTc sestamibi, furifosmin (Q12), or tetrofosmin, only very minimal washout occurs, and separate tracer doses are administered for resting studies. Therefore, washout analysis is not applicable with these agents.

The quantitative polar map approach can be especially useful for novice interpreting physicians in helping them identify true perfusion defects. Perfusion defect

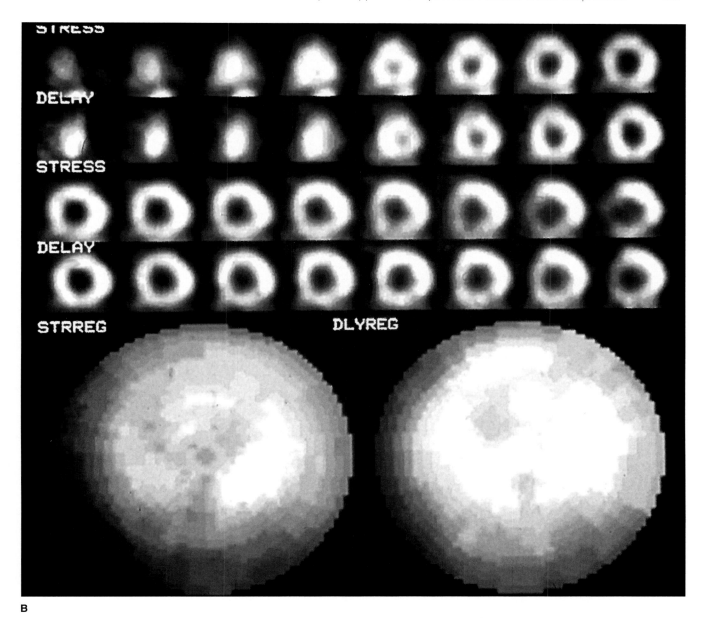

Figure 4-33   (Continued)

extent, severity, and percentage of reversibility all can be quantified as "scores" that can be particularly helpful in evaluating disease progression or the efficacy of medical therapy or intervention (Plate 8). However, for physicians with a moderate or greater degree of experience, the benefit of quantitative analysis is debatable. Experience has shown, in fact, that quantitative analysis is indeed a "doubled-edged sword." Although defects can be more readily identified by quantitative analysis and test sensitivity for coronary artery disease increased, apparent defects due to technical error, instrumentation defects, variations in patient body habitus, etc, can all be accentuated, thereby potentially decreasing test specificity. This pitfall is particularly problematic for the nov-

ice interpreter, since such an inexperienced physician will most likely be least cognizant of all of the potential sources of scan artifacts.

GATED PERFUSION SPECT: VISUAL ANALYSIS

With gated ^{99m}Tc sestamibi SPECT myocardial perfusion and ventricular function can be evaluated simultaneously following a single tracer injection. Although perfusion images obtained following either a stress or rest injection can be gated, the wall motion images are always acquired

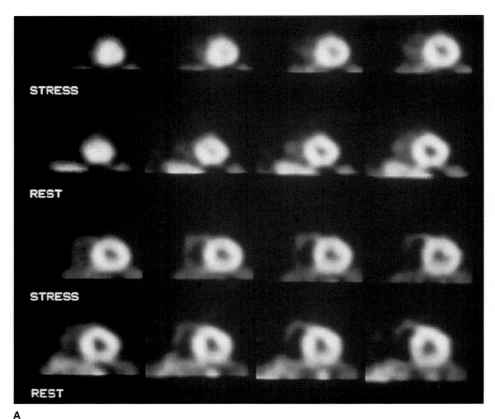

A

Figure 4-34 Stress and rest short axis **(A)** and horizontal long axis **(B)** ^{99m}Tc sestamibi tomograms and quantitative polar plots **(C)** in a patient with long-standing hypertension and borderline left ventricular hypertrophy (LVH) on the electrocardiogram. There is a mild-to-moderate increase in tracer concentration in the distal septum. Since the images are normalized to the "hot" septum, the remainder of the myocardium appears abnormal. Bull's-eye severity plots **(C, bottom row)** demonstrate a characteristic "reverse C-shaped" abnormality. Such findings may be striking in patients with more marked LVH.

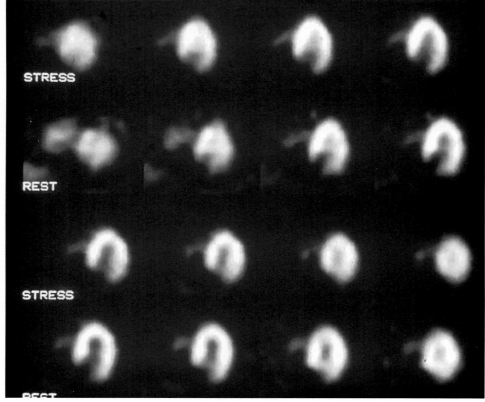

B

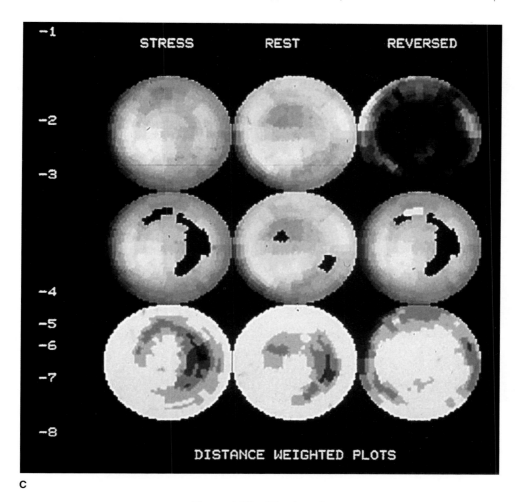

c

Figure 4-34 (*Continued*)

with the patient at rest, so only resting function can be evaluated. Generally, it is preferable to gate the sestamibi SPECT images with the higher count density: the stress images in either a separate-day protocol or a single-day rest/stress protocol, or the resting images obtained with a single-day stress/rest protocol. For adequate gated studies, approximately the same number of cardiac cycles should be acquired for each stop of the tomographic acquisition. Arrhythmias and associated arrhythmic beat rejection software, used routinely for planar gated blood pool imaging, will result in acquisition of a variable number of cardiac cycles during each projection image and can potentially introduce image artifacts (Fig. 4-40, Plate 9). For this reason many laboratories find it more advantageous to accept arrhythmic beats, potentially degrading the integrity of the "end-diastolic" and "end-systolic" frames, but avoiding artifacts due to acceptance of a variable number of cardiac cycles in each projection image. However, considering the fact that most gated SPECT perfusion studies are acquired for only eight frames per cardiac cycle, selected frames seldom truly represent end-diastole and end-systole.

Gated SPECT images are useful to evaluate left ventricular wall motion and wall thickening. Wall motion is best assessed by evaluating endocardial border excursion during systole. Our laboratory has found the black-and-white image display most advantageous for this purpose. Slight image contrast enhancement at the console is helpful in accentuating endocardial borders. A linear gray scale is particularly useful to evaluate areas of markedly decreased count density and is therefore the preferable display to determine wall motion of markedly hypoperfused myocardial regions (Fig. 4-41, Plate 10).

Wall thickening can be evaluated by gated SPECT since for small objects, like the myocardium, owing to the "partial volume effect," an increase in object size is manifested as an increase in image intensity.[65] Therefore, since an observer much more readily appreciates an increase in intensity as a change in color rather than an increase in gray-scale brightness, evaluation of gated SPECT images for wall thickening in color appears to be preferable to black-and-white display (Fig. 4-41, Plate 10). In summary, gated SPECT myocardial perfusion images may be most effectively viewed in dynamic for-

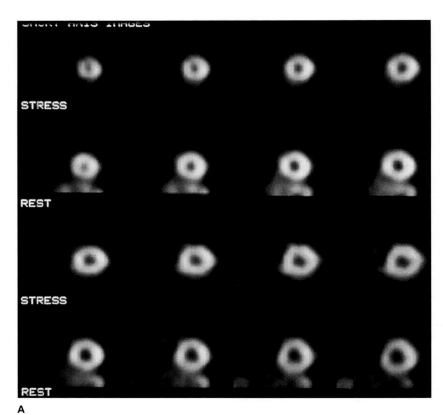

A

Figure 4-35 A posterolateral wall "hot spot" is present in ^{99m}Tc sestamibi short axis (**A**) tomograms and quantitative polar plots (**B**) owing to a prominent posterior papillary muscle. Image normalization to this "hot spot" creates an apparent mild defect in the contralateral anteroseptal wall.

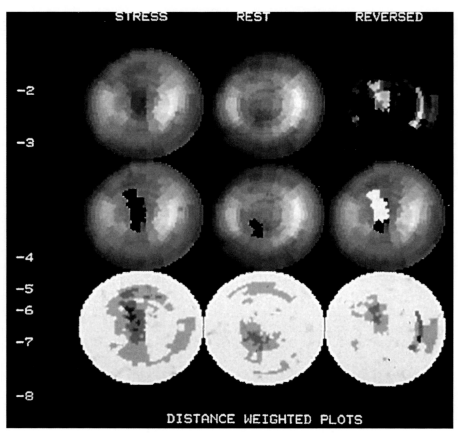

B

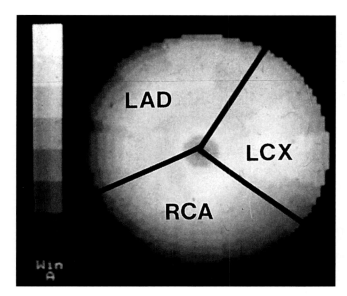

Figure 4-36 Approximate coronary vascular territories superimposed on a normal polar map.

mat, both in black and white to assess wall motion, and in color to assess wall thickening.

The combined assessment of myocardial perfusion and function is of particular value in a number of diseases where ventricular functional abnormalities may coexist with, and often exceed, the severity of perfusion defects. These conditions include valvular heart disease and diffuse small vessel coronary disease, as is observed in diabetics and patients with connective tissue disorders, where epicardial coronary disease and associated regional perfusion defects may be less severe than small vessel disease, which causes a global decrease in left ventricular function (Fig. 4-42). Patients with chest pain referred for perfusion imaging may have an underlying cardiomyopathy that may coexist with coronary disease or may even be the sole cause of the patient's symptoms. Such patients include those with hypertension, renal failure, and drug-related cardiomyopathies.

The value of rest and exercise perfusion imaging in patients with recent myocardial infarction to evaluate infarct size and the presence of additional stress-induced ischemia is well recognized. The incidence of arrhythmias, heart failure, and subsequent cardiac events is related to infarct size. In patients with additional stress-induced ischemia the incidence of death and future cardiac events is significantly greater than in those with normal scans or only fixed perfusion defects. Moreover, it is well known that patient prognosis is directly related to left ventricular ejection fraction.[66] With gated sestamibi SPECT, infarct size, the presence or absence of stress-induced ischemia, and left ventricular ejection fraction (see the following) can all be evaluated using a single study. For many patients this combined assessment can obviate the necessity of a separate echocardiogram

or gated blood pool study to measure ejection fraction and thereby decrease hospitalization cost.

Attenuation artifacts are a significant cause of false-positive perfusion scans, resulting in decreased test specificity and, ultimately, unnecessary expensive cardiac catheterization. As described previously in this chapter, an advantage of gated sestamibi SPECT applicable to a broad spectrum of patients is its ability to differentiate myocardial scar from attenuation artifact as a cause of fixed perfusion defects. Transmural infarcts will demonstrate decreased wall thickening, whereas myocardial segments with diminished tracer activity as a result of attenuation artifacts will move and thicken normally. Although in patients with marked breast or diaphragmatic attenuation both end-diastolic and end-systolic count density may be reduced in the anterior or inferior walls, respectively, the increase in count density from diastole to systole will be equivalent to that in normal myocardium. Thus, by viewing gated tomograms routinely when sestamibi scans are interpreted, test specificity for coronary disease can be improved significantly.[16,17]

Finally, gated sestamibi SPECT has a potential role in the assessment of myocardial viability.[67,68] If a fixed perfusion defect demonstrates relatively preserved wall thickening and motion, this should correspond to the presence of viable myocardium. In contrast, if a myocardial segment containing a perfusion defect does not move or thicken, it may represent scarring, although severely stunned or hibernating, but viable, myocardium cannot be excluded.

Gated Perfusion SPECT: Quantitative Analysis

It is possible to derive quantitative parameters of left ventricular function, including volumes and ejection fraction, from gated sestamibi SPECT. In the horizontal and vertical long axis mid-ventricular tomograms, both at end-diastole and end-systole, the endocardial border can be traced manually or by an automated edge-detection algorithm. From these tracings, the horizontal and vertical dimensions of the ventricular cavity can be determined at each point (pixel) from the apex to the base (Fig. 4-43). After these dimensions are corrected for scatter and the inherent spatial resolution capabilities of the camera/collimator system, left ventricular end-diastolic and end-systolic volumes and ejection fraction are calculated. Ejection fractions determined by this method have correlated closely with those obtained using gated blood pool and first pass RNA techniques.[69-70] Such quantitative methods are particularly useful in assessing changes in ventricular function in patients undergoing sequential studies (Fig. 4-43). Occasionally, in patients with severe perfusion defects it is not possible to define the endocardial border entirely using this method, and thus derivation of quantitative parameters is not possible.

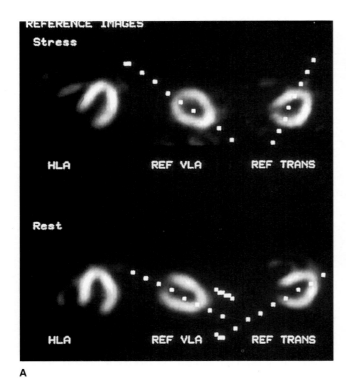

A

Figure 4-37 Incorrect selection of the long axis of the left ventricle in the stress ^{99m}Tc sestamibi transaxial tomogram (**A, upper right image**) is apparent when compared with the correct axis selected in the rest image (**A, lower right**). Resulting stress short axis tomograms (**B**) contain an apparent septal defect due to foreshortening of the septum. Comparing the stress and rest tomograms, differences in the left ventricular cavity configuration are apparent. In the stress vertical long axis tomograms (**C**), in lateral slices the valve plane is lost since the axis transects the lateral wall. Differences in axis alignment are apparent in horizontal long axis tomograms (**D**). As in the short axis tomograms, the stress quantitative polar plots (**E**) contain an artifact involving the base of the septum.

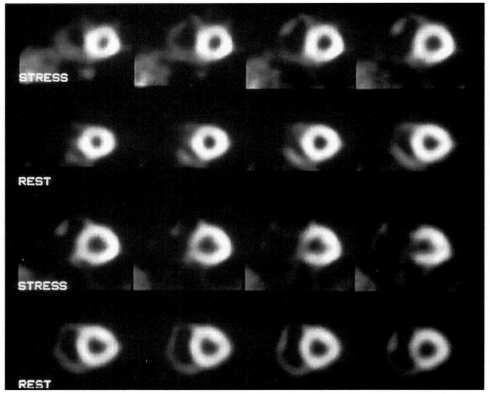

B

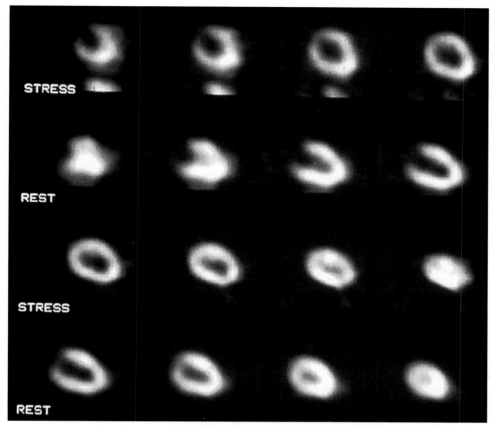

C

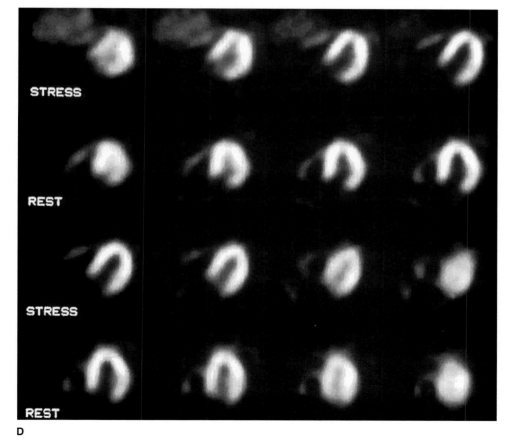

D

Figure 4-37 (*Continued*)

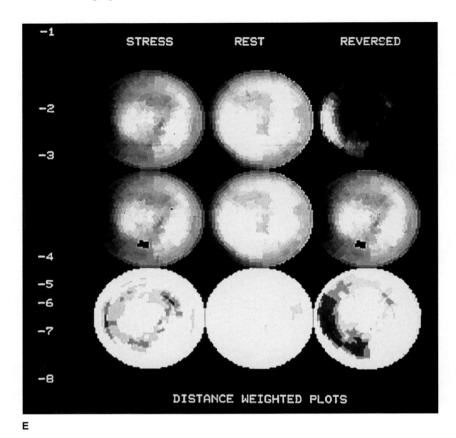

E

Figure 4-37 **(Continued)**

Errors in endocardial border detection can result in significant underestimation or overestimation of left ventricular volumes and ejection fraction. Both manual and automated techniques are subject to particular error at

the valve plane where no myocardium is present and in areas of markedly decreased tracer concentration due to infarction. Therefore, in all cases the interpreting physician should inspect the endocardial borders selected, especially at end-diastole and end-systole. With some automated techniques endocardial borders are computer-determined by searching outward from the left ventricular center until an endocardial edge is detected. Endocardial border detection may be further confounded if the left ventricular center point is placed incorrectly. Therefore, the position of the left ventricular center point should also be reviewed by the physician.

Table 4-2 Reporting of Myocardial Perfusion SPECT Results

When SPECT myocardial perfusion images are viewed in a stepwise, systematic fashion and all of the previous points are considered, results should be reported to include the following:
A) Characterization of defects
 1) Extent
 2) Severity
 3) Vascular territory
 4) Reversibility
 5) Right ventricular myocardial extension
 6) Wall motion (resting)
 7) Wall thickening (resting)
B) Ventricular configuration
 1) Degree of left ventricular dilatation (i.e., volume)
 2) Right ventricular volume
 3) Increased right ventricular tracer uptake or wall thickness
C) Ventricular function
 1) Global left ventricular function (resting)
 2) Global right ventricular function (resting)
D) Ancillary indicators of myocardial ischemia or poor ventricular function
 1) Increased lung uptake
 2) Transient ischemic dilatation

THREE-DIMENSIONAL DISPLAYS

Three-dimensional displays of myocardial perfusion SPECT are available on most nuclear medicine computer systems. Their impact on diagnostic accuracy is poorly documented, and in most laboratories they have not replaced the systematic interpretation of tomographic slices described previously. Presently, most three-dimensional SPECT images are surface maps of myocardial count density (Plates 1, 2, 11). The appearance of the three-dimensional display is therefore dependent on

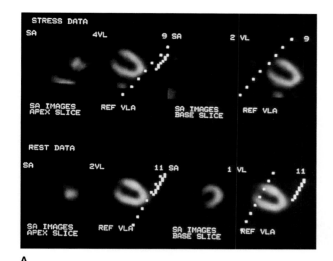

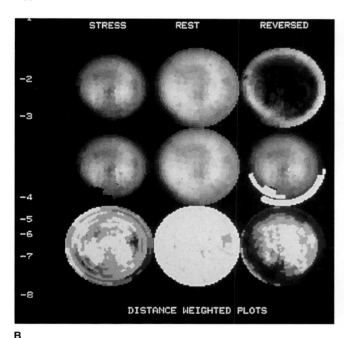

Figure 4-38 The basal limits of the left ventricle are selected too far basally in the stress vertical long axis mid-ventricular tomogram **(upper right)**. The basal limits are selected correctly for the resting study **(lower right) (A)**. In reconstructed polar maps **(B)** there is a resulting "rim" of decreased tracer concentration around the base of the stress study **(upper left)**. The artifact is not present in the resting image. By quantitative analysis a peculiar circumferential reversible basal perfusion abnormality is identified.

the threshold selected to display the myocardial surface. If the threshold is too low, activity immediately adjacent to the heart, such as liver or bowel activity, may blend with the myocardium, rendering these three-dimensional images uninterpretable. Alternately, if the threshold is too high, minimal defects may be greatly accentuated (Plate 12). With more sophisticated reconstruction methods, such as maximum projection im-

aging, three-dimensional images may gain a more important role.[71,72]

CONCLUSION

With a systematic stepwise approach, maximal diagnostic and prognostic information can be obtained from myocardial perfusion SPECT (Table 4-2). In each step of image interpretation the physician should be attentive to possible image artifacts.

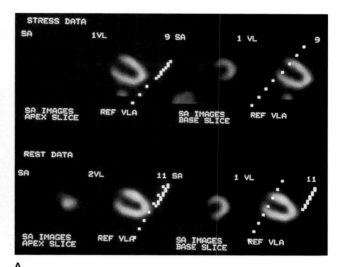

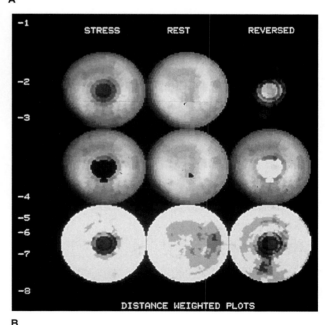

Figure 4-39 The apical limits of the left ventricle are selected too far apically in the stress vertical long axis mid-ventricular tomogram **(upper left)**. The apical limits are selected correctly for the resting study **(lower left) (A)**. In reconstructed polar maps **(B)** there is a resulting artifactual reversible apical perfusion defect.

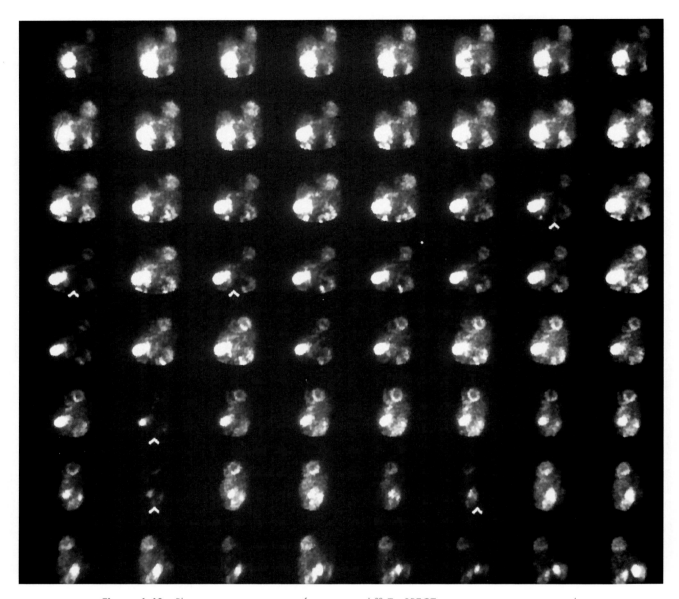

Figure 4-40   Planar projection images from a gated ^{99m}Tc SPECT acquisition in a patient with marked arrhythmia. Despite a 100 percent window (±50 percent) centered over the mean R-R interval, there is considerable rejection of irregular beats. This is manifested by data dropout in individual projection images (arrows). When viewed in endless-loop cinematic format, a "flashing" pattern is apparent.

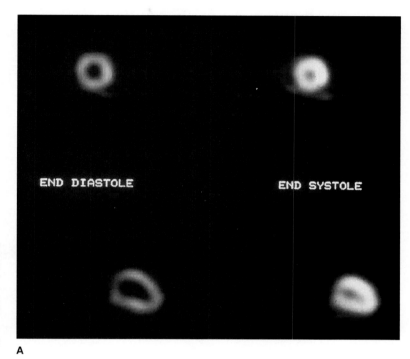

Figure 4-41 A: Normal ⁹⁹ᵐTc sestamibi gated SPECT. Short axis **(top)** and vertical long axis **(bottom)** tomograms are displayed in black and white. **B:** Patient with marked and extensive inferoposterior scarring. In the black-and-white short axis **(top)** and horizontal long axis **(bottom)** tomograms, motion of the severely hypoperfused inferoposterior wall can best be evaluated. (See color plates for corresponding chromatic images.)

A

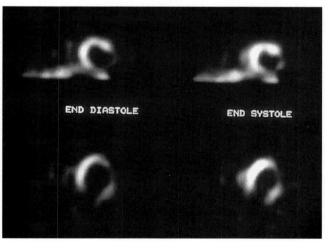

B

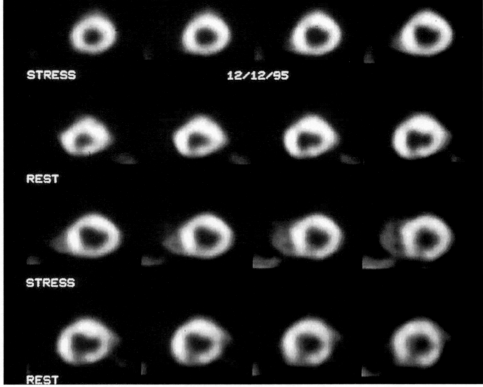

A

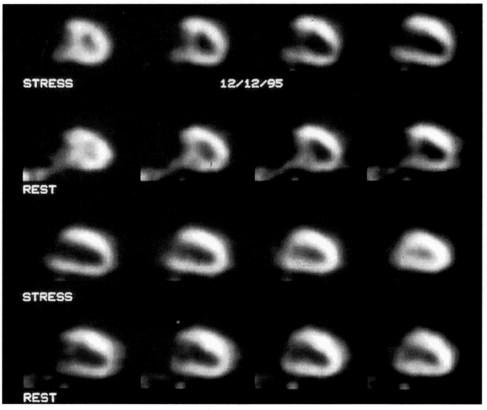

B

Figure 4-42 In this patient with mitral valve insufficiency moderate left ventricular dilation is apparent in stress and rest short axis (A) and vertical long axis (B) ^{99m}Tc-sestamibi tomograms. Myocardial perfusion is normal. End-diastolic and end-systolic images demonstrate normal left ventricular function (C).

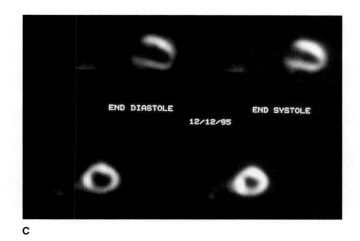

C

Figure 4-42 (*Continued*)

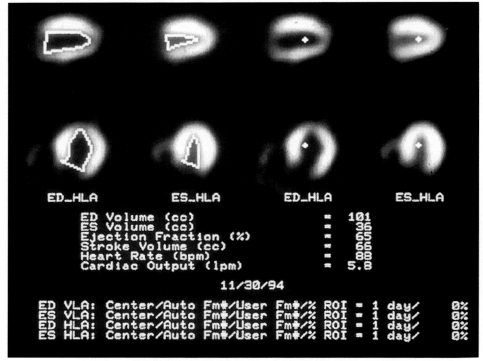

A

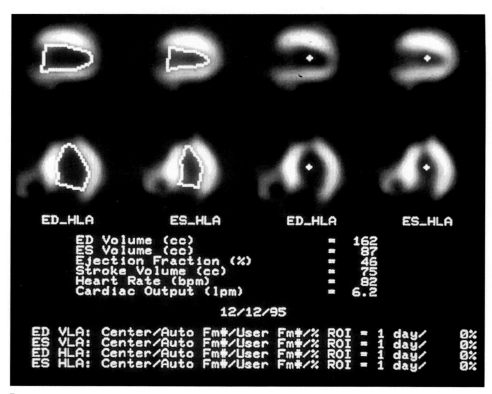

B

Figure 4-43 Quantitative analysis of gated ^{99m}Tc sestamibi SPECT of the case example shown in Fig. 4-42 reveals a borderline increase in left ventricular end-diastolic volume (101 cc), but normal end-systolic volume (35 cc) and ejection fraction (65 percent) **(A)**. Approximately 1 y later the patient presented with worsening dyspnea and atypical chest pain. A follow-up gated stress/ rest ^{99m}Tc sestamibi gated SPECT scan again demonstrated normal perfusion; however, left ventricular function had deteriorated **(B)**. End-diastolic volume had increased (162 cc), end-systolic volume had also increased (87 cc), and ejection fraction had decreased (46 percent). Echocardiography subsequently demonstrated worsening of the patient's mitral and aortic insufficiency.

REFERENCES

1. DePuey EG, Garcia EV: Optimal specificity of thallium-201 SPECT through recognition of imaging artifacts. *J Nucl Med* 30:441, 1989.
2. Standardization of cardiac tomographic imaging. From the Committee on Advanced Imaging and Technology, Council on Clinical Cardiology, American Heart Association; Cardiovascular Imaging Committee, American College of Cardiology; and Board of Directors, Cardiovascular Council, Society of Nuclear Medicine. *J Nucl Med* 33:1434, 1992.
3. Friedman J, Berman DS, Van Train K, et al: Patient motion in thallium-201 myocardial SPECT imaging: An easily identified frequent source of artifactual defect. *Clin Nucl Med* 13:321, 1988.
4. Cooper JA, Neumann PH, McCandles BK: Effect of patient motion on tomographic myocardial perfusion imaging. *J Nucl Med* 13:1566, 1992.
5. Botvinick EH, Yu Yz, O'Connell WJ, Dae MW: A quantitative assessment of patient motion and its effect on myocardial perfusion SPECT images. *J Nucl Med* 34:303, 1993.
6. Prigent FM, Hyun M, Berman DS, Rozanski A: Effect of motion on thallium-201 SPECT studies: A simulation and clinical study. *J Nucl Med* 34:1845, 1993.
7. Cooper JA, Neumann PH, McCandless BK, et al: Detection of patient motion during tomographic myocardial perfusion imaging. *J Nucl Med* 34:1341, 1993.
8. Cooper JA, McCandless BK: Preventing patient motion during tomographic myocardial perfusion imaging. *J Nucl Med* 36:2001, 1995.
9. Friedman J, Van Train K, Maddahi J, et al: "Upward creep" of the heart: A frequent source of false-positive reversible defects during thallium-201 stress-redistribution SPECT. *J Nucl Med* 30:1718, 1989.
10. Germano G, Kavanagh PB, Kiat H, et al: Temporal image fractionation: Rejection of motion artifacts in myocardial SPECT. *J Nucl Med* 35(7):1193, 1994.
11. Eisner RL: Sensitivity of SPECT thallium-201 myocardial perfusion imaging to patient motion. *J Nucl Med* 33:1571, 1992.
12. Eisner RL, Churchwell A, Noever T, et al: Quantitative analysis of the tomographic thallium-201 myocardial bull's-eye display: Critical role of correcting for patient motion. *J Nucl Med* 29:91, 1988.
13. Geckle WJ, Frank TL, Links JM, et al: Correction for patient and organ movement in SPECT: Application to exercise thallium-201 cardiac imaging. *J Nucl Med* 27:899, 1986.
14. Eisner RL, Noever T, Nowak D, et al: Use of cross-correlation function to detect patient motion during SPECT imaging. *J Nucl Med* 28:97, 1987.
15. Germano G, Chua T, Kavanagh PB, et al: Detection and correction of patient motion in dynamic and static myocardial SPECT using a multi-detector camera. *J Nucl Med* 34:1349, 1993.
16. DePuey EG, Rozanski A: Gated Tc-99m sestamibi SPECT to characterize fixed defects as infarct or artifact. *J Nucl Med* 36:952, 1995.
17. Taillefer R, DePuey EG, Udelson J, et al: Comparative diagnostic accuracy of thallium-201 and Tc-99m-sestamibi myocardial imaging in detection of CAD in women. In press.
18. King MA, Tsui BMW, Pan TS, et al: Attenuation compensation for cardiac single-photon emission computed tomographic imaging: Part 2. Attenuation compensation algorithms. *J Nucl Cardiol* 3:55, 1996.
19. Ficaro EP, Fessler JA, Shreve PD, et al: Simultaneous transmission/emission myocardial perfusion tomography: Diagnostic accuracy of attenuation-corrected ^{99m}Tc sestamibi single-photon emission computed tomography. *Circulation* 93:463, 1996.
20. Bailey DL, Hutton BF, Walter PJ: Improved SPECT using simultaneous emission and transmission tomography. *J Nucl Med* 28:844, 1987.
21. Galt JR, Cullum SJ, Garcia EV: SPECT quantification: A simplified method of attenuation and scatter correction for cardiac imaging. *J Nucl Med* 33:2232, 1992.
22. Manglos SH, Bassano DA, Thomas FD: Cone-beam transmission CT for nonuniform attenuation compensation of SPECT images. *J Nucl Med* 32:1813, 1991.
23. Tung C-H, Gullberg GT, Zeng GL, et al: Nonuniform attenuation correction using simultaneous transmission and emission converging tomography, *IEEE Trans Nucl Sci* 39:1134, 1992.
24. Machac J, George T: Effect of 360° SPECT prone imaging on Tl-201 myocardial perfusion studies. *J Nucl Med* 21:812, 1990.
25. Kiat H, Van Train KF, Friedman JD, et al: Quantitative stress-redistribution thallium 201 SPECT using prone imaging: Methodologic development and validation. *J Nucl Med* 33:1509, 1992.
26. O'Connor MK, Bothun ED: Effects of tomographic table attenuation on prone and supine cardiac imaging. *J Nucl Med* 36:1102, 1995.
27. King MA, Xia W, deVries DJ, et al: A Monte Carlo investigation of artifacts caused by liver uptake in single photon emission computed tomography perfusion imaging with technetium 99m labeled agents. *J Nucl Cardiol* 3:18, 1996.
28. Boucher CA, Zir LM, Beller Ga, et al: Increased lung uptake of thallium 201 during exercise myocardial imaging: Clinical, hemodynamic and angiographic implications in patients with coronary artery disease. *Am J Cardiol* 46:189, 1980.
29. Levy R, Rozanski A, Berman DS, et al: Analysis of the degree of pulmonary thallium washout after exercise in patients with coronary artery disease. *J Am Coll Cardiol* 2:719, 1983.
30. Villanueva FS, Kaul S, Smith WH, et al: Prevalence and correlates of increased lung/heart ratio of thallium 201 during dipyridamole stress imaging for suspected coronary artery disease. *Am J Cardiol* 66:1324, 1990.
31. Gill JB, Ruddy TD, Newell JB, et al: Prognostic importance of thallium uptake by the lungs during exercise in coronary artery disease. *N Engl J Med* 317:1486, 1987.
32. Bingham JH, McKusick KA, Strauss HW, et al: Influence of coronary artery disease on pulmonary uptake of thallium 201. *Am J Cardiol* 46:821, 1980.
33. Tamaki N, Itoh H, Ishi Y, et al: Hemodynamic significance

of increased lung uptake of thallium 201. *Am J Roentgenol* 138:223, 1982.

34. Giubbini R, Campini R, Milan E, et al: Evaluation of technetium-99m-sestamibi lung uptake: Correlation with left ventricular function. *J Nucl Med* 36:58, 1995.

35. Saha M, Farrand TF, Brown KA: Lung uptake of technetium 99m sestamibi: Relation to clinical, exercise, hemodynamic, and left ventricular function variables. *J Nucl Cardiol* 1:52, 1994.

36. Hurwitz GA, Fox SP, Driedger AA, et al: Pulmonary uptake of sestamibi on early post-stress images: Angiographic relationships, incidence and kinetics. *Nuclear Medicine Communications* 14:15, 1993.

37. Weiss AT, Berman DS, Lew AS, et al: Transient ischemic dilation of the left ventricle on stress thallium-201 scintigraphy: A marker of severe and extensive coronary artery disease. *J Am Coll Cardiol* 9(4):752, 1987.

38. Stolzenberg J: Dilation of the left ventricular cavity on stress thallium scan as an indicator of ischemic disease. *Clin Nucl Med* 5:289, 1980.

39. Chouraqui P, Rodrigues E, Berman D, Maddahi J: Significance of dipyridamole induced transient dilation of the left ventricle during thallium-201 scintigraphy in suspected coronary artery disease. *Am J Cardiol* 66(7):689, 1990.

40. Alazraki N, Taylor A: "Diverging wall" sign of apical aneurysm on thallium-201 SPECT images. *Clin Nucl Med* 10:13, 1985.

41. Hecht HS, Hopkins JM, Rose JG, et al: Reverse redistribution: Worsening of thallium-201 myocardial images from exercise to redistribution. *Radiology* 140:177, 1981.

42. Silberstein EB, DeVries DF: Reverse redistribution phenomenon in thallium-201 stress tests: angiographic correlation and clinical significance. *J Nucl Med* 26:707, 1985.

43. Weiss AT, Maddahi J, Lew AS, et al: Reverse redistribution of thallium 201: A sign of nontransmural myocardial infarction with patency of the infarct-related coronary artery. *J Am Coll Cardiol* 7:61, 1986.

44. Nishimura T, Uehara T, Hayshida K, Kozuka T: Clinical significance of ^{201}Tl reverse redistribution in patients with aorto-coronary bypass surgery. *Eur J Nucl Med* 13:139, 1987.

45. Popma JJ, Smitherman TC, Walker BS, et al: Reverse redistribution of thallium 201 detected by SPECT imaging after dipyridamole in angina pectoris. *Am J Cardiol* 65:1176, 1990.

46. Pace L, Cuocolo A, Maurea S, et al: Reverse redistribution in resting thallium-201 myocardial scintigraphy in patients with coronary artery disease: Relation to coronary anatomy and ventricular function. *J Nucl Med* 34:1688, 1993.

47. Pace L, Cuocolo A, Marzullo P, et al: Reverse redistribution in resting thallium 201 myocardial scintigraphy in chronic coronary artery disease: An index of myocardial viability. *J Nucl Med* 36:1968, 1995.

48. Brown KA, Benoit L, Clements JP, Wackers FJTh: Fast washout of thallium 201 from area of myocardial infarction: Possible artifact of background subtraction. *J Nucl Med* 28:945, 1987.

49. Leppo J: Thallium washout analysis: Fact or fiction? *J Nucl Med* 28:1058, 1987.

50. DePuey EG, Jones ME, Gasera EV: Evaluation of right ventricular regional perfusion with ^{99m}Tc sestamibi SPECT. *J Nucl Med* 32:1199, 1991.

51. Andersen HR, Falk E, Nielsen D: Right ventricular infarction: Frequency size and topography in coronary disease: A prospective study comprising 107 consecutive autopsies from a coronary care unit. *J Am Coll Cardiol* 10:1223, 1987.

52. Isner JM: Right ventricular myocardial infarction. *JAMA* 259:712, 1988.

53. Isner JM, Roberts WC: Right ventricular infarction complicating left ventricular infarction secondary to coronary heart disease: Frequency, location-associated findings and significance from analysis of 236 necropsy patients with acute of healed myocardial infarction. *Am J Cardiol* 42:885, 1978.

54. Strauss HD, Sobel BE, Roberts R: The influence of occult right ventricular infarction on enzymatically estimated infarct size, hemodynamics and prognosis. *Circulation* 62:503, 1980.

55. Hirzel HO, Senn M, Nuesch K, et al: Thallium-201 scintigraphy in complete left bundle branch block. *Am J Cardiol* 53:1309, 1984.

56. DePuey EG, Krawczynska EG, Robbins WL: Thallium-201 SPECT in coronary artery disease patients with left bundle branch block. *J Nucl Med* 29:1479, 1988.

57. Burns RJ, Galligan L, Wright LM, et al: Improved specificity of myocardial thallium-201 single photon emission computed tomography in patients with left bundle branch block by dipyridamole. *Am J Cardiol* 68:504, 1991.

58. Matzer LA, Kiat H, Friedman JD, et al: A new approach to the assessment of tomographic thallium-201 scintigraphy in patients with left bundle branch block. *J Am Coll Cardiol* 17:1309, 1991.

59. Civelek AC, Gozukara I, Durski K, et al: Detection of left anterior descending coronary artery disease in patients with left bundle branch block. *Am J Cardiol* 70:1565, 1992.

60. Rockett JF, Chadwick W, Moinuddin M, et al: Intravenous dipyridamole thallium-201 SPECT imaging in patients with left bundle branch block. *Clin Nucl Med* 6:401, 1990.

61. Larcos G, Brown ML, Gibbons RJ: Role of dipyridamole thallium-201 imaging in left bundle branch block. *Am J Cardiol* 68:1097, 1991.

62. DePuey EG, Guertler-Krawczynska E, Perkins JV, et al: Alterations in myocardial thallium-201 distribution in patients with chronic systemic hypertension undergoing single photon emission computed tomography. *Am J Cardiol* 62:234, 1988.

63. DePasquale EE, Nody AC, DePuey EG, et al: Quantitative rotational thallium-201 tomography for identifying and localizing coronary artery disease. *Circulation* 77:316, 1988.

64. Sorrell V, Figueroa B, Hansen CL: The "hurricane sign": Evidence of patient motion artifact on cardiac single photon emission computed tomographic imaging. *J Nucl Cardiol* 3:86, 1996.

65. Cooke CD, Garcia EV, Cullom SJ, et al: Determining the accuracy of calculating systolic wall thickening using a fast Fourier transform approximation: A simulation study

based on canine and patient data. *J Nucl Med* 35:1185, 1994.

66. Pryor DB, Harrell FE Jr, Lee KL, et al: An improving prognosis over time in medially treated patients with coronary artery disease. *Am J Cardiol* 52:444, 1993.

67. Chua T, Kiat H, Germano G, et al: Gated technetium-99m sestamibi for simultaneous assessment of stress myocardial perfusion, postexercise regional ventricular function and myocardial viability. *J Am Coll Cardiol* 23:1107, 1994.

68. Hambye AS, VanDen Branden F, Vandevivere J: Diagnostic value of ^{99m}Tc sestamibi gated SPECT to assess viability in a patient after acute myocardial infarction. *Clin Nuc Med* 21(1):19, 1996.

69. DePuey EG, Nichols KN, Dobrinsky C: Left ventricular ejection fraction from gated Tc-99m sestamibi SPECT. *J Nucl Med* 34:1871, 1993.

70. Germano G, Kiat H, Kavanagh PB, et al: Automatic quantification of ejection fraction from gated myocardial perfusion SPECT. *J Nucl Med* 36:2138, 1995.

71. Faber TL, Akers MS, Peshock RM, Corbett JR: Three-dimensional motion and perfusion quantification in gated single-photon emission computed tomograms. *J Nucl Med* 32:2311, 1991.

72. Faber TL, Cooke CD, Peifer JW, et al: Three-dimensional displays of left ventricular epicardial surface from standard cardiac SPECT perfusion quantification techniques. *J Nucl Med* 26:697, 1995.

Myocardial Viability in Chronic Coronary Artery Disease: Perfusion, Metabolism, and Contractile Reserve

Vasken Dilsizian
James A. Arrighi

Over the past two decades, paradigms concerning the relationship between myocardial perfusion and left ventricular function have changed dramatically with the introduction of two pathophysiological states: stunned[1] and hibernating[2] myocardia. Substantial data now exist to indicate that under certain conditions, when viable myocytes are subjected to ischemia, prolonged alterations in regional or global left ventricular function may occur and that this dysfunction may be completely reversible.[3-13] Therefore, contrary to the conventional wisdom, impaired left ventricular function at rest in patients with coronary artery disease is not necessarily an irreversible process.[14-19]

Stunned myocardium refers to the state of persistent regional dysfunction after a transient period of ischemia that has been followed by reperfusion, and is most likely operative in many acute coronary syndromes.[1] Hibernating myocardium refers to persistent regional left ventricular dysfunction arising from prolonged myocardial hypoperfusion at rest.[2] The distinction between these two pathophysiological states may have important clinical implications. In the case of stunning, intervention aimed at reducing the number, severity, or duration of ischemic episodes would be expected to result in improvement in contractile function. In the case of hibernation, interventions that favorably alter the supply-demand relationship of the myocardium, either improvement in blood flow or reduction in demand, would result in functional improvement. If stunned and hibernating states indeed can be altered by therapeutic interventions, then the identification of such states prospectively in a particular patient

may have significant clinical relevance, in part because left ventricular function is a major determinant of survival in coronary artery disease.[20-24]

The goal of myocardial viability assessment, therefore, is to differentiate, prospectively, patients with potentially reversible from irreversible left ventricular dysfunction. Ideally, such information would be used to guide therapeutic decisions for revascularization. This may result in more appropriate utilization of resources and enhanced efficiency of health care delivery.

Currently, there are a number of diagnostic techniques for assessing myocardial viability in patients with stunned and hibernating myocardium.[25] Among them, evaluation of regional perfusion, cell membrane integrity, and metabolism using nuclear techniques, as well as contractile reserve with low-dose dobutamine echocardiography, have gained considerable interest for differentiating viable from nonviable myocardium in asynergic regions. Although more conventional approaches of identifying scarred and necrotic myocardium include presence of occluded coronary artery,[26-32] regional contractile dysfunction,[3-13] and electrocardiographic Q wave,[16,33-35] they have been shown to be less accurate. New modalities on the horizon include the use of metabolic tracers with single photon emission tomography (SPECT), more precise quantitative metabolic evaluations with positron emission tomography (PET), echocardiographic assessment of perfusion with contrast agents, and the use of magnetic resonance imaging. This chapter will focus on the assessment of myocardial ischemia and viability in patients with chronic heart disease and hibernating myocardium. Evaluation of myocardial viability in the setting of acute coronary syndromes will be discussed elsewhere.

Chronic Coronary Artery Disease and Myocardial Ischemia

Unlike acute myocardial syndromes (unstable angina or myocardial infarction) where impairment of coronary blood flow is caused by abrupt plaque rupture, thrombus formation, and vascular occlusion,[36–39] chronic coronary artery syndromes result from a slower progression of atherosclerosis in response to chronic endothelial injury.[37] Clinical manifestations of such slow progression of atherosclerosis include chronic stable angina, silent ischemia or infarction, and chronic hibernation.

CORONARY FLOW RESERVE

Regional myocardial blood flow is critically dependent on the driving pressure gradient and the resistance of the vascular bed. Despite wide fluctuations in coronary perfusion pressure, the coronary vascular bed maintains regional blood flow within a narrow range via autoregulation.[40] Hence, despite chronic, progressive coronary artery stenosis, regional blood flow at rest may be unaffected until the stenosis exceeds 90 percent of the normal vessel diameter.[41] In the absence of flow-limiting coronary artery stenosis, maximum blood flow (coronary flow reserve) in normal subjects is approximately five times that measured under resting conditions.[42] In the presence of subcritical coronary artery stenosis, however, autoregulation is incapable of preserving maximum blood flow during exercise or pharmacological stress. Hence, unlike flow under resting conditions, coronary blood flow reserve may be reduced with only a 50 percent coronary artery stenosis, affecting more the endocardial rather than epicardial layers.[43] Myocardial perfusion imaging, therefore, identifies subcritical coronary artery stenosis when performed in conjunction with exercise or pharmacologic stress but not at rest.

MYOCARDIAL ISCHEMIA

Imbalance between oxygen supply, usually due to reduced regional myocardial perfusion, and oxygen demand, determined primarily by the rate and force of regional contraction, is termed ischemic myocardium. Clinical presentation of such imbalance may be symptomatic (angina pectoris) or asymptomatic (silent ischemia). If the oxygen supply-demand imbalance is transient (i.e., triggered by exertion), it represents reversible ischemia. In the absence of myocardial necrosis, the degree of regional contractile dysfunction has been shown to be proportional to the extent of myocardial isch-

emia.[44–47] On the other hand, if regional oxygen supply-demand imbalance is prolonged (i.e., during myocardial infarction), high energy phosphates will be depleted, regional contractile function will progressively deteriorate,[48] and cell membrane rupture with cell death will ensue (myocardial infarction).

Hibernating Myocardium

The concept that left ventricular dysfunction at rest is not necessarily an irreversible process was proposed by Rahimtoola.[2] Prolonged, subacute or chronic myocardial hypoperfusion, in which myocytes remain viable but regional contractility is reduced to match the reduced blood supply, has been termed hibernating myocardium (Fig. 5-1). The clinical observation that restoration of myocardial blood flow may result in recovery of regional and global left ventricular function (Fig. 5-2) suggests that some asynergic regions at rest may represent hibernating but viable myocardium.[1,2,8–12,14–19] It has been suggested that during hibernation, a new state of equilibrium is reached between blood flow (oxygen supply) and contraction (oxygen demand) whereby myocardial necrosis is prevented. Therefore, hibernation is a protective response of the myocytes to decrease oxygen demand in the setting of decreased oxygen availability, thereby reestablishing perfusion-contraction coupling.[49] Since there are no adequate animal models of hibernation, the precise pathophysiological mechanisms responsible for the reduced contractile function have not been established. In addition, there are no serial studies in patients in whom hibernating myocardium has been shown to be a truly chronic condition. It is conceivable that some cases of presumed hibernation may represent stunning. Other cases may represent intermittent stunning with hibernation, in which chronically underperfused myocardium becomes transiently ischemic (regional oxygen supply-demand imbalance).[50]

Among patients with preoperative left ventricular dysfunction at the National Institutes of Health,[51] nearly one-third exhibited a significant increase in global left ventricular ejection fraction after coronary artery bypass surgery (Fig. 5-3). Of interest, the severity of the left ventricular dysfunction at rest did not predict the results of revascularization. Recently, an identical prevalence of hibernating myocardium (one-third) was reported by investigators at the Mayo Clinic,[52] among patients with coronary artery disease and left ventricular dysfunction referred for coronary artery bypass surgery. In a different group of patients,[18] increase in global left ventricular function at rest was shown to be related to the extent of ischemic regions manifesting an improvement in regional systolic function after revascularization (Fig. 5-4). Hence, prospective distinction of hibernating but

Hibernating Myocardium

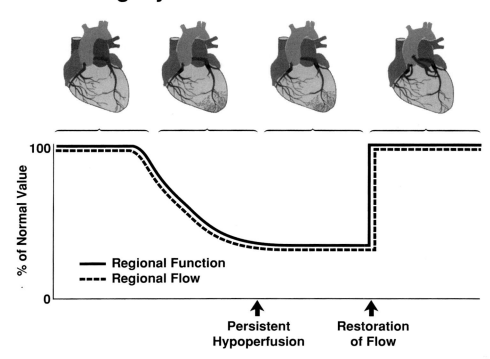

Figure 5-1 A schematic diagram of hibernating myocardium.

viable myocardium from scarred myocardium on the basis of preoperative resting left ventricular function alone can be clinically difficult. Therefore, the utility of thallium-201 (^{201}Tl) scintigraphy, technetium-99m-labeled perfusion tracers, positron emission tomography, and dobutamine echocardiography for the evalua-

**Pre-Operative
Single vessel disease
– Occluded L.A.D.**

LVED = 128
EF = 0.37

**8 Months
Post-Operative
Patent Coronary By-Pass
Graft to L.A.D.**

LVED = 104
EF = 0.76

——— End-diastole
- - - - End-systole

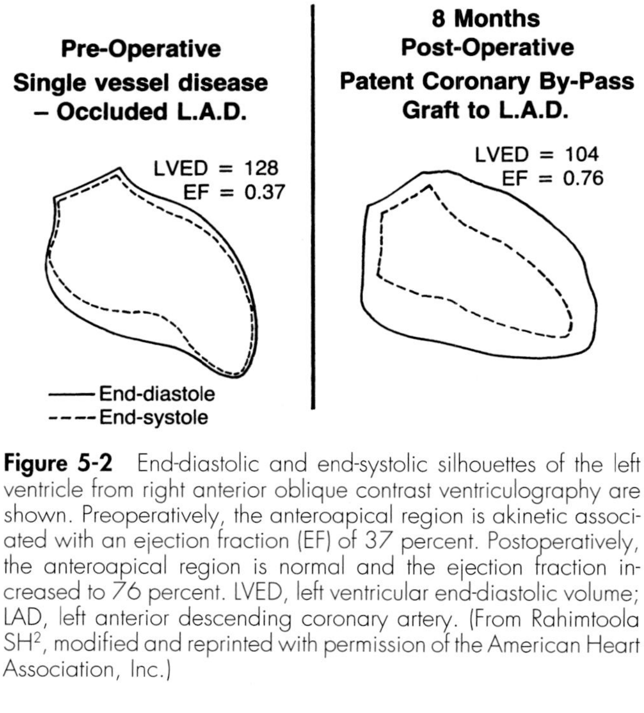

Figure 5-2 End-diastolic and end-systolic silhouettes of the left ventricle from right anterior oblique contrast ventriculography are shown. Preoperatively, the anteroapical region is akinetic associated with an ejection fraction (EF) of 37 percent. Postoperatively, the anteroapical region is normal and the ejection fraction increased to 76 percent. LVED, left ventricular end-diastolic volume; LAD, left anterior descending coronary artery. (From Rahimtoola SH[2], modified and reprinted with permission of the American Heart Association, Inc.)

tion of myocardial viability in patients with chronic coronary artery disease will be discussed.

THALLIUM-201 SCINTIGRAPHY

For the last two decades, ^{201}Tl has been a clinically important tracer with which to assess both regional blood flow and myocardial viability. Myocardial uptake early after intravenous injection of ^{201}Tl is proportional to regional blood flow with a high first-pass extraction fraction in the range of 85 percent.[53] Like potassium, ^{201}Tl is transported across the myocyte sarcolemmal membrane via the Na-K ATPase transport system.[54,55] Experimental studies with ^{201}Tl have demonstrated that the cellular extraction of ^{201}Tl across the cell membrane is unaffected by hypoxia unless irreversible injury is present.[56,57] Similarly, pathophysiologic conditions of chronic hypoperfusion (hibernating myocardium) and postischemic dysfunction (stunned myocardium), in which regional contractile function is impaired in the presence of myocardial viability, do not adversely alter extraction of ^{201}Tl.[58-60] Thus, intracellular uptake of ^{201}Tl across the sarcolemmal membrane is maintained for as long as sufficient blood flow is present to deliver ^{201}Tl to the myocardial cell. ^{201}Tl does not actively concentrate in regions of infarcted or scarred myocardium. Therefore,

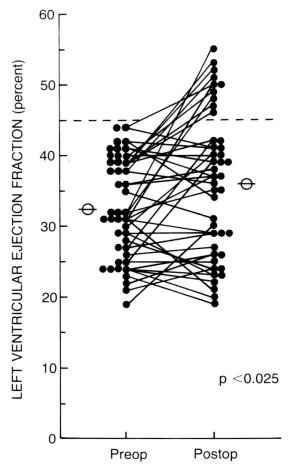

Figure 5-3 The prevalence of improvement in left ventricular ejection fraction at rest in 43 patients with preoperative (preop) left ventricular dysfunction. Left ventricular ejection fraction was assessed 6 mo after (postop) coronary artery bypass surgery. The dashed line at 45 percent indicates the lower limit of normal resting ejection fraction for the authors' laboratory. Substantial increases in ejection fraction were observed in 15 patients (35 percent), and the postoperative ejection fraction was normal in 10 patients (23 percent). (From Bonow et al,[51] reproduced with permission.)

decreased myocardial uptake early after ^{201}Tl injection could be caused either by reduced regional blood flow or infarction.

The period that follows initial myocardial uptake of ^{201}Tl is termed the delayed or redistribution phase. Regional ^{201}Tl activity on redistribution images, acquired either 2–4 h or 8–72 h after stress, has been used to demonstrate the distribution of viable myocytes and the extent of scarred myocardium. Studies in experimental animals have shown that myocardial concentration of ^{201}Tl changes over time. During the redistribution phase, there is a continuous exchange of ^{201}Tl between the myocardium and the extracardiac compartments, driven by the concentration gradient of the tracer and myocyte viability. Thus, the extent of defect resolution, from the

initial to delayed redistribution images over time, termed reversible defect, reflects one index of myocardial viability. When only scarred myocardium is present, the degree of the initial ^{201}Tl defect persists over time without redistribution, and is termed irreversible defect. When both viable and scarred myocardium are present, ^{201}Tl redistribution is incomplete, giving the appearance of partial reversibility on delayed images.

There are a number of ^{201}Tl protocols that are currently used for assessing myocardial viability (Fig. 5-5). Advantages and disadvantages of these various protocols, stress-redistribution, late redistribution, ^{201}Tl reinjection, and rest-redistribution are reviewed in the following sections.

Stress-Redistribution

As the uptake and retention of ^{201}Tl by myocardial cells is an active process, ^{201}Tl scintigraphy has the rather unique potential for distinguishing viable from nonviable myocardium with greater precision than can be achieved by the assessment of regional anatomy or function alone. In 1977, Pohost et al[61] made the observation that ^{201}Tl defects on immediate postexercise images may normalize or redistribute if images were repeated several hours after the initial stress study. In a number of animal studies, redistribution on a delayed image was shown to represent reduced ^{201}Tl concentration in normal segments along with increased ^{201}Tl concentration in ischemic segments.[61–68] Clearance of ^{201}Tl from the normal myocardium mirrored the ^{201}Tl clearance from the blood,

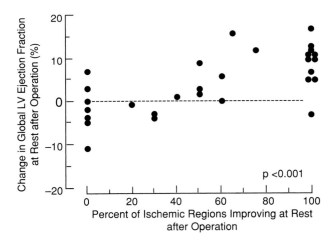

Figure 5-4 Change in left ventricular (LV) ejection fraction after coronary artery bypass surgery as a function of the percentage of ischemic LV regions manifesting improved regional function after operation. The ischemic regions were defined as those in which the ejection fraction decreased during exercise before surgery more than two standard deviations below the mean change observed in that region in normal volunteers during exercise. (From Dilsizian et al,[18] by permission of the *American Journal of Cardiology*.)

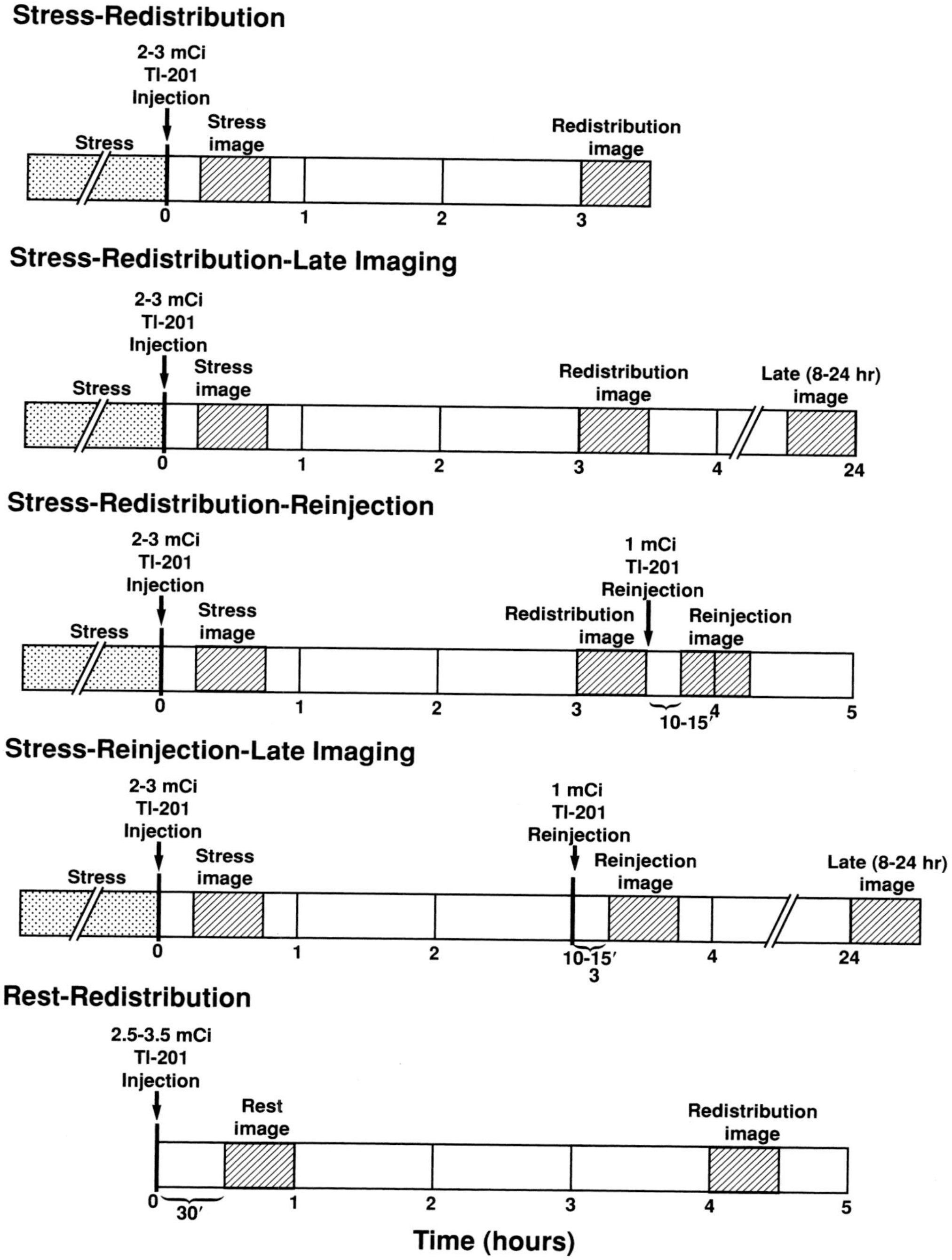

Figure 5-5 Thallium protocols for assessing myocardial viability.

whereas in ischemic segments there was slow accumulation of ^{201}Tl from the recirculating ^{201}Tl within the blood.[63,64] The presence of ^{201}Tl redistribution was subsequently confirmed in patients with coronary artery disease undergoing exercise or pharmacologic stress testing, as well as after the injection of ^{201}Tl at rest. Hence, the acquisition of redistribution images 3–4 h after the administration of intravenous ^{201}Tl at peak stress or at rest became the standard for ^{201}Tl scintigraphic studies. However, further experience indicated that there are limitations of stress followed by 3- to 4-h redistribution imaging for differentiating ischemic but viable myocardium from nonviable myocardium.

Stress-induced ^{201}Tl defects that redistribute on 3- to 4-h delayed images are accurate indicators of ischemic but viable myocardium. However, the converse, abnor-

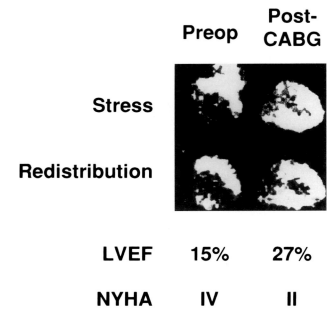

Preop Post-CABG

Stress

Redistribution

LVEF	15%	27%
NYHA	IV	II

Figure 5-6 Evidence for viable myocardium in a region with an irreversible ^{201}Tl defect. Pre- and postoperative anterior planar ^{201}Tl images demonstrate partially reversible inferior and fixed apical ^{201}Tl defects preoperatively that normalize after coronary artery bypass surgery. The left ventricular ejection fraction increased from 15 percent before to 27 percent after surgery. (Modified and reprinted with permission of the publisher, from: Selection of angina-free patients with severe left ventricular dysfunction for myocardial revascularization, Akins et al,[69] *Am J Cardiol*, Vol. 46, pp. 695–700. Copyright 1980 by Excepta Medica Inc.)

mal ^{201}Tl defects during stress that persist on delayed images, does not necessarily indicate myocardial scar. Ischemic but viable regions and regions with mixed viable and scarred myocardium may appear irreversible on stress-redistribution studies (Fig. 5-6). Many patients with irreversible ^{201}Tl defects on stress-redistribution imaging have no evidence of prior myocardial infarction and will have normal ^{201}Tl uptake after revascularization.[69–74] Using ^{201}Tl quantification, Gibson et al[70] demonstrated that 45 percent of segments with irreversible defects had improved ^{201}Tl uptake after coronary artery bypass surgery.[70] Segments that were likely to improve had ^{201}Tl activity that was >50 percent of the activity in normal regions. Similar results were obtained after successful percutaneous coronary angioplasty.[71,74] Thus, standard stress, 3- to 4-h redistribution ^{201}Tl scintigraphy may underestimate the presence of ischemic but viable myocardium in many patients with coronary artery disease.

Late Redistribution

Among patients demonstrating apparent irreversible ^{201}Tl defects on conventional stress-redistribution stud-

ies, the identification of viable myocardium may be improved by allowing a longer period for ^{201}Tl redistribution (Fig. 5-7). In a series of patients with coronary artery disease, 21 percent of the segments with irreversible ^{201}Tl defects on the 3- to 4-h delayed images showed redistribution when late images were obtained 18–24 h after exercise.[75] Myocardial segments demonstrating such late ^{201}Tl redistribution were usually perfused by critically narrowed coronary arteries. These initial observations using planar imaging were subsequently confirmed with SPECT.[72–76] To determine the frequency of late redistribution in a nonselective patient population, Yang et al[76] studied 118 consecutive patients with irreversible ^{201}Tl defects on standard stress-redistribution studies.[76] In this prospective study using SPECT, late redistribution was observed in 53 percent of the patients and in 22 percent of the segments with 4-h irreversible defects (Fig. 5-8). However, despite implementing 50 percent longer imaging time, a number of late redistribution studies had suboptimal count statistics at 24 h.

A possible explanation for late redistribution is that in certain ischemic myocardial regions supplied by critically stenosed coronary arteries, the initial uptake of

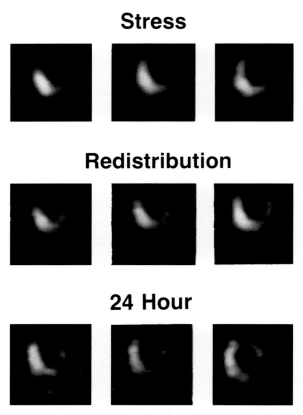

Stress

Redistribution

24 Hour

Figure 5-7 Short axis ^{201}Tl tomograms during stress, redistribution, and 24-h imaging from a patient with coronary artery disease. There are extensive anterior and lateral ^{201}Tl abnormalities during stress, which persist on redistribution images but which improve at 24 h. (Modified and reprinted from Dilsizian et al,[100] with permission of the American Heart Association, Inc.)

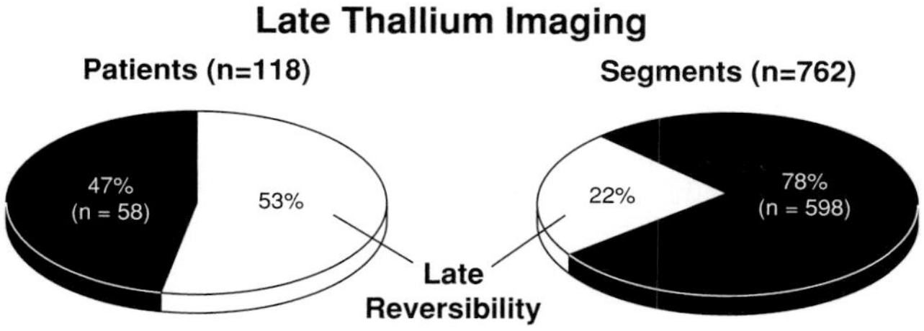

Late Thallium Imaging

Patients (n=118)   **Segments (n=762)**

47%
(n = 58)   53%   22%   78%
(n = 598)

**Late
Reversibility**

Figure 5-8 Pie chart showing the frequency of late reversibility and nonreversibility in 118 consecutive patients. In this prospective study, late redistribution was observed in 53 percent of the patients (on the left) and in 22 percent of the segments with 4-h irreversible defects (on the right). (From Yang et al,[76] modified and reprinted with permission from the American College of Cardiology, *Journal of the American College of Cardiology*, 15:334, 1989.)

[201]Tl is low (because delivery is impaired) and the rate of ^{201}Tl accumulation from the recirculating tracer within the blood over the 3- to 4-h redistribution period is very slow. Thus, ischemic but viable myocardium may mimic the appearance of scarred myocardium. However, if a greater time is allowed for redistribution, then a greater number of viable myocardial regions may be differentiated from scarred myocardium.

Late redistribution in a region with an irreversible ^{201}Tl defect on conventional stress-redistribution studies is an accurate marker of ischemic and viable myocardium. Kiat et al[73] reported that 95 percent of segments that demonstrated late redistribution at 18–24 h showed improved ^{201}Tl uptake after revascularization.[73] However, as with early (2- to 4-h) redistribution imaging, the absence of late (8- to 72-h) redistribution remains an inaccurate marker for scarred myocardium; 37 percent of segments that remained irreversible on both 3- to 4-h and 24-h studies also improved after revascularization.[73] These data suggest that although late ^{201}Tl imaging improves the identification of viable myocardium, it continues to underestimate segmental improvement after revascularization.

Thallium Reinjection

In 1990, we introduced the concept that reinjection of ^{201}Tl at rest after stress 3- to 4-h redistribution imaging improves the assessment of myocardial viability.[77,78] Among 100 patients with coronary artery disease studied using ^{201}Tl SPECT, 33 percent of abnormal myocardial regions on stress appeared to be irreversible on 3- to 4-h redistribution images. However, after reinjecting a second dose of 1 mCi (37 MBq) of ^{201}Tl at rest immediately after redistribution images and followed by image acquisition 10–15 min later, 49 percent of the apparently irreversible defects on 3- to 4-h redistribution images demonstrated improved or normal ^{201}Tl uptake.[77] More-

over, in the subgroup of patients who underwent coronary angioplasty, 87 percent of myocardial regions identified as viable by reinjection studies had normal ^{201}Tl uptake and improved regional wall motion after coronary angioplasty. In contrast, all regions with irreversible defects on reinjection imaging before angioplasty had abnormal regional wall motion after coronary angioplasty. Similar results were obtained subsequently in other medical centers,[78-85] and in a recent multicenter trial undertaken in Italy, involving 402 consecutive patients with ischemic heart disease recruited from 12 hospitals.[86] In the Italian multicenter study, of the 118 patients with irreversible defects on standard stress-redistribution images, 58 (49 percent) showed reversibility of these defects only after ^{201}Tl reinjection. These findings with exercise were confirmed when ^{201}Tl reinjection was performed immediately after pharmacologic stress-redistribution studies.[83,87,88] A patient example demonstrating the ^{201}Tl reinjection effect is shown in Fig. 5-9.

The experience with ^{201}Tl reinjection before and after revascularization now totals 161 patients in the literature, performed in five different medical centers.[77,79,83-85,89] The available data suggest that enhanced ^{201}Tl uptake after reinjection in otherwise irreversible stress-redistri-

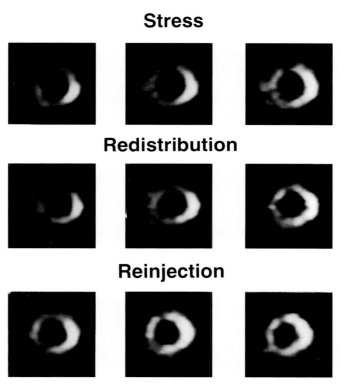

Stress

Redistribution

Reinjection

Figure 5-9 Short axis ^{201}Tl tomograms during stress, redistribution, and reinjection imaging in a patient with coronary artery disease. There are extensive ^{201}Tl abnormalities in the anterior and septal regions during stress that persist on redistribution images but improve markedly on reinjection images. (From Dilsizian et al,[77] with permission of the *New England Journal of Medicine*, 323:141, 1990. Copyright 1990 Massachusetts Medical Society. All rights reserved.)

bution defects predicts improvement in regional function at rest after revascularization in 80 to 91 percent of regions. In contrast, in regions with irreversible defects after reinjection, regional function improved after revascularization in only 0 to 18 percent of myocardial regions.

The following is a possible explanation for the salutary results of ^{201}Tl reinjection clinically. The *initial* myocardial uptake of [201]Tl (postinjection) reflects regional blood flow, whereas *delayed* redistribution of ^{201}Tl in a given defect depends not only on the severity of the initial defects but also on the presence of viable myocytes,[90] the concentration of the tracer in the blood,[91,92] and the rate of decline of ^{201}Tl levels in the blood.[93–96] Thus, the heterogeneity of regional blood flow observed on the initial stress-induced ^{201}Tl defects may be independent of the subsequent extent of ^{201}Tl redistribution.[66,97] If the blood ^{201}Tl level remains the same (or increases) during the period between stress and 3- to 4-h redistribution imaging, then an apparent defect in a region with viable myocytes that can retain ^{201}Tl should improve. On the other hand, if the serum ^{201}Tl concentration decreases during the imaging interval, the delivery of ^{201}Tl may be insufficient, and the ^{201}Tl defect may remain irreversible even though the underlying myocardium is viable.[98] This suggests that some ischemic but viable regions may never redistribute, even with late (24-h) imaging, unless serum levels of ^{201}Tl are increased. This hypothesis is supported by a study where ^{201}Tl reinjection was performed immediately after 24-h redistribution images were obtained.[99] Improved ^{201}Tl uptake after reinjection occurred in 39 percent of defects (representing 44 percent of patients) that appeared irreversible on late (24-h) redistribution images. This percentage is remarkably similar to the 37 percent of irreversible defects at 24 h that improve after revascularization, as previously reported by Kiat et al.[73]

SHOULD LATE REDISTRIBUTION IMAGING BE ACQUIRED AFTER THALLIUM REINJECTION?

If ^{201}Tl reinjection after stress 3- to 4-h redistribution improves detection of ischemic and viable myocardium, it is possible that delaying the redistribution period between reinjection and repeat imaging from 10 min to 24 h may identify additional viable regions. In a study of 50 patients with chronic coronary artery disease who underwent four sets of images (stress, 3- to 4-h redistribution, reinjection, and 24-h redistribution images), only 11 percent of myocardial regions (involving 6 percent of patients) that remained irreversible after both 3- to 4-h redistribution and reinjection showed evidence of late redistribution (Fig. 5-10). It was concluded that all clinically relevant information pertaining to viability was obtained by a stress-redistribution-reinjection protocol.[100] These observations have been confirmed by subse-

quent studies.[101,102] Therefore, late imaging after ^{201}Tl reinjection is not necessary.

STRESS-REINJECTION PROTOCOL: IS 3- TO 4-H REDISTRIBUTION IMAGING NECESSARY?

In view of the clinical success of ^{201}Tl reinjection, many nuclear laboratories have adopted the practice of eliminating 3- to 4-h redistribution imaging. This approach assumes that a stress-reinjection protocol (without the 3- to 4-h redistribution image) provides the same information regarding stress-induced ischemia and viability as a stress-redistribution-reinjection protocol. However, further analysis of data among 50 patients who underwent all four sets of images (stress, 3- to 4-h redistribution, reinjection, and 24-h redistribution) revealed that there are potential limitations in not performing 3- to 4-h redistribution images.[103]

Despite the logistical concerns of performing ^{201}Tl reinjection in all patients after 3- to 4-h redistribution imaging, elimination of the 3- to 4-h redistribution images may incorrectly assign up to 25 percent of reversible ^{201}Tl defects on stress-redistribution images as "irreversible" after reinjection.[77,103] Reversible stress-redistribution defects that appear to wash out after reinjection, and thus appear "fixed" on stress-reinjection images, result from a disproportionately smaller increment in regional ^{201}Tl activity after reinjection in some ischemic regions compared with the uptake in normal regions, a phenomenon we have termed "differential uptake."[77,103] Unlike conventional redistribution imaging, in which washout reflects an actual net loss of ^{201}Tl activity from stress to redistribution imaging, it is the low differential uptake of ^{201}Tl after reinjection that is responsible for the appearance of washout. However, late (24-h) redistribution images acquired after reinjection demonstrated further redistribution in these regions resulting in relative ^{201}Tl activities that were indistinguishable from those observed on 3- to 4-h redistribution images (Fig. 5-11).

These findings in patients with chronic coronary artery disease suggest that elimination of the 3- to 4-h redistribution images and reliance on reinjection images alone would underestimate defect reversibility, and hence, viability in a considerable number of ischemic regions. However, a stress-reinjection protocol appears to be a reasonable alternative to stress-redistribution-reinjection imaging, as long as late (24-h) imaging is performed in those patients with irreversible defects. Thus, high predictive accuracy for ischemic and viable myocardium can be achieved with ^{201}Tl scintigraphy with either a stress-redistribution-reinjection or stress-reinjection–late redistribution imaging. For either of these protocols, the third set of images is only necessary if an irreversible defect exists on the stress-redistribution or the stress-reinjection images.

Myocardial Regions

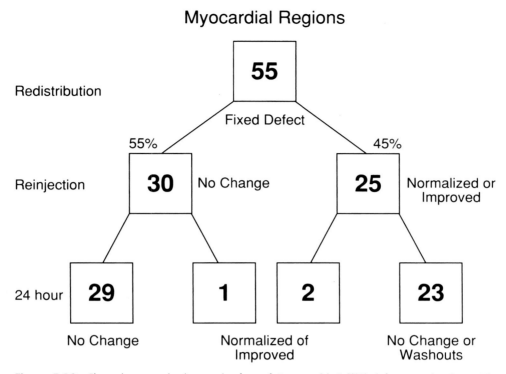

Figure 5-10 Flow diagram displaying the fate of "irreversible" [201]Tl defects on the 3- to 4-h standard redistribution studies after reinjection and at 24 h. (From Dilsizian et al,[100] by permission of the American Heart Association, Inc.)

EARLY THALLIUM REINJECTION: DOES THALLIUM REINJECTION EARLY AFTER STRESS PROVIDE THE SAME INFORMATION AS REINJECTION AFTER 3–4 H REDISTRIBUTION?

An alternative method to stress-redistribution-reinjection imaging would be to reinject ^{201}Tl immediately after the stress images are completed and acquire a modified redistribution image 3–4 h later. Since the modified redistribution image would represent redistribution of both the stress and the reinjected ^{201}Tl doses, this may avoid the acquisition of three sets of images. When Kiat et al[104] applied such an early ^{201}Tl reinjection protocol, 24 percent of irreversible ^{201}Tl defects on stress-modified redistribution images became reversible when a third set of images were acquired 24 h later. Although van Eck-Smit et al[105] reported that there was good agreement between 1-h and 3-h modified redistribution images after early reinjection, an independent validation of the accuracy of the early reinjection technique was not provided. In a subsequent publication, Klingensmith and Sutherland[106] compared stress–early reinjection with conventional stress-redistribution-reinjection ^{201}Tl imaging among two groups of patients with similar clinical parameters. Consistent with previous observations, the frequency of reversible defects was significantly less with early reinjection compared with the standard 3-h reinjection protocol. Recently, in addition to acquiring stress–early reinjection images, a second 1-mCi (37-MBq) dose of ^{201}Tl was reinjected after 3-h modified redistribution

images were completed and a third set of images was acquired.[107] When modified redistribution images after early reinjection were compared with standard 3-h reinjection images, early ^{201}Tl reinjection underestimated myocardial viability in about 25 percent of irreversible defects. These preliminary data suggest, therefore, that a 3–4 h delay after exercise is necessary to accurately determine myocardial ischemia and viability among patients with chronic left ventricular dysfunction.

THALLIUM REINJECTION IN REGIONS WITH REVERSE REDISTRIBUTION

On conventional stress-redistribution imaging, reverse redistribution indicates either the appearance of a new defect on the redistribution images or the worsening of a defect apparent on stress images. It remains unclear, however, whether regions demonstrating the phenomenon of reverse redistribution represent scarred or viable myocardium. Hence, the clinical significance of reverse redistribution in chronic coronary artery disease is uncertain (for additional discussion of reverse redistribution, see Chap. 1).

Since ^{201}Tl reinjection is a valuable technique for detecting myocardial viability, its effect was examined among patients with chronic coronary artery disease, all of whom demonstrated reverse redistribution on stan-

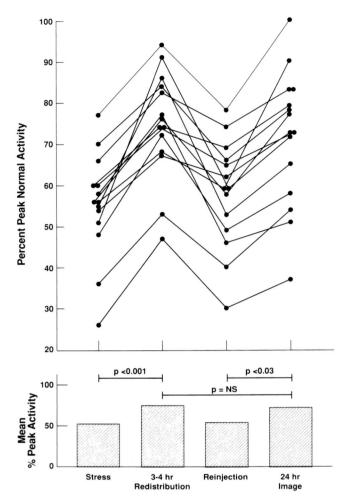

Figure 5-11 Relative regional ^{201}Tl activity (presented as a percentage of normal activity) in 14 regions demonstrating the phenomenon of apparent ^{201}Tl washout due to low differential uptake. **Top panel:** Individual data points are displayed for stress, 3- to 4-h redistribution, reinjection, and 24-h images. **Bottom panel:** Mean ^{201}Tl activity in relation to each of the four corresponding images. If the 3- to 4-h redistribution images were eliminated and the reinjection images were acquired alone, these regions would be incorrectly assigned to be irreversible. On the 24-h images, redistribution is again apparent, indicating reversibility of the defect, and the relative ^{201}Tl activity is similar to that observed on the 3- to 4-h redistribution studies. (From Dilsizian et al,[103] by permission of the American Heart Association, Inc.)

dard stress-redistribution studies.[108] Enhanced ^{201}Tl uptake after reinjection occurred in 82 percent of regions with reverse redistribution (Fig. 5-12). Regions with improved ^{201}Tl uptake after reinjection were associated with absence of electrocardiographic and functional indices of myocardial necrosis, and supplied by severely stenosed coronary arteries with good collaterals. Furthermore, metabolic activity as assessed by ^{18}F fluorodeoxyglucose (^{18}F FDG) was preserved by PET imaging in such regions. In contrast, regions with reverse redistribution in which

^{201}Tl activity failed to increase after reinjection were associated with electrocardiographic Q waves, severely impaired regional contraction, and severely reduced ^{18}F FDG and blood flow (FDG/blood flow match) by PET. These observations indicate that ^{201}Tl reinjection may be helpful in differentiating scarred from viable myocardium in regions with reverse redistribution.[108] Similar results were obtained by other investigators.[109]

SEVERITY AND MAGNITUDE OF CHANGE IN THALLIUM ACTIVITY AFTER REINJECTION DISTINGUISHES VIABLE FROM NONVIABLE MYOCARDIUM

From comparative ^{18}F-FDG PET and ^{201}Tl SPECT studies, among regions considered "irreversible" on redistribution images, the severity of reduction in ^{201}Tl activity correlated with the degree of metabolic activity as assessed by ^{18}F-FDG uptake. ^{18}F-FDG uptake was preserved in 91 percent of mildly reduced (60 to 84 percent of peak activity) and 84 percent of moderately reduced (50 to 59 percent of peak activity) irreversible ^{201}Tl regions.[110] Hence, the level of ^{201}Tl activity itself in mild-to-moderate defects might be a clinically reliable marker of myocardial viability. In a subsequent study of 150 patients with chronic ischemic coronary artery disease who underwent a stress-redistribution-reinjection ^{201}Tl protocol, the increase in regional ^{201}Tl activity from redistribution to reinjection was computed, normalized to the increase observed in a normal region, and termed "differential uptake."[111] A substantial differential uptake was observed after reinjection in regions in which ^{201}Tl defects remain irreversible despite reinjection by using analysis of *relative* regional ^{201}Tl activity. The magnitude of increase in ^{201}Tl activity (differential uptake) was significantly greater in mild-to-moderate defects than in severe irreversible defects, suggesting that these regions represent viable myocardium (Fig. 5-13). This was confirmed by the corresponding PET data.[111]

These initial observations regarding the relation between magnitude of ^{201}Tl activity within irreversible ^{201}Tl defects and viability were supported by a comparative clinicopathological study by Zimmermann et al.[112] Among 37 patients with significant left anterior descending coronary artery disease undergoing coronary artery bypass surgery, the magnitude of ^{201}Tl activity within irreversible preoperative stress-redistribution-reinjection ^{201}Tl images was correlated with the extent of interstitial fibrosis determined from intraoperative transmural left ventricular biopsies of the anterior wall (Fig. 5-14). Although there was a good overall inverse correlation between the percentage of ^{201}Tl activity on redistribution images and the percentage of interstitial fibrosis, the inverse relation was significantly better after ^{201}Tl reinjection. Similar results were obtained at the National Institutes of Health.[113] These data demonstrate that residual ^{201}Tl activity after reinjection

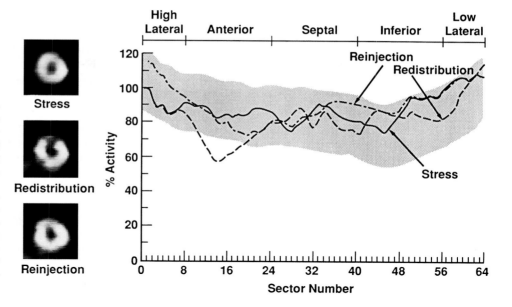

Figure 5-12 An example of reverse redistribution in the anterior region with enhanced ^{201}Tl uptake after ^{201}Tl reinjection. Representative short axis tomograms obtained during stress, redistribution, and reinjection are shown on the left. On the right, plots of quantitative regional ^{201}Tl activity during stress, redistribution, reinjection are compared with the normal range (mean ± 2 SD for normal subjects), represented as the shaded area. (From Marin-Neto et al,[108] by permission of the American Heart Association, Inc.)

is proportional to the mass of preserved viable myocardium and confirm the value of ^{201}Tl reinjection for assessing myocardial viability.

Rest-Redistribution Imaging

The stress-redistribution-reinjection ^{201}Tl protocol provides important diagnostic and prognostic information

regarding both inducible ischemia and myocardial viability. However, if the clinical question to be addressed is one of the presence and extent of viable myocardium within dysfunctional regions and not inducible ischemia, it is reasonable to perform only rest-redistribution ^{201}Tl imaging.

Thallium 201 defects on resting images have been reported during angina-free periods in patients with unstable angina and without myocardial infarction and in

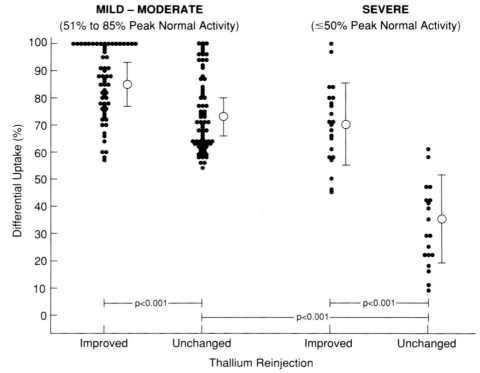

Figure 5-13 Plots show differential regional uptake of ^{201}Tl after reinjection based on analysis of changes in the *magnitude* of regional ^{201}Tl activity in regions with irreversible ^{201}Tl defects on redistribution imaging. **Left panel:** regions with mild-to-moderate reduction in ^{201}Tl activity on redistribution images (ranging from 51 to 85 percent of peak normal activity). **Right panel:** regions with severe reduction in ^{201}Tl activity (≤50 percent of peak activity). Within each panel, regions are further subdivided on the basis of improved or unchanged *relative* [201]Tl activity after reinjection. Mild-to-moderate defects in which relative ^{201}Tl activity was unchanged after reinjection had significantly greater increase in absolute ^{201}Tl activity than similar regions that represented severe irreversible defects. (From Dilsizian et al,[111] by permission of the American Heart Association, Inc.)

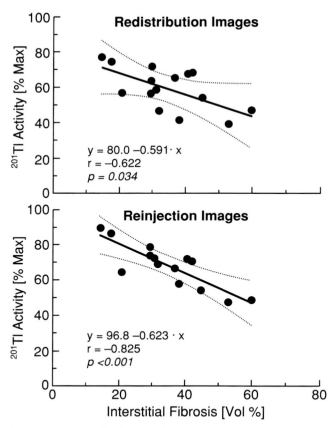

Figure 5-14 Graphs showing the relation between regional ^{201}Tl activity on redistribution (top panel) and reinjection (bottom panel) images and regional volume fraction of interstitial fibrosis in patients with chronic stable coronary artery disease undergoing coronary artery bypass surgery. Two transmural biopsy specimens were taken during surgery, and volume fraction of interstitial fibrosis was assessed by use of light microscopic morphometry. Dotted lines indicate 95 percent confidence limits for the regression line. % Max indicates percentage of maximum normal activity. When compared with redistribution images, regression analysis reveals a significantly improved correlation ($p < 0.01$) between ^{201}Tl reinjection and regional volume fraction of interstitial fibrosis. (From Zimmermann et al,[112] modified and reprinted with permission of the American Heart Association, Inc.)

patients with severe coronary artery disease in the absence of an acute ischemic process or previous myocardial infarction.[114,115] Furthermore, it has been recognized that many of these defects on the initial rest images may redistribute over the next 2–4 h. Since these initial reports, several studies have evaluated the efficacy of rest-redistribution ^{201}Tl imaging in predicting the outcome of myocardial regions after revascularization.[116–118] Among regions with reversible rest-redistribution ^{201}Tl defects preoperatively, 77 to 86 percent had normal ^{201}Tl uptake and improved left ventricular function after revascularization. However, 22 to 38 percent of regions with irreversible rest-redistribution defects preoperatively also showed improved left ventricular contraction

postoperatively. Thallium-201 defects in each of these studies were classified as being reversible, partially reversible, or irreversible. However, the severity of the irreversible ^{201}Tl defects was not assessed.

Recently, improved results were obtained using quantitative analysis in which the severity of reduction in ^{201}Tl activity was assessed within irreversible rest-redistribution ^{201}Tl defects.[89,119] When myocardial viability was defined as ^{201}Tl activity greater than 50 percent of peak activity in normal regions, 57 percent of severely asynergic regions that were viable by ^{201}Tl showed improved wall motion after surgery, compared with only 23 percent of severely asynergic regions that were considered to be nonviable by [201]Tl.[119] Furthermore, the number of asynergic but viable myocardial segments correlated well with postoperative improvement in global left ventricular function.

In another study, quantitative ^{201}Tl scintigraphic findings obtained from patients undergoing both stress-redistribution-reinjection and rest-redistribution SPECT imaging were compared with metabolic activity determined by PET.[89] In these patients, stress-redistribution-reinjection and rest-redistribution imaging provided concordant information regarding myocardial viability (normal/reversible or irreversible) in 72 percent of myocardial regions (Fig. 5-15). However, when the severity of the ^{201}Tl defect was analyzed (mild-to-moderate versus severe) in the irreversible defects, the concordance between stress-redistribution-reinjection and rest-redistri-

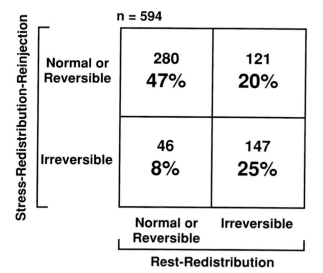

Figure 5-15 Chart showing concordance and discordance between stress-redistribution-reinjection and rest-redistribution ^{201}Tl images in 20 patients who underwent positron emission tomographic studies. Five myocardial regions of interest were drawn on the transaxial tomograms from the five sets of ^{201}Tl images, and ^{201}Tl activities were then computed within each region. Thallium-201 defects were classified as normal/reversible or irreversible. (From Dilsizian et al,[89] by permission of the American Heart Association, Inc.)

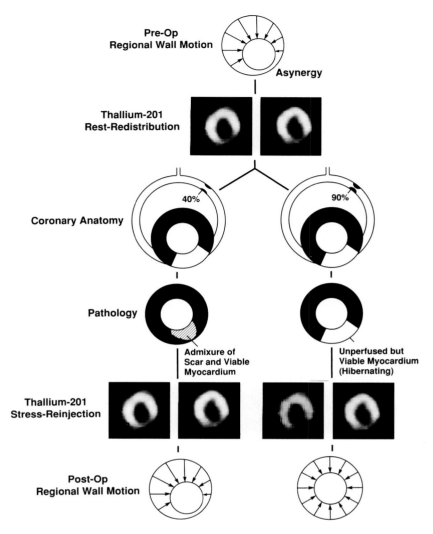

Figure 5-16 A schematic diagram of how exercise stress may produce greater regional myocardial blood flow heterogeneity when compared with rest-redistribution imaging and thereby differenti-ate an asynergic region with mixed scarred and viable myocardium from a region with underperfused but viable (hibernating) myocardium. A preoperative asynergic myocardial region that exhibits reduced ^{201}Tl uptake at rest and remains irreversible on the redistribution study may represent a region with a patent (40 percent stenosis) coronary artery after thrombolytic therapy (on the left) or a region with a critically narrowed (90 percent stenosis) coronary artery without myocardial infarction (on the right). In the case of the patient with 40 percent coronary artery stenosis and prior myocardial infarction, the dysfunctional myocardium (assessed several months after the acute infarction) represents mixed scarred and viable myocardium that will *not* recover after revascularization. In contrast, in the patient with 90 percent coronary artery stenosis without prior myocardial infarction the dysfunctional myocardium perfused by this artery represents underperfused but viable myocardium that will recover completely after revascularization. These two situations can be differentiated by performing a stress-redistribution-reinjection study but not by performing a rest-redistribution study. (From Dilsizian et al,[89] by permission of the American Heart Association, Inc.)

bution imaging regarding myocardial viability increased to 94 percent.[89]

Which Thallium Protocol for Identifying Chronic Heart Disease?

In most cases, the identification of presence and extent of myocardial ischemia is much more important clinically for patient management and risk stratification than knowledge of myocardial viability. The impact of a stress study in differentiating an asynergic region with mixed scarred and viable myocardium from a region with underperfused but viable (hibernating) myocardium is outlined in Fig. 5-16. It has been well recognized that regional contraction itself could influence the appearance of myocardial perfusion images.[120–124] A region with minimal or absent systolic wall thickening may appear to have reduced ^{201}Tl activity on a rest-redistribution study as a result of partial volume and recovery coefficient

effects in the presence of thinned or nonthickening myocardium. An asynergic region with a mild-to-moderate irreversible rest-redistribution ^{201}Tl pattern may be seen in any of the following situations: 1) mixed scarred and viable myocardium in the presence of an open artery, 2) mixed scarred and viable myocardium in the presence of an artery with angiographically intermediate stenosis, which may (2a) or may not (2b) be physiologically significant, and 3) predominantly underperfused but viable (hibernating) myocardium (stenotic artery). Demonstration of stress-induced ischemia will differentiate situations 1 and 2b from situations 2a and 3, and will be particularly helpful when the coronary anatomy is unknown. This has important clinical implications in terms of decisions regarding further invasive diagnostic evaluation and treatment because impaired regional function can be reversed in the presence of hibernating myocardium (situation 3) or stress-induced ischemia (situation 2a) but not in regions supplied by an open artery (situation 1) or an artery with a non-flow-limiting stenosis (2b). In the clinical setting of an asynergic region with a mild-to-moderate irreversible rest-redistribution ^{201}Tl pattern in a distribution of a critically stenosed artery, it is difficult to justify the need for demonstrating stress-induced ischemia before revascularization, particularly in symptomatic patients with multivessel disease and decreased left ventricular function. Demonstration of stress-induced ischemia will be helpful, however, to evaluate the physiologic significance of an angiographically intermediate stenosis in an artery supplying an asynergic region with a mild-to-moderate irreversible rest-redistribution ^{201}Tl defect.

If the clinical question is one of myocardial viability within asynergic regions, then a rest-redistribution ^{201}Tl protocol along with quantitative analysis of the severity of the ^{201}Tl defect may suffice. On the other hand, if the clinical question is one of ischemia and viability, then stress-redistribution-reinjection or stress-reinjection–late-redistribution imaging provides the most comprehensive information.

TECHNETIUM 99m–LABELED PERFUSION TRACERS

Imaging With Technetium-99m Tracers

Despite the excellent physiologic characteristics of ^{201}Tl for imaging myocardial perfusion and viability, its relatively low energy gamma spectrum increases the problems of photon attenuation as a function of tissue depth and is suboptimal for scintillation camera imaging. Following the initial efforts of Deutsch et al[125] for developing cationic ^{99m}Tc complexes, four different classes of ^{99m}Tc-labeled compounds have been developed since 1981 for myocardial perfusion imaging: 1) isonitriles (^{99m}Tc sestamibi), 2) boronic acid adducts of technetium dioxime (BATO) (^{99m}Tc teboroxime), 3) diphosphines (^{99m}Tc tetrofosmin), and 4) mixed ligand complexes (^{99m}Tc furifosmin). These technetium-labeled compounds overcome two major limitations of [201]Tl: low photon energy (69–80 keV mercury x-rays) and long physical half-life (73 h). The short 6-h half-life of ^{99m}Tc permits the administration of doses 10 times higher than ^{201}Tl, thereby improving the resolution of the images (higher photon flux and count statistics) while maintaining a relatively low radiation burden on the patient. Soft tissue attenuation is also less than with ^{201}Tl, resulting in improved spatial resolution and less prominent artifacts. Despite the recognized metabolic or transmembrane trapping of these ^{99m}Tc tracers, the relationship between myocardial tracer uptake and blood flow is not significantly altered except during acute myocardial ischemia, conditions of extremely low pH, or hyperemic flow.

These technetium-labeled tracers are taken up by the myocardium in proportion to regional blood flow, and recent studies have indicated that the accuracy of these tracers for detecting coronary artery disease is similar to that of [201]Tl.[126-128] However, preliminary data with regard to the application of these tracers for the assessment of myocardial viability suggest that they may underestimate defect reversibility and myocardial viability.

Technetium 99m Sestamibi

Technetium 99m sestamibi is a lipophilic cationic complex that is taken up by myocytes across mitochondrial membranes, but at equilibrium it is retained within the mitochondria owing to a large negative transmembrane potential.[129] Like thallium, initial uptake of ^{99m}Tc sestamibi reflects both regional blood flow and myocardial extraction; these vary depending on the retention mechanism involved for each individual tracer. Transcapillary transport and myocardial retention of both ^{99m}Tc sestamibi and ^{201}Tl are affected by the perfusion rate, capillary permeability, and binding characteristics within the myocardium.[130,131] Using a blood-perfused, isolated rabbit heart model, Leppo and Meerdink[130] have shown that the average extraction fraction of ^{99m}Tc sestamibi (39 percent $\pm$ 9 percent) is significantly less than that of [201]Tl (73 percent $\pm$ 10 percent, $p < 0.001$), and that ^{99m}Tc sestamibi has a higher parenchymal cell permeability and higher volume of distribution than [201]Tl. Despite differences in kinetics between ^{99m}Tc sestamibi and ^{201}Tl, the initial regional myocardial uptake of the two tracers is similar, and both agents have similar accuracy for detecting coronary artery disease.[132-135] Various ^{99m}Tc sestamibi protocols that are currently used for assessing myocardial ischemia and viability are shown in Fig. 5-17.

Although published reports to date have demonstrated a good correlation between rest ^{99m}Tc sestamibi uptake and degree of coronary artery stenosis,[136] the correlation between ^{99m}Tc sestamibi uptake and viability as assessed by wall motion is less impressive.[137] Among regions with only moderate (50 to 67 percent of peak activity) reduction in ^{99m}Tc sestamibi activity, 80 percent had improved ^{99m}Tc sestamibi activity after coronary artery bypass surgery. However, 39 percent of regions with severe (<50 percent of peak) reduction in ^{99m}Tc sestamibi activity also showed improved regional perfusion postoperatively.

TECHNETIUM-99m-SESTAMIBI IMAGING IN CHRONIC CORONARY ARTERY DISEASE AND HIBERNATION

In stunned but viable myocardium, in which regional contractility is impaired despite restoration of coronary blood flow, ^{99m}Tc sestamibi uptake should be an accurate marker of cellular viability, and this has been confirmed in several studies.[59,138-144] In patients studied within the

2-Day Sestamibi

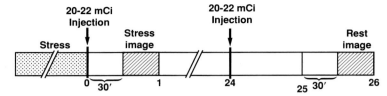

1-Day Sestamibi

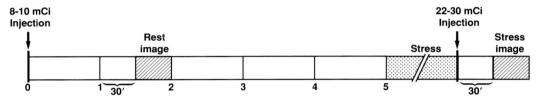

Rest-Redistribution-Stress Sestamibi

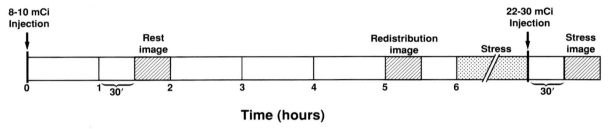

Time (hours)

Figure 5-17 Technetium-99m-sestamibi protocols for assessing myocardial ischemia and viability.

first week of thrombolytic therapy for acute myocardial infarction, ^{99m}Tc sestamibi defect size correlates well with regional wall motion at the time of discharge,[142] with late ejection fraction measurements,[142] and with peak release of creatine kinase.[143] Unlike stunned myocardium, ^{99m}Tc sestamibi imaging for identifying hibernating myocardium in patients with chronic coronary artery disease and left ventricular dysfunction may be less accurate. There are a growing number of studies to suggest that ^{99m}Tc sestamibi underestimates defect reversibility and myocardial viability in patients with chronic coronary artery disease.[137,145–161]

Using conventional planar imaging and qualitative analysis among patients with chronic coronary artery disease, Cuocolo et al[145] reported that 29 percent of reversible myocardial regions by ^{201}Tl reinjection appeared irreversible when a 2-d stress-rest ^{99m}Tc sestamibi protocol was performed. In our laboratory,[152] using SPECT imaging and quantitative analysis, 36 percent of myocardial regions that were classified as ischemic but viable by the ^{201}Tl stress-redistribution-reinjection protocol were misclassified as irreversible defects on the ^{99m}Tc sestamibi rest-stress protocol (Fig. 5-18). PET imaging was used as the gold standard to confirm viability of these regions.[152] These initial observations, both with planar and SPECT

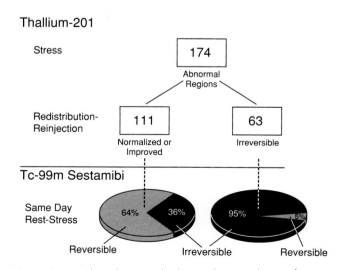

Figure 5-18 Flow diagram displaying the prevalence of reversible and irreversible ^{201}Tl perfusion defects by stress-redistribution-reinjection and same-day rest-stress ^{99m}Tc sestamibi studies in 54 patients with chronic coronary artery disease with a mean left ventricular ejection fraction of 34 ± 14 percent. (From Dilsizian et al,[152] by permission of the American Heart Association, Inc.)

imaging, have been confirmed by subsequent studies.[146-151,153-161]

If the mechanism of the ^{201}Tl reinjection effect is merely that the reinjected ^{201}Tl dose provides a better assessment of resting myocardial perfusion than redistribution images, then ^{201}Tl reinjection results should be equivalent to results obtained when ^{99m}Tc sestamibi is injected at rest. It is likely that the period of ^{201}Tl redistribution after exercise may be the key factor, with the images after reinjection incorporating resting blood flow along with the metabolic information inherent in the redistribution data. These observations imply that perfusion agents that measure coronary blood flow alone may not assess myocardial viability as well as an agent that redistributes, such as [201]Tl. Thus, ^{99m}Tc sestamibi may underestimate viable myocardium in regions with chronic reduction in blood flow, as observed in hibernating myocardium.

SEVERITY OF REGIONAL TECHNETIUM-99m SESTAMIBI DEFECT

One approach that may overcome, in part, the limitations of ^{99m}Tc sestamibi in assessing myocardial viability is to quantify the severity of regional ^{99m}Tc sestamibi activity. Such quantitative methods have been useful in ^{201}Tl imaging for identifying viable myocardium within apparently irreversible ^{201}Tl defects.[89,110,111] In one study, among regions with irreversible ^{99m}Tc sestamibi defects that were considered to be viable by ^{201}Tl imaging and

PET, 78 percent had only mild-to-moderately reduced ^{99m}Tc sestamibi activity.[152] If such mild-to-moderate ^{99m}Tc sestamibi defects are considered to represent nonischemic but viable myocardium, and only severe reduction in activity (<50 percent of normal) is considered evidence of nonviability, then the overall concordance between ^{201}Tl and ^{99m}Tc sestamibi studies was increased to 93 percent (Fig. 5-19). However, despite the application of quantitative techniques, other studies have reported that rest ^{99m}Tc sestamibi imaging underestimates myocardial viability when compared with PET.[149,154,156,159-161] In patients with chronic coronary artery disease undergoing both rest ^{99m}Tc sestamibi SPECT and ^{18}F-FDG PET studies, Altehoefer et al[149,156] found discordance between the severity of ^{99m}Tc sestamibi defects and ^{18}F-FDG uptake (Fig. 5-20). Using the same threshold quantitative values for viability, Sawada et al[154] found that the ^{99m}Tc sestamibi defect size at rest was larger than that from perfusion images with ^{13}N-ammonia and PET. Furthermore, 47 percent of segments with severe ^{99m}Tc sestamibi defects (<50 percent of peak activity) had preserved metabolic activity as assessed by ^{18}F-FDG PET.

It is important to point out, however, that the mere presence of viable myocardium (severity of regional ^{99m}Tc sestamibi defect) does not necessarily indicate ischemic myocardium (stress-induced reversible defect). It is more likely for an ischemic region to improve after revascularization than nonischemic but viable myocardium (mild-to-moderate reduction in tracer activity).[162] In the study

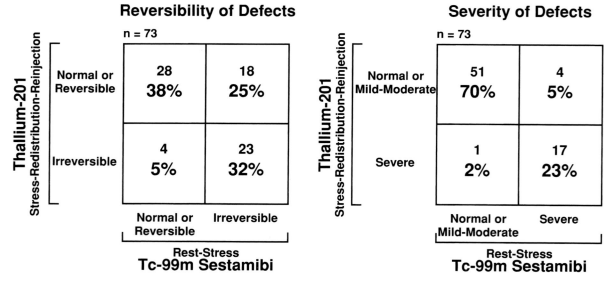

Figure 5-19 Diagram showing concordance and discordance between ^{201}Tl stress-redistribution-reinjection and ^{99m}Tc sestamibi rest-stress images in 25 patients who also underwent PET studies. Data on reversibility of defects (normal/reversible or irreversible) are shown on the left, and severity of defects (normal/mild-to-moderate or severe) is shown on the right. Eighteen of 22 discordant regions between ^{201}Tl and ^{99m}Tc sestamibi studies are reversible by ^{201}Tl redistribution-reinjection studies. Myocardial viability was confirmed in 17 of 18 regions by PET. (From Dilsizian et al,[152] by permission of the American Heart Association, Inc.)

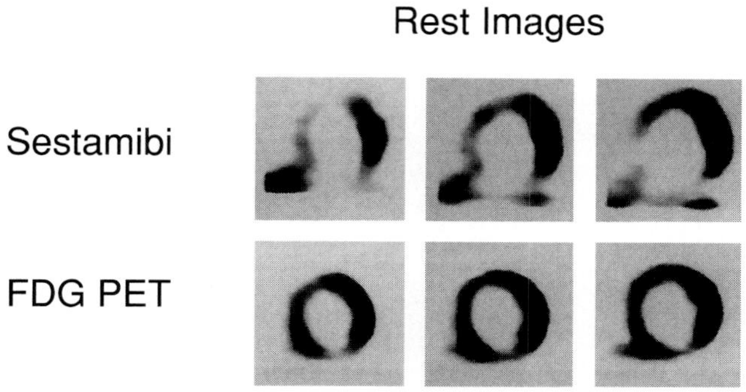

Rest Images

Sestamibi

FDG PET

Figure 5-20 Discordance between PET and rest ^{99m}Tc sestamibi SPECT imaging is demonstrated in this patient with three-vessel coronary artery disease. Three consecutive short axis tomograms are displayed for ^{99m}Tc sestamibi (top), with corresponding ^{18}F-FDG PET tomograms (bottom). Rest ^{99m}Tc sestamibi images reveal extensive perfusion abnormalities involving the anteroapical, septal, and inferior regions with preserved viability in the posterolateral region and mixed viable and scarred myocardium in the septal region. Fluorine-18-FDG uptake in the corresponding regions demonstrates preserved metabolic activity and viability in all three coronary artery vascular territories. The patient had totally occluded but collateralized left anterior descending and right coronary arteries and severe stenosis of the left circumflex artery. (From Altehoefer et al,[156] Significance of defect in technetium-99m-MIBI SPECT at rest to assess myocardial viability: Comparison with fluorine-18-FDG PET, modified and reprinted with permission of the *Journal of Nuclear Medicine*, 35:569, 1994.)

by Marzullo et al,[157] 37 percent of segments exhibiting ^{99m}Tc sestamibi activity of >55 percent of peak normal (viable at rest) showed no improvement in regional contraction after revascularization. Therefore, the distinction between ischemic myocardium (stress-induced reversible defect) and viable myocardium (severity of defect at rest) has important clinical implications (Table 5-1).

TECHNETIUM-99m SESTAMIBI REDISTRIBUTION AND CLINICAL RELEVANCE

Redistribution of ^{99m}Tc sestamibi has been observed both in animal models[163–166] and in patients with chronic coro-

nary artery disease.[152,158,167–169] However, the extent of redistribution with ^{99m}Tc sestamibi is significantly less than that observed with ^{201}Tl. Following transient ischemia and reperfusion in a canine model, Li et al[164] have demonstrated that ^{99m}Tc sestamibi undergoes myocardial redistribution, albeit more slowly and less completely when compared with ^{201}Tl (Fig. 5-21). Technetium-99m sestamibi redistribution over 2.5 h was also observed in an animal model of sustained low flow ischemia.[165] In clinical studies of patients undergoing exercise studies, minimal but clinically relevant redistribution has been observed in ischemic myocardium.[167,168] Among patients with angiographically documented coronary artery disease, significant ^{99m}Tc sestamibi redistribution was ob-

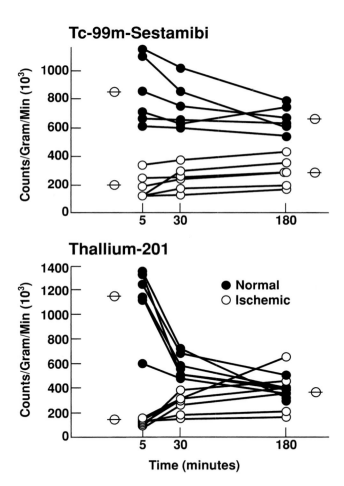

Figure 5-21 Technetium-99m-sestamibi and ^{201}Tl activities in myocardial biopsies from the normal (closed circles) and ischemic zones (open circles) in six dogs 5 min, 30 min, and 180 min after injection of the tracers. The dogs were reperfused just after the 5-min biopsies. The bisected circles represent mean activity values in each zone. For both ^{99m}Tc sestamibi and ^{201}Tl, note the consistent fall in normal zone activity and rise in ischemic zone activity consistent with redistribution. However, by 180 min, redistribution is complete for ^{201}Tl but not for ^{99m}Tc sestamibi. (From Li et al,[164] Myocardial redistribution of technetium-99m-methoxyisobutyl isonitrile (sestamibi), reprinted with permission from the *Journal of Nuclear Medicine*, 31:1069, 1990.)

Table 5-1 Definitions of Myocardial Viability With Single Photon Tracers

Scintigraphic Interpretation	Clinical Interpretation
I. Reversible defect after stress	Ischemic but viable myocardium
II. Irreversible defect after stress	

Mild-moderate
    (51 to 85% of normal
    activity)
	Nonischemic, viable myocardium

Severe (≤50% of normal activity)	Nonischemic, scarred myocardium

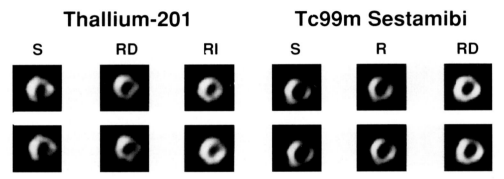

Figure 5-22   An example of a patient with reversible ^{201}Tl defects and irreversible defects on rest-stress ^{99m}Tc-sestamibi imaging. Two consecutive short axis tomograms are displayed for ^{201}Tl stress (S), redistribution (RD), and reinjection (RI) with corresponding ^{99m}Tc-sestamibi tomograms of stress, rest (R), and redistribution. Thallium-201 stress-redistribution images reveal partially reversible inferior and fixed anterolateral defects that improve after reinjection of ^{201}Tl at rest. Same-day rest-stress ^{99m}Tc-sestamibi images incorrectly identified the anterolateral region as being irreversibly impaired and nonviable and the inferolateral region to be only partially reversible when compared with the ^{201}Tl redistribution-reinjection study. However, ^{99m}Tc-sestamibi redistribution images acquired 4 h following injection of the tracer at rest show partial reversibility in the anterolateral region and complete reversibility of the inferolateral region comparable to the ^{201}Tl reinjection image. (From Dilsizian et al,[152] by permission of the American Heart Association, Inc.)

served in 31 percent of SPECT myocardial regions, from 69.9 ± 22.5 percent at 5 min poststress to 74.5 ± 20.8 percent at 120 min after injection of ^{99m}Tc sestamibi at peak stress ($p < 0.01$).[168] Redistribution of ^{99m}Tc sestamibi has also been observed following rest studies.[152,169] When an additional redistribution image was obtained 4 h after injecting the tracer at rest, ^{99m}Tc sestamibi redistribution occurred in 38 percent of regions with perfusion defects on the initial rest image that were identified as viable by ^{201}Tl and PET studies (Fig. 5-22). Such redistribution was observed in 22 percent of patients, and increased the overall concordance between ^{201}Tl and ^{99m}Tc sestamibi imaging regarding defect reversibility.[152]

Comparing SPECT ^{99m}Tc sestamibi imaging with ^{201}Tl imaging, using a rest-redistribution ^{99m}Tc sestamibi protocol, Maurea et al[169] reported that among regions with severe ^{99m}Tc sestamibi defects at rest (mean 43 percent $\pm$ 8 percent) that were identified as viable by ^{201}Tl, 24 percent showed improved ^{99m}Tc sestamibi uptake (mean 60 percent $\pm$ 8 percent) when redistribution images were acquired approximately 5 h later ($p < 0.001$). Such delayed uptake of ^{99m}Tc sestamibi (redistribution) was observed in 65 percent of the patients studied with coronary artery disease and left ventricular dysfunction. Hence, the clinical relevance of rest ^{99m}Tc sestamibi redistribution has been confirmed by other investigators.

REVASCULARIZATION STUDIES

There are a growing number of studies in the literature that have evaluated ^{99m}Tc sestamibi uptake before and

after revascularization.[147,148,157,169,170] In 1992, Lucignani et al[148] reported that among 54 asynergic regions studied before surgery, 42 had normal or reduced perfusion at rest and developed stress-induced ischemia; 11 had markedly reduced or absent perfusion at rest. After revascularization, although recovery of wall motion was observed in 79 percent of regions with stress-induced ischemia, 72 percent of regions with markedly reduced or absent perfusion at rest also showed improved wall motion after surgery. In a recent study, using planar imaging and quantitative analysis, Marzullo et al[157] compared the results of rest ^{99m}Tc sestamibi with rest ^{201}Tl studies before and after revascularization. In this study, the sensitivity and specificity of rest ^{99m}Tc sestamibi for detecting functional recovery after revascularization were 73 percent and 55 percent, respectively. From a total of 105 asynergic regions, 25 had discordant viability information between ^{201}Tl and ^{99m}Tc sestamibi, 12 regions were judged to be normal on ^{99m}Tc sestamibi and abnormal by ^{201}Tl, and 13 regions were abnormal on ^{99m}Tc sestamibi but normal by [201]Tl. After revascularization, 11 of 12 regions with normal ^{99m}Tc sestamibi (abnormal ^{201}Tl) had persistent regional dysfunction, and 11 of 13 regions with abnormal ^{99m}Tc sestamibi (normal ^{201}Tl) showed postoperative improvement in regional function.[157] These results suggest that ^{99m}Tc sestamibi may both over- and underestimate myocardial viability and functional recovery after revascularization when compared with [201]Tl (Fig. 5-23). Among 18 patients with coronary artery disease undergoing revascularization, more favorable positive (80 percent) and negative (96 percent) predictive accuracies were attained by Udelson et al[170] when the severity of ^{99m}Tc sestamibi defect was

Figure 5-23 Evidence for viable myocardium in a region with an irreversible ^{99m}Tc-sestamibi defect. Preoperative anterior planar ^{201}Tl images on the right demonstrate a severe irreversible inferior ^{201}Tl defect on stress-redistribution images that becomes partially reversible after reinjection and improves after coronary artery bypass surgery. Two-d rest-stress ^{99m}Tc-sestamibi images (on the left), performed 5 d after the ^{201}Tl study, show a severe irreversible inferior defect preoperatively that improves after coronary artery bypass surgery. The left ventricular ejection fraction increased from 40 percent before to 55 percent after surgery. (From Maurea et al,[155] Improved detection of viable myocardum with thallium-201 reinjection in chronic coronary artery disease: comparison with technetium-99m-MIBI imaging, modified and reprinted with permission from the *Journal of Nuclear Medicine*, 35:621, 1994.)

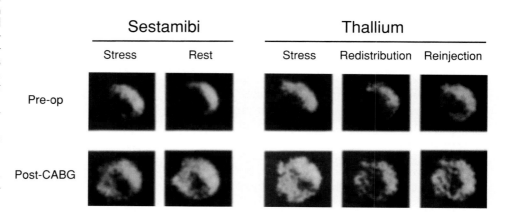

quantified at rest.[170] However, a recent publication by Maurea et al[169] suggests that such high positive and negative predictive accuracies for recovery of function after revascularization can be attained only if a rest-redistribution ^{99m}Tc sestamibi protocol is utilized. In their study, 83 percent of regions with a combination of severely reduced ^{99m}Tc sestamibi uptake at rest and redistribution on 5-h delayed images showed improvement in regional contractile function after revascularization. Global left ventricular ejection fraction increased in these patients from 42 percent ± 7 percent before surgery, to 47 percent ± 7 percent after revascularization ($p < 0.01$). In contrast, 96 percent of segments with severely reduced ^{99m}Tc sestamibi uptake at rest that remained irreversible on 5-h redistribution images had persistent left ventricular dysfunction after revascularization.

In summary, ^{99m}Tc sestamibi appears to underestimate myocardial ischemia and viability in patients with chronic coronary artery disease and left ventricular dysfunction compared with ^{201}Tl scintigraphy and ^{18}F-FDG-PET. To overcome this limitation, Berman et al[171] have proposed dual-isotope imaging that combines rest-redistribution ^{201}Tl with stress ^{99m}Tc sestamibi (Fig. 5-24), thereby taking advantage of the favorable properties of each of the two tracers. Whether measuring redistribution of ^{99m}Tc sestamibi after rest injections will enhance assessment of viable myocardium is a subject of ongoing investigation. Perhaps a more likely improvement could be achieved through combined ^{99m}Tc sestamibi perfusion and functional imaging or ECG gated myocardial perfusion studies.

Technetium-99m-Teboroxime

Technetium-99m-teboroxime is a neutral, lipophilic compound that is extracted by the myocardium in proportion to regional blood flow and its extraction remains linear even at high flow conditions.[172,173] In cultured myocardial cells, the accumulation of teboroxime has been shown to be 4 to 7.5 times greater than that of ^{99m}Tc sestamibi but the differences were not as pronounced for ^{201}Tl.[174,175] In human subjects, teboroxime permits accurate assessment of coronary blood flow even during pharmacologic hyperemia.[176–179] Unlike ^{99m}Tc sestamibi, which is retained within the mitochondria, teboroxime washes out rapidly from the myocardium at a rate proportional to regional blood flow. Therefore, both uptake and washout of teboroxime depend predominantly on regional myocardial blood flow and are not confounded by tissue metabolism or other binding characteristics within the myocardium.[180–185] Despite its rapid washout,

Dual-Isotope (Thallium-Sestamibi) Imaging

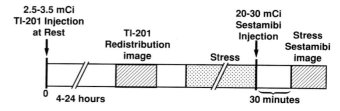

Figure 5-24 Dual-isotope (thallium-sestamibi) myocardial viability protocol.

some reports have suggested that teboroxime underestimates myocardial ischemia and viability when compared with [201]Tl.[176,186–189] Larger series are clearly needed to define the utility of teboroxime for viability assessment.

Technetium-99m-Tetrofosmin

Technetium-99m-tetrofosmin is a lipophilic phosphine dioxo cation that is distributed within the myocardium in proportion to regional blood flow.[190,191] Unlike ^{201}Tl, tetrofosmin does not redistribute significantly over time, thereby necessitating two injections of the tracer—at peak exercise and at rest.[192] Myocardial uptake and blood clearance kinetics of tetrofosmin are similar to ^{99m}Tc sestamibi. However, the clearance of tetrofosmin from lungs and liver is faster than that of ^{99m}Tc sestamibi, which may improve the resolution of early cardiac images and reduce the overall radiation burden.[193] In a recent multicenter trial, when the efficacy of tetrofosmin was compared with ^{201}Tl stress-redistribution scintigraphy, the overall concordance between the two tracers for defining normal or abnormal regions was approximately 80 percent.[128] However, when patients were categorized as showing normal, ischemic, infarction, or mixed (infarction and viable) myocardium, the concordance between tetrofosmin and ^{201}Tl decreased to only 59 percent. Furthermore, when the 2-day stress-rest tetrofosmin protocol was compared with stress-redistribution-reinjection ^{201}Tl among patients with coronary artery disease and left ventricular dysfunction, ^{201}Tl and tetrofosmin provided discordant information in 40 percent of segments; 88 percent appearing irreversible on tetrofosmin images but reversible (ischemic and viable) on ^{201}Tl reinjection images.[194] A patient with discordant ^{201}Tl stress-redistribution-reinjection and 2-day stress-rest as well as 3-h delayed rest tetrofosmin imaging is shown in Fig. 5-25. These data suggest that, like ^{99m}Tc sestamibi, tetrofosmin underestimates myocardial ischemia and viability in patients with chronic coronary artery disease and left ventricular dysfunction.

[99m]Tc-Furifosmin (Q12)

Technetium-99m-furifosmin (Q12) is a mixed-ligand cationic complex that is avidly taken up by the myocardium in relation to regional blood flow, as measured by the radioactive microsphere technique, for flows up to 2 mL/gm/min.[195] However, with pharmacologic stress (blood flow above 2 mL/g/min), Q12 activity does not increase proportionately. Q12 is cleared primarily by the hepatobiliary system and approximately 30 percent by the kidneys. Similar to tetrofosmin, Q12 does not redistribute significantly from the time of injection.[195]

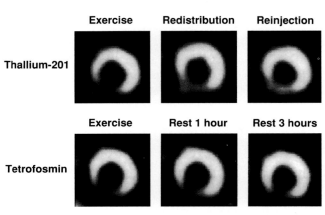

Figure 5-25   An example of a patient with reversible ^{201}Tl and irreversible tetrofosmin defects. Short axis tomograms are displayed for ^{201}Tl stress, redistribution, and reinjection with corresponding tetrofosmin stress, 1-h delayed rest, and 3-h delayed rest injected tomograms. Thallium-201 tomograms reveal a severe inferior perfusion defect during stress with partial reversibility on redistribution and further improvement on reinjection images. Stress, 1-h delayed rest, and 3-h delayed rest tetrofosmin images show a severe irreversible defect in the inferior region. (From Matsunari et al,[194] Myocardial viability assessment with technetium-99m-tetrofosmin and thallium-201 reinjection in coronary artery disease, modified and reprinted with permission from the *Journal of Nuclear Medicine*, 36:1961, 1995.)

In a pilot study, in which Q12 and ^{201}Tl imaging were compared with coronary angiography for detection of 50 percent or greater coronary artery stenosis, the respective diagnostic sensitivities and specificities were 90 percent and 90 percent for ^{201}Tl and 85 percent and 80 percent for Q12 (p = NS).[196] Although there was good overall concordance of Q12 with ^{201}Tl in normal and irreversible regions, agreement between ^{201}Tl stress-redistribution-reinjection and rest-stress Q12 for detecting myocardial ischemia and viability (defect reversibility) was poor. Multicenter clinical trials are currently under way comparing Q12 with ^{201}Tl in the same patients to better define Q12's role in assessing myocardial viability.

POSITRON EMISSION TOMOGRAPHY

Viable myocardium may be identified by PET on the basis of preserved myocardial blood flow or preserved or enhanced myocardial metabolic substrate utilization (Table 5-2). In regions with impaired myocardial blood

Table 5-2   PET Protocols for Assessing Myocardial Viability

^{18}F-FDG blood flow mismatch
Rubidium-82 uptake and washout
Oxidative metabolism with carbon 11 acetate
Water-perfusable tissue index

flow and a modest level of metabolic activity, approximately one-fifth of basal myocardial oxygen consumption is required to sustain sarcolemmal cell membrane integrity.[197] A variety of myocardial blood flow and metabolic tracers are available for the purpose of viability assessment. In general, the definition of myocardial viability with PET involves the assessment of resting flow and metabolic activity using separate tracers, although certain tracers may be used for simultaneous flow and metabolic measurements. In addition to differences in radiotracers compared with SPECT imaging, PET provides an accepted method to correct for attenuation effects, higher spatial resolution, and higher count density images. Therefore, quantitative assessment of regional myocardial blood flow and metabolic activity under various physiologic conditions is possible with PET. However, for clinical assessment of viability, detailed quantitative analysis of absolute blood flow may not be necessary.

Perfusion Imaging with PET

Myocardial blood flow tracers include ^{15}O water, ^{13}N ammonia, ^{82}Rb, and ^{62}Cu-PTSM. In contrast to all other clinically used PET tracers, which are cyclotron produced, ^{82}Rb and ^{62}Cu-PTSM are generator produced; use of the latter is currently being investigated. PET perfusion tracers may be used to quantitate absolute (in milliliters per minute per gram of tissue) or relative regional myocardial blood flow. For purposes of viability assessment, regional myocardial perfusion is usually compared with metabolic activity. Certain radiotracers, however, such as ^{82}Rb, ^{15}O water, and ^{11}C acetate, may give information on both blood flow and myocardial viability as described below.

^{15}O WATER

Oxygen-15-water is a freely diffusible tracer, the kinetics of accumulation and clearance of which are less complicated than tracers that are partially extractable. Quantitative assessment of regional ^{15}O water perfusion correlates closely with perfusion assessed by microspheres.[198] Because ^{15}O water is distributed in both the vascular space and myocardium, visualization of myocardial activity requires correction for activity in the vascular compartment. This is accomplished by acquiring a separate scan that identifies either the intravascular or myocardial compartments. Identification of the intravascular compartment is accomplished after inhalation of ^{15}O-CO, which labels red blood cells. Subtraction of ^{15}O-CO images from ^{15}O water images results in visualization of the myocardium.[198,199] It may be possible to eliminate the ^{15}O-CO by analyzing separately the early phase of ^{15}O

water distribution, which reflects first pass of the tracer through the cardiac blood pool.[200] Alternatively, the myocardium can be identified using the metabolic images, such as with ^{18}F FDG. Regions of interest drawn on the ^{18}F-FDG study then may be applied to corresponding slices of the ^{15}O water study. Myocardial uptake of ^{15}O water parallels regional blood flow even in hyperemic ranges.[200–203]

Water-Perfusable Tissue Index (PTI) Recent studies have explored the ability of ^{15}O water to assess myocardial viability through modification of the blood flow information (Fig. 5-26). This method is based on measurement of perfusable tissue fraction (PTF), which was first introduced by Iida et al[202] as a method to correct for the partial volume effects in ^{15}O water studies. These investigators defined PTF as the fractional volume of a given region of interest occupied by myocardium that is capable of rapidly exchanging water. Using transmission and $C^{15}O$ blood pool images, a quantitative estimate of extravascular tissue density, called anatomical tissue fraction (ATF), is derived. The ratio of PTF/ATF, called the perfusable tissue index (PTI), thus represents the proportion of the extravascular tissue that is perfusable by ^{15}O water. The ratio should be unity in normal myocardium and reduced in scar.

Yamamoto et al[204] applied this technique to patients with acute and chronic ischemic heart disease and in healthy volunteers. In healthy volunteers, PTI was 1.08 ± 0.07 g (perfusable tissue)/g (total anatomical tissue). In the patients with chronic ischemic heart disease, PTI was significantly lower in regions that were nonviable by metabolic (^{18}F FDG/blood flow ratio) than in viable regions (0.75 ± 0.14 vs 0.53 ± 0.12, $p < 0.01$). Among patients who were treated successfully with thrombolysis after an acute myocardial infarction, no segment with a PTI < 0.7 exhibited functional recovery. The same investigators subsequently reported their experience in 12 patients with chronic ischemic heart disease and prior myocardial infarction who were undergoing revascularization.[205] The data showed that regions in which functional recovery was observed after revascularization always had a PTI > 0.7. Functional recovery was not observed in regions with PTI < 0.7. These preliminary data suggest that ^{15}O water may provide information on regional myocardial perfusion and viability without necessitating a separate metabolic assessment.

^{13}N AMMONIA

Nitrogen-13-ammonia is the most commonly used extractable perfusion tracer with PET.[206,207] Its myocardial extraction is nonlinear and inversely related to blood flow, and its uptake is thought to involve a carrier-mediated transport.[208,209] The kinetics of accumulation and clearance from myocardium depend on the conversion

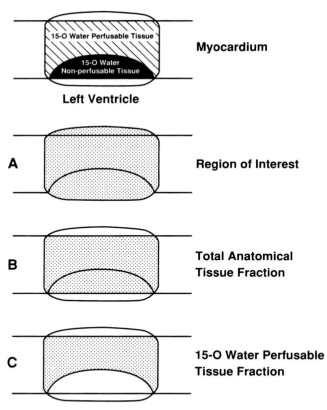

Myocardium

Left Ventricle

A   **Region of Interest**

B   **Total Anatomical Tissue Fraction**

C   **15-O Water Perfusable Tissue Fraction**

C/B = 15-O Water Perfusable Tissue Index (PTI)

Figure 5-26 Schematic of a myocardial region of interest containing a mixture of ^{15}O-water perfusable and nonperfusable tissue. **Panel A:** Volume of the region of interest. **Panel B:** Anatomic tissue fraction for the region of interest produced by subtraction of the blood pool (^{15}O-CO) from the transmission images after normalization of the latter to tissue density (1.04 g/mL). Total anatomic tissue fraction represents the total extravascular tissue and contains both perfusable and nonperfusable tissue components. **Panel C:** ^{15}O-water perfusable tissue fraction for the region of interest that is calculated from the ^{15}O-water data set and identifies the mass of tissue within the region of interest that is capable of rapid transsarcolemmal exchange of water. Note that the nonperfusable or necrotic region is excluded from this parameter. The ^{15}O-water perfusable tissue index is calculated by dividing ^{15}O-water perfusable tissue fraction (panel C) by the total anatomic tissue fraction (panel B) and represents the fraction of the total anatomic tissue that is perfusable by water. (From Yamamoto et al,[204] modified and reprinted by permission of the American Heart Association, Inc.)

of ammonia to glutamine via the glutamine synthetase pathway. Absolute quantification requires two- and three-compartment kinetic models that incorporate extraction and rate constants.[210,211] Experimental studies suggest that myocardial uptake of ^{13}N ammonia reflects absolute blood flows of up to 2 to 2.5 mL/g/min and plateaus in the hyperemic range.[208,209]

Nitrogen-13-ammonia is used most commonly to assess regional myocardial blood flow in relation to meta-

bolic activity, such as ^{18}F FDG. The techniques used to evaluate regional blood flow with ^{13}N ammonia have been either qualitative or semiquantitative (e.g., circumferential profile analysis). However, recent studies indicate that absolute quantification of myocardial blood flow with ^{13}N ammonia may be useful in differentiating viable from nonviable myocardium. Based on experimental data suggesting that a minimum level of myocardial blood flow is necessary to maintain human myocyte viability, Gewirtz et al[212] studied 26 patients with chronic ischemic heart disease with ^{13}N ammonia and ^{18}F FDG. These investigators reported that absolute myocardial blood flow measurements permitted differentiation of viable and nonviable myocardium in asynergic regions. Regions with blood flow < 0.25 mL/g/min were unlikely to be viable by ^{18}F-FDG imaging, and all dyskinetic segments had blood flows < 0.25 mL/g/min. Among patients with chronic coronary artery disease studied before and after revascularization, however, the accuracy of assessing myocardial blood flow alone for viability assessment has been inconsistent.[213–215] Although Tamaki et al[213] reported positive and negative predictive accuracies for improvement in regional asynergy to be only 48 percent and 87 percent, respectively, Grandin et al[214] found absolute ^{13}N ammonia myocardial blood flow to be the best predictor of functional recovery in patients revascularized after anterior myocardial infarction. However, in the latter study, there was a considerable overlap of blood flow values between viable and nonviable segments, and a discriminant function of both blood flow and ^{18}F-FDG uptake was necessary to achieve an overall accuracy of 84 percent.

In most patients referred to PET laboratories for the assessment of myocardial viability, myocardial perfusion imaging is performed before metabolic imaging. In others, in whom inducible ischemia is a clinical concern, perfusion imaging is performed during pharmacologic stress and at rest. Clinical studies from two different laboratories have indicated that asynergic regions with resting ^{13}N ammonia activity less than 40 percent of that in a normal region were unlikely to improve after revascularization.[216,217] In the study by Tamaki et al[217] hypoperfused regions without stress-induced ischemia were highly specific for irreversible myocardial damage. Although the negative predictive values for myocardial viability for these techniques utilizing semiquantitative PET perfusion variables are in the range of 80 to 87 percent, the positive predictive values are low, approximately 48 to 65 percent. In these patients, ^{18}F-FDG metabolic imaging was somewhat better than perfusion imaging in predicting myocardial viability. This may be because the observation that regions with moderate hypoperfusion and reduced metabolic activity (matched defect) may represent regions with admixture of viable and scarred myocardium, but be misclassified as com-

^{13}N-Ammonia/^{18}FDG Imaging

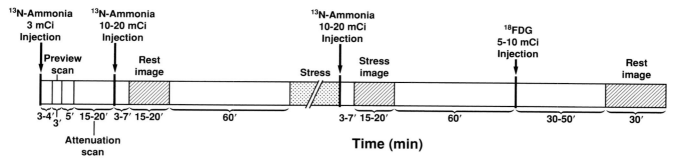

Figure 5-27 Static ^{13}N-ammonia and ^{18}F-FDG PET protocol for assessing myocardial ischemia and viability.

pletely viable by perfusion imaging alone.[218] Thus, at present, metabolic imaging remains the most accurate method to assess myocardial viability with PET. A static ^{13}N ammonia and ^{18}F-FDG PET protocol for assessing myocardial ischemia and viability is shown in Fig. 5-27.

Rubidium 82

Rubidium 82 is a generator-produced cation whose uptake depends on myocardial perfusion.[219] Experimental studies suggest that myocardial uptake of rubidium is proportional to myocardial blood flow up to 2–3 mL/g/min, and that uptake plateaus at hyperemic flows above this range.[220,221] Although the extraction fraction of rubidium may decrease during periods of myocardial ischemia,[220-223] the qualitative assessment of relative rubidium perfusion defects has correlated well with those obtained from microspheres.[224] Clinically, rubidium PET has both high sensitivity and specificity for detecting coronary artery disease.[225-228] As a result, rubidium has received U.S. Food and Drug Administration (FDA) approval for assessment of myocardial perfusion.

The potential utility of rubidium as a marker of myocardial viability is based on its similarities to potassium (as with ^{201}Tl) with regard to membrane transport, trapping, and extraction characteristics.[229,230] Maintenance of the intracellular-extracellular potassium gradient is dependent on cellular viability and intact cell membranes.[231] Myocardial cell necrosis is associated with loss of intracellular potassium,[231] the extent of which is proportional to the extent of necrosis.[232] Experimental studies have demonstrated that rubidium initially distributes in relation to blood flow, and is trapped in normal cells.[233] In necrotic cells, however, the tracer washes out rapidly, and the rate of washout may reliably identify necrotic from viable myocardium.[233] Hence, rubidium is taken up by both viable and necrotic myocardium, but

is not retained by necrotic myocardium. A static rubidium and ^{18}F-FDG PET protocol for assessing myocardial ischemia and viability is shown in Fig. 5-28.

Based on these observations, Gould et al[234] have suggested that the kinetics of rubidium washout may be used clinically as an index of myocardial viability (Fig. 5-29). Using a simple, background-corrected ratio of rubidium activity in the late to early image, the authors estimated that a ratio of 0.825 represented the threshold below which less than 50 percent of viable tissue was present in any given transmural segment. This technique was compared with ^{18}F-FDG PET imaging in 43 patients an average of 27 d post–myocardial infarction. Infarct size assessed by analysis of rubidium kinetics correlated well to infarct size by ^{18}F-FDG PET, independent of infarct age.[234] Furthermore, these authors showed a relationship between quantitative infarct size and viability by PET, left ventricular ejection fraction, and 3-y mortality among patients with and without revascularization.[235] Utilizing dynamic data acquisition, good agreement has also been shown between washout of rubidium (after only a single injection) and ^{18}F-FDG uptake.[236] Thus, the assessment of cell membrane integrity on the basis of rubidium kinetics may be useful for the clinical evaluation of myocardial viability and infarct size.

Relation of coronary flow reserve to myocardial viability The relationship between intact coronary flow reserve and myocardial viability has been demonstrated in experimental and preliminary clinical studies. Several groups of investigators have demonstrated that hypoperfused, functionally impaired myocardium may retain a residual vasodilating capability either transmurally[237,238] or preferentially within the subepicardial vessels.[239] Using direct measurements of microvascular luminal caliber, persistent arteriolar vasomotor tone was demonstrated despite a significant reduction in luminal pressure and flow.[240] Thus, experimental evidence suggests that micro-

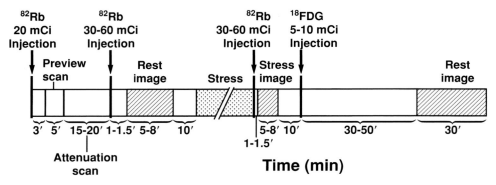

Figure 5-28 Static rubidium and ¹⁸F-FDG PET protocol for assessing myocardial ischemia and viability.

vascular beds distal to a severe, functionally significant coronary stenosis are not maximally vasodilated, and retain some vasodilating capability.

Several clinical studies also have addressed the issue of flow reserve as it related to myocardial viability in chronic coronary artery disease patients. Using ⁹⁹ᵐTc-labeled microsphere scintigraphy, Parodi et al[241] studied 15 patients with isolated left anterior descending coronary artery disease and no prior infarction, five of whom had anterior hypokinesis.[241] Using semiquantitative analysis, these authors demonstrated that patients with resting hypoperfusion had persistent vasodilating capability after papaverine administration, and that

the calculated coronary reserve in these patients was equivalent to that of patients without resting hypoperfusion. In a study of 26 patients with chronic occlusion of a major coronary artery, and no prior myocardial infarction, a significant inverse correlation was observed between wall motion abnormality and collateral flow reserve as assessed by quantitative ¹³N-ammonia PET.[242]

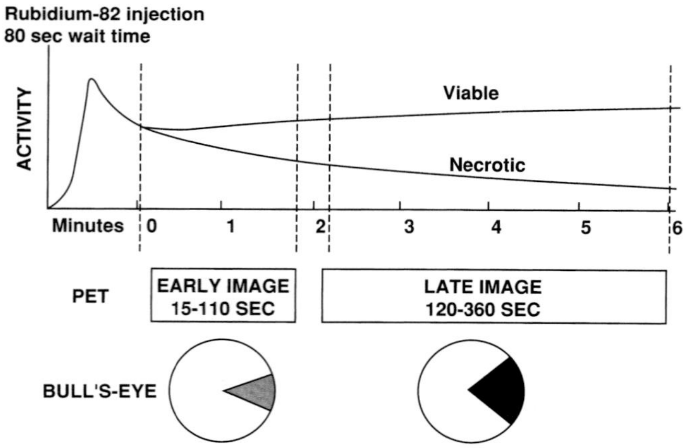

To specifically address the issue of the relation between coronary flow reserve and myocardial viability, Marzullo et al[243] studied 14 patients with prior remote (>3 mo) myocardial infarction and regional ventricular dysfunction with resting and dipyridamole ¹³N-ammonia PET and viability imaging with ¹⁸F-FDG PET. Among myocardial regions with severe resting hypoperfusion, those regions with persistent metabolic activity indicative of viability showed preserved coronary flow reserve, whereas those regions that were metabolically inactive and thus necrotic showed virtually absent flow reserve (2.6 ± 1.3 vs 1.3 ± 0.5, $p < 0.01$). Furthermore, the average flow reserve in the viable, severely hypoperfused segments was similar to that observed in viable segments with only a mild reduction in resting myocardial blood flow (2.6 ± 1.3 vs 2.5 ± 1.6). These data support the concept that persistent coronary flow reserve is a potentially useful and reliable indicator of viable myocardium in patients with previous infarction.

Residual coronary flow reserve may also predict functional recovery after reperfusion of acute myocardial infarction. Suryapranata et al[244] assessed vasodilator reserve using digital subtraction cineangiography at baseline and after intracoronary isosorbide dinitrate in 22 patients who underwent coronary angioplasty within 4 h of acute myocardial infarction. They found that the degree of the hyperemic response immediately after reperfusion was predictive of the degree of functional improvement during follow-up. Thus, residual coronary flow reserve may be an indicator of preserved

Figure 5-29 Schematic protocol utilizing the kinetic changes of rubidium 82 after intravenous injection to assess myocardial viability. As illustrated on the bull's-eye diagram, a new or worsening defect on the late image compared with the early image indicates washout or failure to trap rubidium, and therefore, necrosis. (From Gould et al,[234] Myocardial metabolism of fluorodeoxyglucose compared to cell membrane integrity for the potassium analogue rubidium 82 for assessing infarct size in man by PET, modified and reprinted with permission of the *Journal of Nuclear Medicine,* 32:1, 1991.)

viability in acute myocardial infarction and in chronic coronary artery disease.

Metabolic Imaging with PET

The use of metabolic radiotracers with PET has emerged as a useful approach to investigate the effects of coronary artery disease on myocardial metabolism and viability. At rest, glucose, lactate, and free fatty acids (FFAs) are the primary substrates of myocardial energy production. In the fasting state, FFAs are the primary substrates,[245] accounting for approximately 60 percent of the oxidative metabolic requirements. These FFAs generally undergo complete oxidation in the tricarboxylic acid cycle via β-oxidation, with a small percentage (approximately 15 percent) undergoing reesterification to tissue triglycerides.[246] Myocardial FFA uptake is determined primarily by the arterial FFA concentration.[247] In the fed state, insulin levels increase and result in profound alterations in myocardial metabolism. Glucose metabolism is stimulated, and tissue lipolysis is inhibited, resulting in reduced FFA delivery to the myocardium. The combined effects of insulin on these processes and the increased arterial glucose concentration associated with the fed state result in an increase in myocardial glucose uptake. Under these conditions, glucose becomes the primary substrate for myocardial energy production, accounting for approximately 68 percent of the oxidative metabolic requirements.[248]

Myocardial ischemia is associated with a number of alterations in myocardial metabolism. During ischemia, myocardial lactate uptake may decrease and a net release of lactate may occur.[249] Myocardial glucose extraction increases, the degree of which may correlate to lactate production.[250] Fundamentally, the loss of oxidative potential results in a compensatory shift toward increased glucose utilization through increased glycogen breakdown and increased glucose uptake.[248,251,252] The cells thus may shift to pathways of anaerobic glycolysis (the Pasteur effect), resulting in maintenance of myocyte viability at the expense of less efficient substrate utilization. The tricarboxylic acid cycle, the primary source of high energy phosphates in oxidative metabolism, is inhibited, and its intermediates accumulate.[253] Although the energy produced in this manner may be adequate to maintain the electrochemical gradient across the cell membrane, it may not be sufficient to sustain mechanical work. The sustained reliance on anaerobic metabolism, however, is dependent on coronary flow adequate to wash out the end products of glycolysis (lactate and hydrogen ion).[248,252] In the setting of severe ischemia and markedly reduced coronary flow, the ensuing tissue acidosis ultimately will result in inhibition of phosphofructokinase and glycolysis. Without the production of high energy

phosphates, cell membrane disruption and cell death will occur. Schematic representation of a myocyte with its major metabolic pathways and regulatory steps is shown in Fig. 5-30.

Carbon 11-PALMITATE

Since fatty acids are the primary source of myocardial energy production in the fasted state, early studies focused on the characterization of myocardial kinetics of ^{11}C palmitate. Uptake of ^{11}C palmitate across the sarcolemmal membrane is thought to occur along a concentration gradient, possibly through a facilitated transport. Following myocardial extraction of ^{11}C palmitate, it is cleared biexponentially.[254,255] The initial, rapid-clearance phase represents oxidative metabolism of ^{11}C palmitate through β-oxidation and the tricarboxylic acid cycle. The second, slower-clearance phase of the tracer represents the turnover of ^{11}C palmitate in the endogenous pool of phospholipids and triglycerides.[251,255] During myocardial ischemia or hypoxia, both myocardial extraction and clearance of ^{11}C palmitate are reduced.[256] In a canine model of 3-h coronary artery occlusion and reperfusion, both myocardial extraction and clearance of ^{11}C palmitate were impaired, suggesting reduced fatty acid utilization.[257] However, under ischemic conditions, the kinetics of ^{11}C palmitate are not specific for oxidative metabolism but rather reflect the overall metabolic function of the myocardium. In a reperfused working swine heart model, Liedtke et al[258] reported that fatty acid oxidation actually increases during early reflow. Despite conflicting data in experimental animals, impaired ^{11}C-palmitate oxidation has been demonstrated in patients with acute myocardial ischemia.[259] It is important to keep in mind, however, that the kinetics of myocardial extraction and clearance of fatty acids can be markedly altered by arterial substrate concentration, myocardial ischemia and reperfusion, and hormonal environment.[260–262] As a result, the role of ^{11}C palmitate in the clinical evaluation of patients with chronic coronary artery disease or acute myocardial ischemia has been limited.

FLUORINE-18-FLUORODEOXYGLUCOSE

Fluorine-18-2-fluoro-2-deoxyglucose (^{18}F FDG) is a metabolic marker for glucose uptake that competes with glucose for hexokinase and tracks transmembranous exchange of glucose.[263] Fluorine-18 FDG is phosphorylated by hexokinase into FDG-6-phosphate, a form of deoxyglucose that cannot be metabolized further.[264] Thus, myocardial uptake of ^{18}F FDG reflects the overall rate of transmembrane exchange and phosphorylation of glucose, but its uptake does not selectively track any of the potential metabolic pathways of glucose metabolism such as glycolysis, glycogen synthesis, or the fructose-

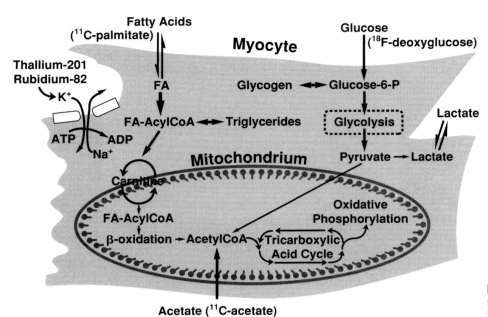

Figure 5-30 Schematic representation of a myocyte with its major metabolic pathways and regulatory steps.

pentose shunt. Because the dephosphorylation rate of glucose is slow, ^{18}F FDG becomes essentially trapped in the myocardium, and measurement of its uptake reflects regional glucose flux.

In addition to the effects of ischemia noted previously, myocardial glucose utilization also is influenced by a number of other factors, including cardiac work, competitive substrates, insulin level, and neurohumoral effects.[251,265,266] The transport of glucose into the cell is facilitated by a family of transmembrane proteins called glucose transporter proteins (GluT). At least five different glucose transporter proteins have been identified, and one of its forms, GluT4, predominates in muscle cells. This particular GluT subtype is quite sensitive to insulin stimulation, and increased insulin levels result in a dramatic increase in the number of GluT4 transporters on the cell membrane surface.

Quantification of regional myocardial glucose metabolism   Although much of the clinical assessment of myocardial viability using ^{18}F FDG is based on comparison of its qualitative or semiquantitative uptake relative to a myocardial perfusion tracer, quantification of myocardial glucose utilization is possible. Quantification requires a correction factor that considers the relationship between the kinetic behavior of ^{18}F FDG to that of naturally occurring glucose with regard to transmembrane transport and phosphorylation. This factor is called the "lumped constant." Experimental studies suggest that the lumped constant is relatively stable under a wide range of physiologic conditions.[267] It is not known, however, whether these experimental data are applicable to humans or whether there may be differences in this constant between patients or regional differences within the

myocardium. Thus, kinetic modeling that attempts to quantify glucose utilization must be interpreted with caution. At present, there are several methods available to quantitate myocardial glucose utilization. Using dynamic PET acquisitions, often coupled with sequential arterial blood sampling, clinically applicable methods include Patlak graphic analysis,[268] measurement of fractional ^{18}F-FDG uptake in relation to delivered dose,[269] and a three-compartment model.[270] Knuuti et al[271] evaluated 70 patients with prior myocardial infarction, 48 of whom also underwent coronary artery bypass surgery, with quantitative (calculation of regional myocardial glucose uptake or rMGU) and semiquantitative (measurement of relative uptake) ^{18}F-FDG PET. They found a substantially greater interindividual variation in rMGU than in normalized ^{18}F-FDG uptake values, and as a result, normalized ^{18}F-FDG uptake measurements were superior to calculation of rMGU for the assessment of myocardial viability. More recently, experimental studies by Hariharan et al[272] identified important potential limitations to the use of ^{18}F FDG for quantification of rMGU.[272] Using an isolated working rat heart model, they determined that the relationship between ^{18}F FDG and [2-3H]glucose uptake and retention may be affected by alterations in substrate availability. Thus, measurement of absolute rMGU with ^{18}F-FDG PET may not be accurate in non–steady state conditions. Additional studies are needed to define the role of absolute quantification of rMGU in clinical practice.

Heterogeneity of ^{18}F-FDG uptake in normals   Several studies have investigated the regional differences in ^{18}F-FDG uptake and rMGU.[273,274] These studies suggest that in both fasting and glucose-loaded states, myocar-

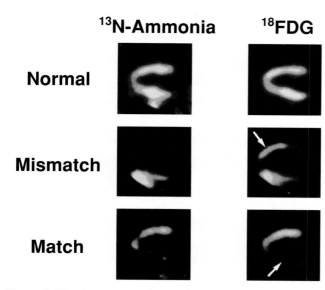

¹³N-Ammonia   ¹⁸FDG

Normal

Mismatch

Match

Figure 5-31 Cross-sectional vertical long axis PET images are shown for ¹³N ammonia and ¹⁸F FDG. Top panel shows examples of normal ¹³N-ammonia and ¹⁸F-FDG uptake. Middle panel shows discordance between ¹⁸F-FDG uptake and ¹³N-ammonia uptake (FDG–blood flow mismatch) in the anterior region indicative of viable myocardium (arrowhead). Lower panel shows concordant severely reduced ¹³N-ammonia and ¹⁸F-FDG uptake (FDG–blood flow match) in the inferior region indicative of myocardial scar.

dial glucose utilization is lower in the anteroseptal region compared with the lateral and inferior regions. The regional differences appear to be more pronounced in the fasting state, where ¹⁸F-FDG uptake may be up to 20 percent lower in the septum and anterior walls.[273] This heterogeneity of rMGU cannot be explained by regional differences in metabolic demand (assessed by ¹¹C-acetate kinetics) or perfusion, and may be minimized by glucose loading.[273,274] Thus, standardization of imaging protocols using some form of glucose loading, sometimes combined with supplemental insulin administration, is recommended for ¹⁸F-FDG viability studies.

Clinical assessment of myocardial viability using ¹⁸F-FDG Metabolic shift from fatty acids to glucose was first characterized in experimental models of ischemia.[275,276] Combined metabolic imaging with ¹⁸F FDG and resting perfusion with ¹³N ammonia was first applied to patients with recent myocardial infarction for the purpose of viability assessment.[277] Among regions with resting hypoperfusion, two patterns of tracer uptake were identified: a concordant reduction in both flow and metabolism (termed a flow-metabolism "match"), which was considered to represent myocardial scar, and a discordant increase in ¹⁸F-FDG uptake compared with flow (termed a flow-metabolism "mismatch") which was considered to represent ischemic, viable myocardium (Fig. 5-31). Subsequently, it was demonstrated that a majority of regions (54 percent) that were associated with chronic

Q waves on electrocardiography were metabolically active by ¹⁸F-FDG PET, and that a significant proportion of these (20 percent) showed flow-metabolism mismatch.[278]

To determine whether enhanced or preserved ¹⁸F-FDG uptake in dysfunctional regions identifies viable myocardium that is capable of functional improvement upon restoration of blood flow, Tillisch et al[35] and Tamaki et al[279] evaluated resting myocardial blood flow and metabolism (using ¹³N ammonia and ¹⁸F FDG) before and after coronary artery revascularization. Metabolic studies were performed with and without glucose loading after an overnight fast. In these two studies, preoperative identification of enhanced ¹⁸F-FDG uptake relative to blood flow was associated with functional improvement in 78 to 85 percent of regions after revascularization. Conversely, contractile function did not improve in 78 to 92 percent of regions demonstrating reduced ¹⁸F-FDG uptake and concomitant reduction in blood flow. In Tillisch's study, 22 (63 percent) of the 35 dysfunctional regions that showed improved contractile function after revascularization had normal blood flow preoperatively.[280] Since dysfunctional regions with preserved blood flow at rest are more likely to represent stunned, rather than hibernating, myocardium, it underscores the importance for consistent definition of "mismatch" regions in various publications (Table 5-3). A correlation between the extent of myocardial mismatch regions and improvement in global left ventricular ejection fraction at 12 to 18 wk after revascularization was also demonstrated in the same study.[35] In patients demonstrating two or more regions of flow-metabolism mismatch, left ventricular ejection fraction improved from a mean of 30 percent before to 45 percent after bypass surgery. Similar improvement in global left ventricular function was reported by other investigators.[281,282]

Subsequently, a number of studies with ¹⁸F-FDG PET before and after revascularization have been performed with fairly consistent results. In general, although the total number of patients studied before and after revascularization is not large, the positive and negative predictive accuracies for functional recovery (or lack

Table 5-3 Definitions and Interpretations of ¹⁸F FDG: Blood Flow Relation with PET

Blood Flow	¹⁸F-FDG Uptake	Interpretation
Normal	Normal	Normal
	Increased	Mismatch—stunned myocardium
	Decreased	Admixture—scar/ viable myocardium
Abnormal	Normal or increased	Mismatch— hibernating myocardium
	Decreased	Match
	Moderate	Admixture (scar/viable)
	Severe	Match—scar

thereof) are in the range of 80 percent.[35,279,281-285] More recently, Tamaki et al[286] evaluated 43 patients with coronary artery disease and regional left ventricular dysfunction with rest/stress ^{13}N-ammonia myocardial perfusion and ^{18}F-FDG metabolic PET imaging. PET viability was determined by three different methods: 1) the magnitude of perfusion at rest, 2) evidence of ischemia by pharmacologic stress (dipyridamole), and 3) the degree of ^{18}F-FDG uptake. Although negative predictive values were similar for each method (87 percent, 87 percent, and 92 percent, respectively), ^{18}F-FDG PET had the best positive predictive accuracy for recovery of function after revascularization (48 percent, 63 percent, and 76 percent, respectively). Similar results were obtained in another study in which [82]Rb was used as the perfusion tracer.[287] However, assessment of viability by the combination of the magnitude of perfusion at rest and ischemia (defect reversibility) versus the ^{18}F-FDG uptake was not provided in either one of the studies. Thus, at present, it appears that PET studies obtained for the purpose of myocardial viability assessment should include a metabolic tracer, such as ^{18}F FDG.

A recent study by vom Dahl et al[288] emphasizes the importance of integrating all available information, including PET, angiographic, and wall motion data, for the optimal selection of patients with coronary artery disease who are being considered for revascularization. Among 33 patients studied with chronic left ventricular dysfunction and no prior coronary artery bypass surgery, the accuracy of PET for the prediction of functional recovery was influenced by the severity of resting regional dysfunction. The positive predictive value for PET ^{18}F-FDG imaging ranged from 37 percent for all regions with perfusion/metabolism mismatch to 88 percent for those regions demonstrating severe hypokinesis or akinesis at rest. The negative predictive accuracy was 86 percent, which is similar to the value reported previously. It is noteworthy that the predictive accuracies reported with PET are quite similar to those reported for ^{201}Tl reinjection; positive predictive value of 80 to 91 percent and negative predictive value of 82 to 100 percent.[77,79,83-85,89]

Although there are several studies that characterize preoperative metabolic alterations in patients with chronic coronary artery disease, only a few studies have reevaluated substrate utilization after revascularization.[289,290] To examine the effects of revascularization on regional coronary blood flow, metabolism and contractile function, Nienaber et al[289] studied patients with PET and echocardiography before, within 72 h, and approximately 2 mo after coronary angioplasty. The authors found that despite restoration of blood flow, both regional contractile function and absolute glucose utilization remained abnormal within 72 h after coronary angioplasty and normalized only during the late follow-up. In a similar study, Marwick et al[290] reported that most

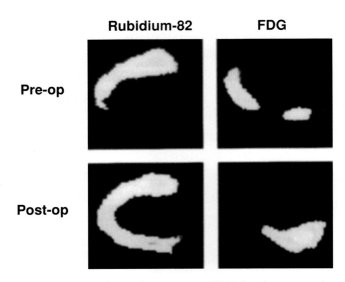

Figure 5-32 Evidence for persistent ^{18}F-FDG utilization in the inferior region despite improved blood flow after revascularization. Preoperative sagittal PET images show severely reduced perfusion defects in the inferoapical and inferior regions associated with enhanced ^{18}F-FDG uptake (mismatch) in both regions. Despite improved perfusion and contraction in the inferoapical and inferior regions after surgery, ^{18}F-FDG activity is reduced in the inferoapical region but not in the inferior region. (From Marwick et al,[285] modified and reprinted by permission of the American Heart Association, Inc.)

preoperative FDG–blood flow mismatch regions that demonstrate improved perfusion and function after revascularization also show reduced ^{18}F-FDG activity, reflecting a metabolic shift back to fatty acids. In the subset of regions in which enhanced ^{18}F-FDG utilization was persistent, as late as 5 mo after the surgery, regional blood flow was severely reduced preoperatively. A patient example with persistent ^{18}F-FDG utilization in a region with improved blood flow after revascularization is shown in Fig. 5-32.

CARBON-11-ACETATE

Carbon-11-acetate is taken up by the myocardium in proportion to blood flow, and its washout rate is directly related to oxidative tricarboxylic acid (TCA) flux.[291-293] Because all major myocardial oxidative fuels are oxidized through conversion to acetyl-CoA and subsequent oxidation through the TCA cycle, there is a consistent relationship between TCA cycle flux and overall myocardial oxygen consumption. Thus, ^{11}C-acetate imaging allows the noninvasive quantification of regional myocardial oxygen consumption, a potentially powerful clinical and experimental technique to evaluate cardiac physiology.

The extraction fraction of ^{11}C acetate after intravenous injection at rest is approximately 65 percent, and decreases to about 50 percent during hyperemia.[294] Gropler et al[295] hypothesized that analysis of the early portion (60 to 180 s after injection of tracer) of the myocardial time–activity curve would reflect primarily delivery and extraction of tracer, and thus may be used as an index of regional myocardial blood flow. Twenty-two subjects with coronary artery disease who were evaluated at rest demonstrated a close correlation between relative early ^{11}C-acetate uptake and relative regional blood flow assessed by [15]O water. Thus, evaluation of the early distribution of ^{11}C acetate at rest may provide a means for assessing relative regional myocardial blood flow. The utility of this approach in hyperemic conditions is unknown.

The noninvasive assessment of regional oxidative metabolism may provide a potentially sensitive index for evaluating myocardial viability. Experimental studies have indicated that measurement of the rate of ^{11}C-acetate clearance from the myocardium is a good index of myocardial oxygen consumption.[296,297] In a canine model, Brown et al[297] showed that the rate constant of the rapid phase of clearance of total ^{11}C activity from the heart was closely correlated with myocardial oxygen consumption ($r = 0.90$) and the rate of [11]CO$_2$ efflux measured directly ($r = 0.95$). Subsequently, it has been determined that this technique may be used clinically as a measure of myocardial oxidative metabolism.[294,298] In normal subjects, there is minimal regional variability in ^{11}C-acetate clearance,[294,298] in contrast to the inhomogeneity often observed with ^{18}F FDG. The feasibility of assessing oxidative metabolic reserve also has been demonstrated and may provide additional insight into the evaluation of patients with myocardial dysfunction.[299]

The clinical applicability of ^{11}C-acetate imaging for viability assessment has been reported in several studies.[300–302] In 11 patients studied soon after myocardial infarction who were subsequently revascularized, viable but dysfunctional myocardium could be distinguished from nonviable myocardium on the basis of ^{11}C-acetate kinetics.[300] Abnormally contracting but viable myocardial regions had oxidative metabolic activity 74 percent that of normal regions, whereas nonviable regions had 45 percent of normal metabolic activity. In 16 patients with chronic coronary artery disease and prior myocardial infarction, viable but dysfunctional myocardium had preserved oxidative metabolism approximately equivalent to that of normal zones.[301] In contrast, nonviable myocardium had only 66 percent of metabolic activity of the normal zones. It should be noted that, based on these studies, threshold values for viability assessment using ^{11}C-acetate may differ between patients studied soon after infarction versus those studied with a history of remote infarction. The same group of investigators subsequently studied 34 patients with chronic coronary artery disease and left ventricular dysfunction with ^{11}C acetate and ^{18}F-FDG PET before revascularization.[302] The

positive and negative predictive values for regional functional recovery in segments that were severely dysfunctional at baseline were 85 percent and 87 percent for acetate, and 72 percent and 82 percent for ^{18}F FDG, respectively, ($p = NS$ between the two tracers). However, preliminary data in patients with recent myocardial infarction suggest that ^{11}C acetate may be more accurate than ^{18}F FDG in predicting recovery of function after revascularization.[303] Other potential advantages of acetate over ^{18}F FDG include its shorter imaging time, the possibility of simultaneous assessment of relative regional myocardial perfusion and metabolism with one tracer, and its more uniform distribution in normals and in diabetic patients who may have a significant number of unintelligible ^{18}F-FDG studies.

Comparison of PET With Thallium SPECT

Since delayed ^{201}Tl images reflect cation flux and sarcolemmal membrane integrity, it is possible that ^{201}Tl may yield comparable viability information as metabolic imaging with ^{18}F FDG. In a canine model of 2 h of coronary occlusion followed by 4 h of reperfusion, ^{201}Tl was injected before reperfusion and ^{18}F FDG was administered 3 h after reflow.[304] Both ^{201}Tl redistribution and preserved ^{18}F-FDG uptake accurately identified viable myocardium after reperfusion. On the other hand, lack of ^{201}Tl redistribution and reduced ^{18}F-FDG uptake identified irreversibly injured, necrotic myocardium.

PET COMPARED WITH 3- to 4-h AND 24-h REDISTRIBUTION IMAGING

Early studies, comparing stress-redistribution ^{201}Tl with PET imaging showed that 38 to 58 percent of regions with apparently "irreversible" [201]Tl defects were viable by PET.[305–308] However, stress-redistribution ^{201}Tl imaging without late (24-h) redistribution or reinjection studies will significantly underestimate myocardial viability.[70,77,79,83–85] In addition, quantitative analysis of the severity of ^{201}Tl activity within irreversible defects may reflect myocardial viability.[70,110–113,309] Among patients with chronic coronary artery disease, when late redistribution ^{201}Tl images were compared with PET, more regions were identified as viable with PET than [201]Tl.[310] However, when the severity of ^{201}Tl activity within fixed 24-h ^{201}Tl defects was assessed, there was an inverse correlation between ^{201}Tl defect score and myocardial viability by PET.[310] Among regions with a significantly reduced 24-h ^{201}Tl score, the probability of PET demonstrating viability was less than 15 percent.

PET COMPARED WITH THALLIUM REINJECTION

In patients with chronic coronary artery disease, the similar predictive accuracies of PET imaging and [201]Tl

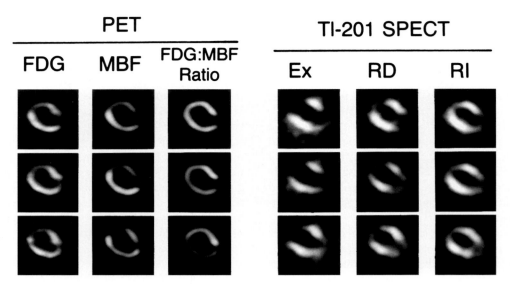

Figure 5-33 Concordance of PET and ^{201}Tl reinjection data. Tomographic ^{18}F FDG, myocardial blood flow (MBF), and ^{18}F-FDG–to–blood flow ratio (FDG:MBF), generated from the quantitative ^{15}O-water data with partial volume and spillover correction are shown on the left panel. The corresponding ^{201}Tl data for exercise (Ex), 3- to 4-h redistribution (RD), and reinjection (RI) are shown on the right panel. Standard exercise-redistribution ^{201}Tl studies demonstrate an apparently irreversible anteroapical defect. Myocardial blood flow is reduced in this region and in the septum according to PET. However, ^{18}F-FDG images demonstrate uptake and, hence, viability in all regions, most notably the anteroapical region. Functional images of ^{18}F-FDG–to–blood flow ratio demonstrate enhanced ^{18}F-FDG uptake relative to blood flow (mismatch) involving the apex and septum. Thallium-201 reinjection images mirror the ^{18}F-FDG images, with evidence of enhanced ^{201}Tl uptake and, hence, viability in the anteroapical region. (From Dilsizian et al,[110] by permission of the American Heart Association, Inc.)

reinjection for differentiating viable from nonviable myocardium have prompted comparative studies of the two imaging techniques in the same patients.[110,311] In the first study, 94 percent of regions demonstrating either complete or partial reversibility on stress-redistribution ^{201}Tl studies were viable by ^{18}F-FDG PET.[110] Furthermore, among regions considered "irreversible" on 3- to 4-h redistribution images, the severity of reduction in ^{201}Tl activity correlated with the likelihood of metabolic activity as assessed by ^{18}F-FDG uptake. In regions with severe irreversible ^{201}Tl defects ($\leq$ 50 percent of peak activity) on redistribution imaging, the results of ^{201}Tl reinjection were comparable to PET, with a concordance between the two techniques of 88 percent for viable or nonviable myocardium.[110] An example of this concordance is demonstrated in Fig. 5-33. These initial observations at the National Institutes of Health were subsequently confirmed by other investigators.[311,312] In Tamaki's study, the concordance between ^{201}Tl reinjection and ^{18}F FDG PET regarding myocardial viability was 85 percent.[311]

There are only limited data comparing rest-redistribution ^{201}Tl imaging with PET.[89,307] In a study in which stress-redistribution-reinjection and rest-redistribution ^{201}Tl imaging were compared with PET (Fig. 5-34), it was concluded that either ^{201}Tl protocol might yield clinically satisfactory information as long as the severity of ^{201}Tl

defects are quantified within rest-redistribution images.[89] However, in the absence of contraindications to stress testing, stress-redistribution-reinjection imaging provides a more comprehensive assessment of the extent and severity of myocardial ischemia, without loss of information on myocardial viability.

PROGNOSTIC VALUE OF PET AND THALLIUM REINJECTION

The prognostic significance of perfusion-metabolism mismatch on PET imaging has been addressed by several nonrandomized, retrospective studies.[313–315] These studies shared certain methodologic flaws in that the nonrandomized designs made it difficult to determine whether the prognostic differences observed in different treatment groups were due to the PET findings or other factors that may have influenced treatment decisions. Each of these three studies, however, comprising 304 total patients and an average follow-up of at least 1 y, have shown remarkably consistent findings. In patients with significant perfusion-metabolism mismatch who were not revascularized, rates for ischemic events and cardiac

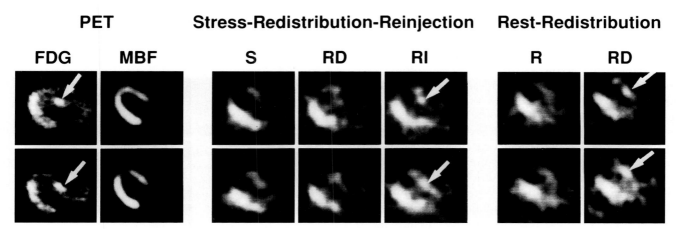

Figure 5-34 Concordance between PET, stress-redistribution-reinjection, and rest-redistribution imaging is demonstrated in this patient example. Two consecutive transaxial tomograms are displayed for ^{18}F FDG and myocardial blood flow (MBF) by PET, with corresponding ^{201}Tl tomograms of stress (S), redistribution (RD), reinjection (RI) and rest (R)-redistribution. On the PET study, myocardial blood flow is reduced in the anteroapical, anteroseptal, and posteroseptal regions. Fluorine-18-FDG uptake in the corresponding regions demonstrate a **mismatch** in the posteroseptal region (arrowhead) and a **match** between ^{18}F-FDG uptake and blood flow in the anteroapical and anteroseptal regions. Corresponding SPECT ^{201}Tl images reveal extensive perfusion abnormalities involving the apical and septal regions during stress, which persist on redistribution images. However, ^{201}Tl reinjection images show improved ^{201}Tl uptake in the posteroseptal region (arrowhead), whereas the apical region remains fixed. On rest-redistribution images, the apical region has severely reduced ^{201}Tl activity that remains fixed, whereas the posteroseptal region that was abnormal on the initial rest study shows significant improvement on 3- to 4-h redistribution study, suggesting viable myocardium. (From Dilsizian et al,[89] with permission of the American Heart Association, Inc.)

deaths were 41 to 50 percent and 14 to 50 percent, respectively. In contrast, patients with perfusion-metabolism mismatch who were revascularized had event and death rates of 8 to 12 percent and 4 to 12 percent, respectively. Thus, the available retrospective data suggest that the particular pattern of perfusion-metabolism mismatch on PET imaging may have important prognostic significance in patients with coronary artery disease and left ventricular dysfunction, and the use of revascularization in such patients is supported.

There are only preliminary data to indicate the prognostic contribution of ^{201}Tl reinjection.[316,317] Miller et al[316] examined the late prognostic value of ^{201}Tl reinjection in patients with coronary artery disease followed for a mean of 9 mo. When the subgroup of patients with cardiac events (death, myocardial infarction, or late coronary revascularization; n = 22) was compared with those without events (n = 38), there were marked differences between the groups in the number of segments with irreversible defects, lung uptake, and transient left ventricular cavity dilatation. Although conventional stress-redistribution studies identified 13 of the 22 patients (59 percent) with cardiac events, ^{201}Tl reinjection predicted additional events in 7 of the 9 patients (78 percent) not identified by stress-redistribution studies alone. Similar observations were reported by Pieri et al.[317] These preliminary data suggest that in addition

to its well-established value as a viability marker, ^{201}Tl reinjection may also help assess risk in patients with chronic coronary artery disease.

Metabolic Imaging With SPECT

The assessment of myocardial metabolism by PET generally is based on quantitative assessments of radiotracer kinetics. Although qualitative approaches to viability assessment using SPECT and more standard tracers may provide valuable information with regard to myocardial viability, PET offers the following potential advantages: 1) accurate quantitation of radiotracer distribution after correction for attenuation; 2) enhanced spatial resolution; and 3) radiotracers that are specifically targeted at defining a certain metabolic parameter (e.g., glucose utilization, FFA oxidation, or oxidative metabolism). Given the technical superiority of PET over SPECT, PET would appear to be the preferred technique to assess both perfusion and metabolism in patients with coronary artery disease. However, by serving as a reference standard, PET has played an important role in recent modifications and improvements of SPECT technology and protocols.

The development of radiopharmaceuticals that measure some aspect of myocardial energy metabolism with single-photon-emitting radioisotopes has proceeded more slowly than that of SPECT perfusion tracers or PET metabolic tracers. The primary limitation has been in labeling; the common single photon radionuclides such as ^{99m}Tc and ^{123}I may alter substrate specificity of those compounds used to track metabolism. Positron emitters, such as ^{18}F, ^{11}C, ^{15}O, and ^{13}N, are less likely to alter the biologic properties of a substrate since these tracers are smaller and, in most cases, substitute for the same corresponding natural element ordinarily found in the biologic compound. Additional difficulties with SPECT imaging are the effects of attenuation, which may be important for any potential quantitative approach to the assessment of metabolism, and its limited spatial resolution. Despite these limitations, the wide availability of SPECT has encouraged the development of suitable metabolic radiotracers that would make the evaluation of myocardial metabolism more available and potentially expand its clinical applications.

^{18}F-FDG SPECT IMAGING

The utility of ^{18}F-FDG imaging using PET is well established, and the clinical demand for ^{18}F-FDG studies, both for cardiac and noncardiac applications, is increasing (see also Chap. 8). Thus, there has been considerable interest in developing methods to image ^{18}F FDG using standard nuclear medicine equipment. Such a concept is not new, and many early bone scans were performed with rectilinear scanners using ^{18}F. While systems are being developed that take advantage of coincidence detection, clinical studies with ^{18}F-FDG SPECT imaging to date have relied on the use of high energy collimators and increased shielding of detector heads. Crystal thickness has not been increased, since such a design would result in a decrease in spatial resolution for standard radiopharmaceuticals. The collimators utilized for ^{18}F-FDG imaging are quite heavy, and modifications of the camera gantry often are necessary to support the added weight.

The feasibility of using a modified SPECT system for imaging with ^{18}F FDG has been reported by several groups.[318,319] The sensitivities of such systems for 511-keV photons is only about 10 percent of that for ^{99m}Tc, and resolution is comparable to ^{201}Tl imaging.[319] Burt et al[320] recently reported their results comparing resting ^{201}Tl SPECT, ^{18}F-FDG PET, and ^{18}F-FDG SPECT in 20 patients with coronary artery disease.[320] They found that approximately 20 percent of regions with severe resting ^{201}Tl defects were viable by ^{18}F-FDG imaging using either SPECT or PET. However, in the latter study, regional contractile function was not assessed. In a subsequent study, in which ^{18}F-FDG SPECT and PET were compared with stress-redistribution-reinjection ^{201}Tl scintigraphy in asynergic myocardial regions, there was a good overall

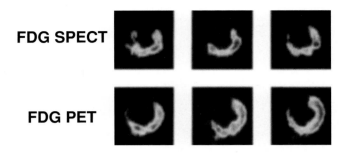

Figure 5-35 Concordance between ^{18}F-FDG SPECT and PET is demonstrated in this patient example. Three short axis tomograms are displayed for ^{18}F-FDG SPECT (top), with corresponding ^{18}F-FDG PET tomograms (bottom). Fluorine-18-FDG uptake is severely reduced in the anterior and anteroseptal regions both on the SPECT and PET studies.

correlation between ^{18}F-FDG uptake and ^{201}Tl reinjection for differentiating viable from nonviable myocardium.[321] Among a total of 33 severely hypokinetic and akinetic or dyskinetic regions, in which viability was a clinical concern, 17 (52 percent) were viable by ^{201}Tl, 22 (67 percent) by ^{18}F-FDG SPECT, and 24 (73 percent) by ^{18}F-FDG PET (p = NS). Regional contractile function, in this study, was assessed using SPECT blood pool imaging for more direct comparison with tomographic ^{18}F-FDG and ^{201}Tl studies.[321]

Fluorine-18-FDG cardiac SPECT, like PET, must be performed in concert with myocardial perfusion imaging, since ischemic regions may have enhanced ^{18}F-FDG uptake, making visualization of normal regions difficult. Thus, SPECT imaging with ^{18}F FDG may be implemented with relatively minor modifications to standard nuclear medicine equipment, and may provide an alternative method for myocardial viability assessment (Fig. 5-35).

ASSESSMENT OF CONTRACTILE RESERVE

Over the past decade, the assessment of myocardial perfusion and viability was primarily accomplished by radionuclide methods. Recently, a growing number of publications have suggested that functional imaging with low-dose dobutamine echocardiography may offer a simple, cost-effective alternative to radionuclide imaging for this indication.

The identification of viable myocardium with functional imaging is based on the principle that whereas regional contractile function may be abnormal at rest, improved contractility with inotropic stimulation may differentiate viable (positive contractile reserve) from nonviable, scarred myocardium (negative contractile reserve).[322] Initial clinical reports of the potential utility of contractile reserve in chronic coronary artery disease patients were made from observations of improved contractile response after premature ventricular beats (postextrasystolic potentiation),[323,324] nitroglycerin,[325] or epinephrine.[326,327] More recent studies have compared directly the results from dobutamine echocardiographic with scintigraphic techniques using ^{201}Tl or ^{18}F-FDG PET.

Echocardiographic Assessment of Myocardial Viability

The utility of echocardiography during dobutamine stimulation in predicting recovery of function after revascularization was first described in patients following acute myocardial infarction.[328–330] In such patients, prolonged but reversible postischemic dysfunction despite restoration of coronary blood flow, termed stunned myocardium, may be prevalent. Data from these studies indicated that dobutamine-responsive improvement in left ventricular wall motion is accurate in predicting functional recovery after infarction,[328,329] even in patients who are not revascularized.[330] Hence, contractile reserve may be unmasked by low-dose catecholamine infusions in regions exhibiting stunned myocardium.

Whether low-dose dobutamine echocardiography is similarly efficacious in the evaluation of the hibernating myocardium is uncertain, as adequate animal models of hibernation are lacking to test this hypothesis. Although contractile reserve may be unmasked by low-dose catecholamine infusions in stunned myocardium, in which coronary flow has been restored, this may not pertain to regions rendered dysfunctional by chronic underperfusion. In patients with critically stenosed coronary arteries, with reduction in coronary blood flow so severe at rest as to produce sustained regional contractile dysfunction, the administration of a positive inotropic agent (even at low doses) may merely increase myocardial demand in the setting of exhausted coronary flow reserve, thereby producing myocardial ischemia and persistent regional dysfunction. Despite this conceptual limitation, there are a number of publications in the literature suggesting that low-dose dobutamine echocardiography may be an accurate predictor of functional recovery after revascularization in patients with chronic left ventricular dysfunction.[331–337]

DOBUTAMINE ECHOCARDIOGRAPHY: EXPERIMENTAL AND CLINICAL STUDIES

To determine whether low-dose dobutamine would be useful in differentiating viable from nonviable myocardium in regions with hibernating myocardium, an animal model of short-term hibernation was developed.[322] Based on promising data from experimental studies, clinical studies have subsequently focused on the application of low-dose dobutamine echocardiography in patients with chronic ischemic heart disease and left ventricular dysfunction.

Cigarroa et al[331] and La Canna et al[332] evaluated contractile reserve with low-dose dobutamine echocardiography before and after revascularization in 25 and 33 patients, respectively, with multivessel coronary disease and left ventricular dysfunction. Resting echocardiography was repeated several weeks after surgery to determine recovery of regional function after revascularization.[331] In these two studies, preoperative identification of contractile reserve, defined as an improvement in regional wall motion and systolic wall thickening during dobutamine infusion, was associated with functional improvement in 82 to 86 percent of regions after revascularization. Conversely, contractile function did not improve in 82 to 87 percent of regions demonstrating lack of contractile reserve.[331,332] However, an important limitation in these studies is that an independent measure of recovery of wall motion after revascularization was not obtained. In Cigarroa's study, a mean index score was used and all 11 patients with a positive contractile response to low-dose dobutamine (left panel of Fig. 5-36) exhibited a mean score of hypokinesis at rest. However, assessment of myocardial viability is a clinical concern among patients with predominantly akinetic and not hypokinetic regions. Whether these favorable results with dobutamine echocardiography also apply to patients with moderate-to-severe left ventricular dysfunction remains unanswered. Since echocardiography was used as the arbiter and standard of myocardial viability (no information on vessel patency postrevascularization), it precludes assessment of the error for this technique on the results obtained. In La Canna's study, up to one-third of patients had technically inadequate transthoracic echocardiographic images. Furthermore, patients with extensive scar and aneurysm, in whom the assessment of viability is of foremost importance, were excluded from the study.

BIPHASIC RESPONSE TO DOBUTAMINE INFUSION

More recently, it has been observed that certain myocardial regions may exhibit a "biphasic" response to graded dobutamine infusion, i.e., improvement in wall motion at low dose but worsening at higher doses of dobutamine.[333,334] When regions with a biphasic response to dobutamine were compared with regions of 1) sustained improvement in wall motion at a low dose of dobutamine that remained improved at high doses, 2) deterioration of resting wall motion upon the administration of dobutamine without any improvement, and 3) persistent wall motion abnormality unaffected by dobutamine, the biphasic response had the most favorable predictive accuracy (72 percent) for recovery of resting function after revascularization.[333] However, since this biphasic dobutamine response was observed in only 23 of 38 segments

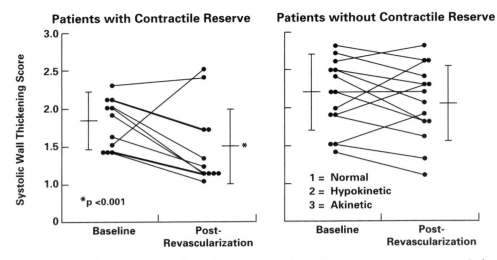

Figure 5-36 Plot of regional echocardiographic systolic wall thickening scores at rest and after revascularization in patients with (left panel) and without (right panel) contractile reserve by low-dose dobutamine echocardiography. (From Cigarroa et al,[331] modified and reprinted by permission of the American Heart Association, Inc.)

that recovered function after angioplasty, the sensitivity of this sign is only 60 percent.[333] Furthermore, among regions that demonstrated persistent improvement of regional contraction at all doses of dobutamine (low and high), only 15 percent of such regions showed recovery of function after revascularization. Clearly, additional studies in larger populations are needed to better define the various patterns of myocardial viability with dobutamine echocardiography.

Comparative Studies of Dobutamine Echocardiography with Radionuclide Techniques

Several studies have compared dobutamine echocardiography with radionuclide techniques for identification of viable myocardium. The relation between contractile response to dobutamine and rest-redistribution ^{201}Tl, stress-redistribution-reinjection ^{201}Tl and, ^{18}F-FDG PET are reviewed.

DOBUTAMINE ECHOCARDIOGRAPHY VERSUS REST-REDISTRIBUTION THALLIUM

Most studies utilizing low-dose dobutamine echocardiography did not provide an assessment of regional blood flow at rest. This has important clinical implications as to whether asynergic regions at rest represent hibernating myocardium (chronic reduction in blood flow) or stunned myocardium (preserved blood flow at rest). Perrone-Filardi et al[335] examined the magnitude of blood flow reduction in such asynergic regions in relation to the efficacy of low-dose dobutamine echocardiography

to predict recovery of function after revascularization. Their results suggest that among asynergic myocardial regions with resting hypoperfusion (hibernating myocardium), low-dose dobutamine predicts improvement in regional function after revascularization with a positive predictive accuracy of 88 percent and negative predictive accuracy of 87 percent.[335] Because only early resting ^{201}Tl images were obtained in this study, for the purpose of defining myocardial perfusion, viability information between ^{201}Tl and dobutamine echocardiography could not be assessed. When Senior et al[336] compared rest-redistribution ^{201}Tl imaging (after nitroglycerin administration) with dobutamine echocardiography in 22 patients undergoing revascularization for chronic coronary artery disease and left ventricular dysfunction, the sensitivity and specificity for detecting viable myocardium were similar for both techniques (87 percent and 82 percent for echocardiography, and 92 percent and 78 percent for ^{201}Tl imaging, respectively).

DOBUTAMINE ECHOCARDIOGRAPHY VERSUS STRESS-REDISTRIBUTION-REINJECTION THALLIUM

At the National Institutes of Health, the relation between ^{201}Tl uptake and contractile response to dobutamine was assessed using transesophageal dobutamine echocardiography and stress-redistribution-reinjection ^{201}Tl protocols.[338] In patients with chronic coronary artery disease and left ventricular dysfunction, a significant relation was observed between ^{201}Tl uptake and response to dobutamine. Of 262 regions considered viable by ^{201}Tl, 167 (64 percent) showed improved contractile function

SEGMENTAL ANALYSIS

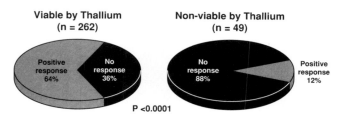

Viable by Thallium
(n = 262)

Positive response 64%
No response 36%

Non-viable by Thallium
(n = 49)

No response 88%
Positive response 12%

P <0.0001

Figure 5-37 Pie chart comparing the proportion of myocardial regions with improved contractile reserve with dobutamine in 262 regions considered to be viable by ^{201}Tl scintigraphy (left panel) and in 49 regions considered to be nonviable by [201]Tl (right panel). (From Panza et al,[338] by permission of the American Heart Association, Inc.)

with dobutamine. In contrast, only 6 of the 49 regions (12 percent) considered nonviable by ^{201}Tl had a positive dobutamine response (Fig. 5-37). Furthermore, among regions with resting wall motion abnormalities (in which viability assessment is a clinical concern), more regions were identified as viable by ^{201}Tl compared with dobutamine echocardiography (84 percent versus 56 percent, respectively, $p < 0.001$) (Fig. 5-38). Patient examples demonstrating concordance and discordance between dobutamine echocardiography and ^{201}Tl scintigraphy are shown in Figs. 5-39 and 5-40. The discordance between the two techniques may reflect differences in the mechanisms by which they detect myocardial viability, and that a positive inotropic response to dobutamine may require a greater number of viable, functional myocytes than is necessary for a particular degree of ^{201}Tl uptake. This hypothesis is supported by the finding that a positive inotropic response to dobutamine was significantly related to the magnitude of ^{201}Tl uptake; the proportion of regions with a positive dobutamine response rose with increasing magnitude of ^{201}Tl uptake. In a subsequent study, frequency distribution of the dobutamine ischemic threshold was analyzed according to the extent of coronary artery disease (Fig. 5-41). In patients with one-

vessel coronary artery disease, the dose of dobutamine at which myocardial ischemia was first detected (ischemic threshold) was 25.4 ± 11.2 μg/kg/min. However, the dobutamine ischemic threshold was significantly lower for patients with two-vessel (14.4 ± 7.9 μg/kg/min) and three-vessel coronary artery disease (9.1 ± 7.9 μg/kg/min, $p < 0.0001$). The induction of ischemia at low doses of dobutamine, observed in a sizable proportion of patients with two- and three-vessel coronary artery disease, may explain why more regions are identified as viable by ^{201}Tl when compared with low-dose dobutamine echocardiography.[339]

Pre- and postrevascularization studies comparing dobutamine echocardiography with dobutamine stress-redistribution-reinjection ^{201}Tl scintigraphy were undertaken by Arnese et al[337] in 38 patients with chronic coronary artery disease and left ventricular dysfunction.[337] Preoperative scintigraphic definition of viability was based on the presence of either normal, complete or partially reversible, and moderately reduced irreversible ^{201}Tl defects. In myocardial segments with severe hypokinesis or akinesis that were successfully revascularized, the sensitivities and specificities for prediction of postoperative improvement in segmental wall motion were 74 percent and 95 percent for dobutamine echocardiography, and 89 percent and 48 percent for dobutamine stress ^{201}Tl imaging. The relative poor specificity of ^{201}Tl may be due to the inclusion of moderately reduced irreversible ^{201}Tl defect as viable regions. Although regions with moderately reduced irreversible ^{201}Tl defects indeed retain viable myocardium, the mere presence of viable myocardium does not necessarily indicate ischemic myocardium.[162]

To determine whether such distinction between ischemic and nonischemic but viable myocardium has implications regarding recovery of function after revascularization, patients with chronic coronary artery disease were studied with pre- and postrevascularization quantitative stress-redistribution-reinjection ^{201}Tl scintigraphy, gated magnetic resonance imaging, and radionuclide angiography.[162] Among 42 asynergic regions demonstrating improved contraction after revascularization, 21 (50 percent) exhibited reversible ^{201}Tl defects and only two had mild-to-moderate irreversible defects. In contrast, of the 20 asynergic regions that did not show improvement after revascularization, 14 (70 percent) demonstrated mild-to-moderate irreversible defects and only three had reversible ^{201}Tl defects ($p < 0.0001$). These data suggest that when performing stress-redistribution-reinjection studies, most mild-to-moderate irreversible ^{201}Tl regions represent an admixture of viable (nonischemic) and scarred myocardium that may not improve after revascularization. On the other hand, the identification of a reversible ^{201}Tl defect on stress images in an asynergic region more accurately predicts recovery of function after surgery.

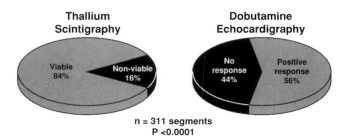

Thallium Scintigraphy

Viable 84%
Non-viable 16%

Dobutamine Echocardigraphy

No response 44%
Positive response 56%

n = 311 segments
P <0.0001

Figure 5-38 Pie chart comparing the proportion of myocardial regions considered to be viable with ^{201}Tl scintigraphy (left) and those showing a positive inotropic response to dobutamine (right) among regions with resting wall motion abnormalities. (From Panza et al,[338] by permission of the American Heart Association, Inc.)

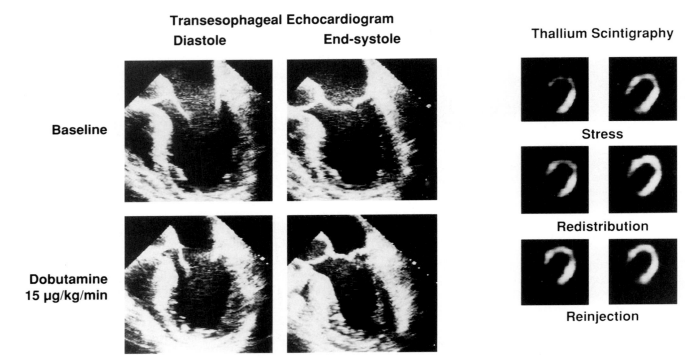

Figure 5-39 Example of concordance between ^{201}Tl scintigraphy with reinjection and low-dose transesophageal echocardiography. Left panels show echocardiographic images obtained from the four-chamber view in diastole (left) and at end-systole (right), at baseline (top), and during low-dose dobutamine infusion (bottom). Right panels show two consecutive transaxial ^{201}Tl tomograms obtained immediately after stress (top), after 3- to 4-h redistribution (middle), and after reinjection (bottom). Echocardiographic images show severe hypokinesis of the basal septum with akinesis of the apical region. With dobutamine, systolic thickening of the septal and apical regions significantly improves. This correlates with ischemic and viable myocardium in the corresponding areas by ^{201}Tl scintigraphy. (From Panza et al,[338] by permission of the American Heart Association, Inc.)

DOBUTAMINE ECHOCARDIOGRAPHY VERSUS PET

Studies comparing dobutamine echocardiography with PET are limited at the present time. Baer et al[340] studied 40 patients with chronic coronary artery disease with dobutamine transesophageal echocardiography and ^{18}F-FDG PET and reported an overall concordance of 90 percent by both techniques. However, regional blood flow was not reported in Baer's study. When both regional blood flow and metabolism were assessed by PET, dobutamine echocardiography significantly underestimated viability in hibernating but not in stunned myocardial regions.[341] Hence, differentiation of stunned from hibernating myocardium in asynergic regions has important implications regarding the predictive accuracy of identifying viable myocardium by dobutamine echocardiography. In 25 patients with ischemic cardiomyopathy, Elsner et al[341] compared low-dose dobutamine echocardiography with PET perfusion and metabolism.[341] Although 42 of 57 (74 percent) asynergic regions identified as stunned myocardium by PET (normal ^{13}N ammonia and normal or increased ^{18}F FDG) improved with dobutamine, only six of 38 (16 percent)

asynergic regions identified as hibernating myocardium by PET (decreased ^{13}N ammonia with normal or increased ^{18}F FDG) showed such improvement with low-dose dobutamine ($p < 0.001$). In a similar study by Hepner et al,[342] involving 35 patients with ischemic cardiomyopathy (mean left ventricular ejection fraction = 29 percent), 70 percent of regions assigned as nonviable by dobutamine echocardiography were determined to be viable by ^{13}N ammonia and ^{18}F-FDG PET.[342] These studies underscore the importance of assessing regional blood flow in asynergic regions when designing comparative studies between dobutamine echocardiography and nuclear techniques.

In a more recent study,[343] when resting myocardial blood flow, assessed by PET, was compared with the myocardial response to dobutamine transesophageal echocardiography,[343] a positive response to dobutamine occurred in 71 percent of regions with preserved myocardial blood flow (≥ 0.6 mL/g/min) compared to only 33 percent of regions with decreased blood flow at rest ($p = 0.0001$). Hence, reduced coronary blood flow at rest is a determinant of myocardial contractile reserve in patients with chronic coronary artery disease and left

Transsophageal Echocardiogram

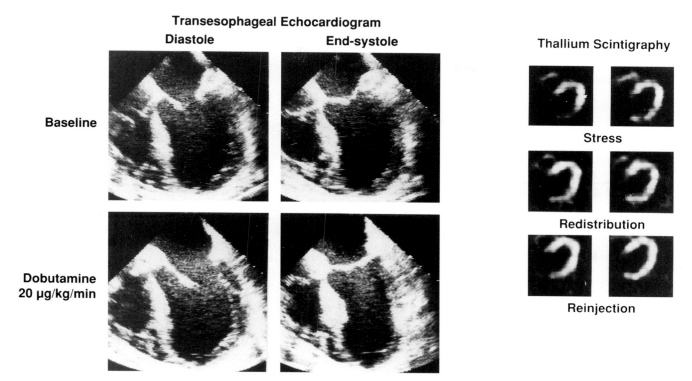

Figure 5-40 Example of discordance between ^{201}Tl scintigraphy and low-dose transesophageal echocardiography. Left panels show echocardiographic images obtained from the four-chamber view in diastole (left) and at end-systole (right), at baseline (top), and during low-dose dobutamine infusion (bottom). Right panels show two consecutive transaxial ^{201}Tl tomograms obtained immediately after stress (top), after 3- to 4-h redistribution (middle), and after reinjection (bottom). Baseline echocardiographic images show akinesis of the apical region with severe hypokinesis of the basal and midwall portions of the interventricular septum. With dobutamine, the systolic thickening of the basal and midwall portions of the septum improves; however, no improvement is seen in the apical region. In contrast, ^{201}Tl scintigraphy shows ischemic and viable myocardium in the apex, septum, and lateral wall. (From Panza et al,[338] by permission of the American Heart Association, Inc.)

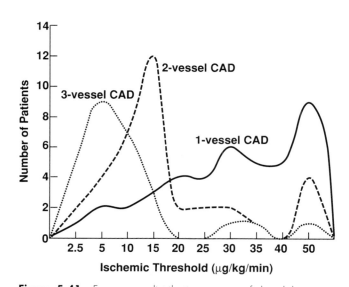

Figure 5-41 Frequency distribution curves of the dobutamine ischemic threshold in patients with one- (solid line), two- (dashed line), and three-vessel (dotted line) coronary artery disease (CAD). (From Panza et al,[338] by permission of the American Heart Association, Inc.)

ventricular dysfunction. Compared with PET perfusion and metabolism, these preliminary data suggest that low-dose dobutamine echocardiography underestimates myocardial viability in hibernating but not in stunned myocardial regions.

Myocardial Contrast Echocardiography

The development of myocardial contrast echocardiography may provide yet another means to assess myocardial viability in chronic coronary artery disease patients. de-Filippi et al[344] compared myocardial contrast echocardiography with dobutamine echocardiography in 35 patients with chronic coronary artery disease.[344] Their findings indicated excellent sensitivity and an acceptable specificity of contrast echocardiography for predicting recovery of function after revascularization (94 percent and 67 percent, respectively), although the specificity of dobutamine echocardiography was better (92 percent). In the future, the utility of contrast echocardiography will likely depend on the development of contrast agents

Table 5-4 Determinants of Regional Myocardial Dysfunction

Local Conditions	Extrinsic Conditions
Degree of subendocardial ischemia	Systolic ventricular pressure
Percentage of myocardial scar	Regional afterload
	Transmural "tethering"
Degree of inotropic stimulation	Interactions with adjacent regions
Mode of electrical activation	

From Ross[6], reprinted with permission of the American Heart Association

that are administered peripherally rather than intracoronary.

DEFINITION OF MYOCARDIAL VIABILITY

A number of important questions still remain operative in the clinical arena. Perhaps the most important questions relate to the definition of myocardial viability itself, the impact of the extent of viability as it relates to improvement in function, the degree to which hibernation and stunning are operative clinically, and the standardization of approaches to viability assessment.

The definition of myocardial viability particularly is problematic. To date, the sine qua non of viable myocardium has been the temporal improvement in contractile function after specific therapeutic interventions, most commonly restoration of blood flow. But this may not be the most appropriate definition. Regional myocardial function can be influenced both by local and extrinsic conditions, as outlined in Table 5-4.[6] The restoration of blood flow to viable myocardium, for example, may not result in significant improvement in regional function in the setting of transmural "tethering" (where an epicardial rim of viable myocardium is tethered to an endocardial scar), but may result in stabilization of the electrical milieu or the prevention of extensive ventricular remodeling in nontransmural infarct zones. These studies raise additional, as yet unanswered questions, with regard to how and why we assess myocardial viability in coronary artery disease patients. The clinical "gold standard" for viability, recovery of global or regional left ventricular dysfunction after revascularization, may underestimate the potential benefits of revascularization and thus the significance of the delineation of viable myocardium. Reperfusion of viable myocardium may have important effects on left ventricular geometry, remodeling, and arrhythmias that may result in potential long-term benefit even in the absence of changes in regional function.

In the future, large clinical trials are needed that evaluate not only recovery of left ventricular function after revascularization, but also left ventricular cavity dilatation, episodes of clinical heart failure, arrhythmias, recurrent ischemic events, and long-term survival.

REFERENCES

1. Braunwald E, Kloner RA: The stunned myocardium: Prolonged, postischemic ventricular dysfunction. *Circulation* 66:1146, 1982.
2. Rahimtoola SH: A perspective on the three large multicenter randomized clinical trials of coronary bypass surgery for chronic stable angina. *Circulation* 72(suppl V):V-123, 1985.
3. Heyndrickx GR, Baig H, Nelkins P, et al: Depression of regional blood flow and wall thickening after brief coronary occlusions. *Am J Physiol* 234:H653, 1978.
4. Rahimtoola SH: Coronary bypass surgery for chronic angina-1981: A perspective. *Circulation* 65:225, 1982.
5. Matsuzaki M, Gallagher KP, Kemper WS, et al: Sustained regional dysfunction, produced by prolonged coronary stenosis: Gradual recovery after reperfusion. *Circulation* 68:170, 1983.
6. Ross J Jr: Assessment of ischemic regional myocardial dysfunction and its reversibility. *Circulation* 74:1186, 1986.
7. Ross J Jr: Mechanisms of regional ischemia and antianginal drug action during exercise. *Prog Cardiovasc Dis* 31:455, 1989.
8. Topol EJ, Weiss JL, Guzman PA, et al: Immediate improvement of dysfunctional myocardial segments after coronary revascularization: Detection by intraoperative transesophageal echocardiography. *J Am Coll Cardiol* 4:1123, 1984.
9. Braunwald E, Rutherford JD: Reversible ischemic left ventricular dysfunction: Evidence for the "hibernating myocardium." *J Am Coll Cardiol* 8:1467, 1986.
10. Cohen M, Charney R, Hershman R, et al: Reversal of chronic ischemic myocardial dysfunction after transluminal coronary angioplasty. *J Am Coll Cardiol* 12:1193, 1988.
11. Carlson EB, Cowley MJ, Wolfgang TC, Vetrovec GW: Acute changes in global and regional rest left ventricular function after successful coronary angioplasty: Comparative results in stable and unstable angina. *J Am Coll Cardiol* 13:1262, 1989.
12. Van den Berg EK, Popma JJ, Dehmer GJ, et al: Reversible segmental left ventricular dysfunction after coronary angioplasty. *Circulation* 81:1210, 1990.
13. Perrone-Filardi P, Bacharach SL, Dilsizian V, et al: Metabolic evidence of viable myocardium in regions with reduced wall thickness and absent wall thickening in patients with chronic ischemic left ventricular dysfunction. *J Am Coll Cardiol* 20:161, 1992.
14. Rees G, Bristow JD, Kremkau EL, et al: Influence of aortocoronary bypass surgery on left ventricular performance. *N Engl J Med* 284:1116, 1971.

15. Chatterjee K, Swan HJC, Parmley WW, et al: Influence of direct myocardial revascularization on left ventricular asynergy and function in patients with coronary heart disease. *Circulation* 47:276, 1973.

16. Rozanski A, Berman DS, Gray R, et al: Use of thallium-201 redistribution scintigraphy in the preoperative differentiation of reversible and nonreversible myocardial asynergy. *Circulation* 64:936, 1981.

17. Brundage BH, Massie BM, Botvinick EH: Improved regional ventricular function after successful surgical revascularization. *J Am Coll Cardiol* 3:902, 1984.

18. Dilsizian V, Bonow RO, Cannon RO, et al: The effect of coronary artery bypass grafting on left ventricular systolic function at rest: Evidence for preoperative subclinical myocardial ischemia. *Am J Cardiol* 61:1248, 1988.

19. Brill DA, Deckelbaum LI, Remetz MS, et al: Recovery of severe ischemic ventricular dysfunction after coronary bypass grafting. *Am J Cardiol* 61:650, 1988.

20. Nesto RW, Cohn LH, Collins JJ Jr, et al: Inotropic contractile reserve: A useful predictor of increased 5-year survival and improved postoperative left ventricular function in patients with coronary artery disease and reduced ejection fraction. *Am J Cardiol* 50:39, 1982.

21. Alderman EL, Fisher LD, Litwin P, et al: Results of coronary artery surgery in patients with poor left ventricular function (CASS). *Circulation* 68:785, 1983.

22. Pigott JD, Kouchoukos NT, Oberman A, Cutter GR: Late results of surgical and medical therapy for patients with coronary artery disease and depressed left ventricular function. *J Am Coll Cardiol* 5:1036, 1985.

23. Mock MB, Ringqvist I, Fisher LD, et al: Survival of medically treated patients in the coronary artery surgery study (CASS) registry. *Circulation* 66:562, 1982.

24. Sheehan FH, Doerr R, Schmidt WG, et al: Early recovery of left ventricular function after thrombolytic therapy for acute myocardial infarction: An important determinant of survival. *J Am Coll Cardiol* 40:633, 1988.

25. Dilsizian V, Bonow RO: Current diagnostic techniques of assessing myocardial viability in hibernating and stunned myocardium. *Circulation* 87:1, 1993.

26. Knoebel SB, Henry PL, Phillips JF, Pauletto FJ: Coronary collateral circulation and myocardial blood flow reserve. *Circulation* 46:84, 1972.

27. Levin DC: Pathways and functional significance of coronary collateral circulation. *Circulation* 50:831, 1974.

28. Schwarz F, Flameng W, Ensslen R, et al: Effects of coronary collaterals on left ventricular function at rest and during stress. *Am Heart J* 95:570, 1978.

29. Goldberg HL, Goldstein J, Borer JS, et al: Functional importance of coronary collateral vessels. *Am J Cardiol* 53:694, 1984.

30. Dilsizian V, Cannon RO, Tracy CM, et al: Enhanced regional left ventricular function after distant coronary bypass via improved collateral blood flow. *J Am Coll Cardiol* 14:312, 1989.

31. DeWood MA, Spores J, Notske R, et al: Prevalence of total coronary occlusion during the early hours of transmural myocardial infarction. *N Engl J Med* 303:897, 1980.

32. Banka VS, Bodenheimer MM, Helfant RH: Determinants of reversible asynergy: The native coronary circulation. *Circulation* 52:810, 1975.

33. Popio KA, Gorlin R, Bechtel D, Levine JA: Postextrasystolic potentiation as a predictor of potential myocardial viability: Preoperative analysis compared with studies after coronary bypass surgery. *Am J Cardiol* 39:944, 1977.

34. Rozanski A, Berman D, Gray R, et al: Preoperative prediction of reversible myocardial asynergy by postexercise radionuclide ventriculography. *N Engl J Med* 307:212, 1982.

35. Tillisch JH, Brunken R, Marshall R, et al: Reversibility of cardiac wall-motion abnormalities predicted by positron tomography. *N Engl J Med* 314:884, 1986.

36. Fuster V, Stein B, Ambrose J, et al: Atherosclerotic plaque rupture and thrombosis: Evolving concepts. *Circulation* 82:II47, 1990.

37. Fuster V, Badimon L, Badimon J, Chesebro J: Mechanisms of disease: The pathogenesis of coronary artery disease and the acute coronary syndromes. Parts I and II. *N Engl J Med* 326:242, 310, 1992.

38. Ambrose J, Winters S, Arora R, et al: Angiographic evolution of coronary artery morphology in unstable angina. *J Am Coll Cardiol* 7:472, 1986.

39. Ambrose J, Tannenbaum M, Alexopoulos D, et al: Angiographic progression of coronary artery disease and the development of myocardial infarction. *J Am Coll Cardiol* 12:56, 1988.

40. Johnson P: Autoregulation of blood flow. *Circ Res* 58:483, 1986.

41. Gould K, Lipscomb K: Effects of coronary stenosis on coronary flow reserve and resistance. *Am J Cardiol* 34:48, 1974.

42. Coffman J, Gregg D: Reactive hyperemia characteristics of the myocardium. *Am J Physiol* 199:1143, 1960.

43. Gewirtz H, Williams D, Ohley W, Most A: Influence of coronary vasodilation on the transmural distribution of myocardial blood flow distal to a severe fixed coronary stenosis. *Am Heart J* 106:674, 1983.

44. Tennant R, Wiggers C: The effect of coronary occlusion on myocardial contractions. *Am J Physiol* 112:351, 1935.

45. Downey J: Myocardial contractile force as a function of coronary blood flow. *Am J Physiol* 230:1, 1976.

46. Vatner S: Correlation between acute reduction in myocardial blood flow and function in conscious dogs. *Circ Res* 47:201, 1980.

47. Lee J, Tajimi T, Guth B, et al: Exercise induced regional dysfunction with subcritical coronary stenosis. *Circulation* 73:596, 1986.

48. Herman M, Heinle R, Klein M, Gorlin R: Localized disorders of myocardial contraction. *N Engl J Med* 227:222, 1967.

49. Ross J Jr: Myocardial perfusion-contraction matching: Implications for coronary heart disease and hibernation. *Circulation* 83:1076, 1991.

50. Bolli R: Myocardial "stunning" in man. *Circulation* 86:1671, 1992.

51. Bonow RO, Dilsizian V: Thallium 201 for assessment of myocardial viability. *Semin Nucl Med* 21:230, 1991.

52. Christian TF, Miller TD, Hodge DO, Gibbons RJ: What

is the prevalence of hibernating myocardium? (abstr). *J Am Coll Cardiol* 27:162A, 1996.

53. Weich HF, Strauss HW, Pitt B: The extraction of thallium 201 by the myocardium. *Circulation* 56:188, 1977.

54. Mullins LJ, Moore RD: The movement of thallium ions in muscle. *J Gen Physiol* 43:759, 1960.

55. Gehring PJ, Hammond PB: The interrelationship between thallium and potassium in animals. *J Pharmacol Exp Ther* 155:187, 1967.

56. Leppo JA, Macneil PB, Moring AF, Apstein CS: Separate effects of ischemia, hypoxia, and contractility on thallium-201 kinetics in rabbit myocardium. *J Nucl Med* 27:66, 1986.

57. Leppo JA: Myocardial uptake of thallium and rubidium during alterations in perfusion and oxygenation in isolated rabbit hearts. *J Nucl Med* 28:878, 1987.

58. Moore CA, Cannon J, Watson DD, et al: Thallium-201 kinetics in stunned myocardium characterized by severe postischemic systolic dysfunction. *Circulation* 81:1622, 1990.

59. Sinusas AJ, Watson DD, Cannon JM, Beller GA: Effect of ischemia and postischemic dysfunction on myocardial uptake of technetium-99m-labeled methoxyisobutyl isonitrile and thallium 201. *J Am Coll Cardiol* 14:1785, 1989.

60. Granato JE, Watson DD, Flanagan TL, Beller GA: Myocardial thallium-201 kinetics and regional flow alterations with 3 hours of coronary occlusion and either rapid reperfusion through a totally patent vessel or slow reperfusion through a critical stenosis. *J Am Coll Cardiol* 9:109, 1987.

61. Pohost GM, Zir LM, Moore RH, et al: Differentiation of transiently ischemic from infarcted myocardium by serial imaging after a single dose of thallium 201. *Circulation* 55:294, 1977.

62. Schwartz JS, Ponto R, Carlyle P, et al: Early redistribution of thallium 201 after temporary ischemia. *Circulation* 57:332, 1978.

63. Beller GA, Watson DD, Ackell P, Pohost GM: Time course of thallium-201 redistribution after transient myocardial ischemia. *Circulation* 61:791, 1980.

64. Okada RD, Pohost GM: Effect of decreased blood flow and ischemia on myocardial thallium clearance. *J Am Coll Cardiol* 3:744, 1984.

65. Pohost GM, Okada RD, O'Keefe DD, et al: Thallium redistribution in dogs with severe coronary artery stenosis of fixed caliber. *Circ Res* 48:439, 1981.

66. Okada RD, Leppo JA, Boucher CA, Pohost GM: Myocardial kinetics of thallium-201 after dipyridamole infusion in normal canine myocardium and in myocardium distal to a stenosis. *J Clin Invest* 69:199, 1982.

67. Okada RD, Leppo JA, Strauss HW, et al: Mechanism and time course of the disappearance of thallium-201 defects at rest in dogs. *Am J Cardiol* 49:699, 1982.

68. Mays AE Jr, Cobb FR: Relationship between regional myocardial blood flow and thallium-201 distribution in the presence of coronary artery stenosis and dipyridamole induced vasodilation. *J Clin Invest* 73:1359, 1984.

69. Akins CW, Pohost GM, Desanctis RW, Block PC: Selection of angina-free patients with severe left ventricular

dysfunction for myocardial revascularization. *Am J Cardiol* 46:695, 1980.

70. Gibson RS, Watson DD, Taylor GJ, et al: Prospective assessment of regional myocardial perfusion before and after coronary revascularization surgery by quantitative thallium-201 scintigraphy. *J Am Coll Cardiol* 1:804, 1983.

71. Liu P, Kiess MC, Okada RD, et al: The persistent defect on exercise thallium imaging and its fate after myocardial revascularization: Does it represent scar or ischemia? *Am Heart J* 110:996, 1985.

72. Cloninger KG, DePuey EG, Garcia EV, et al: Incomplete redistribution in delayed thallium-201 single photon emission computed tomographic images: An overestimation of myocardial scarring. *J Am Coll Cardiol* 12:955, 1988.

73. Kiat H, Berman DS, Maddahi J, et al: Late reversibility of tomographic myocardial thallium-201 defects: An accurate marker of myocardial viability. *J Am Coll Cardiol* 12:1456, 1988.

74. Manyari DE, Knudtson M, Kloiber R, Roth D: Sequential thallium-201 myocardial perfusion studies after successful percutaneous transluminal coronary artery angioplasty: Delayed resolution of exercise-induced scintigraphic abnormalities. *Circulation* 77:86, 1988.

75. Gutman J, Berman DS, Freeman M, et al: Time to completed redistribution of thallium 201 in exercise myocardial scintigraphy: Relationship to the degree of coronary artery stenosis. *Am Heart J* 106:989, 1983.

76. Yang LD, Berman DS, Kiat H, et al: The frequency of late reversibility in SPECT thallium-201 stress-redistribution studies. *J Am Coll Cardiol* 15:334, 1989.

77. Dilsizian V, Rocco TP, Freedman NM, et al: Enhanced detection of ischemic but viable myocardium by the reinjection of thallium after stress-redistribution imaging. *N Engl J Med* 323:141, 1990.

78. Rocco TP, Dilsizian V, McKusick KA, et al: Comparison of thallium redistribution with rest "reinjection" imaging for the detection of viable myocardium. *Am J Cardiol* 66:158, 1990.

79. Ohtani H, Tamaki N, Yonekura Y, et al: Value of thallium-201 reinjection after delayed SPECT imaging for predicting reversible ischemia after coronary artery bypass grafting. *Am J Cardiol* 66:394, 1990.

80. Kuijper AF, Vliegen HW, van der Wall EE, et al: The clinical impact of thallium-201 reinjection scintigraphy for detection of myocardial viability. *Eur J Nucl Med* 19:783, 1992.

81. Bartenstein P, Schober O, Hasfeld M, et al: Thallium-201 single photon emission tomography of myocardium: Additional information in reinjection studies is dependent on collateral circulation. *Eur J Nucl Med* 19:790, 1992.

82. Maublant JC, Lipiecki J, Citron B, et al: Reinjection as an alternative to rest imaging for detection of exercise-induced ischemia with thallium-201 emission tomography. *Am Heart J* 125:330, 1993.

83. Nienaber CA, de la Roche J, Carnarius H, Montz R: Impact of [201]thallium reinjection imaging to identify myocardial viability after vasodilation-redistribution SPECT (abstr). *J Am Coll Cardiol* 21:283A, 1993.

84. Bartenstein P, Hasfeld M, Schober O, et al: Tl-201 reinjection predicts improvement of left ventricular function following revascularization. *Nucl Med* 32:87, 1993.

85. Melin JA, Marwick T, Baudhuin T, et al: Assessment of myocardial viability with thallium-201 imaging and dobutamine echocardiography: A comparative patient analysis (abstr). *Circulation* 88:I, 1993.

86. Inglese E, Brambilla M, Dondi M, et al: Assessment of myocardial viability after thallium-201 reinjection or rest-redistribution imaging: A multicenter study. *J Nucl Med* 36:555, 1995.

87. Lekakis J, Vassilopoulos N, Germanidis J, et al: Detection of viable tissue in healed infarcted myocardium by dipyridamole thallium-201 reinjection and regional wall motion studies. *Am J Cardiol* 71:401,1993.

88. Kennedy NSJ, Cook B, Choy AM, et al: A comparison of the redistribution and reinjection techniques in dipyridamole thallium tomography. *Nuc Med Commun* 14:479, 1993.

89. Dilsizian V, Perrone-Filardi P, Arrighi JA, et al: Concordance and discordance between stress-redistribution-reinjection and rest-redistribution thallium imaging for assessing viable myocardium: Comparison with metabolic activity by PET. *Circulation* 88:941, 1993.

90. Goldhaber SZ, Newell JB, Alpert NM, et al: Effects of ischemic-like insult on myocardial thallium-201 accumulation. *Circulation* 67:778, 1983.

91. Budinger TF, Pohost GM: Indication for thallium reinjection by 3 hour plasma levels (abstr). *Circulation* 88:I, 1993.

92. Budinger TF, Pohost GM: Thallium "redistribution"—an explanation (abstr). *J Nucl Med* 27:996, 1986.

93. Gewirtz H, Sullivan MJ, Shearer DR, et al: Analysis of proposed mechanisms of thallium redistribution: Comparison of a computer model of myocardial thallium kinetics with quantitative analysis of clinical scans. IEEE *Computers in Cardiology*, 1981, pp 75–80.

94. Grunwald AM, Watson DD, Holzgrefe HH Jr, et al: Myocardial thallium-201 kinetics in normal and ischemic myocardium. *Circulation* 64:610, 1981.

95. Okada RD, Jacobs ML, Daggett WM, et al: Thallium-201 kinetics in nonischemic canine myocardium. *Circulation* 65:70, 1982.

96. Nelson CW, Wilson RA, Angello DA, Palac RT: Effect of thallium-201 blood levels on reversible thallium defects. *J Nucl Med* 30:1172, 1989.

97. Leppo JA, Okada RD, Strauss HW, Pohost GH: Effect of hyperaemia on thallium-201 redistribution in normal canine myocardium. *Cardiovasc Res* 19:679, 1985.

98. Budinger TF, Knittel BL: Cardiac thallium redistribution and model (abstr). *J Nucl Med* 28:588, 1987.

99. Kayden DS, Sigal S, Soufer R, et al: Thallium 201 for assessment of myocardial viability: Quantitative comparison of 24-hour redistribution imaging with imaging after reinjection at rest. *J Am Coll Cardiol* 18:1480, 1991.

100. Dilsizian V, Smeltzer WR, Freedman NMT, et al: Thallium reinjection after stress-redistribution imaging: Does 24-hour delayed imaging following reinjection enhance detection of viable myocardium? *Circulation* 83:1247, 1991.

101. Dae MW, Botvinick EH, Starksen NF, et al: Do 4-hour reinjection thallium images and 24-hour thallium images provide equivalent information? (abstr). *J Am Coll Cardiol* 17:29, 1991.

102. McCallister BD, Clemments IP, Hauser MF, Gibbons RJ: The limited value of 24-hour images following 4-hour reinjection thallium imaging (abstr). *Circulation* 84:II, 1991.

103. Dilsizian V, Bonow RO: Differential uptake and apparent thallium-201 "washout" after thallium reinjection: Options regarding early redistribution imaging before reinjection or late redistribution imaging after reinjection. *Circulation* 85:1032, 1992.

104. Kiat H, Friedman JD, Wang FP, et al: Frequency of late reversibility in stress-redistribution thallium-201 SPECT using an early reinjection protocol. *Am Heart J* 122:613, 1991.

105. van Eck-Smit BLF, van der Wall EE, Kuijper AFM, et al: Immediate thallium-201 reinjection following stress imaging: A time-saving approach for detection of myocardial viability. *J Nucl Med* 34:737, 1993.

106. Klingensmith WC III, Sutherland JD: Detection of jeopardized myocardium with ^{201}Tl myocardial perfusion imaging: Comparison of early and late reinjection protocols. *Clin Nuc Med* 18:487, 1993.

107. Dilsizian V, Bonow RO, Quyyumi AA, et al: Is early thallium reinjection after post-exercise imaging a satisfactory method to detect defect reversibility? *Circulation* 88(4):I, 1993.

108. Marin-Neto JA, Dilsizian V, Arrighi JA, et al: Thallium reinjection demonstrates viable myocardium in regions with reverse redistribution. *Circulation* 88:1736, 1993.

109. Soufer R, Dey HM, Lawson AJ, et al: Relationship between reverse redistribution on planar thallium scintigraphy and regional myocardial viability: A correlative PET study. *J Nucl Med* 36:180, 1995.

110. Bonow RO, Dilsizian V, Cuocolo A, Bacharach SL: Identification of viable myocardium in patients with coronary artery disease and left ventricular dysfunction: Comparison of thallium scintigraphy with reinjection and PET imaging with ^{18}F fluorodeoxyglucose. *Circulation* 83:26, 1991.

111. Dilsizian V, Freedman NMT, Bacharach SL, et al: Regional thallium uptake in irreversible defects: Magnitude of change in thallium activity after reinjection distinguishes viable from nonviable myocardium. *Circulation* 85:627, 1992.

112. Zimmermann R, Mall G, Rauch B, et al: Residual Tl-201 activity in irreversible defects as a marker of myocardial viability: Clinicopathological study. *Circulation* 91:1016, 1995.

113. Dilsizian V, Quigg RJ, Shirani J, et al: Histomorphologic validation of thallium reinjection and fluorodeoxyglucose PET for assessment of myocardial viability (abstr). *Circulation* 90:I, 1994.

114. Wackers FJ, Lie KI, Liem KL, et al: Thallium-201 scintigraphy in unstable angina pectoris. *Circulation* 57:738, 1978.

115. Gewirtz H, Beller GA, Strauss HW, et al: Transient defects of resting thallium scans in patients with coronary artery disease. *Circulation* 59:707, 1979.

116. Berger BC, Watson DD, Burwell LR, et al: Redistribution

of thallium at rest in patients with stable and unstable angina and the effect of coronary artery bypass surgery. *Circulation* 60:1114, 1979.

117. Iskandrian AS, Hakki A, Kane SA, et al: Rest and redistribution thallium-201 myocardial scintigraphy to predict improvement in left ventricular function after coronary artery bypass grafting. *Am J Cardiol* 51:1312, 1983.

118. Mori T, Minamiji K, Kurogane H, et al: Rest-injected thallium-201 imaging for assessing viability of severe asynergic regions. *J Nucl Med* 32:1718, 1991.

119. Ragosta M, Beller GA, Watson DD, et al: Quantitative planar rest-redistribution ^{201}Tl imaging in detection of myocardial viability and prediction of improvement in left ventricular function after coronary artery bypass surgery in patients with severely depressed left ventricular function. *Circulation* 87:1630, 1993.

120. Hoffman EJ, Huang SC, Phelps ME: Quantitation in positron emission tomography: 1. Effect of object size. *J Comput Assist Tomogr* 3:299, 1979.

121. Gewirtz H, Grotte GJ, Strauss HW, et al: The influence of left ventricular volume and wall motion on myocardial images. *Circulation* 59:1172, 1979.

122. Parodi AV, Schelbert HR, Schwaiger M, et al: Cardiac emission computed tomography: Estimation of regional tracer concentrations due to wall motion abnormality. *J Comput Assist Tomogr* 8:1083, 1984.

123. Sinusas AJ, Shi QX, Vitols PJ, et al: Impact of regional ventricular function, geometry and dobutamine stress on quantitative ^{99m}Tc-sestamibi defect size. *Circulation* 88:2224, 1993.

124. Eisner RL, Schmarkey S, Martin SE, et al: Defects on SPECT "perfusion" images can occur due to abnormal segmental contraction. *J Nucl Med* 35:638, 1994.

125. Deutsch E, Bushong W, Glavan KA, et al: Heart imaging with cationic complexes of technetium. *Science* 214:85, 1981.

126. Leppo JA, DePuey EG, Johnson LL: A review of cardiac imaging with sestamibi and teboroxime. *J Nucl Med* 32:2012, 1991.

127. Maddahi J, Kiat H, Berman DS: Myocardial perfusion imaging with technetium-99m-labeled agents. *Am J Cardiol* 67:27D, 1991.

128. Zaret BL, Rigo P, Wackers FJT, et al. Myocardial perfusion imaging with ^{99m}Tc tetrofosmin: Comaprison to ^{201}Tl imaging and coronary angiography in a phase III multicenter trial. *Circulation* 91:313, 1995.

129. Piwnica-Worms D, Kronauge JF, Chiu ML: Uptake and retention of hexakis (2-methoxyisobutyl isonitrile) technetium (I) in cultured chick myocardial cells. Mitochondrial and plasma membrane potential dependence. *Circulation* 82:1826, 1990.

130. Leppo JA, Meerdink DJ: Comparison of the myocardial uptake of a technetium-labeled isonitrile analogue and thallium. *Circ Res* 65:632, 1989.

131. Meerdink DJ, Leppo JA: Comparison of hypoxia and ouabain effects on the myocardial uptake kinetics of technetium-99m hexakis 2-methoxy-isobutyl isonitrile and thallium 201. *J Nucl Med* 30:1500, 1989.

132. Wackers FJ, Berman DS, Maddahi J, et al: Technetium-99m hexakis 2-methoxyisobutyl isonitrile: Human bio-

distribution, dosimetry, safety, and preliminary comparison to thallium 201 for myocardial perfusion imaging. *J Nucl Med* 30:301, 1989.

133. Kiat H, Maddahi J, Roy LT, et al: Comparison of technetium-99m methoxy isobutyl isonitrile and thallium 201 for evaluation of coronary artery disease by planar and tomographic methods. *Am Heart J* 117:1, 1989.

134. Kahn JK, McGhie I, Akers MS, et al: Quantitative rotational tomography with Tl-201 and Tc-99m 2-methoxyisobutyl-isonitrile: A direct comparison in normal individuals and patients with coronary artery disease. *Circulation* 79:1282, 1989.

135. Iskandrian AS, Heo J, Kong B, et al: Use of technetium-99m isonitrile (RP-30A) in assessing left ventricular perfusion and function at rest and during exercise in coronary artery disease, and comparison with coronary arteriography and exercise thallium-201 SPECT imaging. *Am J Cardiol* 64:270, 1989.

136. Dilsizian V, Rocco TP, Strauss HW, Boucher CA: Technetium-99m isonitrile myocardial uptake at rest: I. Relation to severity of coronary artery stenosis. *J Am Coll Cardiol* 14:1673, 1989.

137. Rocco TP, Dilsizian V, Strauss HW, Boucher CA: Technetium-99m isonitrile myocardial uptake at rest: II. Relation to clinical markers of potential viability. *J Am Coll Cardiol* 14:1678, 1989.

138. Beanlands RSB, Dawood F, Wen WH, et al: Are the kinetics of technetium-99m methoxyisobutyl isonitrile affected by cell metabolism and viability? *Circulation* 82:1802, 1990.

139. Li QS, Matsumura K, Dannals R, Becker LC: Radionuclide markers of viability in reperfused myocaridum: comparison between ^{18}F-2-deoxyglucose, ^{201}Tl, and ^{99m}Tc-sestamibi (abstr). *Circulation* 82:III, 1990.

140. Verani MS, Jeroudi MO, Mahmarian JJ, et al: Quantification of myocardial infarction during coronary occlusion and myocardial salvage after reperfusion using cardiac imaging with technetium-99m hexakis 2-methoxybutyl isonitrile. *J Am Coll Cardiol* 12:1573, 1988.

141. Sinusas AJ, Trautman KA, Bergin JD, et al: Quantification of "area at risk" during coronary occlusion and degree of myocardial salvage after reperfusion with technetium-99m-methoxyisobutyl-isonitrile. *Circulation* 82:1424, 1990.

142. Gibbons RJ, Verani MS, Behrenbeck T, et al: Feasibility of tomographic technetium-99m hexakis-2-methoxy-2-methylpropyl-isonitrile imaging for the assessment of myocardial area at risk and the effect of acute treatment in myocardial infarction. *Circulation* 80:1277, 1989.

143. Behrenbeck T, Pellikka PA, Huber KC, et al: Primary angioplasty in myocardial infarction: Assessment of improved myocardial perfusion with technetium-99m isonitrile. *J Am Coll Cardiol* 17:365, 1991.

144. Beller GA, Glover DK, Edwards NC, et al: ^{99m}Tc-sestamibi uptake and retention during myocardial ischemia and reperfusion. *Circulation* 87:2033, 1993.

145. Cuocolo A, Pace L, Ricciardelli B, et al: Identification of viable myocardium in patients with chronic coronary artery disease: Comparison of thallium-201 scintigraphy

with reinjection and technetium-99m methoxyisobutyl isonitrile. *J Nucl Med* 33:505, 1992.

146. Bonow RO, Dilsizian V: Thallium-201 and technetium-99m-sestamibi for assessing viable myocardium. *J Nucl Med* 33:815, 1992.

147. Marzullo P, Sambuceti G, Parodi O: The role of sestamibi scintigraphy in the radioisotopic assessment of myocardial viability. *J Nucl Med* 33:1925, 1992.

148. Lucignani G, Paolini G, Landoni C, et al: Presurgical identification of hibernating myocardium by combined use of technetium-99m hexakis-2-methoxyisobutylisonitrile single photon emission tomography and fluorine-18 fluoro-2-deoxy-D-glucose positron emission tomography in patients with coronary artery disease. *Eur J Nucl Med* 19:874, 1992.

149. Altehoefer C, Kaiser HJ, Dorr R, et al: Fluorine-18 deoxyglucose PET for assessment of viable myocardium in perfusion defects in ^{99m}Tc-MIBI SPET: A comparative study in patients with coronary artery disease. *Eur J Nucl Med* 19:334, 1992.

150. Ferreira J, Gil VM, Ventosa A, et al: Reversibility in myocardial perfusion scintigraphy after myocardial infarction: Comparison of SPECT ^{99m}Tc-sestamibi rest-stress single-day protocol and thallium-201 reinjection. *Rev Port Cardiol* 12:1013, 1993.

151. Marzullo P, Parodi O, Reisenhofer B, et al: Value of rest thallium-201/technetium-99m sestamibi scans and dobutamine echocardiography for detecting myocardial viability. *Am J Cardiol* 71:166, 1993.

152. Dilsizian V, Arrighi JA, Diodati JG, et al: Myocardial viability in patients with chronic coronary artery disease: Comparison of ^{99m}Tc-sestamibi with thallium reinjection and ^{18}F-fluorodeoxyglucose. *Circulation* 89:578, 1994.

153. Maurea S, Cuocolo A, Pace L, et al: Left ventricular dysfunction in coronary artery disease: Comparison between rest-redistribution thallium-201 and resting technetium-99m methoxyisobutyl isonitrile cardiac imaging. *J Nucl Cardiol* 1:65, 1994.

154. Sawada SG, Allman KC, Muzik O, et al: Positron emission tomography detects evidence of viability in rest technetium-99m sestamibi defects. *J Am Coll Cardiol* 23:92, 1994.

155. Maurea S, Cuocolo A, Nicolai E, Salvatore M: Improved detection of viable myocardium with thallium-201 reinjection in chronic coronary artery disease: Comparison with technetium-99m-MIBI imaging. *J Nucl Med* 35:621, 1994.

156. Altehoefer C, vom Dahl J, Biedermann M, et al: Significance of defect severity in technetium-99m-MIBI SPECT at rest to assess myocardial viability: Comparison with fluorine-18-FDG PET. *J Nucl Med* 35:569, 1994.

157. Marzullo P, Sambucetti G, Parodi O, et al: Regional concordance and discordance between rest thallium-201 and sestamibi imaging for assessing tissue viability: comparison with postrevascularization functional recovery. *J Nucl Cardiol* 2:309, 1995.

158. Richter WS, Cordes M, Calder D, Eichstaedt H, et al: Washout and redistribution between immediate and two-hour myocardial images using technetium-99m sestamibi. *Eur J Nucl Med* 22:49, 1995.

159. Delbeke D, Videlefsky S, Patton JA, et al: Rest myocardial

perfusion/metabolism imaging using simultaneous dual-isotope acquisition SPECT with technetium-99m-MIBI/fluorine-18-FDG. *J Nucl Med* 36:2110, 1995.

160. Soufer R, Dey HM, Ng CK, Zaret BL: Comparison of sestamibi single-photon emission tomography with positron emission tomography for estimating left ventricular myocardial viability. *Am J Cardiol* 75:1214, 1995.

161. Arrighi JA, Ng CK, Dey H, et al: Resting Tc-99m sestamibi SPECT underestimates myocardial viability in patients with severe ischemic left ventricular dysfunction: comparison with ammonia/FDG PET (abstr). *J Am Coll Cardiol* 27:162A, 1996.

162. Kitsiou AN, Srinivasan G, Quyyumi AA, et al: Stress-induced reversible and mild-moderate irreversible thallium defects: Are they equally accurate for predicting recovery of function after revascularization? (abstr). *J Nucl Med* 37:25P, 1996.

163. Canby RC, Silber S, Pohost GM: Relations of the myocardial imaging agents ^{99m}Tc-MIBI and ^{201}Tl to myocardial blood flow in a canine model of myocardial ischemic insult. *Circulation* 81:289, 1990.

164. Li QS, Solot G, Frank TL, et al: Myocardial redistribution of technetium-99m-methoxyisobutyl isonitrile (sestamibi). *J Nucl Med* 31:1069, 1990.

165. Sinusas AJ, Bergin JD, Edwards NC, et al: Redistribution of ^{99m}Tc-sestamibi and ^{201}Tl in the presence of a severe coronary artery stenosis. *Circulation* 89:2332, 1994.

166. Sansoy V, Glover DK, Watson DD, et al: Comparison of thallium-201 resting redistribution with technetium-99m-sestamibi uptake and functional response to dobutamine for assessment of myocardial viability. *Circulation* 92:994, 1995.

167. Taillefer R, Primeau M, Costi P, et al: Technetium-99m-sestamibi myocardial perfusion imaging in detection of coronary artery disease: Comparison between initial (1-hour) and delayed (3-hour) postexercise images. *J Nucl Med* 32:1961, 1991.

168. Richter WS, Cordes M, Calder D, et al: Washout and redistribution between immediate and two-hour myocardial images using technetium-99m sestamibi. *Eur J Nucl Med* 22:49, 1995.

169. Maurea S, Cuocolo A, Soricelli A, et al: Myocardial viability index in chronic coronary artery disease: Technetium-99m-methoxy isobutyl isonitrile redistribution. *J Nucl Med* 36:1953, 1995.

170. Udelson JE, Coleman PS, Metherall JA, et al: Predicting recovery of severe regional ventricular dysfunction: Comparison of resting scintigraphy with ^{201}Tl and ^{99m}Tc-sestamibi. *Circulation* 89:2552, 1994.

171. Berman DS, Kiat H, Friedman JD, et al: Separate acquisition rest thallium-201/stress technetium-99m sestamibi dual-isotope myocardial perfusion single-photon emission computed tomography: A clinical validation study. *J Am Coll Cardiol* 22:1455, 1993.

172. Weinstein H, Reinhardt CP, Leppo JA: Teboroxime, sestamibi and thallium 201 as markers of myocardial hypoperfusion: Comparison by quantitative dual-isotope autoradiography in rabbits. *J Nucl Med* 34:1510, 1993.

173. DiRocco RJ, Rumsey WL, Kuczynski BL, et al: Measurement of myocardial blood flow using a coinjection tech-

nique for technetium-99m teboroxime, technetium-99m sestamibi and thallium-201. *J Nucl Med* 33:1152, 1992.

174. Maublant JC, Moins N, Gachon P: Uptake and release of two new ^{99m}Tc labeled myocardial blood flow imaging agents in cultured cardiac cells. *Eur J Nucl Med* 15:180, 1989.

175. Kronauge JF, Chiu ML, Cone JS, et al: Comparison of neutral and cationic myocardial perfusion agents: Characteristics of accumulation in cultured cells. *Nucl Med Biol* 19:141, 1992.

176. Seldin DW, Johnson L, Blood DK, et al: Myocardial perfusion imaging with technetium-99m SQ30217: Comparison with thallium 201 and coronary anatomy. *J Nucl Med* 30:312, 1989.

177. Iskandrian AS, Heo J, Nguyen T, Mercuro J: Myocardial imaging with ^{99m}Tc teboroxime: Technique and initial results. *Am Heart J* 121:889, 1991.

178. Iskandrian AS, Heo J, Nguyen T: Tomographic myocardial perfusion imaging with technetium-99m teboroxime during adenosine-induced coronary hyperemia: Correlation with thallium-201 imaging. *J Am Coll Cardiol* 19:307, 1992.

179. Henzlova MJ, Machac J: Clinical utility of technetium-99m teboroxime myocardial washout imaging. *J Nucl Med* 35:575, 1994.

180. Stewart RE, Schwaiger M, Hutchins GD, et al: Myocardial clearance kinetics of technetium-99m SQ30217: A marker of regional myocardial blood flow. *J Nucl Med* 31:1183, 1990.

181. Gray WA, Gewirtz H: Comparison of ^{99m}Tc teboroxime with thallium for myocardial imaging in the presence of a coronary artery stenosis. *Circulation* 84:1796, 1991.

182. Weinstein H, Dahlberg ST, McSherry BA, et al: Rapid redistribution of teboroxime. *Am J Cardiol* 71:848, 1993.

183. Beanlands R, Muzik O, Nguyen N, et al: The relationship between myocardial retention of technetium-99m teboroxime and myocardial blood flow. *J Am Coll Cardiol* 20:712, 1992.

184. Maublant JC, Moins N, Gachon P, et al: Uptake of technetium-99m teboroxime in cultured myocardial cells: Comparison with thallium 201 and technetium-99m sestamibi. *J Nucl Med* 34:225, 1993.

185. Smith AM, Gullberg GT, Christian PE, Data FL: Kinetic modeling of teboroxime using dynamic SPECT imaging of a canine model. *J Nucl Med* 35:484, 1994.

186. Fleming RM, Kirkeeide RL, Taegtmeyer H, et al: Comparison of technetium-99m teboroxime tomography with automated quantitative coronary arteriography and thallium-201 tomographic imaging. *J Am Coll Cardiol* 17:1297, 1991.

187. Hendel RC, Dahlberg ST, Weinstein H, Leppo JA: Comparison of teboroxime and thallium for the reversibility of exercise-induced myocardial perfusion defects. *Am Heart J* 126:856, 1993.

188. Johnson LL, Seldin DW: Clinical experience with technetium-99m teboroxime, a neutral, lipophilic myocardial perfusion imaging agent. *Am J Cardiol* 66:63E, 1990.

189. Bisi G, Sciagra R, Santoro GM, et al: Evaluation of ^{99m}Tc-teboroxime scintigraphy for the differentaition of reversible from fixed defects: Comparison with ^{201}Tl redistribu-

tion and reinjection imaging. *Nucl Med Commun* 14:520, 1993.

190. Kelly JD, Forester AM, Higley B, et al: Technetium-99m tetrofosmin as a new radiopharmaceutical for myocardial perfusion imaging. *J Nucl Med* 34:222, 1993.

191. Sinusas AJ, Shi QX, Saltzberg MT, et al: Technetium-99m tetrofosmin to assess myocardial blood flow: Experimental validation in an intact canine model of ischemia. *J Nucl Med* 35:664, 1994.

192. Jain D, Wackers FJ, Mattera J, et al: Biokinetics of ^{99m}Tc-tetrofosmin, a new myocardial perfusion imaging agent: Implications for a one day imaging protocol. *J Nucl Med* 34:1254, 1993.

193. Higley B, Smith FW, Smith T, et al: Technetium-99m-1,2-bis[bis(2-ethoxyethyl)phosphino]ethane: Human biodistribution, dosimetry and safety of a new myocardial perfusion imaging agent. *J Nucl Med* 34:30, 1993.

194. Matsunari I, Fujino S, Taki J, et al: Myocardial viability assessment with technetium-99m-tetrofosmin and thallium-201 reinjection in coronary artery disease. *J Nucl Med* 36:1961, 1995.

195. Gerson MC, Millard RW, Roszell NJ, et al: Kinetic properties of ^{99m}Tc-Q12 in canine myocardium. *Circulation* 89:1291, 1994.

196. Gerson MC, Lukes J, Deutsch E, et al: Comparison of technetium-99m Q12 and thallium 201 for detection of angiographically documented coronary artery disease in humans. *J Nucl Cardiol* 1:499, 1994.

197. Mckeever NP, Gregg DE, Caney PC: Oxygen uptake of non-working left ventricle. *Circ Res* 6:612, 1958.

198. Bergmann SR, Fox KAA, Rand AL, et al: Quantification of regional myocardial blood flow in vivo with O-15 water. *Circulation* 70:724, 1984.

199. Walsh MN, Bergmann SR, Steele RL, et al: Delineation of impaired regional myocardial perfusion by positron emission tomography with O-15 water. *Circulation* 78:612, 1988.

200. Bacharach SL, Cuocolo A, Bonow RO, et al: Arterial blood concentration curves by cardiac PET without arterial sampling or image reconstruction, in: *Computers in Cardiology*. Washington, D.C.: IEEE Computer Society Press, 1989, p 219.

201. Bergmann SR, Herrero P, Markham J, et al: Noninvasive quantitation of myocardial blood flow in human subjects with oxygen-15-labeled water and positron emission tomography. *J Am Coll Cardiol* 14:639, 1989.

202. Iida H, Kanno I, Takahashi A, et al: Measurement of absolute myocardial blood flow with O-15 water and dynamic positron emission tomography. *Circulation* 78:104, 1988.

203. Araujo LI, Lammertsma AA, Rhodes CG, et al: Noninvasive quantification of regional myocardial blood flow in coronary artery disease with oxygen-15-labeled carbon dioxide inhalation and positron emission tomography. *Circulation* 83:875, 1991.

204. Yamamoto Y, de Silva R, Rhodes CG, et al: A new strategy for the assessment of viable myocardium and regional myocardial blood flow using ^{15}O-water and dynamic positron emission tomography. *Circulation* 86:167, 1992.

205. deSilva R, Yamamoto Y, Rhodes CG, et al: Preoperative

prediction of the outcome of coronary revascularization using positron emission tomography. *Circulation* 86:1738, 1992.

206. Schelbert HR, Wisenberg G, Phelps ME, et al: Noninvasive assessment of coronary stenoses by myocardial imaging during pharmacologic coronary vasodilation. VI. Detection of coronary artery disease by human beings with intravenous N-13 ammonia and positron computed tomography. *Am J Cardiol* 49:1197, 1982.

207. Tamaki N, Senda M, Yonekura Y, et al: Dynamic positron computed tomography of the heart with a high sensitivity positron camera and nitrogen-13 ammonia. *J Nucl Med* 26:567, 1985.

208. Schelbert HR, Phelps ME, Huang S-C, et al: N-13 ammonia as an indicator of myocardial blood flow. *Circulation* 63:1259, 1981.

209. Shah A, Schelbert HR, Schwaiger M, et al: Measurement of regional myocardial blood flow with N-13 ammonia and positron emission tomography in intact dogs. *J Am Coll Cardiol* 5:92, 1985.

210. Krivokapich J, Smith GT, Huang S-C, et al: N-13 ammonia myocardial imaging at rest and with exercise in normal volunteers. *Circulation* 80:1328, 1989.

211. Hutchins GD, Schwaiger M, Rosenspire KC, et al: Noninvasive quantification of regional blood flow in the human heart using N-13 ammonia and dynamic positron emission tomographic imaging. *J Am Coll Cardiol* 15:1032, 1990.

212. Gewirtz H, Fischman AJ, Abraham S, et al: Positron emission tomographic measurements of absolute regional myocardial blood flow permits identification of nonviable myocardium in patients with chronic myocardial infarction. *J Am Coll Cardiol* 23:851, 1994.

213. Tamaki N, Kawamoto M, Tadamura E, et al: Prediction of reversible ischemia after revascularization: Perfusion and metabolic studies with positron emission tomography. *Circulation* 91:1697, 1995.

214. Grandin C, Wijns W, Melin JA, et al: Delineation of myocardial viability with PET. *J Nucl Med* 36:1543, 1995.

215. Kitsiou AN, Bacharach SL, Quyyumi AA, et al: Recovery of function after revascularization is dependent on preservation of myocardial blood flow (abstr). *J Am Coll Cardiol* 27:90A, 1996.

216. Duvernov C, Rothley J, Sitomer J, et al: Relationship of blood flow and functional outcome after coronary revascularization (abstr). *J Nucl Med* 34:155P, 1993.

217. Tamaki N, Kawamoto M, Tadamura E, et al: Prediction of reversible ischemia after revascularization: Perfusion and metabolic studies with positron emission tomography. *Circulation* 91:1697, 1995.

218. Kitsiou AN, Bartlett ML, Bacharach SL, et al: The magnitude of ^{18}F-fluorodeoxyglucose uptake and not O-15-water differentiates recovery of asynergic regions after revascularization (abstr). *Circulation* 90:I, 1994.

219. Love WD, Burch GE: Influence of the rate of coronary plasma flow on the extraction of rubidium-86 from coronary blood. *Circ Res* 7:24, 1959.

220. Selwyn AP, Allan RM, L'Abbate A, et al: Relation between regiona myocardial uptake of rubidium-82 and perfusion: Absolute reduction of cation uptake in ischemia. *Am J Cardiol* 50:112, 1982.

221. Goldstein RA, Mullani NA, Marani SK, et al: Myocardial perfusion with rubidium 82. II: Effects of metabolic and pharmacologic interventions. *J Nucl Med* 24:907, 1983.

222. Fukuyama T, Nakamura M, Nakagaki O, et al: Reduced reflow and diminished uptake of rubidium 86 after temporary coronary occlusion. *Am J Physiol: Heart Circ Physiol* 234:H724, 1978.

223. Wilson RA, Shea M, De Landsheere C, et al: Rubidium-82 myocardial uptake and extraction after transient ischemia: PET characteristics. *J Comput Assist Tomogr* 11:60, 1987.

224. Jeremy RW, Links JM, Becker LC: Progressive failure of coronary flow during reperfusion of myocardial infarction: Documentation of the no reflow phenomenon with positron emission tomography. *J Am Coll Cardiol* 16:695, 1990.

225. Gould KL, Goldstein RA, Mullani NA, et al: Noninvasvie assessment of coronary stenoses by myocardial perfusion imaging during pharmacologic vasodilation. VIII. Clinical feasibility of positron cardiac imaging without a cyclotron using generator-produced rubidium 82. *J Am Coll Cardiol* 7:775, 1986.

226. Demer LL, Gould LK, Goldstein RA, et al: Assessment of coronary artery disease severity by positron emission tomography: Comparison with quantitative arteriography in 193 patients. *Circulation* 79:825, 1989.

227. Go RT, Marwick TH, MacIntyre WJ, et al: A prospective comparison of rubidium-82 PET and thallium-201 SPECT myocardial perfusion imaging utilizing a single dipyridamole stress in the diagnosis of coronary artery disease. *J Nucl Med* 31:1899, 1990.

228. Stewart RE, Schwaiger M, Molina E, et al: Comparison of rubidium-82 positron emission tomography and thallium-201 SPECT imaging for detection of coronary artery disease. *Am J Cardiol* 67:1303, 1991.

229. Ziegler WH, Goresky CA: Kinetics of rubidium uptake in the working dog heart. *Circ Res* 29:208, 1971.

230. Sheehan RM, Renkin EM: Capillary, interstitial, and cell membrane barriers to blood-tissue transport of potassium and rubidium in mammalian skeletal muscle. *Circ Res* 30:588, 1972.

231. Nakaya H, Kimura S, Kanno M: Intracellular K+ and Na+ activities under hypoxia, acidosis, and no glucose in dog hearts. *Am J Physiol* 249:H1078, 1985.

232. Johnson RN, Sammel ML, Norris RM: Depletion of myocardial creatine kinase, lactate dehydrogenase, myoglobin, and K+ after coronary artery ligation in dogs. *Cardiovasc Res* 15:529, 1981.

233. Goldstein RA: Kinetics of rubidium 82 after coronary occlusion and reperfusion: Assessment of patency and viability in open-chested dogs. *J Clin Invest* 75:1131, 1985.

234. Gould KL, Yoshida K, Hess MJ, et al: Myocardial metabolism of fluorodeoxyglucose compared to cell membrane integrity for the potassium analogue rubidium 82 for assessing infarct size in man by PET. *J Nucl Med* 32:1, 1991.

235. Yoshida K, Gould KL: Quantitative relation of myocardial infarct size and myocardial viability by positron

emission tomography to left ventricular ejection fraction and 3-year mortality with and without revascularization. *J Am Coll Cardiol* 22:984, 1993.

236. vom Dahl J, Muzik O, Wolfe ER, et al: Myocardial rubidium-82 tissue kinetics assessed by dynamic positron emission tomography as a marker of myocardial cell membrane integrity and viability. *Circulation* 93:238, 1996.

237. Aversano T, Becker LC: Persistence of coronary vasodilator reserve despite functionally significant flow reduction. *Am J Physiol* 248:H403, 1985.

238. Canty JM, Klocke FJ: Reduced regional myocardial perfusion in the presence of pharmacologic vasodilator reserve. *Circulation* 71:370, 1985.

239. Gallagher KP, Folts JP, Shebuski RJ, et al: Subepicardial vasodilator reserve in the presence of critical coronary stenosis in dogs. *Am J Cardiol* 46:67, 1980.

240. Chilian WM, Layne SM: Coronary microvascular responses to reductions in perfusion pressure: Evidence for a persistent arteriolar vasomotor tone during coronary hypoperfusion. *Circ Res* 66:1227, 1990.

241. Parodi O, Sambuceti G, Roghi A, et al: Residual coronary reserve despite decreased resting blood flow in patients with critical coronary lesions: A study by technetium-99m human albumin microsphere myocardial scintigraphy. *Circulation* 87:330, 1993.

242. Vanoverschelde JJ, Wijns W, Depre C, et al: Mechanisms of chronic regional postischemic dysfunction in humans: New insights from the study of noninfarcted collateral-dependent myocardium. *Circulation* 87:1513, 1993.

243. Marzullo P, Parodi O, Sambuceti G, et al: Residual coronary reserve identifies segmental viability in patients with wall motion abnormalities. *J Am Coll Cardiol* 26:342, 1995.

244. Suryapranata H, Zijlstra F, MacLeod DC, et al: Predictive value of reactive hyperemic response on reperfusion on recovery of regional myocardial function after coronary angioplasty in acute myocardial infarction. *Circulation* 89:1109, 1994.

245. Neely JR, Rovetto MJ, Oram JF: Myocardial utilization of carbohydrate and lipids. *Prog Cardiovasc Dis* 15:289, 1972.

246. Wisneski JA, Gertz EW, Neese RA, et al: Myocardial metabolism of free fatty acids: Studies with ^{14}C-labeled substrates in humans. *J Clin Invest* 79:359, 1987.

247. Opie LH: Metabolism of the heart. I. Metabolism of glucose, glycogen, free fatty acids, and ketone bodies. *Am Heart J* 76:685, 1968.

248. Camici P, Ferrannini E, Opie LH: Myocardial metabolism in ischemic heart disease: Basic principles and application to imaging by positron emission tomography. *Prog Cardiovasc Dis* 32:217, 1989.

249. Gertz EW, Wisneski JA, Neese R, et al: Myocardial lactate metabolism: Evidence of lactate release during net chemical extraction in man. *Circulation* 63:1273, 1981.

250. Most AS, Gorlin R, Soeldner JS: Glucose extraction by the human myocardium during pacing stress. *Circulation* 45:92, 1972.

251. Liedtke AJ: Alterations of carbohydrate and lipid metabolism in the acutely ischemic heart. *Prog Cardiovasc Dis* 23:321, 1981.

252. Opie LH: Effects of regional ischemia on metabolism of glucose and fatty acids: Relative rates of aerobic and anaerobic energy production during myocardial infarction and comparison with effects of anoxia. *Circ Res* 38:I, 1976.

253. Peuhkurinen KJ, Takala TES, Nuutinen EM, Hassinen IE: Tricarboxylic acid cycle metabolites during ischemia in isolated perfused rat heart. *Am J Physiol* 244:H281, 1983.

254. Schon HR, Schelbert HR, Najafi A, et al: C-11 labeled palmitic acid for the noninvasive evaluation of regional myocardial fatty acid metabolism with postiron computed tomography. I. Kinetics of C-11 palmitic acid in normal myocardium. *Am Heart J* 103:532, 1982.

255. Rosamond TL, Abendschein DR, Sobel BE, et al: Metabolic fate of radiolabeled palmitate in ischemic canine myocardium: Implications for positron emission tomography. *J Nucl Med* 28:1322, 1987.

256. Lerch RA, Bergmann SR, Ambos HD, et al: Effect of flow-independent reduction of metabolism on regional myocardial clearance of C-11 palmitate. *Circulation* 65:731, 1982.

257. Schwaiger M, Schelbert HR, Ellison D, et al: Sustained regional abnormalities in cardiac metabolism after transient ischemia in the chronic dog model. *J Am Coll Cardiol* 6:336, 1985.

258. Liedtke AJ, DeMaison L, Eggleston AM, et al: Changes in substrate metabolism and effects of excess fatty acids in reperfused myocardium. *Circ Res* 62:535, 1988.

259. Schelbert HR, Henze E, Schon HR, et al: C-11 palmitic acid for the noninvasive evaluation of regional myocardial fatty acid metabolism wtih positron computed tomography. IV. In vivo demonstration of impaired fatty acid oxidation in acute myocardial ischemia. *Am Heart J* 106:736, 1983.

260. Schelbert HR, Henze E, Schon HR, et al: Carbon-11 palmitate for the noninvasive evaluation of regional myocardial fatty acid metabolism wtih positron computed tomography. III. In vivo demonstration of the effects of substrate availability on myocardial metabolism. *Am Heart J* 105:492, 1983.

261. Fox KAA, Abendschein D, Ambos HD, et al: Efflux of metabolized and nonmetabolized fatty acid from canine myocardium: Implications for quantifying myocardial metabolism tomographically. *Circ Res* 57:232, 1985.

262. Myears DW, Sobel BE, Bergmann SR: Substrate use in ischemic and reperfused canine myocardium: Quantitative considerations. *Am J Physiol: Heart Circ Physiol* 253:H107, 1987.

263. Sokoloff L, Reivich M, Kennedy C, et al: The ^{14}C]-deoxyglucose method for the measurement of local cerebral glucose utilizatio: Theory, procedure and normal values in the conscious and anesthetized albino rat. *J Neurochem* 28:897, 1977.

264. Phelps ME, Schelbert HR, Mazziotta JC: Positron computer tomography for studies of myocardial and cerebral function. *Ann Intern Med* 98:339, 1983.

265. Neely JR, Rovetto MJ, Oram JF: Myocardial utilization of carbohydrate and lipids. *Prog Cardiovasc Dis* 15:289, 1972.

266. Neely JR, Morgan HE: Relationship between carbohy-

drate and lipid metabolism and the energy balance of heart muscle. *Annu Rev Physiol* 36:413, 1974.

267. Marshall RC, Huang SC, Nash WW, Phelps ME: Assessment of the [^{18}F]fluorodeoxyglucose kinetic model in calculations of myocardial glucose metabolism during ischemia. *J Nucl Med* 24:1060, 1983.

268. Gambhir SS, Schwaiger M, Huang SC, et al: Simple noninvasive quantification method for measuring myocardial glucose utilization in humans employing positron emission tomography and fluorine-18 deoxyglucose. *J Nucl Med* 30:359, 1989.

269. Camici P, Araujo LI, Spinks T, et al: Increased uptake of ^{18}F fluorodeoxyglucose in postischemic myocardium of patients with exercise-induced angina. *Circulation* 74:81, 1986.

270. Ratib O, Phelps ME, Huang SC, et al: Positron tomography with deoxyglucose for estimating local myocardial glucose metabolism. *J Nucl Med* 23:577, 1982.

271. Knuuti MJ, Nuutila P, Ruotsalainen U, et al: The value of quantitative analysis of glucose utilization in detection of myocardial viability by PET. *J Nucl Med* 34:2068, 1993.

272. Hariharan R, Bray M, Ganim R, et al: Fundamental limitations of [^{18}F]2-deoxy-2-fluoro-d-glucose for assessing myocardial glucose uptake. *Circulation* 91:2435, 1995.

273. Gropler RJ, Siegel BA, Lee KJ, et al: Nonuniformity in myocardial accumulation of fluorine-18-fluorodeoxyglucose in normal fasted humans. *J Nucl Med* 31:1749, 1990.

274. Hicks RJ, Herman WH, Kalff V, et al: M. Quantitative evaluation of regional substrate metabolism in the human heart by positron emission tomography. *J Am Coll Cardiol* 18:101, 1991.

275. Krivokapich J, Huang SC, Phelps ME, et al: Estimation of rabbit myocardial metabolic rate for glucose using fluorodeoxyglucose. *Am J Physiol* 243:H884, 1982.

276. Ratib O, Phelps ME, Huang SS, et al: Positron tomography with deoxyglucose for estimating local myocardial glucose metabolism. *J Nucl Med* 23:577, 1982.

277. Marshall RC, Tillisch JH, Phelps ME, et al: Identification and differentiation of resting myocardial ischemia and infarction in man with positron emission tomography, F-18 labeled fluorodeoxyglucose and N-13 ammonia. *Circulation* 67:766, 1983.

278. Brunken R, Tillisch J, Schwaiger M, et al: Regional perfusion, glucose metabolism, and wall motion in patients with chronic electrocardiographic Q wave infarctions: Evidence for persistence of viable tissue in some infarct regions by positron emission tomography. *Circulation* 73:951, 1986.

279. Tamaki N, Yonekura Y, Yamashita K, et al: Positron emission tomography using fluorine-18 deoxyglucose in evaluation of coronary artery bypass grafting. *Am J Cardiol* 64:860, 1989.

280. Schelbert HR: Metabolic imaging to assess myocardial viability. *J Nucl Med* 35(suppl):8S, 1994.

281. Luciganani G, Paolini G, Landoni C, et al: Presurgical identification of hibernating myocardium by combined use of technetium-99m hexakis 2-methoxyisobutylisonitrile single photon emission tomography and fluorine-

18-fluoro-2-deoxy-D-glucose positron emission tomography in patients with coronary artery disease. *Eur J Nucl Med* 19:874, 1992.

282. Carrel T, Jenni R, Haubold-Reuter S, et al: Improvement of severely reduced left ventricular function after surgical revascularization in patients with preoperative myocardial infarction. *Eur J Cardiothorac Surg* 6:479, 1992.

283. Nienaber CA, Brunken RC, Sherman CT, et al: Metabolic and functional recovery of ischemic human myocardium after coronary angioplasty. *J Am Coll Cardiol* 18:966, 1991.

284. Tamaki N, Ohtani H, Yamashita K, et al: Metabolic activity in the areas of new fill-in after thallium-201 reinjection: Comparison with positron emission tomography using fluoro-18-deoxyglucose. *J Nucl Med* 32:673, 1991.

285. Marwick TH, MacIntyre WJ, LaFont A, et al: Metabolic responses of hibernating and infarcted myocardium to revascularization: A follow-up study of regional perfusion, function, and metabolism. *Circulation* 85:1347, 1992.

286. Tamaki N, Kawamoto M, Tadamura E, et al: Prediction of reversible ischemia after revascularization: Perfusion and metabolic studies with positron emission tomography. *Circulation* 91:1697, 1995.

287. Go RT, MacIntyre WJ, Saha GB, et al: Hibernating myocardium versus scar: Severity of irreversible decreased myocardial perfusion in prediction of tissue viability. *Radiology* 194:151, 1995.

288. vom Dahl J, Eitzman DT, Al-Aouar ZR, et al: Relation of regional function, perfusion, and metabolism in patients with advanced coronary artery disease undergoing surgical revascularization. *Circulation* 90:2356, 1994.

289. Nienaber CA, Brunken RC, Sherman CT, et al: Metabolic and functional recovery of ischemic human myocardium after coronary angioplasty. *J Am Coll Cardiol* 18:966, 1991.

290. Marwick TH, MacIntyre WJ, LaFont A, et al: Metabolic responses of hibernating and infarcted myocardium to revascularization: A follow-up study of regional perfusion, function, and metabolism. *Circulation* 85:1347, 1992.

291. Taegtmeyer H, Robers AFC, Raine AEG: Energy metabolism in reperfused heart muscle: Metabolic correlates of return of function. *J Am Coll Cardiol* 6:864, 1985.

292. Armbrecht JJ, Buxton DB, Schelbert HR: Validation of [1-^{11}C]acetate as a tracer for noninvasive assessment of oxidative metabolism with positron emission tomography in normal, ischemic, postischemic, and hyperemic canine myocardium. *Circulation* 81:1594, 1990.

293. Vanoverschelde JJ, Melin JA, Bol A, et al: Regional oxidative metabolism in patients after recovery from reperfused anterior myocardial infarction: Relation to regional blood flow and glucose uptake. *Circulation* 85:9, 1992.

294. Armbrecht JJ, Buxton DB, Brunken RC, et al: Regional myocardial oxygen consumption determined noninvasively in humans with [1-^{11}C]acetate and dynamic positron tomography. *Circulation* 80:863, 1989.

295. Gropler RJ, Siegal BA, Geltman EM: Myocardial uptake of carbon-11 acetate as an indirect estimate of regional myocardial blood flow. *J Nucl Med* 32:245, 1991.

296. Brown MA, Marshall DR, Sobel BE, Bergmann SR: De-

lineation of myocardial oxygen utilization with carbon-11 labeled acetate. *Circulation* 76:687, 1987.

297. Brown MA, Myears DW, Bergmann SR: Noninvasive assessment of canine myocardial oxidative metabolism with carbon-11 acetate and positron emission tomography. *J Am Coll Cardiol* 12:1054, 1988.

298. Hicks RJ, Herman WH, Kalff V, et al: Quantitative evaluation of regional substrate metabolism in the human heart by positron emission tomography. *J Am Coll Cardiol* 18:101, 1991.

299. Henes CG, Bergmann SR, Walsh MN, et al: Assessment of myocardial oxidative metabolic reserve with positron emission tomography and carbon-11 acetate. *J Nucl Med* 30:1489, 1989.

300. Gropler RJ, Siegel BA, Sampathkumaran K, et al: Dependence of recovery of contractile function on maintenance of oxidative metabolism after myocardial infarction. *J Am Coll Cardiol* 19:989, 1992.

301. Gropler RJ, Geltman EM, Sampathkumaran K, et al: Functional recovery after coronary revascularization for chronic coronary artery disease is dependent on maintenance of oxidative metabolism. *J Am Coll Cardiol* 20:569, 1992.

302. Gropler RJ, Geltman EM, Sampathkumaran K, et al: Comparison of carbon-11 acetate with fluorine-18-fluorodeoxyglucose for delineating viable myocardium by positron emission tomography. *J Am Coll Cardiol* 22:1587, 1993.

303. Rubin PJ, Lee DS, Geltman EM, et al: The superiority of PET with C-11 acetate compared with F-18 fluorodeoxyglucose for prediction of functional recovery early after myocardial infarction (abstr). *J Nucl Med* 23:39P, 1994.

304. Melin JA, Wijns W, Keyeux A, et al: Assessment of thallium-201 redistribution versus glucose uptake as predictors of viability after coronary occlusion and reperfusion. *Circulation* 77:927, 1988.

305. Brunken R, Schwaiger M, Grover-McKay M, et al: Positron emission tomography detects tissue metabolic activity in myocardial segments with persistent thallium perfusion defects. *J Am Coll Cardiol* 10:557, 1987.

306. Tamaki N, Yonekura Y, Yamashita K, et al: Relation of left ventricular perfusion and wall motion with metabolic activity in persistent defects on thallium-201 tomography in healed myocardial infarction. *Am J Cardiol* 62:202, 1988.

307. Brunken RC, Kottou S, Nienaber CA, et al: PET detection of viable tissue in myocardial segments with persistent defects at Tl-201 SPECT. *Radiology* 65:65, 1989.

308. Tamaki N, Yonekura Y, Yamashita K, et al: SPECT thallium-201 tomography and positron tomography using N-13 ammonia and F-18 fluorodeoxyglucose in coronary artery disease. *Am J Cardiac Imaging* 3:3, 1989.

309. Perrone-Filardi P, Bacharach SL, Dilsizian V, et al: Regional left ventricular wall thickening: Relation to regional uptake of 18-fluorodeoxyglucose and thallium 201 in patients with chronic coronary artery disease and left ventricular dysfunction. *Circulation* 86:1125, 1992.

310. Brunken RC, Mody FV, Hawkins RA, et al: Positron emission tomography detects metabolic viability in myocardium with persistent 24-hour single-photon emission computed tomography TL-201 defects. *Circulation* 86:1357, 1992.

311. Tamaki N, Ohtani H, Yamashita K, et al: Metabolic activity in the areas of new fill-in after thallium-201 reinjection: Comparison with positron emission tomography using fluorine-18-deoxyglucose. *J Nucl Med* 32:673, 1991.

312. Ogiu N, Nakai K, Hiramori K: Thallium-201 reinjection images can identify the viable and necrotic myocardium similarly to metabolic imaging with glucose loading F-18 fluorodeoxyglucose (FDG)-PET. *Ann Nucl Med* 8:171, 1994.

313. Eitzman D, Al-Aouar Z, Kanter HL, et al: Clinical outcome of patients with advanced coronary artery disease after viability studies with positron emission tomography. *J Am Coll Cardiol* 20:559, 1992.

314. DiCarli M, Davidson M, Little R, et al: Value of metabolic imaging with positron emission tomography for evaluating prognosis in patients with coronary artery disease and left ventricular dysfunction. *Am J Cardiol* 73:527, 1994.

315. Lee KS, Marwick TH, Cook SA, et al: Prognosis of patients with left ventricular dysfunction, with and without viable myocardium after myocardial infarction: Relative efficacy of medical therapy and revascularization. *Circulation* 90:2687, 1994.

316. Miller DD, Kemp DL, Armbruster RW, et al: Prognostic synergy of thallium-201 stress/redistribution and reinjection protocols in revascularization candidates (abstr). *J Nucl Cardiol* 2:S70, 1995.

317. Pieri PL, Tisselli A, Moscatelli G, et al: Prognostic value of Tl-201 reinjection in patients with chronic myocardial infarction. *J Nucl Cardiol* 2:S89, 1995.

318. Bax JJ, Visser FC, van Lingen A, et al: Feasibility of assessing regional myocardial uptake of ^{18}F-fluorodeoxyglucose using single photon emission computed tomography. *Eur Heart J* 14:1675, 1993.

319. Drane WE, Abbott FD, Nicole MW, et al: Technology for FDG SPECT with a relatively inexpensive gamma camera. *Radiology* 191:461, 1994.

320. Burt RW, Perkins OW, Oppenheim BE, et al: Direct comparison of fluorine-18-FDG SPECT, fluorine-18-FDG PET and rest thallium-201 SPECT for detection of myocardial viability. *J Nucl Med* 36:176, 1995.

321. Srinivasan G, Kitsiou AN, Bacharach SL, et al: FDG cardiac SPECT versus PET: Relation to SPECT radionuclide angiography and thallium scintigraphy (abstr). *J Nucl Med* 37(5):60P, 1996.

322. Schulz R, Guth BD, Pieper K, et al: Recruitment of an inotropic reserve in moderately ischemic myocardium at the expense of metabolic recovery: A model of short-term hibernation. *Circ Res* 70:1282, 1992.

323. Popio KA, Gorlin R, Bechtel D, Levine JA: Postextrasystolic potentiation as a predictor of potential myocardial viability: Preoperative analysis compared with studies after coronary bypass surgery. *Am J Cardiol* 39:944, 1977.

324. Becker LC, Levine LH, Di Paula AF, et al: Reversal of dysfunction in postischemic stunned myocardium by epinephrine and postextrasystolic potentiation. *J Am Coll Cardiol* 7:580, 1986.

325. Helfant RH, Pine R, Meister SG, et al: Nitroglycerin to unmask reversible asynergy: Correlation with post coronary bypass ventriculography. *Circulation* 50:108, 1974.
326. Horn HR, Teicholz LE, Cohn PF, et al: Augmentation of left ventricular contraction pattern in coronary artery disease by an inotropic catecholamine: The epinephrine ventriculogram. *Circulation* 49:1063, 1974.
327. Bolli R, Zhu WX, Myers ML, et al: Beta-adrenergic stimulation reverses postischemic myocardial dysfunction without producing subsequent functional deterioration. *Am J Cardiol* 56:964, 1985.
328. Barilla F, Gheorghiade KP, Alam M, et al: Low dose dobutamine in patients with acute myocardial infarction identifies viable but not contractile myocardium and predicts the magnitude of improvement in wall motion abnormalities in response to coronary revascularization. *Am Heart J* 122:1522, 1991.
329. Pierard LA, de Landsheere CM, Berthe C, et al: Identification of viable myocardium by echocardiography during dobutamine infusion in patients with myocardial infarction after thrombolytic therapy: Comparison with positron emission tomography. *J Am Coll Cardiol* 15:1021, 1990.
330. Smart SC, Sawasa S, Ryan T, et al: Low-dose dobutamine echocardiography detects reversible dysfunction after thrombolytic therapy of acute myocardial infarction. *Circulation* 88:405, 1993.
331. Cigarroa CG, deFilippi CR, Brickner E, et al: Dobutamine stress echocardiography identifies hibernating myocardium and predicts recovery of left ventricular function after coronary revascularization. *Circulation* 88:430, 1993.
332. La Canna G, Alfieri O, Giubbini R, et al: Echocardiography during infusion of dobutamine for identification of reversible dysfunction in patients with chronic coronary artery disease. *J Am Coll Cardiol* 23:617, 1994.
333. Afridi I, Kleinman NS, Raizner AE, Zoghbi WA: Dobutamine echocardiography in myocardial hibernation: Optimal dose and accuracy in predicting recovery of ventricular function after coronary angioplasty. *Circulation* 91:663, 1995.
334. Senior R, Lahiri A: Enhanced detection of myocardial ischemia by stress dobutamine echocardiography utilizing the "biphasic" response of wall thickening during low and high dose dobutamine infusion. *J Am Coll Cardiol* 26:26, 1995.
335. Perrone-Filardi P, Pace L, Prastaro M, et al: Dobutamine echocardiography predicts improvement of hypoperfused dysfunctional myocardium after revascularization in patients with coronary artery disease. *Circulation* 91:2256, 1995.
336. Senior R, Glenville B, Basu S, et al: Dobutamine echocardiography and thallium-201 imaging predict functional improvement after revascularisation in severe ischaemic left ventricular dysfunction. *Br Heart J* 74:358, 1995.
337. Arnese M, Cornel JH, Salustri A, et al: Prediction of improvement of regional left ventricular function after surgical revascularization: A comparison of low-dose dobutamine echocardiography with ^{201}Tl single-photon emission computed tomography. *Circulation* 91:2748, 1995.
338. Panza JA, Dilsizian V, Laurienzo JM, et al: Relation between thallium uptake and contractile response to dobutamine: Implications regarding myocardial viability in patients with chronic coronary artery disease and left ventricular dysfunction. *Circulation* 91:990, 1995.
339. Panza JA, Curiel RV, Laurienzo JM, et al: Relation between ischemic threshold measured during dobutamine stress echocardiography and known indices of poor prognosis in patients with coronary artery disease. *Circulation* 92:2095, 1995.
340. Baer FM, Voth E, Deutsch HJ, et al: Assessment of viable myocardium by dobutamine transesophageal echocardiography and comparison with fluorine-18 fluorodeoxyglucose positron emission tomography. *J Am Coll Cardiol* 24:343, 1994.
341. Elsner G, Sawada S, Foltz J, et al: Dobutamine stimulation detects stunned but not hibernating myocardium (abstr). *Circulation* 90:I, 1994.
342. Hepner AM, Bach DS, Bolling SF, et al: Positive dobutamine stress echocardiogram predicts viable myocardium in ischemic cardiomyopathy: A comparison with PET (abstr). *Circulation* 90:I, 1994.
343. Panza JA, Dilsizian V, Curiel RV, et al: Relation between myocardial blood flow and contractile reserve in patients with chronic coronary artery disease and impaired left ventricular systolic function. *J Am Coll Cardiol* 27:89A, 1996.
344. deFilippi CR, Willett DL, Irani WN, et al: Comparison of myocardial contrast echocardiography and low-dose dobutamine stress echocardiography in predicting recovery of left ventricular function after coronary revascularization in chronic ischemic heart disease. *Circulation* 92:2863, 1995.

Alternatives to Leg Exercise in the Evaluation of Patients with Coronary Artery Disease: Functional and Pharmacologic Stress Modalities

William P. Follansbee

While the mortality due to coronary artery disease is declining, it remains the largest single cause of death in the United States, accounting for more deaths than all types of cancer combined.[1] Coronary artery disease accounted for nearly 500,000 deaths in the United States in 1990.[2] The Framingham study has shown that coronary artery disease often is initially manifest by a major complication. For example, in men ages 40 to 60 years, the presenting symptom of coronary disease is myocardial infarction in 40 percent and sudden death in 12 percent.[3] Because of the widespread prevalence of the disease, its consequences, and its often catastrophic presentation, there has been intense interest in finding reliable noninvasive techniques to diagnose and quantify the disease in symptomatic or asymptomatic patients.

Exercise has played a central role in the various noninvasive techniques that have been used to evaluate coronary artery disease. Typically this has been in the form of upright, aerobic leg exercise, using either a motorized treadmill or a variably braked bicycle. However, many patients at greatest risk with known or suspected coronary artery disease are unable to perform adequate levels of leg exercise to enable satisfactory evaluation. Furthermore, some testing modalities that involve imaging are not well suited to upright exercise because of the nature of the equipment used. For these reasons, it has been necessary to develop alternative means to stress patients in whom upright leg exercise is not suitable. These alternative stress procedures can be conceptually categorized into three groups. The first uses other forms of exercise instead of upright leg exercise. These include supine leg exercise, arm exercise, and isometric as opposed to aerobic exercise. The second approach uses modalities that simulate exercise effects on the heart, increasing myocardial oxygen demand, without actually requiring the patient to perform exercise. Included in this category are atrial pacing, cold pressor testing, and pharmacologic stress with dobutamine infusion. The third approach uses coronary vasodilators to increase myocardial blood flow pharmacologically, independent of increasing myocardial oxygen demand. The two most commonly used agents in this category have been dipyridamole and adenosine. This chapter examines each of these modalities in terms of their physiology, methodology, and diagnostic efficacy.

Before considering these various stress techniques, however, it is worthwhile to review briefly the physiology of autoregulation of coronary blood flow and the concept of coronary vascular reserve, since these are central to all of the stress methodologies.

AUTOREGULATION OF CORONARY BLOOD FLOW AND THE CONCEPT OF CORONARY VASODILATOR RESERVE

Coronary perfusion pressure is the difference between central aortic blood pressure and right atrial pressure (Fig. 6-1[4]). Since coronary flow to the left ventricle occurs substantially in diastole, it is aortic diastolic pressure

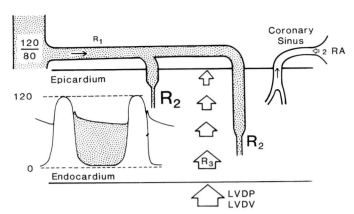

Figure 6-1 The determinants of resting coronary blood flow. The epicardial and large intramyocardial vessels constitute the R1 component of resistance, which in the normal heart contributes comparatively little to the total resistance to flow. Downstream are the small arteries and precapillary arterioles, which proportionally contribute a much greater component of resistance. They are referred to as the R2 vessels. Because the vessels penetrate the myocardial wall, the force transmitted against the wall from the ventricular cavity is also transmitted against the vessels that are contained within the wall. This is the R3 component of resistance, which is unevenly distributed across the muscle, being greatest in the subendocardium and least in the subepicardium. To compensate for the increased R3 resistance in the subendocardium, the R2 vessels vasodilate to maintain normal total resistance and thereby preserve resting blood flow. (From Follansbee,[4] reproduced with permission.)

that defines coronary perfusion pressure. In opposition to this pressure exists resistance, which is present at three levels. First is the resistance of the epicardial and larger intramyocardial coronary arteries, referred to as the R1 component of resistance. In normal arteries greater than 300 μm, the R1 component to resistance is small, although the resistance from vessels in the 200- to 300-μm range has been recently shown to be greater than originally estimated.[5] Downstream are the smaller intramyocardial arteries and the precapillary arterioles, the R2 vessels. Proportionately, these vessels contribute much greater resistance to flow. Finally, the coronary vessels must penetrate the myocardial wall in order to bring blood flow to the myocytes. Any force that is exerted against the muscle is, as a result, also transmitted against the vessels that are contained within it. Wall tension, therefore, constitutes the third component to resistance to flow, the R3 component. Wall tension is unevenly distributed across the myocardial wall, being greatest in the subendocardium and least in the subepicardium. To compensate for this greater R3 resistance in the subendocardium, the R2 vessels in the subendocardium partially vasodilate so that the total resistance remains balanced and flow to the subendocardium is preserved.

Myocardial oxygen demand increases during exercise. The heart is an obligate aerobic organ; to do more work, it must consume more oxygen. Heart rate, blood pressure, left ventricular radius or volume, and contractility are all determinants of myocardial oxygen demand. During exercise, heart rate, blood pressure, and contractility all increase. Ventricular volume may or may not increase, depending on the type and position of exercise. Myocardial oxygen supply must increase to meet the increased oxygen demand. Since oxygen extraction from coronary blood flow is nearly maximal at rest, the heart cannot meaningfully increase its oxygen supply by the mechanism of increasing oxygen extraction. Hence, increased myocardial oxygen consumption can be accomplished only by increasing coronary blood flow. Effective coronary perfusion pressure increases only minimally

during exercise. While systolic blood pressure normally increases during exercise, diastolic blood pressure does not (Fig. 6-2). Therefore, the increase in coronary blood flow needed to meet the increased demand can be achieved only through a decrease in resistance. This primarily occurs through vasodilation of the R2 vessels, which have the capacity to decrease their resistance to approximately 25 percent of the resting level, resulting in an estimated increase in coronary blood flow of approximately 4 times resting levels. The difference between resting and peak coronary blood flow is termed the *coronary vasodilator reserve.*

Measurements of coronary blood flow during exercise have been consistent with these theoretical estimations.[6,7] Kitamura and colleagues noted increases of coronary blood flow of up to 250 to 300 percent in men during strenuous upright bicycle exercise.[8] This peak level would be expected to be lower in less fit individuals or during less extreme levels of exercise. Treadmill exercise in chronically instrumented dogs has been shown to increase coronary blood flow as much as 4 times resting levels.[9] The increase in coronary blood flow with exercise is the intrinsic coronary vascular reserve. Administration of potent pharmacologic direct coronary artery vasodilators can further increase peak coronary blood flow beyond what can be achieved during exercise, with peak flows being as great as 4 to 5 times resting levels.[10,11] Hence, there is a component of coronary vasodilator reserve beyond the intrinsic reserve that can be recruited by pharmacologic as opposed to physiologic stimulation.

Coronary blood flow is typically normal at rest despite the presence of marked stenoses in the R1 vessels, the vessels typically involved in the atherosclerotic process. Gould and coinvestigators noted that, in healthy dogs, resting coronary blood flow was preserved despite progressively increasing coronary stenoses of up to 85 percent of the luminal diameter as induced by an external snare.[12] Only with stenoses beyond 85 percent did resting coronary flow decrease. These observations may not be completely analogous to atherosclerotic coronary dis-

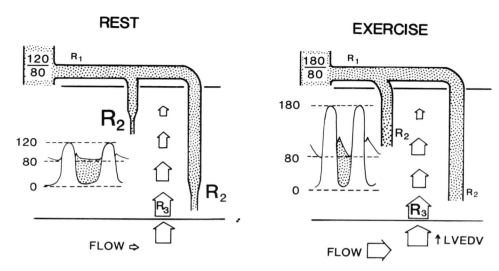

Figure 6-2   Myocardial oxygen demand increases during exercise. Coronary blood flow must increase linearly to meet the increased demand. Perfusion pressure does not increase significantly, since aortic diastolic pressure typically does not increase with aerobic exercise. The increased flow is achieved through a decrease in resistance. The R2 vessels have the capacity to decrease their resistance to approximately 25 percent of resting levels, termed the *coronary vasodilator reserve*. As a result, coronary blood flow can theoretically increase approximately fourfold. (From Follansbee,[4] reproduced with permission.)

ease in humans, since the snare is a very discrete obstruction in an otherwise normal artery, whereas atherosclerosis is a much more diffuse and gradually developing process. Resistance to flow, for example, is directly related to the length of a stenosis. Serial lesions have an impact on flow that is disproportionate to the percent stenosis.[13] Vessel size, variabilities in the measurements of stenosis severity, and the impact of collateral vessels will further confound the estimation of flow relative to percent stenosis of a vessel in humans. Vessel diameter and particularly minimal residual luminal area are better predictors of coronary arterial flow in humans than is percent stenosis.[14] Nevertheless, the concept that resting coronary blood flow is not significantly decreased until stenoses reach approximately 80 to 90 percent of the luminal diameter is well established. The preservation of resting flow in the face of stenoses in the R1 vessels is achieved through vasodilation of the R2 resistance vessels, which serves to keep total resistance normal despite the increased resistance at the R1 vessel level and therefore preserves resting flow at any given perfusion pressure (Fig. 6-3).

In contrast to rest, peak coronary blood flow declines sharply with stenoses of greater than 50 percent (Fig. 6-4).[3,13] The increase in flow that occurs with exercise or pharmacologic vasodilation is primarily achieved through vasodilation of the R2 resistance vessels. Since these vessels have already partially or perhaps completely expended their vasodilator capacity to preserve flow at rest, little or no vasodilator reserve is available to recruit in response to the increased myocardial oxygen demand

associated with exercise. Once the R2 vessels have maximally vasodilated, the autoregulatory reserve is expended and no further increase in flow is possible despite further increases in demand (Fig. 6-3).[15] In addition, since the R3 component of resistance to flow is greatest in the subendocardium, more of the R2 vasodilator reserve capacity is expended at rest to maintain subendocardial perfusion even in normal vessels. As a result, there is less vasodilator reserve in the subendocardium compared to the subepicardium, making the subendocardium particularly vulnerable to ischemia.

In the presence of R1 vessel stenosis, there is the additional potential for a myocardial steal, which can occur in two ways.[16] First, a normal vessel has the capacity to decrease its total resistance to flow substantially during exercise or pharmacologic vasodilation, while an artery with R1 vessel stenosis has less vasodilator reserve. The greater decrease in resistance to flow in the normal vessel will result in it receiving a proportionately greater percent of the coronary flow than the abnormal vessel, i.e., an intramyocardial steal from one vessel's distribution to another's. Second, because the vasodilator reserve is less in the subendocardium compared to the subepicardium, resulting from the greater R3 resistance in the subendocardium, there is also the potential for a steal within an individual vessel's territory, with increased flow to the subepicardium occurring at the expense of the subendocardium.

A final variable in the flow-versus-stenosis relationship is the consideration that coronary stenoses are not fixed but have a variable dynamic component resulting

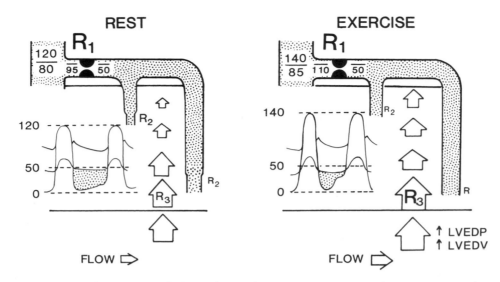

Figure 6-3 In the presence of atherosclerotic obstruction in an extramural coronary artery of up to 80 to 90 percent, resting flow is preserved through the coronary vasodilator reserve. To compensate for the increased R1 resistance, the R2 vessels vasodilate, so that the total resistance in the distribution of the obstructed vessel remains normal and resting flow is preserved. In response to exercise, however, the vessel has limited additional vasodilator reserve, since it has expended its reserve protecting flow at rest. Once the R2 vessels are maximally vasodilated, the system can do nothing more to increase flow. As myocardial oxygen demand increases, flow can not increase to meet the demand and ischemia results. (From Follansbee,[4] reproduced with permission.)

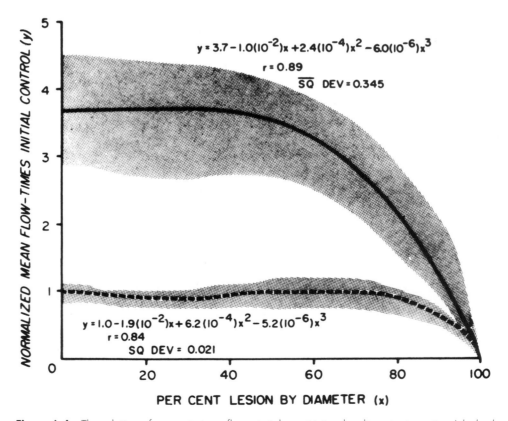

Figure 6-4 The relation of percent circumflex arterial constriction by diameter to resting (*dashed line*) and hyperemic (*solid line*) blood flow. (Reprinted by permission of the publisher from Physiologic basis for assessing critical coronary stenosis: Instantaneous flow response and regional distribution during coronary hyperemia as measures of coronary flow reserve, Gould et al, American Journal of Cardiology, Vol. 33, p. 87. Copyright 1974 by Excerpta Medica Inc.)

Table 6-1   Relationship of Percent Coronary Artery Stenosis to Coronary Artery Flow Under Various Conditions

	Normal *n*	50% Diameter Stenosis		80% Diameter Stenosis	
		n	% of Normal	*n*	% of Normal
Resting blood flow (ml/min/100 g)	80	80	100	80	100
Submaximal exercise					
Increase × resting level	1.5×	1.5×		1.2×	
Blood flow (ml/min/100 g)	120	120	100	96	80
Maximal exercise					
Increase × resting level	2.5×	2.0×		1.2×	
Blood flow (ml/min/100 g)	200	160	80	96	48
Maximum pharmacologic vasodilation					
Increase × resting level	4.0×	2.5×		1.5×	
Blood flow (ml/min/100 g)	320	200	62	120	38

from relative constriction or relaxation of the muscular vessel wall at the site of a stenosis[17,18] Indeed, it has been demonstrated that flow through a coronary vessel might actually decrease during exercise due to worsening of the stenosis severity, rather than increase and then plateau as would be predicted by the previously described paradigm.[19] While it has been postulated that these decreases may be a result of passive changes in stenosis severity as a result of changes in downstream distending pressure within the vessel,[20] this dynamic worsening of stenosis severity can be prevented by the preadministration of nitroglycerin.[21] This implies that the decrease in flow is not passive, but is a result of active exercise-induced coronary vasospasm at the site of the atherosclerotic plaque. The arterial endothelial cell plays a central role in the regulation of local vasomotor tone, and its function is modulated by endothelial cell injury. In the presence of atherosclerosis, stimuli that normally are vasodilating, including exercise, can become vasoconstricting.

Table 6-1 summarizes these concepts, illustrating the relative levels of flow that might be expected in a normal artery and in vessels with 50 percent and 80 percent stenoses, at rest, during submaximal exercise, with maximal exercise, and with pharmacologic coronary vasodilation.

MAXIMAL EXERCISE TESTING

As a reflection of this physiology, exercise has been widely used and extensively validated as a form of stress for the evaluation of patients with known or suspected coronary artery disease. It is used in conjunction with various diagnostic modalities to differentiate the normal from the ischemic response. Exercise electrocardiography primarily assesses the ST-segment response to exercise to identify the presence of ischemia. Ischemia adversely affects regional and typically also global left ventricular function. Exercise echocardiography and ex-

ercise radionuclide ventriculography both assess segmental and global left ventricular function to identify the ischemic response. Myocardial perfusion imaging with thallium-201 (^{201}Tl) chloride, ^{99m}Tc sestamibi, or ^{99m}Tc teboroxime is used to detect a heterogenous flow response to exercise as an indicator of coronary atherosclerotic disease. As such, perfusion imaging has a theoretical advantage over electrocardiographic or myocardial function techniques for detecting disease since these latter techniques require a sufficient limitation of flow relative to demand to cause actual ischemia, while the perfusion indicators only require a heterogenous flow response without necessarily requiring actual ischemia. The uptake of these tracers is flow dependent and relatively linear at lower levels of coronary flow.[22,23] However, only teboroxime maintains linear myocardial uptake relative to flow at high physiologically or pharmacologically induced levels of coronary blood flow, while the uptake of thallium and even more prominently sestamibi becomes nonlinear at higher flow rates.[22-25] While its uptake is linear to flow, teboroxime's washout is so rapid that, within 2 min of injection, thallium activity in the myocardium more accurately reflects flow than does teboroxime.[26] The ratio of maximum flow in the normal vessel relative to the stenotic vessel must be at least 2 to 1 before defects will be apparent with myocardial perfusion imaging using thallium.[10]

In diagnostic testing, it is important that patients be able to achieve a maximal level of myocardial oxygen demand and peak cardiac output. As is illustrated in Table 6-1, with submaximal levels of exercise, the coronary flow response might be completely normal in the presence of stenoses of 50 percent and only mildly reduced even with stenoses as great as 80 percent or more. The limitation in flow relative to peak demand might not be sufficient to cause ischemia or a detectable heterogeneity of flow at submaximal levels of exercise, resulting in either false-negative study results or a study that underestimates the severity of disease.[10]

The degree to which a submaximal peak heart rate achieved during exercise influences sensitivity in diagnostic testing has not yet been clearly established in the literature. With SPECT (single photon emission computed tomography) imaging, for example, Iskandrian and co-workers reported findings from studies of 272 patients whom they divided into two groups: those who had abnormal findings on the exercise electrocardiographic test and/or achieved more than 85 percent of predicted maximum heart rate, and those who achieved less than 85 percent and had a normal electrocardiographic response.[27] The group that achieved a high peak heart rate had a significantly higher frequency of myocardial ischemia detected by SPECT imaging [126 (77 percent) of 164 versus 55 (51 percent) of 108, $p = 0.0001$; overall sensitivity, 88 percent versus 73 percent, $p < 0.002$]. However, the study has an important potential bias since there was a strong correlation between an abnormal electrocardiographic response, which was used to define the groups, and abnormal findings on SPECT study. Supporting this finding, Nyers and co-workers noted a considerable decrease in the sensitivity of both exercise electrocardiography and exercise thallium scintigraphy in patients who were unable to reach a high target heart rate during exercise.[28] In contrast, Mahmarian and co-workers examined findings from 221 patients with coronary disease who had either abnormal or normal results on SPECT exercise study.[29] They noted minimal differences in the exercise parameters achieved by the two groups, which was consistent with findings from a previous study that investigated the effect of exercise level on the sensitivity of planar thallium imaging in asymptomatic patients with coronary artery disease.[30] Nevertheless, there is general agreement that it is desirable to exercise patients to maximal levels in diagnostic testing and, certainly at least in individual patients, a submaximal exercise performance could result in false-negative findings.[31]

Representative data reported from one large department estimated the frequency of a submaximal peak heart rate response to exercise to be approximately 25 percent.[32] This estimation did not include the large number of patients who were not exercised at all, but instead underwent pharmacologic stress testing because they were deemed unsuitable to exercise. There are myriad potential factors that could result in a submaximal exercise performance. Some patients are specifically limited in their ability to perform leg exercise. Included in this group are patients with claudication, degenerative joint disease in the hip or knee, peripheral neuropathy, or spinal cord injuries. In these patients, alternative forms of exercise might be used, sometimes in combination with pharmacologic stress. Other patients might be limited by other organ systems disease, including obstructive lung disease, liver or renal failure, altered levels of consciousness, or generalized debility. For these patients, exercise is not possible at all. Some patients are on medications that block the heart rate response to exercise,

particularly beta blockers, verapamil, or diltiazem. In many cases these medications can be withheld for an exercise test, but in other cases that is not advisable. Finally, patients with intrinsic conduction system disease can have an inadequate heart rate response to exercise. In each of these instances, alternative means of exercise or pharmacologic stress should be utilized.

Upright Leg Exercise

Aerobic or dynamic exercise using large muscle groups achieves the greatest physiologic increase in cardiac output and coronary blood flow. Repetitive alternating contraction of large muscle groups (flexors and extensors) increases total body oxygen consumption while decreasing resistance to perfusion of exercising muscle groups through locally mediated vasodilating mechanisms. Since nonexercising muscle groups vasoconstrict to maximize flow to exercising muscles, use of large muscle groups during exercise has the greatest effect of increasing cardiac output by decreasing resistance in the largest vascular beds. Moreover, exercise can typically be sustained for longer intervals by using large muscle groups. For these reasons, upright aerobic leg exercise is by far the most widely used form of exercise for diagnostic testing. Patients are most familiar and comfortable with this type of exercise and therefore are better able to perform it and sustain it for a sufficiently long period of time to permit meaningful evaluation. Upright exercise testing is most commonly done with graded progressive exercise regimens using treadmill exercise in the United States and upright bicycle exercise in Europe, with equivalent efficacy. Clinically, the *rate–pressure product*, the product of systolic arterial pressure times heart rate, is used as an indicator of the level of myocardial oxygen demand achieved.[33]

Alternative Forms of Exercise

Alternative forms of exercise that can be used instead of upright leg exercise include supine bicycle exercise, aerobic arm exercise, and isometric handgrip exercise.

SUPINE BICYCLE EXERCISE

Certain exercise testing procedures are not readily adaptable to upright exercise, primarily because of limitations of the equipment. For example, while first-pass radionuclide ventriculography can be readily performed during upright exercise, most departments lack multicrystal cameras that are best suited for optimal studies. Equilibrium exercise radionuclide ventriculography examinations using single-crystal Anger scintillation cameras, in contrast, are better suited to supine exercise because it is easier to limit patient motion during study acquisition. The same is true of exercise echocardiography, for similar reasons.

The primary difference between supine bicycle exercise and upright exercise is that venous return is increased in the supine position particularly with elevation of the legs. Left ventricular end-diastolic pressure is increased during supine exercise compared to upright exercise in normals[34] and in patients with coronary artery disease.[35,36] Left ventricular end-diastolic volume is increased both at rest and during exercise in the supine position in patients with coronary artery disease as measured by radionuclide ventriculography.[37-39] End-diastolic volume is also increased at rest in the supine position in normals, although the response during exercise is more variable.[37-39] An increase in end-diastolic volume during exercise in normals appears to occur only at maximal levels of exercise and represents recruitment of Frank–Starling effects.[40] Afterload is increased in supine exercise, both because preload is a determinant of afterload and because blood pressure is higher during supine exercise compared to upright exercise at comparable levels of exercise.[41-43] Wetherbee and colleagues, for example, noted that submaximal supine bicycle exercise resulted in a significantly higher systolic blood pressure and double product than did treadmill exercise.[42] As a result of the increased preload and afterload, myocardial oxygen demand is increased at comparable levels of exercise, heart rate, and double product with supine exercise compared to upright exercise. Reflecting this, cardiovascular stress has been shown to be greater with supine bicycle exercise than it is with upright treadmill exercise at comparable submaximal heart rates.[43]

Peak workloads achieved during exercise are greater during upright exercise than they are during supine exercise.[44] This is likely a manifestation of the mechanical disadvantage of elevating the legs during supine exercise, which leads to accelerated leg fatigue as well as the increased preload and afterload that are associated with supine exercise.[7,35,41,45]

As a manifestation of the increased preload and afterload associated with exercise in the supine position, supine exercise produces more myocardial ischemia at comparable heart rates and rate–pressure products than does upright exercise. Angina pectoris, for example, is produced at lower workloads during supine exercise than it is with upright exercise.[35,36,41,45] The magnitude of ST-segment depression is also greater during supine exercise compared to upright exercise.[36,41,42,45] Currie and coinvestigators noted in their study of 43 subjects with chest pain that the mean maximal ST-segment depression during supine exercise was 2.6 ± 0.2 mm compared to 1.3 ± 0.2 mm with upright exercise ($p < 0.001$), despite the higher workload achieved during upright exercise.[41]

Patients with an abnormal ST-segment response to exercise in the supine position can have a normal ST-segment response to exercise in the upright position.[41,42,46] The supine exercise electrocardiogram has been shown to be a good predictor of triple-vessel or left main coronary disease and of subsequent coronary events, to which the exercise radionuclide ventriculogram added very little.[47,48] This latter finding of the relative predictive power of the supine exercise electrocardiogram compared to the exercise radionuclide ventriculogram from a retrospective analysis requires confirmation in a follow-up prospective study of a different sample population before reliable conclusions can be drawn.

The relative hemodynamic responses of supine exercise compared to upright exercise for normals and patients with coronary artery disease are summarized in Table 6-2.

DYNAMIC ARM EXERCISE

Some patients who can not perform adequate levels of leg exercise to permit diagnostic evaluation can perform meaningful levels of aerobic arm exercise, typically using an arm ergometer.[49] Patients with spinal cord injuries, claudication, peripheral neuropathy, or arthritis involving the hips or knees, for example, may have sufficient mobility of their upper extremities to permit a meaningful evaluation. Because of the lesser muscle mass in the upper extremities and the typical deconditioning of the arms, particularly in the elderly or debilitated populations, fatigue is often a limiting factor in arm exercise performance. Older subjects as a group will reach a lower peak power output than younger subjects.[50] Blood pressure is much more difficult to measure during arm ergometry compared to leg exercise because the arms are involved in the exercise. In some patients with limited but still significant leg function, dynamic arm exercise can be done in conjunction with leg ergometry.[51]

As with upright bicycle exercise, which is non-weight-bearing, work rate with arm ergometry is independent of body weight.[52] Unlike leg ergometry, arm ergometry is not associated with an increase in ventilation or respiratory frequency with increased pedal cycling rate; with increased load, respiratory frequency actually declines, while total ventilation increases, reflecting an increase in tidal volume.[53]

The increase in cardiac output and total body oxygen consumption with arm ergometry is typically only about 60 to 70 percent of an individual's maximum as determined by dynamic leg exercise on a treadmill.[54] However, normal subjects exercising to the same rate–pressure product have the same levels of left ventricular wall stress and increase in contractility with arm exercise compared to leg exercise, despite the lower power output.[55] Arm ergometry is more physiologically stressful than leg er-

Table 6-2 Hemodynamic Responses of Various Forms of Exercise

Hemodynamic Parameter	Upright Dynamic Leg Exercise		Supine Dynamic Leg Exercise		Dynamic Arm Exercise		Isometric Handgrip Exercise	
	Normal	CAD	Normal	CAD	Normal	CAD	Normal	CAD
Heart rate	++++	+++	+++	++/+++	+++	++/+++	+/++	+/++
Systolic blood pressure	+++	++/+++	++++	++++	+++/++++	+++	+++	++/+++
Diastolic blood pressure	0/+	0/+	+	+	++	++	++	++
Rate–pressure product	++++	++/+++	++++	+++	+++/++++	+++	++/+++	++
LVEDV	0/+	+/++	+	++	0	+	0	+
LVEDP	0/+	++	++	+++	+	++	0	++
Cardiac output	++++	++/+++	+++/++++	++/+++	++/+++	++	+/++	+/++
Coronary blood flow	+++	++	+++	++	+++	+/++	+/++	+

CAD, coronary artery disease; LVEDV, left ventricular end-diastolic volume; LVEDP, left ventricular end-diastolic pressure.

gometry at the same level of total body oxygen consumption.[56] Peak heart rate tends to be somewhat lower with arm ergometry compared to treadmill exercise, but peak systolic blood pressure and double product are similar, provided patients have sufficient arm strength to perform a maximal test.[57] In some studies, however, the peak double products achieved during arm exercise have been lower than during leg exercise.[58,59] The heart rate increase relative to total body oxygen demand is greater during arm ergometry in women than in men.[50,55] As noted, the heart rate and blood pressure responses to arm ergometry are more variable than with treadmill exercise, reflecting the variable recruitment of accessory muscles in the chest, back, abdomen, buttocks, and legs for stabilization.[60]

Blood pressure increases linearly with oxygen uptake, but this relationship is steeper with arm exercise than with leg exercise.[61] During exercise, arterial beds in exercising muscle groups vasodilate to increase perfusion to exercising muscles, while there is vasoconstriction in the distribution of nonexercising muscles.[62,63] Because of the comparatively small muscle mass of the upper extremities compared to the lower extremities, total peripheral resistance decreases less with arm exercise than with leg exercise. While there is less increase in cardiac output with arm exercise compared to dynamic leg exercise, mean arterial pressure increases more, reflecting the lesser decrease in peripheral vascular resistance related to the smaller exercising muscle mass.[63] Diastolic blood pressure also tends to be higher with arm exercise, again reflecting the higher peripheral vascular resistance. The lesser increase in cardiac output during arm exercise is a manifestation of a lesser augmentation of stroke volume due to the lesser increase in venous return associated with the smaller exercising muscle mass.[63] The increase in cardiac output, therefore, is substantially dependent on the steep slope of the heart rate response to exercise.

Exercise electrocardiography is less sensitive in the detection of coronary artery disease with arm ergometry than with treadmill testing.[64] Despite the fact that the indices of myocardial oxygen demand, including the peak double product, are similar during arm exercise compared to leg exercise, there is less ischemia, for reasons that are not yet well understood.[55,64] The higher diastolic blood pressure during arm exercise may be responsible, at least in part, by augmenting diastolic coronary perfusion pressure and therefore coronary blood flow at any given level of myocardial oxygen demand.[63] In some studies, the lesser incidence of ischemia during arm exercise has been related to a lower peak double product achieved.[59] Thallium scintigraphy in conjunction with exercise electrocardiography appears to enhance the diagnostic sensitivity of arm ergometry.[65] Thallium scintigraphy was found to have a sensitivity of 83 percent and a specificity of 78 percent in a study of 50 subjects by Balady and co-workers, compared to a sensitivity of 54 percent ($p < 0.01$) and a specificity of 67 percent (p = not significant, NS) for exercise electrocardiography.[65] The study sample in this report was characterized by symptomatically advanced disease with class III or IV angina in 44 percent and prior myocardial infarction in 42 percent, and 98 percent were on cardiac medications (62 percent on beta blockers and 60 percent on calcium channel blockers). It is likely that the sensitivity of arm exercise thallium scintigraphy would be less in a population with less severe disease. While there is limited experience, one small study has suggested that arm exercise thallium scintigraphy has similar sensitivity and specificity for detection of coronary artery disease as does dipyridamole thallium scintigraphy.[66] While experience is again limited and more studies are necessary, arm exercise ergometry has also been found to have prognostic utility in predicting subsequent coronary events in subjects with peripheral vascular disease and claudication.[58]

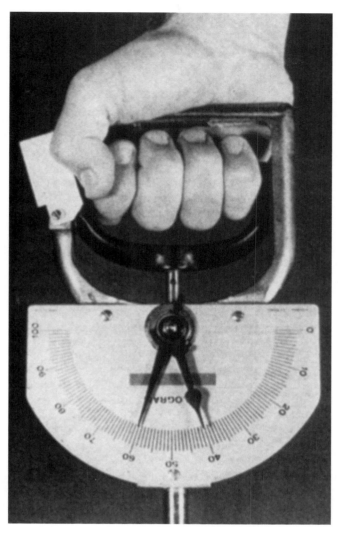

Figure 6-5 A handgrip dynamometer used to perform an isometric handgrip exercise test. Maximum contraction can be measured, after which the patient is asked to perform a sustained contraction at some fraction of their individual maximum. (From Siegel et al,[68] reproduced with permission.)

ISOMETRIC HANDGRIP EXERCISE

Isometric exercise, typically in the form of sustained handgrip stress (although occasionally with more intense upper body exertion[67]), has been investigated as a stress modality for the evaluation of patients with coronary artery disease. Its greatest potential applicability is in similar patient populations who can not perform dynamic leg exercise as was described above with dynamic arm exercise. Isometric handgrip exercise can be standardized and has an advantage in that it is easy to administer and is safe, but it is heavily dependent on patient effort. It is best performed using a hand dynamometer[68] (Fig. 6-5). The subject is asked to perform a maximal squeeze, from which his or her individual maximal forearm compression strength is determined. The individual

is then asked to perform a sustained handgrip maneuver, typically at approximately one-third of his or her maximum level for a period of 3 to 4 min.[69-71] Some studies have used a more intense compression, in the range of 75 to 100 percent of maximum, for 30 to 60 s.[68,72,73] It is important that subjects not perform a Valsalva maneuver during the compression. Handgrip stress has usually been used as an isolated maneuver, but it can also be used in combination with dynamic exercise.[74,75]

The heart rate, blood pressure, and electrocardiographic response to handgrip stress can be readily measured. Handgrip can also be performed in conjunction with radionuclide ventriculography,[69-71,76] echocardiography,[67,77,78] or cardiac catheterization[72,79-83] for more extensive physiologic assessment of the response.

Isometric handgrip exercise differs in many important aspects from aerobic or dynamic exercise (Table 6-2). Isometric exercise is characterized by sustained, tonic muscle contraction. As a result of the sustained muscle contraction, arterial inflow into the exercising muscle is limited, primarily due to compression of the small arteries. Peak heart rate increases approximately 20 to 30 percent during performance of sustained handgrip, an increase that is considerably less than that which occurs with dynamic exercise.[68,72,75,81] Systolic blood pressure increases to a comparable degree as in dynamic exercise, but, in contrast to dynamic exercise, diastolic blood pressure also increases with handgrip.[68,81] This is a reflection of vasoconstriction with isometric exercise, as opposed to the more predominant vasodilation that is associated with dynamic exercise. Mean blood pressure increases more with handgrip exercise than with dynamic exercise, reflecting the increased diastolic pressure. Since peak systolic blood pressure is similar comparing the two modalities but peak heart rate is lower with handgrip, the peak double product and therefore myocardial oxygen demand are also lower with handgrip compared to dynamic exercise. Peak coronary blood flow increases approximately 20 to 45 percent with handgrip at 25 percent of maximum and approximately 70 percent with near maximal handgrip stress.[72,80,83] This increase in coronary blood flow with handgrip is substantially less than that achieved with maximal treadmill exercise.[83]

Cardiac output increases with handgrip exercise, but again the increase is not comparable to that which occurs with dynamic exercise. Laird and coinvestigators, for example, noted that cardiac index increased only 22 percent in healthy adolescents during handgrip.[77] Systemic venous return is less than with dynamic exercise, due to less skeletal muscle pumping of the peripheral venous system and, unless specifically avoided, performance of Valsalva maneuver during isometric exertion. End-diastolic volume and ejection fraction change very little with handgrip in normals.[70,77] The increase in cardiac output, therefore, is primarily mediated through increased heart rate and is modest in degree, reflecting the limited heart rate increment.[70,77] As a group, there is no change in mean ejection fraction in normals in response to handgrip, but individual normals may show a decline of ejection fraction of 5 or more ejection-fraction units.[70,71,77] The decrease in ejection fraction in individual normals may be a reflection of increased afterload or may be due to increased coronary vascular tone.[71,84]

The ejection-fraction and left ventricular end-diastolic pressure (LVEDP) response to handgrip stress is also variable among patients with coronary artery disease.[85] In a hemodynamic study of 72 patients, Fisher and colleagues noted that coronary disease patients with preserved left ventricular function had no significant change in LVEDP with handgrip, whereas LVEDP increased in patients with abnormal left ventricular function.[72] This is consistent with earlier findings described by Kivowitz et al.[80] Helfant and colleagues noted that LVEDP increased more in coronary artery disease patients compared to controls during handgrip.[79] There was no increase in cardiac index and a fall in stroke index in the coronary artery disease patients, whereas cardiac index increased in their normal subjects. Ludbrook and co-workers noted that both LVEDP and right ventricular end-diastolic pressure increase with handgrip while there is no measurable change in left ventricular end-diastolic volume (LVEDV).[82] In their study of 25 patients, left ventricular ejection fraction decreased a mean of 13 percent, but the response was quite variable; in 14 of the 25 subjects, there was no change in ejection fraction. Multiple indices of diastolic function that were measured were all unchanged. The authors hypothesized that the increase in LVEDP was a reflection of increased right ventricular end-diastolic volume and resulting pericardial constraint. This study used a comparatively lower level of handgrip stress (20 percent of maximum), which could have influenced the findings compared to higher levels of stress. Five of their patients, for example, had no increase in blood pressure at all.

Handgrip exercise produces less myocardial ischemia in patients with coronary artery disease than does dynamic leg exercise. This is primarily a manifestation of the lower peak double product achieved with handgrip. In addition, however, the increased diastolic blood pressure associated with handgrip increases coronary perfusion pressure relative to myocardial oxygen demand. Furthermore, because peak heart rate is lower, the diastolic interval is also relatively preserved during handgrip, allowing greater time for coronary perfusion, thereby enhancing myocardial oxygen supply. It is not surprising, therefore, that manifestations of ischemia are less frequent with handgrip exercise than they are with dynamic exercise. Lowe et al noted that only six of 23 patients with greater than 75 percent coronary stenosis had angina with handgrip.[81] Interestingly, all six had a decrease in coronary blood flow with handgrip, whereas none of those without angina decreased coronary flow. Kerber and colleagues found that only three of 90 subjects with coronary artery disease had ST-segment depression during handgrip exercise as opposed to 25 during treadmill exercise.[74] Bodenheimer and co-investigators found that assessment of regional wall motion and regional ejection fraction by radionuclide ventriculography during handgrip stress was associated with a sensitivity of 86 percent and a specificity of 87 percent for detection of coronary artery disease (duplicate report).[69,76] In contrast, Peter and Jones noted the sensitivity of regional wall-motion abnormalities with handgrip radionuclide ventriculographic examination to be only 45 percent.[70] Interestingly, DeBusk and co-workers noted in a study of 30 men that the combination of handgrip exercise with treadmill exercise increases the heart rate and rate–pressure product at the onset of angina or ST-segment depression, and decreases the overall prevalence of angina, compared to dynamic exercise alone.[75] None of their patients had ischemic findings with static exercise alone. This finding was consistent with earlier reports.[73,74] This upward shift of the ischemic threshold by adding static exercise to dynamic exercise appears to be a manifestation of the increased diastolic perfusion pressure associated with isometric stress, with resulting increased coronary blood flow relative to demand.[74,75]

Overall, patients with impaired inotropic reserve are likely to experience an increase in LVEDP and LVEDV, and a decrease in LVEF and left ventricular stroke work in the increased afterload condition associated with sustained handgrip.[80,85] There is general agreement, however, that the prevalence of ischemic responses to handgrip stress is considerably less than with maximal dynamic exercise, and that dynamic exercise is the preferred diagnostic stress modality.[70,73,75] The ejection-fraction response to handgrip is variable and is not a reliable parameter for separating normals from patients with coronary artery disease.[70,86,87] The ejection-fraction response to bicycle exercise as measured by radionuclide ventriculography, in contrast, is considerably more sensitive and specific in detecting coronary artery disease than is the ejection-fraction response to handgrip stress.[70,86,87] Handgrip can be used as an alternative to dynamic exercise in patients or testing conditions in which dynamic exercise is not possible, accepting that there will be some compromise in the sensitivity and specificity that can be expected.

Simulated Exercise

For patients who can not exercise, there are alternative methods to simulate to varying degrees the effects of exercise on the heart, and these methods can be used

Table 6-3   Hemodynamic Responses of Various Forms of Simulated Exercise Compared to Upright Dynamic Leg Exercise

Hemodynamic Parameter	Upright Dynamic Leg Exercise		Atrial Pacing		Cold Pressor		Dobutamine	
	Normal	CAD	Normal	CAD	Normal	CAD	Normal	CAD
Heart rate	++++	+++	++++	++++	+	+	+++/++++	+++/++++
Systolic blood pressure	+++	++/+++	0	0	++	++	++/+++	++/+++
Diastolic blood pressure	0/+	0/+	0	0	+/++	+/++	−/−−	−/−−
Rate–pressure product	++++	++/+++	++	++	+/++	+/++	++/+++	++/+++
LVEDV	0/+	+/++	0	0	0	0/+	0	0/+
LVEDP	0/+	++	−/0	0/++	0	0/+	0	0/+
Cardiac output	++++	++/+++	0	−/0	0	0	++/+++	++/+++
Ejection fraction	+/++	−/−−	0	−/0	+/−	0/−	+/++	+/−
Coronary blood flow	+++	++	+	0/+	+	−	+++	+/++

CAD, coronary artery disease; LVEDV, left ventricular end-diastolic volume; LVEDP, left ventricular end-diastolic pressure.

in conjunction with diagnostic testing. These include electronic atrial pacing, cold pressor provocation, and dobutamine pharmacologic stress.

ELECTRONIC ATRIAL PACING

Heart rate is an important determinant of myocardial oxygen demand and, therefore, of coronary blood flow. Atrial pacing was first used by Sowton et al in 1967 as a potential stress method for detection of coronary artery disease.[88] Atrial pacing not only increases heart rate, but also is an inotropic stimulus.[89] Atrial pacing, via either a right atrial pacing catheter or an esophageal electrode, has been used in conjunction with electrocardiography,[90–92] cardiac catheterization including contrast ventriculography and hemodynamic assessment,[93–96] radionuclide ventriculography,[97–100] myocardial perfusion scintigraphy,[96,101–105] and echocardiography[106–108] as a means of stressing patients with known or suspected coronary artery disease. The experience with atrial pacing has been previously well summarized by Stratmann and Kennedy.[109] Pacing is typically performed beginning at a heart rate of 80 to 100 beats/min and is increased at increments of 10 to 20 beats every 1 to 3 min, to peak rates of 140 to 180 beats/min or until the development of chest pain or marked ST-segment depression. Administration of intravenous atropine (0.5 to 1.5 mg) can be used to facilitate atrioventricular nodal conduction and allow achievement of higher heart rates in patients who develop atrioventricular nodal block.

The hemodynamic responses are quite different comparing atrial pacing to exercise at the same heart rate (Table 6-3). Blood pressure typically does not increase with pacing or increases to a lesser degree than during exercise.[93,96,105,106] Systemic vascular resistance can increase during atrial pacing in patients with coronary artery disease.[98] Nevertheless, both the double product

and afterload are typically lower at a given heart rate during atrial pacing than during exercise. In patients who can achieve only a submaximal peak heart rate during exercise, the peak double product achieved during atrial pacing may be comparable.[104,106] Myocardial oxygen demand is substantially lower during pacing than during exercise at equivalent heart rates. Preload is also less during atrial pacing because the increase in LVEDV that can occur with some forms of exercise does not occur during pacing. LVEDP decreases or remains unchanged in normals during atrial pacing.[93,94,96] The response in patients with coronary artery disease is variable, depending on whether they develop ischemia.[93] During pacing-induced ischemia, both LVEDP and pulmonary capillary wedge pressure increase.[93,94,96,98] Pacing-induced hemodynamic changes in patients with coronary artery disease have been found to correlate with the extent of thallium perfusion defects.[96] Normal subjects have no significant increase in cardiac output during atrial pacing and either no significant change or an increase in left ventricular ejection fraction.[93,94,100] Left ventricular stroke work and stroke volume both decrease during atrial pacing.[93] In contrast, in patients with coronary artery disease, both cardiac index and left ventricular ejection fraction may decrease during atrial pacing.[94,97–100] These changes are frequently accompanied by regional wall-motion abnormalities.[95,97–100]

While it might be hypothesized that the lower levels of myocardial oxygen demand achieved during atrial pacing would result in lower diagnostic sensitivity for detection of coronary artery disease, the reported experience has been somewhat mixed. The sensitivity and specificity of pacing electrocardiography for detection of coronary artery disease have varied widely (20 to 100 percent and 40 to 100 percent, respectively), but have been generally comparable to exercise electrocardiography (Table 6-4).[90–94,102,106,110–113] However, many of these

Table 6-4 Sensitivity and Specificity of Atrial Pacing Electrocardiography in Comparison to Exercise Electrocardiography

	Atrial Pacing		Exercise Testing	
Reference	Sensitivity	Specificity	Sensitivity	Specificity
Lau et al, 1968[110]	78 (28/36)	100 (27–27)	74 (25/34)	100 (27/27)
Brooks and Cuforth, 1971[111]	100 (15/15)	100 (10/10)	67 (7/11)	100 (10/10)
Keleman et al, 1973[90]	74 (36/49)	40 (10/25)	54 (26/48)	96 (23/24)
Linhart, 1972[93]	58 (18/31)	100 (10/10)		
Linhart, 1972[112]	57 (33/58)	100 (10/10)		
Piessens et al, 1974[113]	73 (29/40)	70 (21/30)	60 (24/40)	90 (27/30)
Rios and Hurvitz, 1974[91]	20 (6/29)	95 (20/21)	83 (24/29)	90 (19/21)
Manca et al, 1979[92]	75 (42/75)	64 (22/34)	64 (36/56)	88 (30/34)
Markham et al, 1983[94]	56 (10/18)	80 (8/10)		
Heller et al, 1984[102]	94 (15/16)	83 (5/6)	63 (10/16)	83 (5/6)
Matthews et al, 1989[107]	57 (8/14)	75 (6/8)	64 (9/14)	38 (3/8)
Totals	66 (240/362)	78 (149/191)	65 (161/248)	90 (144/160)

studies have included patients who could not exercise maximally or were on medications that suppressed their heart rate response to exercise, likely biasing the findings against exercise electrocardiography. Based on the physiologic responses to atrial pacing compared to exercise, it is likely that the sensitivity for detection of coronary artery disease is not equivalent to exercise electrocardiography in patients who can exercise maximally. The specificity of atrial pacing also appears to be somewhat less than that of exercise electrocardiography.

Atrial pacing has been used in conjunction with myocardial perfusion scintigraphy. Weiss and co-workers used planar thallium scintigraphy to evaluate 41 patients, 31 of whom had angiographic coronary artery disease (greater than 50 percent narrowing).[100] Thallium scintigraphy had a sensitivity in detection of coronary disease of 94 percent, although two-thirds of the subjects had prior myocardial infarction. Only 52 percent had pacing-induced perfusion abnormalities. Scintigraphy detected 91 percent of patients with right coronary artery disease and 85 percent with left anterior descending disease, but only 33 percent with circumflex coronary disease. Thallium imaging detected only 40 percent of arteries with 50 to 89 percent narrowing, while it detected 75 percent of vessels with 90 to 99 percent obstruction and 88 percent of totally occluded vessels. Heller and colleagues found that the results of exercise thallium scintigraphy were abnormal in 13 (81 percent) of their 16 patients with coronary artery disease, while the results of pacing scintigraphy were abnormal in 15 (94 percent).[102] There was good correlation of perfusion findings comparing individual segments between the two stress modalities. McKay et al found that pacing thallium scintigraphy had a sensitivity of 85 percent and a specificity of 60 percent in their study of 25 subjects.[96] LeFeuvre and coinvestigators performed exercise thallium scintigraphy

in 16 patients with coronary artery disease and no myocardial infarction, in 19 with previous myocardial infarction, and in 14 normals.[104] In patients without infarction, the sensitivity of exercise scintigraphy was 62 percent while it was 87 percent with atrial pacing. In patients with prior infarction, ischemia was detected in 53 percent with exercise and 58 percent with pacing. The specificities were 71 percent and 78 percent, respectively. Since only submaximal exercise was performed, it is likely that the relative sensitivity of exercise scintigraphy might have been underestimated. Nevertheless, these studies indicate that, in patients who can not exercise adequately, pacing thallium scintigraphy appears to be a very suitable alternative.

While little data are yet available, pacing thallium scintigraphy has also been found to have prognostic power in identifying patients at risk of subsequent cardiac events. Stratmann and coinvestigators noted in a study of 210 patients with chest pain that pacing-induced thallium perfusion defects, in particular, identified patients at risk of subsequent cardiac events, including unstable angina, myocardial infarction, and cardiac death.[103]

Atrial pacing stress has also been used in conjunction with radionuclide ventriculography, echocardiography, and contrast ventriculography to examine the left ventricular global and regional functional response to stress and to assess its potential diagnostic value. Johnson and co-workers found that, using atrial pacing in combination with intravenous digital contrast ventriculography, 38 (86 percent) of 44 patients with coronary artery disease but without resting wall-motion abnormalities had new wall-motion abnormalities induced by pacing.[95] One of 17 normals had a resting wall-motion abnormality and none had pacing-induced abnormalities. Stone and coinvestigators compared the findings of pacing contrast ventriculography and radionuclide ventriculography in a study of 13 patients with coronary artery disease.[97] Ejection fraction decreased with pacing, and there was good correlation between the two techniques. The radionuclide study detected all anterior (six) and inferior (four) wall-motion abnormalities detected by contrast ventriculography, although it detected only one of three apical abnormalities. The wall-motion assessment by the nuclear technique correlated well with coronary angiography. Several studies have demonstrated that pacing radionuclide ventriculography has good sensitivity for detection of disease in populations with advanced disease and a high prevalence of resting wall-motion abnormalities.[98,100] More recently, Marangelli and coinvestigators used exercise echocardiography to evaluate 104 consecutive patients undergoing coronary angiography who had no prior myocardial infarction or resting wall-motion abnormalities.[108] Adequate studies were achieved in only 80. Of these 80 patients, 60 (35 with coronary artery disease) underwent successful esophageal pacing echocardiography and dipyridamole echocardiography. Pacing echocardiography had a sensitivity of 83 percent and a specificity of 76 percent in these 60 patients, a finding that was similar to that of the previous study by Iliceto and co-workers.[106]

Cuocolo and colleagues examined the use of atrial pacing scintigraphy with ^{99m}Tc sestamibi, looking at both myocardial perfusion and first-pass left ventricular ejection fraction, compared to exercise scintigraphy in a small study of 10 patients with coronary artery disease.[105] They noted that ejection fraction decreased from 49 percent to 43 percent with pacing and to 42 percent with exercise, and there was good agreement in segmental perfusion analysis comparing the two stress modalities.

Overall, the addition of myocardial perfusion imaging or assessment of global and regional myocardial function appears to add useful diagnostic information in patients undergoing atrial pacing stress evaluation.

COLD PRESSOR STIMULUS

Cold pressor challenge is most commonly performed by immersion of the hand and wrist into ice water (temperature 1° to 4° C) for 1 to 6 min. Alternative approaches have used cold wraps around the neck or applied to the forehead. Cold is a vasoconstricting stimulus, mediated by alpha-adrenergic activation.[114] Heart rate increases only minimally during cold pressor, but both systolic pressure and diastolic blood pressure increase significantly.[115-117] As a result, double product and myocardial oxygen demand increase.[116,117] However, the magnitude of the increase is substantially less than that associated with exercise.[71,117] In normals, there is reflex vasodilation of the coronary resistance vessels during cold pressor that keeps total coronary resistance similar to basal levels, producing an increase in coronary blood flow mediated

by the increase in diastolic perfusion pressure to meet the increased myocardial oxygen demand.[118] In a study using xenon-133 flow measurements in patients on beta-blocker therapy, Malacoff and co-workers noted that normal coronary arteries increase flow by approximately 11 percent during cold pressor stimulation.[114] In contrast, in arteries with stenoses, xenon blood flow was either unchanged or decreased in 14 of 19 vessels. The average decrease in flow was 14 percent. This finding of an absence of an increase or an actual decrease in flow through stenotic coronary arteries in response to cold pressor is consistent with other reports, which have also demonstrated that while cold produces dilation in normal epicardial coronary vessels, it produces vasoconstriction in diseased coronary vessels.[115,118-121] In susceptible individuals, particularly those with a history of variant angina, cold pressor stimulus has the potential to produce frank coronary vasospasm and has been reported in rare cases to cause myocardial infarction.[119,121] Patients with coronary artery disease appear to have an exaggerated systemic blood pressure response to cold pressor compared to normals, which may further predispose them to ischemia.[120]

Cold pressor challenge has been used in conjunction with radionuclide ventriculography,[71,117,121-129] echocardiography,[130] or thallium perfusion imaging[116] to assess its diagnostic utility in the identification and stratification of coronary artery disease. Early studies suggested that the left ventricular ejection fraction response to cold pressor provocation had discriminating value for diagnosis of coronary artery disease. Wainwright and co-workers noted in their study of 50 subjects that ejection fraction increased in all of the normals ($n = 22$), while 19 of 24 abnormals decreased their ejection fraction by more than 8 percent.[122] Cold pressor radionuclide ventriculography was found to be significantly more sensitive than electrocardiography in detecting the presence of coronary artery disease. Verani and colleagues noted in their study of 52 patients (18 normals) that ejection fraction fell significantly in patients with coronary artery disease but did not change in normals during cold pressor, and 79 percent of coronary artery disease patients developed new or worsening wall-motion abnormalities.[126] However, a high percentage of their coronary artery disease patients (21 of 34) had resting wall-motion abnormalities that would bias the findings toward increased sensitivity. Manyari and Kostuk noted that only one of 22 normals decreased their ejection fraction with cold pressor while 11 of 20 coronary artery disease patients decreased their ejection fraction by more than 7 percent, and 12 of 20 developed new wall-motion abnormalities.[39] They found the sensitivity of the ejection-fraction response to be 55 percent, which increased to 70 percent if regional wall-motion analysis was included.

In contrast, multiple subsequent studies reported that

the sensitivity and specificity of cold pressor radionuclide ventriculography were poor, and that the study had little value as a diagnostic tool for coronary artery disease. Wynne and co-workers noted in a study of 20 subjects that the sensitivity of cold pressor radionuclide ventriculography was only 33 percent and the specificity 80 percent.[123] Giles and colleagues noted that nine of 11 normals decreased their ejection fraction with cold pressor, as did 23 of 25 coronary artery disease patients.[125] Wasserman et al found that the mean decrease in ejection fraction among 12 normals subjected to a cold pressor challenge was 5.8 units while it was 5.0 units in 18 patients with coronary artery disease.[127] Jordan and coinvestigators found that ejection fraction dropped in 12 of 20 normals, and that the study had either poor sensitivity or poor specificity for detecting coronary artery disease, depending on the criteria used to define abnormality.[117] Northcote and Cooke noted that ejection fraction decreased from 61 percent to 51 percent in their coronary artery disease patients and from 60 percent to 54 percent in their normals.[129] Multiple studies have demonstrated that exercise radionuclide ventriculography has superior sensitivity and specificity for detection of coronary artery disease compared to cold pressor stress.[39,71,117,126,129]

The variability in findings among the different studies is in part a reflection of the differences in the time course of the cold pressor stimulus and image acquisition, the variability in criteria used to define an abnormal test, and variation in the population samples tested, particularly with regard to the severity of disease and prevalence of resting wall-motion abnormalities. Ejection fraction tends to drop early in the course of cold pressor challenge in healthy individuals and then recover, while it tends to remain depressed longer in patients with coronary artery disease.[71,128] The timing of image acquisition, therefore, will significantly affect specificity. Nevertheless, the weight of the evidence currently available would indicate that cold pressor radionuclide ventriculography lacks sufficient discriminating power to be a useful modality for detection of coronary artery disease.

Cold pressor thallium perfusion scintigraphy may have better diagnostic utility, based on findings of a study by Ahmad and co-workers.[116] The sensitivity of thallium scintigraphy in their study of 36 patients was 77 percent and the specificity was 100 percent. The sensitivity for detection of single-vessel disease was 40 percent, for double-vessel disease was 91 percent, and for triple-vessel disease was 100 percent. These results need to be confirmed by additional studies.

DOBUTAMINE STRESS

Dobutamine hydrochloride is a synthetic catecholamine that has an onset of action of 1 to 2 min after intravenous administration, but requires 5 to 10 min to achieve peak

effect. Its plasma half-life is 2 min, and it is hepatically metabolized both by conjugation and by methylation of the catechol group through the action of the hepatic enzyme catechol-o-methyltransferase.[131] Initially, dobutamine was believed to act primarily on the β_1 receptors, with only secondary effects on the β_2 receptors and the α_1 receptors.[132] Subsequent studies, however, demonstrated that dobutamine has relatively balanced effects on all three receptors.[133] The levo isomer of dobutamine primarily activates the α_1 receptor while the equally prevalent dextro isomer activates both the β_1 and β_2 receptors.

At low to moderate doses (5 to 20 μg/kg/min), dobutamine increases heart rate only modestly, but stroke volume, cardiac output, and inotropy increase substantially.[134,135] Peripheral vascular resistance changes comparatively little due to balanced vasoconstricting effects of direct α_1 stimulation and vasodilating effects of β_2 activation, as well as withdrawal of intrinsic sympathetic tone resulting from the augmentation in stroke volume and cardiac output.[136] Systolic blood pressure increases while diastolic blood pressure decreases; mean arterial pressure, as a result, changes comparatively little.[137] In response to dobutamine, coronary blood flow increases substantially in patients without coronary artery disease.[134] In open-chest dogs, dobutamine at a dose of 10 μg/kg/min increased coronary blood flow 138 percent and increased heart rate 122 percent.[131,138] The increase in coronary blood flow is due both to direct effects of β_2 receptor activation as well as to indirect effects of increasing myocardial oxygen demand with resulting increases in coronary blood flow mediated through the normal autoregulatory mechanisms. At higher doses, do-

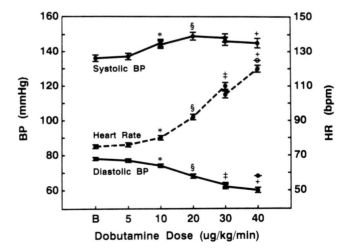

Figure 6-6 The hemodynamic effects of dobutamine at incremental doses up to 40 μg/kg/min. Heart rate increases incrementally at every dose. Systolic blood pressure did not increase after the 20-μg/kg/min dose. Diastolic blood pressure decreased at every dose beyond 5 μg/kg/min. (From Hays et al,[139] *J Am Coll Cardiol* 21:1583, 1993, reproduced with permission of the American College of Cardiology.)

Table 6-5 Side Effects of the Pharmacologic Stress Agents, n (%)

Side Effect	Dobutamine[139] (n = 144)	Dipyridamole[258] (n = 3911)	Adenosine[201] (n = 607)
Chest pain	44 (31)	770 (20)	205 (34)
Headache	20 (14)	476 (12)	125 (21)
Dizziness	5 (4)	460 (12)	40 (7)
Nausea	13 (9)	180 (5)	31 (5)
Hypotension	0	179 (5)	15 (3)
Flushing	20 (14)	132 (3)	211 (35)
Palpitations	42 (30)	127 (3)	
Dyspnea	20 (14)	100 (3)	114 (19)
Paresthesias	18 (12)	49 (1)	
ST changes	72 (50)	292 (8)	76 (13)
Major complication	0	10 (0.3)	1 (0.2)
Fatal MI	0	2 (0.1)	0
Nonfatal MI	0	2 (0.1)	0
Bronchospasm	0	6 (0.2)	1 (0.2)
Total side effects	108 (75)	1830 (47)	481 (80)

MI, myocardial infarction.
Adapted from Mahmarian and Verani,[152] with permission.

butamine further increases heart rate and systolic blood pressure. Hays and coinvestigators noted a dose-dependent increase in systolic blood pressure with doses up to 20 μg/kg/min, while heart rate steadily increased with doses up to the maximum utilized dose of 40 μg/kg/min (Fig. 6-6).[139] Diastolic blood pressure steadily decreased with doses beyond 5 μg/kg/min.

In the distribution of normal coronary arteries, dobutamine increases coronary perfusion evenly to the endocardial and epicardial layers.[140] Predictably, the presence of coronary artery disease blunts the flow response to dobutamine in affected vessels.[134,140,141] Distal coronary vascular resistance decreases with dobutamine infusion while there is an increase in resistance at the site of vascular stenoses, probably due to direct vasoconstricting effects mediated by the abnormal endothelium.[142] Flow may increase in vessels with moderate stenoses in response to dobutamine, although there may be heterogeneity of flow with the primary increase being to the subepicardium with no increase in flow to the subendocardium.[134,140–142] In vessels with severe stenoses, there is no increase in flow at all during dobutamine challenge.[143] The magnitude of increment in heart rate achieved with dobutamine infusion appears to be a defining variable in determining the degree of maldistribution of coronary flow that occurs and the magnitude of the resulting ischemia.[141,143] Implicitly, therefore, achieving a high peak heart rate would be an important variable determining sensitivity of dobutamine stress testing. Overall, however, the heterogeneity of flow that occurs with dobutamine infusion at doses of up to 20 μg/kg/min is less than that which occurs with either adenosine or dipyridamole.[140,144,145]

Side effects with dobutamine infusion are frequent but are generally well tolerated (Table 6-5). Hays and colleagues described side effects in 75 percent of their patients during dobutamine infusion, but only 26 percent could not complete the infusion at the maximum dose of 40 μg/kg/min due to side effects.[139] The most frequent side effects are chest pain; palpitations; headache; flushing; arm, back, or shoulder pain; paresthesias; and nausea.[139] Somewhat in contrast to this, Pennell and coworkers found that only 33 percent of their patients could tolerate a maximum dose of 20 μg/kg/min, with chest pain being the limiting symptom in 78 percent.[146] Mertes and colleagues reported no instances of death, myocardial infarction, or sustained ventricular tachycardia in 1118 patients who underwent dobutamine echocardiography.[147] The primary reason for stopping the test in their subjects was achievement of the target heart rate in 52 percent, achievement of the maximal dose in 23 percent, and angina in 13 percent. Only 3 percent were stopped for noncardiac side effects. Hypersensitivity reactions such as fever, eosinophilia, and bronchospasm have been reported, including anaphylactic or severe bronchospastic reactions to the sodium bisulfite in the preparation.[131] These reactions, however, appear to be rare. ST-segment elevation suggesting severe ischemia has been described with dobutamine infusion in the context of severe coronary obstruction.[148] The half-life of the drug is 2 min, so most side effects resolve within 5 to 10 min after the infusion is stopped. Hypotension can occur in response to dobutamine infusion, but, unlike hypotension associated with exercise, is not related to disease severity and is not associated with worse prognosis.[149,150] Abrupt hypotension can occur and appears to be due to a vasovagal reaction.[149]

Relative contraindications to dobutamine infusion

Table 6-6   Sensitivity and Specificity of Dobutamine Myocardial Perfusion Imaging

Reference	Agent	n	Modality	Sensitivity (%)	Specificity (%)
Mason et al, 1984[156]	^{201}Tl	24	Planar	94	87
Pennell et al, 1991[146]	^{201}Tl	50	SPECT	97	80
Hays et al, 1993[139]	^{201}Tl	144	SPECT	86	90
Pennell et al, 1993[151]	^{201}Tl	30	SPECT	91	79
Warner et al, 1993[157]	^{201}Tl	16	SPECT	93	88
Forster et al, 1993[167]	^{99m}Tc sestamibi	21	SPECT	83	89
Marwick et al, 1993[166]	^{99m}Tc sestamibi	97	SPECT	80	74
Marwick et al, 1993[165]	^{99m}Tc sestamibi	217	SPECT	76	67
Günalp et al, 1993[164]	^{99m}Tc sestamibi	27	SPECT	94	88
Marwick et al, 1994[162]	^{99m}Tc sestamibi	82	SPECT	65	68
Voth et al, 1994[161]	^{99m}Tc sestamibi	35	SPECT	88	—

^{99m}Tc sestamibi, technetium-99m hexakis-2-methoxyisobutyl isonitrile; ^{201}Tl, thallium 201; SPECT, single photon emission computed tomography.

include recent myocardial infarction or unstable angina, hemodynamically significant left ventricular outflow tract obstruction, uncontrolled atrial tachyarrhythmias, ventricular tachycardia, uncontrolled hypertension, aortic dissections, or large aortic aneurysms. Dobutamine can be used safely in patients with asthma.[151]

Dobutamine electrocardiography has high specificity but low sensitivity for detection of coronary artery disease. While the range of sensitivity of dobutamine electrocardiography is wide, overall approximately 35 percent of patients with coronary artery disease will have ST-segment depression on their electrocardiogram in response to dobutamine.[152] The variability in frequency of ST-segment depression is likely due to the populations studied, the severity of disease present, and the doses of dobutamine that were utilized. Dobutamine electrocardiography has been suggested to be more sensitive than exercise electrocardiography despite a lower peak double product achieved, possibly due to the decrease in diastolic perfusion pressure.[137] Dobutamine electrocardiography has been used to detect ischemia in postmyocardial infarction patients[153,154] and to detect coronary restenosis after angioplasty.[155]

Dobutamine stress has been employed in conjunction with myocardial perfusion imaging, using either ^{201}Tl or ^{99m}Tc sestamibi for detection of coronary artery disease (Table 6-6).

Mason and colleagues were the first to use dobutamine in conjunction with thallium scintigraphy for detection of coronary artery disease.[156] The sensitivity of thallium scintigraphy was 94 percent in their population of noninfarct subjects, while the sensitivity of exercise electrocardiography was 60 percent. The specificity of scintigraphy was 87 percent compared to 63 percent for electrocardiography. Several subsequent studies have reported similar results (Table 6-6).[139,146,151,157] Pennell and coinvestigators reported similar experience with dobutamine thallium scintigraphy, noting a sensitivity of 97 percent and specificity of 80 percent, compared to 78 percent and 44 percent, respectively, for exercise electrocardiography in their study of 40 patients.[146] They found a significant relationship between the number of thallium defects and the number of diseased vessels at angiography. Hays and colleagues found a sensitivity of dobutamine thallium scintigraphy of 86 percent and a specificity of 90 percent overall, with a sensitivity of 84 percent in patients with single-vessel disease, 82 percent in those with double-vessel disease, and 100 percent in those with triple-vessel disease.[139] Warner et al reported a sensitivity of 93 percent and a specificity of 88 percent.[157] Based on this reported experience to date, the sensitivity of dobutamine thallium scintigraphy appears to be in the range of approximately 90 percent, and the specificity 85 percent, which is similar to the reported experience with exercise thallium scintigraphy. Liver thallium uptake, however, is higher with dobutamine stress compared to exercise stress, resulting in a less desirable target-to-background ratio.[158] This could potentially affect both sensitivity and specificity. Kumar and co-workers found that dobutamine thallium scintigraphy was less sensitive than dipyridamole thallium scintigraphy in a crossover study of 30 patients, 11 of whom had a prior myocardial infarction, although the maximum administered dose of dobutamine was only 20 μg/kg/min.[159] Dobutamine thallium scintigraphy has also been utilized in patients with syndrome X, in whom it appears to reproduce clinical symptoms reliably and is frequently associated with perfusion abnormalities, suggesting abnormal underlying myocardial physiology possibly at the microvascular level.[160]

The sensitivity and specificity of dobutamine ^{99m}Tc-sestamibi perfusion imaging is similar but perhaps somewhat lower than with dobutamine thallium scintigraphy, possibly related to the more prominent liver uptake with sestamibi (Table 6-6). In a study of 35 patients, Voth and colleagues found the sensitivity of dobutamine sestamibi imaging to be 88 percent compared to 68 percent for exercise electrocardiography.[161] Achievement of a maximal dobutamine dose appears to be an important determinant of sensitivity when used in conjunction with sestamibi imaging. Marwick et al found that a submaximal dobutamine dose was associated with reduced sensitivity (58 percent) compared to maximum dobutamine (73 percent) or maximal exercise (78 percent) sestamibi imaging.[162] Herman and coinvestigators found an excellent segment-by-segment concordance comparing exercise and dobutamine sestamibi images in their study of 24 patients.[163]

Overall, the reported sensitivity and specificity of dobutamine thallium scintigraphy and dobutamine sestamibi imaging appears to be approximately comparable to exercise perfusion imaging, suggesting that dobutamine stress is an acceptable substitute for exercise in patients who are unable to perform adequate levels of exercise and is an acceptable substitute to adenosine or dipyridamole perfusion imaging for patients who are not candidates for that form of stress, particularly because of bronchospastic lung disease.

Thus far, there is only very limited experience addressing the prognostic power of dobutamine perfusion imaging in identifying patients at high or low risk of subsequent cardiac events. Coma-Canella and colleagues found that 45 of their 63 postinfarction patients had additional dobutamine-thallium-induced perfusion defects and that mild to moderate redistributing defects correlated with walls that increased their contractility during dobutamine infusion, while severe redistributing defects were associated with worsening regional wall motion.[168] However, clinical follow-up was not available. Dobutamine thallium scintigraphy has been shown to have prognostic value in a single study in identifying cardiac risk in patients undergoing vascular surgery procedures.[169]

Pharmacologic Coronary Vasodilation

In contrast to maneuvers that simulate the effects of exercise on the heart and thereby secondarily alter myocardial oxygen supply through increased demand, pharmacologic coronary vasodilation can be used directly to increase coronary blood flow independently of myocardial oxygen demand. This has the advantage of not needing the patient to have the physical or mental ability to exercise. The most commonly used agents for clinical imaging are adenosine, which directly produces vasodilation, and dipyridamole, which acts indirectly through its effects on adenosine metabolism. Papaverine is a powerful nonspecific systemic vasodilator with profound coronary artery vasodilating effects on both the R1 and R2 vessels, but it has associated complications that have limited its use.[170] It will not be further considered here.

ADENOSINE AND DIPYRIDAMOLE: PHYSIOLOGY AND HEMODYNAMICS

Adenosine is a naturally occurring, ubiquitous molecule that functions as a physiologic regulator of blood flow in most vascular beds, including the coronary circulation.[171] It is a small, heterocyclic molecule made up of a purine base and ribose. Adenosine is produced intracellularly and is then carried across the sarcolemmal membrane to the outside of the cell via carrier-mediated mechanisms. Once outside the cell, it activates specific, local cell surface receptors. It is then rapidly transported back into the cell and metabolized.

Intracellular adenosine is produced via two predominant pathways: the L-homocysteine adenosine pathway and the adenosine triphosphate (ATP) pathway (Fig. 6-7).[172-174] The ATP pathway generates adenosine through the action of the enzyme 5' nucleotidase on 5' AMP. In the setting of myocardial ischemia, ATP conversion to adenosine diphosphate is accelerated, which results in increased intracellular production of adenosine. Adenosine is transported across the cell membrane via carrier-mediated mechanisms, where it is then able to activate specific adenosine cell surface receptors, A_1 and A_2. Activation of the A_2 receptor on vascular smooth muscle produces activation of adenylate cyclase, which in turn increases cyclic AMP production. In addition, it decreases uptake of calcium across the sarcolemmal membrane and inhibits potassium channels. These effects produce vasodilation and smooth muscle relaxation.[152] There are also A_1 receptors on vascular smooth muscle. Activation of the A_1 receptor by adenosine results in activation of guanylate cyclase to produce guanosine monophosphate, again resulting in vasodilation.[175] There are also A_1 receptors in the sinus and atrioventricular nodes in the heart. Activation of those receptors by adenosine decreases sinus node automaticity, thereby decreasing heart rate, and decreases atrioventricular node conduction (thus the use of adenosine to treat atrioventricular nodal reentrant tachyarrhythmias). Hence, in the presence of myocardial ischemia, there is increased local adenosine production that in turn activates both A_1 and A_2 receptors. This produces coronary artery vasodilation and an increase in myocardial oxygen supply, as well as a decrease in heart rate and myocardial oxygen demand. While the direct effect is one of lowering heart rate, an indirect effect of increasing heart rate can predominate through reflex sympathetic stimulation resulting from a decline in blood pressure. The net effect can then be an increase in myocardial oxygen demand. Adenosine functions as a primary physiologic regulator of autoregulation of coronary blood flow through these mechanisms.

Extracellular adenosine is rapidly transported back into the cells, with an estimated plasma half-life of approximately 2 s.[176] Once intracellular, adenosine is metabolized via three pathways, the predominate one being

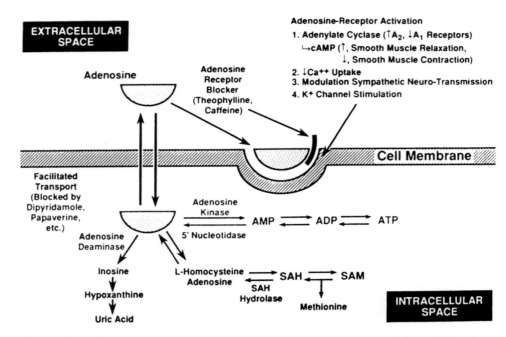

Figure 6-7 Adenosine production, transport, receptor activation, and metabolism. AMP, adenosine monophosphate; ADP, adenosine diphosphate; ATP, adenosine triphosphate; SAH, S-adenosyl homocysteine; SAM, S-adenosyl methionine. (From Verani,[173] reproduced with permission.)

metabolism to inosine through the action of the enzyme adenosine deaminase (Fig. 6-7). Inosine is in turn metabolized to hypoxanthine and then to uric acid. Adenosine can also serve as a metabolic substrate for regeneration of its precursor, ATP, through the action of adenosine kinase. Finally, it can also be conjugated back through the L-homocysteine adenosine pathway to form S-adenosyl homocysteine.

Dipyridamole increases the extracellular concentration of adenosine by blocking its intracellular transport.[177] It also inhibits the intracellular breakdown of adenosine by inhibiting enzymes that are responsible for its metabolism, particularly adenosine deaminase. At high doses, dipyridamole also inhibits the breakdown of cyclic AMP by inhibiting the enzyme phosphodiesterase.[178] Dipyridamole, therefore, acts as an indirect vasodilator primarily through its effects of increasing the concentration of naturally occurring adenosine.

Caffeine and theophylline are both direct competitive blockers of the cell surface A_1 and A_2 receptors. They will therefore inhibit the vasodilating effects of both adenosine and dipyridamole and should be withheld when adenosine or dipyridamole are administered for clinical imaging.[179,180] One double-blind, crossover study of 16 patients suggested that pretreatment with theophylline did not affect adenosine-induced thallium perfusion defects.[181] However, other studies have indicated that caffeine ingestion can result in false-negative results on imaging studies.[182] Current recommendations suggest that caffeine should be withheld for 24 h and theophylline preparations for 72 h prior to clinical studies using

either agent.[183] Aminophylline can be used to reverse side effects of adenosine or dipyridamole administration and has a very rapid action. Because of the extremely short half-life of adenosine, aminophylline administration is primarily applicable to dipyridamole infusion. Pentoxifylline (Trental) is a methylxanthine derivative used in treating patients with claudication, but, unlike theophylline, does not appear to attenuate the hyperemic response to dipyridamole or adenosine and probably does not need to be withheld prior to dipyridamole or adenosine testing.[184]

Dipyridamole is a pyrimidine base that was first introduced in the United States in 1959 as a coronary vasodilator to be used as a possible treatment for angina. Gould and co-workers demonstrated that dipyridamole administered intravenously at a dose of 0.142 mg/kg/min for 4 min (0.56 mg/kg total dose) produced maximal coronary vasodilation with peak flows in the range of 4 to 5 times resting levels.[10,11] Subsequent studies, however, have suggested that a significant percentage of patients may not achieve maximal coronary vasodilation at this dose.[170,185–187] A dipyridamole dose of as high as 0.84 mg/kg infused over 10 min was evaluated by Casanova and co-workers, who noted that this dose resulted in an increase in side effects with no increase in sensitivity of thallium imaging for detection of multiple-vessel coronary artery disease.[188] In contrast, Lalonde and co-workers noted that higher-dose dipyridamole (0.84 mg/kg administered over 6 min) appeared to improve the sensitivity of thallium imaging somewhat.[189] Intravenous adenosine has been approved as a myocardial stress

Table 6-7 Hemodynamic Responses to Dipyridamole and Adenosine Infusion Compared to Upright Leg Exercise

Hemodynamic Parameter	Upright Dynamic Leg Exercise		Dipyridamole Infusion		Adenosine Infusion	
	Normal	CAD	Normal	CAD	Normal	CAD
Heart rate	++++	+++	+/++	+/++	+/++	+/++
Systolic blood pressure	+++	++/+++	−	−	−	−
Diastolic blood pressure	0/+	0/+	−	−	−	−
Rate–pressure product	++++	++/+++	+	+	+	+
LVEDV	0/+	+/++	0	0	0	0
LVEDP	0/+	++	+	++	+	++
Cardiac output	++++	++/+++	++	++	++	++
Ejection fraction	+/++	−/−−	0/+	0/−	0/+	0/−
Coronary blood flow	+++	++	++++	+++/++++	++++	+++/++++

CAD, coronary artery disease; LVEDV, left ventricular end-diastolic volume; LVEDP, left ventricular end-diastolic pressure.

agent. The recommended dose for its administration is also 0.140 mg/kg/min, usually infused over 6 min.[190]

The increase in coronary blood flow achieved with dipyridamole is significantly greater than that achieved with exercise (Table 6-7). Heart rate increases 20 to 40 percent in response to dipyridamole infusion, while systolic blood pressure decreases 4 to 10 percent.[191–196] Diastolic blood pressure and mean blood pressure decrease significantly. Double product increases 11 to 28 percent, which is less than that associated with either isometric or dynamic exercise.[191,195,196] Cardiac output increases approximately 30 percent, and pulmonary capillary wedge pressure may increase slightly.[196,197] Ejection fraction may increase slightly in normals and decrease slightly in patients with coronary disease.[198]

The hemodynamic responses to adenosine infusion are similar to those noted with dipyridamole (Table 6-7). In an investigation of 89 patients, Verani and colleagues noted that heart rate increased incrementally with doses of adenosine above 50 μg/kg/min to a peak increase of 15 beats/min at the maximal dose of 140 μg/kg/min.[199] Systolic and diastolic blood pressure did not decrease significantly until the peak dose (140 μg/kg/min), at which point they decreased 9 and 7 mmHg, respectively. Ogilby and co-workers noted that heart rate increases approximately 20 beats/min during adenosine infusion in normals and patients with coronary artery disease.[200] Abreu and colleagues noted in their study of 607 patients that heart rate with adenosine increased from 75 to 92 beats/min and systolic blood pressure decreased from 138 to 121 mmHg.[201] Cardiac output increased approximately 50 percent in the study by Ogilby et al, primarily due to the increase in heart rate, since stroke volume did not change significantly.[200] Pulmonary capillary wedge pressure increased a mean of 8 mmHg in normals and 14 mmHg in coronary artery disease patients, without development of associated regional wall-motion abnormalities on left ventriculogram and with no change in left

ventricular volume or ejection fraction. This suggested a reduction in diastolic compliance as the mechanism of increase in left ventricular filling pressure, possibly due to engorgement of the myocardial wall resulting from the marked increase in myocardial blood flow, an "erectile" effect.[202] In coronary disease patients, ischemia could also contribute to the increased filling pressures and thus account for the difference in the degree of elevation compared to normals, since diastolic dysfunction is the earliest manifestation of ischemia, occurring before ejection fraction drops.[203,204]

The reported magnitude of increase in coronary blood flow in response to intravenous dipyridamole has varied depending at least in part on the method used to measure the response. Using the inert-gas method, coronary blood flow has been estimated to increase 3½ to 4 times resting levels.[205] Using the Doppler wire technique,[206] dipyridamole infusion, in conjunction with handgrip, increases coronary blood flow velocity 4 to 5 times resting levels.[186] Using thermodilution coronary sinus flow measurements, Brown and colleagues noted an increase of coronary blood flow of 2.8 times baseline in vessels without significant obstruction.[193] If handgrip was used in combination with dipyridamole, they noted that peak coronary blood flow increased to 3.8 times baseline, possibly due to the increase in diastolic perfusion pressure associated with handgrip stress. Others have not noted this increase in peak dipyridamole-induced flow with handgrip.[207] In assessing coronary flow reserve, which can be expressed as a ratio of peak to resting flow, it is also important to take into account variables, such as heart rate and preload, that might increase resting flow, since these variables can cause a decrease in coronary flow reserve without changing peak coronary blood flow.[208]

In a study of 39 patients, Wilson et al demonstrated that intravenous adenosine at doses of 0.070 mg/kg/min increased coronary blood flow a mean of 3.1 times basal rates, and at 0.100 mg/kg/min increased flow 4.4 times.[190] They noted no further increase at the maximal dose of 0.140 mg/kg/min. Maximum hyperemia occurred in a mean of 84 s (range, 23 to 125 s). Hence, a 3- to 4-min infusion before injection of a radioactive tracer is considered to be adequate, with the infusion continued 2 to 3 min longer after injection to allow completion of tracer tissue uptake. At this highest dose, they found the vasodilating effect of adenosine to be comparable to papaverine, with 92 percent of subjects achieving maximum hyperemia. Kern and coinvestigators noted an increase in coronary flow velocity of 64 ± 104 percent, 122 ± 94 percent, and 198 ± 59 percent in normals with adenosine doses of 0.050, 0.100, and 0.150 mg/kg/min, respectively.[209] Hence, there was a further increase between the doses of 0.100 and 0.150 mg/kg/min, although the relatively wide standard deviations indicate a considerable amount of individual variability in response. The response to the highest dose of adenosine was comparable to the response to 10 mg of intracoronary papaverine, similar to the experience of Wilson and colleagues. Based on these findings, the dose of 0.140 mg/kg/min (140 μg/kg/min) has been adopted as the standard clinical dose. Wilson and colleagues noted that coronary flow velocity varied cyclically at lower doses, suggesting fluctuations in myocardial adenosine concentrations and incomplete vasodilation.[190] They did not note this fluctuation at the higher dose of infusion. Even at this dose, however, fluctuation in electrocardiographic ST-segment depression has been described, suggesting that in some patients this dose does not produce maximal vasodilation.[210] An adenosine infusion dose of 200 μg/kg/min has been demonstrated to be well tolerated.[211]

Rossen and coinvestigators examined the coronary vasodilating effects of intravenous dipyridamole compared to intravenous adenosine, using intracoronary papaverine to determine maximal coronary vasodilator reserve.[187] Dipyridamole and adenosine were administered in standard doses (0.56 mg/kg over 4 min for dipyridamole and 0.140 mg/kg/min for adenosine). Heart rate increased a mean of 11 beats/min with both. Mean arterial blood pressure decreased more with adenosine than with dipyridamole (16 ± 5 mmHg versus 10 ± 3 mmHg, respectively, $p < 0.01$). The peak-to-rest coronary blood flow velocity ratio using Doppler measurement was 3.9 ± 1.1 with papaverine, 3.4 ± 1.2 for adenosine, and 3.1 ± 1.2 for dipyridamole. There was a greater decrease in coronary flow resistance with adenosine than with dipyridamole, although the difference in peak-to-rest flow velocity comparing the two did not reach statistical significance. Both were significantly less than that achieved with papaverine. Adenosine had a much faster onset of action than did dipyridamole. In a positron emission tomography coronary flow study of 20 normal volunteers, Chan and coinvestigators noted similar in-

creases in myocardial blood flow from rest (1.1 ± 0.2 ml/min/g) to hyperemia comparing the two agents (4.4 ± 0.9 ml/min/g with adenosine and 4.3 ± 1.3 ml/min/g with dipyridamole), with mean hyperemia-to-rest flow ratios of 4.3 and 4.0, respectively.[212] Importantly, however, they noted marked individual variability in the response to both agents, with individual hyperemia to baseline flow ratios ranging from 2.0 to 8.4 for adenosine and 1.5 to 5.8 for dipyridamole. This observation again suggests that some patients will not achieve maximal coronary vasodilation with the standard doses used with either of these agents.

In the normal coronary vessel, dipyridamole and adenosine increase flow uniformly across the myocardium from the endocardium to the epicardium. The coronary flow response is different, however, in the presence of coronary stenosis. A myocardial steal phenomenon can occur in two ways: a subendocardial to subepicardial steal within the distribution of a single vessel (*vertical steal*) and a steal from one vessel's territory to another's, often mediated at least in part through collateral channels (*horizontal steal*).

A subendocardial steal is a result of the increased R3 component of resistance in the subendocardium compared to the subepicardium. In the presence of an increase in the R2 component of resistance associated with a coronary stenosis, resting flow to the subendocardium is preserved by relative vasodilation of the R2 vessels in the subendocardium compared to the subepicardium, thereby maintaining balanced resistance across the myocardial wall and preserving subendocardial perfusion (Fig. 6-3). As a result, however, there is less coronary vasodilator reserve in the subendocardium compared to the subepicardium in response to dipyridamole or adenosine infusion. Since the subepicardium decreases its resistance more than the subendocardium in response to the vasodilator, there is a relative steal of perfusion toward the subepicardium.[140] This transmural myocardial steal is substantially influenced by the systemic hemodynamic effects of the drug. If dipyridamole is administered intracoronarily instead of intravenously, thereby avoiding the fall in systemic blood pressure, the endocardial to epicardial steal is minimized.[213] The increase in coronary blood flow is also less with intracoronary compared to intravenous dipyridamole infusion.[214]

A myocardial steal phenomenon can also occur from one vessel's distribution to another's by a similar mechanism. A vessel with a stenosis uses part or all of its vasodilator reserve to preserve flow at rest. In response to dipyridamole or adenosine, the normal vessel decreases its resistance markedly while the diseased vessel can not. As a result, flow increases in the normal vessel at the expense of the diseased vessel. This phenomenon is accentuated if flow in the diseased vessel depends on collateral channels, since that flow is directly pressure dependent without autoregulatory capability. Distal perfusion pressure decreases with dipyridamole or adenosine as a result of the decrease in resistance and the decrease in arterial perfusion pressure, which in turn decreases flow through collateral channels. Hence, flow through a diseased artery may actually decrease in response to dipyridamole or adenosine infusion.[215,216] This appears to be a variable finding, however, which was not found in 15 patients with 90 to 100 percent proximal stenosis of the left anterior descending coronary artery studied during dipyridamole infusion by Marchant and co-workers.[217]

Dipyridamole or adenosine infusion would not be expected to cause ischemia, since they are primarily coronary vasodilators.[191,218,219] However, ischemia does occur not infrequently and is multifactorial in etiology. Myocardial oxygen demand increases somewhat as a result of the increased heart rate. Myocardial perfusion pressure decreases due to the decrease in systemic blood pressure. The decrease in perfusion pressure appears to predispose to a myocardial steal, resulting in ischemia in vulnerable areas.[213,220] Ischemia can be manifested by ST-segment depression, angina pectoris, and regional wall-motion abnormalities. Verani and colleagues noted that 12 percent of patients developed ST-segment depression with adenosine infusion.[199] Nishimura and colleagues found that the presence of collateral vessels was the most significant correlate of ischemic ST-segment depression with adenosine infusion in their study of 65 consecutive patients, supporting the hypothesis that a myocardial steal contributes to the development of ischemia.[219] The association of ischemia during adenosine infusion with the presence of collateral vessels suggests that the intercoronary (horizontal) steal is the primary mediator of ischemia rather than the endocardial-to-epicardial (vertical) steal.[221] ST-segment depression during adenosine or dipyridamole infusion has been found in some studies to be a manifestation of multiple-vessel disease.[222] Villanueva and colleagues noted that the most powerful correlate of ST-segment depression during dipyridamole infusion in their study of 204 consecutive patients was the number of segments having thallium redistribution.[223] Marshall and co-workers found in a study of 550 consecutive patients who underwent adenosine stress that ST-segment depression had low sensitivity but high specificity for coronary artery disease.[224] In their study, ST-segment depression correlated with multiple perfusion defects and more severe perfusion defects, again suggesting that it is a marker of more severe disease. In a follow-up report, these investigators noted that 2 mm or more of ST-segment depression during adenosine infusion was the most powerful predictor of subsequent cardiac events by multivariate analysis of the clinical and scintigraphic variables that they assessed in their study of 188 patients (relative risk, 6.5).[225]

Administration of theophylline, a direct antagonist of adenosine, can increase exercise performance in patients with chronic coronary disease, apparently by reducing ischemia.[226] Other studies have indicated that inhibition of adenosine worsens ischemia during exercise.[227]

Angina during dipyridamole or adenosine infusion has been a less predictable indicator of coronary disease.[228] Ando and colleagues described an association between angina during dipyridamole infusion and a drop in systemic blood pressure, multiple-vessel coronary disease, and multiple perfusion defects.[222] Angina also correlated with the occurrence of ST-segment depression in the study by Nishimura et al.[219] In contrast, Homma and co-workers found no difference in the occurrence of chest pain or ST-segment depressions comparing patients with no or single-vessel coronary disease and those with double- or triple-vessel disease.[229] Similarly, Pearlman and Boucher found no difference in the severity of coronary disease comparing patients with chest pain during dipyridamole infusion and those without.[230] Laarman et al also found no difference in the presence of ST-segment depression or angina relative to the severity of coronary disease, but found that ST depression but not chest pain added to the diagnostic information from thallium imaging.[231] Hence, chest pain during adenosine or dipyridamole infusion appears to be a somewhat nonspecific indicator of the presence or severity of coronary disease.

Regional wall-motion abnormalities during dipyridamole were noted by radionuclide ventriculography in 66 percent of 113 patients with coronary disease studied by Klein et al, and 87 percent had a small decrease in ejection fraction.[198] In contrast, Ogilby and co-workers found no regional wall-motion abnormalities or decrease in ejection fraction with adenosine infusion in patients studied by left ventriculography.[200] Jain and colleagues noted that most patients who had transient dipyridamole-induced thallium perfusion abnormalities on SPECT scintigraphy had associated transient wall-motion abnormalities on simultaneous two-dimensional echocardiography.[232] In contrast, Whitfield and co-workers noted that only five of their 24 patients had new wall-motion abnormalities associated with redistributing thallium perfusion defects with dipyridamole.[233] McLaughlin and colleagues performed serial hemodynamic, aortic and coronary sinus lactate, and coronary sinus adenosine measurements in 23 subjects during dipyridamole thallium scintigraphy.[234] They found that dipyridamole-induced perfusion abnormalities were not associated with metabolic or hemodynamic markers of ischemia and argued that the abnormalities were more likely indicators of abnormal coronary flow reserve than of actual ischemia. Studies using dipyridamole echocardiography have demonstrated the development of regional wall-motion abnormalities, although the sensitivity is less than dobutamine echocardiography or myocardial perfusion imaging.[235-239] Similar results have been described with adenosine wall-motion studies that have noted a somewhat variable frequency of wall-motion abnormalities associated with adenosine infusion.[200,240,241] Overall, it appears from these combined data that at least some patients develop sufficient ischemia during dipyridamole or adenosine infusion to develop associated myocardial dysfunction as a result of a myocardial steal phenomenon.

DIPYRIDAMOLE PERFUSION IMAGING

There has now been extensive experience with intravenous dipyridamole utilized as a stress agent for myocardial perfusion imaging, and it is approved in the United States for that use. Prior to the availability of the intravenous preparation, dipyridamole was used in oral form in doses of 300 to 400 mg as a pharmacologic stress agent, with demonstrated efficacy.[242–246] Some studies suggested that the sensitivity and specificity of oral dipyridamole and intravenous dipyridamole were comparable,[247,248] although other studies noted that the results of an oral dipyridamole thallium test were normal in as many as 25 percent of patients who had abnormal exercise thallium test results.[249] Absorption of the oral form of the drug is highly variable, with onset of the peak effects occurring from 30 to 90 min following ingestion.[250,251] Pulverized dipyridamole suspension is somewhat more predictable than dipyridamole tablets.[252] Segal and Davis found no correlation between serum dipyridamole levels and symptoms, the hemodynamic response, or imaging variables after oral dipyridamole administration.[251] Subjects with low dipyridamole blood levels could not be identified clinically, suggesting a risk of false-negative findings. Similar findings have been described by other observers as well.[253] With the availability of intravenous dipyridamole, there is no longer any role for oral dipyridamole testing because of its unpredictable absorption.

As discussed above, the usual dose of intravenous dipyridamole is 0.142 mg/kg/min infused over 4 min (total dose, 0.56 mg/kg). It is distributed within 15 min, with the peak effect occurring 3 to 7 min after completion of the infusion, and is eliminated with a biologic half-life of 88 to 136 min.[254] Radiotracer is typically injected 4 min after completion of the infusion. If handgrip exercise is used in conjunction with dipyridamole stress, it is typically performed between minutes 6 and 10 after initiation of the infusion, at 20 to 30 percent of maximal grip strength.

Safety and side effects Dipyridamole is generally well tolerated with a highly favorable safety profile, although minor side effects are common (approximately 50 to 75 percent; Table 6-5). Noncardiac side effects include headache (5 to 23 percent), dizziness (5 to 21 percent), nausea and vomiting (5 to 12 percent), and flushing (3 to 38 percent).[131] Chest pain occurs in approximately 18

to 42 percent and is a somewhat nonspecific finding. When chest pain is typical angina, however, some studies have found it to be an indicator of severe anatomic disease.[222] Others have not.[229] Atypical chest discomfort is a common and comparatively nonspecific finding. Dipyridamole stress is well tolerated in the elderly.[255,256]

More severe side effects are rare,[257] but have been described. In the registry data report of 3900 patients, four (0.1 percent) suffered myocardial infarction, which was fatal in two.[258] Ventricular arrhythmias can occur, and in some series are related to severity of underlying coronary artery disease.[229,259] Cardiac arrest, myocardial infarction, and death have also been described in other reports.[260–262] The risk of a severe ischemic response is greater in patients with unstable angina than in those with stable angina.[258,261] Persistent severe chest pain and myocardial ischemia have been described after both intravenous and oral dipyridamole.[263–266] Acute bronchospasm can also occur in patients with a history of asthma or severe obstructive lung disease, and in rare cases can lead to respiratory arrest.[258,267] Caution is also necessary in selecting patients with bronchospastic airway disease who can safely discontinue theophylline preparations prior to dipyridamole testing.[229,258]

The side effects of dipyridamole are usually rapidly reversible with the administration of aminophylline in a dose of 100 to 300 mg, which competitively blocks the adenosine receptors.[258,268] Approximately 4 to 18 percent of patients have sufficient symptoms with dipyridamole infusion to warrant administration of aminophylline.[229,255,258] In rare cases, chest pain may not reverse with aminophylline, in which case nitroglycerin is usually but not always effective.[264,268] In patients with underlying variant angina, rapid reversal of dipyridamole-induced coronary artery vasodilation by aminophylline administration can trigger coronary vasospasm with ST-segment elevation.[269] Dipyridamole can be safely administered in selected patients after myocardial infarction, even as early as 1 to 4 days after infarction.[270–275] Dipyridamole can also be safely administered in patients who can not be withdrawn from beta-blocker therapy.[194,195,276]

High-dose dipyridamole (up to 0.84 mg/kg) has been used particularly in echocardiography studies and, while the frequency of side effects increases with increasing dose, side effects remain comparatively minor in severity.[188,189,268,277] High-dose dipyridamole has also been used in conjunction with radionuclide ventriculography.[278] In a multicenter report of over 10,000 patients evaluated with high-dose dipyridamole echocardiography, significant side effects were described in 1.2 percent, including major side effects in 0.07 percent.[268] Major side effects included asystole in three patients, myocardial infarction in three, pulmonary edema in one, ventricular tachycardia in one, and one death. In 60 patients, the infusion was terminated prematurely because of ischemic changes with echocardiographic monitoring. It is important to note, however, that patients were monitored with echocardiography during dipyridamole infusion, and only patients without wall-motion abnormalities at the standard dose of dipyridamole were given the high-dose infusion. Hence, the demonstrated safety of high-dose dipyridamole with echocardiography can not be extrapolated to perfusion imaging where wall motion can not be followed during dipyridamole infusion. Use of high-dose dipyridamole in echocardiographic imaging has been suggested to increase the sensitivity for detection of coronary artery disease.[279]

There are relative contraindications to the use of dipyridamole testing. Patients with a history of intractable wheezing requiring theophylline treatment or those with active wheezing on examination at the time of presentation should not be given dipyridamole (or adenosine) because of the risk of severe bronchospasm. Patients who are hypotensive at baseline (less than approximately 90 mmHg) should be carefully evaluated before administration of dipyridamole because of the risk of a further decline in blood pressure. Patients with high-grade atrioventricular block (second- or third-degree block) should not be given dipyridamole unless they are protected with a pacemaker. In these patient groups, dobutamine is the preferred pharmacologic stress agent. Patients with recent unstable angina or myocardial infarction can receive dipyridamole safely if they are clinically stable, but require careful screening evaluation before proceeding.

Myocardial tracer uptake and target-to-background ratio At rest, the heart receives about 4 percent of cardiac output. Coronary blood flow increases 2 to 2.5 times resting levels at peak exercise, but as a percent of cardiac output, coronary blood flow during exercise is unchanged. The myocardial target-to-background ratio of thallium uptake after exercise is increased not because the heart gets a greater percent of cardiac output than at rest, but because splanchnic blood flow decreases during exercise and lung uptake relative to that of the heart declines. With dipyridamole infusion, coronary blood flow increases substantially more than during maximal exercise, both in absolute terms as well as a percentage of cardiac output (Table 6-7). This higher relative level of coronary blood flow achieved with dipyridamole imaging might be an advantage compared to exercise imaging. However, this potential advantage of increased peak myocardial blood flow may be offset by the fact that myocardial tracer uptake is not linear at high flow rates. At the lower peak levels of coronary blood flow achieved with exercise, thallium uptake is relatively linear in relation to coronary blood flow. At the higher levels of coronary blood flow achieved with dipyridamole, however, there is a sharp drop-off of thallium uptake relative to flow.[280]

Gould and co-workers noted that the ratio of myocardial thallium-to-background uptake with dipyridam-

ole infusion was about 50 percent of that noted with ^{99m}Tc-labeled albumin microspheres, indicating a substantial decrease in thallium extraction fraction at the higher flow rate.[10] The degree of underestimation of flow with maximal vasodilation is greater with ^{99m}Tc sestamibi than with thallium.[281] While this plateauing of myocardial tracer uptake at high levels of coronary blood flow could offset the potential advantages of the higher levels of coronary blood flow achieved with dipyridamole compared to exercise, the marked increase in coronary blood flow relative to cardiac output could compensate for the decreased extraction ratio because of the overall greater thallium delivery.[11,282] Consistent with this finding, myocardial thallium activity has been shown to be greater after dipyridamole or adenosine stress than it is after exercise.[283]

There has been some variability in the reports of the myocardial target-to-background ratio of tracer uptake, an indicator of image quality, with dipyridamole compared to exercise stress. Albro and coinvestigators noted that the myocardial-to-background ratio of thallium uptake was higher for dipyridamole imaging (2.3) than it was for exercise imaging (2.1).[191] In a series of studies, Gould and colleagues concluded that image quality is better with dipyridamole than with exercise as a result of the greater levels of myocardial blood flow achieved.[10,11,191] Other investigators, however, have noted that the myocardial target-to-background ratio of tracer uptake is actually less favorable with dipyridamole than it is with exercise. Pennell and Ell noted that while there is greater myocardial tracer uptake with dipyridamole, the heart-to-background ratio is decreased and is comparatively poor because of the high levels of splanchnic and lung uptake that are present.[284] Several investigators have noted that combining low-level exercise with dipyridamole infusion somewhat increases the peak levels of coronary blood flow achieved, but substantially improves image quality because splanchnic blood flow decreases with a resultant decrease in liver tracer uptake.[231,242,284,313] The myocardial target-to-background ratio is thus improved. Standing or walking in place does not appear to be sufficient to improve image quality appreciably, but low levels of exercise stress either with handgrip or with treadmill or bicycle stress results in increased myocardial blood flow, decreased splanchnic tracer uptake, and substantially improved image quality.[196,284]

The kinetics of thallium washout are also different with dipyridamole infusion compared to exercise stress. The intrinsic myocardial efflux rate of thallium is actually increased in normals with intracoronary infusion of dipyridamole.[285] Even in the setting of a coronary stenosis, intracoronary dipyridamole infusion results in minimal coronary steal, and the intrinsic thallium washout rate is unchanged.[213] In contrast, with intravenous as opposed to intracoronary infusion in the presence of a

Table 6-8 Sensitivity and Specificity of Intravenous Dipyridamole Thallium Scintigraphy

Reference	n	Method	n (%) Sensitivity	n (%) Specificity
Albro et al, 1978[191]	62	Planar	34/51 (67)	10/11 (91)
Narita et al, 1981[289]	50	Planar	24/35 (69)	15/15 (100)
Leppo et al, 1982[195]	60	Planar	37/40 (93)	16/20 (80)
Francisco et al, 1982[290]	86	Planar	41/51 (80)	16/24 (67)
Wilde et al, 1982[291]	27	Planar	16/21 (76)	6/6 (100)
Harris et al, 1982[292]	38	Planar	19/21 (88)	11/17 (65)
Okada et al, 1983[293]	30	Planar	21/23 (91)	7/7 (100)
Sochor et al, 1984[294]	194	Planar	137/149 (92)	36/45 (80)
Okada et al, 1983[293]	66	Planar	36/40 (90)	21/26 (81)
Schmoliner et al, 1984[296]	60	Planar	32/43 (74)	17/17 (100)
Benjelloun et al, 1985[297]	58	Planar	42/51 (82)	7/7 (100)
Taillefer et al, 1986[247]	50	Planar	32/39 (82)	10/11 (91)
Ruddy et al, 1987[298]	80	Planar	45/53 (85)	25/27 (93)
Lam et al, 1988[299]	141	Planar	93/111 (84)	22/31 (71)
Laarman et al, 1988[300]	101	Planar	46/59 (78)	19/22 (86)
Boudreau et al, 1990[301]	40	Planar	19/22 (86)	13/18 (72)
Zhu et al, 1991[304]	170	Planar	129/142 (91)	22/28 (79)
Kong et al, 1992[305]	114	Planar	86/94 (92)	12/20 (60)
Mendelson et al, 1992[306]	79	Planar	51/76 (67)	NA
Francisco et al, 1982[290]	86	SPECT	46/51 (90)	23/24 (96)
Huikuri et al, 1988[303]	93	SPECT	78/81 (96)	9/12 (75)
DePuey et al, 1990[302]	76	SPECT	54/61 (89)	7/15 (47)
Mendelson et al, 1992[306]	79	SPECT	68/76 (89)	NA
Totals	1506	Planar	939/1121 (84)	285/352 (81)
	334	SPECT	247/269 (92)	39/51 (76)

NA, not available; SPECT, single photon emission computed tomography.

coronary stenosis, the decrease in coronary perfusion pressure in conjunction with subnormal endocardial blood flow and resultant ischemia slows thallium efflux, resulting in delayed thallium redistribution.[285] Thallium levels in the circulating blood pool are increased with dipyridamole stress compared to exercise as a result of the larger splanchnic and lung thallium pools. This also has an effect of slowing thallium efflux from the heart down the concentration gradient into the circulating blood pool.[279] Accordingly, different normal standards for thallium washout are necessary compared to exercise imaging.[286,287] Quantitating regional washout does nevertheless help to differentiate normal from abnormal regions in a similar fashion to exercise imaging.[288]

Sensitivity and specificity of dipyridamole thallium imaging The sensitivity and specificity of intravenous dipyridamole thallium imaging have been extensively investigated (Table 6-8).[191,195,247,289–306] The sensitivity of planar dipyridamole thallium scintigraphy is approximately 84 percent and the specificity is 81 percent. While there is less reported experience with SPECT dipyridam-

ole thallium scintigraphy, its sensitivity of 92 percent appears to be somewhat better than with planar imaging, with a somewhat lower specificity of 76 percent. Popma and coinvestigators used receiver–operator characteristic curves to derive regional cutoff criteria for abnormality with quantitative SPECT dipyridamole scintigraphy.[307] The sensitivity of dipyridamole thallium scintigraphy increases relative to the extent of disease and the number of vessels involved. The sensitivity and specificity of dipyridamole thallium imaging are similar in women compared to men.[305] Dipyridamole perfusion scintigraphy has been shown to be useful in differentiating ischemic from nonischemic cardiomyopathy.[308,309] Beta-blocker therapy does not appear significantly to affect defect size or reliability of dipyridamole thallium imaging.[196,310]

Several studies have demonstrated that the sensitivity and specificity of dipyridamole thallium imaging are similar to those of exercise thallium imaging.[194,303,311] Varma and colleagues performed a segment-by-segment quantitative analysis of scintigrams on 21 patients who underwent both studies within several weeks of one another and noted the agreement to be 87 percent.[311] The correlations with coronary angiography were also comparable in the 15 patients who underwent angiography. Martin and co-workers noted that thallium defects are less marked and less frequent with dipyridamole imaging compared to exercise thallium imaging, but they did not have angiographic findings in their patients for correlation.[312] In a randomized crossover study, Kumar and associates found that dipyridamole thallium scintigraphy was more effective than dobutamine thallium scintigraphy in producing perfusion defects, primarily in the lateral wall and apex, and correlated better with angiographic findings.[159] However, the study may have limited clinical relevance because the maximum dose of dobutamine infused was only 20 μg/kg/min.

Combining low-level exercise with dipyridamole stress thallium scintigraphy improves image quality by increasing the myocardial target-to-background ratio, which is likely to enhance diagnostic accuracy.[313–317] While handgrip exercise appears to have some effectiveness, walking on a treadmill for 3 min is preferable in patients who can do it in terms of the overall enhancement of image quality.[315,318] Combining low-level exercise with the dipyridamole infusion also has the potential advantage of improving disease detection in dipyridamole nonresponders. Combining low-level exercise with dipyridamole infusion is safe and well tolerated; indeed, the side effects of the dipyridamole infusion appear to be decreased by exercise.[242,313,314,316,317] Based on these findings, it is preferable that all patients who are undergoing dipyridamole thallium scintigraphy perform low-level exercise, if they are able, preferably by walking but, if not, with handgrip stress.

Increased lung thallium uptake with dipyridamole scintigraphy has been repeatedly shown to be a useful predictor of both the presence and severity of coronary disease. In a small, early series, Okada and co-workers noted that increased lung thallium uptake with dipyridamole scintigraphy increased the probability that coronary artery disease was present, but lung uptake was not related to the severity of disease.[319] In contrast, Villanueva and colleagues noted that the prevalence of an increased ratio of lung thallium uptake was similar with dipyridamole imaging compared to exercise imaging and suggested that it was a potential marker of more severe disease in that it was associated with other scintigraphic findings of disease severity, including the presence of fixed or redistributing defects and left ventricular cavity dilation.[320] However, angiographic data were not available in these patients. Other studies have noted similar findings, but again without angiographic correlation.[321] In a series of 94 patients with angiographic correlation, Hurwitz and co-workers documented a relationship between lung uptake of ^{201}Tl with dipyridamole and the number of critical coronary stenoses. These authors also found that when dipyridamole imaging was combined

with low-level exercise, the implication of increased lung thallium uptake was similar to exercise imaging.[322]

Transient left ventricular cavity dilatation is a related potential marker of disease severity with dipyridamole thallium scintigraphy. Several studies using planar[323–325] or SPECT[326] imaging have demonstrated that transient left ventricular dilatation during dipyridamole infusion is a marker of multiple-vessel disease, critical disease, and increased prognostic risk. The mechanism of transient cavity dilation may not be actual ventricular dilatation, but rather diffuse subendocardial ischemia with subendocardial hypoperfusion resulting in less subendocardial thallium uptake and a larger appearing cavity.[326] In a follow-up study, Veilleux and colleagues demonstrated that patients with transient left ventricular cavity dilation had an increased incidence of fatal and nonfatal myocardial infarctions and cardiac death.[325] Hurwitz and coinvestigators noted that indices of ventricular contraction during gated dipyridamole testing correlated better with anatomically severe disease at angiography than did either increased lung uptake or transient left ventricular cavity dilation, and recommended gated imaging whenever possible.[327]

Patients with left ventricular hypertrophy may have thallium perfusion defects in the absence of coronary artery disease. Of 48 patients with clinical ischemic heart disease but no significant coronary stenoses who were studied by Houghton and colleagues, 40 had left ventricular hypertrophy or diabetes.[328] The authors found that thallium perfusion defects with dipyridamole infusion were a manifestation of abnormal coronary vasodilator reserve, which was predicted by the presence of left ventricular hypertrophy measured by echocardiography. In hypertensive patients with perfusion defects, abnormal vasodilator reserve was typically, but not always, a manifestation of an increased basal coronary flow velocity. Despite this, dipyridamole thallium scintigraphy has been found to be a useful predictor of coronary artery disease in patients with aortic stenosis, although considerable caution is warranted in stressing this population.[329,330] Dipyridamole thallium scintigraphy has also been shown to be an indicator of impaired coronary vasodilator reserve in the subset of patients with hypertrophic cardiomyopathy who have thallium perfusion defects.[331,332] In those patients, the impaired reserve may be a direct manifestation of the underlying disease process, in that it does not appear to correlate with the degree of hypertrophy that is present.[332] Patients with chest pain and normal coronary arteries may also have impaired coronary vasodilator reserve with dipyridamole infusion, but interestingly may have normal vasodilator reserve if infused with papaverine or adenosine.[333] This suggests that the limitation in vasodilator reserve in these patients could be a result of an as-yet-undefined abnormality in adenosine metabolism.

Patients with left bundle branch block may have exercise-induced thallium perfusion abnormalities in the septal region in the absence of coronary artery disease.[334] These defects may represent functional ischemia, or at least hypoperfusion, of the septum as a result of the asynchronous septal contraction. They can be produced in dogs by pacing the right ventricle to simulate left bundle branch block.[334] Multiple reports have indicated that dipyridamole thallium scintigraphy has improved diagnostic accuracy for detection of left anterior descending coronary artery disease in patients with left bundle branch block, compared to exercise scintigraphy.[335-338] One explanation proposed by Hirzel et al,[334] based on the induction of perfusion defects in the septum during moderately rapid right ventricular pacing in dogs, is that the septum is hypoperfused as a result of inadequate diastolic coronary perfusion time, which is a consequence of asynchronous septal contraction complicated by tachycardia. A second proposed explanation for this observation is that, compared to exercise stress, dipyridamole stress is associated with substantially lower systolic blood pressure. The resulting lower systolic wall tension may favorably influence septal perfusion in the presence of asynchronous contraction and decrease the probability of a thallium perfusion abnormality in the absence of coronary artery disease.

Prognostic power of dipyridamole thallium scintigraphy Dipyridamole thallium scintigraphy has been shown to be a useful predictor of subsequent cardiac events in diverse clinical settings. In a study of 516 consecutive patients referred for dipyridamole thallium examination and followed over an average of 21 months, Hendel and colleagues found that history of congestive heart failure, diabetes mellitus, or abnormal scan findings were predictors of subsequent cardiac events, either death or myocardial infarction.[339] Using logistic regression analysis, abnormal scan results were found to be an independent predictor of outcome, identifying a patient subset at a threefold increased risk for cardiac death or nonfatal myocardial infarction over 21 ± 8 months of follow-up. Stratmann and co-workers found similar results in their study of dipyridamole scintigraphy in 373 patients with chest pain.[340] In their study, a fixed thallium perfusion abnormality but not a reversible defect was a predictor of subsequent cardiac events. Only a fixed perfusion abnormality and a history of coronary bypass surgery were independent predictors of outcome. In the Stratmann study, ^{201}Tl reinjection was not used, so the full extent of reversible myocardial ischemia in those patients with fixed perfusion defects and increased cardiac risk was not established. Nevertheless, in other studies using dipyridamole myocardial perfusion imaging to assess cardiac prognosis, the presence of ^{201}Tl redistribution has been a powerful predictor without the addition of thallium reinjection. Younis and coinvestigators found that a reversible defect by dipyridamole thallium imaging has prognostic utility in patients with asymptomatic coronary artery disease.[341] In their study of 107 patients followed over an average of 14 months, using stepwise logistic regression analysis, a reversible thallium perfusion defect was the only significant predictor of subsequent cardiac events of the 18 clinical, scintigraphic, and angiographic variables assessed. Shaw and colleagues demonstrated that dipyridamole thallium scintigraphy is also a powerful predictor of risk of cardiac events in the elderly, a population that often can not exercise sufficiently for diagnostic testing.[342] In their study of 348 patients over the age of 70 years, the presence of fixed, reversible, or combined thallium perfusion defects was significantly associated with occurrence of subsequent cardiac death or myocardial infarction, identifying a subgroup at approximately a sevenfold increased risk. Of note, myocardial infarction or cardiac death occurred in only 5 percent of elderly patients with normal scan findings over a 2-year follow-up period. Abnormal dipyridamole scan results were the single most powerful predictor of outcome of the clinical and radionuclide variables assessed. Gal and coinvestigators also found that a normal dipyridamole thallium study was associated with a low incidence of cardiac events in their 42-month follow-up study of 84 patients with normal scan results.[343]

Dipyridamole thallium scintigraphy has also been used to identify high-risk coronary anatomy. In a study of 466 consecutive patients who underwent dipyridamole thallium scintigraphy, Chikamori and colleagues observed the scintigraphic correlates in 38 patients with a 50 percent or greater stenosis of the left main coronary artery.[344] Nine (24 percent) of the 38 patients had a left main scintigraphic pattern, compared to 9 percent of the remainder. The pattern was present in six of nine with left main disease without right coronary disease and in only three of 29 with coexisting right coronary artery disease. Left main pattern was specific and sensitive for detecting left main disease without right coronary disease. A combination of clinical markers of ischemia during dipyridamole infusion, diffuse slow washout on the scintigram, extensive fixed perfusion defects, and left main pattern were the best predictors of left main disease in the presence of concomitant right coronary disease (72 percent sensitivity and 80 percent specificity).

Dipyridamole thallium scintigraphy has been shown to be a useful predictor of outcome in patients with acute myocardial infarction.[345] In addition, it has been a useful predictor of perioperative cardiac complications in patients who undergo noncardiac surgical procedures. These applications of myocardial perfusion imaging following dipyridamole infusion are discussed in Chap. 23.

Dipyridamole technetium-99m–sestamibi scintigraphy While there is less reported experience using dipyridamole stress with ^{99m}Tc-sestamibi imaging, the findings suggest that it is at least comparable to thallium imaging. This can not be assumed because of the different characteristics of the perfusion agent. Sestamibi, for example, has lower myocardial extraction, particularly at the high flow rates achieved with dipyridamole, than does thallium, which might result in an underestimation of disease.[346] Nevertheless, the sensitivity of dipyridamole sestamibi imaging has compared favorably to thallium scintigraphy. Tartagni and coinvestigators performed SPECT stress dipyridamole sestamibi scintigraphy followed by a same-day rest injection in 30 patients and compared the results to exercise and redistribution thallium scintigraphy.[347] The sensitivity and specificity for detection of coronary artery disease defined by angiography were 100 percent and 75 percent for both tracers. The sensitivities for disease detection in individual vessels with sestamibi imaging were 75 percent for left anterior descending disease, 89 percent for right coronary artery disease, and 80 percent for left circumflex distribution disease. Yang and colleagues noted a sensitivity of 95 percent and specificity of 100 percent for dipyridamole SPECT sestamibi imaging compared to coronary angiography in a study of 44 patients.[348] In their experience, the sensitivity for detection of left circumflex distribution disease was lower (45 percent) than for detection of disease in the left anterior descending (96 percent) or right coronary artery distribution (88 percent). Bisi et al compared exercise versus dipyridamole stress and planar versus SPECT imaging in 20 patients who underwent coronary angiography.[349] They found good agreement in segmental analysis comparing dipyridamole imaging to exercise imaging (sensitivity for detection of individual vessel disease was 49 percent with a specificity of 90 percent for both types of stress using planar imaging). SPECT imaging was significantly better than planar imaging in their experience (SPECT dipyridamole sensitivity and specificity were 74 percent and 100 percent, and exercise sensitivity and specificity were 79 percent and 95 percent, respectively). The sensitivity of planar exercise imaging in their study (49 percent) was lower than expected based on other studies, however, which may have favored SPECT imaging. Further investigation of this question in larger numbers of patients is required. As expected, the sensitivity of stress imaging was less in patients with less severe anatomic disease. Myocardial defect size does not change significantly over 4 h after exercise or dipyridamole stress, so isotope injection and imaging can be temporally uncoupled.[350] The sequence of same-day rest and then dipyridamole stress sestamibi imaging improves the detection of ischemia compared to stress and then rest imaging.[351]

High-dose dipyridamole (in this case, 0.7 mg/kg) has been used in combination with handgrip exercise in an effort to enhance the sensitivity with sestamibi imaging. In a study of 42 patients, Kettunen and colleagues noted a sensitivity of dipyridamole SPECT scintigraphy of 95

percent, with correct identification of significant disease (50 percent or more) in 82 percent of lesions in the left anterior descending, 61 percent in the left circumflex, and 90 percent in the right coronary artery.[352] Again the sensitivity for disease detection was greater in vessels with more severe disease. In the subgroup of 22 patients who also underwent thallium scintigraphy, the sensitivity for identification of individual diseased vessels was not significantly different compared to sestamibi (76 percent thallium and 83 percent sestamibi, p = NS). Minor side effects occurred in just 5 percent of patients with high-dose dipyridamole, possibly because the combination with handgrip exercise tended to preserve blood pressure during dipyridamole infusion. Assessment of ventricular wall motion and ejection fraction by first-pass imaging after high-dose dipyridamole infusion does not appear to add significantly to the information content of the sestamibi perfusion study.[353] Dipyridamole ^{99m}Tc-sestamibi imaging also provides considerable prognostic information, and this is reviewed in Chap. 23.

ADENOSINE PERFUSION IMAGING

There are theoretical advantages to using adenosine instead of dipyridamole as a myocardial stress agent because of its rapid onset of action, ultrashort half-life, and its potentially more potent and predictable coronary vasodilating effects.[354-356] Adenosine produces maximal coronary vasodilation in a significantly greater percentage of patients than does dipyridamole.[356] Its shorter half-life compared to dipyridamole should theoretically decrease its potential risks since adverse reactions would resolve rapidly. The shorter half-life of adenosine can also be a theoretical disadvantage with some imaging protocols, particularly if it is desired to combine pharmacologic vasodilation with low-level exercise.[355] While the experience with adenosine perfusion imaging is not yet as extensive as with dipyridamole imaging, it has nevertheless now been utilized in large numbers of patients with excellent results.

Adenosine infusion results in increased myocardial counts of ^{201}Tl compared to exercise. The heart-to-lung count ratio is similar while the heart-to-liver ratio is lower with adenosine than with exercise as a result of increased liver uptake of ^{201}Tl with adenosine.[357] In a study of 40 patients who underwent both imaging procedures, however, Takeishi and colleagues found that the increased liver activity with adenosine did not result in any reduced accuracy in detecting right coronary artery disease.[357] Performing exercise during adenosine infusion may reduce liver tracer uptake by decreasing splanchnic blood flow, but may at the same time decrease peak coronary blood flow by increasing coronary vascular resistance.[358] The reduction in liver tracer uptake with exercise combined with adenosine or dipyridamole infu-

Table 6-9 Side Effects with Adenosine Infusion, n (%)

Side Effect	Abreu et al[201] (n = 607)	Coyne et al[361] (n = 100)	Iskandrian et al[218] (n = 148)	Gupta et al[362] (n = 144)	Nishimura et al[363] (n = 175)	Total (n = 1174)
Flushing	211 (35)	61 (61)	91 (61)	59 (41)	104 (59)	526 (45)
Chest pain	205 (34)	57 (57)	71 (48)	35 (24)	93 (53)	461 (39)
Dyspnea	114 (19)	62 (62)	36 (24)	33 (23)	81 (46)	326 (28)
Headache	125 (21)	15 (15)	22 (15)	17 (12)	34 (19)	213 (18)
Throat tightness	57 (5)	17 (17)	NA	29 (20)	43 (25)	146 (14)
Dizziness	29 (5)	4 (4)	10 (7)	29 (20)	28 (16)	100 (9)
Atrioventricular block						
First degree	58 (10)	NA	NA	12 (8)	4 (2)	74 (8)
Second or third degree	22 (4)	3 (3)	4 (3)	1 (1)	7 (4)	37 (3)
ST-segment depression	76 (13)	NA	33 (22)	12 (8)	16/120 (13)	137 (13)
Infusion decreased or stopped prematurely	6 (1)	0 (0)	NA	3 (2)	12 (7)	21 (2)
Aminophylline administration	3 (0.5)	0 (0)	7 (5)	4 (3)	4 (2)	18 (2)
Any adverse effect	481 (79)	94 (94)	135 (91)	118 (82)	NA	828 (83)

NA, not available.

sion has been a variable finding.[284] The peak heart-to-lung ratio of thallium uptake increases in patients with advanced coronary artery disease with adenosine infusion and is correlated with the severity and extent of myocardial perfusion defects.[359] Redistribution of thallium perfusion defects with adenosine infusion appears to be a result of loss of thallium activity over time from areas of normal perfusion.[360]

Safety and side effects   Multiple series have examined the frequency and severity of side effects with adenosine infusion (Table 6-9).[201,218,361–363] Of approximately 1170 patients studied, 83 percent experienced some side effect. Flushing was the most common side effect, occurring in approximately 45 percent of patients. Chest pain was the second most common side effect, occurring in 39 percent, whereas dyspnea occurred in 28 percent and ST-segment depression occurred in 13 percent. In the series reported by Abreu and colleagues, 482 patients underwent adenosine perfusion imaging for evaluation of possible coronary artery disease, and 125 underwent evaluation for postmyocardial infarction risk stratification.[201] Chest pain occurred in 34 percent of their patients, and ST-segment depression occurred in 13 percent. However, only 17 percent of the patients with chest pain had associated ST-segment depression. Chest pain with ST-segment depression occurred in only 6 percent of the total study sample. Only 36 percent of the patients who had the adenosine study for evaluation of coronary artery disease and who had chest pain during adenosine infusion had a reversible perfusion abnormality on the scintigram, compared to 61 percent of the patients being examined after myocardial infarction. However, 73 percent of the patients who had chest pain with ST-segment depression during adenosine infusion had reversible per-

fusion defects on scintigraphy. Somewhat in contrast to this experience, in the study by Gupta and co-workers, 11 of 12 patients who had ST-segment depression also had concomitant chest pain.[362] Iskandrian and colleagues compared the 32 coronary disease patients in their study who had ST-segment depression to the 100 patients who had coronary disease but did not have ST-segment depression during adenosine infusion.[218] Patients with ST-segment depression had a higher peak heart rate (91 versus 84 beats/min) and had a greater incidence of chest pain during the adenosine infusion (63 percent versus 43 percent). However, there were no significant differences in either the angiographic extent of disease or in the extent of the perfusion defects on SPECT thallium scintigraphy in the patients with ST-segment depression. In contrast, Marshall and co-workers found that marked ST-segment depression (2 mm or more) was a predictor of subsequent cardiac events.[225] Hence, chest pain and ST-segment depression during adenosine infusion may be manifestations of coronary artery disease, but are comparatively nonspecific. When they occur concomitantly, or when there is marked ST-segment depression, their implication is more significant.

The side effects of adenosine administration can be decreased by exercise during the infusion. Pennell and colleagues randomized 407 patients to one of three groups: adenosine infusion alone, adenosine combined with submaximal exercise, and adenosine combined with symptom-limited exercise.[364] They found that concomitant exercise decreased the noncardiac side effects as well as the frequency of arrhythmias.

First-degree atrioventricular block occurs in approximately 8 percent of patients during adenosine infusion (Table 6-9). Second- or third-degree block occurs in approximately 3 percent, but is virtually always transient

Table 6-10   Sensitivity and Specificity of Adenosine Perfusion Imaging

Reference	n	Method	Sensitivity (%)	Specificity (%)
Verani et al, 1990[199]	89	SPECT	24/29 (83)	15/16 (94)
Nguyen et al, 1990[241]	60	SPECT	49/53 (92)	7/7 (100)
Coyne et al, 1991[361]	100	SPECT	39/47 (83)	40/53 (75)
Iskandrian et al, 1991[218]	148	SPECT	121/132 (92)	14/16 (88)
Nishimura et al, 1991[368]	101	SPECT	61/70 (87)	28/31 (90)
Gupta et al, 1992[362]	123	SPECT	55/66 (83)	35/40 (87)
Ogilby et al, 1992[200]	45	SPECT	31/33 (94)	12/12 (100)
Totals	666		380/430 (88)	151/175 (86)

SPECT, single photon emission computed tomography.

in its duration. It appears to be more common in patients on calcium channel blocker or beta-blocker therapy.[363] Adenosine infusion has been found to be safe in patients with left bundle branch block.[365,366]

While the frequency of side effects is high, they are almost always transient and are well tolerated by patients. None of the patients in the five series summarized in Table 6-9 suffered myocardial infarction, prolonged heart block, significant ventricular arrhythmia, or death. Bronchospasm requiring treatment was rare, being described in approximately seven (0.1 percent) of the 1174 patients. In only 2 percent of patients was it necessary to decrease or terminate the adenosine infusion prematurely because of side effects, and only 1 percent of patients received an aminophylline infusion.

The safety of adenosine infusion has been preliminarily established in patients with moderate to severe aortic stenosis. Samuels and colleagues studied 35 patients with adenosine infusion and redistribution thallium imaging or with rest thallium and adenosine sestamibi imaging.[367] Adenosine was well tolerated in their patients.

Sensitivity and specificity of adenosine thallium perfusion imaging   The sensitivity and specificity of adenosine thallium perfusion imaging for detection of coronary artery disease has been established in numerous studies (Table 6-10).[199,200,218,241,361,362,368] The overall sensitivity of adenosine SPECT thallium imaging is approximately 88 percent and the specificity is 86 percent. The sensitivity increases relative to the number of diseased vessels. Verani and colleagues noted that the sensitivity of adenosine imaging was 73 percent in patients with single-vessel disease, 90 percent in those with double-vessel disease, and 100 percent in those with triple-vessel disease.[199] Iskandrian and coinvestigators noted the diagnostic sensitivity to be 87 percent in patients with single-vessel disease, 92 percent in those with double-vessel disease, and 98 percent in those with triple-vessel disease.[218] Patients who had thallium reinjection had fewer fixed perfusion defects than did patients who underwent traditional redistribution imaging. In a study of 101 consecutive patients who underwent adenosine thallium

perfusion imaging and coronary angiography, Nishimura and colleagues noted that the sensitivity for diagnosing coronary disease in patients without prior myocardial infarction was 76 percent for single-vessel disease, 86 percent for double-vessel disease, and 90 percent for triple-vessel disease.[368] The sensitivity of adenosine SPECT thallium scintigraphy is not significantly different in patients who have a hemodynamic response to the infusion with a decrease in blood pressure, compared to those who do not. Aksut and colleagues noted a sensitivity of 87 percent in 102 hemodynamic nonresponders compared to 91 percent in responders ($p = $ NS).[369]

Samuels and colleagues examined the diagnostic utility of either adenosine thallium scintigraphy or rest thallium and adenosine sestamibi scintigraphy in patients with moderate or severe aortic stenosis.[367] In a study of 20 patients who underwent coronary angiography, they noted that the sensitivity of scintigraphy was 92 percent and the specificity was 71 percent. This is a clinical group in whom there has previously been no reliable and safe means of diagnosing concomitant coronary artery disease. The results of this preliminary study are encouraging, but additional study is needed to establish the safety and efficacy of the procedure in this population.

Combining adenosine infusion with either submaximal or symptom-limited exercise decreases side effects and improves image quality, including the lung-to-heart ratio of thallium uptake.[364,372] In a randomized study of 407 patients, Pennell and colleagues noted that there was a nonsignificant trend toward improved sensitivity by combining adenosine infusion with exercise (sensitivity 98 percent versus 93 percent without exercise, $p = $ 0.07), and image quality was clearly improved.[364] While maximal exercise produced optimal images, the difference compared to submaximal exercise was minor. Since submaximal exercise during the 6-min infusion is logistically much easier, it is considered to be the preferred approach.

In a retrospective, unblinded study, O'Keefe and co-workers examined the comparative diagnostic accuracy of SPECT thallium scintigraphy in patients who received a standard 6-min infusion of adenosine ($n = 233$) compared to those who received a 4-min infusion ($n = 174$).[370] They found no difference in diagnostic accuracy (93 percent for the 6-min protocol and 92 percent for the 4-min protocol), but fewer side effects in patients who received the 4-min infusion. These findings need to be confirmed in a prospective study. Villegas et al found that there was a higher incidence of thallium redistribution after a 6-min adenosine infusion compared to a 3-min infusion.[371]

Several studies have directly compared the sensitivity and specificity of adenosine thallium imaging with exercise thallium imaging in the same patients. Nguyen and co-workers found that the predictive accuracy of adenosine thallium imaging was slightly but not significantly higher than that of exercise thallium imaging (90 percent versus 80 percent, respectively) in 30 patients who underwent both studies.[241] Coyne and colleagues found a sensitivity of exercise thallium scintigraphy of 81 percent and of adenosine thallium scintigraphy of 83 percent ($p = NS$) in their study of 100 patients.[361] In patients without evidence of myocardial infarction on left ventriculography, the sensitivities were again comparable between the two techniques (75 percent versus 79 percent, respectively, $p = NS$). The specificity of the exercise study was 75 percent versus 74 percent for the adenosine study. In a multicenter crossover study, Nishimura and coinvestigators performed exercise and adenosine myocardial perfusion scintigraphy in 175 patients.[363] Using quantitative analysis, the authors found agreement concerning the presence or absence of normal tomogram results in 86 percent of cases. There was also excellent agreement in localizing a perfusion defect to a specific vessel territory (range, 83 to 91 percent). Thallium defect size was significantly larger on the adenosine images compared to the exercise scintigrams. Gupta et al reported a sensitivity of 83 percent and specificity of 87 percent for adenosine SPECT imaging and 82 percent and 80 percent, respectively, for exercise imaging.[362] Most false-negative results occurred in patients with single-vessel disease.

Iskandrian and co-workers examined their experience with exercise thallium scintigraphy ($n = 143$) compared to adenosine thallium scintigraphy ($n = 41$) in patients with chronic occlusion of either the left anterior descending or right coronary artery but without prior infarction.[373] They noted that the sensitivity of adenosine imaging was significantly better than that of exercise imaging (100 percent versus 87 percent, respectively, $p < 0.02$), and the size of the defects was larger, although the study was limited by being a retrospective, nonrandomized review, and studies were not compared in the same patients.

As was noted earlier for dipyridamole perfusion imaging, adenosine thallium scintigraphy is safe in patients with left bundle branch block and appears to be superior to exercise thallium scintigraphy, primarily because of

improved specificity.[365,366] In their study of 173 consecutive patients with left bundle branch block who underwent either exercise ($n = 56$) or adenosine ($n = 117$) thallium scintigraphy, O'Keefe and colleagues noted that the overall predictive accuracy of exercise imaging was 68 percent and of adenosine imaging was 93 percent ($p = 0.01$).[364,366] This was a result of the fact that the specificity of exercise thallium imaging was only 42 percent, whereas it was 82 percent with adenosine scintigraphy ($p < 0.0002$). The frequency of false-positive septal perfusion abnormalities in patients with left bundle branch block who are examined with adenosine thallium scintigraphy has been estimated recently to be no greater than 4 percent.[374]

Many data are currently available regarding the prognostic accuracy of adenosine imaging, although it is likely to be similar to that of dipyridamole imaging and initial reports are encouraging.[375-379] For example, Shaw and colleagues assessed perioperative cardiac events in 60 consecutive patients who underwent adenosine thallium imaging prior to noncardiac surgical procedures.[376] Stepwise logistic regression analysis revealed that, of the clinical, scintigraphic, and angiographic variables assessed, the presence of a combined (fixed and redistributing) adenosine perfusion defect ($p = 0.0007$), triple-vessel coronary artery disease ($p = 0.001$), and left bundle branch block ($p = 0.02$) was predictive of perioperative events. The relative risk for perioperative cardiac events of the thallium defects was 4.9. Marshall and colleagues demonstrated that 2-mm or greater ST-segment depression on electrocardiography during adenosine infusion was the most powerful predictor of cardiac events of the clinical and scintigraphic variables that they assessed in their study of 188 patients.[225] Takeishi and co-workers noted that a left ventricular dilation ratio (comparing left ventricular cavity size between adenosine infusion images and the rest study) and perfusion defect size were significant and independent predictors of anatomically advanced coronary artery disease.[377] More studies will be necessary, however, to confirm the prognostic utility of adenosine thallium perfusion imaging. Studies evaluating the prognostic implications of findings from adenosine myocardial perfusion images performed after acute myocardial infarction are discussed in Chap. 23.

Adenosine sestamibi or dual-isotope perfusion imaging   Leon and coinvestigators compared adenosine SPECT perfusion images with ^{201}Tl to images with ^{99m}Tc sestamibi in dogs.[380] They noted that sestamibi underestimated defect size relative to ^{201}Tl or to the pathologic reference standard. With moderately severe partial coronary occlusion, defect contrast was sharper with ^{201}Tl than with ^{99m}Tc sestamibi.

Amanullah and colleagues examined adenosine SPECT sestamibi in 40 patients with angina pectoris.[381] They noted the sensitivity of sestamibi to be 94 percent, the specificity 100 percent, and the predictive accuracy 95 percent, which was significantly better than wall-motion assessment using adenosine echocardiography in the same patients.

The concordance of findings was assessed comparing adenosine SPECT sestamibi imaging to exercise sestamibi imaging in 22 patients with angiographically documented coronary artery disease studied by Cuocolo and colleagues.[382] They noted that the concordance between the two studies in identification of perfusion status in 484 segments was 90 percent, and agreement on localization of the perfusion defect to a specific vessel territory was 92 percent.

Miller and coinvestigators used a Doppler flow wire to assess coronary flow velocity in response to intracoronary infusion of adenosine in patients with an angiographic coronary artery stenosis that was of intermediate anatomic severity. They found an excellent correlation between the coronary flow velocity distal to the coronary stenosis during adenosine infusion and the presence of a perfusion defect using either adenosine ($n = 20$) or dipyridamole ($n = 13$) sestamibi scintigraphy.[383] All 14 patients with abnormal distal hyperemic flow-velocity values had corresponding reversible ^{99m}Tc-sestamibi defects on SPECT imaging.

Similar to the previously described experience with adenosine thallium scintigraphy, Ebersole and colleagues found that adenosine sestamibi imaging is associated with fewer false-positive scan results than is exercise sestamibi imaging in patients with left bundle branch block.[384] In their study of 11 patients, they found that the specificity of left anterior descending distribution perfusion defects with adenosine imaging was 88 percent compared to only 25 percent for exercise imaging.

The sensitivity and specificity of dual-isotope (rest thallium–stress sestamibi) imaging has been investigated with adenosine ($n = 82$) or dipyridamole ($n = 50$) infusion. The dual-isotope technique has the advantage of faster patient throughput. In 51 consecutive patients with coronary angiography and no prior myocardial infarction, Matzer and coinvestigators noted that the sensitivity was 92 percent and the specificity was 85 percent for determining the presence or absence of coronary disease when disease was defined as stenosis severity of 50 percent of more.[385] Defining significant disease as stenosis severity of 70 percent or greater, they noted a sensitivity of 97 percent and a specificity of 81 percent. The normalcy rate in 58 patients with a low probability of disease was 96 percent.

CONCLUSION

When the purpose of a myocardial perfusion imaging study is to determine (1) the presence or absence of coronary artery disease, (2) the extent or location of coronary disease, or (3) the physiologic severity of an anatomic stenosis, an adequate level of stress is essential. In patients who are unlikely to reach a target level of dynamic exercise, a pharmacologic stress should be substituted for exercise in nearly all cases. Pharmacologic coronary artery vasodilation, with intravenous dipyridamole or adenosine, or pharmacologic inotropic and chronotropic stimulation, with a drug such as dobutamine, provides a powerful adjunct for myocardial perfusion imaging in these and other settings.

REFERENCES

1. World Health Organization (WHO): Cardiovascular diseases: Trends in ischemic heart disease mortality, 1980–1988. *Weekly Epidemiol Rec WHO* 68:49, 1993.
2. Gallium RF: Trends in acute myocardial infarction and coronary heart disease death in the United States. *J Am Coll Cardiol* 23:1273, 1993.
3. Gordon T, Kanel WB: Premature mortality from coronary heart disease: The Framingham study. *JAMA* 215:1617, 1971.
4. Follansbee WP: The heart in vasculitis, in LeRoy EC (ed): *Systemic Vasculitis.* New York: Marcel Dekker; 1992:303–379.
5. Marcus ML, Chilian WM, Kanatsuka H, et al: Understanding the coronary circulation through studies at the microvascular level. *Circulation* 82:1, 1990.
6. Klocke FJ: Coronary blood flow in man. *Prog Cardiovasc Dis* 19:117, 1976.
7. Bache RJ, Dymek DJ: Local and regional regulation of coronary vascular tone. *Prog Cardiovasc Dis* 24:191, 1981.
8. Kitamura K, Jorgensen CR, Gobel FL, et al: Hemodynamic correlates of myocardial oxygen consumption during upright exercise. *J Appl Physiol* 32:516, 1972.
9. Ball RM, Bache RJ: Distribution of myocardial blood flow to the exercising dog with restricted coronary artery inflow. *Circ Res* 38:60, 1976.
10. Gould KL: Noninvasive assessment of coronary stenoses by myocardial perfusion imaging during pharmacologic coronary vasodilation. I. Physiologic basis and experimental validation. *Am J Cardiol* 41:267, 1978.
11. Gould KL, Westcott RJ, Albro PC, et al: Noninvasive assessment of coronary stenoses by myocardial imaging during pharmacologic coronary vasodilation. II. Clinical methodology and feasibility. *Am J Cardiol* 41:279, 1978.
12. Gould KL, Lipscomb K, Hamilton GW: Physiologic basis for assessing critical coronary stenosis: Instantaneous flow response and regional distribution during coronary hyperemia as measures of coronary flow reserve. *Am J Cardiol* 33:87, 1974.
13. Gould KL, Lipscomb K: Effects of coronary stenoses on coronary flow reserve and resistance. *Am J Cardiol* 34:48, 1974.

14. Kirkeeide RL, Gould KL, Parsel L: Assessment of coronary stenoses by myocardial perfusion imaging during pharmacologic coronary vasodilation. VII. Validation of coronary flow reserve as a single integrated functional measure of stenosis severity reflecting all its geometric dimensions. *J Am Coll Cardiol* 7:103, 1986.

15. Parker JO, West RO, DiGiorgi S: The effect of nitroglycerin on coronary blood flow and the hemodynamic response to exercise in coronary artery disease. *Am J Cardiol* 27:59, 1971.

16. Epstein SE, Cannon RO III, Talbot TL: Hemodynamic principles in the control of coronary blood flow. *Am J Cardiol* 56:4E, 1985.

17. Mudge GH, Grossman W, Mills RM Jr, et al: Reflex increase in coronary vascular resistance in patients with ischemic heart disease. *N Engl J Med* 295:1333, 1976.

18. Epstein SE, Talbot TL: Dynamic coronary tone in precipitation, exacerbation and relief of angina pectoris. *Am J Cardiol* 48:797, 1981.

19. Schwartz JS, Tockman B, Cohn JN, et al: Exercise-induced decrease in flow through stenotic coronary arteries in the dog. *Am J Cardiol* 50:1409, 1982.

20. Santamore WP, Walinsky P: Altered coronary flow responses to vasoactive drugs in the presence of coronary arterial stenosis in the dog. *Am J Cardiol* 45:276, 1980.

21. Gage JE, Hess OM, Murakami T, et al: Vasoconstriction of stenotic coronary arteries during dynamic exercise in patients with classic angina pectoris: Reversibility by nitroglycerin. *Circulation* 73:865, 1986.

22. Leppo JA, Meerdink DJ: Comparison of the myocardial uptake of a technetium-labeled isonitrile analogue and thallium. *Circ Res* 65:632, 1989.

23. Marshall RC, Leidholdt EM Jr, Zhang D, et al: Technetium-99m hexakis 2-methoxy-2-isobutyl isonitrile and thallium-201 extraction, washout, and retention at varying coronary flow rates in rabbit heart. *Circulation* 82:998, 1990.

24. Smith AM, Gullberg GT, Christian PE, et al: Kinetic modeling of teboroxime using dynamic SPECT imaging of a canine model. *J Nucl Med* 35:484, 1994.

25. Weinstein H, Reinhardt CP, Leppo JA: Teboroxime, sestamibi and thallium-201 as markers of myocardial hypoperfusion: Comparison by quantitative dual-isotope autoradiography in rabbits. *J Nucl Med* 34:1510, 1993.

26. Glover DK, Ruiz M, Bergmann EE, et al: Myocardial technetium-99m–teboroxime uptake during adenosine-induced hyperemia in dogs with either a critical or mild coronary stenosis: Comparison to thallium-201 and regional blood flow. *J Nucl Med* 36:476, 1995.

27. Iskandrian AS, Heo J, Kong B, et al: Effect of exercise level on the ability of thallium-201 tomographic imaging in detecting coronary artery disease: Analysis of 461 patients. *J Am Coll Cardiol* 14:1477, 1989.

28. Nyers DG, Hankins JH, Keller DM, et al: Effect of exercise level on the diagnostic accuracy of thallium-201 SPECT scintigraphy. *Nebr Med J* 77:26, 1992.

29. Mahmarian JJ, Boyce TM, Goldberg RK, et al: Quantitative exercise thallium-201 single-photon emission computed tomography for the enhanced diagnosis of ischemic heart disease. *J Am Coll Cardiol* 15:318, 1990.

30. Esquivel L, Pollock SG, Beller GA, et al: Effect of the degree of effort on the sensitivity of the exercise thallium-201 stress test in asymptomatic coronary artery disease. *Am J Cardiol* 63:160, 1989.

31. Mahmarian JJ, Verani MS: Exercise thallium-201 perfusion scintigraphy in the assessment of coronary artery disease. *Am J Cardiol* 67:2D, 1991.

32. Verani MS, Mahmarian JJ: Myocardial perfusion scintigraphy during maximal coronary artery vasodilation with adenosine. *Am J Cardiol* 67:12D, 1991.

33. Robinson BF: Relation of heart rate and systolic blood pressure to the onset of pain in angina pectoris. *Circulation* 35:1073, 1967.

34. Thadani U, Parker JO: Hemodynamics at rest and during supine and sitting bicycle exercise in normal subjects. *Am J Cardiol* 41:52, 1978.

35. Bygdeman S, Wahren J: Influence of body position on the anginal threshold during leg exercise. *Eur J Clin Invest* 4:201, 1974.

36. Thadani U, West RO, Mathew TM, Parker JO: Hemodynamics at rest and during supine and sitting bicycle exercise in patients with coronary artery disease. *Am J Cardiol* 39:776, 1977.

37. Poliner LR, Dehmer GJ, Lewis SE, et al: Left ventricular performance in normal subjects: A comparison of the responses to exercise in the upright and supine positions. *Circulation* 62:528, 1980.

38. Freeman MR, Berman DS, Staniloff H, et al: Comparison of upright and supine bicycle exercise in the detection and evaluation of extent of coronary artery disease by equilibrium radionuclide ventriculography. *Am Heart J* 102:182, 1981.

39. Manyari DE, Kostuk WJ: Left and right ventricular function at rest and during bicycle exercise in the supine and sitting positions in normal subjects and patients with coronary artery disease: Assessment by radionuclide ventriculography. *Am J Cardiol* 51:36, 1983.

40. Weiss JL, Weisfeldt ML, Mason SJ, et al: Evidence of Frank–Starling effect in man during severe semisupine exercise. *Circulation* 59:655, 1979.

41. Currie PJ, Kelly MJ, Pitt A: Comparison of supine and erect bicycle exercise electrocardiography in coronary heart disease: Accentuation of exercise-induced ischemic ST depression by supine posture. *Am J Cardiol* 52:1167, 1983.

42. Wetherbee JN, Bamrah VS, Ptacin MJ, et al: Comparison of ST segment depression in upright treadmill and supine bicycle exercise testing. *J Am Coll Cardiol* 11:330, 1988.

43. Coplan NL, Sacknoff DM, Stachenfeld NS, et al: Comparison of submaximal treadmill and supine bicycle exercise. *Am Heart J* 128:416, 1994.

44. Lecerof H: Influence of body position on exercise tolerance, heart rate, blood pressure and respiration rate in coronary insufficiency. *Br Heart J* 33:78, 1971.

45. Levey M, Rozanski A, Valovis R, et al: Comparative ability of upright and supine bicycle exercise electrocardiography to detect coronary artery disease. *Am J Cardiol* 49:945, 1982 (abstr).

46. Currie PJ, Kelly MJ, Kalff V, et al: Detection and localization of single vessel coronary disease: Biplane exercise radionuclide ventriculography or Tl-201 myocardial imaging? *J Nucl Med* 24:36, 1983 (abstr).

47. Gibbons RJ, Zinsmeister AR, Miller TD, et al: Supine exercise electrocardiography compared with exercise radionuclide angiography in noninvasive identification of severe coronary artery disease. *Ann Intern Med* 112: 743, 1990.

48. Simari RD, Miller TD, Zinsmeister AR, et al: Capabilities of supine exercise electrocardiography versus exercise radionuclide angiography in predicting coronary events. *Am J Cardiol* 67:573, 1991.

49. Celli BR: The clinical use of upper extremity exercise, in Wiesman IM, Zeballos RJ (eds): *Clinics in Chest Medicine: Clinical Exercise Testing.* Philadelphia: WB Saunders; 1994:339–349.

50. Balady GJ, Weiner DA, Rose L, et al: Physiologic responses to arm ergometry exercise relative to age and gender. *J Am Coll Cardiol* 16:130, 1990.

51. Lamont LS, Finkelhor RS, Rupert SJ, et al: Combined arm–leg ergometry exercise testing. *Am Heart J* 124: 1102, 1992.

52. Hagberg JM: Exercise assessment of arthritic and elderly individuals, in Panush RS, Lane NE (eds): *Balliere's Clinical Rheumatology: International Practice and Research.* London: Balliere Tindall, 8:1, 1994:29–52.

53. Takano N: Ventilatory responses during arm and leg exercise at varying speeds and forces in untrained female humans. *J Physiol* 468:413, 1993.

54. Stenberg J, Astrand P, Bjorn E, et al: Hemodynamic response to work with different muscle groups, sitting and supine. *J Appl Physiol* 22:61, 1967.

55. Balady GJ, Schick EC Jr, Weiner DA, et al: Comparison of determinants of myocardial oxygen consumption during arm and leg exercise in normal persons. *Am J Cardiol* 57:1385, 1986.

56. Hooker SP, Wells CL, Manore MM, et al: Differences in epinephrine and substrate responses between arm and leg exercise. *Med Sci Sports* 22:779, 1990.

57. Shaw DJ, Crawford MH, Karliner JS, et al: Arm-crank ergometry: A new method for the evaluation of coronary artery disease. *Am J Cardiol* 33:801, 1974.

58. Goodman S, Rubler S, Bryk H, et al: Arm exercise testing with myocardial scintigraphy in asymptomatic patients with peripheral vascular disease. *Chest* 95:740, 1989.

59. Ishii M, Ogawa T, Ushiyama K, et al: Cardiorespiratory responses to standing arm ergometry in patients with ischemic heart disease: Comparison with the results of treadmill exercise. *Jpn Heart J* 32:425, 1991.

60. Balady GJ: Types of exercise: Arm–leg and static–dynamic, in Fletcher GF (ed): *Cardiology Clinics: Exercise Testing and Cardiac Rehabilitation.* Philadelphia: WB Saunders; 1993:29–52.

61. Astrand PO, Ekblom B, Messin R, et al: Intra-arterial blood pressure during exercise with different muscle groups. *J Appl Physiol* 20:253, 1965.

62. Caru B, Colombo E, Santoro F, et al: Regional flow responses to exercise. *Chest* 100(suppl):223S, 1992.

63. Clausen JP, Klausen K, Rasmussen B, et al: Central and peripheral circulatory changes after training in the arms and legs. *Am J Physiol* 225:675, 1972.

64. Balady GJ, Weiner DA, McCabe CH, et al: Value of arm exercise testing in detecting coronary artery disease. *Am J Cardiol* 55:37, 1985.

65. Balady GJ, Weiner DA, Rothendler JA, et al: Arm exercise–thallium imaging testing for the detection of coronary artery disease. *J Am Coll Cardiol* 9:84, 1987.

66. Grover-McKay M, Milne N, Atwood E, et al: Comparison of thallium-201 single-photon emission computed tomographic scintigraphy with intravenous dipyridamole and arm exercise. *Am Heart J* 127:1516, 1994.

67. Fisman EZ, Ben-Ari E, Pines A, et al: Usefulness of heavy isometric exercise echocardiography for assessing left ventricular wall motion patterns late (≥6 months) after acute myocardial infarction. *Am J Cardiol* 70:1123, 1992.

68. Siegel W, Gilbert CA, Nutter DO, et al: Use of isometric handgrip for the indirect assessment of left ventricular function in patients with coronary atherosclerotic heart disease. *Am J Cardiol* 30:48, 1972.

69. Bodenheimer MM, Banka VS, Fooshee CM, et al: Comparison of wall motion and regional ejection fraction at rest and during isometric exercise: concise communication. *J Nucl Med* 20:724, 1979.

70. Peter CA, Jones RH: Effects of isometric handgrip and dynamic exercise on left-ventricular function. *J Nucl Med* 21:1131, 1980.

71. Stratton JR, Halter JB, Hallstrom AP, et al: Comparative plasma catecholamine and hemodynamic responses to handgrip, cold pressor and supine bicycle exercise testing in normal subjects. *J Am Coll Cardiol* 2:93, 1983.

72. Fisher ML, Nutter DO, Jacobs W, et al: Haemodynamic responses to isometric exercise (handgrip) in patients with heart disease. *Br Heart J* 35:422, 1973.

73. Haissly J, Messin R, Degre S, et al: Comparative response to isometric (static) and dynamic exercise tests in coronary disease. *Am J Cardiol* 33:791, 1974.

74. Kerber RE, Miller RA, Najjar SM: Myocardial ischemic effects of isometric dynamic and combined exercise in coronary artery disease. *Chest* 67:388, 1975.

75. DeBusk R, Pitts W, Haskell W, et al: Comparison of cardiovascular responses to static–dynamic effort and dynamic effort alone in patients with chronic ischemic heart disease. *Circulation* 59:977, 1979.

76. Bodenheimer MM, Banka VS, Fooshee CM, et al: Detection of coronary heart disease using radionuclide determined regional ejection fraction at rest and during handgrip exercise: Correlation with coronary arteriography. *Circulation* 58:640, 1978.

77. Laird WP, Fixler DE, Huffines FD: Cardiovascular response to isometric exercise in normal adolescents. *Circulation* 59:651, 1979.

78. Leosco D, Ferrara N, Abete P, et al: Echocardiographic vs hemodynamic monitoring during isometric exercise in patients with coronary artery disease. *G Ital Cardiol* 23:119, 1993.

79. Helfant RH, de Villa MA, Meister SG: Effect of sustained isometric handgrip exercise on left ventricular performance. *Circulation* 44:982, 1971.

80. Kivowitz C, Parmley WW, Donoso R: Effects of isometric exercise on cardiac performance: The grip test. *Circulation* 44:994, 1971.

81. Lowe DK, Rothbaum DA, McHenry PL, et al: Myocardial blood flow response to isometric (handgrip) and treadmill exercise in coronary artery disease. *Circulation* 51:126, 1975.

82. Ludbrook PA, Byrne JD, Reed FR, et al: Modification of left ventricular diastolic behavior by isometric handgrip exercise. *Circulation* 62:357, 1980.

83. Ferguson RJ, Cote P, Bourassa MG, et al: Coronary blood flow during isometric and dynamic exercise in angina pectoris patients. *J Cardiac Rehabil* 1:1, 1981.

84. Brown BG, Josephson MA, Peterson RB, et al: Intravenous dipyridamole combined with isometric handgrip for near maximal acute increase in coronary flow in patients with coronary artery disease. *Am J Cardiol* 48:1077, 1981.

85. Painter P, Hanson P: Isometric exercise: Implications for the cardiac patients. *Cardiovasc Rev Rep* 5:261, 1984.

86. Bodenheimer MM, Banka VS, Agarwal JB, et al: Relative value of isotonic and isometric exercise radionuclide angiography to detect coronary artery disease. *J Am Coll Cardiol* 1:790, 1983.

87. Kaul S, Hecht HS, Hopkins J, et al: Superiority of supine bicycle over isometric handgrip exercise in the assessment of ischemic heart disease: An evaluation of left ventricular ejection fraction response using radionuclide angiography. *Clin Cardiol* 7:547, 1984.

88. Sowton GE, Balcon R, Cross D, et al: Measurement of the angina threshold using atrial pacing: A new technique for the study of angina pectoris. *Cardiovasc Res* 1:301, 1967.

89. Ricci DR, Orlick AE, Alderman EL, et al: Role of tachycardia as an inotropic stimulus in man. *J Clin Invest* 63:695, 1979.

90. Kelemen MH, Gillilan RE, Bouchard RJ, et al: Diagnosis of obstructive coronary disease by maximal exercise and atrial pacing. *Circulation* 48:1227, 1973.

91. Rios JC, Hurwitz LE: Electrocardiographic responses to atrial pacing and multistage treadmill exercise testing: Correlation with coronary arteriography. *Am J Cardiol* 34:661, 1974.

92. Manca C, Bianchi G, Effendy FN, et al: Comparison of five different stress testing methods in the ECG diagnosis of coronary artery disease: Correlation with coronary arteriography. *Cardiology* 64:325, 1979.

93. Linhart JW: Atrial pacing in coronary artery disease. *Am J Med* 53:64, 1972.

94. Markham RV, Winniford MD, Firth BG, et al: Symptomatic, electrocardiographic, metabolic, and hemodynamic alterations during pacing-induced myocardial ischemia. *Am J Cardiol* 51:1590, 1983.

95. Johnson RA, Wasserman AG, Leiboff RH, et al: Intravenous digital left ventriculography at rest and with atrial pacing as a screening procedure for coronary artery disease. *J Am Coll Cardiol* 2:905, 1983.

96. McKay RG, Aroesty JM, Heller GV, et al: The pacing stress test reexamined: Correlation of pacing-induced hemodynamic changes with the amount of myocardium at risk. *J Am Coll Cardiol* 6:1469, 1984.

97. Stone D, Dymond D, Elliott AT, et al: Use of first-pass radionuclide ventriculography in assessment of wall motion abnormalities induced by incremental atrial pacing in patients with coronary artery disease. *Br Heart J* 43:369, 1980.

98. Hecht HS, Chew CY, Burnam M, et al: Radionuclide ejection fraction and regional wall motion during atrial pacing in stable angina pectoris: Comparison with metabolic and hemodynamic parameters. *Am Heart J* 101:726, 1981.

99. Tzivoni D, Weiss AT, Solomon J, et al: Diagnosis of coronary artery disease by multigated radionuclide angiography during right atrial pacing. *Chest* 80:562, 1981.

100. Weiss AT, Gotsman MS, Tzivoni D, et al: Nuclear left ventriculography at rest and during atrial pacing in the evaluation of coronary artery disease. *Isr J Med Sci* 19:1075, 1983.

101. Weiss AT, Tzivoni D, Sagie A, et al: Atrial pacing thallium scintigraphy in the evaluation of coronary artery disease. *Isr J Med Sci* 19:495, 1983.

102. Heller GV, Aroesty JM, Parker JA, et al: The pacing stress test: Thallium-201 myocardial imaging after atrial pacing—Diagnostic value in detecting coronary artery disease compared with exercise testing. *J Am Coll Cardiol* 3:1197, 1984.

103. Stratmann HG, Mark AL, Walter KE, et al: Prognostic value of atrial pacing and thallium-201 scintigraphy in patients with stable chest pain. *Am J Cardiol* 64:985, 1989.

104. LeFeuvre C, Bacheron A, Metzger JPh, et al: Comparison of thallium myocardial scintigraphy after exercise and transesophageal atrial pacing in the diagnosis of coronary artery disease. *Eur Heart J* 13:794, 1992.

105. Cuocolo A, Santomauro M, Pace L, et al: Comparison between exercise and transesophageal atrial pacing in patients with coronary artery disease: Technetium-99m methoxy isobutyl isonitrile simultaneous evaluation of ventricular function and myocardial perfusion. *Eur J Nucl Med* 19:119, 1992.

106. Iliceto S, Sorino M, D'Ambrosio G, et al: Detection of coronary artery disease by two-dimensional echocardiography and transesophageal atrial pacing. *J Am Coll Cardiol* 5:1188, 1985.

107. Matthews RV, Haskell RJ, Gintzon LE, et al: Usefulness of esophageal pill electrode atrial pacing with quantitative two-dimensional echocardiography for diagnosing coronary artery disease. *Am J Cardiol* 64:730, 1989.

108. Marangelli V, Iliceto S, Piccinni G, et al: Detection of coronary artery disease by digital stress echocardiography: Comparison of exercise, transesophageal atrial pacing and dipyridamole echocardiography. *J Am Coll Cardiol* 24:117, 1994.

109. Stratmann HG, Kennedy HL: Evaluation of coronary artery disease in the patient unable to exercise: Alternatives to exercise stress testing. *Am Heart J* 117:1344, 1989.

110. Lau SH, Cohen SI, Stein E, et al: Controlled heart rate by atrial pacing in angina pectoris. *Circulation* 38:711, 1968.

111. Brooks PM, Cutforth R: The value of the atria pacing test. *Med J Aust* 1:470, 1971.

112. Linhart JW: Atrial pacing in coronary artery disease, including preinfarction angina and postoperative studies. *Am J Cardiol* 30:603, 1972.

113. Piessens J, Van Mieghem W, Kesteloot H, et al: Diagnostic value of clinical history, exercise testing and atrial pacing in patients with chest pain. *Am J Cardiol* 33:351, 1974.

114. Malacoff RF, Mudge GH Jr, Holman L, et al: Effect of the cold pressor test on regional myocardial blood flow in patients with coronary artery disease. *Am Heart J* 106:78, 1983.

115. Neill WA, Duncan DA, Kloster F, et al: Response of coronary circulation to cutaneous cold. *Am J Med* 56:471, 1974.

116. Ahmad M, Dubiel JP, Haibach H: Cold pressor thallium-201 scintigraphy in the diagnosis of coronary artery disease. *Am J Cardiol* 50:1253, 1982.

117. Jordan LJ, Borer JS, Zullo M, et al: Exercise versus cold temperature stimulation during radionuclide cineangiography: Diagnostic accuracy in coronary artery disease. *Am J Cardiol* 51:1091, 1983.

118. Nabel EG, Ganz P, Gordon JB, et al: Dilation of normal and constriction of atherosclerotic coronary arteries caused by the cold pressor test. *Circulation* 77:43, 1988.

119. Shea DJ, Ockene IS, Greene HL: Acute myocardial infarction provoked by a cold pressor test. *Chest* 80:649, 1981.

120. Voudoukis IJ: Cold pressor test: A new application as a screening test for arteriosclerosis. *Angiology* 24:472, 1973.

121. Raizner AE, Chahine RA, Ishmori T, et al: Provocation of coronary artery spasm by the cold pressor test: Hemodynamic, arteriographic and quantitative angiographic observations. *Circulation* 62:925, 1980.

122. Wainwright RJ, Brennand-Roper, Cueni TA, et al: Cold pressor test in detection of coronary heart-disease and cardiomyopathy using technetium-99m gated blood-pool imaging. *Lancet* 320:Aug, 1989.

123. Wynne J, Holman L, Mudge GH, et al: Clinical utility of cold pressor radionuclide ventriculography in coronary artery disease. *Am J Cardiol* 47:444, 1981 (abstr).

124. Manyari DE, Nolewajka AJ, Purves P, et al: Comparative value of the cold-pressor test and supine bicycle exercise to detect subjects with coronary artery disease using radionuclide ventriculography. *Circulation* 65:571, 1982.

125. Giles R, Marx P, Commerford P, et al: Rapid sequential changes in left ventricular function during cold pressor and isometric handgrip: Relationship to blood pressure and mechanistic implications. *Am J Cardiol* 49:1002, 1982.

126. Verani MS, Zacca NM, DeBauche TL, et al: Comparison of cold pressor and exercise radionuclide angiocardiography in coronary artery disease. *J Nucl Med* 23:770, 1982.

127. Wasserman AG, Reiss L, Katz RJ, et al: Insensitivity of the cold pressor stimulation test for the diagnosis of coronary artery disease. *Circulation* 67:1189, 1983.

128. Dymond DS, Caplan JL, Platman W, et al: Temporal evolution of changes in left ventricular function induced by cold pressor stimulation: An assessment with radionuclide angiography and gold 195m. *Br Heart J* 51:557, 1984.

129. Northcote RJ, Cooke MBD: How useful are the cold pressor test and sustained isometric handgrip exercise with radionuclide ventriculography in the evaluation of patients with coronary artery disease? *Br Heart J* 57:319, 1987.

130. Gondi B, Nanda NC: Cold pressor test during two-dimensional echocardiography: Usefulness in detection of patients with coronary disease. *Am Heart J* 107:278, 1984.

131. Verani MS: Pharmacologic stress myocardial perfusion imaging. *Curr Probl Cardiol* 18:483, 1993.

132. Sonnenblick EH, Frishman WH, LeJemtel TH, et al: A new synthetic cardioactive sympathetic amine. *N Engl J Med* 300:17, 1979.

133. Ruffolo RR Jr, Sjpradlin TA, Pollock GD, et al: Alpha and beta-adrenergic effects of the stereoisomers of dobutamine. *J Pharmacol Exp Ther* 219:447, 1981.

134. Meyer SL, Curry GC, Consky MS, et al: Influence of dobutamine on hemodynamics and coronary blood flow in patients with and without coronary artery disease. *Am J Cardiol* 38:103, 1976.

135. Iskandrian AS, Verani MS, Heo J: Pharmacologic stress testing: Mechanism of action, hemodynamic responses, and results in detection of coronary artery disease. *J Nucl Cardiol* 1:94, 1994.

136. Liang CS, Hood WB Jr: Dobutamine infusion in conscious dogs with and without autonomic nervous system inhibition: Effects of systemic hemodynamics, regional blood flows and cardiac metabolism. *J Pharmacol Exp Ther* 211:698, 1979.

137. Coma-Canella I, Ortuno F: Comparison of diastolic blood pressure changes with dobutamine and exercise test. *Eur Heart J* 13:1245, 1992.

138. Chatterjee K: Effects of dobutamine on coronary hemodynamics and myocardial energetics, in *Dobutamine: A Ten Year Review*. New York, NCM, 1989, p 49.

139. Hays JT, Mahmarian JJ, Cochran AJ, et al: Dobutamine thallium-201 tomography for evaluating patients with suspected coronary artery disease unable to undergo exercise or vasodilatory pharmacologic testing. *J Am Coll Cardiol* 21:1583, 1993.

140. Fung AY, Gallagher KP, Buda AJ: The physiologic basis of dobutamine as compared with dipyridamole stress interventions in the assessment of critical coronary stenosis. *Circulation* 76:943, 1987.

141. Willerson JT, Hutton I, Watson JT, et al: Influence of dobutamine on regional myocardial blood flow and ventricular performance during acute and chronic myocardial ischemia in dogs. *Circulation* 53:828, 1976.

142. Warltier DC, Zyvoloski M, Gross GJ, et al: Redistribution of myocardial blood flow distal to a dynamic coronary arterial stenosis by sympathomimetic amines: Comparison of dopamine, dobutamine and isoproterenol. *Am J Cardiol* 48:269, 1981.

143. Vatner SF, Gaig H: Importance of heart rate in determining the effects of sympathomimetic amines on regional myocardial function and blood flow in conscious dogs with acute myocardial ischemia. *Circ Res* 45:793, 1979.

144. Knabb RM, Gidday JM, Ely SW, et al: Effects of dipyridamole on myocardial adenosine and active hyperemia. *Am J Physiol* 247:H804, 1984.

145. Wilson RF, Wyche K, Christensen BV, et al: Effects of adenosine on human coronary arterial circulation. *Circulation* 82:1595, 1990.

146. Pennell DJ, Underwood R, Swanton RH, et al: Dobutamine thallium myocardial perfusion tomography. *J Am Coll Cardiol* 18:1471, 1991.

147. Mertes H, Sawada SG, Ryan T, et al: Symptoms, adverse

effects, and complications associated with dobutamine stress echocardiography: Experience in 1118 patients. *Circulation* 88:15, 1993.

148. Previtali M, Lanzarini L, Mussini A, et al: Dobutamine-induced ST segment elevation in a patient with angina at rest and critical coronary lesions. *Eur Heart J* 13:997, 1992.

149. Mazeika PK, Nadazdin A, Oakley CM: Clinical significance of abrupt vasodepression during dobutamine stress echocardiography. *Am J Cardiol* 69:1484, 1992.

150. Marcovitz PA, Bach DS, Mathias W, et al: Paradoxic hypotension during dobutamine stress echocardiography: Clinical and diagnostic implications. *J Am Coll Cardiol* 21:1080, 1993.

151. Pennell DJ, Underwood R, Ell PJ: Safety of dobutamine stress for thallium-201 myocardial perfusion tomography in patients with asthma. *Am J Cardiol* 71:1346, 1993.

152. Mahmarian JJ, Verani MS: Myocardial perfusion imaging during pharmacologic stress testing. *Cardiol Clin* 12:223, 1994.

153. Mannering D, Cripps T, Leech G, et al: The dobutamine stress test as an alternative to exercise testing after acute myocardial infarction. *Br Heart J* 59:521, 1988.

154. Coma-Canella I: Significance of ST segment changes induced by dobutamine stress test after acute myocardial infarction: Which are reciprocal? *Eur Heart J* 12:909, 1991.

155. Coma-Canella I, Daza NS, Orbe LC: Detection of restenosis with dobutamine stress test after coronary angioplasty. *Am Heart J* 124:1196, 1992.

156. Mason JR, Palac RT, Freeman ML, et al: Thallium scintigraphy during dobutamine infusion: Nonexercise-dependent screening test for coronary disease. *Am Heart J* 107:481, 1984.

157. Warner MF, Pippin JJ, DiSciascio G, et al: Assessment of thallium scintigraphy and echocardiography during dobutamine infusion for the detection of coronary artery disease. *Cathet Cardiovasc Diagn* 29:122, 1993.

158. Wallbridge DR, Twekkel AC, Martin W, et al: A comparison of dobutamine and maximal exercise as stress for thallium scintigraphy. *Eur J Nucl Med* 20:319, 1993.

159. Kumar EB, Steel SA, Howey S, et al: Dipyridamole is superior to dobutamine for thallium stress imaging: A randomized crossover study. *Br Heart J* 71:129, 1994.

160. Baig MW, Sheard K, Thorley PJ, et al: The use of dobutamine stress thallium scintigraphy in the diagnosis of syndrome X. *Postgrad Med J* 68:S20, 1992.

161. Voth E, Baer FM, Theissen P, et al: Dobutamine ^{99m}Tc-MIBI single-photon emission tomography: Non-exercise-dependent detection of haemodynamically significant coronary artery stenoses. *Eur J Nucl Med* 21:537, 1994.

162. Marwick TH, D'Hondt AM, Mairesse GH, et al: Comparative ability of dobutamine and exercise stress in inducing myocardial ischaemia in active patients. *Br Heart J* 72:31, 1994.

163. Herman SD, LaBresh KA, Santos-Ocampo CD, et al: Comparison of dobutamine and exercise using technetium-99m sestamibi imaging for the evaluation of coronary artery disease. *Am J Cardiol* 73:164, 1994.

164. Günalp B, Dokumaci B, Uyan C, et al: Value of dobuta-mine technetium-99m–sestamibi SPECT and echocardiography in the detection of coronary artery disease compared with coronary angiography. *J Nucl Med* 34:889, 1993.

165. Marwick T, D'Hondt A, Baudhuin T, et al: Optimal use of dobutamine stress for the detection and evaluation of coronary artery disease: Combination with echocardiography or scintigraphy, or both? *J Am Coll Cardiol* 22:159, 1993.

166. Marwick T, Willemart B, D'Hondt A, et al: Selection of the optimal nonexercise stress for the evaluation of ischemic regional myocardial dysfunction and malperfusion: Comparison of dobutamine and adenosine using echocardiography and ^{99m}Tc-MIBI single photon emission computed tomography. *Circulation* 87:345, 1993.

167. Forster R, McNeill AJ, Salustri A, et al: Simultaneous dobutamine stress echocardiography and technetium-99m isonitrile single-photon emission computed tomography in patients with suspected coronary artery disease. *J Am Coll Cardiol* 21:1591, 1993.

168. Coma-Canella I, del Val Gomez Martinez M, Rodrigo F, et al: The dobutamine stress test with thallium-201 single-photon emission computed tomography and radionuclide angiography: Postinfarction study. *J Am Coll Cardiol* 22:399, 1993.

169. Elliott BM, Robinson JG, Zellner JL, et al: Dobutamine–^{201}Tl imaging: Assessing cardiac risks associated with vascular surgery. *Circulation* 84(suppl III):III-54, 1991.

170. Wilson RF, White CW: Intra coronary papaverine: An ideal coronary vasodilator for studies of the coronary circulation in conscious humans. *Circulation* 73:444, 1986.

171. Berne RM: The role of adenosine in the regulation of coronary blood flow. *Circ Res* 47:807, 1980.

172. Belardinelli L, Linden J, Berne RM: The cardiac effects of adenosine. *Prog Cardiovasc Dis* 32:73, 1989.

173. Verani MS: Adenosine thallium-201 myocardial perfusion scintigraphy. *Am Heart J* 122:269, 1991.

174. Iskandrian AS: Adenosine myocardial perfusion imaging. *J Nucl Med* 35:734, 1994.

175. Kurtz A: Adenosine stimulates guanylate cyclase activity in vascular smooth muscle cells. *J Biol Chem* 262:6296, 1987.

176. Moser GH, Schrader J, Deussen A: Turnover of adenosine in plasma of human and dog blood. *Am J Physiol (Cell Physiol 25)* 256:C799, 1989.

177. Knabb RM, Gidday JM, Ely SW, et al: Effects of dipyridamole on myocardial adenosine and active hyperemia. *Am J Physiol (Heart Circ Physiol 16)* 247:H804, 1984.

178. Fitzgerald GA: Dipyridamole. *N Engl J Med* 316:1247, 1987.

179. Daley PJ, Mahn TH, Zielonka JS, et al: Effect of maintenance oral theophylline on dipyridamole–thallium-201 myocardial imaging using SPECT and dipyridamole-induced hemodynamic changes. *Am Heart J* 115:1185, 1988.

180. Stanek EJ, Melko GP, Charland SL: Xanthine interference with dipyridamole–thallium-201 myocardial imaging. *Ann Pharmacother* 29:425, 1995.

181. Heller GV, Dweik RB, Barbour MM, et al: Pretreatment

with theophylline does not affect adenosine-induced thallium-201 myocardial imaging. *Am Heart J* 126:1077, 1993.

182. Smits P, Corstens FHM, Aengevaeren WRM, et al: False-negative dipyridamole–thallium-201 myocardial imaging after caffeine ingestion. *J Nucl Med* 32:1538, 1991.

183. Jacobson AF, Cerqueira MD, Taisys V, et al: Serum caffeine levels after 24 hours of caffeine abstention: Observations on clinical patients undergoing myocardial perfusion imaging with dipyridamole or adenosine. *Eur J Nucl Med* 21:23, 1994.

184. Brown KA, Slinker BK: Pentoxifylline (Trental) does not inhibit dipyridamole-induced coronary hyperemia: Implications for dipyridamole–thallium-201 myocardial imaging. *J Nucl Med* 31:1020, 1990.

185. O'Byrne GT, Makkahi J, Rozanski A, et al: Myocardial washout of thallium-201 following dipyridamole infusion varies with the infused dose: Implication that adequate myocardial hyperemia may not be achieved by standard dipyridamole dose. *Clin Nucl Med* 11:17, 1986 (abstr).

186. Wilson RF, Laughlin DE, Ackell PH, et al: Transluminal, subselective measurement of coronary artery blood flow velocity and vasodilator reserve in man. *Circulation* 72:82, 1985.

187. Rossen JD, Quillen JE, Lopez AG, et al: Comparison of coronary vasodilation with intravenous dipyridamole and adenosine. *J Am Coll Cardiol* 18:485, 1991.

188. Casanova R, Patroncini A, Guidalotti PL, et al: Dose and test for dipyridamole infusion and cardiac imaging early after uncomplicated acute myocardial infarction. *Am J Cardiol* 70:1402, 1992.

189. Lalonde D, Taillefer R, Lambert R, et al: Thallium-201–dipyridamole imaging: Comparison between a standard dose and a high dose of dipyridamole in the detection of coronary artery disease. *J Nucl Med* 35:1245, 1994.

190. Wilson RF, Wyche K, Christensen BV, et al: Effects of adenosine on human coronary arterial circulation. *Circulation* 82:1595, 1990.

191. Albro PC, Gould KL, Westcott RJ, et al: Noninvasive assessment of coronary stenoses by myocardial imaging during pharmacologic coronary vasodilation. III. Clinical trial. *Am J Cardiol* 42:751, 1978.

192. Gould KL, Schelbert HR, Phelps ME, et al: Noninvasive assessment of coronary stenoses with myocardial perfusion imaging during pharmacologic coronary vasodilation. V. Detection of 47 percent diameter coronary stenosis with intravenous nitrogen-13 ammonia and emission-computed tomography in intact dogs. *Am J Cardiol* 43:200, 1979.

193. Brown BG, Josephson MA, Peterson RB, et al: Intravenous dipyridamole combined with isometric handgrip for near maximal acute increase in coronary flow in patients with coronary artery disease. *Am J Cardiol* 48:1077, 1981.

194. Josephson MA, Brown BG, Hecht HS, et al: Noninvasive detection and localization of coronary stenoses in patients: Comparison of resting dipyridamole and exercise thallium-201 myocardial perfusion imaging. *Am Heart J* 103:1008, 1982.

195. Leppo J, Boucher CA, Okada RD, et al: Serial thallium-201 myocardial imaging after dipyridamole infusion: Diagnostic utility in detecting coronary stenoses and relationship to regional wall motion. *Circulation* 66:649, 1982.

196. Bonaduce D, Muto P, Morgano G, et al: Effect of beta-blockade on thallium-201 dipyridamole myocardial scintigraphy. *Acta Cardiol* 39:399, 1984.

197. Tavazzi L, Previtali M, Salerno JA, et al: Dipyridamole test in angina pectoris: Diagnostic value and pathophysiological implications. *Cardiology* 69:34, 1982.

198. Klein HO, Ninio R, Eliyahu S, et al: Effects of the dipyridamole test on left ventricular function in coronary artery disease. *Am J Cardiol* 69:482, 1992.

199. Verani MS, Mahmarian JJ, Hixson JB, et al: Diagnosis of coronary artery disease by controlled coronary vasodilation with adenosine and thallium-201 scintigraphy in patients unable to exercise. *Circulation* 82:80, 1990.

200. Ogilby JD, Iskandrian A, Untereker WJ, et al: Effect of intravenous adenosine on myocardial perfusion and function: Hemodynamic/angiographic and scintigraphic study. *Circulation* 86:887, 1992.

201. Abreu A, Mahmarian JJ, Nishimura S, et al: Tolerance and safety of pharmacologic coronary vasodilation with adenosine in association with thallium-201 scintigraphy in patients with suspected coronary artery disease. *J Am Coll Cardiol* 18:730, 1991.

202. Vogel WM, Apstein CS, Briggs LL, et al: Acute alterations in left ventricular diastolic chamber stiffness: Role of the "erectile" effect of coronary arterial pressure and flow in normal and damaged hearts. *Circ Res* 51:465, 1982.

203. Chierchia S, Lazzari M, Freedman B, et al: Impairment of myocardial perfusion and function during painless myocardial ischemia. *J Am Coll Cardiol* 1:924, 1983.

204. Poliner LR, Farber SH, Glaeser DH, et al: Alteration of diastolic filling rate during exercise radionuclide angiography: A highly sensitive technique for detection of coronary artery disease. *Circulation* 70:942, 1984.

205. Heiss HW, Barmeyer J, Wink K, et al: Studies on the regulation of myocardial blood flow in man. I. Training effects on blood flow and metabolism of the healthy heart at rest and during standardized heavy exercise. *Basic Res Cardiol* 71:658, 1976.

206. Cole JS, Hartley CJ: The pulsed Doppler coronary artery catheter: Preliminary report of a new technique for measuring rapid changes in coronary artery flow velocity in man. *Circulation* 56:18, 1977.

207. Rossen JD, Simonetti I, Marcus ML, et al: Coronary dilation with standard dose dipyridamole and dipyridamole combined with handgrip. *Circulation* 79:566, 1989.

208. McGinn AL, White CW, Wilson RF: Interstudy variability of coronary flow reserve: Influence of heart rate, arterial pressure, and ventricular preload. *Circulation* 81:1319, 1990.

209. Kern MJ, Deligonul U, Tatineni S, et al: Intravenous adenosine: Continuous infusion and low-dose bolus administration for determination of coronary vasodilator reserve in patients with and without coronary artery disease. *J Am Coll Cardiol* 18:718, 1991.

210. Lapeyre AC III, Gibbons RJ: Electrocardiographic fluc-

tuations during adenosine stress testing. *Mayo Clin Proc* 69:587, 1994.

211. Mohiuddin SM, Esterbrooks DJ, Gupta NC, et al: Safety of different dosages of intravenous adenosine used in conjunction with diagnostic myocardial imaging techniques. *Pharmacotherapy* 13:476, 1993.

212. Chan SY, Brunken RC, Czernin J, et al: Comparison of maximal myocardial blood flow during adenosine infusion with that of intravenous dipyridamole in normal men. *J Am Coll Cardiol* 20:979, 1992.

213. Beller GA, Granato JE, Cannon JM, et al: Effects of intra coronary dipyridamole infusion on regional myocardial blood flow and intrinsic thallium-201 washout in dogs with a critical coronary stenosis. *Am Heart J* 124:56, 1992.

214. Marchant E, Pichard A, Rodriguez JA, et al: Acute effect of systemic versus intracoronary dipyridamole on coronary circulation. *Am J Cardiol* 57:1401, 1986.

215. Arrotti J, Gunnar RM, Ward J, et al: Comparative effects of intravenous dipyridamole and sublingual nitroglycerin on coronary hemodynamics and myocardial metabolism at rest and during atrial pacing in patients with coronary artery disease. *Clin Cardiol* 3:365, 1980.

216. Feldman RL, Nichols WW, Pepine CJ, et al: Acute effect of intravenous dipyridamole on regional coronary hemodynamics and metabolism. *Circulation* 64:333, 1981.

217. Marchant E, Pichard AD, Casanegra P, et al: Effect of intravenous dipyridamole on regional coronary blood flow with 1-vessel coronary artery disease: Evidence against coronary steal. *Am J Cardiol* 53:718, 1984.

218. Iskandrian AS, Heo J, Nguyen T, et al: Assessment of coronary artery disease using single-photon emission computed tomography with thallium-201 during adenosine-induced coronary hyperemia. *Am J Cardiol* 67:1190, 1991.

219. Nishimura S, Kimball KT, Mahmarian JJ, et al: Angiographic and hemodynamic determinants of myocardial ischemia during adenosine thallium-201 scintigraphy in coronary artery disease. *Circulation* 87:1211, 1993.

220. Straat E, Henriksson P, Edlund A: Adenosine provokes myocardial ischaemia in patients with ischaemic heart disease without increasing cardiac work. *J Intern Med* 230:319, 1991.

221. Iskandrian AS: Myocardial ischemia during pharmacological stress testing. *Circulation* 87:1415, 1993.

222. Ando J, Yasuda H, Kobayashi T, et al: Conditions for "coronary steal" caused by coronary vasodilator in man. *Jpn Heart J* 23:79, 1982.

223. Villanueva FS, Smith WH, Watson DD, et al: ST-segment depression during dipyridamole infusion, and its clinical, scintigraphic and hemodynamic correlates. *Am J Cardiol* 69:445, 1992.

224. Marshall ES, Raichlen JS, Tighe DA, et al: ST-segment depression during adenosine infusion as a predictor of myocardial ischemia. *Am Heart J* 127:305, 1994.

225. Marshall ES, Raichlen JS, Kim SM, et al: Prognostic significance of ST-segment depression during adenosine perfusion imaging. *Am Heart J* 130:58, 1995.

226. Barbour MM, Garber CE, Ahlberg AW, et al: Effects of intravenous theophylline on exercise-induced myocardial

ischemia. II. A concentration-dependent phenomenon. *J Am Coll Cardiol* 22:1155, 1993.

227. Laxson DD, Homans DC, Bache RJ: Inhibition of adenosine-mediated coronary vasodilation exacerbates myocardial ischemia during exercise. *Heart Circ Physiol* 34:H1471, 1993.

228. Sylven C, Beermann B, Jonzon B, et al: Angina pectoris-like pain provoked by intravenous adenosine in healthy volunteers. *BMJ* 293:227, 1986.

229. Homma S, Gilliland Y, Guiney TE: Safety of intravenous dipyridamole for stress testing with thallium imaging. *Am J Cardiol* 59:152, 1987.

230. Pearlman JD, Boucher CA: Diagnostic value for coronary artery disease of chest pain during dipyridamole-thallium stress testing. *Am J Cardiol* 61:43, 1988.

231. Laarman GJ, Serruys PW, Verzijlbergen JF, et al: Thallium-201 scintigraphy after dipyridamole infusion with low-level exercise. III. Clinical significance and additional diagnostic value of ST segment depression and angina pectoris during the test. *Eur Heart J* 11:705, 1990.

232. Jain A, Suarez J, Mahmarian JJ, et al: Functional significance of myocardial perfusion defects induced by dipyridamole using thallium-201 single-photon emission computed tomography and two-dimensional echocardiography. *Am J Cardiol* 66:802, 1990.

233. Whitfield S, Aurigemma G, Pape L, et al: Two-dimensional Doppler echocardiographic correlation of dipyridamole–thallium stress testing with isometric handgrip. *Am Heart J* 121:1367, 1991.

234. McLaughlin DP, Beller GA, Linden J, et al: Hemodynamic and metabolic correlates of dipyridamole-induced myocardial thallium-201 perfusion abnormalities in multivessel coronary artery disease. *Am J Cardiol* 74:1159, 1994.

235. Picano E, Masini M, Lattanzi F, et al: Role of dipyridamole–echocardiography test in electrocardiographically silent effort myocardial ischemia. *Am J Cardiol* 58:235, 1986.

236. Margonato A, Chierchia S, Cianflone D, et al: Limitations of dipyridamole–echocardiography in effort angina pectoris. *Am J Cardiol* 59:225, 1987.

237. Perin EC, Moore W, Blume M, et al: Comparison of dipyridamole–echocardiography with dipyridamole–thallium scintigraphy for the diagnosis of myocardial ischemia. *Clin Nucl Med* 16:418, 1991.

238. Pirelli S, Danzi GB, Massa D, et al: Exercise thallium scintigraphy versus high-dose dipyridamole echocardiography testing for detection of asymptomatic restenosis in patients with positive exercise tests after coronary angioplasty. *Am J Cardiol* 71:1052, 1993.

239. Ciliberto GR, Massa D, Mangiavacchi M, et al: High-dose dipyridamole echocardiography test in coronary artery disease after transplantation. *Eur Heart J* 14:48, 1993.

240. Zoghbi WA: Use of adenosine echocardiography for diagnosis of coronary artery disease. *Am Heart J* 122:285, 1991.

241. Nguyen T, Heo J, Ogilby JD, et al: Single photon emission computed tomography with thallium-201 during adenosine-induced coronary hyperemia: Correlation with coronary angiography, exercise thallium imaging

and two-dimensional echocardiography. *J Am Coll Cardiol* 16:1375, 1990.

242. Walker PR, James MA, Wilde RPH, et al: Dipyridamole combined with exercise for thallium-201 myocardial imaging. *Br Heart J* 55:321, 1986.

243. Borges-Neto S, Mahmarian JJ, Jain A, et al: Quantitative thallium-201 single photon emission computed tomography after oral dipyridamole for assessing the presence, anatomic location and severity of coronary artery disease. *J Am Coll Cardiol* 11:962, 1988.

244. Beer SG, Heo J, Kong B, et al: Use of oral dipyridamole SPECT thallium-201 imaging in detection of coronary artery disease. *Am Heart J* 118:1022, 1989.

245. Jain A, Hicks RR, Myers GH, et al: Comparison of coronary angiography and early oral dipyridamole thallium-201 scintigraphy in patients receiving thrombolytic therapy for acute myocardial infarction. *Am Heart J* 120: 839, 1990.

246. Jain A, Myers GH, Rowe MW, et al: Comparison of coronary angiographic features and oral dipyridamole thallium 201 tomography. *Angiology* 42:99, 1991.

247. Taillefer R, Lette J, Phaneuf D-C, et al: Thallium-201 myocardial imaging during pharmacologic coronary vasodilation: Comparison of oral and intravenous administration of dipyridamole. *J Am Coll Cardiol* 8:76, 1986.

248. Boudreau RJ, Strony JT, du Cret RP, et al: Perfusion thallium imaging of type I diabetes patients with end stage renal disease: Comparison of oral and intravenous dipyridamole administration. *Radiology* 175:103, 1990.

249. Gould KL, Sorenson SG, Caldwell JH, et al: Thallium-201 myocardial imaging during coronary vasodilation induced by oral dipyridamole. *J Nucl Med* 27:31, 1986.

250. Homma S, Callahan RJ, Ameer B, et al: Usefulness of oral dipyridamole suspension for stress thallium imaging without exercise in the detection of coronary artery disease. *Am J Cardiol* 57:503, 1986.

251. Segall GM, Davis MJ: Variability of serum drug level following a single oral dose of dipyridamole. *J Nucl Med* 29:1662, 1988.

252. Lavie E, Gergans G, Somberg JC: A comparison of tablets with oral suspension formulation of dipyridamole in thallium myocardial imaging. *J Clin Pharmacol* 32:546, 1992.

253. Kahn D, Argenyi EA, Berbaum K, et al: The incidence of serious hemodynamic changes in physically-limited patients following oral dipyridamole challenge before thallium-201 scintigraphy. *Clin Nucl Med* 15:678, 1990.

254. Nielsen-Kudsk F, Pedersen AK: Pharmacokinetics of dipyridamole. *Acta Pharmacol Toxicol* 44:391, 1979.

255. Gerson MC, Moore EN, Ellis K: Systemic effects and safety of intravenous dipyridamole in elderly patients with suspected coronary artery disease. *Am J Cardiol* 60:1399, 1987.

256. Ando S, Ashihara T, Ando H, et al: Safety and accuracy of dipyridamole thallium myocardial scintigraphy in elderly patients. *Jpn Heart J* 34:245, 1993.

257. Johnston DL, Daley JR, Hodge DO, et al: Hemodynamic responses and adverse effects associated with adenosine and dipyridamole pharmacologic stress testing: A comparison in 2000 patients. *Mayo Clin Proc* 70:331, 1995.

258. Ranhosky A, Kempthorne-Rawson J, and the Intrave-nous Dipyridamole Thallium Imaging Study Group: The safety of intravenous dipyridamole thallium myocardial perfusion imaging. *Circulation* 81:1205, 1990.

259. Bayliss BJ, Pearson M, Sutton GC: Ventricular dysrhythmias following intravenous dipyridamole during "stress" myocardial imaging. *Br J Radiol* 56:686, 1983.

260. Friedman HZ, Goldberg SF, Hauser AM, et al: Death with dipyridamole–thallium imaging. *Ann Intern Med* 109:990, 1988.

261. Blumenthal MS, McCauley CS: Cardiac arrest during dipyridamole imaging. *Chest* 93:1103, 1988.

262. Dubrey SW, Bomanji JB, Noble MIM, et al: Safety of intravenous dipyridamole thallium myocardial perfusion imaging: Experience in 435 patients. *Nucl Med Commun* 14:303, 1993.

263. Keitz TN, Innerfield M, Gitler B, et al: Dipyridamole-induced myocardial ischemia. *JAMA* 257:1515, 1987.

264. Lewen MK, Labovitz AJ, Kern MJ, et al: Prolonged myocardial ischemia after intravenous dipyridamole thallium imaging. *Chest* 92:1102, 1987.

265. Kwai AH, Jacobson AF, McIntyre KM, et al: Persistent chest pain following oral dipyridamole for thallium 201 myocardial imaging. *Eur J Nucl Med* 16:745, 1990.

266. Perper EJ, Segall GM: Safety of dipyridamole–thallium imaging in high risk patients with known or suspected coronary artery disease. *J Nucl Med* 32:2107, 1991.

267. Cushley MJ, Tattersfield AE, Holgate ST: Inhaled adenosine and guanosine on airway resistance in normal and asthmatic subjects. *Br J Clin Pharmacol* 15:161, 1983.

268. Picano E, Marini C, Pirelli S, et al: Safety of intravenous high-dose dipyridamole echocardiography. *Am J Cardiol* 70:252, 1992.

269. Picano E, Lattanzi F, Masini M, et al: Aminophylline termination of dipyridamole stress as a trigger of coronary vasospasm in variant angina. *Am J Cardiol* 62:694, 1988.

270. Leppo JA, O'Brien J, Tothendler JA, et al: Dipyridamole thallium-201 scintigraphy in the prediction of future cardiac events after acute myocardial infarction. *N Engl J Med* 310:1014, 1984.

271. Gimple LW, Hutter AM, Guiney TE, et al: Prognostic utility of predischarge dipyridamole–thallium imaging compared to predischarge submaximal exercise electrocardiography and maximal exercise thallium imaging after uncomplicated acute myocardial infarction. *Am J Cardiol* 64:1243, 1989.

272. Jain A, Hicks RR, Frantz DM, et al: Comparison of early exercise treadmill test and oral dipyridamole thallium-201 tomography for the identification of jeopardized myocardium in patients receiving thrombolytic therapy for acute Q-wave myocardial infarction. *Am J Cardiol* 66:551, 1990.

273. Brown KA, O'Meara J, Chambers CE, et al: Ability of dipyridamole–thallium-201 imaging one to four days after acute myocardial infarction to predict in-hospital and late recurrent myocardial ischemic events. *Am J Cardiol* 65:160, 1990.

274. Okada RD, Glover DK, Leppo JA: Dipyridamole ^{201}Tl scintigraphy in the evaluation of prognosis after myocardial infarction. *Circulation* 84(suppl I):I-132, 1991.

275. Hendel RC, Gore JM, Alpert JS, et al: Prognosis following

interventional therapy for acute myocardial infarction: Utility of dipyridamole thallium scintigraphy. *Cardiology* 79:73, 1991.

276. Okada RD, Bendersky R, Strauss HW, et al: Comparison of intravenous dipyridamole thallium cardiac imaging with exercise radionuclide angiography. *Am Heart J* 114:524, 1987.

277. Lette J, Tatum JL, Fraser S, et al: Safety of dipyridamole testing in 73,806 patients: The multicenter dipyridamole safety study. *J Nucl Cardiol* 2:3, 1995.

278. Cates CU, Kronenberg MW, Collins HW, et al: Dipyridamole radionuclide ventriculography: A test with high specificity for severe coronary artery disease. *J Am Coll Cardiol* 13:841, 1989.

279. Picano E, Lattanzi F, Masini M, et al: High dose dipyridamole echocardiography test in effort angina pectoris. *J Am Coll Cardiol* 8:848, 1986.

280. Weich HF, Strauss HW, Pitt B: The extraction of thallium-201 by the myocardium. *Circulation* 56:188, 1977.

281. Glover DK, Ruiz M, Edwards NC, et al: Comparison between ^{201}Tl and ^{99m}Tc sestamibi uptake during adenosine-induced vasodilation as a function of coronary stenosis severity. *Circulation* 91:813, 1995.

282. Mays AE, Cobb FR: Relationship between regional myocardial blood flow and thallium- 201 distribution in the presence of coronary artery stenosis and dipyridamole-induced vasodilation. *J Clin Invest* 73:1359, 1984.

283. Lee J, Chae SC, Lee K, et al: Biokinetics of thallium-201 in normal subjects: Comparison between adenosine, dipyridamole, dobutamine and exercise. *J Nucl Med* 35:535, 1994.

284. Pennell DJ, Ell PJ: Whole-body imaging of thallium-201 after six different stress regimens. *J Nucl Med* 35:425, 1994.

285. Beller GA, Holzgrefe HH, Watson DD: Intrinsic washout rates of thallium-201 in normal and ischemic myocardium after dipyridamole-induced vasodilation. *Circulation* 71:378, 1985.

286. O'Byrne GT, Rodrigues EA, Maddahi J, et al: Comparison of myocardial washout rate of thallium-201 between rest, dipyridamole with and without aminophylline, and exercise states in normal subjects. *Am J Cardiol* 64:1022, 1989.

287. Munck O, Madsen PV, Kelbaek H, et al: Comparison between reference values for ^{201}thallium uptake and washout from the myocardium after exercise and after dipyridamole. *Clin Physiol* 13:419, 1993.

288. Okada RD, Dai Y, Boucher CA, et al: Serial thallium-201 imaging after dipyridamole for coronary disease detection: Quantitative analysis using myocardial clearance. *Am Heart J* 107:475, 1984.

289. Narita M, Kurihara T, Usami M: Non-invasive detection of coronary artery disease by myocardial imaging with thallium-201: The significance of pharmacologic interventions. *Jpn Circ J* 45:127, 1981.

290. Francisco DA, Collins SM, Go RT, et al: Tomographic thallium-201 myocardial perfusion scintigrams after maximal coronary artery vasodilation with intravenous dipyridamole: Comparison of qualitative and quantitative approaches. *Circulation* 66:370, 1982.

291. Wilde P, Walker P, Watt I, et al: Thallium myocardial imaging: Recent experience using a coronary vasodilator. *Clin Radiol* 33:43, 1982.

292. Harris D, Taylor D, Condon B, et al: Myocardial imaging with dipyridamole: Comparison of the sensitivity and specificity of ^{201}Tl versus MUGA. *Eur J Nucl Med* 7:1, 1982.

293. Okada RD, Lim YL, Rothendler J, et al: Split-dose thallium-201 dipyridamole imaging: A new technique for obtaining thallium images before and immediately after an intervention. *J Am Coll Cardiol* 1:1302, 1983.

294. Sochor H, Pachinger O, Orgis E, et al: Radionuclide imaging after coronary vasodilation: Myocardial scintigraphy with thallium-201 and radionuclide angiography after administration of dipyridamole. *Eur Heart J* 5:500, 1984.

295. Iskandrian AS: What is the optimum dose of dipyridamole for cardiac imaging? *Am J Cardiol* 70:1485, 1992.

296. Schmoliner R, Dudczak R, Kronik G, et al: Impact of thallium-201 imaging on clinical assessment and management of patients with chest pain. *Clin Cardiol* 7:660, 1984.

297. Benjelloun L, Benjelloun H, Laudet M, et al: Discriminant analysis of thallium-201 myocardial scintigrams. *Nucl Med Commun* 6:149, 1985.

298. Ruddy TD, Dighero HR, Newell JB, et al: Quantitative analysis of dipyridamole–thallium images for the detection of coronary artery disease. *J Am Coll Cardiol* 10:142, 1987.

299. Lam JYT, Chaitman BR, Glaenzer M, et al: Safety and diagnostic accuracy of dipyridamole–thallium imaging in the elderly. *J Am Coll Cardiol* 11:585, 1988.

300. Laarman GJ, Bruschke AVG, Verzijlbergen FJ, et al: Efficacy of intravenous dipyridamole with exercise in thallium-201 myocardial perfusion scintigraphy. *Eur Heart J* 9:1206, 1988.

301. Boudreau RJ, Strony JT, du Cret RP, et al: Perfusion thallium imaging of type I diabetes patients with end stage renal disease: Comparison of oral and intravenous dipyridamole administration. *Radiology* 175:103, 1990.

302. DePuey EG, Guertler-Krawczynska E, D'Amato PH, et al: Thallium-201 single photon emission computed tomography with intravenous dipyridamole to diagnose coronary artery disease. *Coronary Artery Dis* 1:75, 1990.

303. Huikuri HV, Korhonen UR, Airaksinen J, et al: Comparison of dipyridamole–handgrip test and bicycle exercise test for thallium tomographic imaging. *Am J Cardiol* 61:264, 1988.

304. Zhu YY, Chung WS, Botvinick EH, et al: Dipyridamole perfusion scintigraphy: The experience with its application in one hundred seventy patients with known or suspected unstable angina. *Am Heart J* 121:33, 1991.

305. Kong BA, Shaw L, Miller D, et al: Comparison of accuracy for detecting coronary artery disease and side-effect profile of dipyridamole thallium-201 myocardial perfusion imaging in women versus men. *Am J Cardiol* 70:168, 1992.

306. Mendelson MA, Spies SM, Spies WG, et al: Usefulness of single-photon emission computed tomography of thallium-201 uptake after dipyridamole infusion for detection of coronary artery disease. *Am J Cardiol* 69:1150, 1992.

307. Popma JJ, Dehmer GJ, Walker BS, et al: Analysis of thallium-201 single-photon emission computed tomography after intravenous dipyridamole using different quantitative measures of coronary stenosis severity and receiver operator characteristic curves. *Am Heart J* 124:65, 1992.

308. Eichhorn EJ, Kosinski EJ, Lewis SM, et al: Usefulness of dipyridamole–thallium-201 perfusion scanning for distinguishing ischemic from nonischemic cardiomyopathy. *Am J Cardiol* 62:945, 1988.

309. Chikamori T, Doi Y, Yonezawa Y, et al: Value of dipyridamole thallium-201 imaging in noninvasive differentiation of idiopathic dilated cardiomyopathy from coronary artery disease with left ventricular dysfunction. *Am J Cardiol* 69:650, 1992.

310. Bridges AB, Kennedy N, McNeil GP, et al: The effect of atenolol on dipyridamole ^{201}Tl myocardial perfusion tomography in patients with coronary artery disease. *Nucl Med Commun* 13:41, 1992.

311. Varma SK, Watson DD, Beller GA: Quantitative comparison of thallium-201 scintigraphy after exercise and dipyridamole in coronary artery disease. *Am J Cardiol* 64:871, 1989.

312. Martin W, Tweddel AC, Main G, et al: A comparison of maximal exercise and dipyridamole thallium-201 planar gated scintigraphy. *Eur J Nucl Med* 19:258, 1992.

313. Walker PR, James MA, Wilde RPH, et al: Dipyridamole combined with exercise for thallium-201 myocardial imaging. *Br Heart J* 55:321, 1986.

314. Calale PN, Guiney TE, Strauss HW, et al: Simultaneous low level treadmill exercise and intravenous dipyridamole stress thallium imaging. *Am J Cardiol* 62:799, 1988.

315. Stern S, Greenberg D, Corne R: Effect of exercise supplementation on dipyridamole thallium-201 image quality. *J Nucl Med* 32:1559, 1991.

316. Ignaszewski AP, McCormick LX, Heslip PG, et al: Safety and clinical utility of combined intravenous dipyridamole/symptom-limited exercise stress test with thallium-201 imaging in patients with known or suspected coronary artery disease. *J Nucl Med* 34:2053, 1993.

317. Pennell DJ, Mavrogeni S, Anagnostopoulos C, et al: Thallium myocardial perfusion tomography using intravenous dipyridamole combined with maximal dynamic exercise. *Nucl Med Commun* 14:939, 1993.

318. Stern S, Greenberg D, Corne R: Quantification of walking exercise required for improvement of dipyridamole thallium-201 image quality. *J Nucl Med* 33:2061, 1992.

319. Okada RD, Dai YH, Boucher CA, et al: Significance of increased lung thallium-201 activity on serial cardiac images after dipyridamole treatment in coronary heart disease. *Am J Cardiol* 53:470, 1984.

320. Villanueva FS, Kaul S, Smith WH, et al: Prevalence and correlates of increased lung/heart ratio of thallium-201 during dipyridamole stress imaging for suspected coronary artery disease. *Am J Cardiol* 66:1324, 1990.

321. Movahed A, Reeves WC, Batts J, et al: Significance of increased Tl-201 uptake by the lungs in patients undergoing oral dipyridamole–thallium myocardial imaging. *Clin Nucl Med* 17:489, 1992.

322. Hurwitz GA, O'Donoghue P, Powe JE, et al: Pulmonary thallium-201 uptake following dipyridamole–exercise combination compared with single modality stress testing. *Am J Cardiol* 69:320, 1992.

323. Lette J, Lapointe J, Waters D, et al: Transient left ventricular cavitary dilation during dipyridamole–thallium imaging as an indicator of severe coronary artery disease. *Am J Cardiol* 66:1163, 1990.

324. Chouraqui P, Rodrigues EA, Berman DS, et al: Significance of dipyridamole-induced transient dilation of the left ventricle during thallium-201 scintigraphy in suspected coronary artery disease. *Am J Cardiol* 66:689, 1990.

325. Veilleux M, Lette J, Mansur A, et al: Prognostic implications of transient left ventricular cavitary dilation during exercise and dipyridamole–thallium imaging. *Can J Cardiol* 10:259, 1994.

326. Takeishi Y, Tono-oka I, Ikeda K, et al: Dilation of the left ventricular cavity on dipyridamole thallium-201 imaging: A new marker of triple-vessel disease. *Am Heart J* 121:466, 1991.

327. Hurwitz GA, O'Donoghue JP, MacDonald AC, et al: Markers of left ventricular dysfunction induced by exercise, dipyridamole or combined stress on ECG-gated myocardial perfusion scans. *Nucl Med Commun* 14:318, 1993.

328. Houghton JL, Frank MJ, Carr AA, et al: Relations among impaired coronary flow reserve, left ventricular hypertrophy and thallium perfusion defects in hypertensive patients without obstructive coronary artery disease. *J Am Coll Cardiol* 15:43, 1990.

329. Huikuri HV, Korhonen UR, Ikaheimo MJ, et al: Detection of coronary artery disease by thallium imaging using a combined intravenous dipyridamole and isometric handgrip test in patients with aortic valve stenosis. *Am J Cardiol* 59:336, 1987.

330. Rask P, Karp K, Edlund B, et al: Computer-assisted evaluation of dipyridamole thallium-201 SPECT in patients with aortic stenosis. *J Nucl Med* 35:983, 1994.

331. Koga Y, Yamaguchi R, Ogata M, et al: Decreased coronary vasodilator capacity in hypertrophic cardiomyopathy determined by split-dose thallium–dipyridamole myocardial scintigraphy. *Am J Cardiol* 65:1134, 1990.

332. Takata J, Counihan PJ, Gane JN, et al: Regional thallium-201 washout and myocardial hypertrophy in hypertrophic cardiomyopathy and its relation to exertional chest pain. *Am J Cardiol* 72:211, 1993.

333. Holdright DR, Lindsay DC, Clarke D, et al: Coronary flow reserve in patients with chest pain and normal coronary arteries. *Br Heart J* 70:513, 1993.

334. Hirzel HO, Senn M, Nuesch K, et al: Thallium-201 scintigraphy in complete left bundle branch block. *Am J Cardiol* 53:764, 1984.

335. Rockett JF, Wood WC, Moinuddin M, et al: Intravenous dipyridamole thallium-201 SPECT imaging in patients with left bundle branch block. *Clin Nucl Med* 15:401, 1990.

336. Larcos G, Brown ML, Gibbons RJ: Role of dipyridamole thallium-201 imaging in left bundle branch block. *Am J Cardiol* 68:1097, 1991.

337. Burns RJ, Galligan L, Wright LM, et al: Improved specificity of myocardial thallium-201 single-photon emission computed tomography in patients with left bundle

branch block by dipyridamole. *Am J Cardiol* 68:504, 1991.

338. Jukema JW, van der Wall EE, van der Vis-Melsen MJE, et al: Dipyridamole thallium-201 scintigraphy for improved detection of left anterior descending coronary artery stenosis in patients with left bundle branch block. *Eur Heart J* 14:53, 1993.

339. Hendel RC, Layden JJ, Leppo JA: Prognostic value of dipyridamole thallium scintigraphy for evaluation of ischemic heart disease. *J Am Coll Cardiol* 15:109, 1990.

340. Stratmann HG, Younis LT, Kong B: Prognostic value of dipyridamole thallium-201 scintigraphy in patients with stable chest pain. *Am Heart J* 123:317, 1992.

341. Younis LT, Byers S, Shaw L, et al: Prognostic importance of silent myocardial ischemia detected by intravenous dipyridamole thallium myocardial imaging in asymptomatic patients with coronary artery disease. *J Am Coll Cardiol* 14:1635, 1989.

342. Shaw L, Chaitman BR, Hilton TC, et al: Prognostic value of dipyridamole thallium-201 imaging in elderly patients. *J Am Coll Cardiol* 19:1390, 1992.

343. Gal RA, Gunasekera J, Massardo T, et al: Long-term prognostic value of a normal dipyridamole thallium-201 perfusion scan. *Clin Cardiol* 14:971, 1991.

344. Chikamori T, Doi YL, Yonezawa Y, et al: Noninvasive identification of significant narrowing of the left main coronary artery by dipyridamole thallium scintigraphy. *Am J Cardiol* 68:472, 1991.

345. Okada RD, Glover DK, Leppo JA: Dipyridamole ^{201}Tl scintigraphy in the evaluation of prognosis after myocardial infarction. *Circulation* 84(suppl I):I-132, 1991.

346. Melon PG, Beanlands RS, DeGrado TR, et al: Comparison of technetium-99m sestamibi and thallium-201 retention characteristics in canine myocardium. *J Am Coll Cardiol* 20:1277, 1992.

347. Tartagni F, Dondi M, Limonetti P, et al: Dipyridamole technetium-99m-2-methoxy isobutyl isonitrile tomoscintigraphic imaging for identifying diseased coronary vessels: Comparison with thallium-201 stress–rest study. *J Nucl Med* 32:369, 1991.

348. Yang C, Wu C, Jong S, et al: Intravenous dipyridamole technetium-99m myocardial perfusion scintigraphy for detection of coronary artery disease. *Kaohsiung J Med Sci* 8:59, 1992.

349. Bisi G, Sciagra R, Santoro GM, et al: Evaluation of coronary artery disease extent using ^{99m}Tc-sestamibi: Comparison of dipyridamole versus exercise and of planar versus tomographic imaging. *Nucl Med Commun* 14:946, 1993.

350. Villanueva-Meyer J, Mena I, Diggles L, et al: Assessment of myocardial perfusion defect size after early and delayed SPECT imaging with technetium-99m–hexakis 2-methoxyisobutyl isonitrile after stress. *J Nucl Med* 34:187, 1993.

351. Taillefer R: Technetium-99m sestamibi myocardial imaging: Same-day rest–stress studies and dipyridamole. *Am J Cardiol* 66:80E, 1990.

352. Kettunen R, Huikuri HV, Heikkala J, et al: Usefulness of technetium-99m–MIBI and thallium-201 in tomographic imaging combined with high-dose dipyridamole

and handgrip exercise for detecting coronary artery disease. *Am J Cardiol* 68:575, 1991.

353. Sciagra R, Bisi G, Santoro GM, et al: Evaluation of coronary artery disease using technetium-99m–sestamibi first-pass and perfusion imaging with dipyridamole infusion. *J Nucl Med* 35:1254, 1994.

354. Wackers FJT: Adenosine–thallium imaging: Faster and better? *J Am Coll Cardiol* 16:1384, 1990.

355. Wackers FJT: Adenosine or dipyridamole: Which is preferred for myocardial perfusion imaging? *J Am Coll Cardiol* 17:1295, 1991.

356. Gupta NC, Esterbrooks D, Mohiuddin S, et al: Adenosine in myocardial perfusion imaging using positron emission tomography. *Am Heart J* 122:293, 1991.

357. Takeishi Y, Abe S, Chiba J, et al: Organ distribution of thallium-201 during intravenous adenosine infusion: Comparison with exercise. *Am Heart J* 127:1268, 1994.

358. Muller P, Czernin J, Choi Y, et al: Effect of exercise supplementation during adenosine infusion on hyperemic blood flow and flow reserve. *Am Heart J* 128:52, 1994.

359. Iskandrian AS, Heo J, Nguyen T, et al: Left ventricular dilatation and pulmonary thallium uptake after single-photon emission computer tomography using thallium-201 during adenosine-induced coronary hyperemia. *Am J Cardiol* 66:807, 1990.

360. Leppo J, Rosenkrantz J, Rosenthal R, et al: Quantitative thallium-201 redistribution with a fixed coronary stenosis in dogs. *Circulation* 63:632, 1981.

361. Coyne EP, Belvedere DA, Vande PR, et al: Thallium-201 scintigraphy after intravenous infusion of adenosine compared with exercise thallium testing in the diagnosis of coronary artery disease. *J Am Coll Cardiol* 17:1289, 1991.

362. Gupta NC, Esterbrooks DJ, Hilleman DE, et al: Comparison of adenosine and exercise thallium-201 single-photon emission computed tomography (SPECT) myocardial perfusion imaging. *J Am Coll Cardiol* 19:248, 1992.

363. Nishimura S, Mahmarian JJ, Boyce TM, et al: Equivalence between adenosine and exercise thallium-201 myocardial tomography: A multicenter, prospective, crossover trial. *J Am Coll Cardiol* 20:265, 1992.

364. Pennell DJ, Mavrogeni SI, Forbat SM, et al: Adenosine combined with dynamic exercise for myocardial perfusion imaging. *J Am Coll Cardiol* 25:1300, 1995.

365. O'Keefe JH Jr, Bateman TM, Silvestri R, et al: Safety and diagnostic accuracy of adenosine thallium-201 scintigraphy in patients unable to exercise and those with left bundle branch block. *Am Heart J* 124:614, 1992.

366. O'Keefe JH, Bateman TM, Barnhart CS: Adenosine thallium-201 is superior to exercise thallium-201 for detecting coronary artery disease in patients with left bundle branch block. *J Am Coll Cardiol* 21:1332, 1993.

367. Samuels B, Kiat H, Friedman JD, et al: Adenosine pharmacologic stress myocardial perfusion tomographic imaging in patients with significant aortic stenosis: Diagnostic efficacy and comparison of clinical, hemodynamic and electrocardiographic variables with 100 age-matched control subjects. *J Am Coll Cardiol* 25:99, 1995.

368. Nishimura S, Mahmarian JJ, Boyce TM, et al: Quantitative thallium-201 single-photon emission computed to-

mography during maximal pharmacologic coronary vasodilation with adenosine for assessing coronary artery disease. *J Am Coll Cardiol* 18:736, 1991.

369. Aksut SV, Pancholy S, Cassel C, et al: Results of adenosine single photon emission computed tomography thallium-201 imaging in hemodynamic nonresponders. *Am Heart J* 130:67, 1995.

370. O'Keefe JH, Batemann TM, Handlin LR, et al: Four-versus 6-minute infusion protocol for adenosine thallium-201 single photon emission computed tomography imaging. *Am Heart J* 129:482, 1995.

371. Villegas BJ, Hendel RC, Dahlberg ST, et al: Comparison of 3- versus 6-minute infusions of adenosine in thallium-201 myocardial perfusion imaging. *Am Heart J* 126:103, 1993.

372. Takeishi Y, Abe S, Chiba J, et al: Organ distribution of thallium-201 during intravenous adenosine infusion: Comparison with exercise. *Am Heart J* 127:1268, 1994.

373. Iskandrian AS, Kegel J, Heo J, et al: The perfusion pattern in coronary artery occlusion: Comparison of exercise and adenosine. *Cathet Cardiovasc Diagn* 27:255, 1992.

374. Patel R, Bushnell DL, Wagner R, et al: Frequency of false-positive septal defects on adenosine/^{201}Tl images in patients with left bundle branch block. *Nucl Med Commun* 16:137, 1995.

375. Verani MS: Exercise and pharmacologic stress testing for prognosis after acute myocardial infarction. *J Nucl Med* 35:716, 1994.

376. Shaw L, Miller D, Kong BA, et al: Determination of perioperative cardiac risk by adenosine thallium-201 myocardial imaging. *Am Heart J* 124:861, 1992.

377. Takeishi Y, Chiba J, Abe S, et al: Noninvasive identification of left main and three-vessel coronary artery disease by thallium-201 single photon emission computed tomography during adenosine infusion. *Ann Nucl Med* 8:1, 1994.

378. Mahmarian JJ, Mahmarian AC, Marks GF, et al: Role of adenosine thallium-201 tomography for defining long-term risk in patients after acute myocardial infarction. *J Am Coll Cardiol* 25:1333, 1995.

379. Mahmarian JJ, Pratt CM, Nishimura S, et al: Quantitative adenosine ^{201}Tl single-photon emission computed tomography for the early assessment of patients surviving acute myocardial infarction. *Circulation* 87:1197, 1993.

380. Leon AR, Eisner RL, Martin SE, et al: Comparison of single-photon emission computed (SPECT) myocardial perfusion imaging with thallium-201 and technetium-99m sestamibi in dogs. *J Am Coll Cardiol* 20:1612, 1992.

381. Amanullah AM, Bevegard S, Lindvall K, et al: Assessment of left ventricular wall motion in angina pectoris by two-dimensional echocardiography and myocardial perfusion by technetium-99m sestamibi tomography during adenosine-induced coronary vasodilation and comparison with coronary angiography. *Am J Cardiol* 72:983, 1993.

382. Cuocolo A, Soricelli A, Pace L, et al: Adenosine technetium-99m–methoxy isobutyl isonitrile myocardial tomography in patients with coronary artery disease: Comparison with exercise. *J Nucl Med* 35:1110, 1994.

383. Miller DD, Donohue TJ, Younis LT, et al: Correlation of pharmacological ^{99m}Tc-sestamibi myocardial perfusion imaging with poststenotic coronary flow reserve in patients with angiographically intermediate coronary artery stenoses. *Circulation* 89:2150, 1994.

384. Ebersole DG, Heironimus J, Toney MO, et al: Comparison of exercise and adenosine technetium-99m sestamibi myocardial scintigraphy for diagnosis of coronary artery disease in patients with left bundle branch block. *Am J Cardiol* 71:450, 1993.

385. Matzer L, Kiat H, Wang FP, et al: Pharmacologic stress dual-isotope myocardial perfusion single-photon emission computed tomography. *Am Heart J* 128:1067, 1994.

SINGLE-PHOTON IMAGING OF MYOCARDIAL METABOLISM

Myocardial Metabolic Imaging with Radiolabeled Fatty Acids

Christopher L. Hansen

Fatty acids are the principal source of energy for the heart under resting conditions; their metabolism is greatly influenced by ischemia and other pathologic states. This has stimulated research into the diagnostic utility of employing radiolabeled fatty acids for myocardial metabolic imaging.

Some of the earliest attempts at imaging the heart were performed using labeled fatty acids (Fig. 7-1). Initial investigators were interested in using fatty acids for diagnosing coronary artery disease (CAD)—a task that has become the mainstay of nuclear cardiology. However, with the widespread acceptance of myocardial perfusion imaging with thallium-201 and technetium-99m agents, interest in the use of fatty acid tracers for this indication has waned. The importance of identifying myocardial viability for the purpose of selecting patients most likely to benefit from coronary revascularization is an indication that has renewed interest in these agents.

The most commonly investigated fatty acids are shown in Fig. 7-2. Almost all of the fatty acid research done with positron emission tomography (PET) has involved the use of ^{11}C palmitate; this work has contributed greatly to the basic understanding of fatty acid metabolism in health and disease. The evolution of the single photon emitting fatty acids, available today, is a process that has required the close interaction of basic scientists, radiopharmacists, and clinicians. Early investigators, using mostly straight-chain fatty acids, developed a body of knowledge regarding the metabolism and handling of fatty acids. Problems caused by the release of free isotope after metabolism limited their utility, and interest

in these agents faded. Currently, interest has focused on phenyl-fatty acids, the most important being ^{123}I phenylpentadecanoic acid (IPPA), as markers of metabolism, or in modified fatty acids, such as [123]I β-methyl phenylpentadecanoic acid (BMIPP), which have been designed to block metabolism in order to produce higher-quality images.

METABOLISM OF FATTY ACIDS

There are many good reviews of myocardial fatty acid metabolism[1-9]; it will only be reviewed briefly here. The heart has high energy requirements and consequently is very active metabolically. It derives most of its energy requirements from glucose, fatty acids, and lactate but will oxidize many substrates, including ketones, amino acids, pyruvate, and acetate. Fatty acids supply 60 to 85 percent of the heart's resting metabolic requirements because fatty acids inhibit the metabolism of glucose and only trace amounts of lactate are present at rest. Fatty acids are superior to glucose for supplying the large energy flux required by the heart.[5]

Figure 7-3 summarizes fatty acid transfer and metabolism. Fatty acids circulate in the plasma either as free fatty acids (FFA) bound to albumin or incorporated into triglycerides. The binding energy with albumin comes from hydrophobic interactions between the fatty acid

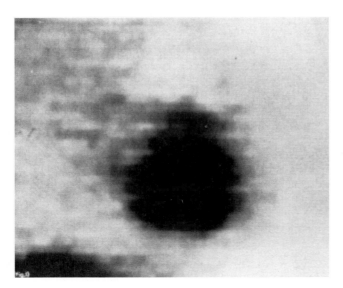

Figure 7-1 This image, published in 1965, represents the first attempt at imaging the heart with a radiolabeled fatty acid. Dogs were imaged with oleic acid that had been labeled across the double bond with [131]I. (From Evans et al,[88] with permission from the American Heart Association, Inc.)

and pockets in the albumin that are lined with nonpolar amino acid side chains.[10] The endothelium contains lipoprotein lipase, which hydrolyzes triacylglycerols in chylomicrons and very low density lipoprotein (VLDL) to provide fatty acids.[11] In some animals, triglycerides provide a significant fraction of the fatty acids metabolized by the myocardium,[12] but it is not clear how important they are in humans.

Transfer of fatty acids from the capillaries into the myocardium requires crossing a series of membranes and aqueous phases, a task made more complicated by the fact that fatty acids are insoluble in water. The endothelium is a major barrier to fatty acid uptake.[13] Extraction of fatty acids is variable; it is a function of fatty acid concentration, the FFA-albumin molar ratio, chain length, and the degree of saturation.[14,15] There appears to be a threshold below which fatty acid uptake will not occur.[16] The identification of albumin receptors on uncoated pits and plasmalemmal vesicles of mouse endothelium suggested that fatty acid transport across the endothelium is effected by transcytosis.[17] Fatty acids cross the interstitial space bound to albumin.[9,18] The mechanism of uptake of fatty acids by the myocytes is not clear. Some investigators have suggested that fatty acid uptake is a non-energy-dependent, mass-action effect with the rapid fatty acid metabolism inside the myocyte creating a strong inward gradient.[19] Others have suggested a dual mechanism involving both passive diffusion and a saturable (ie, receptor-based) process.[20,21] More recently, the importance of passive diffusion for fatty acid uptake has been challenged.[22] Intramyocardial transport of fatty acids is assisted by fatty acid binding

protein (FABP), a 40-kd protein present in high concentration in the cytosol.[23–26] FABP may be involved in carrier mediated transport of fatty acids across the sarcolemma.[27,28]

In the cytosol, fatty acids can either back-diffuse out of the cell,[29,30] or become activated via the enzyme acyl coenzyme A synthetase, also known as thiokinase. Activation is an energy-dependent process that leaves the fatty acid polar and thus trapped inside the cell. Activated fatty acids are either transported to the mitochondria via a complex carnitine dependent system or are incorporated into intracellular lipids, mainly phospholipids or triglycerides. The first step for fatty acids entering the lipid pool is esterification, which requires the presence of alpha-glycerol phosphate. The lipid pools and the carnitine system compete for activated fatty acids[31]; the relative fraction of fatty acids going through either pathway depends on many factors including the energy demands of the cell and presence of sufficient oxygen.

The carnitine system is composed of several proteins including carnitine, carnitine palmitoyltransferase I (CPT I), carnitine acetyltransferase I, the carnitine carrier, carnitine palmitoyltransferase II, and carnitine acetyltransferase II.[32] Inside the mitochondrion, the fatty acid undergoes β-oxidation where two carbon fragments are removed from the caroboxyl side of the fatty acid as acetyl-CoA. This fragment then undergoes oxidation in the Krebs cycle, which generates 12 molecules of ATP. The total amount of energy produced from a fatty acid will depend on the number of acetyl-CoA fragments, which is a function of the chain length. The oxidation of a molecule palmitate, as an example, produces 129 molecules of ATP.

The metabolism of fatty acids has been shown to be biexponential—reflecting the half-lives of fatty acids undergoing β-oxidation and those being incorporated into the myocardial lipid pools.[33,34] Beta-oxidation is very rapid; fatty acids in this phase have a half-life of only a few minutes. Intracellular triglycerides represent a reservoir of fatty acids available for β oxidation.[35] The half-life of the lipid pool is much longer, on the order of 1–2 h.

Myocardial fatty acid consumption increases with myocardial work or catecholamine stimulation.[33,36–39] This is probably due to a reduction in the NADH/NAD ratio and consequent stimulation of the Krebs cycle and hence β-oxidation.[38] Myocardial extraction of fatty acids will increase in the setting of decreased coronary blood flow in order to maintain adequate myocardial energy supplies.[40]

Fatty acids block myocardial glucose metabolism at several points; these include hexokinase, phosphofructokinase, and pyruvate dehydrogenase.[5,6,41] Since there are only trace amounts of lactate in the circulating plasma under resting conditions, its contribution to myocardial energy production is negligible. However, lactate levels

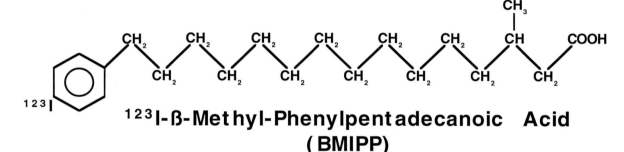

Figure 7-2 The four most thoroughly investigated fatty acids are the positron emitter ^{11}C palmitate, the straight chain fatty acid iodoheptadecanoic acid, iodophenylpentadecanoic acid (IPPA), and its β-methylated version BMIPP.

increase substantially with moderate and higher levels of exercise. Lactate inhibits the oxidation both of glucose and fatty acids and can provide as much as 87 percent of myocardial oxidative energy production.[42–46] Lactate may block fatty acid metabolism by inhibiting activation.[13]

Early evaluations of the drug clofibrate led to the observation that it caused an increase in hepatic peroxisomes. Further evaluation led to the discovery that these peroxisomes contained a cyanide-insensitive fatty acyl-CoA oxidizing system.[47] Other researchers have demonstrated that myocardial peroxisomes also contain this system.[48,49] Several investigators have suggested that α-oxidation of fatty acids occurs in peroxisomes,[50–52] but

their contribution to normal fatty acid metabolism is probably not important.

METABOLISM OF FATTY ACIDS IN DISEASE

Ischemia and Infarction

Myocardial fatty acid metabolism is extremely sensitive to ischemia[7]; the important effects are summarized in Fig. 7-4. Different investigators have found varying responses of fatty acid uptake with ischemia; some describe

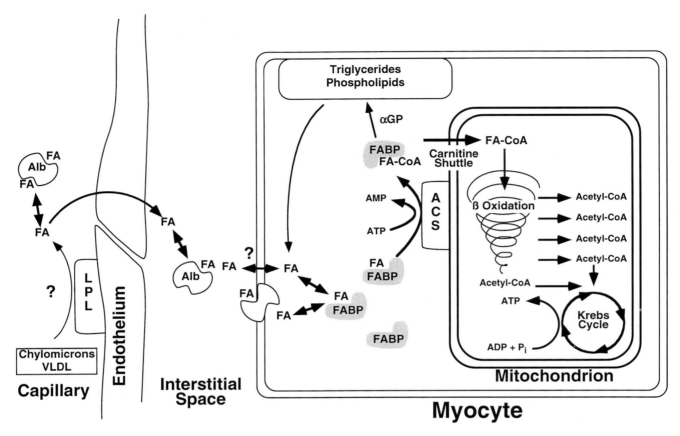

Figure 7-3 Summary of myocardial fatty acid metabolism. See text for details. Abbreviations: FA—Fatty acid; Alb—Albumin; VLDL—Very low density lipoprotein; LPL—Lipoprotein lipase; FABP—Fatty acid binding protein; ACS—Acyl Coenzyme A synthetase; αGP—alpha glycerol phosphate.

decreased uptake[53,54] and others report an increase.[40,55] Ischemia has two components: a decrease in perfusion and an inadequate delivery of oxygen. Lerch et al compared the effects of ischemia versus hypoxia in a dog model[56]; they found comparable changes in fatty acid metabolism with these two interventions and concluded that these changes were an effect of decreased oxygen delivery, not decreased blood flow.

Inadequate delivery of oxygen will rapidly reduce β-oxidation and the flux of fatty acids in this pathway.[57,58] Lower levels of ATP result in less fatty acids being activated by acyl-CoA synthetase, allowing more back-diffusion out of the cell.[29,59] During ischemia, fatty acids lose their ability to inhibit glycolysis,[60] and anaerobic glycolysis becomes the predominant source of energy. Accelerated glycolysis increases levels of alpha-glycerol phosphate, which helps drive intracellular fatty acids into the TG pool.[61] The net effect is an absolute increase in the amount of fatty acid retained in the TG pool.

Many of the effects of myocardial infarction on fatty acid metabolism are predictable.[62] There is a decrease in the amount of viable myocardium with consequent decrease in myocardial uptake and metabolism of fatty acids.[63] The size of the defect, not surprisingly, correlates with the size of the infarction.[64–66] Bilheimer and associates demonstrated that there was an increase in fatty acid accumulation in the areas adjacent to the infarct.[67]

Cardiomyopathy

Disturbances of fatty acid metabolism may be the primary cause or a secondary effect of a cardiomyopathy. Diphtheria toxin produces myocardial dysfunction by inhibiting the synthesis of carnitine.[68] Carnitine deficiency, caused by renal carnitine wasting, has been described as a cause of congestive cardiomyopathy.[69] Kubota and associates found that abnormalities of fatty acid metabolism were an early finding in a Syrian hamster model of cardiomyopathy and preceded metabolic abnormalities of glucose or perfusion.[70]

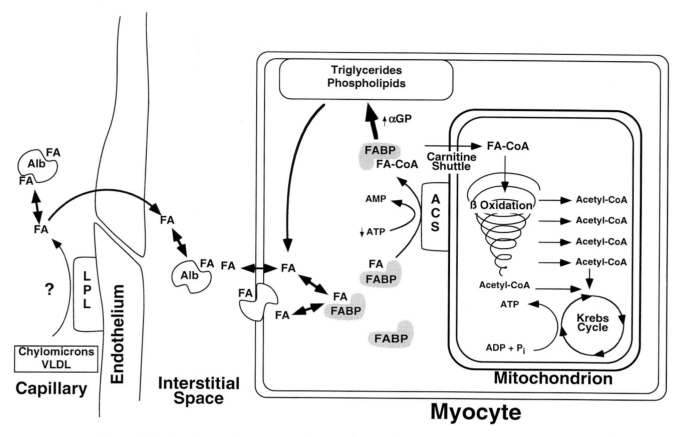

Figure 7-4 The effects of ischemia on fatty acid metabolism are summarized here. Hypoxia inhibits β-oxidation and the Krebs cycle; there is a decrease in transfer of fatty acids into the mitochondria. Increased anaerobic glycolysis increases intracellular alpha glycerol phosphate, which increases flux of activated fatty acids into the triglyceride pool. Decreased ATP will reduce the amount of fatty acid that is activated. There is an increase in back-diffusion of unactivated fatty acid. Overall, there is an increase in esterification of fatty acids compared to lipolysis of triglycerides, and retention of the fatty acid is prolonged. Abbreviations are the same as in Fig. 7-3.

Stunning and Hibernation

Myocardial stunning refers to prolonged mechanical dysfunction after a transient ischemic insult.[71,72] Myocardial hibernation refers to an adaptive down regulation of myocardial contractile function in the setting of chronic ischemia.[73] The clinical recognition of these conditions is important because they reflect the presence of myocardium that is still viable despite decreased contractility. The hallmark of stunning is a region of the myocardium that has an intact blood supply and gradually recovers contractile function. The hallmark of myocardial hibernation is myocardial dysfunction that recovers after restoration of blood flow.

Aerobic metabolism decreases or ceases with both of these conditions, and the main source of myocardial energy is glycolysis. It has been suggested that ATP derived from glycolysis is used mainly to support membrane integrity, whereas ATP derived from oxidative metabolism is used to support contractile function.[74] This may act as a protective mechanism that optimizes the ability of the myocardium to survive ischemic insults. In the clinical setting, there may be areas of myocardial stunning intermixed with areas of necrosis. Myocardial hibernation can also coexist with areas of myocardial necrosis.

In animal models of myocardial stunning, the severity and duration of the contractile dysfunction have been shown to be a function of the duration of the ischemic insult. Shorter periods of ischemia produce wall motion abnormalities that improve after minutes to hours; longer episodes may result in dysfunction that persists for weeks.

It is simpler to create animal models of stunning than of hibernation; consequently, most of the available research has dealt with stunning. Stunning appears to produce changes in metabolism similar to ischemia. Schwaiger and associates demonstrated in a dog model that after 20 min of coronary artery occlusion myocar-

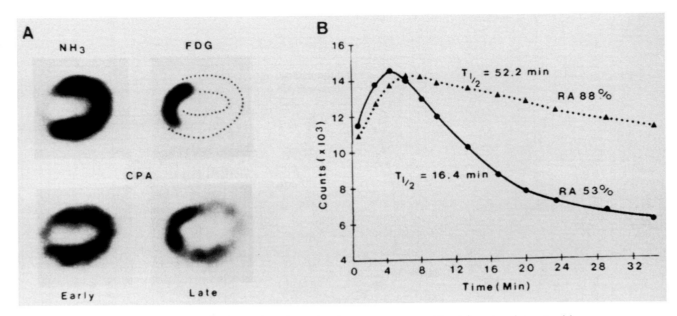

Figure 7-5 This study shows the relationship between coronary blood flow (as determined by ^{13}N, NH$_3$), glucose metabolism (as measured by ^{18}F fluorodeoxyglucose, FDG) and fatty acid metabolism (as measured by ^{11}C palmitate, CPA) in a dog model after 3 h of coronary occlusion followed by reperfusion. **A:** All four images represent the same cross-sectional region of the heart. The ammonia image shows decreased perfusion. The FDG image shows increased glucose metabolism in this region. The palmitate images show an initial decrease in uptake that largely reflects reduced perfusion to this region with much slower clearance on the late image. This reflects delayed metabolism of fatty acids in this region and is consistent with a higher proportion of the fatty acid in the triglyceride pool. **B:** These are the time activity curves from the same dog. The activity in the normal section is shown by the solid curve; the reperfused region is shown by the dotted curve. Initially there is lower activity in the reperfused region consistent with decreased perfusion to this area. The delayed metabolism in this region results in much slower clearance of activity. (From Schwaiger et al,[76] reprinted with permission from the American College of Cardiology.)

dial metabolism of palmitate was affected for more than 3 h after the restoration of blood flow.[75] There was marked reduction in the amount of palmitate entering the rapid β-oxidation pool and an increase in the triglyceride pool, which resulted in prolonged myocardial retention of this fatty acid. In a similar model, which used 3 h of coronary occlusion, the same group showed that myocardial metabolism of palmitate was again delayed.[76] At the same time, there was an increase in glucose metabolism, which they were able to demonstrate with ^{18}F fluorodeoxyglucose (FDG) (Fig. 7-5). In this latter model, which had both stunning and necrosis, they were able to demonstrate that wall motion improved most between 24 h and 1 wk after the insult but milder abnormalities persisted for up to 4 wk. Both delayed metabolism of palmitate and increased uptake of FDG were seen in regions of the myocardium that recovered. Their data suggested that palmitate was a better indicator of the amount of necrosis than FDG. Chatelain et al found in a rat model of severe transient ischemia that myocardial oxidation of fatty acids was markedly depressed and that the recovery of fatty acid oxidation paralleled the recovery of wall motion.[77] Buxton and co-workers investigated a canine model of stunning using PET imaging.[78]

They reported increased FDG uptake and delayed palmitate metabolism in reversibly injured regions. They also noted that oxidative metabolism and wall motion demonstrated parallel recovery in time.

Several investigators have reported that reperfused myocardium has an increased preference for fatty acids. Liedtke and associates explored a swine model of transient ischemia and discovered that reperfused myocardium had a higher rate of oxidation of palmitate when compared with the control.[79] This occurred despite persistent wall-motion abnormalities. They postulated a metabolic uncoupling between substrate metabolism and either energy production or transfer to contractile proteins to explain this finding. Lopaschuk and associates investigated the relative contributions of palmitate and glucose in a rat heart model of stunning.[80] They found that palmitate retained its inhibitory effect on glucose metabolism and that over 90 percent of the ATP produced from exogenous substrates was generated from palmitate. They also reported that the amount of fatty acid incorporated into TG was nearly twice that of controls. Görge and colleagues investigated a retrogradely perfused rat heart model of severe ischemia and reperfusion.[81] They demonstrated the pattern of increased glucose and decreased palmitate, but this pattern rapidly normalized. Their data suggested that the same pattern of altered metabolism could be seen in some irreversibly injured regions of the myocardium. The inhibitory effects lactate has on fatty acid metabolism may be attenuated after myocardial stunning.[82,83]

FATTY ACID IMAGING

All forms of nuclear imaging rely on either the biologic behavior of the administered isotope (as with ^{201}Tl or [82]Rb) or on incorporating a suitable radioisotope into a biologically active molecule. The most commonly used positron emitters, such as ^{11}C or ^{13}N, are isotopes of atoms that occur naturally in biologic compounds. Although there is some suggestion of different biologic behavior with different isotopes,[84] it can be assumed, for practical purposes, that such a labeled molecule has behavior that is indistinguishable from the unlabeled molecule. Compared to positron emitters, single-photon-emitting isotopes tend to be larger and heavier, so labeling a biologically active molecule with one changes its shape and may significantly alter its biochemical properties.

The chemistry of organohalides is well known; this has led to the preference for isotopes of iodine when labeling fatty acids. Iodine 131 was used initially, but is now rarely used because of its unfavorable energy profile and dosimetry. Iodine 123 is a cyclotron product that has much more favorable dosimetry and imaging characteristics. Earlier problems with contaminants have been successfully resolved, and it can now be produced in high purity at an acceptable cost. The advantages of the isotope technetium 99m, both in imaging characteristics and cost, are well appreciated. Despite several attempts, no satisfactory technetium-based fatty acid has yet been developed.[85–87]

In 1965, Evans and associates became the first group to image the heart with a fatty acid by labeling oleic acid with ^{131}I across the double bond (Fig. 7-1).[88] They later studied myocardial fatty acid uptake in 21 patients with a history of heart disease and 21 controls.[89] The image quality of these early studies was variable. Later, investigators at UCLA emphasized that labeling across the double bond left the iodine atom protruding from the side of the fatty acid.[90,91] This created steric hindrance, which reduced the uptake approximately 50 percent compared with the unlabeled molecule and altered the metabolism.[90] The size of an iodine atom—2.15 Å—is very close to that of a methyl group—2.0 Å.[92] It was suggested that by labeling the omega (terminal) carbon of a long chain fatty acid, the iodine atom would have the same biochemical properties as a terminal methyl group and

thus avoid the problems of steric hindrance.[91] Further research with these compounds was encouraging. Investigators showed that the metabolic fate of a fatty acid was a function of chain length[15,93] and led to the "odd-even" rule: The end product of metabolism of halogenated fatty acids with an odd number of carbons was free halogen, and for even numbers of carbons it was the halo-acetic acid.[93]

Several investigators began to focus on ^{123}I hexadecenoic acid, an analogue of oleic acid, and compared its ability to diagnose coronary disease with thallium 201.[94–97] They investigated hexadecenoic acid's behavior as a perfusion agent but did not explore its potential for identifying metabolic effects of ischemia. Okada and colleagues studied the closely related ^{123}I hexadecanoic acid in a dog model of coronary ligation.[98] Surprisingly, they found no significant difference in metabolism between the ischemic and non-ischemic regions of the ventricle.

Other investigators studied heptadecanoic acid, a stearic acid analog, and concluded that its metabolism was similar to palmitate.[92,99] Van der Wall et al showed that heptadecanoic acid had 40 percent greater uptake than hexadecenoic acid and concluded that it would be a superior agent.[100] Visser et al showed that in a canine model of ischemia, higher amounts of heptadecanoic acid were incorporated into intracellular TG pools.[101] Van der Wall and colleagues showed that ischemia caused delayed metabolism of heptadecanoic acid in patients with both stable and unstable angina pectoris.[102,103] Other investigators demonstrated abnormal fatty acid metabolism post infarction.[104–106]

The "odd-even" rule would predict that metabolism of straight chain fatty acids results in either free iodine or iodoacetate (for odd- or even-numbered chains, respectively).[94] As the metabolites accumulate there is a steady increase in background activity, which results in significant image degradation.[107] An early solution involved injecting free [123]I NaI 30 min after the isotope was injected and performing a background correction.[104,108] This improved image quality and permitted metabolic analysis, but imaging was restricted to one planar view and it precluded SPECT imaging (Fig. 7-6).

Further experience with these isotopes led to doubts about their ability to measure fatty acid metabolism. Schön et al demonstrated that the uptake of heptadecanoic acid was in fact slightly less than that of palmitate and that the early phase of metabolism did not reflect myocardial oxygen consumption, as it did with palmitate.[109,110] Other researchers also expressed doubts about the ability to accurately measure abnormalities of fatty acid metabolism with heptadecanoic acid.[111–113] Visser et al obtained serial myocardial biopsies for 30 min after injecting dogs with ^{131}I heptadecanoic acid. They demonstrated that as early as 5 min after injection, 61 percent of the activity was due to free iodine.[114] They concluded

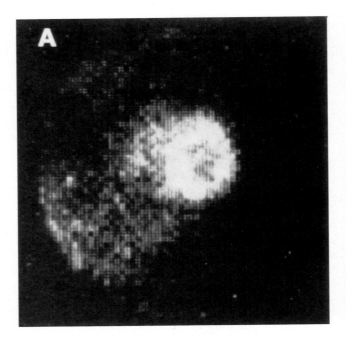 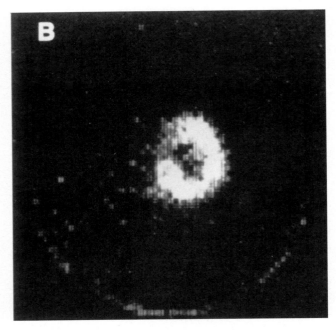

Before Correction   After Correction

Figure 7-6 Anterior heptadecanoic acid images from a normal control both before and after background correction. The background correction method requires a second injection of [123]I NaI. (From Freundlieb et al,[108] reprinted by permission of the Society of Nuclear Medicine.)

that the observed clearance of the isotope was due more to diffusion of free iodine out of the cell than to metabolism of the fatty acid.

Phenyl Fatty Acids

Machulla and associates reevaluated the original research into β-oxidation performed by Knoop in 1904, which showed that phenyl fatty acids underwent β-oxidation in the same manner as straight chain fatty acids.[115] They focused on ω-(p-^{123}I-phenyl)-pentadecanoic acid (IPPA). The end product of β-oxidation of IPPA is iodobenzoic acid, which is rapidly converted to hippuric acid and excreted by the kidneys, thereby avoiding the problem of background contamination by free iodine or iodoacetic acid. They demonstrated that the initial myocardial uptake of this fatty acid was high and that there was no significant release of free iodine. Kulkarni et al modified the synthesis of IPPA by employing an organothallium intermediate and markedly improved the synthetic yield.[116]

The metabolism of IPPA has been extensively explored. The initial myocardial uptake of IPPA is proportional to coronary blood flow.[117] Westera and associates found evidence for a dual uptake mechanism.[21] Their

data suggested a carrier-mediated mechanism that decreased with ischemia and also passive diffusion. Schmitz et al showed by gas-liquid chromatographic-mass spectrometric analysis that 73 percent of recovered activity was in myocardial triglycerides.[118] They found phenylproprionic, phenylpropenoic, and benzoic acids, breakdown products consistent with β-oxidation. Chien et al showed that end products of IPPA metabolism accounted for less than 5 percent of all myocardial activity and that the incorporaton of IPPA into intracellular lipids was similar to palmitate.[119] Reske and associates demonstrated in both murine and canine models that IPPA had a biexponential metabolism and myocardial distribution very similar to palmitate.[120–122] Other researchers have reported, however, that there is a higher percentage of IPPA incorporated into triglycerides when compared to palmitate.[123]

There has been considerable clinical experience thus far with IPPA.[124–126] Kennedy and associates studied the ability of sequential IPPA planar images to diagnose CAD.[127] They found that perfusion defects and clearance abnormalities correlated well with the presence of coronary artery disease. Hansen et al looked at a larger series of patients with documented CAD with exercise IPPA SPECT imaging; a subgroup underwent imaging also with thallium 201.[128] A normal database was constructed from a group of younger, healthy patients (Fig. 7-7).

8 Minutes

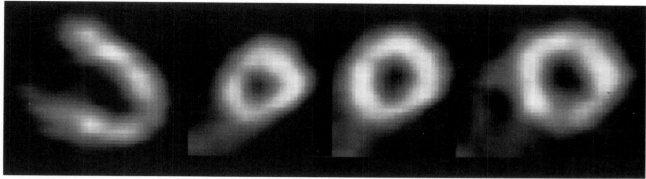

40 Minutes

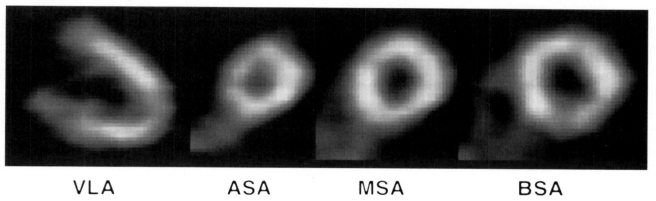

VLA   ASA   MSA   BSA

Figure 7-7   SPECT IPPA images in a normal control. There is homogeneous uptake throughout the myocardium on the initial (8-min) images. Activity remains homogeneous on the delayed images, reflecting homogeneous metabolism of the radiopharmaceutical in all regions of the myocardium. (VLA, vertical long axis; ASA, apical short axis; MSA, middle short axis; BSA, basal short axis.)

Twenty-seven of the 33 patients with coronary artery disease had decreased uptake or clearance of IPPA that was more than two standard deviations from the mean of the normals. The ability of IPPA to identify CAD was slightly higher than thallium in the subgroup that underwent testing with both isotopes, though this difference was not statistically significant. Schad et al performed rapid sequential imaging with a multicrystal camera in patients with coronary artery disease.[129] They were able to show abnormalities of metabolism of IPPA in patients with exercise-induced ischemia. The abnormalities of IPPA metabolism induced by ischemia have been shown to improve with antianginal medication.[130]

Studies that evaluate myocardial fatty acid metabolism after maximal exercise to diagnose coronary artery disease are confounded by the problem of lactate competing with fatty acids. Arterial lactate concentration rises quickly at levels of exercise above the anaerobic threshold and begins to inhibit myocardial metabolism of fatty acids; the degree of the inhibition will be variable and will depend on the lactate level. The implications of this problem can be seen in data published by Pippen

et al, who evaluated 19 normal volunteers studied at rest, during submaximal exercise (average of 69 percent of the maximal predicted heart rate), and during maximal exercise (average 94 percent of the maximal predicted heart rate).[131] They found that initial uptake of IPPA increased with increasing levels of exercise and was highest in the maximal exercise group. This finding would be expected from increasing blood flow with higher levels of exercise. They also showed that the clearance of IPPA was highest in the submaximal exercise group. This finding is explained by fatty acid metabolism increasing with the increasing work loads up to the anaerobic threshold (which occurs at approximately 70 percent of the maximal predicted heart rate) and then decreasing at higher levels of exercise owing to rising levels of lactate. It appears, therefore, that at maximal levels of exercise, fatty acids will behave consistently like perfusion agents but give inconsistent results for metabolic analysis. Therefore, the use of fatty acid imaging agents for the detection of CAD would optimally require a form of stress that does not generate lactate. Figure 7-8 shows the images from a patient studied using

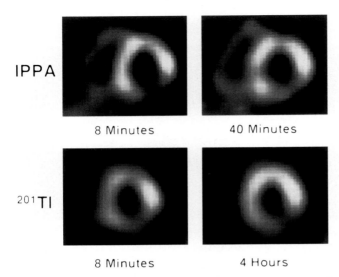

IPPA

8 Minutes   40 Minutes

^{201}Tl

8 Minutes   4 Hours

Figure 7-8 The patient whose images are shown here received streptokinase shortly after developing an inferior wall MI. Catheterization revealed an 80 percent circumflex lesion. Shown are the results of a submaximal thallium test and a stress IPPA study performed with respiratory gas exchange monitoring to exercise the patient up to the anaerobic threshold. The thallium study shows an inferior wall defect that demonstrates reverse redistribution—a common finding in patients with an open artery after infarction but not accepted as evidence for ischemia. The IPPA shows an inferolateral wall defect that shows delayed clearance, strongly suggesting the presence of residual ischemia in this region.

a protocol in which the patient was exercised up to the anaerobic threshold as determined by respiratory gas exchange monitoring and confirmed with lactate measurements. Other possible forms of stress would be atrial pacing or pharmacologic stress with dobutamine. Tamaki and associates have evaluated palmitate metabolism using PET after dobutamine stress,[132] but further experience will be necessary. The higher cost of ^{123}I will probably prevent acceptance of these radiolabeled fatty acids for routine diagnosis of CAD.

Abnormal IPPA metabolism after infarction has been demonstrated in both animal models and patients. Rellas and colleagues showed that there was decreased uptake and delayed metabolism in a region of experimentally induced infarction in a canine model.[133] Hansen et al evaluated 14 patients shortly after acute myocardial infarction.[134] They also demonstrated decreased uptake and reduced metabolism of IPPA in the region of the infarct. An unexpected finding in this study was increased metabolism of IPPA in regions remote from the infarct. Walamies et al showed improvement in IPPA metabolism in patients who maintained arterial patency after receiving thrombolysis for an acute myocardial infarction.[135]

Abnormal fatty acid metabolism has been demonstrated in other causes of cardiac disease. Ugolini et al demonstrated abnormal fatty acid metabolism in 19 patients with nonischemic cardiomyopathy.[136] They demonstrated patchy uptake of IPPA and more rapid metabolism, when compared to controls. Abnormal fatty acid metabolism has also been demonstrated in patients with left ventricular hypertrophy and with syndrome X.[137,138]

Myocardial Viability

Murray and associates used sequential planar imaging with a multicrystal camera in a group of 15 patients with severe CAD who were scheduled to undergo bypass grafting.[139] They found that IPPA markers of myocardial viability agreed with histologic evidence of viability obtained from intraoperative biopsies. Kuikka et al performed metabolic imaging with IPPA and perfusion imaging with MIBI on a group of 31 patients with severe CAD.[140] They derived an index of IPPA activity divided by perfusion that they called a "metabolic reserve." They showed that this correlated with resting ejection fraction and proposed that it represented viability. This study did not confirm viability or show improvement after revascularization.

Hansen et al reported the results of a phase I/II study of IPPA in patients with CAD undergoing revascularization. Sequential SPECT imaging was performed, and changes in left ventricular function after revascularization were documented by radionuclide ventriculography. In a preliminary report, they demonstrated that the metabolism of IPPA could be modeled as a monoexponential decay and that delayed metabolism may be an indicator of viability and predict improvement (Fig. 7-9).[141] In a later study, this analysis was advanced where parametric images were derived that showed regions of intermediate metabolism of IPPA.[142] The amount of myocardium with intermediate metabolism was shown to be a good predictor of which patients would improve after revascularization (Fig. 7-10). Iskandrian et al, evaluating a subgroup of patients in this protocol who had also undergone rest thallium perfusion imaging, found that IPPA more often showed evidence of ischemia than did thallium 201.[143]

Modified Fatty Acids

The problem of free iodine accumulation led to another strategy: the development of modified fatty acids. By modified, it is meant to encompass those fatty acids that are structurally altered in a manner that slows or completely blocks β-oxidation and thus prolongs myocardial retention of the fatty acid. Prolonging retention in this manner results in improved image quality but sacrifices metabolic information.

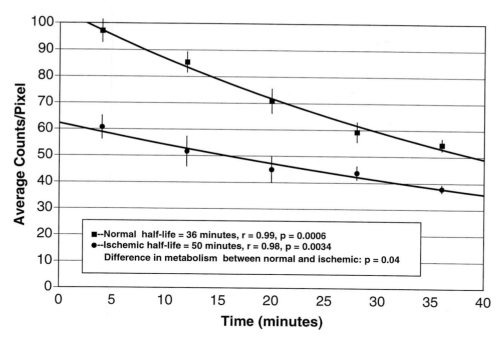

Figure 7-9   These are time activity curves from sequential SPECT images from a resting IPPA study in a patient who presented with unstable angina, three-vessel coronary artery disease, and inferior hypokinesis on radionuclide ventriculography. The top curve represents activity in the anterior wall; the bottom curve represents activity in the inferior wall. There is reduced uptake and delayed metabolism in the inferior wall. After bypass grafting the patient had an improvement in the wall motion of the inferior wall. (From Hansen,[141] reprinted by permission of the Society of Nuclear Medicine.)

Beta-oxidation is the most common but not the only way that myocytes can catabolize fatty acids; both α- and ω-oxidation systems have been described.[144,145] Although these pathways make a minimal contribution under normal conditions,[146] they become more important when β-oxidation is inhibited. Many of the modified fatty acids will undergo initial α-oxidation followed by β-oxidation. Since α-oxidation is a much slower process than β-oxidation,[147,148] the retention of these fatty acids is significantly prolonged. It is also possible to modify fatty acids in such a way as to completely block all oxidation and even further prolong myocardial retention.

Knapp, noting the biochemical similarity between tellurium and the $-CH=CH-$ moiety, proposed 9-telluraheptadecanoic acid.[149] The presence of tellurium in the carbon chain completely blocks β-oxidation. They introduced the "tellurium heteroatom" into several long chain fatty acids using ^{123m}Te as the radioisotope.[150,151] However, partly because of ^{123m}Te's half-life of 119 d, interest in this class of fatty acids faded.

Another approach was the addition of a methyl group at the β carbon. It was felt that this modification would block β-oxidation without severely affecting uptake. Early experience with ^{11}C isotopes comparing β-methylheptadecanoic with palmitic acid confirmed this.[152,153]

Otto et al demonstrated that chain length also affects the myocardial uptake of modified fatty acids.[154] Researchers at Oak Ridge evaluated several modified aryl fatty acids and proposed β-methyl iodophenylpentadecanoic acid (BMIPP or BMIPPA).[155–157] Beta-methylation blocks the initial step of β-oxidation and the terminal phenyl group blocks omega oxidation. It has been shown that the metabolism of these fatty acids in the cell begins with α-oxidation, which removes the β-methyl group; the remaining fragment then undergoes β-oxidation.[158] Humbert and associates compared the metabolism of BMIPP with IPPA using both iodinated and carbon-14 labeled versions.[159] They found that there was less uptake of the β-methylated fatty acid. They also reported that a lower percentage of the β-methylated fatty acids was incorporated into intracellular lipid pools.

Other types of modifications have been investigated. The addition of a second β-methyl group (dimethyl-iodophenylpentadecanoic acid or DMIPP) appears to block both α- and β-oxidation completely and results in a fatty acid that undergoes no significant myocardial oxidation.[123,160–162] The effect of moving the methyl group further down the carbon chain was explored with iodine-123-iodophenyl-9-methyl-pentadecanoic acid. This was compared to thallium using dual isotope imaging after maximal exercise in 11 patients with CAD.[163] There was complete concordance between the two studies. Other

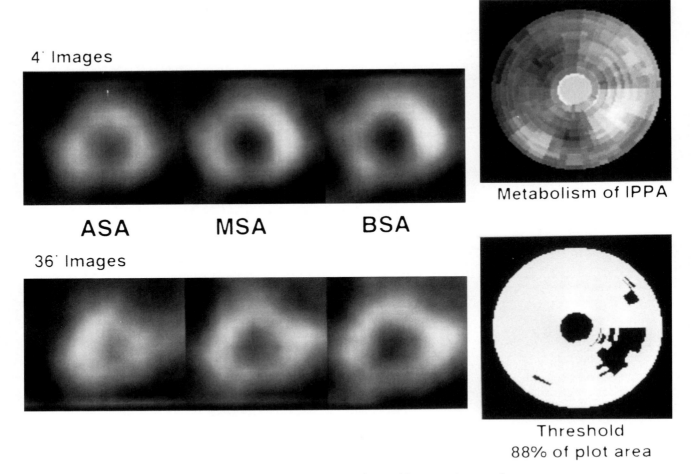

4' Images

ASA   MSA   BSA

36' Images

Metabolism of IPPA

**Threshold
88% of plot area**

Figure 7-10   Five sequential resting IPPA images obtained from 4 to 36 min after injection were used to create a parametric image demonstrating metabolism. The first and last short axis images and parametric images are shown. In this study the amount of myocardium in an intermediate metabolic range was found to correlate with improvement in ejection fraction after revascularization. Visually, delayed metabolism can be appreciated in the anteroseptal region; the parametric image shows most of the ventricle in the intermediate range. This patient had two-vessel coronary artery disease; his ejection fraction improved from 18 percent to 28 percent after revascularization. (From Hansen et al,[142] reprinted by permission of the Society of Nuclear Medicine.)

investigators have explored the ortho isotope of phenyl pentadecanoic acid (oPPA), which does not undergo β-oxidation.[164,165] Both animal and human studies have shown abnormal fatty acid uptake in various forms of cardiomyopathy.[70,166]

Myocardial Viability

Tamaki et al compared results of BMIPP and thallium imaging in 28 patients with myocardial infarction and 4 normal controls.[167] They showed homogeneous uptake of both tracers in the normals and decreased uptake in regions of infarction. They found that BMIPP uptake was relatively lower than thallium in patients who had

recent infarction or who had undergone revascularization (Fig. 7-11). They proposed that this pattern of relatively decreased uptake of BMIPP may represent viable myocardium. Franken et al looked at 22 patients who had received thrombolysis for acute myocardial infarction.[168] They found that the pattern of relatively decreased BMIPP compared to sestamibi was seen more often in patients with preserved wall motion or in those that demonstrated inotropic reserve with dobutamine stimulation. Matsunari et al used an imaging protocol with rapid sequential SPECT imaging to study 26 patients with a history of MI.[169] They also showed a relative decrease in BMIPP uptake; their results suggested that this may be due to increased back-diffusion of unactivated isotope. Research has suggested that BMIPP up-

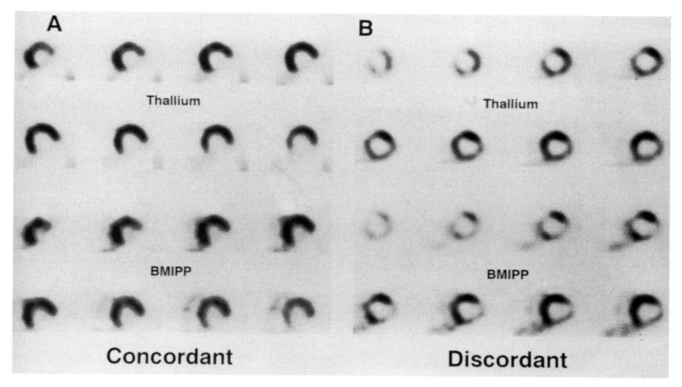

Figure 7-11 **A:** These images show corresponding short axis slices from thallium and BMIPP studies in a patient with an inferior wall MI. Both the thallium and BMIPP slices show a severe inferolateral defect. These images are concordant and are felt to reflect nonviable myocardium in the inferolateral wall. **B:** This is the same orientation as **A.** This is a different patient who had an old anterior wall MI and a recent (2½ wk) inferior wall MI. Both the thallium and BMIPP images show a concordant decrease in uptake in the anterior wall. However, there is much less uptake of BMIPP in the inferolateral wall when compared with thallium. This discordant uptake is felt to reflect viability in this region. (From Tamaki et al,[167] Figs. 2 and 3, reprinted by permission of the Society of Nuclear Medicine.)

take has correlated with intracellular ATP levels[170]; this, when taken in combination with the observation that a relatively higher proportion of BMIPP is in the cytosol as free fatty acid,[159] would suggest that these observations may be due to rapid washout of unactivated fatty acids in regions of stunning or hibernation.

However, the uptake of BMIPP in regions of ischemia or stunning appears to be inconsistent. Miller et al, when studying a canine model of infarction and reperfusion, showed a relative increase in BMIPP compared to perfusion, as measured by ^{201}Tl, in viable myocardial regions.[171] Nishimura et al reported a relative increase in BMIPP uptake compared to thallium in a canine occlusion/reperfusion model.[172] Saito et al evaluated 7 patients with unstable angina who had preserved wall motion and 6 patients with acute myocardial infarction treated with thrombolysis. Half of the infarct patients showed the described pattern of relatively decreased uptake of BMIPP.[173] However, 5 out of 7 patients with unstable angina had relatively increased BMIPP uptake compared with thallium. If the identification of viability

using this technique depends on the presence of thallium uptake in a region (combined with the relative absence of BMIPP), it could be argued that the thallium uptake alone is sufficient for identifying viability and thus obviating the need for the BMIPP. This issue has not been settled, and further investigation will need to be performed.

CONCLUSION

The last 30 years have witnessed a tremendous research effort into developing effective radiolabeled fatty acids for myocardial metabolic imaging. Without a substantial reduction in the cost of ^{123}I, or development of an effective technetium-based fatty acid, their use for the routine diagnosis of coronary disease will probably be limited. Their utility in the identification of viable myocardium is a new indication that shows great promise but requires further investigation.

REFERENCES

1. Bing RJ: Cardiac metabolism. *Phys Rev* 45:171, 1965.
2. Opie LH: Metabolism of the heart in health and disease. I. *Am Heart J* 76:685, 1968.
3. Opie LH: Metabolism of the heart in health and disease. II. *Am Heart J* 77:100, 1969.
4. Opie LH: Metabolism of the heart in health and disease. III. *Am Heart J* 77:383, 1969.
5. Neely JR, Rovetto MJ, Oram JF: Myocardial utilization of carbohydrate and lipids. *Prog Cardiovasc Dis* 15:289, 1972.
6. Neely JR, Morgan HE: Relationship between carbohydrate and lipid metabolism and the energy balance of heart muscle. *Ann Rev Phys* 36:413, 1974.
7. Liedtke AJ: Alterations of carbohydrate and lipid metabolism in the acutely ischemic heart. *Prog Cardiovasc Dis* 23:321, 1981.
8. Opie LH: Substrate and energy metabolism of the heart, in Sperelakis N (ed): *Physiology and Pathophysiology of the Heart*. Boston, Martinus Nijhoff Publishing, 1984, pp 301–336.
9. van der Vusse GJ, Glatz JF, Stam HC: Myocardial fatty acid homeostasis. *Mol Cell Biochem* 88:1, 1989.
10. Spector AA: Fatty acid binding to plasma albumin. *J Lipid Res* 16:165, 1975.
11. Cryer A: The role of the endothelium in myocardial lipoprotein dynamics. *Mol Cell Biochem* 88:7, 1989.
12. Wolfe RR, Durkot MJ: Role of very low density lipoproteins in the energy metabolism of the rat. *J Lipid Res* 26:210, 1985.
13. Rose CP, Goresky CA: Constraints on the uptake of labeled palmitate by the heart: The barriers at the capillary and sarcolemmal surfaces and the control of intracellular sequestration. *Circ Res* 41:534, 1977.
14. Evans JR: Importance of fatty acid in myocardial metabolism. *Circ Res* XIV & XV (suppl II):II96, 1964.
15. Otto CA, Brown LE, Wieland DM, Beierwaltes WH: Radioiodinated fatty acids for myocardial imaging: Effects on chain length. *J Nucl Med* 22:613, 1981.
16. Carlsten A, Hallgren B, Jagenburg R, et al: Myocardial arteriovenous differences of individual free fatty acids in healthy human individuals. *Metabolism* 12:1063, 1963.
17. Ghitescu L, Fixman A, Simionescu M, Simionescu N: Specific binding sites for albumin restricted to plasmalemmal vesicles of continuous capillary endothelium: Receptor-mediated transcytosis. *J Cell Biol* 102:1304, 1986.
18. Bassingthwaighte JB, Noodleman L, van der Vusse G, Glatz JF: Modeling of palmitate transport in the heart. *Mol Cell Biochem* 88:51, 1989.
19. Fournier NC: Uptake and transport of lipid substrates in the heart. *Basic Res Cardiol* 82:11, 1987.
20. Paris S, Samuel D, Jacques Y, et al: The role of serum albumin in the uptake of fatty acids by cultured cardiac cells from chick embryo. *Eur J Biochem* 83:235, 1978.
21. Westera G, Van der Wall EE, Visser FC, et al: The uptake of iodinated free fatty acids in the (ischemic) dog heart: Indications for a dual uptake mechanism. *Int J Nucl Med Biol* 10:231, 1983.
22. Stremmel W: Transmembrane transport of fatty acids in the heart. *Mol Cell Biochem* 88:23, 1989.
23. Fournier N, Geoffroy M, Deshusses J: Purification and characterization of a long chain, fatty-acid-binding protein supplying the mitochondrial beta-oxidative system in the heart. *Biochimica et Biophysica Acta* 533:457, 1978.
24. Veerkamp JH, van Moerkerk HT: Fatty acid-binding protein and its relation to fatty acid oxidation. *Mol Cell Biochem* 123:101, 1993.
25. Glatz JF, van der Vusse GJ: Intracellular transport of lipids. *Mol Cell Biochem* 88:37, 1989.
26. Peeters RA, Veerkamp JH: Does fatty acid-binding protein play a role in fatty acid transport? *Mol Cell Biochem* 88:45, 1989.
27. Vyska K, Meyer W, Stremmel W, et al: Fatty acid uptake in normal human myocardium. *Circ Res* 69:857, 1991.
28. Fujii S, Kawaguchi H, Yasuda H: Purification of high affinity fatty acid receptors in rat myocardial sarcolemmal membranes. *Lipids* 22:544, 1987.
29. Fox KA, Abendschein DR, Ambos HD, et al: Efflux of metabolized and nonmetabolized fatty acid from canine myocardium: Implications for quantifying myocardial metabolism tomographically. *Circ Res* 57:232, 1985.
30. Duwel CM, Visser FC, van Eenige MJ, Roos JP: Variables of myocardial backdiffusion, determined with 17-iodo-131 heptadecanoic acid in the normal dog heart. *Mol Cell Biochem* 88:191, 1989.
31. Borrebaek B, Christiansen R, Christophersen BO, Bremer J: The role of acyltransferases in fatty acid utilization. *Circ Res* 38:I16, 1976.
32. Scholte HR, Luyt-Houwen IE, Vaandrager-Verduin MH: The role of the carnitine system in myocardial fatty acid oxidation: Carnitine deficiency, failing mitochondria and cardiomyopathy. *Basic Res Cardiol* 82:63, 1987.
33. Schön HR, Schelbert HR, Robinson G, et al: C-11 labeled palmitic acid for the noninvasive evaluation of regional myocardial fatty acid metabolism with positron-computed tomography. I. Kinetics of C-11 palmitic acid in normal myocardium. *Am Heart J* 103:532, 1982.
34. Schelbert HR, Henze E, Schön HR, et al: C-11 palmitate for the noninvasive evaluation of regional myocardial fatty acid metabolism with positron computed tomography. III. In vivo demonstration of the effects of substrate availability on myocardial metabolism. *Am Heart J* 105:492, 1983.
35. Nellis SH, Liedtke AJ, Renstrom B: Fatty acid kinetics in aerobic myocardium: Characteristics of tracer carbon entry and washout and influence of metabolic demand. *J Nucl Med* 33:1864, 1992.
36. Crass MFd, McCaskill ES, Shipp JC: Effect of pressure development on glucose and palmitate metabolism in perfused heart. *Am J Physiol* 216:1569, 1969.
37. Oram JF, Bennetch SL, Neely JR: Regulation of fatty acid utilization in isolated perfused rat hearts. *J Biol Chem* 248:5299, 1973.
38. Neely JR, Whitmer M, Mochizuki S: Effects of mechanical activity and hormones on myocardial glucose and fatty acid utilzation. *Circ Res* 38:I22, 1976.
39. Klein MS, Goldstein RA, Welch MJ, Sobel BE: External assessment of myocardial metabolism with [^{11}C]palmitate in rabbit hearts. *Am J Physiol* 237:H51, 1979.

40. Fox KA, Nomura H, Sobel BE, Bergmann SR: Consistent substrate utilization despite reduced flow in hearts with maintained work. *Am J Physiol* 244:H799, 1983.

41. Lassers BW, Kaijser L, Wahlqvist ML, Carlson LA: Relationship in man between plasma free fatty acids and myocardial metabolism of carbohydrate substrates. *Lancet* 2:448, 1971.

42. Issekutz B Jr, Miller HI, Paul P, Rodahl K: Effect of lactic acid on free fatty acids and glucose oxidation in dogs. *Am J Physiol* 209:1137, 1965.

43. Drake AJ: Preferential uptake of lactate by normal myocardium. *J Physiol* 289:89P, 1979.

44. Drake AJ, Haines JR, Noble MI: Preferential uptake of lactate by the normal myocardium in dogs. *Cardiovasc Res* 14:65, 1980.

45. Wyns W, Schwaiger M, Huang SC, et al: Effects of inhibition of fatty acid oxidation on myocardial kinetics of ^{11}C-labeled palmitate. *Circ Res* 65:1787, 1989.

46. Spitzer JJ: Effect of lactate infusion on canine myocardial free fatty acid metabolism in vivo. *Am J Physiol* 226:213, 1974.

47. Lazarow PB, De Duve C: A fatty acyl-CoA oxidizing system in rat liver peroxisomes: Enhancement by clofibrate, a hypolipidemic drug. *Proc Nat Acad Sciences U.S.A.* 73:2043, 1976.

48. Kang ES, Mirvis DM, James C, et al: Induction of fatty acid oxidation in the canine myocardium by clofibrate (abstr). *Clin Res* 31:461a, 1983.

49. Kang ES, Mirvis DM: Reversible, highly localized alterations in fatty acid metabolism in the chronically ischemic canine myocardium. *Am J Cardiol* 54:411, 1984.

50. Poulos A, Sharp P, Singh H, et al: Formic acid is a product of the alpha-oxidation of fatty acids by human skin fibroblasts: Deficiency of formic acid production in peroxisome-deficient fibroblasts. *Biochem J* 292:457, 1993.

51. Singh I, Pahan K, Singh AK, Barbosa E: Refsum disease: A defect in the alpha-oxidation of phytanic acid in peroxisomes. *J Lipid Res* 34:1755, 1993.

52. Wanders RJ, Van Roermund CW: Studies on phytanic acid alpha-oxidation in rat liver and cultured human skin fibroblasts. *Biochimica et Biophysica Acta* 1167:345, 1993.

53. Gould KL, Kelley KO, Halter JB: Changes in regional myocardial metabolism during partial stenosis in the presence of coronary vasodilators. *J Cardiovasc Pharm* 3:936, 1981.

54. Weiss ES, Hoffman EJ, Phelps ME, et al: External detection and visualization of myocardial ischemia with ^{11}C-substrates in vitro and in vivo. *Circ Res* 39:24, 1976.

55. Lerch RA, Ambos HD, Bergmann SR, et al: Localization of viable, ischemic myocardium by positron-emission tomography with ^{11}C-palmitate. *Circulation* 64:689, 1981.

56. Lerch RA, Bergmann SR, Ambos HD, et al: Effect of flow-independent reduction of metabolism on regional myocardial clearance of ^{11}C-palmitate. *Circulation* 65:731, 1982.

57. Schön HR, Schelbert HR, Najafi A, et al: C-11 labeled palmitic acid for the noninvasive evaluation of regional myocardial fatty acid metabolism with positron-computed tomography. II. Kinetics of C-11 palmitic acid in acutely ischemic myocardium. *Am Heart J* 103:548, 1982.

58. Schelbert HR, Henze E, Keen R, et al: C-11 palmitate for the noninvasive evaluation of regional myocardial fatty acid metabolism with positron-computed tomography. IV. In vivo evaluation of acute demand-induced ischemia in dogs. *Am Heart J* 106:736, 1983.

59. Rosamond TL, Abendschein DR, Sobel BE, et al: Metabolic fate of radiolabeled palmitate in ischemic canine myocardium: Implications for positron emission tomography. *J Nucl Med* 28:1322, 1987.

60. Neely JR, Bowman RH, Morgan HE: Effects of ventricular pressure development and palmitate on glucose transport. *Am J Physiol* 216:804, 1969.

61. Scheuer J, Brachfeld N: Myocardial uptake and fractional distribution of palmitate-1 C-14 by the ischemic dog heart. *Metabolism: Clinical & Experimental* 15:945, 1966.

62. Opie LH: Metabolism of free fatty acids, glucose and catecholamines in acute myocardial infarction: Relation to myocardial ischemia and infarct size. *Am J Cardiol* 36:938, 1975.

63. Sobel BE, Weiss ES, Welch MJ, et al: Detection of remote myocardial infarction in patients with positron emission transaxial tomography and intravenous ^{11}C-palmitate. *Circulation* 55:853, 1977.

64. Weiss ES, Ahmed SA, Welch MJ, et al: Quantification of infarction in cross sections of canine myocardium in vivo with positron emission transaxial tomography and ^{11}C-palmitate. *Circulation* 55:66, 1977

65. Ter-Pogossian MM, Klein MS, Markham J, et al: Regional assessment of myocardial metabolic integrity in vivo by positron-emission tomography with ^{11}C-labeled palmitate. *Circulation* 61:242, 1980.

66. Geltman EM, Biello D, Welch MJ, et al: Characterization of nontransmural myocardial infarction by positron-emission tomography. *Circulation* 65:747, 1982.

67. Bilheimer DW, Buja LM, Parkey RW, et al: Fatty acid accumulation and abnormal lipid deposition in peripheral and border zones of experimental myocardial infarcts. *J Nucl Med* 19:276, 1978.

68. Molstad P, Bohmer T: The effect of diphtheria toxin on the cellular uptake and efflux of L-carnitine: Evidence for a protective effect of prednisolone. *Biochimica et Biophysica Acta* 641:71, 1981.

69. Waber LJ, Valle D, Neill C, et al: Carnitine deficiency presenting as familial cardiomyopathy: A treatable defect in carnitine transport. *J Pediatrics* 101:700, 1982.

70. Kubota K, Som P, Oster ZH, et al: Detection of cardiomyopathy in an animal model using quantiative autoradiography. *J Nucl Med* 29:1697, 1988.

71. Heyndrickx GR, Millard RW, McRitchie RJ, et al: Regional myocardial functional and electrophysiological alterations after brief coronary artery occlusion in conscious dogs. *J Clin Invest* 56:978, 1975.

72. Braunwald E, Kloner RA: The stunned myocardium: Prolonged, postischemic ventricular dysfunction. *Circulation* 66:1146, 1982.

73. Rahimtoola SH: The hibernating myocardium. *Am Heart J* 117:211, 1989.

74. Weiss J, Hiltbrand B: Functional compartmentation of glycolytic versus oxidative metabolism in isolated rabbit heart. *J Clin Invest* 75:436, 1985.

75. Schwaiger M, Schelbert HR, Keen R, et al: Retention and clearance of C-11 palmitic acid in ischemic and reperfused canine myocardium. *J Am Coll Cardiol* 6:311, 1985.

76. Schwaiger M, Schelbert HR, Ellison D, et al: Sustained regional abnormalities in cardiac metabolism after transient ischemia in the chronic dog model. *J Am Coll Cardiol* 6:336, 1985.

77. Chatelain P, Papageorgiou I, Luthy P, et al: Free fatty acid metabolism in "stunned" myocardium. *Basic Res Cardiol* 82:169, 1987.

78. Buxton DB, Mody FV, Krivokapich J, et al: Quantitative assessment of prolonged metabolic abnormalities in reperfused canine myocardum. *Circulation* 85:1842, 1992.

79. Liedtke AJ, DeMaison L, Eggleston AM, et al: Changes in substrate metabolism and effects of excess fatty acids in reperfused myocardium. *Circ Res* 62:535, 1988.

80. Lopaschuk GD, Spafford MA, Davies NJ, Wall SR: Glucose and palmitate oxidation in isolated working rat hearts reperfused after a period of transient global ischemia. *Circ Res* 66:546, 1990.

81. Gorge G, Chatelain P, Schaper J, Lerch R: Effect of increasing degrees of ischemic injury on myocardial oxidative metabolism early after reperfusion in isolated rat hearts. *Circ Res* 68:1681, 1991.

82. Renstrom B, Nellis SH, Liedtke AJ: Metabolic oxidation of pyruvate and lactate during early myocardial reperfusion. *Circ Res* 66:282, 1990.

83. Mickle DAG, del Nido PJ, Wilson GJ, et al: Exogenous substrate preference of the post-ischaemic myocardium. *Cardiovasc Res* 20:256, 1986.

84. Ciais P, Tans PP, Trolier M, et al: A large northern hemisphere terrestrial CO_2 sink indicated by the ^{13}C-^{12}C ratio of atmospheric CO_2. *Science* 269:1098, 1995.

85. Bonte JF, Graham KD, Moore JG, et al: Preparation of ^{99m}Tc-oleic acid complex for myocardial imaging (abstr). *J Nucl Med* 14:381, 1973.

86. Astheimer L, Linse KH, Ramamoorthy N, Schwochau K: Synthesis, characterization and evaluation of ^{99}Tc/^{99m}Tc DIARS and DMPE complexes containing pentadecanoic acid. *Int J Radiation Applic Instr—Part B, Nucl Med Biol* 14:545, 1987.

87. Mach RH, Kung HF, Jungwiwattanaporn P, Guo YZ: Synthesis and biodistribution of a new class of ^{99m}Tc-labeled fatty acid analogs for myocardial imaging. *Int J Radiation Applic Instr—Part B, Nucl Med Biol* 18:215, 1991.

88. Evans JR, Gunton RW, Baker RG, et al: Use of radioiodinated fatty acid for photoscans of the heart. *Circ Res* 26:1, 1965.

89. Gunton RW, Evans JR, Baker RG, et al: Demonstration of myocardial infarction by photoscans of the heart in man. *Am J Cardiol* 16:482, 1965.

90. Poe ND, Robinson GD, MacDonald NS: Myocardial extraction of labeled long-chain fatty acid analogs. *Proc Soc Exp Biol & Med* 148:215, 1975.

91. Robinson GD Jr, Lee AW: Radioiodinated fatty acids for heart imaging: Iodine monochloride addition compared with iodide replacement labeling. *J Nucl Med* 16:17, 1975.

92. Feinendegen LE, Vyska K, Freundlieb C, et al: Noninvasive analysis of metabolic reactions in body tissues: The case of myocardial fatty acids. *Eur J Nucl Med* 6:191, 1981.

93. Knust EJ, Kupfernagel C, Stocklin G: Long-chain F-18 fatty acids for the study of regional metabolism in heart and liver: Odd-even effects of metabolism in mice. *J Nucl Med* 20:1170, 1979.

94. Poe ND, Robinson GD Jr, Graham LS, MacDonald NS: Experimental basis of myocardial imaging with ^{123}I-labeled hexadecenoic acid. *J Nucl Med* 17:1077, 1976.

95. Poe ND, Robinson GD Jr, Zielinski FW, et al: Myocardial imaging with ^{123}I-hexadecenoic acid. *Radiology* 124:419, 1977.

96. van der Wall EE, Heidendal GA, den Hollander W, et al: I-123 labeled hexadecenoic acid in comparison with thallium 201 for myocardial imaging in coronary heart disease: A preliminary study. *Eur J Nucl Med* 5:401, 1980.

97. Westera G, van der Wall EE, Heidendal GA, van den Bos GC: A comparison between terminally radioiodinated hexadecenoic acid (I-HA) and ^{201}Tl-thallium chloride in the dog heart: Implications for the use of I-HA for myocardial imaging. *Eur J Nucl Med* 5:339, 1980.

98. Okada RD, Elmaleh D, Werre GS, Strauss HW: Myocardial kinetics of ^{123}I-labeled-16-hexadecanoic acid. *Eur J Nucl Med* 8:211, 1983.

99. Machulla HJ, Stöcklin G, Kupfernagel C, et al: Comparative evaluation of fatty acids labeled with ^{11}C, ^{34}Cl, ^{77}Br, and ^{123}I for metabolic studies of the myocardium: Concise communication. *J Nucl Med* 19:298, 1978.

100. van der Wall EE, Westera G, Heidendal GA, den Hollander W: A comparison between terminally radioiodinated hexadecenoic acid (^{125}I-HA) and heptadecanoic acid (^{131}I-HOA) in the dog heart. *Eur J Nucl Med* 6:581, 1981.

101. Visser FC, van Eenige MJ, Westera G, et al: Kinetics of radioiodinated heptadecanoic acid and metabolites in the normal and ischaemic canine heart. *Eur Heart J* 6:97, 1985.

102. van der Wall EE, Heidendal GA, den Hollander W, et al: Metabolic myocardial imaging with ^{123}I-labeled heptadecanoic acid in patients with angina pectoris. *Eur J Nucl Med* 6:391, 1981.

103. van der Wall EE, Heidendal GA, den Hollander W, et al: Myocardial scintigraphy with ^{123}I-labeled heptadecanoic acid in patients with unstable angina pectoris. *Postgrad Med J* 59:38, 1983.

104. van der Wall EE, den Hollander W, Heidendal GA, et al: Dynamic myocardial scintigraphy with ^{123}I-labeled free fatty acids in patients with myocardial infarction. *Eur J Nucl Med* 6:383, 1981.

105. Visser FC, Westera G, Van Eenige MJ, et al: Free fatty acid scintigraphy in patients with successful thrombolysis after acute myocardial infarction. *Clin Nucl Med* 10:35, 1985.

106. Chappuis F, Meier B, Belenger J, et al: Early assessment

of tissue viability with radioiodinated heptadecanoic acid in reperfused canine myocardium: Comparison with thallium 201. *Am Heart J* 119:833, 1990.

107. Luthy P, Chatelain P, Papageorgiou I, et al: Assessment of myocardial metabolism with iodine-123 heptadecanoic acid: Effect of decreased fatty acid oxidation on deiodination. *J Nucl Med* 29:1088, 1988.

108. Freundlieb C, Hock A, Vyska K, et al: Myocardial imaging and metabolic studies with [17–^{123}I]iodoheptadecanoic acid. *J Nucl Med* 21:1043, 1980.

109. Schön HR, Senekowitsch R, Berg D, et al: Measurement of myocardial fatty acid metabolism: Kinetics of iodine-123 heptadecanoic acid in normal dog hearts. *J Nucl Med* 27:1449, 1986.

110. Schön HR: I-123 heptadecanoic acid—value and limitations in comparison with C-11 palmitate. *Eur J Nucl Med* 12:S16, 1986.

111. van der Wall EE: Myocardial imaging with radiolabeled free fatty acids: Applications and limitations. *Eur J Nucl Med* 12:S11, 1986.

112. Visser FC, Westera G, van Eenige MJ, et al: The myocardial elimination rate of radioiodinated heptadecanoic acid. *Eur J Nucl Med* 10:118, 1985.

113. Visser FC, van Eenige MJ, van der Wall EE, et al: The elimination rate of ^{123}I-heptadecanoic acid after intracoronary and intravenous administration. *Eur J Nucl Med* 11:114, 1985.

114. Visser FC, van Eenige MJ, Westera G, et al: Metabolic fate of radioiodinated heptadecanoic acid in the normal canine heart. *Circulation* 72:565, 1985.

115. Machulla HJ, Marsmann M, Dutschka K: Biochemical concept and synthesis of a radioiodinated phenyl fatty acid for in vivo metabolic studies of the myocardium. *Eur J Nucl Med* 5:171, 1980.

116. Kulkarni PV, Parkey RW: A new radioiodination method utilizing organothallium intermediate radioiodination of phenylpentadecanoic acid (IPPA) for potential application in myocardial imaging (abst). *J Nucl Med* 23:105, 1982.

117. Caldwell JH, Martin GV, Link JM, et al: Iodophenylpentadecanoic acid-myocardial blood flow relationship during maximal exercise with coronary occlusion. *J Nucl Med* 31:99, 1990.

118. Schmitz B, Reske SN, Machulla HJ, et al: Cardiac metabolism of omega-(p-iodo-phenyl)-pentadecanoic acid: A gas-liquid chromatographic-mass spectrometric analysis. *J Lipid Res* 25:1102, 1984.

119. Chien KR, Han A, White J, Kulkarni P: In vivo esterification of a synthetic ^{125}I-labeled fatty acid into cardiac glycerolipids. *Am J Physiol* 245:H693, 1983.

120. Reske SN, Sauer W, Machulla HJ, Winkler C: 15(p-[^{123}I]iodophenyl)pentadecanoic acid as tracer of lipid metabolism: Comparison with [1-^{14}C]palmitic acid in murine tissues. *J Nucl Med* 25:1335, 1984.

121. Reske SN, Sauer W, Machulla HJ, et al: Metabolism of 15 (p ^{123}I iodophenyl-)pentadecanoic acid in heart muscle and noncardiac tissues. *Eur J Nucl Med* 10:228, 1985.

122. Reske SN: ^{123}I-phenylpentadecanoic acid as a tracer of cardiac free fatty acid metabolism: Experimental and clinical results. *Eur Heart J* 6:39, 1985.

123. Sloof GW, Visser FC, Teerlink T, et al: Incorporation of radioiodinated fatty acids into cardiac phospholipids of normoxic canine myocardium. *Mol Cell Biochem* 116:79, 1992.

124. Reske SN, Knapp FF Jr, Winkler C: Experimental basis of metabolic imaging of the myocardium with radioiodinated aromatic free fatty acids. *Am J Physiol Imaging* 1:214, 1986.

125. Jansen DE, Pippin J, Hansen C, et al: Use of radioactive iodine-labeled fatty acids for myocardial imaging. *Am J Cardiac Imaging* 1:132, 1987.

126. Kulkarni PV, Corbett JR: Radioiodinated tracers for myocardial imaging. *Sem Nucl Med* 20:119, 1990.

127. Kennedy PL, Corbett JR, Kulkarni PV, et al: Iodine 123-phenylpentadecanoic acid myocardial scintigraphy: Usefulness in the identification of myocardial ischemia. *Circulation* 74:1007, 1986.

128. Hansen CL, Corbett JR, Pippin JJ, et al: Iodine-123 phenylpentadecanoic acid and single photon emission computed tomography in identifying left ventricular regional metabolic abnormalities in patients with coronary heart disease: Comparison with thallium-201 myocardial tomography. *J Am Coll Cardiol* 12:78, 1988.

129. Schad N, Wagner RK, Hallermeier J, et al: Regional rates of myocardial fatty acid metabolism: Comparison with coronary angiography and ventriculography. *Eur J Nucl Med* 16:205, 1990.

130. Zimmermann R, Tillmanns H, Kapp M, et al: Reduction of myocardial ischemia by gallopamil: A dual-isotope study with thallium 201 and iodine 123 phenylpentadecanoic acid. *J Cardiovasc Pharm* 20:S40, 1992.

131. Pippen JJ, Jansen DE, Henderson EB, et al: Myocardial fatty acid utilization at various workloads in normal volunteers: Iodine 123 phenylpentadecanoic acid and single photon emission computed tomography to investigate myocardial metabolism. *Am J Cardiac Imaging* 6:99, 1992.

132. Tamaki N, Kawamoto M, Takahashi N, et al: Assessment of myocardial fatty acid metabolism with positron emission tomography at rest and during dobutamine infusion in patients with coronary artery disease. *Am Heart J* 125:702, 1993.

133. Rellas JS, Corbett JR, Kulkarni P, et al: Iodine-123 phenylpentadecanoic acid: Detection of acute myocardial infarction and injury in dogs using an iodinated fatty acid and single-photon emission tomography. *Am J Cardiol* 52:1326, 1983.

134. Hansen CL, Kulkarni PV, Ugolini V, Corbett JR: Detection of alterations in left ventricular fatty acid metabolism in patients with acute myocardial infarction by 15-(p-^{123}I-phenyl)-pentadecanoic acid and tomographic imaging. *Am Heart J* 129:476, 1995.

135. Walamies M, Virtanen V, Koskinen M, Uusitalo A: Patency of the infarct-related coronary artery—a pertinent factor in late recovery of myocardial fatty acid metabolism among patients receiving thrombolytic therapy? *Eur J Nucl Med* 21:968, 1994.

136. Ugolini V, Hansen CL, Kulkarni PV, et al: Abnormal myocardial fatty acid metabolism in dilated cardiomyopathy detected by iodine-123 phenylpentadecanoic acid and tomographic imaging. *Am J Cardiol* 62:923, 1988.

137. Wolfe CL, Kennedy PL, Kulkarni PV, et al: Iodine-123 phenylpentadecanoic acid myocardial scintigraphy in patients with left ventricular hypertrophy: Alterations in left ventricular distribution and utilization. *Am Heart J* 119:1338, 1990.

138. Walamies M, Koskinen M, Uusitalo A, Niemela K: Inhomogeneous exercise uptake and accelerated washout of a radioiodinated fatty acid analogue in syndrome X: A SPECT study of the left ventricle. *Int J Cardiac Imaging* 10:123, 1994.

139. Murray G, Schad N, Ladd W, et al: Metabolic cardiac imaging in severe coronary disease: Assessment of viability with iodine-123-iodophenylpentadecanoic acid and multicrystal gamma camera, and correlation with biopsy. *J Nucl Med* 33:1269, 1992.

140. Kuikka JT, Mussalo H, Hietakorpi S, et al: Evaluation of myocardial viability with technetium-99m hexakis-2-methoxyisobutyl isonitrile and iodine 123 phenylpentadecanoic acid and single photon emission tomography. *Eur J Nucl Med* 19:882, 1992.

141. Hansen CL: Preliminary report of an ongoing phase I/II dose range, safety and efficacy study of iodine-123-phenylpentadecanoic acid for the identification of viable myocardium. *J Nucl Med* 35:38S, 1994.

142. Hansen CL, Heo J, Oliner C, et al: Prediction of improvement of left ventricular function with iodine-123 IPPA after coronary revascularization. *J Nucl Med* 36:1987, 1995.

143. Iskandrian AS, Powers J, Cave V, et al: Assessment of myocardial viability by dynamic tomographic iodine 123 iodophenylpentadecanoic acid imaging: Comparison with rest-redistribution thallium 201 imaging. *J Nucl Cardiol* 2:101, 1995.

144. Mead JF, Levis GM: A 1 carbon degradation of the long chain fatty acids of brain sphingolipids. *J Biol Chem* 238:1634, 1963.

145. Preiss B, Bloch K: Omega-oxidation of long chain fatty acids in rat liver. *J Biol Chem* 239:85, 1964.

146. Antony GJ, Landau BR: Relative contributions of alpha-, beta-, and omega-oxidative pathways to in vitro fatty acid oxidation in rat liver. *J Lipid Res* 9:267, 1968.

147. Huang S, Van Veldhoven PP, Vanhoutte F, et al: Alpha-oxidation of 3-methyl-substituted fatty acids in rat liver. *Arch Biochem Biophys* 296:214, 1992.

148. Takahashi T, Takahashi H, Takeda H, Shichiri M: Alpha-oxidation of fatty acids in fasted or diabetic rats. *Diabetes Res Clin Prac* 16:103, 1992.

149. Knapp FF Jr: Selenium and tellurium as carbon substitutes, in Spencer R (ed): *Radiopharmaceuticals: Structure-Activity Relationships.* New York, Grune & Stratton, 1981, pp 345–391.

150. Goodman MM, Knapp FF Jr, Callahan AP, Ferren LA: Synthesis and biological evaluation of 17-[^{131}I]iodo-9-telluraheptadecanoic acid, a potential imaging agent. *J Med Chem* 25:613, 1982.

151. Goodman MM, Knapp FF Jr, Callahan AP, Ferren LA: A new, well-retained myocardial imaging agent: Radioiodinated 15-(p-Iodophenyl)-6-tellurapentadecanoic acid. *J Nucl Med* 23:904, 1982.

152. Livni E, Elmaleh DR, Levy S, et al: Beta-methyl[1-^{11}C]heptadecanoic acid: A new myocardial metabolic tracer for positron emission tomography. *J Nucl Med* 23:169, 1982.

153. Elmaleh DR, Livni E, Levy S, et al: Comparison of ^{11}C and ^{14}C-labeled fatty acids and their beta-methyl analogs. *Int J Nucl Med Biol* 10:181, 1983.

154. Otto CA, Brown LE, Scott AM: Radioiodinated branched-chain fatty acids: Substrates for beta oxidation? Concise communication. *J Nucl Med* 25:75, 1984.

155. Goodman MM, Kirsch G, Knapp FF Jr: Synthesis and evaluation of radioiodinated terminal p-iodophenyl-substituted alpha- and beta-methyl-branched fatty acids. *J Med Chem* 27:390, 1984.

156. Knapp FF Jr, Goodman MM: The design and biological properties of iodine-123 labeled beta-methyl-branched fatty acids. *Eur Heart J* 6:71, 1985.

157. Knapp FF Jr, Goodman MM, Callahan AP, Kirsch G: Radioiodinated 15-(p-iodophenyl)-3,3-dimethylpentadecanoic acid: A useful new agent to evaluate myocardial fatty acid uptake. *J Nucl Med* 27:521, 1986.

158. Yamamichi Y, Kusuoka H, Morishita K, et al: Metabolism of iodine-123-BMIPP in perfused rat hearts. *J Nucl Med* 36:1043, 1995.

159. Humbert T, Keriel C, Batelle DM, et al: Intramyocardial fate of 15-p-iodophenyl-beta-methylpentadecanoic acid (IMPPA): Is it a good tracer of fatty acid myocardial uptake? *Mol Cell Biochem* 88:195, 1989.

160. Ambrose KR, Owen BA, Goodman MM, Knapp FF Jr: Evaluation of the metabolism in rat hearts of two new radioiodinated 3-methyl-branched fatty acid myocardial imaging agents. *Eur J Nucl Med* 12:486, 1987.

161. Demaison L, Dubois F, Apparu M, et al: Myocardial metabolism of radioiodinated methyl-branched fatty acids. *J Nucl Med* 29:1230, 1988.

162. Sloof GW, Visser FC, van Eenige MJ, et al: Comparison of uptake, oxidation and lipid distribution of 17-iodoheptadecanoic acid, 15-(p-iodophenyl)pentadecanoic acid and 15-(p-iodophenyl)-3,3-dimethylpentadecanoic acid in normal canine myocardium. *J Nucl Med* 34:649, 1993.

163. Chouraqui P, Maddahi J, Henkin R, et al: Comparison of myocardial imaging with iodine-123-iodophenyl-9-methyl pentadecanoic acid and thallium-201-chloride for assessment of patients with exercise-induced myocardial ischemia. *J Nucl Med* 32:447, 1991.

164. Henrich MM, Vester E, von der Lohe E, et al: The comparison of 2-^{18}F-2-deoxyglucose and 15-(ortho-^{123}I-phenyl)-pentadecanoic acid uptake in persisting defects on thallium 201 tomography in myocardial infarction. *J Nucl Med* 32:1353, 1991.

165. Kaiser KP, Geuting B, Grossmann K, et al: Tracer kinetics of 15-(ortho-$^{123/131}$I-phenyl)-pentadecanoic acid (oPPA) and 15-(para-$^{123/131}$I-phenyl)-pentadecanoic acid (pPPA) in animals and man. *J Nucl Med* 31:1608, 1990.

166. Kurata C, Tawarahara K, Taguchi T, et al: Myocardial emission computed tomography with iodine-123-labeled beta-methyl-branched fatty acid in patients with hypertrophic cardiomyopathy. *J Nucl Med* 33:6, 1992.

167. Tamaki N, Kawamoto M, Yonekura Y, et al: Regional metabolic abnormality in relation to perfusion and wall

motion in patients with myocardial infarction: Assessment with emission tomography using an iodinated branched fatty acid analog. *J Nucl Med* 33:659, 1992.

168. Franken PR, De Geeter F, Dendale P, et al: Abnormal free fatty acid uptake in subacute myocardial infarction after coronary thrombolysis: Correlation with wall motion and inotropic reserve. *J Nucl Med* 35:1758, 1994.

169. Matsunari I, Saga T, Taki J, et al: Kinetics of iodine-123-BMIPP in patients with prior myocardial infarction: Assessment with dynamic rest and stress images compared with stress thallium-201 SPECT. *J Nucl Med* 35:1279, 1994.

170. Fujibayashi Y, Yonekura Y, Takemura Y, et al: Myocardial accumulation of iodinated beta-methyl-branched fatty acid analogue, iodine-125-15-(p-iodophenyl)-3-(R,S)methylpentadecanoic acid (BMIPP), in relation to ATP concentration. *J Nucl Med* 31:1818, 1990.

171. Miller DD, Gill JB, Livni E, et al: Fatty acid analogue accumulation: A marker of myocyte viability in ischemic-reperfused myocardium. *Circ Res* 63:681, 1988.

172. Nishimura T, Sago M, Kihara K, et al: Fatty acid myocardial imaging using ^{123}I-beta-methyl-iodophenyl pentadecanoic acid (BMIPP): Comparison of myocardial perfusion and fatty acid utilization in canine myocardial infarction (occlusion and reperfusion model). *Eur J Nucl Med* 15:341, 1989.

173. Saito T, Yasuda T, Gold HK, et al: Differentiation of regional perfusion and fatty acid uptake in zones of myocardial injury. *Nucl Med Com* 12:663, 1991.

SPECT Imaging of Fluorodeoxyglucose

Robert W. Burt

This chapter discusses the use of single photon emission computed tomography (SPECT) applied to imaging the uptake of fluorine-18 fluorodeoxyglucose (^{18}F FDG) in the myocardium. The technical details of tomographic imaging of myocardial perfusion with single-photon agents, which also apply to this use, are found in Chap. 3 on myocardial perfusion imaging. A detailed discussion of the cellular physiology involved with the use of ^{18}F FDG in myocardial ischemia and detection of potential viability can be found in Chap. 9 on positron emission tomography (PET) of the heart. The present chapter is not intended as a discussion of the merits of ^{18}F FDG imaging as related to cardiac viability determination but as an introduction to the feasibility of using near-standard SPECT instrumentation for this purpose.

The use of ^{18}F FDG in combination with PET imaging has become an established technique for the evaluation of myocardium compromised by severe ischemia.[1] The conversion of myocardial cellular metabolism from the use of fatty acids as the primary substrate to the use of glucose has been well described. The administration of the glucose analog ^{18}F FDG and subsequent demonstration of its preferential accumulation in ischemic segments detects and confirms this metabolic change and demonstrates that the segment is viable.

This procedure is used to identify myocardial segments with impaired regional contraction that have a high likelihood of functional improvement with revascularization. Characterization of the contractile function of these segments is made during contrast ventriculography or with noninvasive procedures, including echocar-diography or radionuclide ventriculography. If a segment with vascular compromise shows clear evidence of intrinsic wall motion, a ^{18}F FDG procedure is redundant. Practically, however, demonstration of intrinsic regional wall motion may not be clear-cut because hypokinesis may be mimicked by "tethering" of an akinetic scarred segment by adjacent segments.

The availability of ^{18}F FDG imaging has been restricted by the lack of PET tomographs easily available for clinical applications, the limited availability of the ^{18}F FDG tracer, and the reluctance of many third-party payers to reimburse providers for the procedure because of its costs. The problem of limited availability of PET tomographs could be averted if ^{18}F FDG imaging is adapted successfully to conventional nuclear medicine instrumentation. Several investigators have shown the successful application of standard nuclear medicine instrumentation, usually with multiheaded SPECT instruments, for this purpose.[2-8]

Imaging ^{18}F FDG in the heart for viability studies is a different problem than imaging the heart with a perfusion agent to detect ischemia. Perfusion imaging requires very high sensitivity and the ability to resolve small areas of myocardium with low or no uptake. Imaging the heart using ^{18}F FDG is technically a much simpler task. The goal is to detect uptake of ^{18}F FDG in a myocardial segment or segments of clinically significant size. These are relatively large targets and the presence of only minimal uptake is not relevant. The answer to the clinical question of myocardial viability is typically "yes" or "no" based on glucose uptake in a segment. In some areas, SPECT devices are superior to the more specialized PET instruments. Most present PET tomographs have no easy method for centering the heart in a fairly narrow field of view. The PET instrument used in our laboratory has approximately a 4-inch field of view; however, the exact position of the heart in the field is seen only after reconstruction of the images. This causes difficulties in both accurate positioning of the heart and in failure to visualize all segments of dilated hearts. Neither is a problem with SPECT instruments with their associated viewing devices. Typical three-headed SPECT cameras have a 10- or 20-inch field of view and persistence displays to aid in patient positioning. This allows easy positioning and imaging of even the largest or most dilated heart.

Usually PET cardiac viability procedures include a transmission scan to determine tissue attenuation followed by an image of myocardial blood flow, and then by an image of ^{18}F FDG metabolism. Following ^{18}F FDG injection there is a 45 to 120 min delay to allow for incorporation of tracer into the myocardium. During the PET study period, which may take as long as 2 h or more, the patient should remain immobile in the scanner. The patient is instructed not to move; however, this is difficult and if movement is not noticed, portions of the heart may not be visualized on the resultant images. SPECT ^{18}F FDG images typically require the patient to be in the scanner no more than 30 min as no transmission scan is done. Patients are positioned in the instrument just before imaging and all preparation can be done elsewhere, even in a coronary care unit.

Images of the myocardium produced with modern PET will nearly always be superior in technical quality to those obtained with a SPECT system. With PET, more and thinner sections will be obtained and hearts with relatively poor ^{18}F FDG uptake may produce satisfactory clinical images for diagnosis. The greatest advantages of the SPECT approach are the availability of the SPECT devices and their uses in other applications. The imaging techniques are similar to those used for cardiac perfusion imaging with single-photon tracers and require little or no additional technical effort or training.

INSTRUMENTATION

Imaging ^{18}F FDG has been performed on a variety of gamma cameras. Initial studies used planar imaging with single-head instruments.[9-13] It seems clear, however, that ^{18}F FDG images are best performed with instruments producing tomographic images that are easily compared with SPECT perfusion images. These images provide high contrast resolution compared to planar studies. Although successful ^{18}F FDG imaging has been performed

with single head, dual-head, or triple-head systems; the latter two methods produce superior results.[2,4] A three-head camera will provide 50 percent more sensitivity when compared to a similar dual-head camera.

Until recently most standard cameras had important limitations when 511-keV imaging was performed. They can be grouped into specific considerations:

1. Collimator design
2. Crystal
3. Detector head shielding
4. Gantry strength
5. Electronics

Collimation

Collimators designed for 511-keV SPECT imaging are heavy, thick, clumsy to handle, and insensitive. For cardiac ^{18}F FDG imaging, the collimator design should give equal weight to resolution and sensitivity. Currently described systems for SPECT imaging of ^{18}F FDG have used collimators with hole lengths of 78 to 100 mm, hole diameters of 3.8 to 6.6 mm, and septal thickness of 1.7 to 3.3 mm. These systems have yielded full width at half-maximum resolution in air at 10 cm from the collimator face of 11.9 to 15.2 mm.[2-4,7,10] Although resolution is less than that obtained with SPECT imaging of thallium 201 (^{201}Tl) or technetium 99m (^{99m}Tc), the 511-keV emissions of ^{18}F FDG are less influenced by Compton scatter. The net result is acceptable image resolution with SPECT imaging of ^{18}F FDG on the systems described. An additional major consideration is septal penetration of the 511-keV emissions. Some septal penetration is acceptable and the system that we use has 8 to 10 percent (Fig. 8-1).

Although satisfactory design of high energy collimators is not a particularly difficult task, handling them is. Some of these collimators may weigh more than 200 kg each. A clinical system must provide a convenient and reliable method of handling the collimators and changing them on the camera heads.

Crystal

A standard ⅜-inch sodium iodide crystal provides limited capability for interaction with 511-keV positrons. The efficiency of a ⅜-inch (9-mm) sodium iodide crystal for 511-keV photons is approximately 30 percent of the efficiency for 140-keV photons of ^{99m}Tc. Nevertheless, the photon yield of ^{18}F FDG is twice that of single-photon tracers and Compton scatter rejection by the energy window is highly effective at 511 keV. The net result is satisfactory detection of 511-keV photons with a stan-

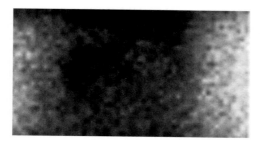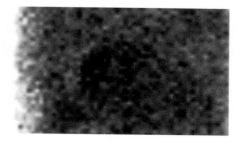

Figure 8-1 Anterior SPECT projections. **Left:** Poorly shielded camera with scatter from brain and bladder reducing effective field of view. Diabetic patient with poor sugar control producing poor contrast. **Right:** Well shielded camera without scatter. Diabetic patient with good sugar control, but abnormal FDG distribution in heart.

dard ⅜-inch crystal. The additional sensitivity associated with increasing the crystal thickness to ½ inch has been reported to be only 5 to 10 percent and this small improvement in sensitivity for positron detection often does not justify the adverse effects of the thicker crystal when the same camera is used for other standard nuclear medicine procedures.

The 30 percent lower efficiency of a ⅜-inch sodium iodide crystal combined with the approximately threefold loss of sensitivity with the use of a high energy collimator results in detection of approximately 9 percent of counts per unit of radioactivity for ^{18}F FDG compared to ^{201}Tl.[3] This potential limitation of SPECT imaging of ^{18}F FDG is overcome by administering more activity (e.g., 10 mCi, 370 MBq) of ^{18}F FDG in comparison to a 3-mCi dose of ^{201}Tl.

Camera Head

The camera head should be well shielded, especially on the side facing the patient's head, to prevent photon penetration. When ^{18}F FDG is injected, a large portion of the dose goes to the brain, much more than to the heart or surrounding tissues. This is a "hot" source and can produce an arc of scatter at the top of the images. With most devices the heart size is such that interference from scatter can be avoided by centering the heart in the field of view. It is easier to locate the heart for imaging correctly if this arc of scatter is not present. Scatter is also present from the lower torso and bladder, but it is not of the same magnitude.

Gantry

The gantry should be strong and stable to handle the collimator weight with safety and without bowing. If the gantry or collimator support should slip or break during a study, the possible consequences to a patient are obvious. Bowing of the gantry may produce distor-

tions in reconstruction if collimator angles and distances from the camera head to the patient change during rotation. Other considerations from routine SPECT image acquisition such as accurate center of rotation (COR) correction and stable angular incremental motions also apply but may be more difficult to achieve because of collimator weight. If the gantry does not perform angular rotation in accurate increments or if the collimators do not follow a predictable arc during rotation, both the COR corrections and reconstructions may be unsatisfactory. The system should be designed to support this extra collimator weight. High energy collimators should not be added to systems not designed to support their weight.

Camera Electronics

The camera electronics should be stable and capable of correctly positioning the 511-keV photons without modification, which would limit other camera uses. This can be demonstrated by the usual quality control techniques except using a 511-keV source for the measurements. A flood-correction map to be used in reconstruction should be acquired and stored. Presently, sheet sources producing 511-keV photons are just becoming commercially available. An alternative approach is to produce ^{18}F maps without a collimator in place, using a ^{18}F point source at a distance. This approach is not entirely satisfactory; however, given the resolution of the system as a whole, it seems acceptable. One should avoid filling a plastic sheet fluid source with ^{18}F. It is quite reactive and will fix to the plastic randomly. The ^{18}F FDG sheet sources seem to work satisfactorily but are difficult to handle, especially for large field systems.

IMAGING PROTOCOLS

A ^{18}F FDG study should be performed in conjunction with images of a myocardial perfusion marker used to demonstrate hypoperfused areas.[2,4,14,15] A ^{201}Tl image set, preferably with the tracer injected at rest, can be used. Alternatively, the ^{18}F FDG images may be reviewed in conjunction with a previous stress-redistribution ^{201}Tl examination. If akinetic or severely hypokinetic myocardial segments are identified by other methods, then images obtained at 15 min following injection of ^{201}Tl, and again at 3 h, can provide useful information concerning both myocardial perfusion and viability. A 3- to 5-mCi dose of ^{201}Tl is used to ensure adequate images. If persistent defects of the suspect segments are present on the 3-h rest thallium image set, this defines the segments to be further evaluated with FDG (Plates 13, 14, and 15). In many cases the rest (or reinjection) thallium images alone will provide the necessary viability information and the ^{18}F FDG study will not be required.[16-19] Locally, the cost of an ^{18}F FDG dose is about eight times that of a ^{201}Tl dose.

Others have used ^{99m}Tc sestamibi for identification of myocardial hypoperfusion in conjunction with FDG viability assessment with good results.[13,14] Sawada, however, compared rest ^{99m}Tc sestamibi alone to ^{18}F FDG for viability estimates and found a greater discrepancy than reported with ^{201}Tl alone.[20] Rest-injected ^{99m}Tc sestamibi appears to be a satisfactory substitute for [13]NH$_3$ as a primary perfusion marker. It may be less satisfactory when given only during stress. In theory, if multiple segments have reduced perfusion at stress, and one is very hypermetabolic for glucose, an accurate evaluation of the others may not be possible. Reports using the ^{99m}Tc sestamibi/^{18}F FDG technique are early in development but it appears to be useful in reducing actual imaging time.[13,14] The ability to do simultaneous imaging with ^{18}F FDG and ^{99m}Tc sestamibi or ^{201}Tl also clearly demonstrates the capabilities of modern SPECT cameras.

Injection of the FDG tracer should be done under carefully controlled conditions after the patient has fasted for at least 6 h, preferably overnight. Glucose management is key to producing satisfactory clinical images and is accomplished by glucose loading and blood glucose control with insulin.[21,22] Detailed description of these protocols is beyond the scope of this chapter and should be developed in individual laboratories; however, administration of ^{18}F FDG when the blood glucose is elevated will nearly always produce poor quality SPECT images. Glucose and ^{18}F FDG accumulate slowly and only the ^{18}F FDG is trapped in the myocardium. Later images may improve FDG delineation.[19] The PET protocols usually begin image acquisition 45 to 60 min after FDG injection. We routinely begin SPECT imaging no sooner than 1 h after injection and have obtained useful images as much as 2.5 to 3 h after injection.

Imaging Parameters

The systems that we have available for ^{18}F FDG cardiac imaging are three-head devices. Our acquisition parameters are identical to those used for rest thallium imaging and require about 19 min to complete. We have found that using a continuous acquisition technique with narrow angles of "binning" routinely produces superior images as 10 to 15 percent more counts are acquired in the same time. The Butterworth filters used for thallium imaging can also be applied for processing ^{18}F FDG images. However, the global uptake of ^{18}F FDG in the myocardium varies; when ^{18}F FDG activity is lower than expected a filter modification can be made to "soften" the images. Because filters are not identical from manufacturer to manufacturer, trials of filters on individual systems should be done by the user. If attenuation correction is used, the attenuation coefficient should be set to 0.089 for the 511-keV photons and not to the default setting used for ^{201}Tl or [99m]Tc.

Low FDG uptake is a severe handicap to SPECT imaging and is somewhat less of a problem with PET. PET cameras have much higher sensitivity than SPECT cameras with high energy collimators.[8,23] Though degraded, PET images are more likely to be of useful technical quality in this circumstance because of the superior sensitivity of the instrument. Careful management of the glucose levels will improve uptake and is the single most important portion of the SPECT protocols.[24,25]

Image Evaluation

The fairly simple evaluation schema for these ^{201}Tl/FDG image sets is summarized in Table 8-1.

Quantitative comparison of the relative uptakes of ^{18}F FDG and a perfusion tracer can be accomplished by using standard tomographic slice formats that place normalized sections (short axis, horizontal long axis, and vertical long axis) as adjacent slices. The 50 percent of maximum ^{18}F FDG uptake level is typically used as a separation point that defines segments likely viable from those not likely to respond to revascularization.

A recent study reported on the comparison of the distribution of ^{201}Tl and ^{18}F FDG uptake in normal subjects.[26] Without known flow disturbances in the heart, the uptake of both tracers was concordant. Applying this information to the comparison of ^{201}Tl and ^{18}F FDG images might allow detection of resting ischemia by showing focal hypermetabolism in segments of relatively

Table 8-1   FDG and Thallium Uptake in Myocardial Segments

	FDG No Uptake	FDG Uptake
Thallium no uptake	Probably not viable	Ischemic but viable
Thallium uptake	Normal not ischemic[a]	Normal

[a] This is seen when other segments are hypermetabolic.

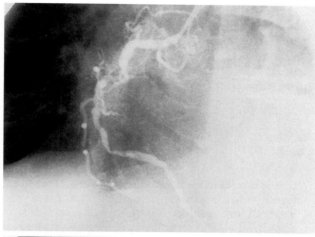

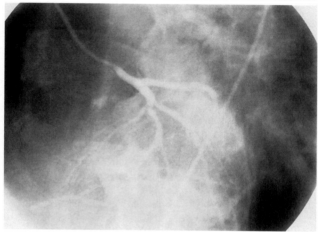

Figure 8-2 **Top:** Selective right coronary arteriogram in the left anterior oblique projection for the patient whose ^{201}Tl and ^{18}F FDG images are shown in Plate 16. This shows a diffusely diseased right coronary artery that is totally occluded proximally filling anterogradely via bridging collaterals. The posterior descending branch fills from the right coronary artery. The angiographic distribution corresponds to the matched perfusion and metabolism defects (indicative of myocardial scar) demonstrated in the inferior left ventricular wall in Plate 16. **Bottom:** Selective left coronary arteriogram in the left anterior oblique projection for the same patient. This demonstrates a left anterior descending coronary artery lesion less than 50 percent stenotic between the first and second diagonal branches. The first diagonal branch has hemodynamically insignificant disease at its origin. The left circumflex is abruptly occluded in its early course posteriorly. Left-to-left collaterals are noted filling the distal left circumflex distribution in the atrioventricular groove. Left-to-right collaterals are seen to fill the distal right coronary artery distribution. The left circumflex distribution corresponds to a region of preserved myocardial perfusion on the ^{201}Tl images and an area of apparent hypermetabolism on the ^{18}F FDG SPECT images. (Courtesy of James V. Faris, M.D.)

normal thallium uptake (Plate 16 and Fig. 8-2). We have encountered this combination of findings clinically and this area is under investigation.

Large studies directly validating ^{18}F FDG SPECT imaging against recovery of regional myocardial contraction following coronary artery revascularization are not available at the time of writing. Nevertheless, early re-

ports showing a high correlation of ^{18}F FDG activity detection by SPECT and PET methods show the need for further studies. In a recent study[2] of 20 patients with a total of 61 myocardial segments with fixed ^{201}Tl defects, ^{18}F FDG SPECT and ^{18}F FDG PET uptake were concordant in 56 of 61 segments (92 percent).

LIMITATIONS AND FUTURE DIRECTIONS OF FDG SPECT IMAGING

This technique has limitations. They mainly are related to sensitivity of the imaging systems, especially those systems with less than three detectors. When ^{18}F FDG uptake is low, then reconstruction of resulting low count images will produce marginal results. The availability of ^{18}F FDG is presently limited; however, it is now being distributed in some metropolitan areas.

Nearly all SPECT camera manufacturers are pursuing the technology required for imaging ^{18}F FDG. Most appear to be concentrating on improving collimator design and camera shielding; however, there are now efforts to "design in" coincidence counting capability in large field opposed detector cameras. Sensitivity appears to be reduced but resolution is improved. It seems likely that these devices will produce images rivaling those from PET tomographs; however, imaging times may be much longer and lower doses of FDG may be necessary because of system dead times.

SUMMARY AND CONCLUSIONS

The work of several investigators, all relatively recent, has shown that it is clinically practical to image ^{18}F FDG in the myocardium with satisfactory clinical results using fairly standard modern multihead gamma cameras.[27] To do this successfully, the instrumentation must be capable of imaging high energy photons and able to support heavy collimators. The imaging techniques are not exotic; however, attention to detail and careful glucose management are integral to good results. Integration of ^{18}F FDG imaging with cardiac perfusion imaging with single-photon agents extends the capability of nuclear imaging techniques. Further, fairly simple camera development should produce even better images. When a wider clinical need for ^{18}F FDG follows, commercial supplies of ^{18}F FDG will emerge.

REFERENCES

1. Tillisch J, Brunken R, Marshall R, et al: Reversibility of cardiac wall motion abnormalities predicted by positron tomography. *N Engl J Med* 314:884, 1986.

2. Burt RW, Perkins OW, Oppenheim BE, et al: Direct comparison of F-18 FDG SPECT, F-18 FDG PET and rest thallium SPECT for detection of myocardial viability. *J Nucl Med* 36:176, 1995.

3. Drane WE, Abbott FD, Nicole MW, et al: Technology for FDG SPECT with a relatively inexpensive gamma camera. *Radiology* 191:461, 1994.

4. Stoll H-P, Helwig N, Alexander C, et al: Myocardial metabolic imaging by means of fluorine-18 deoxyglucose/technetium-99m sestamibi dual-isotope single photon emission tomography. *Eur J Nucl Med* 21:1085, 1994.

5. Huitnik JM, Visser FC, van Lingen A, et al: Feasibility of planar fluorine-18-FDG imaging after recent myocardial infarction to assess myocardial viability. *J Nucl Med* 36:975, 1995.

6. Martin WH, Delbeke D, Patton JA, et al: FDG-SPECT: correlation with FDG-PET. *J Nucl Med* 36:988, 1995.

7. Bax JJ, Visser FC, Van Lingen A, et al: Myocardial F-18 fluorodeoxyglucose imaging by SPECT. *Clin Nucl Med* 20:486, 1995.

8. Leichner PK, Morgan HT, Holdeman KP, et al: SPECT imaging of fluorine-18. *J Nucl Med* 36:1471, 1995.

9. Williams KA, Taillon LA, Stark VJ: Quantitative planar imaging of glucose metabolic activity in myocardial segments with exercise thallium-201 perfusion defects in patients with myocardial infarction: Comparison with late (24-hour) redistribution in thallium imaging for detection of hibernating myocardium. *Am Heart J* 124:294, 1992.

10. van Lingen A, Huijgens PC, Visser FC, et al: Performance characteristics of a 511-keV collimator for imaging positron emitters with a standard gamma-camera. *Eur J Nucl Med* 19:315, 1992.

11. Every JL, Barton HJ, Leaney P, et al: Planar F-18 fluorodeoxyglucose (FDG) imaging for viable myocardium with an anger gamma camera. *Eur J Nucl Med* 20:851, 1993 (abstr).

12. Hoflin F, Ledermann H, Noelpp U, et al: Routine 18F-2-deoxy-2-fluoro-D- glucose (18F-FDG) myocardial tomography using a normal large field of view gamma camera. *Angiology* 40:1058, 1989.

13. Kalff V, Berlangier SU, Van Every B, et al: Is planar thallium-201/fluorine-18 fluorodeoxyglucose imaging a reasonable clinical alternative to positron emission tomographic myocardial viability scanning? *Eur J Nucl Med* 22:625, 1995.

14. Sandler MP, Videlefsky S, Delbeke D, et al: Evaluation of myocardial ischemia using a rest metabolism/stress perfusion protocol with fluorine-18 deoxyglucose/technetium-99m MIBI and dual-isotope simultaneous-acquisition single-photon emission computed tomography. *J Am Coll Cardiol* 26:870, 1995.

15. Delbeke D, Videlefsky S, Patton JA, et al: Rest myocardial perfusion/metabolism imaging using simultaneous dual-isotope acquisition SPECT with technetium-99m-MIBI/fluorine-18-FDG. *J Nucl Med* 36:2110, 1995.

16. Dilsizian V, Perrone-Filardi P, Arrighi JA, et al: Concordance and discordance between stress-redistribution-reinjection and rest-redistribution thallium imaging for assessing viable myocardium. Comparison with metabolic activity by positron emission tomography. *Circulation* 88:941, 1993.

17. Tamaki N, Ohtani H, Yamashita K, et al: Metabolic activity in the areas of new fill-in after thallium-201 reinjection: Comparison with positron emission tomography using fluorine-18-deoxyglucose. *J Nucl Med* 32:673, 1991.

18. Inglese E, Brambilla M, Dondi M, et al: Assessment of myocardial viability after thallium-201 reinjection of rest-redistribution imaging: A multicenter study. *J Nucl Med* 36:555, 1995.

19. Maddahi J, Schelbert H, Brunken R, et al: Role of thallium-201 and PET imaging in evaluation of myocardial viability and management of patients with coronary artery disease and left ventricular dysfunction. *J Nucl Med* 35:707, 1994.

20. Sawada SG, Allman KC, Muzik O, et al: Positron emission tomography defects evidence of viability in rest technetium-99m sestamibi defects. *J Am Coll Cardiol* 23:92, 1994.

21. Knuuti MJ, Nuutila P, Ruotsalainen U, et al: Euglycemic hyperinsulinemic clamp and oral glucose load in stimulating myocardial glucose utilization during positron emission tomography. *J Nucl Med* 33:1255, 1992.

22. Huitink JM, Visser FC, van Leeuwen GR, et al: Influence of high and low plasma insulin levels on the uptake of fluorine-18 fluorodeoxyglucose in myocardium and femoral muscle, assessed by planar imaging. *Eur J Nucl Med* 22:1141, 1995.

23. Macfarlane DJ, Cotton L, Ackermann RJ, et al: Triple-head SPECT with 2-[fluorine-18]fluoro-2-deoxy-D-glucose (FDG): Initial evaluation in oncology and comparison with FDG PET. *Radiology* 194:425, 1995.

24. Gropler RJ, Siegel BA, Lee KJ, et al: Nonuniformity in myocardial accumulation of fluorine-18-fluorodeoxyglucose in normal fasted humans. *J Nucl Med* 31:1749, 1990.

25. Hicks RJ, Herman WH, Kalff V, et al: Quantitative evaluation of regional substrate metabolism in the human heart by positron emission tomography. *J Am Coll Cardiol* 18:101, 1991.

26. Bax J, Visser F, van Lingen A, et al: Relation between myocardial uptake of thallium-201 chloride and fluorine-18 fluorodeoxyglucose imaged with single-photon emission tomography in normal individuals. *Eur J Nucl Med* 22:56, 1995.

27. Kelly MJ, Kalff V: Fluorine 18-labeled fluorodeoxyglucose myocardial scintigraphy with anger gamma cameras for assessing myocardial viability. *J Nucl Cardiol* 2:360, 1995 (review).

POSITRON EMISSION TOMOGRAPHY

Positron Emission Tomography of the Heart

Steven R. Bergmann

Physicians and researchers have a number of diverse approaches for assessment of the anatomy, function, perfusion, and metabolism of the human heart. In this era of cost containment, however, new technologies must provide superior information on which clinical decisions are made or provide unique insights into pathophysiologic processes. Positron emission tomography (PET) has evolved as a noninvasive approach for the assessment of myocardial perfusion, metabolism, and function of the heart. As with all new techniques, rational use requires knowledge of the relative strengths and limitations of the approach.

It is clear that PET, with its intrinsic quantitative capabilities, can provide estimates of both myocardial perfusion and metabolism in absolute terms. With the use of labeled compounds of physiologic interest, valuable insights into the physiology of cardiac disease of diverse etiologies can be obtained, and PET has proven extremely valuable for research applications. However, it remains to be determined whether PET will provide direct clinical diagnostic advantages over existing, and generally less expensive, approaches for the diagnosis and assessment of treatment efficacy of diseases of the heart.

This chapter reviews the basic principles of PET and summarizes the major clinical observations made to date in order to assist physicians in identifying patients who are most likely to benefit from this specialized procedure.

THE EVOLUTION OF PET OF THE HEART

At the most basic level, the heart can be viewed as a pump, and the end point of almost all cardiac disease is the inability of the heart to maintain pump function. This view belies the marvelous and complex dependence of pump function on myocardial blood flow and on the biochemical reactions that support myocyte homeostasis, electrophysiologic integrity, energy production, and contractile performance.

Because myocardial metabolism and function are intimately coupled with flow, noninvasive nuclear medicine techniques with extractable flow tracers such as ^{201}Tl or ^{99m}Tc sestamibi constitute the mainstay for evaluation of coronary artery disease. Noninvasive assessments of metabolism with iodinated fatty acids have also been applied in patients. Nonetheless, limitations inherent to the use of nonphysiologic single-photon-emitting radiotracers—even with the use of single photon emission computed tomography (SPECT)—have limited the quantitative power of these approaches.

PET is capable of providing quantitative estimates of the distribution of positron-emitting radionuclides within the body within the defined limitations of the spatial resolution of the particular tomographic instrument used. Since substances of physiologic interest can be labeled, perfusion and metabolically important biochemical pathways can be assessed with PET. In addition, regional function can be determined concomitantly.

PET has developed rapidly over the 20 years since the first whole-body tomograph was developed and built by Ter-Pogossian and colleagues[1] because of the availability of cyclotrons necessary to produce the short-half-life positron-emitting radionuclides within medical centers and the ability of radiochemists to develop rapid synthetic procedures for incorporation of these radionuclides into compounds. Advances in computer and mathematical procedures as well as the entrance of committed industrial concerns have facilitated the development of the technology.

Despite considerable progress, PET of the heart remains a complex procedure because of the multifaceted need for cyclotron or generator production of radioisotopes and radiochemical synthesis, the demands of the detection system, and the complex biological behaviors of tracers.

BASIC CONCEPTS OF PET

Radiotracers Used in PET of the Heart

One of the most fundamental attractions of PET is the ability to label compounds of physiologic interest.[2-4] The positron-emitting isotopes of oxygen, carbon, nitrogen, and fluorine exhibit chemical and physical properties identical to naturally occurring compounds and make them particularly attractive for incorporation into substrates that participate in physiologically important processes (Table 9-1). The short physical half-life of positron-emitting radionuclides avoids high-radiation burdens for most studies. Use of the shorter half-life tracers, such as ^{82}Rb and ^{15}O, enables sequential studies under rapidly changing conditions. Some positron-emitting radionuclides, such as ^{18}F, are amenable to remote radiopharmaceutical production and scheduled delivery.

The development of generator-produced positron-emitting radionuclides should diminish the requirements for on-site cyclotrons and synthetic chemistry labora-

tories. Generators employ relatively long half-life parent compounds and obviate the need for an on-site cyclotron. For instance, ^{68}Ga is prepared from a ^{68}Ge generator, which has a half-life of 287 days. Rubidium 82, another generator-produced isotope, is produced from ^{82}Sr, which has a half-life of 25 days. The use of these and other generators makes it feasible for institutions without cyclotrons to participate in PET.

Localization of Positron Emission

Wrenn et al[5] and Brownell and Sweet[6] demonstrated almost 40 years ago that a positron-emitting radionuclide within the body could be localized accurately because of the nature of the emitted radiation. Positron-emitting radionuclides are inherently unstable. When the high-energy positron is emitted from a nucleus, it rapidly loses energy and, after traveling a distance, interacts with an electron to yield two photons emitted at an angle of approximately 180°, each with an energy of 511 keV (Fig. 9-1). Coincidence counting, i.e., the detection of two photons by opposing detectors within a given time window (typically 5 to 20 ns), compensates for attenuation regardless of the location of the emission and electronically collimates the field of view to enable precise localization of the annihilation event.[7-9]

Tomographic Instrumentation

A number of tomographic systems are currently in use.[7-9] All are expansions of the concept of a single-coincidence

Table 9-1 Positron-Emitting Compounds Used for PET of the Heart

Radionuclide	Half-life	Compound	Use
Cyclotron produced			
Oxygen 15	2.1 min	H_2O	Blood flow
		CO	Blood volume
		CO_2	Blood flow
		O_2	Metabolism
		Butanol	Blood flow
Nitrogen 13	10.0 min	NH_3	Blood flow/metabolism
		Various amino acids	Metabolism
Carbon 11	20.4 min	Palmitate	Metabolism
		Acetate	Metabolism
		Glucose	Metabolism
		Microspheres	Blood flow
		BMHDA	Metabolism
		Hydroxyephedine	Adrenergic receptors
		Amino acids	Metabolism
Fluorine 18	110 min	Deoxyglucose	Metabolism
		Fluoromisonidazole	Hypoxic myocardium
		Fluorodopamine	Adrenergic receptors
Generator produced			
Rubidium 82	76 s	RbCl	Blood flow/cell viability
Gallium 68	68 min	Microspheres	Blood flow
		Transferrin	Plasma volume
Copper 62	9.7 min	PTSM	Blood flow

BMHDA, β-methyl-heptadecanoic acid; PTSM, pyruvaldehyde *bis*(N⁴-methylthiosemicarbazone).

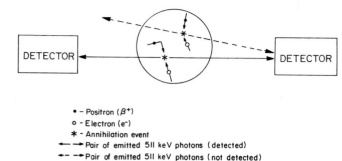

• – Positron (β⁺)
○ – Electron (e⁻)
∗ – Annihilation event
←—→ Pair of emitted 511 keV photons (detected)
←– –→ Pair of emitted 511 keV photons (not detected)

Figure 9-1 Schematic diagram of positron emission and annihilation photon detection. When a positron (β⁺) is emitted from the nucleus, it travels a short distance, rapidly loses kinetic energy, and interacts with an electron. This results in the emission of two *annihilation* photons emitted at an angle of approximately 180° from each other, each with an energy of 511 keV. If the two photons are detected in coincidence (within a prespecified time window, generally 5 to 20 ns), an annihilation event is "detected." Electronic collimation limits the field of view to the region between opposing detectors.

field of view and consist of a ring of detectors around the body (Fig. 9-2). Most have at least three and some have up to five or more rings in the axial direction to enable the simultaneous acquisition of multiple trans-

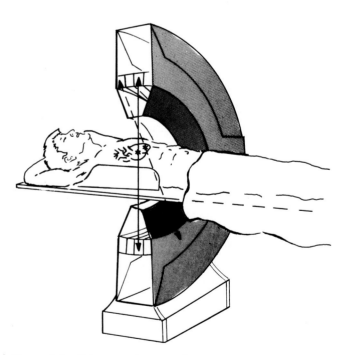

Figure 9-2 Schematic diagram of a PET instrument. Most tomographs employ multiple rings around the patient, which enables the simultaneous acquisition of data in multiple transverse planes. The fidelity of the reconstructed image depends on multiple factors, including the number of lines of coincidence recorded. Accordingly, most detectors are operated in coincidence with multiple opposing detectors as well as detectors with adjacent rings. Typically, several million coincidence events are recorded.

verse "slices" of the myocardium. More recent, commercially available tomographs use "blocks" of scintillation detectors such as bismuth germanate and Anger logic to provide a large axial field of view and greater numbers of transaxial cuts. Since the fidelity of the reconstruction in relation to the actual distribution of the positron-emitting radionuclides within the tissue depends on the number of projections obtained, each detector is typically operated in coincidence with multiple opposing detectors, thus providing numerous coincidence lines through the imaged object. Some systems use rotation or wobble of the detector ring to increase the number of acquisition planes further. Cross-coincidence between rings is often used to increase the number of reconstructed transverse planes.

A number of different scintillation detectors are used based predominantly on the major application of the particular tomographic instrument. Cesium-fluoride crystals enable the most rapid data acquisition and least detector *dead time* because they have the shortest fluorescence decay time (5-ns decay constant). This allows the use of short coincidence resolving times, making these crystals particularly useful for applications with high counting rates and fast dynamic events. Bismuth germanate crystals are used in most commercially available tomographs. They are relatively "slow" (300-ns decay constant) but have high stopping power for photons, making them efficient. Barium-fluoride detectors lie in between these two extremes.

Acquired coincidence data are stored and processed with a computer system after correction for photon attenuation that occurs despite the relatively high energy of the annihilation photons. Attenuation correction factors are typically measured directly by acquisition of an attenuation scan, using an external ring or rod source of radioactivity prior to collection of emission data.

Reconstruction Algorithms

Consideration of the algorithms used for construction of tomographic images is beyond the scope of this chapter. Several approaches can be employed, including backprojection and confidence weighting.[7-10] Some tomographic instruments incorporate *time of flight*, the small difference (in the order of 300 to 500 ps) in the time of arrival of a pair of photons at two opposing detectors to ascertain more precisely the locus of the emission and to reduce scatter and detection of "accidental" events (detection of a coincidence event by simultaneous arrival of two unrelated photons at opposing detectors).[10] Additional considerations in the fidelity of data include the effects of incorrect attenuation factors, scattered radiation, accidental coincidences, and machine and computer dead time, among others.[9-11] Future mathematical reconstruction schemes will undoubtedly improve the quantitative aspects of PET.

Image Display

In virtually all PET tomographs, emission data are collected from transverse rings surrounding the patient. Results are most typically displayed as count-based tomograms (Fig. 9-3). Reconstruction schemes allow transverse data to be reformatted and displayed in sagit-

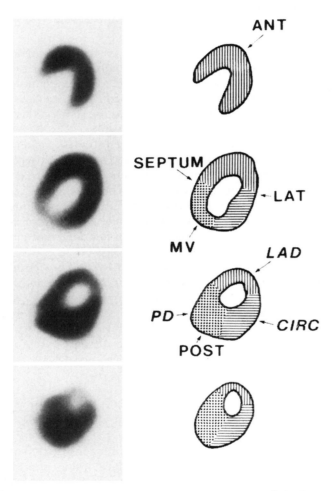

Figure 9-3 Contiguous transverse reconstructions of the heart obtained after the intravenous administration of ^{13}N ammonia in a normal human subject. The cross sections of the left ventricle are displayed as if viewed from below. The right ventricular myocardium is not usually visualized because the resolution of current PET instruments is not sufficiently high to resolve the thin wall. Reconstructions are routinely made at multiple levels from the base (*top*) to the apex (*bottom*). The schematic representation on the right delineates the anterior (ANT), lateral (LAT), and posterior (POST) myocardium and the mitral valve (MV) plane. The distributions of the left anterior descending (LAD), left circumflex (CIRC), and posterior descending (PD) coronary arteries are indicated by the different *cross-hatching*. (From Schelbert et al,[50] reproduced with permission of the American College of Cardiology.)

tal, coronal, short-axis, or "bull's-eye" projections.[12-14] Dynamic scanning (i.e., collection of sequential emission data to enable analysis of the temporal change in tracer content in regions of interest with time) coupled to a physiologically appropriate mathematical model can provide estimates of myocardial perfusion or metabolism that can then be displayed as parametric images (images of actual perfusion in milliliters per gram per minute or of substrate utilization in moles per gram per minute).[15]

Spatial Resolution

Spatial resolution is typically reported in terms of the line-spread function of a capillary tube of radioactivity to describe the full-width at half-maximum (FWHM) or full-width at tenth-maximum (FW0.1M). Typical values in the current generation of instruments are from 4 to 9 mm FWHM in "raw" reconstructions and 6 to 13 mm FWHM in filtered reconstructed images. The ultimate spatial resolution of PET imaging systems may be limited by the distance traversed by the high-energy positrons in tissue prior to their interaction with electrons (Table 9-2),[11,16,17] modest angular deviations from 180° of the emitted photons, physical constraints of the dimension of the detector rings, and statistical considerations.[7-11,16,17]

The spatial resolution of PET is more limited than that of other imaging modalities such as x-ray computed tomography, cardiac ultrasound, or magnetic resonance imaging. For tomography of the heart, quantification of the distribution of tracers is further limited by physical considerations including cardiac and respiratory motion, partial volume effects, and spillover of radioactivity from adjacent regions.[11]

EFFECTS OF MOTION

Absolute quantification requires that the imaged object be stationary throughout the imaged interval. This criterion is not met for the heart because of the complex motion during the cardiac and respiratory cycles. A number of studies have demonstrated that cardiac PET images are degraded by the effects of cardiac and respiratory motion.[18,19] Strategies to overcome the effects of motion have been proposed, such as electrocardiographic gating and breath holding or respiratory gating to account for the effects of respiratory motion. Nonetheless, these corrections have not been employed routinely, since these maneuvers decrease the amount of usable data that can be obtained in a given scan interval, thereby degrading image and statistical data quality or extending the total scan interval needed to achieve adequate count statistics. This latter option is impractical in studies using kinetic dynamic data for modeling. Accordingly, other strategies will need to be employed such

Table 9-2   Positron Energies and Path Lengths Prior to Annihilation of Commonly Used Positron-Emitting Radionuclides

Isotope	$\beta^+ E_{MAX}$ (meV)	$\beta^+ E_{AVE}$ (meV)	Range (FWHM, mm)	Range (FW01.M, mm)
Cyclotron produced				
Fluorine 18	0.633	0.203	1.0	1.8
Carbon 11	0.959	0.326	1.1	2.2
Nitrogen 13	1.197	0.432	1.4	2.8
Oxygen 15	1.738	0.696	1.5	3.6
Generator produced				
Gallium 68	1.898	0.783	1.7	4.0
Copper 62	2.93	1.28	NA	NA
Rubidium 82	3.148	1.385	1.7	5.8

$\beta^+ E_{MAX}$, maximum positron energy; $\beta^+ E_{AVE}$, average positron energy; FWHM, full-width at half-maximum range in water; FW0.1M, full-width at tenth-maximum range in water; NA, not available.

Adapted with permission from Cho et al.,[17] Positron ranges obtained from biomedically important positron-emitting radionuclides, *J Nucl Med* 16:1174, 1975; and from Graham and Lewellen.[217] Reproduced with permission and modified from Ter-Pogossian.[218]

as accounting for the effects of motion within mathematical models.

PARTIAL VOLUME EFFECTS

Partial volume effects can profoundly influence the results obtained with cardiac PET.[11,20-22] When the dimensions of an imaged object are less than twice the FWHM spatial resolution of the particular instrument used, the actual radioactivity in the region is not registered faithfully. The impact of this phenomenon is inversely and nonlinearly proportional to the dimensions of the imaged object.[20] Since the thickness of the myocardium (0.8 to 1.2 cm) is close to the FWHM of most instruments, true tracer content within the heart is typically underestimated by 40 to 80 percent.[20] This effect can become critical when imaging thinned structures, as may occur during ischemia or with infarction, since tissue with the same amount of radiotracer per gram as normal myocardium can appear as a defect simply based on partial volume effects (Fig. 9-4).

Correction for effects of partial volume can be made by independent assessments of wall thickness with techniques such as echocardiography, x-ray computed tomography, or magnetic resonance imaging, but difficulties are encountered in translating measurements made with these independent modalities to ungated PET data, especially when obtained at different times (when loading conditions or regional function may be different) or with modalities that quantify thickness in different planes of interrogation. Although average wall thickness measurements have been used for partial volume corrections and may suffice for some applications,[21,22] more recent approaches have employed correction for these effects within specific mathematical schemes.[23-25]

SPILLOVER

Spillover of counts is also a direct consequence of the limited spatial resolution of PET instruments and refers

to the apparent radioactivity in a region of interest due to cross-contamination from an adjacent region. This is most marked, for instance, when looking at a region devoid of tracer in which regional radiotracer content may be overestimated because of radioactivity in adjacent normal regions of myocardium or adjacent blood pool. These effects become critical when PET is being used for quantitative applications. Corrections for spillover from blood-pool radioactivity can be made using administration of a tracer of the blood pool (such as ^{15}O-labeled carbon monoxide)[24] or with mathematical techniques.[24-26]

Despite these considerable physical limitations, quantitative estimates of the true tissue tracer content

CONTROL   OCCLUSION

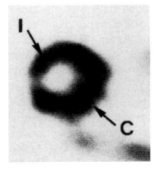 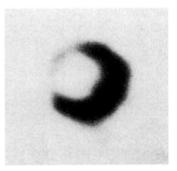

Figure 9-4 Two midventricular tomographic reconstructions obtained after the administration of ^{13}N ammonia to a dog and demonstrating the profound influence of partial volume effects on PET reconstructions. On the *left* is a tomogram obtained under "control" circumstances and delineating the relatively homogeneous distribution of tracer. Three minutes after the control data had been acquired, the left anterior descending coronary artery was occluded (*right*). After occlusion, despite the fact that the actual counts per gram have not changed, a large defect appears in the ischemic zone due to the wall thinning and partial volume effects, diminishing apparent radioactivity. I, region to be made ischemic; C, normal (control) region. (From Parodi et al,[21] reproduced with permission.)

are achievable when appropriate correction schemes are employed. These have enabled quantitative regional estimates of myocardial perfusion and metabolism.

MEASUREMENT OF MYOCARDIAL PERFUSION WITH PET

Measurement of myocardial perfusion is the cornerstone for the diagnosis of coronary artery disease and assessment of its severity and for evaluation of the efficacy of pharmacologic or mechanical therapies designed to improve nutritive perfusion. Although coronary arteriography provides valuable delineation of coronary artery anatomy, even with "quantitative" assessments of stenosis severity, nutritive myocardial perfusion, assessed by measurement of perfusion reserve after maximum coronary vasodilatation, does not readily correlate with anatomic stenosis severity.[27]

Qualitative Imaging Versus Quantitative Estimates of Perfusion

Assessment of perfusion reserve provides a sensitive indicator of the physiologic significance of coronary artery disease.[28] Most investigators use intravenous dipyridamole or adenosine to augment myocardial perfusion and delineate flow reserve. Such estimates improve the specificity and sensitivity for detection of coronary artery disease and have been used to quantify the effects of interventions designed to augment perfusion. Although conventional nuclear medicine studies with single-photon-emitting tracers and detection techniques enable delineation of the relative distribution of tracers at rest and after exercise or pharmacologic coronary vasodilatation, only PET provides absolute quantification of regional myocardial perfusion. Even without absolute quantitation of flow, PET may be more sensitive and specific than conventional scintigraphy for the identification of coronary artery disease (Table 9-3).

Qualitative identification of absolute perfusion defects is relatively straightforward in patients with single-vessel coronary disease in whom a region of heart supplied by nondiseased coronary arteries enables comparisons of net uptake. Heterogeneity of accumulation of tracer, indicative of disparities in regional perfusion, have been observed in subjects at rest or after hyperemic stress induced with intravenous dipyridamole. All PET tracers for estimates of myocardial perfusion have enabled identification of coronary artery disease in patients with stenoses from 40 to 70 percent. Although some investigators have indicated that PET detects coronary

artery disease with a higher sensitivity and specificity than ^{201}Tl,[29,30] others have observed only a modest improvement in sensitivity with PET compared with ^{201}Tl SPECT scintigraphy, and overall specificity was slightly better with SPECT.[31] Stewart et al showed a comparable sensitivity for the detection of coronary artery disease between PET (using [82]Rb) and ^{201}Tl SPECT, but superior specificity with PET (88 percent compared with 53 percent). The superiority of PET disappeared when patients with prior infarction were excluded from the analysis.[32] Detailed studies of diagnostic sensitivity and specificity for coronary disease detection comparing estimates made with PET to those made with ^{99m}Tc-sestamibi SPECT have not yet been published.

A major unresolved issue is the clinical need for quantitative assessments of myocardial perfusion in absolute terms (milliliters per gram per minute) available with PET as opposed to qualitative imaging (i.e., simple visual assessment of static images).[33,34] It appears that for some applications, such as the diagnosis of coronary artery disease or assessment of the success of myocardial revascularization, qualitative imaging may be sufficient, although clearly the influence of partial volume effects must be considered (Fig. 9-4) when qualitative assessments are made. For other applications—such as evaluation of patients with chest pain and normal coronary arteries or of patients with cardiac transplantation in whom uptake of flow tracers may be homogeneous despite the presence of diffuse coronary intimal hyperplasia (see below) and for evaluation of myocardial perfusion reserve—quantitative estimates of perfusion with PET will be necessary. Patients with balanced lesions or with multivessel disease may also require absolute quantification of perfusion in order to assess the physiologic significance of their disease and of therapies designed to augment perfusion. Clearly, for research applications in which absolute quantification of perfusion is needed to answer fundamental questions, PET is unsurpassed.

Assessment of Myocardial Perfusion with Microspheres

Radiolabeled microspheres have long been the "gold standard" for experimental studies of myocardial blood flow, despite indications that microspheres may underestimate flow in ischemic regions.[35,36] Microspheres are labeled particles, generally ranging from 9 to 30 μm, that are trapped virtually completely in arteriolar or capillary vessels during the first pass through the vascular bed in the organ of interest. Microspheres need to be injected systemically to obviate trapping in the venous circulation. In experimental studies, a reference flow is obtained by withdrawing arterial blood at a known flow rate with a withdrawal pump and counting the radioactivity of the microspheres in the arterial blood sample.

Table 9-3 Selected Studies Using PET for Detection of Coronary Artery Disease

	Number of Subjects	Percent		Comments
		Sensitivity	Specificity	
Rubidium 82				
Gould et al.[72]	27[a]	95	100	Visual interpretation of perfusion images compared with angiographic measures of CFR. Sensitivty 31% in patients with mild CAD.
Stewart et al.[32]	60	87	82	Sensitivity of PET and ^{201}Tl SPECT similar, but specificity of PET higher than ^{201}Tl SPECT.
Demer et al.[53]	82	NP	NP	Visual interpretation of perfusion images correlated with quantitative angiographic measures of stenosis severity.
Go et al.[30]	202	93	78	Sensitivity of PET higher than ^{201}Tl SPECT; however, study design may have been biased against ^{201}Tl SPECT.
Nitrogen-13 ammonia				
Schelbert et al.[50]	45	97	100	Patients with angiographic documentation of CAD; ^{13}N-ammonia PET correctly localized 90% of stenoses.
Gould et al.[72]	23[a]	95	100	Same as for [82]Rb.
Yonekura et al.[55]	60	97	99	Patients with angiographic documentation of CAD. Circumferential profiles used to analyze perfusion images.
Tamaki et al.[31]	51	88	90	Similar sensitivity and specificity as ^{201}Tl SPECT (81% and 94%).
Demer et al.[53]	111[a]	NP	NP	Same as [82]Rb.
Oxygen-15 water				
Iida et al.[24]	15	NP	NP	Measurements of regional perfusion in absolute terms demonstrated diffuse reductions in regional perfusion in patients with three-vessel CAD.
Walsh et al.[96]	33	93	NP	Estimates of relative regional perfusion compared with quantitative angiographic measures of stenosis severity.

[a] Separate estimates of sensitivity and specificity for [82]Rb and ^{13}N-ammonia not provided.
CAD, coronary artery disease; CFR, coronary flow reserve; NP, not provided.
Reproduced with permission from Gropler et al.[170]

Flow is then quantitated by comparing the number of radioactive spheres in the arterial blood sample with the number of radioactive spheres counted in the organ of interest.[35]

The microsphere technique has been used extensively with great accuracy in experimental studies and to a much more limited extent in patients. For routine practice, the technique is limited by several factors, most notably, the necessity for microspheres to be administered in the arterial circulation. For use to assess myocardial perfusion, the microspheres need to be administered into the left atrium. Although, clinically, microspheres have been shown to be extremely safe and not lead to further arterial compromise, there is some concern that the radiolabeled microspheres can physically occlude vascular beds that may already be at risk.

Macroaggregated albumin microspheres labeled with either ^{68}Ga or ^{11}C have been used for measurement of myocardial perfusion in vivo with PET.[37-39] Normal and ischemic myocardium have been identified after left atrial or ventricular administration as well as with intracoronary administration of microspheres at the time of cardiac catheterization. Quantitative assessments of myocardial blood flow have been possible when corrections were made for cardiac motion and partial volume effects.[37-39] Nonetheless, because of the requirement for systemic arterial administration and therefore for invasive catheterization, radiolabeled microspheres are not used routinely.

Assessment of Perfusion with Extracted Tracers

A second approach for the measurement of myocardial perfusion is the fractional distribution approach using tracers (usually cations) that are extracted and retained by the heart. This is the most commonly used approach both in conventional nuclear medicine (i.e., with ^{201}Tl or ^{99m}Tc sestamibi) and also with PET. PET tracers, which are used with this approach, include ^{13}N ammonia, [82]Rb chloride, and [62]Cu pyruvaldehyde *bis* [N^4-methylthiosemicarbazone] (PTSM) . The approach is widely used because of its convenience. It assumes that the intravenously injected radiopharmaceutical is taken up and released by cells throughout the body in a uniform way and that the kinetics are independent of regional flow or the metabolic status of the particular tissue under study.

NITROGEN-13 AMMONIA

Nitrogen-13 ammonia has been extensively used for assessment of myocardial perfusion with PET.

Kinetics Although ammonia is a gas, ^{13}N ammonia falls into the category of cation-type tracers, since at physiologic pH the major form is NH_4^+.

Although the exact mechanism of transport of NH_4^+ across the myocardial sarcolemma is not definitively known, it is thought to be carrier mediated. Because of the high single-pass extraction fraction (approximately 70 to 80 percent at physiologic flow rates), the relatively prolonged retention of tracer by the heart (biological half-life of 80 to 400 min) after intravenous administration and rapid blood-pool clearance, ^{13}N ammonia provides excellent quality images of the myocardium. Of interest, several investigators have demonstrated heterogeneity in the uptake of ^{13}N ammonia in the hearts of healthy volunteers, which reflects regional differences in the metabolism of ^{13}N ammonia rather than true flow discrepancies.[40,41]

Since the extraction fraction of ^{13}N ammonia is inversely and nonlinearly related to flow, net uptake of ^{13}N ammonia into tissue plateaus at flows above 2.0 to 2.5 ml/g/min (Fig. 9-5).[42,43] In isolated perfused hearts, both extraction fraction and myocardial retention of ^{13}N

ammonia were shown to be related not only to flow but also to myocardial oxygenation per se.[44,45] In addition, since ^{13}N ammonia trapping by the myocardium depends on conversion of ammonia to glutamine via the glutamine synthetase pathway, factors that can influence this pathway can also influence the kinetics of tracer in the myocardium.[44] Metabolic interventions can also influence the extraction and retention of ammonia and its intermediates by factors independent of flow.[44-46] Accordingly, for myocardial quantitation, mathematical models to account for extraction and retention of ammonia were developed and have been used to quantify flow in absolute terms in human subjects.[47,48]

An additional factor complicating quantitation of myocardial perfusion with ^{13}N ammonia is the observed breakdown of ^{13}N ammonia after administration in humans. Rosenspire et al found that, within 2 min after intravenous administration in humans, ^{13}N ammonia circulates in the blood as metabolic intermediates, predominantly urea and amino acids,[49] although the influence of this breakdown on flow quantitation appears to be minimal.

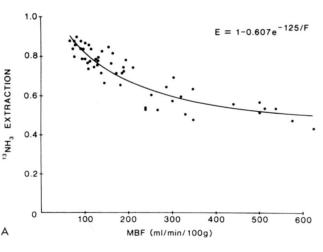

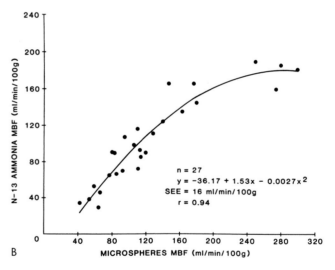

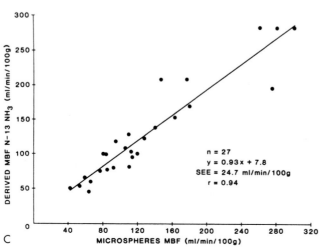

Figure 9-5 A: Relationship between the single-pass extraction fraction of ^{13}N ammonia and flow obtained after intracoronary bolus administration in dogs and demonstrating the inverse, nonlinear relationship. (From Schelbert et al,[42] reproduced with permission of the American Heart Association, Inc.) **B:** Relationship between regional myocardial blood flow determined with ^{13}N ammonia and PET in comparison with radiolabeled microspheres. With flows greater than approximately 2 ml/g/min, net uptake plateaus. Accordingly, without correction for decreased extraction at high flow, ^{13}N ammonia is relatively insensitive to flow at hyperemic flow rates. **C:** After correction for the nonlinear relationship between flow and uptake of ^{13}N ammonia, quantitative estimates of flow can be obtained. (From Shah et al,[43] reproduced with permission of the American College of Cardiology.)

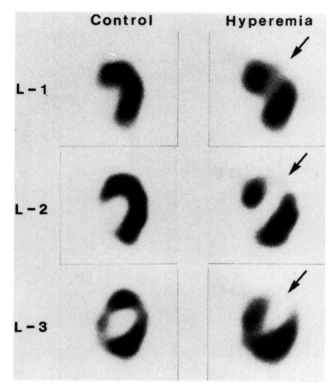

Control   **Hyperemia**

L–1

L–2

L–3

Figure 9-6 Three midventricular tomographic reconstructions obtained under resting conditions after administration of ¹³N ammonia to a patient with single-vessel left anterior descending coronary artery disease (*left*), showing relatively homogeneous tracer distribution throughout the left ventricular myocardium. After administration of intravenous dipyridamole to induce coronary hyperemia (*right*), an anterior defect is observed. Without quantitation of flow in absolute terms (or another tracer that showed uptake), it would be impossible to know whether this deficit was due to a true disparity in flow in the anterior region compared with flow in normal regions or due to wall thinning in response to the primary or secondary effects of the drug (see Fig. 9-4). (From Schelbert et al,[50] reproduced with permission of the American College of Cardiology)

Clinical observations Nitrogen-13 ammonia has been used extensively in qualitative imaging of myocardial perfusion in patients with coronary artery disease.[47–58] Typically, 10 to 15 mCi of ¹³N ammonia is injected intravenously and static images, 5 to 10 min long, are acquired beginning 3 to 10 min after tracer administration to enable clearance of tracer from the blood. Smokers or patients with lung disease have been noted to have increased lung uptake of ¹³N ammonia, thereby degrading myocardial images. Use of ¹³N ammonia has enabled identification of patients with coronary artery disease (Fig. 9-6) in a number of clinical studies with a sensitivity and specificity of greater than 90 percent (Table 9-3).[50,55] Scans are usually made at rest and after coronary hyperemia induced with intravenous dipyridamole. However, it must be recalled that "defects" can be caused by wall-thinning or wall-motion abnormalities per se induced by pharmacologic agents and may not

reflect actual decreases in flow. However, use of quantitative estimates of flow with the mathematical models developed, which accounts for partial volume and spillover effects, has greatly added to the utility of flow measurements with ¹³N ammonia. A simplified method for quantification of myocardial perfusion with ¹³N ammonia employing graphical analysis has been proposed and validated in experimental studies.[56]

Several interesting clinical observations have been made with ¹³N ammonia by using absolute quantification. Dayanikli et al demonstrated that asymptomatic men with a family history of coronary artery disease and a high-risk lipid profile had absolute flow at rest that was not different from age-matched, low-risk controls.[57] However, blood flow in response to intravenous adenosine was diminished (perfusion reserve of 2.93 ± 0.86 compared with the normal response, 4.27 ± 0.52, $p < 0.001$), suggesting that absolute quantification of myocardial perfusion enables detection of abnormal vasodilatory responses in a high-risk group prior to the development of clinical symptoms and thus may enable detection of atherosclerotic coronary artery disease prior to clinical manifestations. Di Carli et al demonstrated an inverse, nonlinear relationship between the severity of coronary artery stenosis by quantitative coronary arteriography and perfusion reserve assessed with ¹³N ammonia and PET. The latter successfully separated coronary lesions of an intermediate severity (<70 percent) from those with a greater severity, although substantial overlap was observed.[58] Gould et al demonstrated that intense, short-term cholesterol-lowering medical therapy diminished the size and severity of perfusion abnormalities after infusion of dipyridamole in patients with coronary artery disease, suggesting that PET could be used to monitor the efficacy of such interventions.[59] Finally, Neglia et al demonstrated that patients with dilated cardiomyopathy have diminished myocardial perfusion at rest and during either atrial pacing or intravenous dipyridamole, despite normal systemic hemodynamics.[60] Taken together, these studies demonstrate the utility of quantitative estimates of myocardial perfusion using ¹³N ammonia.

RUBIDIUM-82 CHLORIDE

Rubidium-82 chloride is an attractive tracer for assessment of myocardial perfusion because it is generator produced and because its short physical half-life (76 s) enables rapid sequential scans with minimal radiation burden to the patient.

Kinetics Love and Burch first suggested that the uptake of ⁸²Rb measured by direct analysis of myocardial samples reflected myocardial perfusion,[61] and a number of other studies demonstrated that the externally detectable fraction of myocardial uptake of rubidium correlated well with the distribution of radiolabeled microspheres early after administration. Similar to the case for ^{13}N ammonia, the single-pass extraction of rubidium by the heart is inversely and nonlinearly related to myocardial blood flow.[62-66]

Selwyn et al showed that regional myocardial uptake of ^{82}Rb assessed with PET correlated only poorly with the distribution of radiolabeled microspheres in dogs and that, in patients, extraction fraction of ^{82}Rb was inversely related to flow.[62] Goldstein and co-workers demonstrated that net uptake of tracer plateaued at flow rates greater than 2.5 to 3 ml/g/min, indicating that accumulation of ^{82}Rb in the myocardium was relatively insensitive to changes in flows that would normally occur with exercise or after pharmacologic coronary hyperemia with dipyridamole.[64] Fukuyama et al demonstrated that the extraction of rubidium decreases with ischemic intervals of greater than 60 min in experimental animals,[65] and Wilson et al demonstrated that the uptake and net extraction of ^{82}Rb are profoundly influenced by as few as 10 min of transient occlusion.[63] Accordingly, in order to quantify myocardial perfusion in absolute terms with ^{82}Rb, the kinetics of both extraction and retention of tracer by the myocardium must be considered.[66] Although challenging because of the short physical half-life of ^{82}Rb, a two-compartment model was implemented for use with PET and shown to correlate well with flow measured with concomitantly administered radiolabeled microspheres over the flow range from 0.14 to 4.25 ml/g/min.[67] This approach has not yet been implemented in humans, and studies using ^{82}Rb clinically employ simple net uptake for assessments.

Based on the observation of decreased trapping of rubidium by injured myocardium, Goldstein et al proposed that analysis of the myocardial time–activity curves may enable delineation between viable and irreversibly injured myocardium.[68,69] Herrero et al showed that this backdiffusion rate constant increased significantly in regions with severe ischemia.[67]

Clinical observations Rubidium-82 chloride has been used extensively for clinical assessments of myocardial perfusion in patients with coronary artery disease[30,32,53,70-74] and is the only Food and Drug Administration–approved PET tracer. The quality of myocardial images obtained after intravenous administration of ^{82}Rb depends on the tracer infusion duration and imaging protocol. Since ^{82}Rb is generator produced, it must be eluted from the generator prior to infusion. Typically 30 to 50 mCi is administered as an infusion over 30 to 60 s and, after allowing 1 to 3 min for arterial clearance, images are obtained over a 3- to 5-min interval. Although disappearance of tracer from the arterial blood is rapid, infusion systems with prolonged administration times result in high myocardial blood-pool activity. The short half-life of this tracer allows sequential studies (i.e., every

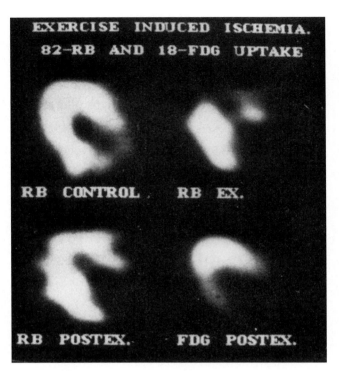

Figure 9-7 PET reconstructions obtained in a patient with coronary artery disease after intravenous administration of ^{82}Rb before exercise (*top left*), showing homogeneous uptake of tracer, and during exercise (*top right*), showing diminished apparent radioactivity in the anterior myocardium. Six minutes after the end of exercise (*bottom left*), after a third administration of tracer, the disparity is no longer present. On the *bottom right* is the distribution of ^{18}F FDG (administered 8 min after the end of exercise and recorded 60 min after tracer administration), showing enhanced FDG accumulation in the area that was ischemic during exercise. In this set of reconstructions, lateral myocardium is to the left, septum is to the right, and anterior is uppermost. (From Camici et al,[71] reproduced with permission of the American Heart Association, Inc.)

8 min) (Fig. 9-7). After provocative stimulation with exercise or intravenous dipyridamole, sensitivity and specificity for detection of coronary artery disease exceed 84 to 90 percent[30,32,53] but may be diminished in patients without prior infarction[32] or in patients with left ventricular hypertrophy.[75] In a large, community-hospital-based study, the average sensitivity was 87 percent with a specificity of 88 percent when the coronary artery was narrowed by greater than 67 percent diameter.[76] Gould et al have recently demonstrated that decreased retention of ^{82}Rb correlates with increased uptake of ^{18}F fluorodeoxyglucose (FDG), suggesting that the dynamic kinetics of ^{82}Rb may be used to delineate cellular viability.[77] Viability was not assessed directly. Nonetheless, the approach warrants further exploration. Goldstein et al also demonstrated the ability of this agent to delineate improved perfusion reserve after successful angioplasty.[74]

COPPER-62 PTSM

Because of the limitations of ^{13}N ammonia and ^{82}Rb, other tracers have been sought for the quantitation of myocardial perfusion. Copper-62 PTSM, is a lipophilic compound that can be labeled with generator-produced ^{62}Cu as well as with a number of other positron and single-photon-emitting copper radionuclides. The tracer exhibits a high single-pass extraction by the myocardium and, once extracted, essentially irreversible binding by the heart. Although initial studies in isolated hearts and intact dogs were promising[78-80] and initial images of the human myocardium were of high quality, more recent studies have demonstrated high incorporation of tracer into liver (impairing assessment of the inferior wall) and diminished net uptake (relative to flow) in response to dipyridamole, suggesting attenuation of tracer uptake at high flow rates.[81-83] This was subsequently shown to be related to increased binding of ^{62}Cu PTSM to human albumin, thereby limiting "free" tracer accessible for extraction by the heart.[84] It is possible that newer substituted ^{62}Cu-labeled thiosemicarbazones such as copper ethylglyoxal or *n*-propyl-glyoxal thiosemicarbazone, which have been shown in in vitro studies to have diminished avidity for human albumin but still avid myocardial extraction and retention, may be superior candidates for generator-produced perfusion agents for quantification of regional myocardial perfusion in humans.

Measurement of Myocardial Perfusion with Diffusible Tracers

Because of the inverse and nonlinear relationship between myocardial extraction and flow and also the partial dependence of extraction and retention of these tracers on myocardial metabolism, a number of groups have evaluated the utility of diffusible tracers for assessment of myocardial perfusion. Positron-emitting tracers that have been used include ^{11}C butanol and ^{15}O butanol and ^{15}O-labeled water ($H_2^{15}O$). Perfusion is quantified using a modification of the approach developed by Kety to describe the exchange of inert gas between blood and tissue.[85] Although the use of this technique has a long history, only with the development of tomographic instruments able to acquire data with short temporal scans (i.e., 2 to 5 s per scan) did the ability to quantify myocardial perfusion with this approach become feasible. The approach requires that the time–activity curve of arterial blood (obtained in dynamic studies by placing a region of interest within the left atrial or left ventricular blood pool) as well as the time–activity curve of the myocardium be measured.

KINETICS OF ^{15}O-LABELED WATER

Because of the short physical half-life of ^{15}O (2.1 min) and its rapid, automated production, $H_2^{15}O$ has been the focus of most studies using the diffusible tracer approach. Direct comparison between flow estimated with radiolabeled water and by assessments with microspheres showed that the approach is valid over a wide range of flows as well as with the metabolic alterations that occur with ischemia and reperfusion.[25,86-91]

To assess myocardial blood flow in quantitative terms completely noninvasively with PET, dynamic scans are obtained in short frames (i.e., 2 to 5 s) over 1 to 5 min after bolus intravenous administration of 15 to 25 mCi of tracer, and the time–activity curve of tracer in arterial blood and in multiple myocardial regions of interest is measured.[24,25] In a direct comparison between the accuracy of estimates of myocardial perfusion with $H_2^{15}O$ and ^{13}N ammonia, estimates made with radiolabeled water correlated more closely with microspheres than estimates made with ^{13}N ammonia.[91] More recently, the approach has been modified for use with scanners with slower crystals, whereby ^{15}O-labeled CO_2 is administered by inhalation over 3 to 4 min and scanning performed during the inhalation period as well as for several minutes after the inhalation is stopped. The labeled CO_2 is converted to $H_2^{15}O$ by the ubiquitous carbonic anhydrase enzyme. Although there is some concern that this quasi–steady-state approach may be less sensitive to high flow rates, it has been validated in experimental animals.[90] Corrections for partial volume and spillover effects are incorporated within the operational flow equation obviating the need for independent assessments.[24,25]

CLINICAL ASSESSMENTS OF MYOCARDIAL PERFUSION WITH ^{15}O-LABELED WATER

Because $H_2^{15}O$ resides in the vascular pool as well as diffusing into myocardium, for visualization of the heart, tomograms obtained after administration of labeled water require correction for radioactivity in the vascular compartment.[24,25] This is accomplished under most circumstances with a separate scan involving the inhalation of ^{15}O-labeled carbon monoxide (40 to 50 mCi), which rapidly labels erythrocytes and provides accurate delineation of the vascular blood pool. Tomographic images obtained after $H_2^{15}O$ are corrected on a pixel-by-pixel basis for labeled water residing in the blood pool and provide an image of the myocardium (Plate 17). Although the quality of these corrected images is usually quite satisfactory for clinical assessments, images are of generally poorer quality than those obtained with extractable tracers and are especially compromised if the patient moves during the scanning procedure.

Bergmann et al demonstrated that quantitation of perfusion in absolute terms was achievable in human subjects.[25] Myocardial perfusion reserve evaluated by assessing myocardial perfusion at rest and after intravenous dipyridamole averaged 4.1 (Fig. 9-8). Senneff et al demonstrated that older adults (with a mean age of 55)

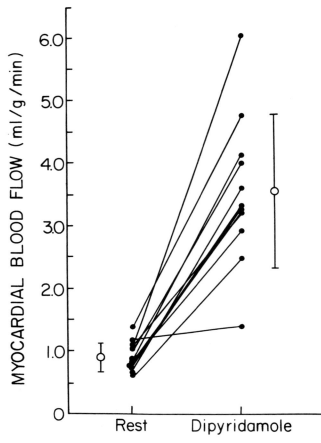

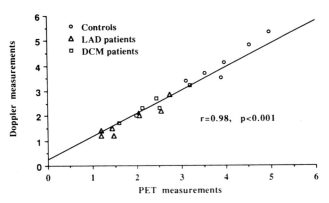

Figure 9-9 Correlation between estimates of myocardial perfusion reserve made with PET using $H_2^{15}O$ compared with coronary flow velocity reserve obtained with invasive assessments made with an intracoronary Doppler catheter. Included are six "control" patients who underwent angiography for atypical chest pain but who had angiographically normal coronary arteries, eight patients with coronary artery disease (stenoses ranging from 70 to 90 percent), and six patients with idiopathic dilated cardiomyopathy (but without coronary stenoses greater than 50 percent). As shown, correlation between the two approaches was excellent. The PET approach also provides estimates of perfusion in absolute terms (i.e., milliliters per gram per minute). (From Merlet et al,[98] reproduced with permission.)

Figure 9-8 Estimates of myocardial perfusion at rest and after coronary hyperemia induced with intravenous dipyridamole in 11 healthy human volunteers with a low likelihood of coronary artery disease. Estimates were obtained with $H_2^{15}O$ and a mathematical model that calculates not only perfusion but that accounts for partial volume and spillover effects. Estimates of myocardial perfusion reserve (the ratio between flow after maximum hyperemia compared with flow at rest) obtained with the PET approach agree closely with measurements of flow reserve obtained with other modalities (see Fig. 9-9). (From Bergmann et al,[25] reproduced with permission of the American College of Cardiology.)

at low risk for cardiovascular disease had a diminished hemodynamic response to dipyridamole and had a diminished hyperemic response compared with younger adults. These results suggested that age-related norms for the perfusion response to pharmacologic agents may be important.[92] These results have recently been corroborated,[93,94] although Czernin et al found no decrease in the hyperemic response in older adults using ^{13}N ammonia as the flow tracer.[95]

Walsh et al demonstrated the utility of $H_2^{15}O$ for delineation of coronary artery disease in patients at rest and after provocative stimulation with intravenous dipyridamole.[96] Iida et al also showed decreased myocardial blood flow in patients with coronary artery disease using $H_2^{15}O$ and PET.[24] Quantitative assessments of coronary flow reserve made with $H_2^{15}O$ and PET have corre-

lated extremely closely with invasive measurements of coronary flow reserve in patients (Fig. 9-9).[97,98] Uren et al assessed the relationship between the severity of coronary stenoses and myocardial perfusion reserve with $H_2^{15}O$ in 35 patients with single-vessel artery disease and normal left ventricular function and compared results with those obtained in 21 age-matched controls.[99] Flow was measured at rest and after intravenous adenosine or dipyridamole. At rest, there was no difference in flow between patients and normal volunteers; during hyperemia, however, myocardial perfusion was diminished in patients and perfusion reserve correlated inversely with the degree of stenosis (Fig. 9-10). Diminished perfusion reserve was noted in some regions remote from macroscopically diseased vessels.[100]

The approach has also been used to identify the efficacy of therapeutic strategies. Walsh et al demonstrated that myocardial perfusion reserve was impaired in regions distal to stenosis prior to single-vessel coronary angioplasty but normalized after successful angioplasty.[101] In contrast, Uren et al found somewhat blunted perfusion reserve early after coronary angioplasty that normalized sometime between 7 days and 3 months after the procedure.[102] The reason for the differences observed in these two studies is unclear. In another study, Uren et al found a diminished response to dipyridamole in both reperfused as well as remote (normal) myocardium in patients studied after myocardial infarction.[103] PET using $H_2^{15}O$ has also shown the efficacy of reperfusion strategies. Henes et al showed effective restoration of myocardial perfusion in patients suffering

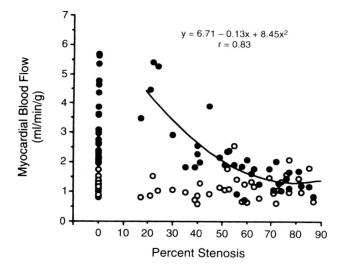

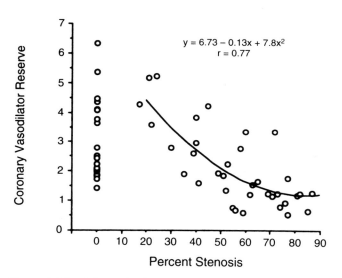

Figure 9-10 Relationship between myocardial blood flow (*top*) and perfusion reserve (the ratio of hyperemic flow to rest flow) in relation to stenosis diameter in 21 control subjects with a low likelihood of coronary artery disease and in 35 patients with single-vessel coronary artery disease and normal left ventricular function. Under resting conditions (*open circles*), myocardial perfusion is normal in patients but, with hyperemia (*solid circles*), peak flow achieved decreases significantly with the severity of the stenosis. Thus, PET enables quantification of the physiologic significance of coronary stenoses in absolute terms. (From Uren et al,[99] reproduced with permission.)

from evolving myocardial infarction treated with thrombolytic therapy and demonstrated that flow in the reperfused zone, studied under resting conditions, was normal[104] (Plate 18).

The value of quantitative assessment of myocardial perfusion has been demonstrated in studies of patients with chest pain but angiographically normal coronary arteries and in the evaluation of patients with cardiac allografts. In these patients, the distribution of perfusion can be homogeneous, but abnormalities in perfusion at rest and after hyperemic provocation can be ascertained by quantitative estimates of flow. Geltman et al demonstrated that approximately 50 percent of patients with chest pain but angiographically normal coronary arteries had abnormal (high) flow at rest and impaired (low) flow reserve in response to intravenous dipyridamole.[105] Cardiac transplant recipients were noted to have high resting perfusion (associated with their increased heart rates and hypertension) but unimpaired response to vasodilatory stress.[106,107]

One of the most interesting areas for use of $H_2^{15}O$ and PET has been the putative utility of the *perfusible tissue index* (PTI) as a prospective measure of myocardial viability.[108-110] In patients with left ventricular dysfunction due to chronic coronary artery disease, the level of myocardial perfusion under resting conditions is reduced in viable myocardium compared with that observed in normal tissue but is higher than that observed in nonviable myocardium. Nonetheless, significant overlap exists (Fig. 9-11).[110] PTI has been introduced to differentiate viable from nonviable myocardium based on the concept that areas of infarction (scar) cannot rapidly exchange $H_2^{15}O$. Iida et al showed that PTI decreased significantly in infarcted regions in patients with previous infarction compared with values obtained in remote regions.[108] Yamamoto et al showed that PTI was decreased in reversibly injured myocardium compared with remote normal myocardium and decreased to a greater extent in irreversibly injured myocardium, and demonstrated that PTI was a useful prognostic indicator of recovery of contractile function after successful thrombolysis.[109] De Silva et al demonstrated that contractile function recovered after coronary artery bypass surgery only in segments where PTI was greater than 0.7 (Fig. 9-11).[110] These studies suggest that $H_2^{15}O$ can be used to assess not only myocardial perfusion but also potentially myocardial viability. Herrero et al recently demonstrated that PTI likely reflects tissue heterogeneity and absolute levels of flow rather than the ability of $H_2^{15}O$ to diffuse to infarcted versus noninfarcted tissue.[111] Should these clinical studies be corroborated in a larger number of patients, the approach would have obvious application and would enable rapid prospective assessments of myocardial viability using PET with $H_2^{15}O$.

ASSESSMENT OF MYOCARDIAL METABOLISM WITH PET

Although assessment of myocardial perfusion and perfusion reserve remains the cornerstone for the diagnosis of coronary artery disease and for assessment of the efficacy of therapies designed to augment nutritive perfu-

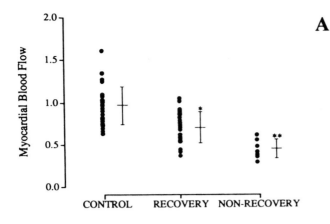

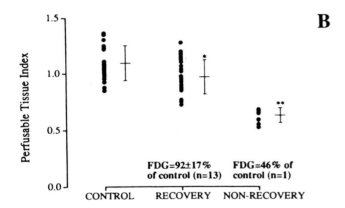

Figure 9-11 **A:** Values for myocardial blood flow (milliliters per gram per minute) obtained before coronary revascularization from 12 patients with chronic coronary artery disease in segments with normal function (control), in segments with reversible dysfunction (recovery), and in segments with persistent dysfunction (nonrecovery). Although average flow is higher in segments that recovered function compared with those that did not, there is marked overlap. **B:** Estimates of the perfusible tissue index (PTI) in the same regions separated viable from nonviable myocardium. *Significant difference compared with control. **Significant difference compared with control and recovery groups. (From De Silva et al,[110] reproduced with permission of the American Heart Association, Inc.)

sion, derangements in contractile function reflect abnormalities in myocardial metabolism, whether due to primary metabolic abnormalities or secondarily due to diminished perfusion (and therefore reflecting decreased oxygen and substrate supply in relation to energy demands). Accordingly, detection of metabolic dysfunction with PET may provide early and/or more specific identification of derangements in the relationship between myocardial perfusion and metabolism. Since the metabolic perturbations that occur with ischemia have been characterized extensively, they have served as the initial focus for studies with PET.

The positron-emitting radionuclides ^{15}O, ^{11}C, ^{13}N, and ^{18}F all have been particularly useful in assessing myocardial metabolism with PET because of the ability to incorporate these tracers within compounds of physiologic interest.

General Scheme of Myocardial Metabolism

The myocardium uses a variety of substrates, including fatty acids and glucose, and to a lesser extent lactate, pyruvate, ketones, and amino acids.[112-115] The particular pattern of substrate use depends on arterial substrate content, myocardial perfusion and oxygenation, the metabolic status of the myocardium, and other factors such as hormonal milieu. Thus, the behavior of any one tracer provides only partial insight regarding overall intermediary metabolism.[116] In addition, under almost all circumstances, assessment of myocardial metabolism must be coupled with either qualitative or quantitative assessments of myocardial perfusion, since metabolism is so tightly coupled to perfusion.

The heart is an aerobic organ that has high-energy flux necessary for the production of high-energy phosphates essential for contraction as well as for maintenance of normal cellular homeostasis and the electrophysiologic properties of the heart. Under normal physiologic conditions, oxidative metabolism of nonesterified (free) fatty acids (NEFAs) provides 40 to 60 percent of the energy used by the heart (Fig. 9-12).[112-115] Glucose provides an important alternate fuel and accounts for approximately 20 to 40 percent of the energy needs of the heart under fasting conditions. After a meal or after an oral or intravenous glucose load, more than 60 percent of the energy needs of the heart can be supplied by aerobic, oxidative metabolism of glucose.

Determinants of NEFA uptake by the heart include the arterial concentration, fatty-acid chain length, the ratio of NEFA to albumin, and the hormonal milieu. Under normoxic conditions, metabolism of NEFA occurs by β-oxidation in the mitochondria, although a fraction of extracted fats are incorporated into neutral lipid storage forms such as triglycerides as well as into membrane phospholipids (Fig. 9-12). Following a carbohydrate load, the utilization of NEFA is diminished due to the peripheral actions of insulin, which diminishes fat lipolysis and results in a decreased plasma NEFA content. Additionally, insulin directly stimulates myocardial glucose utilization (Fig. 9-13).

Glucose transport into the myocyte is regulated by a stereospecific carrier system, which is accelerated in the presence of insulin. Once extracted, glucose is phosphorylated to glucose-6-phosphate by hexokinase. The well-regulated glycolytic pathway controls conversion of glucose-6-phosphate to pyruvate. Normally pyruvate undergoes conversion to acetyl-coenzyme A (CoA),

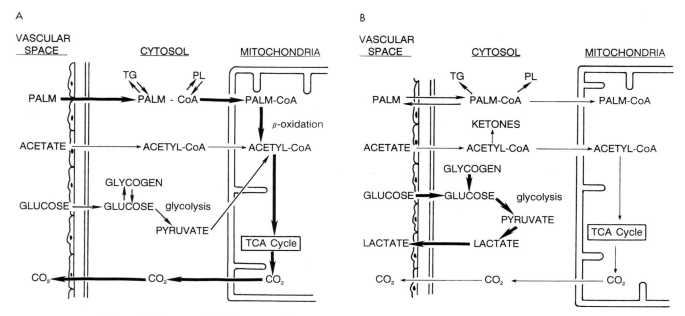

Figure 9-12 Simplified diagrams of myocardial metabolism under normoxic conditions **(A)** and after ischemia **(B)**. During normoxia, fatty acid represents the major source for energy production, although glucose utilization is enhanced after a glucose load. With ischemia, β-oxidation is inhibited and extracted fatty acids are shunted into triglyceride and phospholipid pools. Backdiffusion is increased as well. Glucose metabolism is enhanced through anaerobic glycolysis to lactate. This pathway cannot supply sufficient energy for maintenance of function, although it may be sufficient to maintain cell viability for a while. With reperfusion, fatty acid again becomes the major substrate for energy supply, although glycolytic flux can remain enhanced. PALM, palmitate; TG, triglyceride; PL, phospholipid; CoA, coenzyme A; TCA, tricarboxylic acid.

which is then oxidized aerobically in the tricarboxylic acid (TCA) cycle. Oxidation of glucose is inhibited by fatty acids at several regulatory levels. Under postprandial circumstances, glucose can be stored as myocardial glycogen. The activity of the glycogen synthesis pathway is stimulated by increased intracellular levels of glucose-6-phosphate and insulin.

The TCA cycle is the final common pathway for oxidative metabolism by the heart. Substrates are converted by β-oxidation or glycolysis to acetyl-CoA, which under aerobic circumstances undergoes metabolism to CO_2 in the TCA cycle. The TCA cycle provides $NADH_2$, which yields hydrogen atoms that then enter the electron transport chain where adenosine diphosphate (ADP) is converted to the high-energy adenosine triphosphate (ATP) by oxidative phosphorylation.

During myocardial ischemia, profound alterations in metabolism occur (Fig. 9-12).[112–116] β-Oxidation of fatty acid is diminished early after hypoxia because the activity of several enzymes involved in the fatty-acid oxidation pathway are inhibited by lactate and/or hydrogen ions that accumulate in ischemic tissue. Since β-oxidation is diminished, fatty acids are shunted into neutral and phospholipid.[117,118] Long-chain acyl-CoA and acyl-carnitines, which may be arrhythmogenic or may be negative inotropes, can accumulate. The diminished availability

of unesterified CoA decreases thioesterification of NEFA and increases backdiffusion. Glucose becomes the predominant source for energy production through anaerobic metabolism to lactate, although aerobic glucose metabolism may still be important. Increased intracellular lactate is a relatively specific marker for ischemia. The initial augmentation of anaerobic glycolysis stimulated by ischemia is short-lived because lactate, NADH, and hydrogen ions accumulate and depress the regulatory enzymes of the glycolytic pathway. Although anaerobic glycolysis can partially compensate for impaired metabolism, it cannot meet the high-energy demands of the myocardium. It is estimated that glycolysis during ischemia limits overall energy supply to 10 to 30 percent of the energy needs of the heart, which is perhaps sufficient to maintain cellular viability.[115]

With reperfusion after brief intervals of ischemia, oxidation of fatty acids is restored and serves as the major substrate for energy supply although glucose utilization remains enhanced.[116] With prolonged periods of ischemia followed by reperfusion, restoration of fatty-acid oxidation may be delayed and, under these circumstances, enhanced glycolysis may be important in maintaining cellular viability.[119] It appears that recovery of oxidative metabolism is a prerequisite for recovery of myocardial function after reperfusion.[120,121]

GLUCOSE UTILIZATION

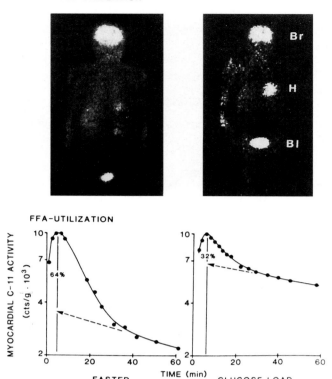

Figure 9-13   Effects of substrate availability on the myocardial uptake of ¹⁸F FDG (*top*) and on the kinetics of myocardial time–activity curves after administration of ¹¹C palmitate (*bottom*) in a normal human subject. Data on the *left* were obtained after an overnight fast and data on the *right* were obtained after administration of oral glucose. Under fasted conditions, myocardial uptake of ¹⁸F FDG is minimal but is enhanced after a glucose load. Under fasted conditions, a large proportion of extracted palmitate enters a rapidly turning over pool, predominantly representative of β-oxidation. After the glucose load, a smaller proportion enters this pool, and the slope of clearance of ¹¹C is diminished. This figure graphically demonstrates the dependence of the kinetics of tracers of myocardial metabolism on the arterial substrate concentration and pattern of myocardial substrate use. Br, brain; H, heart; Bl, bladder. (From Schelbert and Schwaiger,[220] reproduced with permission.)

Tracer Strategies for Assessment of Myocardial Metabolism with PET

Two general strategies have evolved for assessment of myocardial metabolism with PET. The first characterizes the dynamic myocardial time–activity data of positron-emitting radionuclides incorporated into physiologic substrates. This approach assumes that the metabolism of the radiopharmaceutical is identical to the native compound. The use of this approach is the most physiologically appropriate but is limited in some instances because metabolism of the tracer gives rise to numerous labeled intermediary compounds (which may differ under different flow or metabolic conditions). Accordingly, assess-

ments with tracers using this approach require knowledge of the metabolic pathways of the substance being traced and use of appropriate mathematical models to account for the appearance and disposition of labeled metabolites. Analysis is simplified if the tracer's metabolism can be characterized by a single end product (such is the case for ¹⁵O oxygen or for ¹¹C acetate; see below) or if measurements are made prior to production of labeled metabolites.

The alternative approach uses substrate analogs. Tracers employed are selected to be metabolically trapped in tissue as a result of a particular pathway or intermediate that renders the tracer refractory to further metabolism. The use of analogs requires a factor known as a *lumped constant* to account for differences between the behavior of the analog and that of the natural substrate. Lumped constants must be verified under the particular physiologic or pathophysiologic condition under study.

Specific Tracers of Myocardial Metabolism

CARBON-11 PALMITATE

Under physiologic circumstances, palmitate comprises approximately 25 to 30 percent of circulating fatty acid in blood. Accordingly, its oxidation accounts for approximately 50 percent of the overall myocardial energy production attributable to fatty-acid oxidation. Because of the central role of fatty-acid metabolism in overall energy production of the heart and because the changes in fatty-acid metabolism during ischemia have been well characterized, the myocardial kinetics of ¹¹C palmitate were the initial focus for the differentiation by PET of ischemic from normal tissue.

Kinetics   The metabolic fate of ¹¹C palmitate has been characterized extensively. After bolus administration of tracer into the coronary artery of experimental animals, single-pass extraction averages 30 to 60 percent. The myocardial time–activity curve, monitored externally, exhibits several components.[117,122,123] Clearance from the heart occurs in three identifiable phases. The first reflects primarily vascular washout of nonextracted or backdiffused tracer. The second (with a biological half-life of approximately 20 min in humans) reflects primarily β-oxidation. The third phase (with a biological half-life of hours) reflects predominantly incorporation of tracer into triglyceride and phospholipid pools and subsequent turnovers of these pools.[117,118] Under normoxic conditions, 90 to 95 percent of the extracted palmitate is metabolized to ¹¹C-labeled CO_2 that then egresses from the myocardium. Experimental studies have demonstrated that the rate of clearance of the second phase is directly coupled to β-oxidation under aerobic conditions and, since myocardial work is the predominant determinant of oxygen demand, to contractile function.[123]

With ischemia, backdiffusion of nonmetabolized fatty acid increases, and the clearance of the second portion of the time–activity curve diminishes.[117,118] This decrease has been shown to correlate with decreased fatty-acid oxidation and is related to diminished mitochondrial oxidation due to diminished delivery of oxygen rather than to diminished flow per se.[122] Lerch et al demonstrated that diminished clearance from the myocardium was indicative of jeopardized but viable myocardium in regions distal to stenoses.[124] Under these conditions, assessment of the early portion of the time–activity curve may overestimate β-oxidation and cannot be interpreted unambiguously.[117]

Schelbert et al demonstrated that the kinetics of myocardial time–activity curves after administration of ^{11}C palmitate are markedly altered by arterial substrate supply (Fig. 9-13).[125,126] This sensitivity makes the unambiguous interpretation of time–activity curves by simple analysis of clearance under varying substrate conditions problematic. Accordingly, although analysis of the kinetic time–activity curves after administration of ^{11}C palmitate can be used to identify myocardium at risk, careful attention must be given to substrate conditions. Because of the central role of fatty-acid metabolism in the heart, Bergmann et al recently demonstrated that myocardial palmitate metabolism can be quantified in absolute terms (i.e., nanomoles per gram per minute) in experimental animals by using a four-compartment mathematical model, which accounts for the various pathways of metabolism under varying conditions. Preliminary results with this model appear promising.[127]

Clinical observations Despite the limitations of estimates of palmitate metabolism based on either net uptake or exponential clearance analysis, this tracer has proved useful for the detection of ischemic heart disease. In patients with transmural infarction, defects of accumulation of ^{11}C palmitate are recognized consistently and their location correlates closely with the location identified with the electrocardiogram or by regional wall-motion abnormalities.[128,129] Diminished accumulation of ^{11}C palmitate detected tomographically correlated closely with depletion of myocardial creatine phosphate in dogs[130] and, in subsequent clinical studies, tomographic estimates obtainable 15 to 30 min after intravenous administration of 20 mCi ^{11}C palmitate in patients with myocardial infarction correlated closely to enzymatic estimates of infarction size based on analysis of plasma creatine curves.[129] Cardiac PET with ^{11}C palmitate also proved useful in characterizing the efficacy of interventions designed to salvage ischemic myocardium.[131-133] Sobel et al evaluated 19 patients with acute, evolving myocardial infarction immediately and 48 to 72 h after thrombolytic therapy.[134] In patients with suc-

cessful recanalization, the extent of the uptake defect decreased by 29 percent, whereas no change was observed in eight patients with persistent occlusion.

Analysis of time–activity curves after intravenous administration of ^{11}C palmitate has proved useful in delineating jeopardized but viable myocardium in patients. Grover-McKay et al demonstrated in patients with coronary artery disease that, at rest, tissue uptake and clearance of ^{11}C palmitate did not differ between myocardium supplied by normal arteries compared with those supplied by arteries with significant stenosis.[135] With pacing, however, diminished uptake and delayed clearance in myocardium distal to areas supplied by stenotic vessels suggested impaired β-oxidation (Fig. 9-14). Although pacing provoked no electrocardiographic evidence of ischemia nor angina, echocardiography detected mild wall-motion abnormalities in five of ten patients. These studies suggested that subtle abnormalities in energy metabolism could be detected with a metabolic tracer even in the absence of usual criteria of ischemia. Despite these observations, the approach has not been used routinely because of the difficulties in quantitative assessment of the kinetic curves after administration of ^{11}C palmitate, the influence on such curves of numerous factors, and the time necessary to perform this type of metabolic study (2 to 3 h). In addition, it is not clear that the diagnostic or prognostic values of this approach surpass single-photon scintigraphy. Based on the studies using ^{11}C palmitate and PET, a number of centers have used iodinated fatty acids for delineation of ischemic heart disease in patients. Although the myocardial kinetics of the iodinated compounds differ from those of naturally occurring fatty acids, identification of jeopardized but viable myocardium may be possible with iodinated fatty acids and single photon emission detection techniques.[136] Single-photon imaging of iodinated fatty acids is reviewed in detail in Chap. 7.

Carbon-11 palmitate has also been used to study the metabolism of patients with cardiomyopathy. Sochor et al demonstrated that the washout kinetics of ^{11}C palmitate are different in patients with cardiomyopathy.[137] However, these results may simply reflect a tomographic manifestation of myocardial injury giving rise to spatially heterogeneous normal and abnormal tissue. Using exponential analysis of washout curves, Kelly et al recently demonstrated that patients with inherited disorders of critical enzymes in the fatty-acid oxidation pathway can be identified by diminished clearance of extracted ^{11}C palmitate (Fig. 9-15).[138] More recently, using the compartmental model developed and validated in experimental animals,[127] it has been demonstrated that specific abnormalities of uptake and metabolism can be delineated in patients with both inherited and acquired cardiomyopathy.[139,140] Utilization of this approach should facilitate an improved understanding of the biochemical abnormalities that underlie inherited and acquired cardiomy-

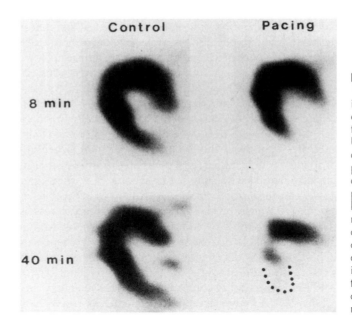

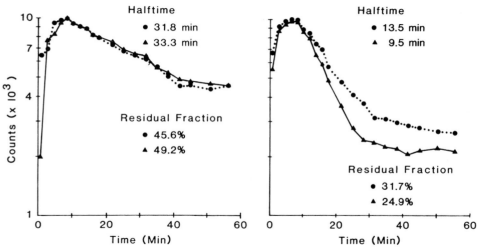

Figure 9-14 Midventricular reconstructions after administration of ^{11}C palmitate under control conditions (*left*) and during pacing (*right*) in a patient with a 90 percent stenosis of the left anterior descending coronary artery. The 8-min images (*top*) reflect initial uptake, whereas the 40-min images (*bottom*) reflect tracer residualizing in myocardium. Uptake is homogeneous at rest and during pacing. Although clearance was homogeneous at rest, it became heterogeneous during pacing with delayed clearance (greater myocardial retention) in the anteroseptal myocardium, reflecting impairment of β-oxidation during pacing in myocardium supplied by the stenotic coronary artery. The kinetic curves are shown on the *bottom*. Normal myocardium is represented by the *triangles* and the anteroseptal myocardium (myocardium at risk) by the *closed circles*. Under control circumstances, the clearance half-times and residual fractions were similar. In contrast, during pacing, the clearance half-time was protracted in the jeopardized region compared with normal myocardium. Note, however, that during pacing, overall clearance, reflective of myocardial metabolism of fatty acids, was increased. (From Grover-McKay et al,[135] reproduced with permission of the American Heart Association, Inc.)

opathies and provide an approach for the assessment of pharmacologic and, ultimately, gene-replacement therapy.

FLUORINE-18 FLUORODEOXYGLUCOSE

This has been the most extensively studied tracer for use with PET. Although many have accepted the utility of this tracer for the identification of viable myocardium, the metabolism of FDG is complex, and interpretation of results obtained with this tracer are controversial.

Basis for the use of glucose for assessment of myocardial ischemia and viability Early after ischemia, when aerobic metabolism becomes limited, energy supply from glucose increases. Extraction of glucose from plasma is accelerated, as is glycolytic flux.[112–115] Although energy

production from glycolysis during ischemia limits energy supply to approximately 30 percent of the overall energy needs of the working heart, sustained energy metabolism from glucose may be sufficient to provide high-energy phosphates to maintain cellular viability although not contractile function.[112–115]

Because of the central role of glucose, ^{11}C-labeled glucose as well as the glucose analog, ^{18}F FDG, were evaluated to characterize myocardial metabolism in ischemic myocardium. In studies in isolated perfused hearts, single-pass extraction of ^{11}C-labeled glucose was found to increase fivefold with ischemia. However, as duration of ischemia became prolonged, glucose uptake declined.[141] These results underscore the complex behavior of glucose kinetics with respect to the severity and duration of ischemia, potentially limiting interpretations of tomograms obtained. Although initial studies demonstrated the potential utility of tomography with ^{11}C glu-

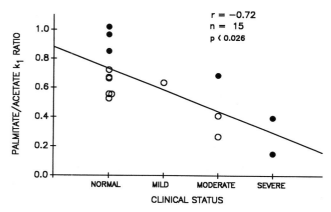

Figure 9-15 Relationship between clinical severity associated with long-chain acyl-CoA dehydrogenase deficiency and the ratio of myocardial clearance of ^{11}C palmitate to ^{11}C acetate (which is an index of the percent of total oxidative metabolism accounted for by palmitate oxidation) in normal subjects and in patients with long-chain acyl-CoA dehydrogenase deficiency with mild, moderate, and severe symptomology. The *open circles* represent data from those older than 16 years of age, whereas the *closed circles* represent data from subjects younger than age 12. It was observed that the more severe deficits were associated with a greater impairment of palmitate oxidation (a lower palmitate–acetate clearance ratio). In addition, children had a higher reliance on fatty-acid metabolism than did adults, which may explain why children with this disease are more severely affected. Thus, PET can assess the phenotypic expression of inherited diseases involving metabolic pathways and may be useful in defining the efficacy of therapeutic interventions, including, ultimately, gene-replacement therapy. (From Kelly et al,[138] reproduced with permission.)

cose after ischemia to identify jeopardized but viable myocardium,[85] quantitative interpretation with this tracer is limited because ^{11}C glucose is metabolized to numerous labeled intermediates. Accordingly, ^{18}F FDG has been the focus of study.

Kinetics Fluorine-18 2-fluoro-2-deoxyglucose is transported across the sarcolemma and can either backdiffuse or be phosphorylated.[142,143] Fluorine-18 FDG-6-phosphate is not available for further metabolism to either glycogen or to pyruvate (Fig. 9-16). The phosphorylated compound is thought to remain trapped intracellularly because of the relative impermeability of the sarcolemma to this intermediate and because dephosphorylation is thought to be modest in the heart. Using a tracer model originally developed by Sokoloff for the estimation of glucose utilization rate in brain with deoxyglucose, Ratib et al noted a close correlation between estimates of glucose metabolism using FDG compared with rates measured directly.[143]

After intravenous administration, ^{18}F FDG accumulates only slowly in the myocardium but remains trapped over several hours. Myocardial accumulation of tracer is markedly dependent on the nutritional status of the subject. Under fasted conditions, arterial fatty-acid con-

tent is high and uptake of ^{18}F FDG is markedly suppressed (Fig. 9-13). After a carbohydrate meal or glucose load, however, myocardial ^{18}F-FDG accumulation is augmented. Utilization of glucose by the heart is also affected either directly or indirectly by catecholamines.[144] In addition, Sease et al suggested that FDG accumulation in myocardium reflects uptake of glucose by leukocytes or other vascular cellular elements,[145] although this interpretation is controversial.[146] Monitoring of arterial and myocardial time–activity curves, employing correction for spillover effects, enables calculation of regional glucose metabolic rates.[143] However, because FDG is not a physiologic substrate and because its metabolic fate is different from that of native glucose, calculation of metabolic rates requires the use of a lumped constant to account for differences between tracer kinetics of the analog and that of glucose. Recent studies have demonstrated the sensitivity of the uptake of FDG to levels of glucose, insulin, and other competing substrates.[147–149] In addition, the uptake of FDG during ischemia and with reperfusion is complex and can either be decreased or increased, depending on levels of ischemia, arterial substrate, and time.[147–151] Finally, although uptake of FDG appears to correlate somewhat with the degree of fibrosis,[152] experimental studies have demonstrated that FDG is taken up in areas of infarction, even though it is apparent that admixtures of viable with nonviable cells are difficult to eliminate completely as the cause for this concerning observation.[151,153,154]

Clinical observations For most imaging procedures, ^{18}F FDG is administered intravenously, and myocardium is scanned 45 to 60 min after tracer administration—a time sufficient for accumulation of tracer in the heart and clearance of tracer from blood. Nearly all studies have used qualitative assessments of glucose uptake related to an assessment of perfusion (made with a separate tracer—typically ^{13}N ammonia, $H_2^{15}O$, or ^{82}Rb). Although some investigators have advocated the performance of studies in fasted subjects since this, at times, enhances identification of ischemic myocardium,[155] it has been shown that there are marked regional inhomogeneities of uptake in ^{18}F-FDG uptake when studied under fasting conditions (Plate 19), despite normal levels of myocardial perfusion and uptake and utilization of other substrates.[156,157] Obviously, this lack of homogeneity seriously compromises interpretations made under fasting conditions. Thus, in nearly all reports, patients have been studied after an oral glucose load, and euglycemic insulin-clamp conditions have been added to improve image quality further.[158,159] Pharmacologic alternatives have also been proposed for improving image quality—thus, nicotinic acid, which lowers serum fatty acids and enhances glucose uptake by the heart, has also been used.[160] Use of euglycemic insulin-clamp techniques also

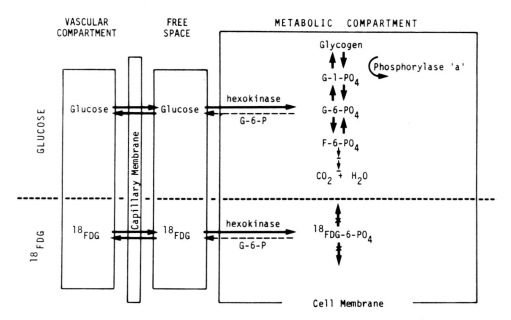

Figure 9-16 Schematic diagram for metabolism for native glucose (*top*) and for the glucose analog, ^{18}F FDG (*bottom*). The analog is handled similarly to the native substrate initially, but FDG-6-PO$_4$ is not a substrate for glycogen synthesis or for glycolytic metabolism. Using a *lumped constant* to account for differences in the handling of the two compounds, steady-state glucose uptake can be estimated with ^{18}F FDG, although the lumped constant may be sensitive to changes in plasma substrate, insulin, and other metabolic factors (see the text). (From Phelps et al,[142] reproduced with permission.)

improves uptake of FDG in diabetic patients, although glucose uptake is still diminished.[161]

Identification of jeopardized but viable myocardium, which may benefit from pharmacologic or mechanical intervention, is key in clinical decision making in cardiology and is an area in which PET offers considerable promise. Jeopardized but viable myocardium is defined as regions that demonstrate contractile dysfunction as a result of either acute or multiple intermittent episodes of ischemia or because of limited nutritive perfusion, but that manifests improved contractile function after appropriate therapy. Definitive evidence of myocardial viability is the temporal improvement in contractile function irrespective of the etiology of the dysfunction or the specific therapeutic intervention employed.[162] Nonetheless, considerable effort has been devoted to defining prospective approaches to delineate jeopardized but viable myocardium.

Results from a number of studies of patients with coronary artery disease have suggested that PET with FDG can identify viable myocardium in zones of contractile dysfunction. Four patterns of ^{18}F-FDG uptake have been observed. In normal myocardium, uptake of a perfusion tracer and of ^{18}F FDG are relatively uniform. In areas of myocardial infarction, a deficit of flow is "matched" with a deficit in ^{18}F-FDG accumulation (Fig. 9-17). Regions with a decrease in flow but with maintained accumulation of ^{18}F FDG (a flow–metabolism

"mismatch") are felt to represent jeopardized but viable myocardium amenable to interventional strategies. A fourth pattern of preserved perfusion but reduced glucose metabolism has also been identified and appears to be associated with myocardial viability. Improvement in regional function after revascularization was evident in 75 to 85 percent of dysfunctional segments that exhibited FDG accumulation, whereas 78 to 92 percent of segments with diminished flow and concomitantly reduced FDG uptake failed to exhibit functional improvement after surgery[163–169] (Table 9-4). In contrast to these results, in patients studied within 72 h of acute myocardial infarction and treated conservatively (i.e., no pharmacologic or mechanical revascularization), only 50 percent of segments demonstrating uptake of FDG improved functionally over time.[165] These contrasting results are likely caused by the inability of FDG to determine the metabolic fate of glucose in the myocardium (anaerobic versus aerobic metabolism or glycogen synthesis). In addition, the pattern of glucose use is related to the duration of time after ischemia, as well as the fate of jeopardized myocardium that in turn depends on collateral flow, loading conditions, and adjunctive therapy.[170–172] The problem of prospectively identifying jeopardized but viable myocardium is especially important in patients with severe left ventricular dysfunction in whom significant benefit can be achieved with revascularization but who are at a higher risk of perioperative morbidity and mor-

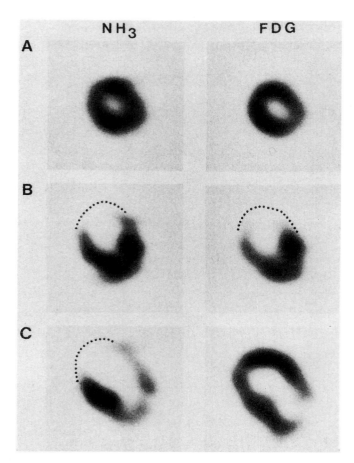

Figure 9-17 Distribution of myocardial perfusion evaluated with ¹³N ammonia (*left*) and of glucose metabolism evaluated with ¹⁸F FDG (*right*) in a normal volunteer, at the *top* **(A)**, showing matched distribution of tracers. In the *middle* **(B)** are tomograms obtained from a patient with myocardial infarction. Blood flow is diminished in the anterior wall (*broken line*), associated with a proportional decrease in FDG accumulation. Shown in **C** (*bottom*) are tomograms from a patient in whom myocardial perfusion is diminished in the anterior wall, whereas glucose utilization in the hypoperfused segment is markedly enhanced. This flow–FDG "mismatch" is felt to represent viable myocardium. (From Schelbert,²²¹ reproduced with permission.)

tality. Recent studies have confirmed that concordantly decreased flow and ¹⁸F-FDG accumulation represent nonviable myocardium.¹⁷³⁻¹⁷⁵ However, Gropler et al found the utility of normal or increased levels of ¹⁸F FDG in predicting myocardial recovery after revascularization to be lower than that reported by others. In a recent study by Gropler et al, 34 patients were evaluated with both ¹⁸F FDG and ¹¹C acetate (which measures myocardial oxygen consumption; see below) both before and after coronary artery revascularization. Estimates of oxidative metabolism were superior to estimates made with ¹⁸F FDG especially in segments with severe dysfunction.¹⁷⁵ Piérard et al similarly found that uptake of FDG was not necessarily predictive of viability.¹⁷⁶ A pattern of normal myocardial perfusion with reduced FDG up-

take in regions of left ventricular function appears to represent admixtures of infarction and reversibly ischemic myocardium.¹⁷⁶,¹⁷⁷

In comparing the results of flow–FDG mismatches with thallium scintigraphy, Brunken et al found that nearly 50 percent of segments with fixed defects by conventional ²⁰¹Tl criteria were viable according to PET criteria.¹⁷⁸,¹⁷⁹ These results would imply that thallium scintigraphy underestimates the extent of viable tissue in hypoperfused segments. In a follow-up study, evaluating 24-h redistribution ²⁰¹Tl images, Brunken et al found uptake of ¹⁸F FDG in the majority of fixed ²⁰¹Tl defects. Severe defects were less likely to exhibit metabolic activity on PET images than defects with less pronounced reductions in ²⁰¹Tl activity¹⁸⁰ (Fig. 9-18). Again, it should be remembered that the presence of FDG in a hypoperfused region is not always indicative of myocardium that will improve after revascularization, and postrevascularization studies were not performed. However, a series of reports indicated that ²⁰¹Tl reinjection at 4 h may improve the delineation of viable myocardium. In two studies from the National Institutes of Health, thallium scintigraphy with reinjection was shown to be nearly equal to PET FDG studies in identifying viable myocardium when the absolute amount of thallium uptake was considered.¹⁸¹,¹⁸² Accordingly, the incremental value of PET with FDG compared with more conventional single-photon scintigraphy has not been completely elucidated. Thallium-201 redistribution/reinjection was shown to be better than ⁹⁹ᵐTc sestamibi as compared with PET using ¹⁸F FDG for identification of viable myocardium.¹⁸³ Assessment of FDG uptake with quantitative techniques appears to be no better than estimates made by visual inspection, due to the larger variability of quantitative estimates of myocardial glucose uptake.¹⁸⁴

In summary, assessment of myocardial viability is possible with PET and ¹⁸F FDG. Dysfunctional areas with diminished perfusion and diminished FDG uptake represent scar and are unlikely to recover with revascularization. Dysfunctional areas with diminished flow but preserved FDG uptake are more variable in their response but in many cases appear to reflect viable myocardium. Recent data from Gropler et al suggest that measurements of oxidative metabolism by using ¹¹C acetate may be better in the prospective distinction of viable from nonviable myocardium. It should be remembered that metabolic patterns should not be misconstrued as a new "gold standard" for delineation of viability, since myocardial viability can be determined only in retrospect based on improvement of function with therapy. Since experimental studies have demonstrated that deoxyglucose can accumulate in infarcted tissue and since uptake of FDG depends on multiple factors, including patterns of flow, oxygen, and substrate availability, interpretation should be made cautiously. The changing patterns of metabolism early after infarction and reperfusion have

Table 9-4 Accuracy of PET Metabolic Criteria for Detecting Viable Myocardium

Study	Subjects, n	Predictive Value, %[a] Viable	Nonviable	Comments
Fluorine-18 fluorodeoxyglucose				
Tillisch et al.[167]	17	85[b]	92[b]	Patients with chronic CAD studied before CABG. Improvement in left ventricular ejection fraction related to number of viable segments present initially.
Tamaki et al.[168]	28	78[b]	80[b]	PET and echocardiographic studies performed before and after CABG. Functional recovery associated with resolution of perfusion and metabolic abnormalities.
Schwaiger et al.[214]	13	50	90	Patients studied 72 h after MI. No thrombolytic agents given or further revascularization procedures implemented.
Piérard et al.[176]	17	55[c]	100[c]	Patients studied 9 days after MI. Functional improvement occurred in 100% of patients with normal flow and metabolism but in only 17% of patients with "flow-metabolism mismatch."
Marwick et al.[215]	16	71	76	PET studies performed before and after revascularization. FDG imaging performed after exercise under fasting conditions. Metabolic abnormalities present after revascularization in 29% of viable regions.
Lucignani et al.[216]	14	95	80	Perfusion studies performed with the use of 99mTc MIBI. FDG studies performed under fasting conditions.
Gropler et al.[175]	34	52[d] 72[e]	81[d] 82[e]	Criteria for viability compared with those with PET and 11C acetate.
Carbon-11 acetate				
Gropler et al.[175]	34	67[d] 85[e]	89[d] 87[d]	Criteria for viability compared favorably with those using PET and FDG.
Henes et al.[104]	8	NP	NP	Sequential PET studies performed in patients early after thrombolysis. Functional recovery associated with improvement in oxidative metabolism.
Gropler et al.[173]	11	NP	NP	PET with 11C acetate and FDG performed before and after CABG or PTCA in patients with recent MI. Maintenance of oxidative metabolism was more reliable than preserved glucose metabolism in determining functional recovery. Metabolic improvement associated with functional recovery.
Gropler et al.[174]	16	NP	NP	PET with 11C acetate and FDG studies performed in patients with stable CAD before CABG or PTCA. Functional recovery dependent on maintenance of oxidative metabolism and not glucose metabolism.

[a] Predictive value = true positives/(true positives + false positives).
[b] Predictive values based on numbers of regions analyzed.
[c] Predictive values based on numbers of patients analyzed.
[d] Predictive values of criteria for mild and moderately dysfunctional segments.
[e] Predictive values of criteria for severely dysfunctional segments.
CABG, coronary artery bypass grafting; CAD, coronary artery disease; FDG, 18F fluorodeoxyglucose; MI, myocardial infarction; MIBI, sestamibi; NP, not provided; PET, positron emission tomography; PTCA, percutaneous transluminal coronary angioplasty.
Reproduced with permission from Gropler and Bergmann.[169]

limited the utility of FDG under these circumstances. Since the uptake of FDG by the myocardium does not distinguish between aerobic and anaerobic metabolism, the finding of enhanced 18F-FDG activity may under certain circumstances be ambiguous, since anaerobic metabolism cannot provide sufficient energy to sustain myocardium for prolonged periods of time.

Despite these caveats, an important study from Eitzman et al demonstrated that the pattern of 18F-FDG uptake is strongly predictive of future clinical events. Fifty percent of patients with a pattern indicative of viable myocardium who did not undergo revascularization suffered myocardial infarction or death within 1 year of the time of the PET scan. Less than 4 percent of patients with viable myocardium by PET who did undergo revascularization died or suffered an infarction.[185]

During the same period, 5 percent of patients died who did not have viable myocardium as determined by PET (and who did not undergo revascularization). A similar high predictive value was found by Tamaki et al.[186] In an analysis of the cost effectiveness of PET in comparison with angiography, with the exercise electrocardiogram, and with SPECT, Patterson et al (using a mathematical model based on Bayes' theorem) found that, in patients with a probability of coronary artery disease (<70 percent stenosis), PET is the most cost-effective modality for delineating disease amenable to treatment, followed by SPECT, the exercise electrocardiogram, and angiography.[187] Obviously, this model is quite dependent on the designated cost of each test and other model parameters. Recent studies have also demonstrated that SPECT imaging of 18F- FDG uptake is feasible, and should studies

ISCHEMIC CARDIOMYOPATHY

Figure 9-18 Cross-sectional transaxial data from a patient with ischemic cardiomyopathy that demonstrate uptake of ^{18}F FDG in a region with a persistent ^{201}Tl defect. The patient's 24-h ^{201}Tl image is shown in the *left panel,* and the corresponding ^{13}N-ammonia perfusion and ^{18}F-FDG reconstructions are shown in the *middle* and *rightmost panels,* respectively. A fixed thallium defect is observed in the anterior myocardium, and diminished perfusion is also evident in the ^{13}N-ammonia scan. FDG uptake is apparent in the anteroseptal segments, suggesting myocardial viability. Some investigators have suggested that reinjection of ^{201}Tl provides results that are concordant with those obtained with ^{18}F FDG (see the text). In addition, uptake of ^{18}F FDG in areas of diminished perfusion does not always indicate true viability (i.e., recovery of function after revascularization; see the text). (From Brunken et al,[180] reproduced with permission of the American Heart Association, Inc.)

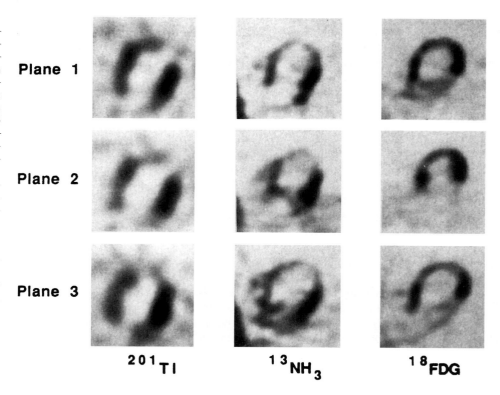

Plane 1   Plane 2   Plane 3

[201]Tl   [13]NH3   [18]FDG

demonstrate the utility of this approach, it may provide an alternative to PET scanning.[188,189]

CARBON-11 ACETATE

Because of the complexities of interpretation of ^{11}C palmitate and of ^{18}F FDG and because experimental studies have demonstrated that assessment of myocardial metabolism with only one of these agents does not provide a picture of overall myocardial energy use, a tracer for estimation of overall oxidative metabolism was sought. Additional impetus was prompted by the observation that functional recovery of reperfused myocardium is determined by the recovery of its ability to metabolize oxidatively.[120,121] Although oxygen participates in the final common pathway for aerobic metabolism of all substrates, delineation of the utilization of myocardial oxygen consumption with ^{15}O-labeled oxygen is more complex, since the conversion of molecular oxygen to water is so rapid and because administration of ^{15}O-labeled oxygen by inhalation results in radioactivity within the lungs.

Brown et al demonstrated that ^{11}C acetate, a short-chain fatty acid oxidized by the myocardium virtually exclusively in the mitochondria, can be used to assess overall oxidative metabolism because oxidation of acetate is so tightly linked to oxidative phosphorylation.[190,191]

Kinetics In 1982, the group at Hammersmith Hospital performed preliminary studies with ^{11}C acetate.[192] These workers demonstrated that the clearance of extracted tracer from the heart after exercise was accelerated in normal myocardium and decreased in ischemic myocardium. Brown et al demonstrated that the slope of clearance of ^{11}C from the heart after initial extraction was directly linked to oxidation of acetate and production of ^{11}C-labeled CO_2 and directly linked to oxidative metabolism over a wide range of flow and metabolic conditions.[190,191,193] Single-pass extraction of ^{11}C acetate ranges between 30 and 60 percent and is virtually independent of the pattern of substrate utilization. With ischemia, the slope of clearance is diminished and reflects diminished oxidative metabolism.[190] These results were corroborated by others.[194,195] Although compartmental mathematical models have been proposed for assessment of regional myocardial oxygen consumption with ^{11}C acetate,[196] they have not been widely used and they appear to offer a relatively small incremental benefit compared with analysis of the exponential clearance alone. Use of estimates of regional myocardial oxygen consumption with ^{11}C acetate in experimental preparations combined with estimates of wall function have been used to generate estimates of regional efficiency[197,198] and have permitted important insights into pathophysiologic processes. For example, Bergmann et al demonstrated that stunned myocardium maintains significant oxidative reserve following short periods of transient myocardial ischemia.[197]

Clinical observations After intravenous administration, extraction of ^{11}C acetate by human myocardium is avid and blood-pool clearance rapid yielding excellent images of the myocardium (Plates 18 and 19). After initial extraction, clearance of ^{11}C activity from the heart at rest is monoexponential with a biological half-life of approximately 12 to 14 min.[199-201] With exercise or with dobutamine, the slope of the clearance is enhanced, reflecting the increase in oxidative metabolism.[200,201] This approach may enable assessment of *metabolic reserve*, analogous to the assessment of flow reserve after maximum coronary vasodilatation.

In patients with infarction, diminished oxidative metabolism is distinct (Plate 20) and does not change with time in patients treated conservatively.[199] Early after reperfusion, although myocardial perfusion may be near normal, myocardial oxidative metabolism is diminished (Plate 18).[104] This may be a consequence of myocardial "stunning" or may reflect a primary defect in energy production. After thrombolysis, recovery of acetate metabolism is delayed but predicts regional functional recovery.[104,173] Since maintenance of the ability of myocardium to metabolize oxidatively appears to be a necessary prerequisite for cell viability and ultimately to provide adequate energy for contractile function, recent studies have explored the utility of ^{11}C acetate for delineating viable from nonviable myocardium. In patients with stable coronary artery disease, the level of oxidative metabolism in viable myocardium (assessed by functional measurements before and after revascularization) was similar to that of normally functioning myocardium and significantly greater than observed in nonviable myocardium. Discrimination between viable and nonviable myocardium was more accurate based on estimates of oxidative metabolism made with ^{11}C acetate than based on estimates of perfusion or glucose metabolism.[169,174,175] Approximately 15 percent of nonviable segments exhibited increased uptake of FDG relative to flow but markedly diminished oxidative metabolism, suggesting anaerobic glycolysis in these segments. Twenty percent of viable segments exhibited reduced myocardial glucose metabolism in the presence of normal oxidative metabolism, suggesting that alternative substrates were being used for sustained oxidative metabolism. Estimates of regional myocardial oxidative metabolism by PET and ^{11}C acetate were more accurate than estimates of glucose metabolism in both patients with acute infarction as well as those with chronic coronary artery disease (Table 9-4

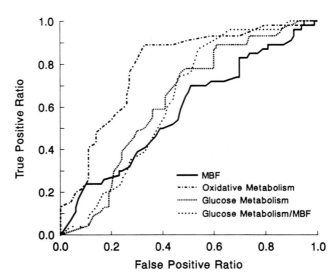

Figure 9-19   Receiver operating characteristic (ROC) curves for prediction of functional recovery based on measurements of regional myocardial blood flow (MBF), oxidative metabolism assessed with ^{11}C acetate, glucose metabolism (^{18}F FDG), and glucose metabolism normalized to flow. Measurements of oxidative metabolism were the most accurate, as evidenced by the left and upward shift of the ROC curve for these measurements (area under the curve = 0.79) compared with curves reflecting estimates of MBF (0.58), ^{18}F FDG (0.63), or glucose metabolism normalized to flow (0.63, $p < 0.02$ for each compared with estimates obtained with acetate alone). These data, obtained in 34 patients with chronic coronary artery disease, demonstrate that estimates of oxidative metabolism are the best predictor of the recovery of function after revascularization. (Gropler et al,[175] *J Am Coll Cardiol* 22:1587, 1993, reproduced with permission of the American College of Cardiology.)

and Fig. 9-19). The accuracy was even better in segments that exhibited severe dysfunction where differentiation of viable from nonviable myocardium is most important clinically. These results have been corroborated by others.[202,203] Accordingly, use of ^{11}C acetate holds great promise for delineation of viable from nonviable myocardium because of its strong predictive accuracy, the fact that its kinetics are not influenced by substrate environment or patterns of myocardial substrate use, and its ability to correlate with overall regional myocardial oxygen consumption, a critical determinant of myocardial viability. In addition, two studies have suggested that the initial uptake of acetate by the myocardium, which is anticipated to be flow dependent, can be used to estimate regional myocardial perfusion,[204,205] which would further streamline imaging protocols, if verified.

OTHER TRACERS OF METABOLISM

A number of other intermediate metabolites, including ^{11}C-labeled lactate, pyruvate, and amino acid, have been proposed for use in the assessment of myocardial metabolism.[85,206] The kinetics of the individual amino acids vary markedly with the position of the label within the molecule. The labeled carbon atoms in these intermediates are rapidly exchanged with constituents of numerous other metabolic pathways, the interpretation of results obtained is complex and these agents have not been used extensively, and their use clinically remains to be defined.

Fluorine-18 fluoromisonidazole An alternative approach to the detection of viable myocardium has been proposed by Shelton et al and by Martin et al using a class of compounds known as *hypoxic sensitizers,* of which ^{18}F fluoromisonidazole has been most extensively studied.[207,208] These tracers diffuse readily into myocardium. With normal levels of oxygen, they are metabolized in a cycle back to the parent compound, which can diffuse back out of the cell. With tissue hypoxia, however, they are reduced and incorporated into insoluble protein constituents. The accumulation of these compounds depends on low oxygen content in myocardial tissue and not on low flow per se. Infarcted myocardium does not accumulate these tracers, since it lacks the enzymes needed to participate in the intermediary reactions. Tracer uptake was observed in regions with low flow[207] as well as in myocardium that showed improved contractile function following reperfusion.[208] Recently, iodinated as well as ^{99m}Tc-labeled congeners of misonidazole have been prepared and may offer the possibility of use of this tracer with conventional imaging approaches.

ASSESSMENT OF MYOCARDIAL RECEPTORS WITH PET

An additional capability of PET is the delineation of myocardial drug and receptor distribution, density, and kinetic flux. A wide variety of ligands have been produced, but only a limited number have been tested clinically. The utility of receptor imaging is covered elsewhere in the monograph, and several recent reviews regarding assessment of receptor function with PET have been published.[209,210] Problems approachable with receptor imaging include evaluations of the role of receptors in the failing heart and their response to therapeutic interventions such as β-blockade as well as evaluation of drugs and their effect on receptor number and function. Mapping receptors may enable delineation of foci of receptor inhomogeneities that may be arrhythmogenic, thereby guiding management in patients with intractable, life-threatening arrhythmias. The clinical utility of the assessment of myocardial receptors with PET has not been clearly defined, although its use for defining a number of biological questions is clear.

ASSESSMENT OF MECHANICAL FUNCTION

Although PET is unlikely to serve as a primary diagnostic tool for the assessment of mechanical cardiac function, it is often useful to couple assessment of myocardial perfusion and metabolism with regional function. A number of approaches have been utilized to delineate mechanical function with PET. Most tracers that are extracted by the myocardium can be used to assess regional function by employing cardiac gating.[211] In addition, regional function can be quantified with ^{15}O-labeled carbon monoxide analogously to conventional radionuclide ventriculograms.[212] Accordingly, when patients undergo PET studies, assessments of mechanical functions can be made routinely, obviating the need for a second assessment of function with a different modality.

THE ROLE OF PET IN CLINICAL DECISION MAKING

PET of the heart enables noninvasive quantification of regional myocardial metabolism and perfusion. The importance of any diagnostic test, however, is its impact on clinical diagnosis and patient management.[213–221]

Quantitative assessment of myocardial perfusion with PET clearly is sensitive and specific for the diagnosis of coronary artery disease and for assessment of the efficacy of therapies designed to restore nutritive perfusion. Although PET has several theoretical advantages over conventional scintigraphy and marked quantitative superiority, proven benefit in the management of patients has not been unequivocal, especially when results of conventional scintigraphy are interpreted by experienced observers. Nonetheless, PET does appear to delineate perfusion defects in the inferior wall more effectively.

PET studies of myocardial perfusion are best reserved for patients with equivocal findings with conventional scintigraphy or for use in those in whom more accurate quantitative estimates of perfusion may be necessary to assist clinicians in decision making for selection of specific interventions. In addition, several groups of patients may require estimates of perfusion with PET rather than with conventional approaches, including those patients with cardiac transplants, patients with cardiomyopathy, patients with chest pain but angiographically normal coronary arteries, and patients with balanced or multivessel coronary artery disease in whom abnormalities of myocardial perfusion may be homogeneous (i.e., without regional disparity). Since PET enables measurement of perfusion in quantitative terms, it can delineate flow deficits despite their homogeneity in such patients.

Metabolic studies with PET can delineate fatty-acid, glycolytic, and oxidative metabolism and thereby aid in the definition of metabolically active, viable tissue that will improve functionally after coronary revascularization. Such assessments are particularly beneficial in patients with severe ventricular dysfunction in whom surgical risk is high but in whom revascularization is potentially extremely beneficial. PET metabolic studies are also very helpful in patients with equivocal results of conventional imaging. Further studies will be necessary to determine whether delayed ^{201}Tl imaging or reinjection protocols can adequately define regions of hypoperfused but viable myocardium in a more cost-effective manner. Comparison between PET and single-photon-emitting tracers of flow and metabolism will be needed to determine whether the quantitative power of PET adds measurably to clinical decisions under routine circumstances.

Although PET is an expensive technology, it offers the potential for delineating the perfusion and biochemical derangements underlying myocardial disease. Characterization by PET of underlying specific biochemical derangements is likely to facilitate understanding of the pathogenesis of cardiac disorders and promote assessment of potential therapeutic interventions. PET is a powerful technology that is clearly superior to conventional nuclear imaging for answering specific biological questions in appropriately selected patients.

REFERENCES

1. Ter-Pogossian MM, Phelps ME, Hoffman EJ, Mullani NA: A positron-emission transaxial tomograph for nuclear imaging (PETT). *Radiology* 114:89, 1975.

2. Welch MJ, Shaikh AM: Radiopharmaceuticals for cardiac positron emission tomography, in Bergmann SR, Sobel BE (eds): *Positron Emission Tomography of the Heart.* Mount Kisco, NY, Futura, 1992, pp 77–96.

3. Fowler JS, Wolf AP: Positron emitter-labeled compounds: Priorities and problems, in Phelps ME, Mazziotta MC, Schelbert HR (eds): *Positron Emission Tomography and Autoradiography: Principles and Applications for the Brain and Heart.* New York, Raven, 1986, pp 391–450.

4. Barrio JR: Biochemical principles in a radiopharmaceutical design and utilization, in Phelps ME, Mazziotta MC, Schelbert HR (eds): *Positron Emission Tomography and Autoradiography: Principles and Applications for the Brain and Heart.* New York, Raven, 1986, pp 451–492.

5. Wrenn FR, Jr, Good ML, Handler P: The use of positron-emitting radioisotopes for the localization of brain tumors. *Science* 113:525, 1951.

6. Brownell GL, Sweet WH: Localization of brain tumors with positron emitters. *Nucleonics* 11:40, 1953.

7. Ter-Pogossian MM: Positron emission tomography instrumentation, in Reivich M, Alavi A (eds): *Positron Emission Tomography.* New York, Alan R Liss, 1985, pp 43–61.

8. Huang S-C, Phelps ME: Principles of tracer kinetic modeling in positron emission tomography and autoradiography, in Phelps ME, Mazziotta MC, Schelbert HR (eds): *Positron Emission Tomography and Autoradiography: Principles and Applications for the Brain and Heart.* New York, Raven, 1986, pp 287–346.

9. Volkow ND, Mullani NA, Bendriem B: Positron emission tomography instrumentation: An overview. *Am J Physiol Imaging* 3:142, 1988.

10. Budinger TF: Time-of-flight positron emission tomography: Status relative to conventional PET. *J Nucl Med* 24:73, 1982.

11. Bacharach SL: The physics of positron emission tomography, in Bergmann SR, Sobel BE (eds): *Positron Emission Tomography of the Heart.* Mount Kisco, NY, Futura, 1992, pp 13–44.

12. Senda M, Yonekura Y, Tamaki N, et al: Interpolating scan and oblique-angle tomograms in myocardial PET using nitrogen-13 ammonia. *J Nucl Med* 27:1830, 1986.

13. Miller TR, Starren JB, Grothe RA Jr: Three-dimensional display of positron emission tomography of the heart. *J Nucl Med* 29:530, 1988.

14. Hicks K, Ganti G, Mullani N, Gould KL: Automated quantitation of three-dimensional cardiac positron emission tomography for routine clinical use. *J Nucl Med* 30:1787, 1989.

15. Miller TR, Wallis JW, Geltman EM, Bergmann SR: Three-dimensional functional images of myocardial oxygen consumption from positron tomography. *J Nucl Med* 31:2064, 1990.

16. Phelps ME, Hoffman EJ, Huang S-C, Ter-Pogossian MM: Effect of positron range on spatial resolution. *J Nucl Med* 16:649, 1975.

17. Cho ZH, Chan JK, Ericksson L, et al: Positron ranges obtained from biomedically important positron-emitting radionuclides. *J Nucl Med* 16:1174, 1975.

18. Hoffman EJ, Phelps ME, Wisenberg G, et al: Electrocardiographic gating in positron emission computed tomography. *J Comput Assist Tomogr* 3:733, 1979.

19. Ter-Pogossian MM, Bergmann SR, Sobel BE: Influence of cardiac and respiratory motion on tomographic reconstructions of the heart: Implications for quantitative nuclear cardiology. *J Comput Assist Tomogr* 6:1148, 1982.

20. Hoffman EA, Huang S-C, Phelps ME: Quantitation in positron emission computed tomography. 1. Effect of object size. *J Comput Assist Tomogr* 3:299, 1979.

21. Parodi O, Schelbert HR, Schwaiger M, et al: Cardiac emission computed tomography: Underestimation of regional tracer concentrations due to wall motion abnormalities. *J Comput Assist Tomogr* 8:1083, 1984.

22. Henze E, Huang S-C, Ratib O, et al: Measurements of regional tissue and blood-pool radiotracer concentrations from serial tomographic images of the heart. *J Nucl Med* 24:987, 1983.

23. Herrero P, Markham J, Myears DW, et al: Measurement of myocardial blood flow with positron emission tomography: Correction for count spillover and partial volume effects. *Math Comput Model* 11:807, 1988.

24. Iida H, Kanno I, Takahashi A, et al: Measurement of

absolute myocardial blood flow with $H_2^{15}O$ and dynamic positron-emission tomography. *Circulation* 78:104, 1988.

25. Bergmann SR, Herrero P, Markham J, et al: Noninvasive quantitation of myocardial blood flow in human subjects with oxygen-15-labeled water and positron emission tomography. *J Am Coll Cardiol* 14:639, 1989.

26. Herrero P, Markham J, Bergmann SR: Quantitation of myocardial blood flow with $H_2^{15}O$ and positron emission tomography: Assessment and error analysis of a mathematical approach. *J Comput Assist Tomogr* 13:862, 1989.

27. Marcus ML, Harrison DG, White CW, et al: Assessing the physiologic significance of coronary obstructions in patients: Importance of diffuse undetected atherosclerosis. *Prog Cardiovasc Dis* 31:39, 1988.

28. Gould KL: Identifying and measuring severity of coronary artery stenosis: Quantitative coronary arteriography and positron emission tomography. *Circulation* 78:237, 1988.

29. Gould KL: How accurate is thallium exercise testing for the diagnosis of coronary artery disease? *J Am Coll Cardiol* 14:1487, 1989.

30. Go RT, Marwick TH, MacIntyre WJ, et al. A prospective comparison of rubidium-82 PET and thallium-201 SPECT myocardial perfusion imaging utilizing a single dipyridamole stress in the diagnosis of coronary artery disease. *J Nucl Med* 31:1899, 1990.

31. Tamaki N, Yonekura Y, Senda M, et al: Value and limitation of stress thallium-201 single photon emission computed tomography: Comparison with nitrogen-13 ammonia positron tomography. *J Nucl Med* 29:1181, 1988.

32. Stewart RE, Schwaiger M, Molina E, et al: Comparison of rubidium-82 positron emission tomography and thallium-201 SPECT imaging for detection of coronary artery disease. *Am J Cardiol* 67:1303, 1991.

33. Di Chiro G, Brooks RA: PET quantitation: Blessing and curse. *J Nucl Med* 29:1603, 1988 (editorial).

34. Rottenberg DA, Strother SC, Moeller JR: In defense of quantitative PET techniques. *J Nucl Med* 30:564, 1989 (letter).

35. Heymann MA, Payne BD, Hoffman JIE, Rudolph AM: Blood flow measurements with radionuclide-labeled particles. *Prog Cardiovasc Dis* 20:55, 1977.

36. Yoshida S, Akizuki S, Gowski D, Downey JM: Discrepancy between microsphere and diffusible tracer estimates of perfusion to ischemic myocardium. *Am J Physiol: Heart Circ Physiol* 249:H255, 1985.

37. Wisenberg G, Schelbert HR, Hoffman EA, et al: In vivo quantitation of regional myocardial blood flow by positron-emission computed tomography. *Circulation* 63:6:1248, 1981.

38. Wilson RA, Shea MJ, De Landsheere CM, et al: Validation of quantitation of regional myocardial blood flow in vivo with ^{11}C-labeled human albumin microspheres and positron emission tomography. *Circulation* 70:717, 1984.

39. Selwyn AP, Shea MJ, Foale R, et al: Regional myocardial and organ blood flow after myocardial infarction: Application of the microsphere principle in man. *Circulation* 73:433, 1986.

40. De Jong RM, Blanksma PK, Willemsen ATM, et al: Posterolateral defect of the normal human heart investigated with nitrogen-13–ammonia and dynamic PET. *J Nucl Med* 36:581, 1995.

41. Beanlands RSB, Muzik O, Hutchins GD, et al: Heterogeneity of regional nitrogen 13-labeled ammonia tracer distribution in the normal human heart: Comparison with rubidium 82 and copper 62-labeled PTSM. *J Nucl Cardiol* 1:225, 1994.

42. Schelbert HR, Phelps ME, Huang S-C, et al: N-13 ammonia as an indicator of myocardial blood flow. *Circulation* 63:1259, 1981.

43. Shah A, Schelbert HR, Schwaiger M, et al: Measurement of regional myocardial blood flow with N-13 ammonia and positron-emission tomography in intact dogs. *J Am Coll Cardiol* 5:92, 1985.

44. Bergmann SR, Hack S, Tewson T, et al: The dependence of accumulation of $^{13}NH_3$ by myocardium on metabolic factors and its implications for quantitative assessment of perfusion. *Circulation* 61:34, 1980.

45. Krivokapich J, Huang S-C, Phelps ME, et al: Dependence of $^{13}NH_3$ myocardial extraction and clearance on flow and metabolism. *Am J Physiol: Heart Circ Physiol* 242:H536, 1982.

46. Rauch B, Helus F, Grunze M, et al: Kinetics of ^{13}N-ammonia uptake in myocardial single cells indicating potential limitations in its applicability as a marker of myocardial blood flow. *Circulation* 71:387, 1985.

47. Krivokapich J, Smith GT, Huang S-C, et al: ^{13}N ammonia myocardial imaging at rest and with exercise in normal volunteers. *Circulation* 80:1328, 1989.

48. Hutchins GD, Schwaiger M, Rosenspire KC, et al: Noninvasive quantification of regional blood flow in the human heart using N-13 ammonia and dynamic positron emission tomographic imaging. *J Am Coll Cardiol* 15:1032, 1990.

49. Rosenspire KC, Schwaiger M, Mangner TJ, et al: Metabolic fate of [^{13}N]ammonia in human and canine blood. *J Nucl Med* 31:163, 1990.

50. Schelbert HR, Wisenberg G, Phelps ME, et al: Noninvasive assessment of coronary stenoses by myocardial imaging during pharmacologic coronary vasodilation. VI. Detection of coronary artery disease in human beings with intravenous N-13 ammonia and positron computed tomography. *Am J Cardiol* 49:1197, 1982.

51. Konishi Y, Ban T, Okamoto Y, et al: Myocardial positron tomography with N-13 ammonia in assessment of aortocoronary bypass surgery. *Jpn Circ J* 52:411, 1988.

52. Tamaki N, Yonekura Y, Senda M, et al: Myocardial positron computed tomography with ^{13}N-ammonia at rest and during exercise. *Eur J Nucl Med* 11:246, 1985.

53. Demer LL, Gould KL, Goldstein RA, et al: Assessment of coronary artery disease severity by positron emission tomography: Comparison with quantitative arteriography in 193 patients. *Circulation* 79:825, 1989.

54. Tamaki N, Senda M, Yonekura Y, et al: Dynamic positron computed tomography of the heart with a high sensitivity positron camera and nitrogen-13 ammonia. *J Nucl Med* 26:567, 1985.

55. Yonekura Y, Tamaki N, Senda M, et al: Detection of coronary artery disease with ^{13}N-ammonia and high-res-

olution positron-emission computed tomography. *Am Heart J* 113:645, 1987.

56. Choi Y, Huang S-C, Hawkins RA, et al: A simplified method for quantification of myocardial blood flow using nitrogen-13–ammonia and dynamic PET. *J Nucl Med* 34:488, 1993.

57. Dayanikli F, Grambow D, Muzik O, et al: Early detection of abnormal coronary flow reserve in asymptomatic men at high risk for coronary artery disease using positron emission tomography. *Circulation* 90:808, 1994.

58. Di Carli M, Czernin J, Hoh CK, et al: Relation among stenosis severity, myocardial blood flow, and flow reserve in patients with coronary artery disease. *Circulation* 91:1944, 1995.

59. Gould KL, Martucci JP, Goldberg DI, et al: Short-term cholesterol lowering decreases size and severity of perfusion abnormalities by positron emission tomography after dipyridamole in patients with coronary artery disease: A potential noninvasive marker of healing coronary endothelium. *Circulation* 89:1530, 1994.

60. Neglia D, Parodi O, Gallopin M, et al: Myocardial blood flow response to pacing tachycardia and to dipyridamole infusion in patients with dilated cardiomyopathy without overt heart failure: A quantitative assessment by positron emission tomography. *Circulation* 92:796, 1995.

61. Love WD, Burch GE: Influence of the rate of coronary plasma flow on the extraction of Rb[86] from coronary blood. *Circ Res* 7:24, 1959.

62. Selwyn AP, Allan RM, l'Abbate A, et al: Relation between regional myocardial uptake of rubidium-82 and perfusion: Absolute reduction of cation uptake in ischemia. *Am J Cardiol* 50:112, 1982.

63. Wilson RA, Shea M, De Landsheere C, et al: Rubidium-82 myocardial uptake and extraction after transient ischemia: PET characteristics. *J Comput Assist Tomogr* 11:60, 1987.

64. Goldstein RA, Mullani NA, Marani SK, et al: Myocardial perfusion with rubidium-82. II. Effects of metabolic and pharmacologic interventions. *J Nucl Med* 24:907, 1983.

65. Fukuyama T, Nakamura M, Nakagaki O, et al: Reduced reflow and diminished uptake of ^{86}Rb after temporary coronary occlusion. *Am J Physiol: Heart Circ Physiol* 234:H724, 1978.

66. Mullani NA, Gould KL: First-pass measurements of regional blood flow with external detectors. *J Nucl Med* 24:577, 1983.

67. Herrero P, Markham J, Shelton ME, Bergmann SR: Implementation and evaluation of a two-compartment model for quantification of myocardial perfusion with rubidium-82 and positron emission tomography. *Circ Res* 70:496, 1992.

68. Goldstein RA: Kinetics of rubidium-82 after coronary occlusion and reperfusion: Assessment of patency and viability in open-chested dogs. *J Clin Invest* 75:1131, 1985.

69. Goldstein RA: Rubidium-82 kinetics after coronary occlusion: Temporal relation of net myocardial accumulation and viability in open-chested dogs. *J Nucl Med* 27:1456, 1986.

70. Goldstein RA, Mullani NA, Wong W-H, et al: Positron imaging of myocardial infarction with rubidium-82. *J Nucl Med* 27:1824, 1986.

71. Camici P, Araujo LI, Spinks T, et al: Increased uptake of ^{18}F-fluorodeoxyglucose in postischemic myocardium of patients with exercise-induced angina. *Circulation* 74:81, 1986.

72. Gould KL, Goldstein RA, Mullani NA, et al: Noninvasive assessment of coronary stenoses by myocardial perfusion imaging during pharmacologic coronary vasodilation. VIII. Clinical feasibility of positron cardiac imaging without a cyclotron using generator-produced rubidium-82. *J Am Coll Cardiol* 7:775, 1986.

73. Goldstein RA, Kirkeeide RL, Demer LL, et al: Relation between geometric dimensions of coronary artery stenoses and myocardial perfusion reserve in man. *J Clin Invest* 79:1473, 1987.

74. Goldstein RA, Kirkeeide RL, Smalling RW, et al: Changes in myocardial perfusion reserve after PTCA: Noninvasive assessment with positron tomography. *J Nucl Med* 28:1262, 1987.

75. Marwick TH, Cook SA, Lafont A, et al: Influence of left ventricular mass on the diagnostic accuracy of myocardial perfusion imaging using positron emission tomography with dipyridamole stress. *J Nucl Med* 32:2221, 1991.

76. Williams BR, Mullani NA, Jansen DE, Anderson BA: A retrospective study of the diagnostic accuracy of a community hospital-based PET center for the detection of coronary artery disease using rubidium-82. *J Nucl Med* 35:1586, 1994.

77. Gould KL, Yoshida K, Hess MJ, et al: Myocardial metabolism of fluorodeoxyglucose compared to cell membrane integrity for the potassium analogue rubidium-82 for assessing infarct size in man by PET. *J Nucl Med* 32:1, 1991.

78. Shelton ME, Green MA, Mathias CJ, et al: Kinetics of copper-PTSM in isolated hearts: A novel tracer for measuring blood flow with positron emission tomography. *J Nucl Med* 30:1843, 1989.

79. Shelton ME, Green MA, Mathias CJ, et al: Assessment of regional myocardial and renal blood flow with copper-PTSM and positron emission tomography. *Circulation* 82:990, 1990.

80. Herrero P, Markham J, Weinheimer CJ, et al: Quantification of regional myocardial perfusion with generator-produced [62]Cu-PTSM and positron emission tomography. *Circulation* 87:173, 1993.

81. Beanlands RSB, Muzik O, Mintun M, et al: The kinetics of copper-62–PTSM in the normal human heart. *J Nucl Med* 33:684, 1992.

82. Melon PG, Brihaye C, Degueldre C, et al: Myocardial kinetics of potassium-38 in humans and comparison with copper-62–PTSM. *J Nucl Med* 35:1116, 1994.

83. Herrero P, Hartman JJ, Green, MA, et al: Assessment of regional myocardial perfusion with generator-produced [62]Cu-PTSM and PET in human subjects. *J Nucl Med*, in press

84. Mathias CJ, Bergmann SR, Green MA: Species-dependent binding of copper(II) *bis*(thiosemicarbazone) radiopharmaceuticals to serum albumin. *J Nucl Med* 36:1451, 1995.

85. Bergmann SR, Fox KAA, Geltman EM, Sobel BE: Posi-

tron emission tomography of the heart. *Prog Cardiovasc Dis* 28:165, 1985.

86. Bergmann SR, Fox KAA, Rand AL, et al: Quantification of regional myocardial blood flow in vivo with $H_2^{15}O$. *Circulation* 70:724, 1984.

87. Tripp MR, Meyer MW, Einzig S, et al: Simultaneous regional myocardial blood flows by tritiated water and microspheres. *Am J Physiol: Heart Circ Physiol* 232:H173, 1977.

88. Knabb RM, Fox KAA, Sobel BE, Bergmann SR: Characterization of the functional significance of subcritical coronary stenoses with $H_2^{15}O$ and positron-emission tomography. *Circulation* 71:1271, 1985.

89. Huang SC, Schwaiger M, Carson RE, et al: Quantitative measurement of myocardial blood flow with oxygen-15 water and positron computed tomography: An assessment of potential and problems. *J Nucl Med* 26:616, 1985.

90. Araujo LI, Lammertsma AA, Rhodes CG, et al: Noninvasive quantification of regional myocardial blood flow in coronary artery disease with oxygen-15-labeled carbon dioxide inhalation and positron emission tomography. *Circulation* 83:875, 1991.

91. Bol A, Melin JA, Vanoverschelde J-L, et al: Direct comparison of [¹³N]ammonia and [¹⁵O]water estimates of perfusion with quantification of regional myocardial blood flow by microspheres. *Circulation* 87:512, 1993.

92. Senneff MJ, Geltman EM, Bergmann SR: Noninvasive delineation of the effects of moderate aging on myocardial perfusion. *J Nucl Med* 32:2037, 1991.

93. Uren NG, Camici PG, Wijns W, et al: The effect of aging on coronary flow reserve in man. *Circulation* 88:I-171, 1993 (abstr).

94. Bergmann SR, Herrero P, Geltman EM: Blunted response of myocardial perfusion to dipyridamole in older adults (Revisited). *J Nucl Med* 36:1137, 1995 (letter).

95. Czernin J, Müller P, Chan S, et al: Influence of age and hemodynamics on myocardial blood flow and flow reserve. *Circulation* 88:62, 1993.

96. Walsh MN, Bergmann SR, Steele RL, et al: Delineation of impaired regional myocardial perfusion by positron emission tomography with $H_2^{15}O$. *Circulation* 78:612, 1988.

97. Shelton ME, Senneff MJ, Ludbrook PA, et al: Concordance of nutritive myocardial perfusion reserve and flow velocity reserve in conductance vessels in patients with chest pain with angiographically normal coronary arteries. *J Nucl Med* 34:717, 1993.

98. Merlet P, Mazoyer B, Hittinger L, et al: Assessment of coronary reserve in man: Comparison between positron emission tomography with oxygen-15-labeled water and intracoronary Doppler technique. *J Nucl Med* 34:1899, 1993.

99. Uren NG, Melin JA, De Bruyne B, et al: Relation between myocardial blood flow and the severity of coronary-artery stenosis. *N Engl J Med* 330:1782, 1994.

100. Uren NG, Marraccini P, Gistri R, et al: Altered coronary vasodilator reserve and metabolism in myocardium subtended by normal arteries in patients with coronary artery disease. *J Am Coll Cardiol* 22:650, 1993.

101. Walsh MN, Geltman EM, Steele RL, et al: Augmented

myocardial perfusion reserve after angioplasty quantified by positron emission tomography with $H_2^{15}O$. *J Am Coll Cardiol* 15:119, 1990.

102. Uren NG, Crake T, Lefroy DC, et al: Delayed recovery of coronary resistive vessel function after coronary angioplasty. *J Am Coll Cardiol* 21:612, 1993.

103. Uren NG, Crake T, Lefroy DC, et al: Reduced coronary vasodilator function in infarcted and normal myocardium after myocardial infarction. *N Engl J Med* 331:222, 1994.

104. Henes CG, Bergmann SR, Perez JE, et al: The time course of restoration of nutritive perfusion, myocardial oxygen consumption, and regional function after coronary thrombolysis. *Coronary Artery Dis* 1:687, 1990.

105. Geltman EM, Henes CG, Walsh MN, et al: The pathogenesis of chest pain with normal coronary arteries delineated by positron emission tomography and $H_2^{15}O$. *J Am Coll Cardiol* 15:159A, 1990 (abstr).

106. Senneff MJ, Hartman JJ, Sobel BE, et al: Persistence of coronary vasodilator responsivity after cardiac transplantation. *Am J Cardiol* 71:333, 1993.

107. Rechavia E, Araujo LI, de Silva R, et al: Dipyridamole vasodilator response after human orthotopic heart transplantation: Quantification by oxygen-15-labeled water and positron emission tomography. *J Am Coll Cardiol* 19:100, 1992.

108. Iida H, Rhodes CG, de Silva R, et al: Myocardial tissue fraction: Correction for partial volume effects and measure of tissue viability. *J Nucl Med* 32:2169, 1991.

109. Yamamoto Y, de Silva R, Rhodes CG, et al: A new strategy for the assessment of viable myocardium and regional myocardial blood flow using ¹⁵O-water and dynamic positron emission tomography. *Circulation* 86:167, 1992.

110. De Silva R, Yamamoto Y, Rhodes CG, et al: Preoperative prediction of the outcome of coronary revascularization using positron emission tomography. *Circulation* 86:1738, 1992.

111. Herrero P, Staudenerz A, Walsh JF, et al: Heterogeneity of myocardial perfusion provides the physiological basis of "perfusable tissue index." *J Nucl Med* 36:320, 1995.

112. Bing RJ: Cardiac metabolism. *Physiol Rev* 45:171, 1965.

113. Neely JR, Morgan HE: Relationship between carbohydrate and lipid metabolism and the energy balance of heart muscle. *Annu Rev Physiol* 36:413, 1974.

114. Liedtke AJ: Alterations of carbohydrate and lipid metabolism in the acutely ischemic heart. *Prog Cardiovasc Dis* 23:321, 1981.

115. Camici P, Ferrannini E, Opie LH: Myocardial metabolism in ischemic heart disease: Basic principles and application to imaging by positron emission tomography. *Prog Cardiovasc Dis* 32:217, 1989.

116. Myears DW, Sobel BE, Bergmann SR: Substrate use in ischemic and reperfused canine myocardium: Quantitative considerations. *Am J Physiol: Heart Circ Physiol* 253:H107, 1987.

117. Fox KAA, Abendschein DR, Ambos HD, et al: Efflux of metabolized and nonmetabolized fatty acid from canine myocardium: Implications for quantifying myocardial metabolism tomographically. *Circ Res* 57:232, 1985.

118. Rosamond TL, Abendschein DR, Sobel BE, et al: Meta-

bolic fate of radiolabeled palmitate in ischemic canine myocardium: Implications for positron emission tomography. *J Nucl Med* 28:1322, 1987.

119. Schwaiger M, Schelbert HR, Ellison D, et al: Sustained regional abnormalities in cardiac metabolism after transient ischemia in the chronic dog model. *J Am Coll Cardiol* 6:336, 1985.

120. Taegtmeyer H, Roberts AFC, Raine AEG: Energy metabolism in reperfused heart muscle: Metabolic correlates to return of function. *J Am Coll Cardiol* 6:864, 1985.

121. Weinheimer CJ, Brown MA, Nohara R, et al: Functional recovery after reperfusion is predicated on recovery of myocardial oxidative metabolism. *Am Heart J* 125:939, 1993.

122. Lerch RA, Bergmann SR, Ambos HD, et al: Effect of flow-independent reduction of metabolism on regional myocardial clearance of ^{11}C-palmitate. *Circulation* 65:731, 1982.

123. Schon HR, Schelbert HR, Najafi A, et al: C-11 labeled palmitic acid for the noninvasive evaluation of regional myocardial fatty acid metabolism with positron-computed tomography. II. Kinetics of C-11 palmitic acid in acutely ischemic myocardium. *Am Heart J* 103:548, 1982.

124. Lerch RA, Ambos HD, Bergmann SR, et al: Localization of viable, ischemic myocardium by positron-emission tomography with ^{11}C-palmitate. *Circulation* 64:689, 1981.

125. Schelbert HR, Henze E, Schon HR, et al: C-11 palmitate for the noninvasive evaluation of regional myocardial fatty acid metabolism with positron computed tomography. III. In vivo demonstration of the effects of substrate availability on myocardial metabolism. *Am Heart J* 105:492, 1983.

126. Schelbert HR, Henze E, Sochor H, et al: Effects of substrate availability on myocardial C-11 palmitate kinetics by positron emission tomography in normal subjects and patients with ventricular dysfunction. *Am Heart J* 111:1055, 1986.

127. Bergmann SR, Weinheimer CJ, Markham J, Herrero P: Quantitation of myocardial fatty acid metabolism using positron emission tomography. *J Nucl Med,* in press.

128. Sobel BE, Weiss ES, Welch MJ, et al: Detection of remote myocardial infarction in patients with positron emission transaxial tomography and intravenous ^{11}C-palmitate. *Circulation* 55:853, 1977.

129. Ter-Pogossian MM, Klein MS, Markham J, et al: Regional assessment of myocardial metabolic integrity in vivo by positron-emission tomography with ^{11}C-labeled palmitate. *Circulation* 61:242, 1980.

130. Weiss ES, Ahmed SA, Welch MJ, et al: Quantification of infarction in cross sections of canine myocardium in vivo with positron emission transaxial tomography and ^{11}C-palmitate. *Circulation* 55:66, 1977.

131. Bergmann SR, Lerch RA, Fox KAA, et al: Temporal dependence of beneficial effects of coronary thrombolysis characterized by positron tomography. *Am J Med* 73:573, 1982.

132. Bergmann SR, Fox KAA, Ter-Pogossian MM, et al: Clot-selective coronary thrombolysis with tissue-type plasminogen activator. *Science* 220:1181, 1983.

133. Knabb RM, Rosamond TL, Fox KAA, et al: Enhance-

134. Sobel BE, Geltman EM, Tiefenbrunn AJ, et al: Improvement of regional myocardial metabolism after coronary thrombolysis induced with tissue-type plasminogen activator or streptokinase. *Circulation* 69:983, 1984.

135. Grover-McKay M, Schelbert HR, Schwaiger M, et al: Identification of impaired metabolic reserve by atrial pacing in patients with significant coronary artery stenosis. *Circulation* 74:281, 1986.

136. Hansen CL, Corbett JR, Pippin JJ, et al: Iodine-123 phenylpentadecanoic acid and single photon emission computed tomography in identifying left ventricular regional metabolic abnormalities in patients with coronary heart disease: Comparison with thallium-201 myocardial tomography. *J Am Coll Cardiol* 12:78, 1988.

137. Sochor H, Schelbert HR, Schwaiger M, et al: Studies of fatty acid metabolism with positron emission tomography in patients with cardiomyopathy. *Eur J Nucl Med* 12:S66, 1986.

138. Kelly DP, Mendelsohn NJ, Sobel BE, et al: Detection and assessment by positron emission tomography of a genetically determined defect in myocardial fatty acid utilization (long-chain acyl-CoA dehydrogenase deficiency). *Am J Cardiol* 71:738, 1993.

139. Bergmann SR, Rubin PJ, Hartman JJ, Herrero P: Detection of abnormalities in fatty acid metabolism in patients with cardiomyopathy using PET. *J Nucl Med* 36:142P, 1995 (abstr).

140. Bergmann SR, Herrero P, Hartman JJ, et al: Quantitative assessment of myocardial fatty acid metabolism in pediatric patients with inherited cardiomyopathy. *Circulation* 92(Suppl I):I-444, 1995 (abstr).

141. Weiss ES, Hoffman EJ, Phelps ME, et al: External detection and visualization of myocardial ischemia with ^{11}C-substrates in vitro and in vivo. *Circ Res* 39:24, 1976.

142. Phelps ME, Schelbert HR, Mazziotta JC: Positron computed tomography for studies of myocardial and cerebral function. *Ann Intern Med* 98:339, 1983.

143. Ratib O, Phelps ME, Huang S-C, et al: Positron tomography with deoxyglucose for estimating local myocardial glucose metabolism. *J Nucl Med* 23:577, 1982.

144. Merhige ME, Ekas R, Mossberg K, et al: Catecholamine stimulation, substrate competition, and myocardial glucose uptake in conscious dogs assessed with positron emission tomography. *Circ Res* 61(suppl II):II-124, 1987.

145. Sease D, Garza D, Merhige ME, Gould KL: Does myocardial uptake of F-18–fluorodeoxyglucose by positron emission tomography reliably indicate myocardial viability in acute myocardial infarction? *Circulation* 80:II-378, 1989.

146. Wijns W, Melin JA, Leners N, et al: Accumulation of polymorphonuclear leukocytes in reperfused ischemic canine myocardium: Relation with tissue viability assessed by fluorine-18–2-deoxyglucose uptake. *J Nucl Med* 29:1826, 1988.

147. Ng CK, Holden JE, DeGrado TR, et al: Sensitivity of myocardial fluorodeoxyglucose lumped constant to glucose and insulin. *Am J Physiol: Heart Circ Physiol* 260:H593, 1991.

148. Hariharan R, Bray M, Ganim R, et al: Fundamental

limitations of [^{18}F]2-deoxy-2-fluoro- D-glucose for assessing myocardial glucose uptake. *Circulation* 91:2435, 1995.

149. Liedtke AJ, Renstrom B, Nellis SH: Correlation between [5-^{3}H]glucose and [U-^{14}C]deoxyglucose as markers of glycolysis in reperfused myocardium. *Circ Res* 71:689, 1992.

150. McFalls EO, Ward H, Fashingbauer P, et al: Myocardial blood flow and FDG retention in acutely stunned porcine myocardium. *J Nucl Med* 36:637, 1995.

151. Buxton DB, Schelbert HR: Measurement of regional glucose metabolic rates in reperfused myocardium. *Am J Physiol: Heart Circ Physiol* 261:H2058, 1991.

152. Maes A, Flameng W, Nuyts J, et al: Histological alterations in chronically hypoperfused myocardium: Correlation with PET findings. *Circulation* 90:735, 1994.

153. Sebree L, Bianco JA, Subramanian R, et al: Discordance between accumulation of C-14 deoxyglucose and Tl-201 in reperfused myocardium. *J Mol Cell Cardiol* 23:603, 1991.

154. Yaoita H, Fischman AJ, Wilkinson R, et al: Distribution of deoxyglucose and technetium-99m–glucarate in the acutely ischemic myocardium. *J Nucl Med* 34:1303, 1993.

155. Tamaki N, Yonekura Y, Konishi J: Myocardial FDG PET studies with fasting, oral glucose-loading or insulin clamp methods. *J Nucl Med* 33:1263, 1992 (editorial).

156. Gropler RJ, Siegel BA, Lee KJ, et al: Nonuniformity in myocardial accumulation of fluorine-18-fluorodeoxyglucose in normal fasted humans. *J Nucl Med* 31:1749, 1990.

157. Hicks RJ, Herman WH, Kalff V, et al: Quantitative evaluation of regional substrate metabolism in the human heart by positron emission tomography. *J Am Coll Cardiol* 18:101, 1991.

158. Knuuti MJ, Nuutila P, Ruotsalainen U, et al: Euglycemic hyperinsulinemic clamp and oral glucose load in stimulating myocardial glucose utilization during positron emission tomography. *J Nucl Med* 33:1255, 1992.

159. Schelbert HR: Euglycemic hyperinsulinemic clamp and oral glucose load in stimulating myocardial glucose utilization during positron emission tomography. *J Nucl Med* 33:1263, 1992 (editorial).

160. Knuuti MJ, Yki-Järvinen H, Voipio-Pulkki L-M, et al: Enhancement of myocardial [fluorine-18]fluorodeoxyglucose uptake by a nicotinic acid derivative. *J Nucl Med* 35:989, 1994.

161. Ohtake T, Yokoyama I, Watanabe T, et al: Myocardial glucose metabolism in noninsulin-dependent diabetes mellitus patients evaluated by FDG-PET. *J Nucl Med* 36:456, 1995.

162. Gropler RJ, Bergmann SR: Myocardial viability: What is the definition? *J Nucl Med* 32:10, 1991 (editorial).

163. Marshall RC, Tillisch JH, Phelps ME, et al: Identification and differentiation of resting myocardial ischemia and infarction in man with positron computed tomography, ^{18}F- labeled fluorodeoxyglucose and N-13 ammonia. *Circulation* 67:766, 1983.

164. Brunken R, Tillisch J, Schwaiger M, et al: Regional perfusion, glucose metabolism, and wall motion in patients with chronic electrocardiographic Q wave infarctions:

Evidence for persistence of viable tissue in some infarct regions by positron emission tomography. *Circulation* 73:951, 1986.

165. Schwaiger M, Brunken R, Grover-McKay M, et al: Regional myocardial metabolism in patients with acute myocardial infarction assessed by positron emission tomography. *J Am Coll Cardiol* 8:800, 1986.

166. Schwaiger M, Brunken RC, Krivokapich J, et al: Beneficial effect of residual anterograde flow on tissue viability as assessed by positron emission tomography in patients with myocardial infarction. *Eur Heart J* 8:981, 1987.

167. Tillisch J, Brunken R, Marshall R, et al: Reversibility of cardiac wall-motion abnormalities predicted by positron tomography. *N Engl J Med* 314:884, 1986.

168. Tamaki N, Yonekura Y, Yamashita K, et al: Positron emission tomography using F-18 deoxyglucose in evaluation of coronary-artery bypass-grafting. *Am J Cardiol* 64:860, 1989.

169. Gropler RJ, Bergmann SR: Flow and metabolic determinants of myocardial viability assessed by positron-emission tomography. *Coronary Artery Dis* 4:495, 1993.

170. Gropler RJ, Geltman EM, Sobel BE: Clinical applications of cardiac positron emission tomography, in Bergmann SR, Sobel BE (eds): *Positron Emission Tomography of the Heart.* Mount Kisco, NY, Futura, 1992, pp 255–292.

171. Bergmann SR: Use and limitations of metabolic tracers labeled with positron-emitting radionuclides in the identification of viable myocardium. *J Nucl Med* 35(Suppl):15S, 1994.

172. Schwaiger M, Neese RA, Araujo L, et al: Sustained nonoxidative glucose utilization and depletion of glycogen in reperfused canine myocardium. *J Am Coll Cardiol* 13:745, 1989.

173. Gropler RJ, Siegel BA, Sampathkumaran K, et al: Dependence of recovery of contractile function on maintenance of oxidative metabolism after myocardial infarction. *J Am Coll Cardiol* 19:989, 1992.

174. Gropler RJ, Geltman EM, Sampathkumaran K, et al: Functional recovery after coronary revascularization for chronic coronary artery disease is dependent on maintenance of oxidative metabolism. *J Am Coll Cardiol* 20:569, 1992.

175. Gropler RJ, Geltman EM, Sampathkumaran K, et al: Comparison of carbon-11–acetate with fluorine-18–fluorodeoxyglucose for delineating viable myocardium by positron emission tomography. *J Am Coll Cardiol* 22:1587, 1993.

176. Piérard LA, De Landsheere CM, Berthe C, et al: Identification of viable myocardium by echocardiography during dobutamine infusion in patients with myocardial infarction after thrombolytic therapy: Comparison with positron emission tomography. *J Am Coll Cardiol* 15:1021, 1990.

177. Perrone-Filardi P, Bacharach SL, Dilsizian V, et al: Clinical significance of reduced regional myocardial glucose uptake in regions with normal blood flow in patients with chronic coronary artery disease. *J Am Coll Cardiol* 23:608, 1994.

178. Brunken R, Schwaiger M, Grover-McKay M, et al: Positron emission tomography detects tissue metabolic activ-

ity in myocardial segments with persistent thallium perfusion defects. *J Am Coll Cardiol* 10:557, 1987.

179. Brunken RC, Kottou S, Nienaber CA, et al: PET detection of viable tissue in myocardial segments with persistent defects at Tl-201 SPECT. *Radiology* 172:65, 1989.

180. Brunken RC, Vaghaiwalla Mody F, Hawkins RA, et al: Positron emission tomography detects metabolic viability in myocardium with persistent 24-hour single-photon emission computed tomography ^{201}Tl defects. *Circulation* 86:1357, 1992.

181. Bonow RO, Dilsizian V, Cuocolo A, Bacharach SL: Identification of viable myocardium in patients with chronic coronary artery disease and left ventricular dysfunction: Comparison of thallium scintigraphy with reinjection and PET imaging with [18]F- fluorodeoxyglucose. *Circulation* 83:26, 1991.

182. Dilsizian V, Perrone-Filardi P, Arrighi JA, et al: Concordance and discordance between stress–redistribution–reinjection and rest–redistribution thallium imaging for assessing viable myocardium: Comparison with metabolic activity by positron emission tomography. *Circulation* 88:941, 1993.

183. Dilsizian V, Arrighi JA, Diodati JG, et al: Myocardial viability in patients with chronic coronary artery disease: Comparison of ^{99m}Tc-sestamibi with thallium reinjection and [^{18}F]fluorodeoxy-glucose. *Circulation* 89:578, 1994.

184. Knuuti MJ, Nuutila P, Ruotsalainen U, et al: The value of quantitative analysis of glucose utilization in detection of myocardial viability by PET. *J Nucl Med* 34:2068, 1993.

185. Eitzman D, Al-Aouar Z, Kanter HL, et al: Clinical outcome of patients with advanced coronary artery disease after viability studies with positron emission tomography. *J Am Coll Cardiol* 20:559, 1992.

186. Tamaki N, Kawamoto M, Takahashi N, et al: Prognostic value of an increase in fluorine-18 deoxyglucose uptake in patients with myocardial infarction: Comparison with stress thallium imaging. *J Am Coll Cardiol* 22:1621, 1993.

187. Patterson RE, Eisner RL, Horowitz SF: Comparison of cost-effectiveness and utility of exercise ECG, single photon emission computed tomography, positron emission tomography, and coronary angiography for diagnosis of coronary artery disease. *Circulation* 91:54, 1995.

188. Kelly MJ, Kalff V: Fluorine 18-labeled fluorodeoxyglucose myocardial scintigraphy with Anger gamma cameras for assessing myocardial viability. *J Nucl Cardiol* 2:360, 1995.

189. Burt RW, Perkins OW, Oppenheim BE, et al: Direct comparison of fluorine-18–FDG SPECT, fluorine-18–FDG PET and rest thallium-201 SPECT for detection of myocardial viability. *J Nucl Med* 36:176, 1995.

190. Brown MA, Marshall DR, Sobel BE, Bergmann SR: Delineation of myocardial oxygen utilization with carbon-11 labeled acetate. *Circulation* 76:687, 1987.

191. Brown MA, Myears DW, Bergmann SR: Noninvasive assessment of canine myocardial oxidative metabolism with carbon-11 acetate and positron emission tomography. *J Am Coll Cardiol* 12:1054, 1988.

192. Pike VW, Eakins MN, Allan RM, Selwyn AP: Preparation of [1-^{11}C]acetate: An agent for the study of myocardial metabolism by positron emission tomography. *Int J Appl Radiat Isot* 33:505, 1982.

193. Brown MA, Myears DW, Bergmann SR: Validity of estimates of myocardial oxidative metabolism with carbon-11 acetate and positron emission tomography despite altered patterns of substrate utilization. *J Nucl Med* 30:187, 1989.

194. Ng CK, Huang S-C, Schelbert HR, Buxton DB: Validation of a model for [1-^{11}C]acetate as a tracer of cardiac oxidative metabolism. *Am J Physiol: Heart Circ Physiol* 266:H1304, 1994.

195. Armbrecht JJ, Buxton DB, Schelbert HR: Validation of [1-^{11}C]acetate as a tracer for noninvasive assessment of oxidative metabolism with positron emission tomography in normal, ischemic, postischemic, and hyperemic canine myocardium. *Circulation* 81:1594, 1990.

196. Buck A, Wolpers HG, Hutchins GD, et al: Effect of carbon-11–acetate recirculation on estimates of myocardial oxygen consumption by PET. *J Nucl Med* 32:1950, 1991.

197. Bergmann SR, Weinheimer CJ, Brown MA, Perez JE: Enhancement of regional myocardial efficiency and persistence of perfusion, oxidative and functional reserve with paired pacing of stunned myocardium. *Circulation* 89:2290, 1994.

198. Wolpers HG, Buck A, Nguyen N, et al: An approach to ventricular efficiency by use of carbon 11–labeled acetate and positron emission tomography. *J Nucl Cardiol* 1:262, 1994.

199. Walsh MN, Geltman EM, Brown MA, et al: Noninvasive estimation of regional myocardial oxygen consumption by positron emission tomography with carbon-11 acetate in patients with myocardial infarction. *J Nucl Med* 30:1798, 1989.

200. Henes CG, Bergmann SR, Walsh MN, et al: Assessment of myocardial oxidative metabolic reserve with positron emission tomography and carbon-11 acetate. *J Nucl Med* 30:1489, 1989.

201. Armbrecht JJ, Buxton DB, Brunken RC, et al: Regional myocardial oxygen consumption determined noninvasively in humans with [1-^{11}C]acetate and dynamic positron tomography. *Circulation* 80:863, 1989.

202. Czernin J, Porenta G, Brunken R, et al: Regional blood flow, oxidative metabolism, and glucose utilization in patients with recent myocardial infarction. *Circulation* 88:884, 1993.

203. Hicks RJ, Melon P, Kalff V, et al: Metabolic imaging by positron emission tomography early after myocardial infarction as a predictor of recovery of myocardial function after reperfusion. *J Nucl Cardiol* 1:124, 1994.

204. Gropler RJ, Siegel BA, Geltman EM: Myocardial uptake of carbon-11–acetate as an indirect estimate of regional myocardial blood flow. *J Nucl Med* 32:245, 1991.

205. Chan SY, Brunken RC, Phelps ME, Schelbert HR: Use of the metabolic tracer carbon-11–acetate for evaluation of regional myocardial perfusion. *J Nucl Med* 32:665, 1991.

206. Krivokapich J: Assessment of myocardial amino acid and protein metabolism with the use of amino acids labeled with positron-emitting radionuclides, in Bergmann SR,

Sobel BE (eds): *Positron Emission Tomography of the Heart.* Mount Kisco, NY, Futura, 1992, pp 185–208.

207. Shelton ME, Dence CS, Hwang D-R, et al: Myocardial kinetics of fluorine-18 misonidazole: A marker of hypoxic myocardium. *J Nucl Med* 30:351, 1989.

208. Martin GV, Caldwell JH, Graham MM, et al: Noninvasive detection of hypoxic myocardium using fluorine-18–fluoromisonidazole and positron emission tomography. *J Nucl Med* 33:2202, 1992.

209. Syrota A: Cardiac receptors studied by positron emission tomography. *Acta Radiol* 374(Suppl):85, 1990.

210. Schwaiger M, Hutchins GD, Wieland DM: Noninvasive evaluation of the cardiac sympathetic nervous system with positron emission tomography, in Bergmann SR, Sobel BE (eds): *Positron Emission Tomography of the Heart.* Mount Kisco, NY, Futura, 1992, pp 231–254.

211. Yamashita K, Tamaki N, Yonekura Y, et al: Quantitative analysis of regional wall motion by gated myocardial positron emission tomography: Validation and comparison with left ventriculography. *J Nucl Med* 30:1775, 1989.

212. Miller TR, Wallis JW, Landy BR, et al: Measurement of global and regional left ventricular function by cardiac PET. *J Nucl Med* 35:999, 1994.

213. Bergmann SR: Positron emission tomography in cardiology: A clinical procedure, a research tool, or both? *Coronary Artery Dis* 3:439, 1992 (editorial).

214. Schwaiger M, Brunken R, Grover-McKay M, et al: Regional myocardial metabolism in patients with acute myocardial infarction assessed by positron emission tomography. *J Am Coll Cardiol* 8:800, 1986.

215. Marwick TH, MacIntyre WJ, Lafont A, et al: Metabolic responses of hibernating and infarcted myocardium to revascularization. *Circulation* 85:1347, 1992.

216. Lucignani G, Paolinin G, Landoni C, et al: Presurgical identification of hibernating myocardium by combined use of technetium-99m hexakis 2-methoxyisobutylisonitrile single photon emission tomography and fluorine-18 fluoro-2-deoxy-D-glucose positron emission tomography in patients with coronary artery disease. *Eur J Nucl Med* 19:874, 1992.

217. Graham MM, Lewellen TK: PET and its role in metabolic imaging. *Mayo Clin Proc* 64:725, 1989.

218. Ter-Pogossian MM: Instrumentation for cardiac positron emission tomography: Background and historical perspective, in Bergmann SR, Sobel BE (eds): *Positron Emission Tomography of the Heart.* Mount Kisco, NY, Futura, 1992, pp 2–12.

219. Herrero P, Bergmann SR: Assessment of myocardial perfusion with ^{15}O-water, in Schwaiger M (ed): *Cardiac Positron Emission Tomography.* Norwell, MA: Kluwer, 1996, pp. 147–160.

220. Schelbert HR, Schwaiger M: PET studies of the heart, in Phelps ME, Mazziotta JC, Schelbert HR (eds): *Positron Emission Tomography and Autoradiography.* New York, Raven, 1986, pp 581–661.

221. Schelbert HR: Current status and prospects of new radionuclides and radiopharamaceuticals for cardiovascular nuclear medicine. *Semin Nucl Med* 17:145, 1987.

BLOOD-POOL IMAGING

First-Pass Radionuclide Angiocardiography

Frans J. Th. Wackers

The technique of first-pass radionuclide angiocardiography involves the passage of a radionuclide bolus through the central circulation, which is then monitored by a gamma camera having high count rate capability.[1-6] This approach allows for assessment of cardiac function on the basis of only a few heartbeats and therefore is ideally suited to situations in which cardiac function is expected to change rapidly, as during exercise or acute interventions. Another practical aspect of first-pass studies is that the acquisition can be completed within a 30-s time interval and does not require major patient cooperation. For reliable assessment and calculation of right and left ventricular ejection fractions by this technique, equipment with high count rate capability is a first requirement. Until recently, only the multicrystal camera could provide such count density. However, a new generation of single-crystal gamma cameras has been developed that approaches the count rate capability of the multicrystal gamma camera. Therefore, it is conceivable that in the future the decision whether or not to perform first-pass radionuclide angiocardiography will be determined more by the specific clinical problem to be addressed than by the availability of particular equipment. We anticipate that first-pass radionuclide angiography will be more widely used with further development of gamma cameras and new radiopharmaceuticals.

CONCEPT OF FIRST-PASS RADIONUCLIDE ANGIOCARDIOGRAPHY

In first-pass radionuclide angiocardiography, a radioactive bolus is injected rapidly in a peripheral arm vein

and a time–activity curve generated over a precordial region of interest. Assessment of right and left ventricular function is possible since there is temporal separation of right and left ventricular phases on the time–activity curve[7] (Figs. 10-1 and 10-2). This temporal separation is essential for data analysis and depends to an important extent on adequate injection technique. For assessment of cardiac function, it is assumed that homogeneous mixing of the radioactive tracer within the blood has occurred and that changes in count rate are therefore proportional to changes in volume of the cardiac chambers during contraction. This assumption of complete mixing is probably correct for the left ventricle; however, for the right ventricle, streaming of the bolus can occasionally be a problem. Nevertheless, reliable and reproducible clinical results have been obtained also for right ventricular ejection fraction.[8-10]

ADMINISTRATION OF THE RADIONUCLIDE

In most cardiovascular nuclear laboratories, a peripheral antecubital arm vein is considered to be appropriate for first-pass studies, although some investigators prefer and routinely use an external jugular vein. In our laboratory, we found an antecubital vein injection adequate in most instances. The patient, in either a supine or upright position in front of the gamma camera, is injected in either the right anterior oblique or the anterior position. Although other views are possible, we believe that the anterior position is preferred because it brings the heart closest to the detector, thereby maximizing photon detection. In addition, this position is the easiest to use during

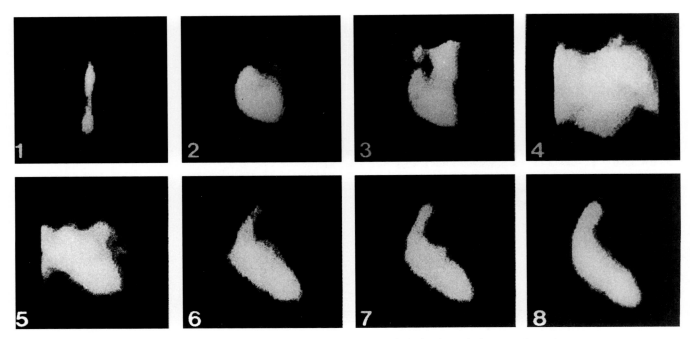

Figure 10-1 Flow study of the first transit of a radionuclide bolus through the central circulation. Note the temporal separation of right (*frame 3*) and left (*frame 7*) ventricular phases. (From Berger et al,[7] reproduced with permission.)

upright bicycle exercise. If serial studies are performed, it is important that this position be duplicated.

The quality of the first-pass time–activity curve depends to a large extent on the quality of the injection. A very tight bolus, i.e., less than 2 s in duration, is absolutely necessary for shunt detection.[11] Although a tight bolus is also required for assessment of right and left ventricular ejection fractions, it is more important that the radionuclide be injected smoothly and that it arrive in the central circulation as a single *front*.[12]

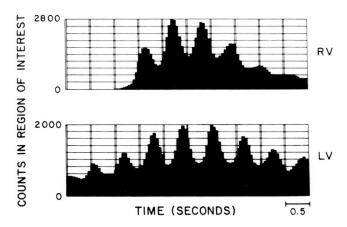

Figure 10-2 Right ventricular (RV) and left ventricular (LV) time–activity curves. Note the temporal separation of RV and LV phases. Each high-frequency oscillation in the time–activity curve corresponds to one cardiac cycle. The *peaks* (maximal counts) and *valleys* (minimal counts) represent diastole and systole, respectively. (From Berger et al,[7] reproduced with permission.)

For the injection, usually a 19- or 20-gauge ½-inch indwelling polyethylene catheter is inserted in the arm vein. Subsequently, the catheter is attached to an extension tube of approximately 3 ml with a three-way stopcock attached to one end. The tube is filled with normal saline, and a radioactive bolus of less than 1 mL in volume is introduced into the tubing, with 0.1 mL of air bubbles on either side of it. The radioactive bolus is actually administered by flushing this tubing system very rapidly with at least 10 mL of normal saline. This injection should be smooth and continuous so as to avoid a broken bolus. It is important to inject the radioactive bolus into a large antecubital vein and not a more distal, smaller vein, which would result in a fractionated bolus. For this reason, the Oldendorf technique is not recommended as an alternative means of bolus injection. Quality control of the injection technique can be achieved quantitatively by analysis of a time–activity curve over the superior caval vein or by visual inspection of serial images of the cardiac flow study. A broken bolus can be detected as the arrival of two waves of radioactivity in the central circulation.

TECHNETIUM 99m

The conventional radionuclide employed for first-pass studies is technetium 99m (^{99m}Tc). If only one assessment of left ventricular function is required, ^{99m}Tc pertechnetate is used. If multiple studies are to be performed, other ^{99m}Tc-labeled compounds may be used to reduce residual background activity. For example, when two sequential studies are performed, as at rest and during exercise, the injection at rest usually is done with ^{99m}Tc diethylene triamine pentaacetic acid (DTPA), which is cleared rapidly by the kidneys and allows a repeat injection of ^{99m}Tc pertechnetate 20 min later during peak exercise. It is possible to combine a first-pass study with an equilibrium study. For this purpose, the patient is given stannous pyrophosphate prior to the second injection of free ^{99m}Tc pertechnetate. Usually 10 to 25 mCi of ^{99m}Tc is used for each injection, and since the total daily dose should not exceed 30 mCi for an adult, a maximum of three injections (each of 10 mCi) can be given using ^{99m}Tc. The total body and target organ radiation exposure from ^{99m}Tc is within accepted limits based on known dosimetry.

Recently, new ^{99m}Tc-labeled myocardial perfusion agents have been developed. Because of the higher dose (20 to 25 mCi) that can be administered in comparison to thallium 201, injection during peak exercise can be utilized for first-pass radionuclide angiocardiography. This modality will make it truly feasible to evaluate myocardial perfusion and function during one exercise session (Fig. 10-3).[13,14]

SHORT-LIVED RADIOISOTOPES

The relatively long half-life (6 h) of ^{99m}Tc and the patient's dosimetry considerations limit the total number of first-pass studies that can be performed in sequence, as well as the dose per study. Recently, short-lived radioisotopes have been proposed for first-pass angiocardiography. Tantalum 178 (half-life, 9.3 min) has been proposed as a generator-produced short-lived radionuclide.[15] Using a single-crystal gamma camera, however, the initial clinical results have been disappointing because of the low energy of major photon emissions (x-rays at 55 to 65 keV) and the substantial background activity resulting from high energy 500-keV photon emissions. More promising results have been reported with the use

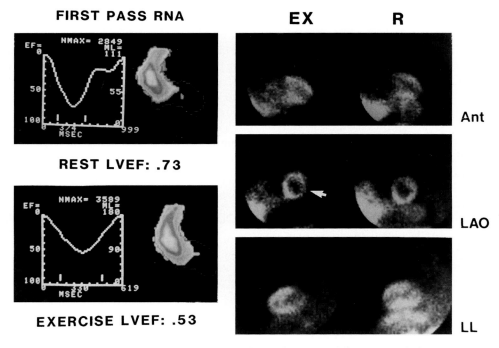

FIRST PASS RNA

REST LVEF: .73

EXERCISE LVEF: .53

EX   R

Ant

LAO

LL

Figure 10-3 First-pass radionuclide angiocardiography (RNA) (*left*) at rest and during exercise, and myocardial perfusion imaging (*right*) at rest (R) and after exercise (EX) using ^{99m}Tc sestamibi. Resting left ventricular ejection fraction (LVEF) was obtained by a rapid bolus injection of ^{99m}Tc DTPA. Peak exercise LVEF was obtained by injection of 20 mCi of ^{99m}Tc sestamibi. Exercise myocardial perfusion imaging was performed 1 h later. The resting myocardial perfusion images were obtained 24 h later after a repeat injection of 20 mCi ^{99m}Tc sestamibi. Thus, one dose of ^{99m}Tc sestamibi provided peak exercise LVEF as well as images of myocardial perfusion at peak exercise. Resting LVEF and myocardial perfusion were normal. During exercise, however, LVEF decreased, an abnormal LVEF response. The myocardial perfusion images showed evidence of exercise-induced ischemia in the inferolateral wall (*arrow*). (From Wackers et al,[14] reproduced with permission.)

of a multiwire proportional gamma camera, which operates extremely well with low energy photons.[16] Another ultra-short-lived generator-produced radionuclide that has been proposed is iridium 191m.[17] This tracer has optimal photon energy (129 keV). Because of its short half-life of 4.9 s, initial clinical results have been reported in pediatric patients. Although it was felt that the half-life would be too short for use in adults, recent reports have demonstrated its feasibility for performing first-pass angiocardiography in the adult population.

We have investigated the use of gold 195m (^{195m}Au).[18,19] Its half-life of 30.5 s appears to be ideally suited for application in adults. In normal adult subjects, radioactivity reaches the left heart chamber within approximately 10 to 15 s after a rapid bolus injection into the basilic vein. This interval may be considerably longer in seriously ill cardiac patients but rarely exceeds 25 s. The half-life of the parent mercury 195m is long enough (41.6 h) to allow shipment of the generator to relatively remote places. The yield of this generator is approximately 40 percent, and adequate dosage (15 to 30 mCi) of ^{195m}Au can be obtained per elution. The initial results with first-pass studies using ^{195m}Au have been extremely satisfactory. The quality of images and the count rate statistics are comparable to an equivalent dose of ^{99m}Tc. The advantages of the use of ^{195m}Au are as follows:

1. There is considerably reduced patient radiation dose per injection compared with ^{99m}Tc: 20 times less to the whole body and 5 times less to the target organ, the kidneys.
2. The short-lived radionuclide allows for a more extensive analysis of ventricular function in patients with coronary artery disease. Instead of evaluating ejection fraction only at baseline and at peak exercise, ^{195m}Au allows for rapid serial assessments of left ventricular function at the intermediate stages of exercise (Fig. 10-4). The pattern of left ventricular dysfunction during exercise may be of relevance for management of these patients.
3. Probably a more important practical application is the possibility of combining assessment of cardiac function with evaluation of myocardial perfusion[20] (Fig. 10-5).

By performing these studies simultaneously, this approach may provide a means of assessing more reliably the functional significance of coronary artery stenosis. This combined technique also has obvious advantages as far as the cost effectiveness of patient evaluation is concerned, since only one exercise test is needed to obtain this information. Nevertheless, the role of the short-lived radioisotopes in first-pass radionuclide angiocardiography remains investigative at the time of writing.

MULTICRYSTAL AND SINGLE-CRYSTAL CAMERAS

Since reliable first-pass angiocardiography depends on accumulation of sufficient count density, only the multicrystal camera with a count rate capability of over 1,000,000 cps was, until recently, well suited for this imaging technique. As mentioned above, conventional single-crystal cameras were limited in count rate capability (maximal 60,000 cps) for acquiring sufficient counts for first-pass studies. However, newer-generation digital single-crystal cameras can acquire considerably higher count rates (up to 150,000 cps), which will allow adequate count density for first-pass studies.

DATA STORAGE

Depending on the scintillation camera and computer used, image data are usually stored in list mode or frame mode on a high speed magnetic disk. In general, studies at rest are obtained at 40- to 50-ms intervals to enable accurate analysis of the high-frequency components of the time–activity curve generated over the cardiac region. The optimal framing interval has been shown to be greatly dependent on heart rate. At resting heart rates, the framing rates noted above are adequate. However, at increased heart rates, as during exercise, higher framing rates (10- to 30-ms intervals) are needed. It is important to realize that although improved temporal resolution is achieved with progressive decrease of the frame interval, counts per frame and hence the statistical reliability decrease.

COUNTING STATISTICS AND EJECTION FRACTION

The calculation of ejection fraction is affected by counting statistics, i.e., absolute counts obtained in end diastole and end systole. The statistical error is related to the value of ejection fraction.[21] The lower the counts and the lower the ventricular ejection fraction, the greater the potential statistical error. For a background-corrected end-diastolic count rate of 100 counts per frame, an ejection fraction of 50 percent would have a propagated error of $\pm$ 14 percent. In contrast, for a count rate of 1000 counts per frame, the same ejection fraction would have an error of 5 percent. These two count densities are in the range of those routinely encountered for a single beat with single-crystal and multicrystal cameras, respectively. The *representative* cardiac cycle on first-pass studies using a multicrystal camera typically has

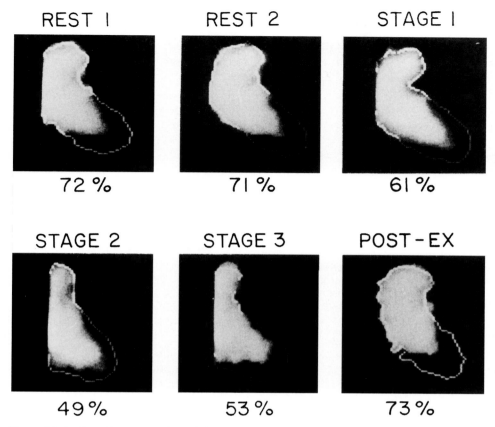

Figure 10-4 Serial first-pass radionuclide angiocardiography with ^{195m}Au. The end-systolic images are superimposed over the end-diastolic perimeter. Images are obtained at rest, at the end of each stage of exercise, and within 1 min of termination of exercise. Calculated left ventricular ejection fraction is displayed below each image. (From Wackers et al,[19] reproduced with permission.)

a background-corrected end-diastolic count density of approximately 5000 counts per frame. The statistical error with this count density is in the range of 2 percent. This count rate and statistical error are comparable to those obtained with equilibrium radionuclide angiocardiography.

Table 10-1 shows the percentage error in ejection fraction for different values of ejection fraction and end-diastolic counts. If the statistical error is to be kept within 3 percent in a patient with 80 percent ejection fraction, at least 2000 background-corrected counts should be present in end diastole. For the same statistical reliability in a patient with a 30 percent ejection fraction, 30,000 counts are required (Fig. 10-6). Fortunately, most patients with low ejection fraction have large, dilated ventricles and, therefore, satisfactory counting statistics are relatively easily obtained. The additional use of smoothing algorithms and root mean square analysis may reduce statistical errors and is particularly important for low count rate data obtained with the single-crystal gamma camera. Although the final statistical error for such studies can be decreased to an acceptable low level, the results

become dependent on the assumption imposed by the curve-fitting techniques employed.

QUANTITATIVE ANALYSIS OF FIRST-PASS DATA

Processing of a first-pass radionuclide study usually involves the following steps: (1) generation of an initial time–activity curve over the cardiac region, (2) identification of right and left ventricular phases, (3) generation of final time–activity curves over regions of interest corresponding to the left and right ventricles, (4) background subtraction, (5) generation of a representative cardiac cycle, and (6) calculation of left or right ventricular ejection fraction.

1. Analysis of the initial time–activity curve serves as a quality control (see p. 312) and permits inspection of the temporal separation of right and left ventricular phases, estimation of the peak count density achieved, and determination of the presence of irregular beats.

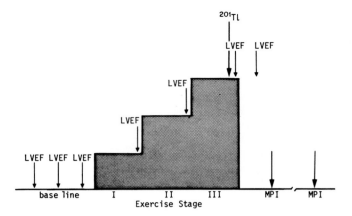

Figure 10-5 Protocol of combined [195m]Au and ^{201}Tl stress imaging. Serial left ventricular ejection fraction (LVEF) is determined at baseline and at the end of each 3-min stage of exercise. When the patient appears to approach the end point of exercise, ^{201}Tl is injected. The patient is encouraged to exercise at least 1 min more. At the very peak of exercise, LVEF is determined again, after which the patient stops exercising. Within 1 min of discontinuation of the stress test, LVEF determination is repeated. Subsequently, postexercise and delayed ^{201}Tl myocardial perfusion imaging (MPI) is performed. (From Wackers,[20] reproduced with permission.)

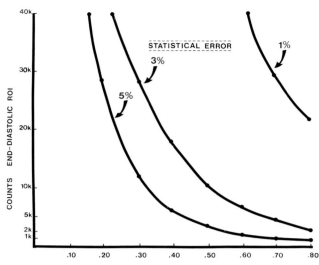

Figure 10-6 Effect of count density in the end-diastolic region of interest (ROI) over the left ventricle and statistical error in the calculation of ejection fraction. Considerably higher count density is required in patients with abnormal ventricular function than in patients with normal ventricular function for identical statistical reliability. Typical radionuclide angiocardiography studies are required with approximately 3 percent statistical error. (From Wackers,[21] reproduced with permission.)

2. The selection of the portion of the time–activity curve containing data of either the right or the left ventricular phase simplifies processing and focuses on only those frames that contain useful data. Moreover, overlapping structures (right or left ventricle) are excluded (Fig. 10-2).

3. Subsequently, the processing focuses on the image of the ventricle under study. For the left ventricle, a fixed region of interest corresponding to the end-diastolic image of the left ventricle is chosen using, for example, color-coded isocount images to standardize definition of

Table 10-1   Percentage Statistical Error in Ejection Fraction for Different Ejection Fractions and End-Diastolic Counts

End-Diastolic Counts	Ejection Fraction						
	.20	.30	.40	.50	.60	.70	.80
100	88	54	38	28	22	18	15
200	62	38	27	20	16	12	10
500	39	24	17	13	10	8	6.5
800	31	19	13	10	8	6	5
1,000	28	17	12	9	7	5.5	4.5
2,000	20	12	9	6	5	4	3
5,000	12	8	6	4	3	2.5	2
8,000	10	6	5	3.5	2.5	2	1.6
10,000	9	5	4	3	2	1.5	1.5
20,000	6	4	3	2	1.5	1	1
30,000	5	3	2	1.5	1	1	0.8

From Wackers,[20] reproduced with permission.

the region of interest. A most critical aspect of identifying the left ventricular region of interest is appropriate exclusion of the proximal aorta. For the right ventricle, the stroke-volume image (derived by subtraction of the end-systolic image from the end-diastolic image) is used to define a fixed region of interest. With the use of this method, identification of the tricuspid and pulmonary valve planes is facilitated. Alternatively, a varying region of interest can be used in end diastole and end systole when valve planes can be recognized with sufficient confidence.

4. Background subtraction for left ventricular function can be performed using several approaches. In our laboratory we select from the time–activity curve the frame immediately prior to the first recognizable left ventricular beat (Fig. 10-7). The image in this frame (background image) represents overlying and scattered radiation from the left atrium and lungs at a time when all the radionuclide is in these structures. This image is then subtracted from each of the subsequent frames that make up the left ventricular phase. An alternative approach involves placement of a horseshoe-shaped region of interest around the apex of the left ventricle, from which a time–activity curve is generated that is to be subtracted from the ventricular time–activity curve. A third method involves subtraction of a constant percentage based on average counts measured in a region of interest surrounding the left ventricle. It is important to realize that no method of background correction is perfect and that the purpose of any such method is to intro-

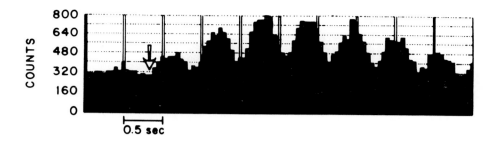

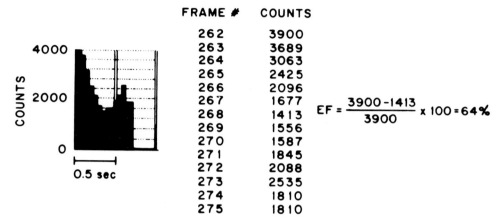

FRAME #	COUNTS
262	3900
263	3689
264	3063
265	2425
266	2096
267	1677
268	1413
269	1556
270	1587
271	1845
272	2088
273	2535
274	1810
275	1810

$$EF = \frac{3900 - 1413}{3900} \times 100 = 64\%$$

Figure 10-7 Time–activity curve and representative cycle used to calculate left ventricular ejection fraction (EF) in a normal patient. The time–activity curve is shown in the *top panel*, and EF calculation is in the *bottom panel*. The *arrow* in the time–activity curve indicates the frame of background selection. The counts in the representative cycle are the summed counts of four background-corrected beats. In this study, end-diastolic counts were 3900, end-systolic counts were 1413, and calculated EF was 64 percent. (From Marshall et al,[6] reproduced with permission of the American Heart Association, Inc.)

duce a correction factor so that the radionuclide ejection fraction correlates with the contrast-derived ejection fraction. Therefore, background correction should be well standardized and not arbitrarily varied. For example, for the method employed in our laboratory, the choice of the correct background frame is essential: if it is chosen too early, background activity is underestimated, resulting in a lower ejection fraction; when the frame is chosen too late, left ventricular ejection fraction may be overestimated because of erroneously increased background activity.

For calculation of right ventricular ejection fraction using a fixed region of interest, the generated time–activity curve has to be corrected for overlying right atrial activity. This has been done empirically by generating an atrial time–activity curve at the interface of the right atrium and right ventricle, which is then subtracted from the initial time–activity curve (Fig. 10-8). When a varying region of interest is employed, no background subtraction is usually necessary.[10]

5. Ventricular ejection fraction is determined from a *summed cardiac cycle*. On inspection of the time–activity curve during the ventricular phase, peaks and valleys are

discerned. The peaks represent end-diastolic counts (ED) and the valleys end-systolic counts (ES). Left ventricular ejection fraction is calculated from the background-corrected data:

$$\frac{ED - ES}{ED} \times 100$$

It is assumed that during peak left ventricular activity complete mixing of the blood in this chamber has occurred. During the earliest discernible ventricular contraction, not all radioactive blood has filled the chamber and, during the latest beats, most of the radioactive blood has already left the chamber. Only beats around the peak of the time–activity curve (i.e., those with 80 percent or more of maximal activity) are therefore used for data analysis. According to these criteria, usually one or two beats during the right ventricular phase and four to five beats during the left ventricular phase are available for analysis (Figs. 10-7 and 10-8). As mentioned above, the overall statistical accuracy of the calculated ejection fraction can be increased by averaging several individual beats by forming a so-called summed representative cy-

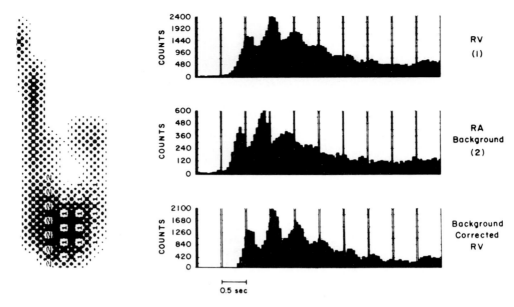

Figure 10-8 Right ventricular (RV) image (*left*) and RV and right atrial (RA) and background-corrected time–activity curves (*right*). The numerals "1" represent the RV region of interest, and the numerals "2" represent the standardized background zone. Note that peak RV activity (*right*) occurs when RA activity is lowest. The background-corrected RV time–activity curve was obtained by subtracting the RA curve from the RV curve. (From Berger et al,[8] reproduced with permission.)

cle. Although the count density on studies acquired with a multicrystal camera is relatively high, the "summing" of peaks and valleys by visual inspection of the time–activity curve may not be entirely correct because of statistical noise in the count data. By simultaneously recording the electrocardiographic (ECG) signal (*gated first pass*), improved superimposition of identical phases of the cardiac cycle may be achieved.

VALIDATION OF FIRST-PASS TECHNIQUE

Numerous studies have demonstrated good agreement between left ventricular ejection fraction measured by first-pass radionuclide angiocardiography and by contrast angiocardiography.[6,22–27] First-pass data also correlate closely with ejection fractions obtained by equilibrium radionuclide angiocardiography (Fig. 10-9).[22,23] The variation resulting from reprocessing the same study and restudying the same patient on different occasions has been shown to be well within an acceptable range.[3,6,22,28] First-pass right ventricular ejection fraction has been validated against cine-magnetic resonance imaging.[10]

REGIONAL WALL MOTION

Left ventricular regional wall motion can be evaluated from first-pass studies. However, since these studies are

usually performed in only one view, the extent of wall motion that can be analyzed is limited. Again, statistical considerations play dominant roles in determining the adequacy of the first-pass data for assessment of regional

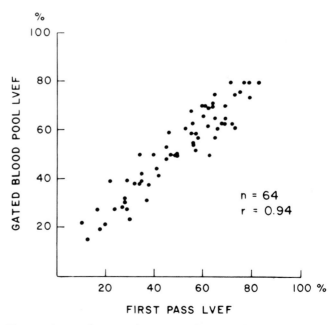

Figure 10-9 Left ventricular ejection fraction (LVEF) obtained in 64 patients initially by first-pass technique and then by equilibrium radionuclide angiocardiography. An excellent correlation exists between the two methods over a wide range of LVEF. (From Wackers et al,[22] reproduced with permission.)

REST

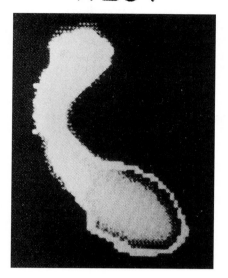

EXERCISE

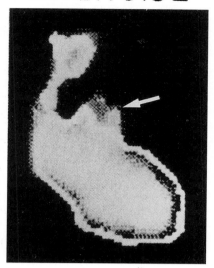

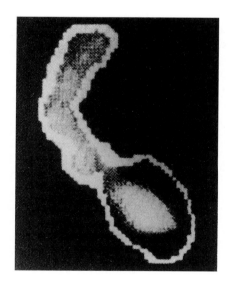

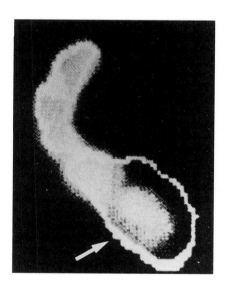

Figure 10-10 Regional wall-motion studies by first-pass angio-cardiography at rest and exercise in two patients with coronary artery disease. *Top:* At rest, diffuse hypokinesis is present; during exercise, the left ventricle dilates and mitral regurgitation becomes evident (*arrow*). *Bottom:* At rest, the left ventricle is normal in size and contraction; during exercise, inferior hypokinesis is apparent (*arrow*). Left ventricular ejection fraction decreased during exercise in both patients. (From Berger et al,[7] reproduced with permission.)

wall motion. Images of relatively high count rate density are available from the summed representative cycle obtained with the multicrystal camera. The regional wall motion can be analyzed in a number of different ways. The end-diastolic outline can be superimposed on the end-systolic image, which will visualize local contraction abnormalities (Fig. 10-10).[6,27] It is also possible to view all frames from the representative cycle as an endless-loop movie, similar to the method employed for viewing equilibrium radionuclide studies. Quantitative analysis can be carried out by measuring chord shortening, simi-

lar to that used in contrast angiography.[25,26] In addition, functional images can be generated based on count differences between end diastole and end systole.[29] For example, regional ejection-fraction images display the relative contribution of different regions to total left ventricular ejection fraction and allow detection of diminished motion in nontangential wall segments.[30] Each of these radionuclide approaches has been shown to agree closely with contrast angiocardiographic assessment of wall motion. However, detailed evaluation of wall motion, especially in patients with coronary artery disease, should be carried out in more than one position. This is presently more easily achieved by the equilibrium technique than by the first-pass technique. However, future use of short-lived radioisotopes will enable serial and multiple-view studies employing first-pass angiocardiography.

POTENTIAL PROBLEMS WITH ASSESSMENT OF RIGHT VENTRICULAR FUNCTION

There are theoretical considerations that make the right ventricle a less than ideal chamber for analysis by first-pass technique. It is conceivable that in some patients the radionuclide bolus does not completely mix with blood before entering the right ventricle. Mixing has to take place in the right atrium, which is relatively close to the injection site, and the passive flow of blood from right atrium to right ventricle may limit adequate mixing. Moreover, there can be streaming in the right ventricle, i.e., the blood enters and leaves the ventricle via the shortest route without mixing with blood in the apex. One of the disadvantages of right ventricular first-pass studies is that these two potential sources of error are difficult to control or even to recognize. For these reasons, it is useful to check the morphology and contraction pattern of the right ventricle by equilibrium radionuclide angiocardiography for each patient. Streaming can occur in a variety of conditions: hyperdynamic state, severely impaired regional right ventricular function, and left-to-right shunt by ventricular septal defect. In spite of these considerations, ample clinical experience has shown the feasibility and usefulness of the assessment of right ventricular function by first-pass angiocardiography.[7,9,10]

QUALITY CONTROL

Patient Positioning

In first-pass angiocardiography, the patient must be positioned in front of the camera before any radionuclide is injected. In patients with enlarged hearts, it is conceivable that portions of the chambers will be "cut off" and not in the field of view, which will make it impossible to determine the ejection fraction accurately. The patient's optimum position can be determined easily from a transmission scan with a cobalt-57 flood. By holding the source behind the patient's back, a negative image of the heart is acquired and appropriate adjustments in position can be made.

Quality of Injection

A first important quality control of a first-pass study consists of analysis of the radionuclide bolus. This can be done by generating a time–activity curve over the superior caval vein or, as mentioned above, by visual inspection of the flow of the radionuclide as it enters the central circulation (see Fig. 10-1). A broken bolus will be detected in this analysis. Of the two parameters, a broken bolus is far more damaging to the quality of the study than is a slightly spread out bolus.

Counts

Counts are essential for the statistical reliability of the study. In a typical first-pass study, a peak count density in the right ventricular phase (without background correction) should be at least 3000 to 4000 counts per 50-ms frame, whereas the peak counts during the left ventricular phase (without background correction) should be around 1000 counts per 50-ms frame.

Inspection of the Time–Activity Curve

Ventricular arrhythmias can render a first-pass study useless for the calculation of ejection fraction. If possible, one should exclude premature beats and postpremature beats from analysis. However, since only a limited number of beats with adequate count density are available for analysis during the left ventricular phase and even fewer beats during the right ventricular phase, premature beats prove to be a serious limitation of this technique. An extreme example of irregular rhythm is offered by the patient with atrial fibrillation. In this situation, one can either analyze the beats with the lowest and the highest ejection fractions, to assess the range of contraction, or calculate the average of all beats. If numerous irregular beats are present, analysis may be impossible and equilibrium radionuclide angiocardiography is the preferred method. The latter technique offers several options for dealing with the effect of arrhythmia (see Chap. 11).

As mentioned above, the time–activity curve should also be inspected for adequate temporal separation of the right and left ventricular phases. In cases of poor temporal separation, background activity is overestimated and the value for left ventricular ejection fraction will be erroneously high.

Regions of Interest

The regions of interest should be defined with good understanding of the cardiac anatomy. Most errors are made in identification of the valve planes. The generation of functional images can be extremely helpful in recognizing these anatomic landmarks.

FUTURE DIRECTIONS FOR FIRST-PASS ANGIOCARDIOGRAPHY

Assessment of right and left ventricular function at rest or during exercise has been shown to have a major impact on clinical decision making and patient management.[27] First-pass radionuclide angiocardiography offers a distinct advantage over exercise equilibrium radionuclide angiocardiography. Because data are acquired over a short time period, utilizing only three to five cardiac cycles, it is likely that they approximate true left ventricular function during peak exercise more closely than data acquired over several hundreds of heartbeats, as is done in equilibrium radionuclide angiocardiography. Unavoidable body motion during exercise has a major degrading effect on the quality of exercise equilibrium studies, which is reflected in poor reproducibility of data processing. It can be expected that with further improvement of the count rate capability of gamma cameras, it will be possible to acquire reliable first-pass studies on most commercially available equipment.[31] In addition, short-lived radionuclides would make it feasible to perform many repeat injections. The latter imaging agents potentially can be used in combination with myocardial perfusion imaging agents, such as thallium 201.[20] Other unexplored territories for first-pass radionuclide angiocardiography are, for example, the cardiothoracic intensive care unit or operating room, where prolonged imaging would interfere with patient care. Rapidly performed serial first-pass studies could provide extremely useful clinical and pathophysiologic information in these settings.

Combined Assessment of Perfusion and Function

In recent years, a number of ^{99m}Tc-labeled myocardial perfusion imaging agents have been introduced for clinical imaging. Because of the relatively high dose (10 to 30 mCi) of radioactivity that can be administered, combined assessment of myocardial perfusion and myocardial function has become feasible. Present state-of-the-art single-crystal gamma cameras have sufficiently high count sensitivity to enable reliable first-pass angiocardiography, in particular when data are acquired in list mode with ECG gating. Thus, a rest injection of a ^{99m}Tc-labeled myocardial perfusion imaging agent can be used readily for simultaneous assessment of resting left ventricular

ejection fraction. However, since exercise is best performed on upright bicycle or treadmill, and since single-crystal SPECT (single photon emission computed tomography) cameras generally are designed for imaging with patients in the supine position, the multicrystal gamma camera remains the equipment of choice for exercise first-pass angiocardiography. Several investigators have demonstrated the feasibility of this combined approach.[32,33] Palmas et al[34] recently showed that combined assessment of myocardial perfusion and first-pass ventricular function yields incremental diagnostic value over that of myocardial perfusion imaging alone. Thus, first-pass angiocardiography has become extremely promising as a complementary noninvasive diagnostic modality for efficient and complete evaluation of patients with suspected coronary artery disease.

REFERENCES

1. Van Dyke D, Anger HO, Sullivan RW, et al: Cardiac evaluation from radioisotope dynamics. *J Nucl Med* 13:585, 1972.
2. Weber PM, dos Remedios LV, Jasko IA: Quantitative radioisotopic angiocardiography. *J Nucl Med* 13:815, 1972.
3. Schelbert HR, Verba JW, Johnson AD, et al: Nontraumatic determination of left ventricular ejection fraction by radionuclide angiocardiography. *Circulation* 51:902, 1975.
4. Steele PP, Kirch D, Matthews M, et al: Measurement of left heart ejection fraction and end-diastolic volume by a computerized, scintigraphic technique using a wedged pulmonary arterial catheter. *Am J Cardiol* 34:179, 1974.
5. Steele P, Van Dyke D, Trow RS, et al: Simple and safe bedside method for serial measurement of left ventricular ejection fraction, cardiac output, and pulmonary blood volume. *Br Heart J* 36:122, 1974.
6. Marshall RC, Berger HJ, Costin JC, et al: Assessment of cardiac performance with quantitative radionuclide angiocardiography: Sequential left ventricular ejection fraction, normalized left ventricular ejection rate, and regional wall motion. *Circulation* 56:820, 1977.
7. Berger HJ, Matthay RA, Pytlik LM, et al: First-pass radionuclide assessment of right and left ventricular performance in patients with cardiac and pulmonary disease. *Semin Nucl Med* 9:275, 1979.
8. Berger HJ, Matthay RA, Loke J, et al: Assessment of cardiac performance with quantitative radionuclide angiocardiography: Right ventricular ejection fraction with reference to findings in chronic obstructive pulmonary disease. *Am J Cardiol* 41:897, 1978.
9. Tobinick E, Schelbert HR, Henning H, et al: Right ventricular ejection fraction in patients with acute inferior and anterior myocardial infarction assessed by radionuclide angiography. *Circulation* 57:1078, 1978.
10. Johnson LL, Lawson MA, Blackwell GG, et al: Optimizing the method to calculate right ventricular ejection fraction

from first-pass data acquired with a multicrystal camera. *J Nucl Cardiol* 2:372, 1995.

11. Maltz DL, Treves S: Quantitative radionuclide angiocardiography: Determination of Qp:Qs in children. *Circulation* 47:1049, 1973.

12. Dymond DS, Elliott A, Stone D, et al: Factors that affect the reproducibility of measurements of left ventricular function from first-pass radionuclide ventriculograms. *Circulation* 65:311, 1982.

13. Baillet GY, Mena IG, Kuperus JH, et al: Simultaneous technetium-99m MIBI angiography and myocardial perfusion imaging. *J Nucl Med* 30:38, 1989.

14. Wackers FJ: New horizons for myocardial perfusion imaging with technetium-99m-labeled isonitriles, in Pohost GM, Higgins CB, Nanda NC, et al (eds): *New Concepts in Cardiac Imaging 1989*. Chicago, Year Book Medical, 1989, pp 93–108.

15. Holman BL, Neirinckx RD, Treves S, Tow DE: Cardiac imaging with tantalum-178. *Radiology* 131:525, 1979.

16. Lacy JL, Verani MS, Ball ME, et al: First-pass radionuclide angiography using a multiwire gamma camera and tantalum-178. *J Nucl Med* 29:293, 1988.

17. Treves S, Cheng C, Samuel A, et al: Iridium-191 angiocardiography for the detection and quantitation of left-to-right shunting. *J Nucl Med* 21:1151, 1980.

18. Wackers FJTh, Giles RW, Hoffer PB, et al: Gold-195m, a new generator-produced short-lived radionuclide for sequential assessment of ventricular performance by first pass radionuclide angiocardiography. *Am J Cardiol* 50:89, 1982.

19. Wackers FJTh, Stein R, Pytlik L, et al: Gold-195m for serial first pass radionuclide angiocardiography during upright exercise in patients with coronary artery disease. *J Am Coll Cardiol* 2:497, 1983.

20. Wackers FJ: Characteristics of radiopharmaceuticals in nuclear cardiology: Implications for practical cardiac imaging, in Simoons ML, Reiber JHC (eds): *Nuclear Imaging in Clinical Cardiology*. The Hague, Martinus Nijhoff, 1984, pp 19–37.

21. Wackers FJ: Radionuclide techniques for assessment of cardiac function in man, in Linden RJ (ed): *Techniques in Cardiovascular Physiology. II. Techniques in Life Sciences*. Shannon, Elsevier Ireland, 1984, P320, pp 1–26.

22. Wackers FJTh, Berger HJ, Johnstone DE, et al: Multiple gated cardiac blood pool imaging for left ventricular ejection fraction: Validation of the technique and assessment of variability. *Am J Cardiol* 43:1159, 1979.

23. Folland ED, Hamilton GW, Larson SM, et al: The radionuclide ejection fraction: A comparison of three radionuclide techniques with contrast angiography. *J Nucl Med* 18:1159, 1977.

24. Ashburn WL, Schelbert HR, Verba JW: Left ventricular ejection fraction: A review of several radionuclide angiographic approaches using the scintillation camera. *Prog Cardiovasc Dis* 20:267, 1978.

25. Hecht HS, Mirell SG, Rolett EL, et al: Left ventricular ejection fraction and segmental wall motion by peripheral first pass radionuclide angiography. *J Nucl Med* 19:17, 1978.

26. Bodenheimer MM, Banka VS, Fooshee CM, et al: Quantitative radionuclide angiography in the right anterior oblique view: Comparison with contrast ventriculography. *Am J Cardiol* 41:718, 1978.

27. Rerych SK, Scholz PM, Newman GE, et al: Cardiac function at rest and during exercise in normals and in patients with coronary heart disease. *Ann Surg* 187:449, 1978.

28. Marshall RC, Berger HJ, Reduto LA, et al: Variability in sequential measures of left ventricular performance assessed with radionuclide angiocardiography. *Am J Cardiol* 41:531, 1978.

29. Schad N: Nontraumatic assessment of left ventricular wall motion and regional stroke volume after myocardial infarction. *J Nucl Med* 18:333, 1977.

30. Bodenheimer MM, Banka VS, Fooshee CM, et al: Comparison of wall motion and regional ejection fraction at rest and during isometric exercise: Concise communication. *J Nucl Med* 20:724, 1979.

31. Nichols K, DePuey EG, Gooneratne N, et al: First-pass ventricular ejection fraction using a single-crystal nuclear camera. *J Nucl Med* 35:1292, 1994.

32. Villanueva-Meyer J, Mena I, Narahara KA: Simultaneous assessment of left ventricular wall motion and myocardial perfusion with technetium-99m–methoxy isobutyl isonitrile at stress and rest in patients with angina: Comparison with thallium-201 SPECT. *J Nucl Med* 31:457, 1990.

33. Williams KA, Taillon LA, Draho JM, Foisy MF: First-pass radionuclide angiographic studies of left ventricular function with technetium-99m–teboroxime, technetium-99m–sestamibi and technetium-99m–DTPA. *J Nucl Med* 34:394, 1993.

34. Palmas W, Friedman JD, Diamond GA, et al: Incremental value of simultaneous assessment of myocardial function and perfusion with technetium-99m sestamibi for prediction of extent of coronary artery disease. *J Am Coll Cardiol* 25:1024, 1995.

Equilibrium Radionuclide Angiocardiography

Frans J. Th. Wackers

Equilibrium radionuclide angiocardiography (ERNA), also known as radionuclide ventriculography (RVG) or gated blood pool imaging, was developed in the mid 1970s as a radionuclide-imaging technique to evaluate cardiac function using conventional single crystal gamma cameras.[1] The methodology depends on three components: (1) stable radionuclide labeling of the intravascular blood pool; (2) electrocardiographic (ECG) gating of the gamma camera/computer system; and (3) computer processing of digitized radionuclide-imaging data. Until the late 1980s ERNA was ubiquitously used as a noninvasive means to assess cardiac function. In recent years, in many institutions two-dimensional echocardiography has taken over this role. This is an unfortunate shift in use of technology because radionuclide angiography has been demonstrated to be the most accurate and most reproducible method to assess noninvasively right and left ventricular function.

BLOOD POOL LABELING

The purpose of blood pool labeling is to retain a radiotracer within the intravascular space. This was initially successfully achieved by binding ^{99m}Tc pertechnetate to human serum albumin (HSA).[1-3] However, this labeling method has been abandoned because the radiolabel is relatively unstable. Adequate quality blood pool imaging

using ^{99m}Tc-HSA was feasible for only a limited period of time. Presently three efficient methods exist to label the patient's own red blood cells (RBCs) with ^{99m}Tc pertechnetate: the in vivo labeling method, the modified in vivo labeling method, and the in vitro labeling method.

In vivo labeling The most commonly used method is the in vivo labeling method.[4] Cold (nonradiolabeled) stannous pyrophosphate (2 to 3 mg) is injected intravenously. The tin (i.e., stannous) diffuses passively through the RBC membrane. After a 10-to-30-min interval 20 to 30 mCi (740 to 1110 MBq, or 10 to 13 MBq/kg body weight)[5] ^{99m}TcO$_4$- (pertechnetate) is injected intravenously. Negatively charged ^{99m}Tc pertechnetate enters RBCs actively through the band-3 anion transport system and is reduced by the positively charged tin and binds to the beta chain of hemoglobin.[6,7] This relatively stable binding retains ^{99m}Tc pertechnetate within the RBCs for hours. We have been able to perform adequate quality clinical ERNA imaging for up to 8 h after labeling. This in vivo labeling method yields in general acceptable labeling efficiency of the RBCs in most patients (85 to 95 percent).

Modified in vivo labeling Labeling efficiency can be further improved using the modified in vivo technique.[8] The patient is again injected with cold stannous pyrophosphate similar to the in vivo method. After 10 to 30 min, 3.0 ml blood is withdrawn into a syringe that contains 25 to 30 mCi ^{99m}Tc pertechnetate. To prevent

Table 11-1 Causes of Poor Red Blood Cell Labeling

Cause	Mechanism
Hydralazine	Oxidation of stannous ion
Prazosin	Decreases labeling rate
Propranolol	Increases dissociation
Digoxin	Decreases labeling rate
Doxorubicin	?
Iodinated contrast	?
Heparin	Complexes with ^{99m}Tc Oxidation of stannous ion
Dextrose	Complexes with ^{99m}Tc
Methyldopa	Induces RBC antibodies Oxidation of stannous ion
Penicillin	Induces RBC antibodies
Quinidine	Induces RBC antibodies
Immune disorders	Induces RBC antibodies
Prolonged generator ingrowth	Increased carrier
Decreased hematocrit	Relative increase in plasma which oxidizes stannous ion (?)
Excess stannous ion	^{99m}Tc reduced outside the RBC
Insufficient stannous ion	Incomplete reduction with free ^{99m}Tc pertechnetate

(From Parker DA, et al. Gerson's *Cardiac Nuclear Medicine*, 2nd ed., reproduced with permission.)

clotting, 0.5 ml acid–citrate-dextrose (ACD) is drawn into the syringe. Heparin is not used because it reduces RBC labeling efficiency.[9] Stannous-primed blood is incubated within the syringe for approximately 20 min and is then reinjected into the patient. Using this method, labeling efficiency is consistently higher then 90 percent.

In vitro labeling For the in vitro labeling method RBC labeling is performed in a sterile kit (Ultratag®).[10–12] Using a large-bore needle 1.0 to 3.0 ml blood is collected using ACD as anticoagulant. The whole blood is transferred to a 10-ml closed-system sterile kit lyophilized reaction vial containing 50 μg stannous chloride dihydrate. After 5 min of incubation, 0.6 ml 0.1% sodium hypochlorite solution is added and mixed. Subsequently, after adding 1.0 ml ACD, 30 to 35 mCi ^{99m}Tc is added. A dose of 25 to 30 mCi ^{99m}Tc-labeled RBCs is then withdrawn and reinjected into the patient. Labeling efficiency has been reported to be greater than 98 percent.

Causes for poor ^{99m}Tc labeling efficiency A number of frequently used drugs and solutions interfere with RBC labeling[13–16] (Table 11-1). Because heparin unfavorably affects labeling efficiency,[9] if at all possible, ^{99m}Tc pertechnetate should not be injected in heparinized intravenous lines, or the lines should be flushed thoroughly. Similarly,

intravenous lines containing dextrose solution may alter labeling efficiency. In addition antibodies against RBC may inhibit labeling.[17] Antibodies may develop secondary to drugs such as methyldopa and penicillin. Antibodies may also be present in patients with chronic lymphocytic leukemia, non-Hodgkin's lymphoma, and systemic lupus erythematosus. Labeling efficiency is also diminished when "old" ^{99m}Tc pertechnetate is used.[18] Technetium 99m decays to ^{99}Tc, which is no longer useful for imaging, but nevertheless competes with the radioactive form for stannous ions. To prevent the presence of carrier ^{99}Tc, the ^{99m}Tc dose should be taken from relatively fresh (less than 24 h after elution) eluate. Poor labeling can easily be recognized on an ERNA image: free ^{99m}Tc pertechnetate accumulates in the mucosa of the stomach and in the thyroid gland.

Gamma Camera-Computer System

Equilibrium radionuclide angiocardiography is best performed using a small field of view gamma camera. A typical small field of view cardiac camera has an approximately 25-cm diameter crystal. This conveniently allows for imaging of the heart and its surroundings without the need for magnification. Using larger field of view cameras, such as standard single photon emission computed tomography (SPECT) cameras, the image of the heart is frequently too small, occupying relatively few pixels in the computer matrix, and requires the use of magnification or zoom. Usually a 1.2 zoom factor is sufficient. An optimal quality ERNA image of the heart occupies approximately one third of the field of view. Occasionally, in particular using a large field of view camera, intense extracardiac activity (e.g., spleen) may cause a problem with image display. Computer images are usually normalized to the hottest pixel within the image. In the presence of intense extracardiac activity, radioactivity in the heart is at the darker end of the gray scale and may be almost invisible. Rather than using lead shielding as recommended by some, normalization of the image to the hottest pixel *within the heart* usually deals adequately with this display problem.

Cardiac cameras may have a crystal thickness of ¼ or ⅜ inch (0.63 or 0.95 cm). A sodium iodide crystal of ⅜-inch thickness stops 90 percent of the gamma rays emitted by ^{99m}Tc. Although a thinner, 0.63-cm crystal can provide slightly better resolution, it captures only 78 percent of the incoming ^{99m}Tc gamma rays. This decreased efficiency results in slightly increased acquisition times. This is a consideration when exercise ERNA studies are acquired. The thin crystal detectors are optimal for thallium 201 (^{201}Tl) imaging.

The use of a parallel-hole general all-purpose collimator is standard for ERNA imaging. For exercise studies, with otherwise marginal count density, the use of high sensitivity collimation may improve image quality. A 20 percent gamma camera energy window is set symmetrically over the 140-keV photon peak of ^{99m}Tc. The gamma camera is interfaced with a computer and ECG gating device. The ERNA studies are acquired on computer using a 64 × 64 matrix and word mode. Acquisition software allows predefinition of acquisition parameters, such as the number of frames per cardiac cycle, time length of each frame, beat rejection, and acquisition stopping parameters. Most commercially available computers have well validated software for calculation of left ventricular function parameters.

ECG-Synchronized Gating

Although a relatively high dose of radioactivity is used for RBC labeling, radioactivity is distributed over the entire vascular space of the body. Consequently, count density over the heart may be relatively low. To acquire adequate count density images, data should be collected over multiple cardiac cycles.[19,20] Simply imaging the heart for an extended period of time would result in images that are importantly blurred by cardiac motion. To circumvent this problem, gamma camera acquisition is synchronized, or "gated," to the patient's R wave on the ECG (Fig. 11-1). When an R wave is detected, the gating device sends a signal to the computer to start an acquisition sequence. The cardiac cycle is divided into multiple intervals. A separate image is acquired for each interval. If the intervals are short enough, cardiac motion during each interval becomes insignificant and multiple sharp images, each during a different portion of the cardiac cycle, are acquired. Using the ECG R wave to indicate the start of the cardiac cycle, the computer directs incoming image data from the gamma camera to appropriate memory locations (bins) in computer memory. Image data corresponding to the first interval are placed into a first memory bin, image data from the second interval are placed in a second memory bin, and so on. This is repeated for each cardiac cycle until sufficient counts have been accumulated in each bin. Each bin or frame then holds an image of the heart at a different portion of the cardiac cycle. An adequate study contains 250,000 to 500,000 counts per frame, acquired in approximately 5 min from 300 to 400 heartbeats. This series of images acquired during the cardiac cycle can be displayed in rapid sequence on the computer screen. This cine display creates the illusion of a beating heart. By observing this closed-loop cinematic display, the size of cardiac chambers, right and left ventricular wall motion, and great vessels can be evaluated.

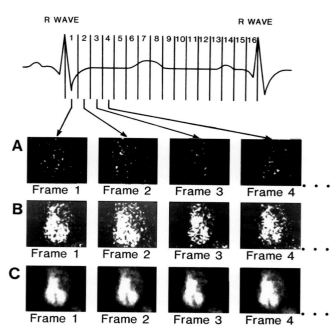

Figure 11-1 Computer acquisition of ERNA. The computer uses the R wave of the ECG to signal the computer to start an acquisition sequence. The cardiac cycle is divided into 16 equal intervals. Gamma camera counts occurring during the first interval are stored in frame 1 in computer memory. Those counts occurring during the second interval are stored in frame 2, and so on for all 16 intervals. Only the first four frames are illustrated. Row A demonstrates the contents of the first four computer frames after image data from one cardiac cycle have been collected. Because of the low count rate (750 counts per frame), there is not enough statistical information within any frame to form a usable image. If image data from additional cardiac cycles are acquired and added to the data already within computer memory, sufficient count statistics eventually will be accumulated to produce recognizable images. Row B shows the contents of the first computer frames after 20 cardiac cycles (15,000 counts per frame). Further accumulation of counts can additionally improve image quality as demonstrated in row C, which displays the contents of the same for computer frames after counts of 400 cardiac cycles (300,000 counts per frame) have been collected. (From Parker DA, et al. Gerson's *Cardiac Nuclear Medicine*, 2nd ed., reproduced with permission.)

FRAMING REQUIREMENTS

Use of ERNA relies on dividing the cardiac cycle into multiple time intervals or frames.[19,21] When the cardiac cycle is divided into a greater number of frames, greater temporal resolution is achieved. However with an increased number of frames per cycle, the frames are of shorter duration and longer acquisition times are needed for adequate counts and image quality. Doubling the number of frames per cardiac cycle will double acquisition time. Computer setup may give the option to either divide the R-R interval in a preset number of frames or preset the time length of each frame. Presently, the most common practice is that each R-R cycle is divided into 16 frames, which provides adequate temporal resolution for the average normal resting heart rate. Less than 50 ms/frame is preferred for resting ERNA studies. Calculation of ejection fraction imposes lesser demands on temporal resolution than calculation, for example, of ventricular filling parameters. Depending on the software used, assessment of diastolic filling requires high temporal resolution acquisition. However, some software packages achieve comparable accurate measurements of diastolic filling using 16-frame acquisition and Fourier curve fitting.

BEAT REJECTION

The ERNA data are acquired over many cardiac cycles, 250 or more. This assumes that the patient's heart rate is stable during the entire duration of acquisition. However, some cardiac cycles may be longer and some may be shorter than the average cycle length. When irregular heartbeats constitute more than 10 percent of the total accumulated cycles, errors are introduced into the shape of the ventricular time–activity curve.[22] Most of these errors are introduced during the diastolic portion of the left ventricular volume curve, with minimal effect on the systolic portion.

Several computer methods have been developed to selectively reduce or eliminate irregular heartbeats. One method is *postbeat filtration*. As the computer acquires each cardiac cycle, it checks the R-R interval and compares it to predetermined acceptable limits. If the R-R interval is within these limits, the computer proceeds to acquire the next cardiac cycle. If the R-R interval falls outside these limits, no further cardiac cycles are required until the R-R interval returns to an acceptable value. Because irregular beats often occur in quick succession, this method "filters out" short bursts of irregularity. Unfortunately, the initial irregular beat that triggered the filter is included in the study. Because of this, postbeat filtration deals poorly with frequent isolated irregular beats. Ejection fraction calculation may be inaccurate by as much as 5 to 10 percentage points as a result of these beats.

Another similar method of rejecting irregular beats is *dynamic beat filtration*. With this method, the data from each cardiac cycle are first placed in a temporary storage buffer within the computer, rather than being added to the image frames. The computer then checks to see if the R-R interval falls within predetermined acceptable limits. If the beat is acceptable the data in the temporary buffer are added to the image frames. If the R-R interval is not acceptable, the data in the temporary buffer are discarded. This method of beat filtration will eliminate every irregular beat falling outside the user-specified limits. The only drawback with dynamic beat filtration is the need for more sophisticated computer software including a large memory capacity and high speed disk storage.

A third method dealing with irregular beats is the *list mode acquisition*. This method differs from the others in that the image data from the camera are not processed as they are acquired. Instead, the position of every count coming from the camera is stored on a high speed disk together with the timing data of the ECG. This information is acquired over several minutes and can quickly fill even a large capacity disk. Once the acquisition is complete, the operator can analyze the recorded data at leisure. Limits for the R-R intervals are set and the data are reconstructed into images in a fashion similar to that used for dynamic beat filtration. The advantage of list mode acquisitions is that the data can be analyzed in different ways. Various R-R intervals can be selected to correspond to a specific type of beat, for example, a sinus beat, premature ventricular beat, or postextrasystolic beat. The disadvantages of list mode acquisitions are the need for a large disk storage capacity and increased processing time.

R-R INTERVAL SELECTION

All three methods of arrhythmia filtration require the operator to select an acceptable range of R-R intervals. This is best accomplished by generating an R-R interval histogram before image acquisition, in which the computer measures multiple R-R intervals and plots their relative frequency. The dominant R-R interval is then usually chosen for acquisition. Once the R-R interval has been determined, a window of allowable intervals is selected. Generally a window of 10 to 15 percent is used. If the window is too narrow, few beats will meet the acceptable limits and acquisition time may become excessively long. If the window is made too wide, undesirable irregular beats might be accepted and affect the overall quality of image data.

Effect of arrhythmias on image display and calculation of left ventricular ejection fraction   Acquisition parameters are chosen with the patient at rest, preferably comfortable and relaxed lying on the imaging table. Normally all cardiac cycles at rest are of approximately the same duration, with slight variation during the respiratory cycle. Slowing of the heart rate after acquisition parameters are entered into the computer may result in a typical artifact on cine image display: "blinking" at the end of the cycle. This is caused by a slower heart rate during acquisition than the preset R-R interval (Fig. 11-2). During the long R-R intervals (slow heart rate) not all frames at the end of an acquisition cycle are filled with image data, resulting in frames with lower count density, which in turn result in the blinking effect (darker images) on

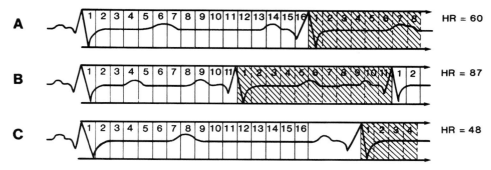

Figure 11-2 Effect of changing heart rate on ERNA acquisition. **A:** In this example the cardiac cycle is divided into 16 equal frames with a heart rate of 60 beats/min. Each frame is 62.5 ms long. This interval is fixed for the entire acquisition. If heart rate does not change during acquisition, data are consistently acquired for all frames. This is assumed to be the case when ERNA is acquired over many heartbeats. **B:** If the heart rate increases during the acquisition there is not enough time between R waves to fill all 16 frames. For example, a new R wave occurred after only 11 frames were collected. The R wave causes the computer to begin a new sequence of acquisitions. Frames 12 to 16 fail to receive any counts. **C:** If the heart rate slows during acquisition the computer uses up all 16 frames before the cardiac cycle is finished. The last portion of the cycle is not recorded. The information recorded on each frame does not exactly correspond to the same portion of the cardiac cycle as in **A.** (from Parker DA, et al. Gerson's *Cardiac Nuclear Medicine*, 2nd ed., reproduced with permission.)

cine display. When one encounters such a study, inspection of the shape of the left ventricular time–activity curve is an important step of quality assurance. If the time–activity curve shows that only one or two of the last frames are involved, the clinical usefulness of the ERNA study is unaffected. Left ventricular ejection fraction (LVEF) can still be determined reliably. The above-described minor effect by slowing of the heart rate occurs relatively frequently and does not seriously affect the clinical usefulness of ERNA studies. Atrial fibrillation represents an extreme situation of irregular heart rhythm, in particular in patients who are not yet treated with digoxin. Inspection of the left ventricular time–activity curve is in this situation of crucial importance (Figs. 11-3 and 11-4). Only when a predominant cycle length exists (i.e., a well defined trough is present in the time–activity curve) can a meaningful LVEF be calculated from such data. Contrary to what is generally believed, ERNA LVEF can be calculated in most patients with atrial fibrillation. This LVEF represents the *average* LVEF of many cardiac cycles. However, to provide clinically meaningful information, the window of accepted R-R intervals must be relatively narrow to avoid averaging cardiac cycles with widely varying timing of end-systole.

Image Acquisition

Data acquisition depends on adequate ECG gating. After preparation of the patient's skin, three radiolucent chest lead electrodes are placed. Electrode placement should be adjusted, if needed, for maximal ECG R-wave amplitude.

ELECTROCARDIOGRAPHIC-GATED FIRST-PASS ANGIOCARDIOGRAPHY

The injection of labeled RBCs can be used for the performance of ECG-gated first-pass radionuclide angiocardiography to assess right ventricular ejection fraction (RVEF).[23,24] The gated first-pass study is performed with the patient lying supine and the camera in either the right anterior oblique (RAO) or, more commonly, in the anterior position. The radioactive dose is injected rapidly as a bolus. Immediately before the injection, the computer is started for acquisition of an ERNA study (either in frame mode or list mode) and terminated as soon as the radioactive bolus is seen entering the pulmonary artery.

EQUILIBRIUM ANGIOCARDIOGRAPHY

After injection of the ^{99m}Tc-labeled RBCs, with or without first-pass angiographic acquisition, radioactivity equilibrates within the cardiovascular space and equilibrium radionuclide images can be acquired within a few minutes. Usually at least three views are acquired for complete evaluation of all cardiac chambers—the anterior view, the left anterior oblique (LAO) view (i.e., the obliquity that provides best separation between right and left ventricles), and the left lateral view.[24,25] The latter is acquired with the patient lying on the right side. Although caudal angulation of the detector head is often

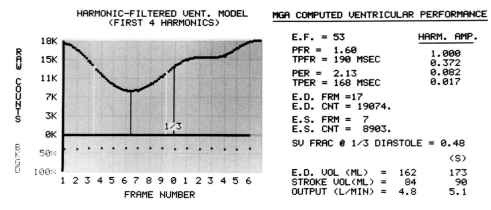

Figure 11-3 Computer-generated time–activity curve (left ventricular volume curve) from ERNA study. **Left panel:** The left ventricular volume curve is generated from a 16-frame ERNA acquisition using Fourier curve fitting (first 4 harmonics). **Right panel:** Automated calculation of left ventricular ejection fraction (EF), peak filling rate (PFR), time to peak filling rate (TPFR), peak ejection rate (PER), and time to peak ejection rate (TPER). The end-diastolic frame number (ED FRM) and end-diastolic counts (ED CNT), as well as the end-systolic frame number and systolic counts are shown. Furthermore the stroke volume (SV) fraction at one third diastole is calculated. Finally end-diastolic volume, stroke volume, and cardiac output are calculated as indicated.

recommended for the LAO view for better separation of left atrium and left ventricle, this has very little effect on determination of ejection fraction. It is important to keep the gamma camera as close to the chest as possible in all views. The acquisition of a gated first-pass study takes only 15 s, whereas the acquisition of equilibrium images usually takes approximately 5 min. These acqui-

sition times may have to be adjusted, depending on actual counts acquired in the whole image.

COUNT REQUIREMENTS

The more counts that are acquired within a frame, the better the image and the smaller the statistical error in

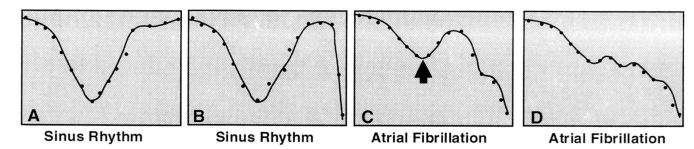

A	B	C	D
Sinus Rhythm	**Sinus Rhythm**	**Atrial Fibrillation**	**Atrial Fibrillation**

Figure 11-4 Effect of heart rate irregularity on left ventricular time–activity curve. **A:** Left ventricular time–activity curve of a patient with perfectly regular sinus rhythm. The left ventricular volume curve returns at the end of the cardiac cycle to the same count level, as at the beginning of the acquisition cycle. **B:** Left ventricular volume curve of a patient in sinus rhythm and multiple premature ventricular beats. Because of earlier occurring R waves, the last two frames of the acquisition cycle contain fewer counts (see Fig. 11-2). The lesser counts of these two frames create "blinking" on cine display of the ERNA study. **C:** Left ventricular volume curve in a patient with atrial fibrillation on digoxin. Although the heart rate is totally irregular, there is a predominant R-R interval resulting in a definite trough at systole (*arrow*). From this curve LVEF can be calculated. However, because the timing of end-systole will vary with each beat, the calculated LVEF will not necessarily correspond to the LVEF of a single beat with an average R-R interval length unless a very narrow window of R-R intervals is accepted. **D:** A patient with atrial fibrillation without digoxin therapy. The R-R intervals are extremely irregular and no predominant R-R interval is present. From this curve no ejection fraction can be calculated. It should be noted that in most patients with atrial fibrillation ERNA curves similar to those in **C** are obtained; a curve as in **D** is the exception rather than rule.

calculating LVEF. If the heart is contributing most of the counts, at least 250,000 counts per frame, or a total of 5 million counts in 16 frames, should be acquired for a resting ERNA study. One should be aware that count density within a *frame* does not always reflect count density within the *left ventricle*. Relative count distribution within the image should be inspected before defining acquisition parameters. Occasionally excessive extracardiac activity may be present, for example in the spleen. For these circumstances some gamma cameras allow predefinition of count density to be acquired within the left ventricle rather than in the entire frame. A count density of 250 counts/cm² within the left ventricle is optimal for good quality image data.

Computer Processing

The underlying principle of quantitative radionuclide angiography is that the amount of radioactivity registered by the gamma camera is proportional to the volume of blood in the cardiac ventricles. Thus, changes in ventricular count density parallel changes in ventricular volume. This allows for calculation of LVEF.

LEFT VENTRICULAR EJECTION FRACTION

The most important quantitative parameter derived by computer processing from ERNA studies is global LVEF. The LVEF can be calculated from the LAO view because in this projection the left ventricular cavity is projected without significant overlap by other cardiac structures. In the anterior view the right ventricle is superimposed on a portion of the left ventricle, whereas in the left lateral view the left ventricle is superimposed on the right ventricle. With a correctly angulated LAO view, the thickness of the myocardium provides a natural "shielding" from radioactivity in the right ventricle and the left atrium.

Many versions of computer software exist on different commercially available computer systems to determine LVEF.[26,27] Some software packages are completely automated; most are semiautomated and allow operator interaction. Despite differences in software details, the basic computerized approach to derive LVEF from ERNA studies is the same. Changes in count density are assessed from varying regions of interest that define the edges of left ventricular endocardial borders throughout the cardiac cycle (Fig. 11-5). Left ventricular counts are then corrected for extracardiac background activity. From the background-corrected counts (that are proportional to left ventricular volume changes) a left ventricular time–activity curve is generated. The LVEF is calculated as follows:

$$\frac{\text{End-Diastolic Counts} - \text{End-Systolic Counts}}{\text{End-Diastolic Counts}}$$

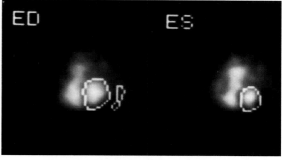

End Diastolic Counts 13,980

LVEF .56

Figure 11-5 Regions of interest to calculate LVEF. To calculate LVEF the computer generates regions of interest that define left ventricular endocardial edges in end-diastole (ED) and end-systole (ES). A crescent-shaped region adjacent to the lateral border of the left ventricle in ED provides an estimate of background radioactivity.

Using most commercially available computer software, the lower limit of normal LVEF is approximately 0.50. Regardless of the software used, the following quality assurance checks should be performed before reporting LVEF.

1. Are the automatically or semiautomatically generated left ventricular edges correct (see Fig. 11-5)? Most importantly, is the left atrium appropriately excluded from the left ventricular systolic frames?
2. Is the background region correctly chosen? The background region usually is a 2- to 3-pixel-wide crescent-shaped region positioned 1 to 3 pixels away from the posterolateral wall. Does the background region incorporate excessive extracardiac activity that could cause an artifactually high LVEF?
3. Is the shape of the time–activity curve appropriate (see Figs. 11-3 and 11-4)? Is there a well defined systolic trough, with appropriate increase in counts during diastole? Is there a "drop-off" in counts in the last diastolic frames that could affect calculation of diastolic filling parameters?
4. Are left ventricular end-diastolic counts adequate to ensure statistical reliability? When LVEF is normal, end-diastolic counts should be at least 3000, whereas when LVEF is abnormal end-diastolic counts should be at least 15,000 to 20,000.

Radionuclide-derived LVEF is highly accurate and extremely reproducible, substantially better than that of the echocardiographic LVEF (Fig. 11-6).[28,29] Resting LVEF has been shown in many studies to be the single most important quantifiable clinical parameter that de-

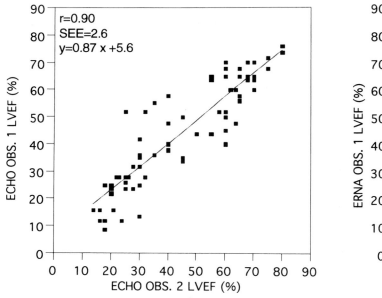

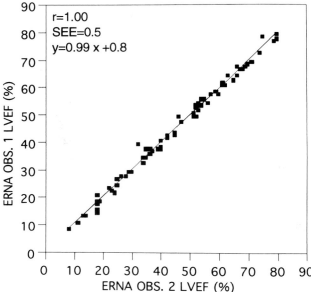

Figure 11-6 Interobserver variability of quantitative radionuclide LVEF by ERNA (right) and visual LVEF by two-dimensional echocardiography (left). Mean interobserver variability is minimal (3.8 percent) with ERNA and substantially greater (18.1 percent) with echocardiography. (From Van Royen et al,[29] by permission of Excerpta Medica, Inc.)

termines prognosis in patients with coronary artery disease.[30,31]

Regional left ventricular ejection fraction Regional LVEF can be calculated by determining the geometric center of the left ventricle and dividing the left ventricle into five zones, corresponding to the basal septal, apical septal, inferoapical, inferolateral, and posterolateral regions (Fig. 11-7).[32] The area involving the valve planes is excluded. Regional LVEF is computed from count density changes during the cardiac cycle. Because

changes in count density reflect three-dimensional volume changes, these measurements are more meaningful than one-dimensional methods, such as regional chord shortening.

Diastolic filling parameters (See Chap. 15).

Left ventricular volumes (See Chap. 12).

RIGHT VENTRICULAR EJECTION FRACTION

Because of overlap with other cardiac chambers RVEF (see Chap. 14) cannnot be determined routinely from an ERNA study. Frequently there is overlap of right atrial activity during right ventricular systole, which will lead to an erroneously low calculated RVEF. For studies acquired on a single crystal gamma camera, the above-described combination of first-pass technique and ECG gating or "gated first-pass radionuclide angiocardiography" is usually the best approach.[23,24] This technique provides the temporal and anatomic separation of the first-pass technique and uses the R-wave signal of the ECG as a means to correctly sum relatively noisy scintillation data. The (re-)injection of [99mTc]-labeled RBCs can conveniently be used for gated first-pass angiocardiography. For a typical gated first-pass study, data from 5 to 10 heartbeats are usually accumulated. No background correction is required when the study is performed in the RAO or anterior projection because there is virtually

Normal Regional LVEF

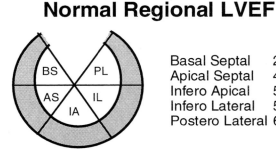

Basal Septal	26%
Apical Septal	41%
Infero Apical	50%
Infero Lateral	54%
Postero Lateral	61%

Figure 11-7 Schematic diagram of left ventricular regions in the LAO view for calculation of regional LVEF. The area of the valve planes is excluded. Lower limits of normal regional LVEF, derived in 40 normal individuals, are shown for the basal septal (BS), apical septal (AS), inferoapical (IA), inferolateral (IL), and posterolateral (PL) regions.

no overlap of right atrium and right ventricle and data collection is terminated before radioactivity enters the lung. A time–activity curve is generated over the right ventricle using an end-diastolic and end-systolic region of interest. Using this method the lower limit of normal RVEF is approximately 0.40.

Qualitative Image Analysis

In addition to calculation of the above-described left ventricular and right ventricular global function parameters, clinically meaningful qualitative and morphologic information can be derived by visual qualitative evaluation of ERNA images.[24] The multiframe digitized scintigraphic data are spatially and temporally smoothed and displayed on a computer screen as endless-loop movies. Multiple-view ERNA images are preferably reviewed simultaneously on the computer screen.

Characterization of Cardiac Structures on Multiple Views

RIGHT ANTERIOR OBLIQUE VIEW (Fig. 11-8)

Gated first-pass angiography in the RAO or anterior view permits visualization of right ventricular contraction without superimposition of other cardiac structures. The superior vena cava is visualized as a vertically running vessel from the top of the image down to the right atrium. The size of the right atrium cannot always be judged reliably from the gated first-pass study because of "streaming" of the radioactive bolus and incomplete mixing with right atrial blood. The inferior vena cava is only visualized in the presence of tricuspid regurgitation. Tricuspid regurgitation can be recognized only on a first-pass study. The right ventricle is triangular in shape in this projection; the pulmonary outflow tract extends cranially and connects with the main pulmonary artery. The ascending aortic is often visualized as a "negative image" between the right atrium and pulmonary artery.

ANTERIOR VIEW (Fig. 11-9)

On the anterior view, the border-forming contour on the right side of the heart (left side of image) is the right atrium. Assessment of contraction pattern and size of the right atrium can be made only from the anterior view. On the other projections, the right atrium is either not seen (left lateral) or may move passively (LAO). One boundary of the right ventricle (tricuspid valve plane) can be recognized as a linear photopenic area distal to the right atrium. This photopenic reference area is caused by attenuation by fatty tissue in the atrioventricular groove. Of the remainder of the right ventricle, usually only the inferior wall and sometimes the apex can be seen. However, most of the right ventricular contour

is obscured by underlying left ventricular blood pool activity. To the viewer's right, the border-forming contour of the heart on the anterior view is the left ventricle. Because of the overlying activity of the right ventricle, only the anterolateral wall and apex can be evaluated. Many times, the inferior wall is completely obscured by the right ventricular blood pool. Further structures that can be evaluated on the anterior view are the pulmonary artery and the ascending aorta.

LEFT ANTERIOR OBLIQUE VIEW (Fig. 11-10)

The LAO view is the projection that best separates right and left ventricular blood pools. The angle of optimal ventricular separation varies in each individual patient. Usually, this is not a standard 45° angulation, but has to be searched for by the technologist. On a correctly angulated LAO projection, the photopenic area of the septum is vertical. To the left is the foreshortened right ventricle. The right atrium is partially hidden behind and superior to the right ventricle. On cine display of the LAO view, the right atrium almost always appears to contract. However, even in patients with atrial fibrillation, this motion may be observed and is an optical illusion. The twisting motion of the heart during ventricular systole causes the right atrium to move passively. To the right side, the left ventricular blood pool is well isolated from the surrounding structures by the myocardium as a photopenic halo. Although the left atrial radioactivity is behind the left ventricle, the distance from the left atrium to the detector head is too large for left atrial activity to contribute significantly to left ventricular blood pool activity. Therefore, an area of interest selected over the left ventricle in this particular view will almost exclusively contain count density changes from the left ventricular blood pool. The appendage of the left atrium can occasionally be seen superior to the left ventricle, usually separated from the left ventricular blood pool by the photopenic area of myocardium. As a rule, the left ventricular blood pool is projected as a "short axis" view. In other words, one looks "down the barrel" of the left ventricle. In some patients, the heart is vertical in position. This anatomic variant can be recognized because of the elongated shape of both ventricles and visualization of both the right atrium and left atrium superior to the ventricles.

LEFT LATERAL VIEW (Fig. 11-11)

This view is taken with the patient lying on the right side. This patient position is important because it makes it possible to bring the detector head close to the patient's chest, which is almost impossible with the patient lying supine. Secondly, when the patient is lying on the right side, the orientation of the long axis of the heart shifts from angulated to the left chest wall toward a vertical

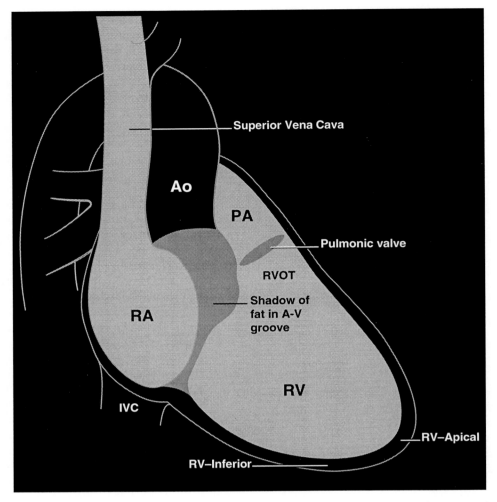

Figure 11-8 Schematic representation of cardiac anatomy in the RAO view used for the gated first-pass study (see text). RVOT, right ventricular outflow tract; A-V, atrioventricular; Ao, aorta; PA, pulmonary artery; RA, right atrium; RV, right ventricle; IVC, inferior vena cava. (Courtesy Patrick J. Lynch, 1992).

position, parallel to the long axis of the body. Consequently, the left lateral view shows the long axis of the left ventricle best. Because of individual variations among patients, either the straight left lateral or the left posterior oblique view will usually show the long axis of the left ventricle best. "Long axis" is defined as the longest dimension from valve plane to apex and best separation of left atrium from left ventricle. In the left lateral projection, the left ventricle is superimposed on activity of the right ventricle. However, because of the distance of the right ventricle from the detector and radiation attenuation, this does not interfere with analysis of regional wall motion of the left ventricle. Anterior and superior to the left ventricle, the right ventricular outflow tract and the pulmonary artery can be noted. The anterior wall (anteroseptal portion) and the inferoposterior wall of the left ventricle are well visualized. In fact, the left lateral view is the

only view in which the posterobasal segment of the left ventricle can be analyzed. The mitral valve plane is often well demarcated by a linear photopenic area caused by attenuation by fatty tissue in the atrioventricular groove. Posterior to the left ventricle are the left atrium and the descending aorta.

Visual assessment of chamber size and myocardial thickness   High quality multiple-view ERNA studies contain considerably more clinically useful information than LVEF alone. For example, one can qualitatively assess the relative sizes of various cardiac chambers (assuming that the same camera and magnification are used). Because in many patients the right ventricle is normal in size and function, right ventricular end-diastolic size may be a useful bench mark for qualitative assessment of the relative size of other cardiac structures. On a normal study, the right ventricle is usually somewhat larger than

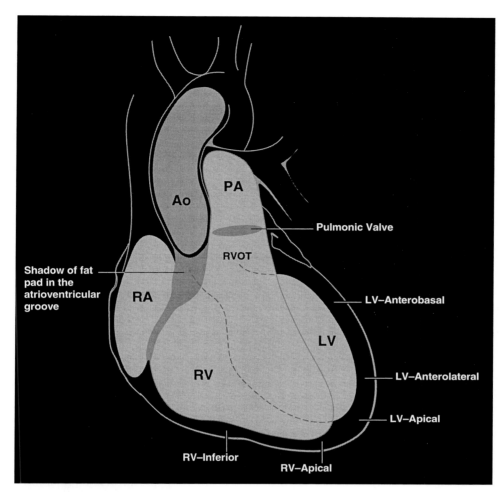

Figure 11-9 Schematic representation of cardiac anatomy on equilibrium radionuclide angiocardiography in the anterior view (see text). LV, left ventricle. Other abbreviations as in Fig. 11-8. (Courtesy Patrick J. Lynch, 1992).

the left ventricle. The size of the ventricles should be compared in the end-diastolic phase of the cardiac cycle.

The presence or absence of marked left ventricular hypertrophy can be estimated by qualitative assessment of the thickness of the septum. The septum is well delineated by right and left ventricular blood pool and thus the thickness of the myocardium can be appreciated. In severe left ventricular hypertrophy, a thick photopenic halo may surround the left ventricular blood pool.

Regional wall-motion analysis Radionuclide angiographic evaluation of ventricular regional wall-motion abnormalities requires acquisition of multiple good quality views, thereby allowing detailed analysis of each myocardial segment. The left lateral views are extremely useful for complete regional wall-motion analysis. Regional

wall motion is usually graded as normal, mildly hypokinetic, severely hypokinetic, or akinetic.

Left ventricle On the anterior view, there is substantial overlap of right ventricular and left ventricular blood pools. Hence only the anterior, lateral, and apical segments of the left ventricle can be analyzed without interference due to superimposed structures on the anterior view. On the LAO view, the posterolateral, inferolateral, inferoapical, and septal segments can be evaluated. It must be noted, however, that this projection produces substantial left ventricular foreshortening. For example, septal excursion may be minimized because major systolic motion occurs perpendicular to the field of view. Contractility of the apex and posterolateral wall is best evaluated in this perspective.

The most important projections for detection of regional wall motion abnormalities are the left lateral

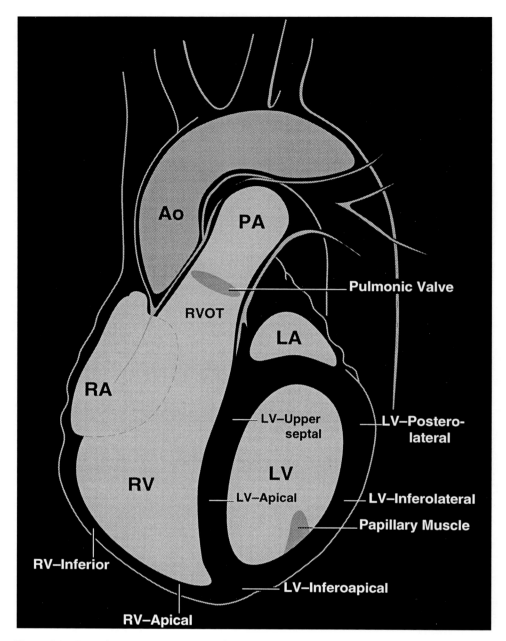

Figure 11-10   Schematic representation of cardiac anatomy on equilibrium radionuclide angiocardiography in the LAO view (see text). LA, left atrium. Other abbreviations as in Figs. 11-8 and 11-9. (Courtesy Patrick J. Lynch, 1992).

views. These show the long axis of the left ventricle with excellent delineation of both the anterior wall and inferoposterior wall.

Right ventricle   Regional wall motion of the right ventricle is difficult to assess even on multiple projections because of (1) the overlap of left ventricular blood pool activity on the anterior projection; (2) foreshortening of the right ventricular motion and atrial blood pool overlap on the LAO projection; and

(3) superimposition and overlap of the left ventricle on the right ventricular blood pool on the left lateral projection. Global and regional wall motion of the right ventricle is best evaluated on the anterior view or from the RAO gated first-pass study.

Atria   The right atrium forms the left lower border on the anterior view of the cardiac image. Size and contractility of the right atrium can be evaluated in this view during ventricular systole. The left atrium is best evalu-

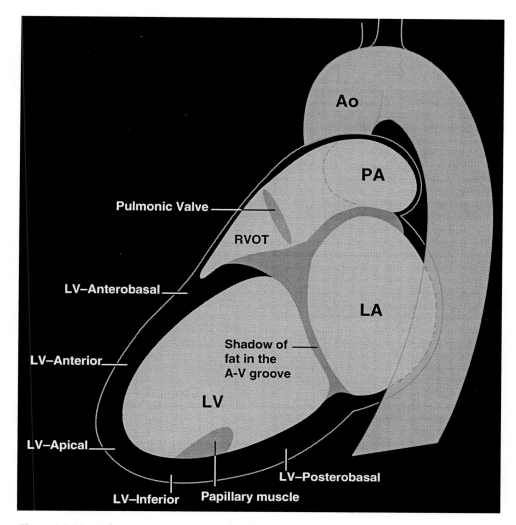

Figure 11-11 Schematic representation of cardiac anatomy on equilibrium radionuclide angiocardiography in the left lateral view (see text). Abbreviations as in Figs. 11-8, 11-9, and 11-10.

ated on the left lateral view during ventricular systole. Because of overlying and surrounding radioactivity, frequently no outline of the left atrium is present. However, the general size and contractility of the left atrium usually can be appreciated. The size of the left atrium should be judged in comparison to the long axis of the left ventricle. The contraction of the left atrium can be recognized as a change in count density (displayed as changing brightness) during the cardiac cycle. The contraction of both atria is usually easily discernible on radionuclide studies. Atrial contraction does, however, occur at the very end of the acquisition cycle. Atrial contraction is considerably shorter than the ventricular cycle. In the presence of ventricular ectopy or irregular rhythm, the last couple of frames have lower count density, resulting in "flicker" of the endless-loop cine. The technologist often "cuts off" one or two frames at the end of the cycle for aesthetic reasons. As a result, atrial contraction may no longer be visible.

Great vessels The pulmonary artery and the ascending and descending aorta can also be evaluated visually on good quality ERNA studies. Only qualitative assessments, such as dilatation of the pulmonary artery and dilatation and tortuosity of the ascending aorta, aortic arch, or descending aorta, can be made.

INTERPRETATION OF EQUILIBRIUM RADIONUCLIDE ANGIOCARDIOGRAPHIC STUDIES

Visual qualitative interpretation of ERNA studies should be performed from the computer screen by viewing ERNA studies in endless-loop cine display. It is preferred to display multiple views simultaneously using the four quadrants of the screen to facilitate three-dimensional interpretation of findings. The following static end-diastolic and end-systolic images depict incompletely the visual information that can be derived from ERNA movie display. The reader is referred to commercially available educational material for a more realistic learning experience.[33,34]

Normal Images

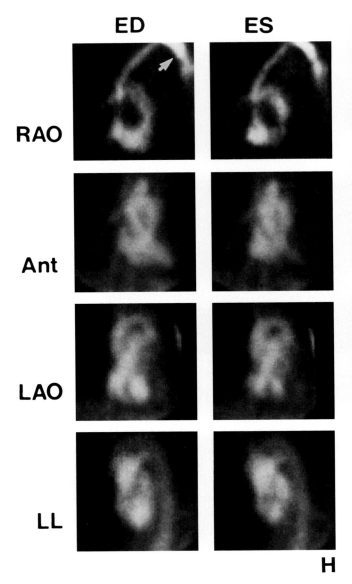

Figure 11-12 Normal ERNA. The end-diastolic (ED) and end-systolic (ES) frames are shown for the right anterior oblique view (RAO), the anterior view (ANT), the left anterior oblique view (LAO), and the left lateral view (LL). For gated first-pass angiography (RAO view) the radioactive bolus was injected in the left antecubital vein. The usual site of injection is in the right antecubital vein. Unlike on routine first-pass studies, the left subclavian vein (*arrow*) is visualized on this image. Compare these images with the schematic drawings in Figs. 11-8 through 11-11. Shown abbreviations are used for all following images.

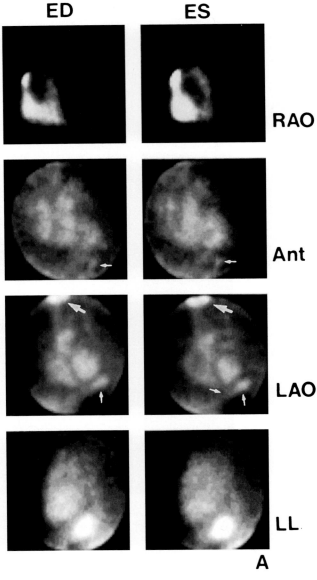

Figure 11-13 Example of poor RBC labeling with ^{99m}Tc. A substantial amount of free (unlabeled) ^{99m}Tc pertechnetate was injected. This can be recognized from intense radiopharmaceutical uptake in the mucosa of the stomach (*small arrows*). Free ^{99m}Tc pertechnetate is also accumulated in the thyroid gland (*large arrows*).

ED   ES

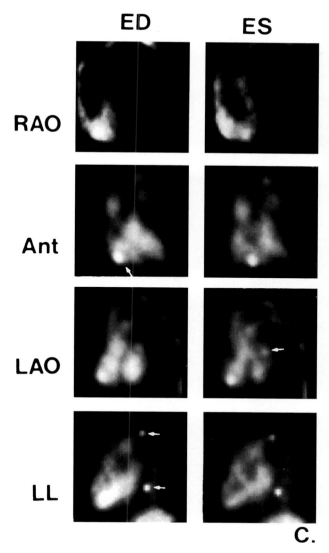

RAO

Ant

LAO

LL

C.

Figure 11-14 Red blood cell microclots. The modified in vivo RBC labeling method involves drawing the patient's blood into a syringe. Occasionally microclots of labeled RBCs may form within the syringe due to inadequate mixing with ACD. When radiolabeled blood is then reinjected in the patient, small RBC clots with high specific radioactivity are injected as well. On these images several microclots can be noted: one in the right ventricle and several in the lungs (*arrows*).

Coronary Artery Disease

ED   ES

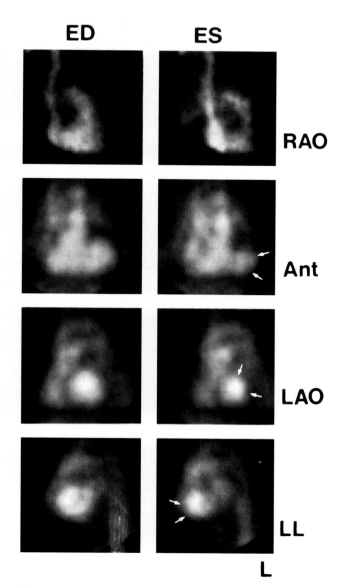

RAO

Ant

LAO

LL

L

Figure 11-15 Studies of a patient with an anterolateral and posterolateral myocardial infarction. The right atrium and right ventricle are normal. The RVEF is 0.48. The left ventricle is enlarged and shows an extensive regional wall motion abnormality involving the anterolateral, posterolateral, and apical walls (*arrows*). Global LVEF is depressed at 0.35.

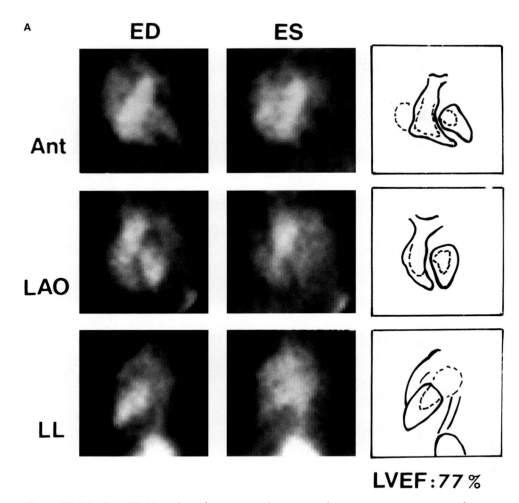

A

ED   ES

Ant

LAO

LL

LVEF: 77%

Figure 11-16   Rest ERNA studies of a patient who sustained a perioperative anterior infarction. **A:** Resting ERNA study acquired before coronary bypass surgery. The RVEF is 0.65. Global LVEF is normal at 0.77. **B:** Resting ERNA study acquired after coronary bypass surgery. The right ventricle is normal in size and contractility. The left ventricle is enlarged and shows an extensive anteroapical and septal area of akinesia (*arrows*). Global LVEF is severely depressed at 0.33.

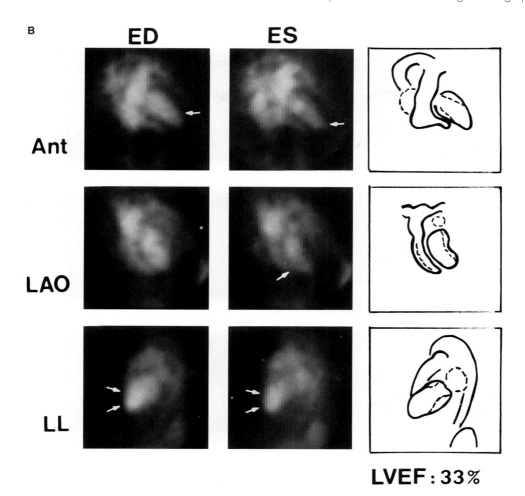

Figure 11-16 *(Continued)*

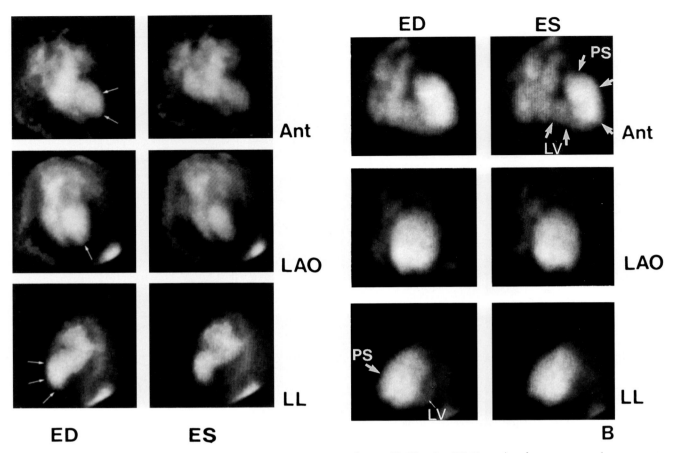

Figure 11-17   An ERNA study of a patient with extensive antero-septal myocardial infarction and a left ventricular aneurysm. The right ventricle is normal in size and contractility. The left ventricle is markedly enlarged and shows severe akinesia of the anterolateral wall, septum, and apex. In the left lateral view distortion of the left ventricular contour in end-diastole (ED), consistent with an ante-roapical aneurysm, can be appreciated. (From Kelley et al,[25] reproduced with permission.)

Figure 11-18   An ERNA study of a patient with an anterior wall left ventricular pseudoaneurysm. The right atrium is enlarged. The right ventricle is enlarged but shows normal contractility in the anterior and LAO view. The left ventricle is markedly enlarged and seems to consist of two chambers. This is particularly clear on the anterior view (*arrows*). This patient sustained an anterolateral wall left ventricular (LV) myocardial infarction with rupture, that was retained by pericardium, resulting in a large pseudoaneurysm (PS).

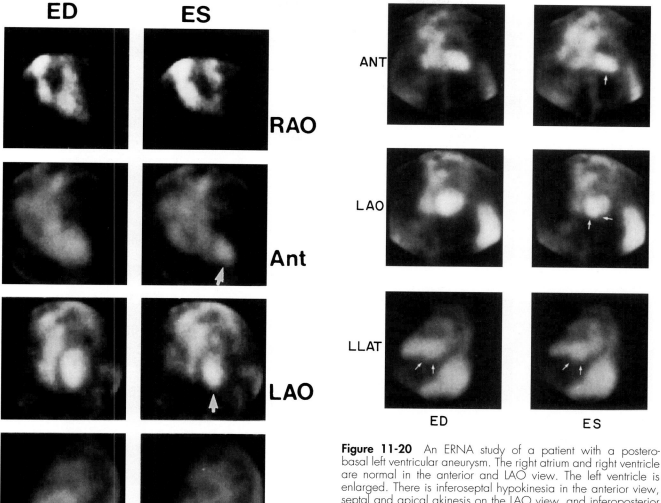

ED   **ES**

RAO

Ant

LAO

LL

D

Figure 11-19 An ERNA study of a patient with inferior wall myocardial infarction. The gated first-pass study in the RAO view is normal. The RVEF was 0.42. Also on the anterior view, the right ventricle is normal. The left ventricle is enlarged and shows inferoapical hypokinesia in the LAO view (*arrow*) and inferoposterior akinesia in the left lateral view (*arrows*). The LVEF is markedly depressed at 0.39.

ANT

LAO

LLAT

ED   **ES**

Figure 11-20 An ERNA study of a patient with a posterobasal left ventricular aneurysm. The right atrium and right ventricle are normal in the anterior and LAO view. The left ventricle is enlarged. There is inferoseptal hypokinesia in the anterior view, septal and apical akinesis on the LAO view, and inferoposterior akinesia on the left lateral view (*arrows*). There is a distortion of the left ventricular contour in end-diastole (ED), consistent with a posterobasal aneurysm. (From Kelly et al,[25] reproduced with permission.)

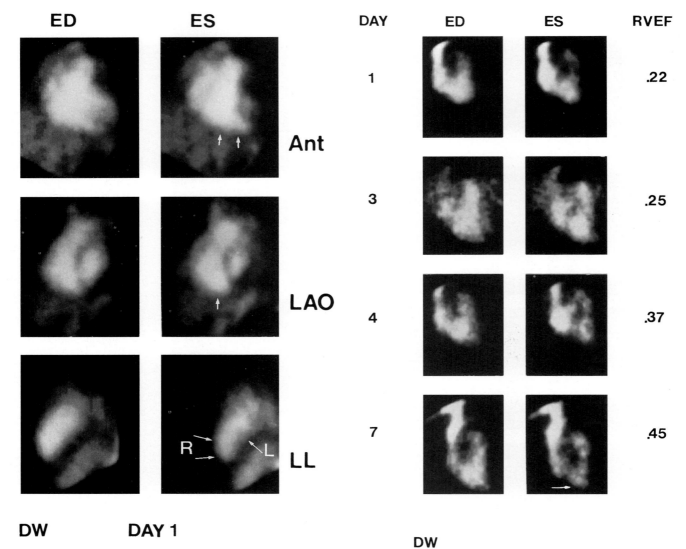

Figure 11-21 An ERNA study of a patient with inferior wall myocardial infarction and right ventricular infarction. On the anterior view, the right ventricle (*arrows*) is massively enlarged and severely hypokinetic. This can also be appreciated on the LAO view. On the LAO view the left ventricle is slightly enlarged but shows normal contractility. On the left lateral view the predominant structure is the enlarged right ventricle (R), which is severely hypokinetic. The left ventricle (L, *arrow*) is barely visible against the large right ventricular volume of radioactivity. This is a typical image of a patient with a relatively small left ventricular inferior wall myocardial infarction and a large right ventricular infarction. The LVEF is preserved at 0.51. Global RVEF, by gated first-pass technique, is severely depressed at 0.22.

Figure 11-22   Serial RVEF by gated first-pass technique in the same patient as in Fig. 11-21. On day 1 of the acute infarct, global RVEF is severely depressed at 0.22. During the following days, RVEF improves to 0.45, although inferior right ventricular hypokinesia (*arrow*) remains present at hospital discharge.

ED   ES   LVEF

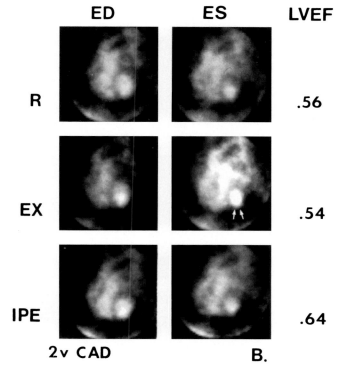

R   .56

EX   .54

IPE   .64

2v CAD   **B.**

Figure 11-23 Rest (R) and exercise (EX) ERNA in a patient with double-vessel coronary artery disease. At rest the right ventricle is normal in size and contractility; the left ventricle is slightly enlarged and shows inferoapical hypokinesis. Resting global LVEF is preserved at 0.56. At peak exercise (EX) there is poor contractility of the right ventricle. The left ventricle is further enlarged and shows inferoapical hypokinesis. The response of the LVEF to exercise is abnormal: no significant (> 0.05) increase in LVEF. LVEF at peak supine bicycle exercise is 0.54. Immediately postexercise (IPE), LVEF normalizes to 64 percent. These images are representative for the quality of images that can be obtained with ERNA during stress testing.

Valvular Heart Disease

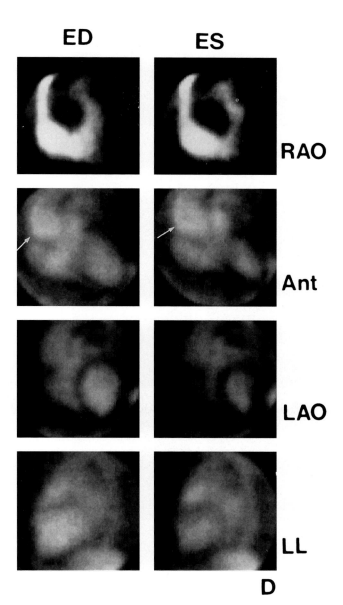

ED   ES

RAO

Ant

LAO

LL

D

Figure 11-24 An ERNA study of a patient with aortic regurgitation. The right atrium and right ventricle are normal on the gated first-pass study in the RAO view. The "black hole" between the right atrium and the pulmonary artery is the "negative image" of a markedly dilated aortic root. On the anterior view, the aortic root and ascending aorta are now visible as a positive image (*arrow*). Right atrium and right ventricle are normal in size and contractility. The left ventricle is enlarged and elongated and shows contraction mainly along the short axis, but not along the long axis. This is a typical image pattern in patients with aortic regurgitation. On the LAO view the right ventricle again can be appreciated to contract normally. The left ventricle shows evidence of left ventricular volume overload. Overall left ventricular contraction is only moderately depressed. Global LVEF is 0.48. The left lateral image further confirms enlargement of the left ventricle with moderately depressed LVEF. No regional wall motion abnormalities are present

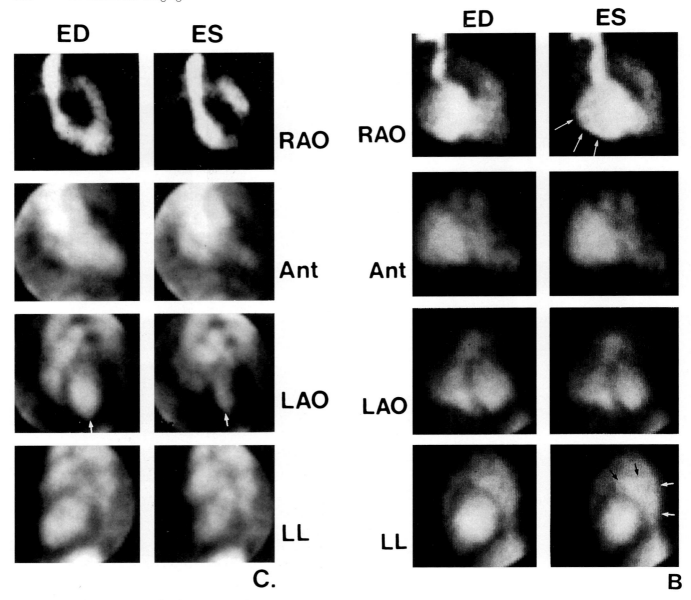

ED   **ES**

RAO

Ant

LAO

LL

C.

ED   **ES**

RAO

Ant

LAO

LL

B

Figure 11-25   An ERNA study of a patient with aortic regurgitation. Similar to the image in Fig. 11-24, the right ventricle is normal in size and contractility. The left ventricle is enlarged and elongated and shows contraction along the short axis and not along the long axis, resulting in apical hypokinesis (*arrow*). Global LVEF in this patient is 0.56.

Figure 11-26   An ERNA study of a patient with aortic regurgitation and atrial fibrillation. On the gated first-pass study in the RAO view, the right atrium (*long arrows*) is remarkably enlarged and does not contract. The right ventricle is normal in size and contractility. On the anterior view again a very large akinetic right atrium can be noted. On the LAO view the left ventricle is enlarged and shows diminished contractility without particular regional contraction abnormalities. Similarly on the left lateral view, the enlarged left ventricle is diffusely hypokinetic (LVEF 0.42) . The left atrium (*short arrows*) is markedly enlarged and does not contract. Even in the absence of valvular heart disease, atrial fibrillation may result in biatrial enlargement.

ED   ES

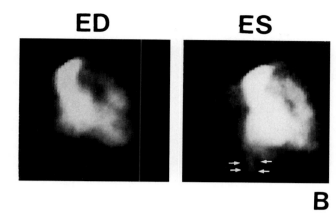

B

Figure 11-27 Gated first-pass study of a patient with tricuspid valve regurgitation. The gated first-pass study shows a large right atrium with regurgitation (arrows) into the inferior caval vein during systole. The right ventricle is enlarged but shows overall normal contractility.

ED   ES

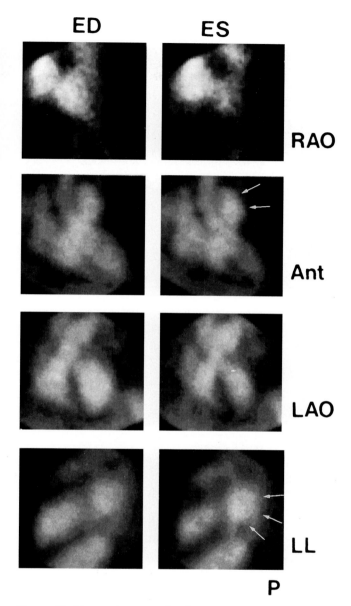

RAO

Ant

LAO

LL

P

Figure 11-28 An ERNA study of a patient with mitral stenosis and mitral regurgitation. On the gated first-pass study in the RAO view the right ventricle is normal in size and contractility. The right atrium is probably enlarged. On the anterior view the right atrium is again enlarged but shows normal contractility; the right ventricle is enlarged with normal contractility; the pulmonary artery (arrows) is dilated. On the LAO view the left ventricle is enlarged and shows diminished contractility. Global LVEF is 0.43. On the left lateral view a large left ventricle with the diminished contractility and an enlarged left atrium are present. This constellation of findings is consistent with mitral regurgitation and mitral stenosis.

Miscellaneous

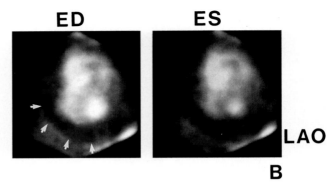

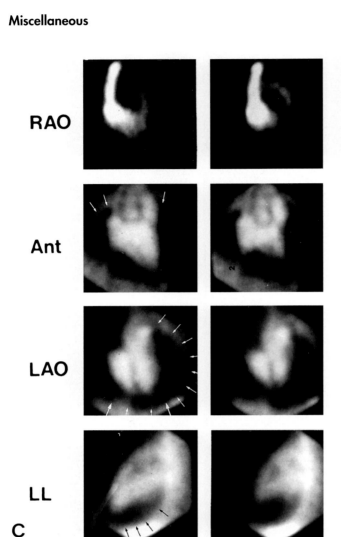

Figure 11-29 An ERNA study in a patient with a pericardial effusion. The gated first-pass study in the RAO view shows normal right atrial and right ventricular size and contractility. This is confirmed on the anterior view and LAO view. Remarkable is the photopenic area (*arrows*) surrounding the heart, extending up to the roots of the great vessels. On the cine display swinging motion of the heart can be appreciated. This image is characteristic of a large pericardial infusion.

Figure 11-30 This image shows a photopenic area (*arrows*) surrounding the heart, apparently comparable to that in Figure 11-29. However, it should be noted the photopenic area is not as dense as in the previous figure; neither is there a sharp contour, nor does the photopenic area extend to the roots of the large vessels. In this patient the shadow is caused by attenuation of radioactivity by overlying breast tissue. The diagnosis of pericardial effusion on ERNA studies should be made with caution and should be confirmed by echocardiography.

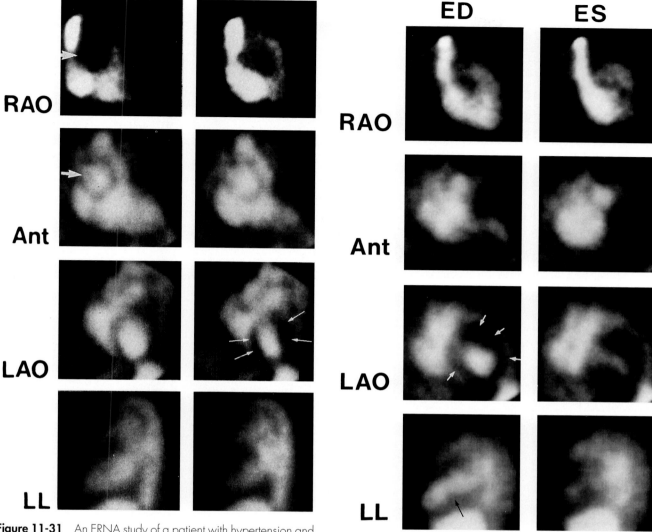

ED   **ES**

RAO

Ant

LAO

LL

G.

Figure 11-31 An ERNA study of a patient with hypertension and moderate left ventricular hypertrophy. On the gated first-pass study in the RAO position the right atrium and right ventricle are normal in size and contractility. The aortic root is dilated and is visualized as a negative image on the RAO view (*thick arrow*) and as a positive image on the anterior view (*thick arrow*). On the LAO view the right ventricle is normal in size and contractility. The left ventricle is enlarged and shows a photopenic area (*thin arrows*) surrounding the left ventricle. This is evidence of the presence of moderate left ventricular hypertrophy. Global LVEF is moderately depressed with apical akinesia.

Figure 11-32 An ERNA study of a patient with severe left ventricular hypertrophy. The gated first-pass study in the RAO position shows a normal right ventricle and right atrium. On the anterior view the left ventricular cavity can be seen clearly in end-diastole but not in end-systole. On the LAO view the left ventricle is surrounded by a massive photopenic area (*arrows*), which indicates left ventricular hypertrophy. During systole there is almost complete obliteration of the left ventricluar cavity. On the left lateral view a typical feature of left ventricular hypertrophy can be seen; the left ventricle has an hourglass appearance. The indentation in the inferior wall (*black arrow*) is caused by a hypertrophied papillary muscle.

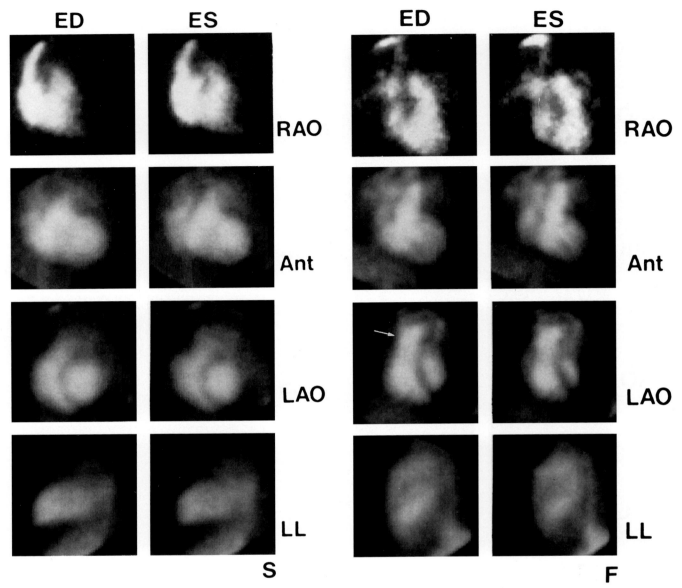

ED **ES**

RAO

Ant

LAO

LL

S

ED **ES**

RAO

Ant

LAO

LL

F

Figure 11-33 An ERNA study of a patient with alcoholic cardiomyopathy. On the gated first-pass study in the RAO position the right atrium and right ventricle are enlarged and show diminished contractility. This is confirmed on the anterior and the LAO views. The left ventricle is markedly enlarged and shows diffusely diminished contractility. This is further confirmed in the left lateral view. The RVEF is depressed at 0.35; LVEF is severely depressed at 0.23.

Figure 11-34 ERNA study of a patient with severe obstructive pulmonary disease. On the gated first-pass study the right ventricle is enlarged and shows severely diminished contractility. Global RVEF is 0.27. On the anterior view the image is dominated by the enlarged right ventricle; the left ventricle cannot be discerned well. On the LAO view the right ventricle is enlarged and shows diminished contractility. The pulmonary artery is dilated (*arrow*). The left ventricle is slightly enlarged but shows normal contractility. On the left lateral view the left ventricle is projected against the background of the enlarged and hypokinetic right ventricle.

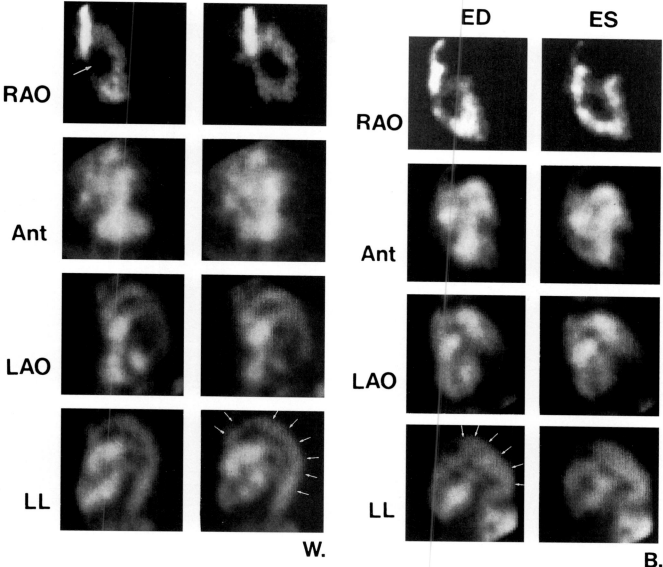

Figure 11-35 An ERNA study of a patient with dilation of the aortic arch. On the gated first-pass study the right atrium and right ventricle are normal in contractility. The RVEF fraction is 0.47. A negative image (*arrow*) of the ascending aorta is noted. On the anterior view the right atrium and right ventricle are normal in size and contractility. The left ventricle is normal in size and shows normal regional contractility. On the LAO view there is evidence of left ventricular hypertrophy. On the LAO and the lateral views it can be appreciated that the ascending and descending aorta (*arrows*) is markedly dilated.

Figure 11-36 An ERNA study of a patient with an aneurysm of the thoracic aorta. On the gated first-pass study the right atrium and right ventricle are normal in size and contractility. This is confirmed on the anterior view. The left ventricle is normal and shows normal regional contractility, as also can be seen on the LAO and left lateral views. The most abnormal feature on these images is best seen in the left lateral view. The ascending aorta is wide and torturous and shows a massive aneurysm (*arrows*) in the aortic arch and descending aorta.

A

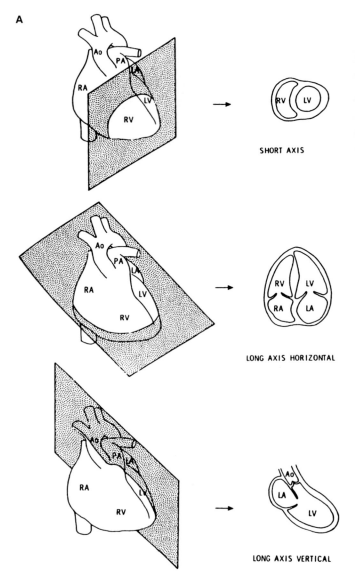

SHORT AXIS

LONG AXIS HORIZONTAL

LONG AXIS VERTICAL

B

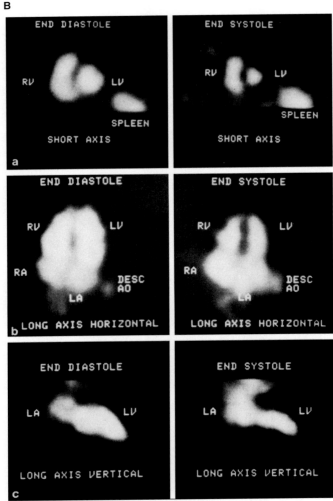

Figure 11-37 (*Continued*)

Figure 11-37 **A:** Standard planes orthogonal to the long axis of the left ventricle (LV) for display of gated blood pool tomograms. RV, right ventricle; LA, left atrium; RA, right atrium; Ao, aorta; PA, pulmonary artery. **B:** End-diastolic and end-systolic blood pool tomographic slices. Short axis (*top*), horizontal long axis (*middle*), vertical long axis (*bottom*). (From Underwood et al,[41] reproduced with permission.)

Gated Blood Pool Tomography

Planar radionuclide angiography is limited inherently because it displays and analyzes three-dimensional structures with a two-dimensional method. The planar approach results in extensive overlap of cardiac structures. For example, with planar blood pool imaging, the left ventricle is only well isolated spatially from other cardiac structures in a "best septal" LAO projection. However, in this projection, the septum and lateral wall may be foreshortened, the inferior wall and apex cannot be dis-

tinguished, and the anterior and posterior walls are not visualized at all. Additional planar blood pool projections are used in an attempt to isolate specific left ventricular walls but the entire left ventricle cannot be isolated, making quantitative assessment of regional left ventricular wall motion difficult.

Increasing capacity and speed of nuclear medicine computers are making the tomographic approach to gated blood pool imaging clinically relevant. The tomographic approach permits reconstruction of gated blood pool data oriented along the long axis of the left ventricle. Gated blood pool data formatted along the left ventricular long axis are optimal for quantitation of left ventricular regional wall motion and also facilitate direct comparisons to contrast left ventriculography, gated magnetic resonance imaging, and two-dimensional echocardiography.

Following RBC labeling by one of the methods described earlier, a series of planar projections is acquired at 3° to 6° angular increments over a 180° orbit with a rotating gamma camera system. At each stop on the camera orbit, data are sorted into 8 or 16 sequential temporal frames based on the elapsed time following the patient's last ECG R wave. For each of the 8 or 16 time increments, the planar projections are backprojected to form a three-dimensional data set that can then be re-registered along the long-axis of the left ventricle (Fig. 11-37). The resultant 8 or 16 sequential tomographic data sets can be displayed in a cinematic format using volume rendering[35] to yield a three-dimensional representation of the blood pools. Alternatively, the endocardial surfaces of the left ventricle can be identified by an automated computer method and the left ventricle can be presented as a cinematic display of the motion of the left ventricular endocardial surface through the cardiac cycle.[36]

Data from gated blood pool tomograms can also be analyzed quantitatively. Early methods selected a central left ventricular long axis slice, divided the left ventricle into two-dimensional sectors, and measured a shortening fraction along each cord extending from the left ventricular centroid in diastole to the left ventricular edge.[37,38] This approach limits analysis of the three-dimensional motion of the left ventricle to two-dimensional analysis in a single plane. Subsequently, methods were developed to analyze motion of the endocardial surface of the left ventricle in all directions.[36] Motion of the left ventricle during the cardiac cycle also involves substantial rotational and translational displacement. This results in greater apparent displacement of the lateral wall compared to the interventricular septum because the center of the left ventricular cavity rotates toward the left side of a short axis blood pool image from the viewer's perspective. To correct for cardiac rotational and translational movement, the centroid of the left ventricle is identified separately in diastole and systole. For each point on the endocardial surface of the left ventricle, the distance from the left ventricle centroid to the endocardial surface is calculated in diastole. A corresponding distance from the location of the left ventricle centroid in systole to the same endocardial location in systole is made. The difference represents regional left ventricular wall motion and is relatively independent of cardiac rotational and translational motion.[39] Regional wall motion and regional ejection fraction can be quantitated for all segments of the left ventricle.[39]

The tomographic approach to gated blood pool imaging has been validated in comparison to ventricular phantoms[37] and in comparison to motion of radioactive sources implanted on the endocardial surface of the left ventricle in a canine model.[36] Gill et al[37] found a good correlation of left ventricular regional wall motion on the long axis oblique view of the gated blood pool tomogram to wall motion on the RAO contrast ventriculogram [$r = 0.82$, $p < 0.0001$, standard error of the estimate (SEE), 14%]. Favorable comparisons of gated

blood pool tomography to contrast ventriculography for detection of left ventricular regional wall-motion abnormalities have been confirmed by others.[38,40–42] In addition, assessments of regional wall motion by gated blood pool tomography have been compared to assessments by planar equilibrium radionuclide angiography[40,41,43] and echocardiography.[42] Planar and tomographic radionuclide ventriculography have been directly compared in the assessment of regional left ventricular function in patients with a left ventricular aneurysm before and after aneurysmectomy. Tomographic radionuclide angiography appeared to provide information that was more accurately predictive of results after aneurysmectomy compared to planar imaging.[44]

Global LVEF by gated blood pool tomography compares favorably to LVEF by planar equilibrium radionuclide angiography ($r = 0.92$, SEE 4.2) and by contrast ventriculography ($r = 0.79$, SEE 7.0).[40] Calculation of left ventricular volumes from gated blood pool tomography is discussed in Chap. 12.

Gated blood pool tomography is becoming increasingly feasible as a clinical approach to the assessment of global and regional left ventricular function. As noted in Chap. 4, global and regional left ventricular function have also been estimated from gated myocardial perfusion tomograms. However, as a result of limitations in edge detection from gated tomographic perfusion images in regions of severe myocardial hypoperfusion, gated blood pool tomography is likely to become a noninvasive standard against which other measurements of left ventricular function will be compared.

CONCLUSION

Equilibrium radionuclide angiocardiography is an important and clinically well validated technique to assess noninvasively cardiac function. The technique provides reliable and reproducible quantitative measurements of ventricular systolic and diastolic function. In addition, from good quality ERNA images a comprehensive qualitative assessment of cardiac morphology and function can be made. Appropriate clinical application of ERNA imaging can have an important impact on patient management.[45]

ACKNOWLEDGMENT

The author wishes to acknowledge Doctors David A. Parker, Kastytis C. Karvelis, James H. Thrall, and Jerry W. Froelich, authors of this chapter in the second edition of *Cardiac Nuclear Medicine*, some of whose text he has retained in this edition.

REFERENCES

1. Strauss W, Zaret BL, Hinley RJ, et al: A scintiphotographic method for measuring left ventricular ejection fraction in man without cardiac catheterization. *Am J Cardiol* 28:575, 1971.
2. Secker-Walter RH, Resnick L, Kunz H, et al: Measurement of left ventricular ejection fraction. *J Nucl Med* 14:798, 1973.
3. Thrall JH, Freitas JE, Swanson DP, et al: Clinical comparison of cardiac blood pool visualization with technetium-99m red blood cells labeled in vivo and with technetium-99m human serum albumin. *J Nucl Med* 19:796, 1978.
4. Pavel DG, Zimmer M, Patterson VN: In vivo labeling of red blood cells with 99m Tc: A new approach to blood pool visualization. *J Nucl Med* 18:305, 1977.
5. Atkins HL, Thomas SR, Buddemeyer U, et al: MIRD dose estimate report no. 14: Radiation absorbed dose from technetium-99m-labeled red blood cells. *J Nucl Med* 31:378, 1990.
6. Rehani MM, Sharma SK: Site of Tc-99m binding to the red blood cell: Concise communication. *J Nucl Med* 21:676, 1980.
7. Callahan RJ, Rabito CA: Radiolabeling of erythrocytes with technetium-99m: Role of band-3 protein in the transport of pertechnetate across the cell membrane. *J Nucl Med* 31:2004, 1990.
8. Callahan RJ, Froelich JW, McKusick KA, et al: A modified method for the in vivo labeling of red blood cells with Tc-99m: Concise communication. *J Nucl Med* 23:315, 1982.
9. Porter WC, Dees SM, Freitas JE, et al: Acid-citrate dextrose compared with heparin in the preparation of in vivo/in vitro technetium-99m red blood cells. *J Nucl Med* 24:383, 1983.
10. Hegge FN, Hamiliton GW, Larson SM, et al: Cardiac chamber imaging: A comparison of red blood cells labeled with Tc-99m in vitro and in vivo. *J Nucl Med* 19:129, 1978.
11. Kelbaek H: Technetium-99m labeling of red blood cells: In vitro evaluation of a new approach. *J Nucl Med* 271:1770, 1986.
12. Patrick ST, Glowniak JV, Turner FE, et al: Comparison of in vitro RBC labeling with the Ultratag® RBC kit versus in vivo labeling. *J Nucl Med* 32:242, 1991.
13. Hladik WB, Ponto JA, Stathis VJ: Drug-radiopharmaceutical interactions, in Thrall JH, Swanson DP (eds): *Diagnostic Interventions in Nuclear Medicine*. Chicago, Year Book Medical Publishers, 1985, pp 226–246.
14. Zanelli GD: Effect of certain drugs used in the treatment of cardiovascular disease on the "in vitro" labelling of red blood cells with Tc-99m. *Nucl Med Commun* 3:155, 1982.
15. Lee HB, Wexler JP, Scharf SC, et al: Pharmacologic alterations in Tc-99m binding by red blood cells: Concise communication. *J Nucl Med* 24:397, 1983.
16. Pauwels EK, Feitsma RIJ, Blom J: Influence of Adriamycin on red blood cell labeling: A pitfall in scintigraphic blood pool imaging. *Nucl Med Comm* 4:290, 1983.
17. Leitl GP, Drew HM, Kelly ME, et al: Interference with Tc-99m labeling of red blood cells by RBC antibodies. *J Nucl Med* 21:P44, 1980 (abstr).
18. Kelly MJ, Cowie AR, Antonino A, et al: An assessment of factors which influence the effectiveness of the modified in vivo technetium-99m-erythrocyte labeling technique in clinical use. *J Nucl Med* 33:2222, 1992.
19. Bacharach SL, Green MV, Borer JS, et al: Beat-by-beat validation of ECG gating. *J Nucl Med* 21:307, 1980.
20. Borer JS, Kent KM, Bacharach SL, et al: Sensitivity, specificity and predictive accuracy of radionuclide cineangiography during exercise in patients with coronary artery disease: Comparison with exercise electrocardiography. *Circulation* 60:572, 1979.
21. Hamilton GW, Williams DL, Caldwell JH: Frame rate requirements for recording time-activity curves by radionuclide angiography, in Sorenson JA (book coordinator): *Nuclear Cardiology: Selected Computer Aspects*. New York, Society Nuclear Medicine, 1978, pp 75–83.
22. Brash HM, Wraith PK, Hannan WJ, et al: The influence of ectopic heart beats in grated ventricular blood pool studies. *J Nucl Med* 21:391, 1980.
23. Winzelberg GG, Boucher CA, Pohost GM, et al: Right ventricular function in aortic and mitral valve disease: Relation of gated first-pass radionuclide angiography to clinical and hemodynamic findings. *Chest* 79:520, 1981.
24. Wackers FJTh, Mattera JA: Evaluation of cardiac function by radionuclide angiocardiography: In particular of the right ventricle. *Dynamic Cardiovascular Imaging* 1:292, 1988.
25. Kelly MJ, Giles RW, Simon TR, et al: Multigated equilibrium radionuclide angiocardiography: Improved detection of left ventricular wall motion abnormalities and aneurysms by the addition of the left lateral view. *Radiology* 139:167, 1981.
26. Reiber JHC, Lie SP, Simoons ML, et al: Clinical validation of fully automated computation of ejection fraction from gated, equilibrium blood-pool scintigrams. *J Nucl Med* 24:1099, 1983.
27. Lee FA, Fetterman R, Zaret BL, Wackers FJTh: Rapid radionuclide derived systolic and diastolic cardiac function using cycle-dependent background correction and Fourier analysis. In: *Proceedings of Computers in Cardiology*. IEEE Computer Society, Linkoping, Sweden, September 8–11, 1985, pp. 443–446.
28. Wackers FJTh, Berger HJ, Johnstone DE, et al: Multiple gated cardiac blood pool imaging for left ventricular ejection fraction: Validation of the technique and assessment of variability. *Am J Cardiol* 43:1159, 1979.
29. van Royen N, Jaffe CC, Krumholz HK, et al: Comparison and reproducibility of visual echocardiographic and quantitative radionuclide left ventricular ejection fraction: Clinical implications. *Am J Cardiol* 77:843, 1996.
30. The Multicenter Postinfarction Research Group. Risk stratification and survival after myocardial infarction. *N Engl J Med* 309:331, 1983.
31. Zaret BL, Wackers FJTh, Terrin ML, et al: Value of radionuclide rest and exercise left ventricular ejection fraction

in assessing survival of patients after thrombolytic therapy for acute myocardial infarction: Results of thrombolysis in myocardial (TIMI) phase II study. *J Am Coll Cardiol* 26:73, 1995.

32. Zaret BL, Wackers FJTh, Terrin ML, et al, for the TIMI investigators: Assessment of global and regional left ventricular performance at rest and during exercise following thrombolytic therapy for acute myocardial infarction: Results of the thrombolysis in myocardial infarction (TIMI) II study. *Am J Cardiol* 69:1, 1992.

33. Wackers FJTh: Gated blood pool imaging. Audiovisual Program. Continuing Education Lecture # 140, (video). Society of Nuclear Medicine, Reston, VA, 1988.

34. Wackers FJTh, Jaffe CC, Lynch PJ: Equilibrium and gated first pass radionuclide angiocardiography, (video laser disk). St. Louis, Mosby-Year Book, 1992.

35. Miller TR, Wallis JW, Sampathkumaran KS: Three-dimensional display of gated cardiac blood-pool studies. *J Nucl Med* 30:2036, 1989.

36. Faber TL, Stokely EM, Templeton GH, et al: Quantification of three-dimensional left ventricular segmental wall motion and volumes from gated tomographic radionuclide ventriculograms. *J Nucl Med* 30:638, 1989.

37. Gill JB, Moore RH, Tamaki N, et al: Multigated blood-pool tomography: New method for the assessment of left ventricular function. *J Nucl Med* 27:1916, 1986.

38. Barat J-L, Brendel AJ, Colle J-P, et al: Quantitative analysis of left-ventricular function using gated single photon emission tomography. *J Nucl Med* 25:1167, 1984.

39. Cerqueira MD, Harp GD, Ritchie JL: Quantitative gated blood pool tomographic assessment of regional ejection fraction: Definition of normal limits. *J Am Coll Cardiol* 20:934, 1992.

40. Corbett JR, Jansen DE, Lewis SE, et al: Tomographic gated blood pool radionuclide ventriculography: Analysis of wall motion and left ventricular volumes in patients with coronary artery disease. *J Am Coll Cardiol* 6:349, 1985.

41. Underwood SR, Walton S, Ell PJ, et al: Gated blood-pool emission tomography: A new technique for the investigation of cardiac structure and function. *Eur J Nucl Med* 10:332, 1985.

42. Honda N, Machida K, Takishima T, et al: Cinematic three-dimensional surface display of cardiac blood pool tomography. *Clin Nucl Med* 16:87, 1991.

43. Tamaki N, Mukai T, Ishii Y, et al: Multiaxial tomography of heart chambers by gated blood-pool emission computed tomography using a rotating gamma camera. *Radiology* 147:547, 1983.

44. Lu P, Liu X, Shi R, et al: Comparison of tomographic and planar radionuclide ventriculography in the assessment of regional left ventricular function in patients with left ventricular aneurysm before and after surgery. *J Nucl Cardiol* 1:537, 1994.

45. Port SC, Wackers FJTh: Clinical application of radionuclide angiography. *J Nucl Cardiol* 2:551, 1995.

Radionuclide Ventriculography: Left Ventricular Volumes and Pressure–Volume Relations

Myron C. Gerson
Ronald Rohe

In this chapter, radionuclide assessment of ventricular volumes and pressures is discussed. These measurements provide useful information for the assessment of cardiac performance. Systolic cardiac performance is determined by four major factors: (1) frequency of contraction, (2) preload, (3) afterload, and (4) contractile state. For clinical assessment of cardiac hemodynamics, these determinants are often represented by (1) heart rate, (2) left ventricular end-diastolic volume, (3) systolic arterial blood pressure or systemic vascular resistance, and (4) ejection- or preejection-phase indices of the rate or degree of cardiac pressure or volume change. The left ventricular ejection fraction though widely used to measure left ventricular performance, does not provide an isolated assessment of the inotropic state of the left ventricle but, rather, is influenced by preload and afterload conditions. To further characterize the contractile state of the left ventricle, radionuclide ventriculography may be used to measure noninvasively left ventricular volumes. The rationale for making such measurements is discussed, as are the methods employed. Practical clinical aspects of these measurements are also considered. Finally, the use of indirect radionuclide measures of left ventricular filling pressure is discussed.

RELEVANCE OF LEFT VENTRICULAR VOLUME AND PRESSURE MEASUREMENT IN THE EVALUATION OF CARDIAC PERFORMANCE

Starling described the active tension of muscle fibers as a function of fiber length.[1] In vivo, the output of the heart in volumes per minute may be expressed as a function of the cardiac volume prior to ejection. For each individual patient, the heart can produce a range of cardiac outputs over a range of preejection volumes.

In the resting state, cardiac output is often indistinguishable in the normal and the diseased heart. Resting cardiac output in the diseased heart may be maintained by an increase in left ventricular end-diastolic volume, a reduction in afterload, or an increase in heart rate. Since the diseased heart may compensate for an imbalance between systemic cardiac output and systemic oxygen requirements by dilating (i.e., utilizing preload reserve), it is helpful to measure the end-diastolic volume to identify the contribution of augmented preload to the compensation of a failing heart. For example, a left ventricular ejection fraction of 55 percent may be normal if cardiac volumes are normal. If the left ventricle is dilated and impedance to ejection is low, as in mitral regurgitation, a left ventricular ejection fraction of 55 percent may correspond to depressed ventricular contractility.[2]

Systolic left ventricular function may also be expressed as a function of afterload. If this is expressed as a relationship of systolic arterial pressure or systemic vascular resistance versus left ventricular ejection fraction, the contribution of preload to measured left ventricular performance remains undefined. If left ventricular end-systolic volume is used in place of ejection fraction, however, contractility may be assessed more directly, because the end-systolic volume has been found to be independent of preload.[3] Increasing levels of left ventricular end-systolic pressure (Fig. 12-1, upper left corner of the loop) produce a linear increase in end-systolic volume if contractility is not altered. Therefore, the con-

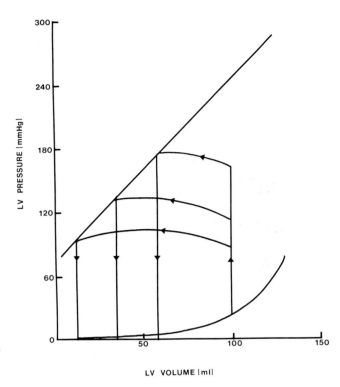

Figure 12-1 Three left ventricular pressure–volume loops generated at varying levels of afterload when ventricular preload is artificially held constant. The curvilinear relationship of diastolic pressure and volume forms the lower segment of each loop. Since preload is constant, each loop shares the end-diastolic volume illustrated by the line with an upward arrow at 100 ml. However, varying systolic pressures (illustrated by lines with horizontal arrows) produce varying levels of end-systolic volume when left ventricular contractility remains unchanged. Points locating the end-systolic pressure and volume of the left ventricle can be connected by a straight line. The slope of this straight line reflects left ventricular contractility independent of loading conditions. (Adapted from Ross,[2] reprinted with permission of the American College of Cardiology, *Journal of the American College of Cardiology,* 5:811, 1985.)

ejection fraction but the contractile state of the myocardium may be normal.

Drug interventions in patients with cardiac disease often produce changes in both loading conditions and myocardial contractility. To assess the influence of such interventions on preload, serial radionuclide measurements of left ventricular end-diastolic volume can be used. To assess the effect of a drug directly on myocardial contractility, radionuclide measurement of left ventricular end-systolic volume can be used to measure the end-systolic pressure–volume relationship.

Limitations of ejection-phase indices, including the ejection fraction, are also shown by the response to physiologic interventions. In a patient with a resting left ventricular ejection fraction of 60 percent, a severely hypertensive response to exercise may be accompanied by an exercise ejection fraction of 60 percent. Although an increase in ejection fraction with exercise in response to catecholamine stimulation might be expected, failure of the ejection fraction to rise might result from diminished contractility or from an abnormal rise in afterload. The latter factor would be considered in measurement of the end-systolic pressure–volume relationship during exercise. Therefore, clinical application of the left ventricular ejection fraction as a measure of ventricular contractility must be interpreted in the context of preload, afterload, and heart rate. The left ventricular end-systolic pressure–volume relationship offers a potential measure of left ventricular contractility independent of loading conditions.

METHODS FOR LEFT VENTRICULAR VOLUME MEASUREMENT BY RADIONUCLIDE VENTRICULOGRAPHY

Geometric Methods

Ventricular volumes measured from contrast ventriculography by length-area methods[7,8] have served as a standard for noninvasive volume measurements. These methods require the assumption that the shape of the left ventricle can be approximated by the shape of a prolate ellipse. Then the left ventricular volume (vol_{LV}) may be approximated from a single-plane angiogram by the formula

$$vol_{LV} = LD^2 (\pi/6)CF^3 \qquad (1)$$

where L = longest measured left ventricular axis
D = short axis measurement derived from length (L) and a planimetered area of the ventricle ($D = 4A/\pi L$)
CF^2 = correction factor relating a 1-cm² grid to an observed measurement of the grid on film

tractile state of the left ventricle can be related to the slope of the end-systolic pressure–volume relationship.[4,5] Assessment of the contractile state of the ventricle by systolic pressure–volume relationships is illustrated by considering a normal subject who is subjected to a pharmacologic increase in afterload. As the systemic arterial pressure rises with phenylephrine infusion in normal subjects pretreated with atropine, the ejection fraction of the left ventricle falls.[6] The left ventricle dilates in diastole and in systole, tending to maintain a normal end-systolic pressure–volume relationship.[6] In a patient with heart disease, the left ventricular end-diastolic volume may already be increased prior to drug infusion, limiting the extent to which the heart can further dilate (limited preload reserve) in response to afterload stress. As a further example, in a patient with severe aortic stenosis, abnormally elevated afterload may depress the left ventricular

The correction factor is then modified for volume measurement (CF³).

Similar geometric approaches have been applied to the measurement of volumes by first-pass radionuclide angiography (usually using a multicrystal gamma camera) and to equilibrium radionuclide ventriculography.[9-11] These measurements have been limited by the poor resolution of standard gamma cameras. Limited resolution of equilibrium blood-pool images can lead to unacceptable interobserver and intraobserver variability in the detection of left ventricular edges. Commercially available semiautomated edge-detection routines available for the determination of left ventricular ejection fraction provide improved reproducibility but appear to underestimate the area of the left ventricle by incorrectly locating the left ventricular edges within the left ventricular contour. Modification of the second derivative method of edge detection may provide improved edge-detection reproducibility without underestimating volumes,[12,13] but further validation is needed.

The assumption that the shape of the left ventricle can be approximated by a prolate ellipse becomes increasingly tenuous when segmental disorders of the ventricle are present in coronary artery disease or when the ventricle dilates, as in valvular regurgitation. Approximation of the shape of the right ventricle from a geometric figure is even more problematic.

Massie and associates[11] compared single and biplane area–length measurements of left ventricular volumes obtained by radionuclide methods to those obtained by a nongeometric counts-based method. The radionuclide volume measurements were compared with contrast angiography volumes in 20 patients. Volumes from the nongeometric counts-based method correlated most closely with volume measurements from contrast ventriculography ($r = 0.98$). Standard errors of the estimates for geometric techniques were high relative to nongeometric methods ($p < 0.05$), and the 95 percent confidence levels for geometric volumes were wide.

With the advent of gated single photon emission computed tomography (SPECT), a geometric method incorporating three-dimensional volume-rendered images might be used to assess left ventricular (LV) volume directly.[14,15] The practical use of such techniques is, perhaps, most hampered by the decreased spatial resolution of SPECT images as compared with their planar counterparts. Also, with gating, each three-dimensional volume-rendered cardiac time phase will likely suffer from poor count statistics, resulting in ill-defined volume boundaries. The recent introduction of fan-beam and cone-beam SPECT, together with dual- and triple-headed cameras, may improve overall count sensitivity to a degree sufficient to overcome these shortcomings.

For the sake of convenience, these three-dimensional volume studies might be combined with perfusion imaging; however, there then appears the possibility of an ill-defined wall boundary, owing to myocardial perfusion defects. These defects must be "patched" before volume determinations are made.

In a later section, estimation of left ventricular volumes by *gated SPECT* is revisited under the heading of *blood-pool tomography*.

Nongeometric Techniques: Preliminary Considerations

With adequate mixing in the blood, the concentration of radionuclide blood tracers is inversely proportional to the total circulating blood volume. Under stable conditions, blood contained in a vascular structure such as the heart will emit a constant amount of activity per unit of volume. Measurement of intravascular volume in an organ by blood-pool tracers is fundamentally based on the premise that the measured volume is directly proportional to the radioactivity emitted from that organ and inversely proportional to the concentration of radioactivity in the blood contained in the organ:

Intravascular volume of an organ

$$\propto \frac{\text{emitted radioactivity from the organ}}{\substack{\text{concentration of radioactivity} \\ \text{in blood in the organ}}} \quad (2)$$

The actual radionuclide measurement of ventricular volumes by this relationship involves a number of variables, which may be summarized by the following relation:

$$\text{vol}_{LV}\,(\text{ml}) = \frac{R\,(\text{cps})}{S\,(\text{cps/mCi})\,D\,(\text{mCi/ml})} \quad (3)$$

where R = observed net count rate from the ventricular chamber, expressed as

$$\frac{\text{net LV counts}}{\text{time per frame} \times \text{no. of cardiac cycles}}$$

S = Sensitivity for detecting activity in the heart (i.e., count rate expected per unit activity from the ventricle),
expressed as
(cps/mCi for a standard counted in air) × (an attenuation correction)
D = activity density in blood in the left ventricle determined from a blood sample, expressed as mCi activity/ml blood.

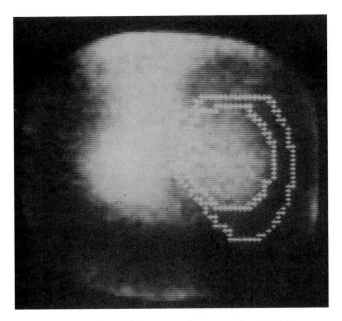

Figure 12-2 Radionuclide ventriculogram in the 40° left anterior oblique projection. Manual and semiautomated regions of interest are drawn around the left ventricular activity on the end-diastolic frame. The manually drawn region of interest is the larger of the two. (From Links et al,[16] reproduced with permission of the American Heart Association, Inc.)

MEASUREMENT OF COUNTS FROM THE VENTRICLE

Measurement of the observed count rate (R) from the ventricular chamber requires the separation of counts originating from the ventricular chamber (net counts) from counts originating from superimposed activity from other blood-containing organs (e.g., lung) and from scattered counts (*tissue cross talk*). Collectively these last two factors are imprecisely referred to as *background* activity. Identification of counts in the ventricle requires the generation of a region of interest enclosing the chamber (Fig. 12-2). This may be done using a manually drawn region of interest or an automated mathematically determined outline (usually using a second derivative edge-detection program). Links and associates[16] found that the regions created by a commercially available computer program led to underestimation of left ventricular end-diastolic volume by an average of 41 percent. Similar underestimation did not occur using larger, manually selected regions of interest (Fig. 12-2). One disadvantage of manually selected regions of interest is their limited reproducibility.[17] Links and associates found a 12 percent intraobserver variability in volume measurements using manually selected regions of interest. In addition, Fearnow and associates,[18] using an elliptical phantom, found that larger regions of interest surrounding the left ventricle overestimated left ventricular counts, apparently by including an increased number of scattered photons.

It is likely that the use of a *best septal* left anterior oblique projection would improve the selection of a region of interest around the left ventricle, particularly when cardiac rotation is present.[19] This may improve measurement of counts from the left ventricle. The selected angle would then be used in calculating the depth of the center of the ventricle in the chest (see discussion of attenuation distance below). Further validation of this modification of the Links method is needed.

Counts acquired from the region of interest surrounding the left ventricle may be corrected for background activity by a computer program that selects a background region of interest adjacent to the ventricle. Although reproducible, this approach incorrectly presumes that background activity in the region of the heart is uniform[20] and also that activity in a background region of interest adjacent to the heart is equivalent to background activity superimposed on the heart. Because background activity behind the heart is attenuated by cardiac contents, this assumption is not valid. Nevertheless, several authors have found good correlation of radionuclide ventricular volumes with volumes obtained by contrast ventriculography, using a paracardiac region for background correction.

SENSITIVITY FOR DETECTING ACTIVITY IN THE HEART

Sensitivity of the detector   The sensitivity (S) for detecting activity in the heart depends on the sensitivity of the detector and the magnitude of photon attenuation by tissues between the heart and the detector. Detector sensitivity is maintained constant from study to study by monitoring constancy of gamma-camera performance, collimation, and photopeak width. For some older gamma cameras, a correction of the ventricular count rate for camera dead time may be advisable.[21]

Attenuation distance   The effect of attenuation on the observed count rate depends on the attenuation coefficient and the attenuation distance of tissues located between the cardiac blood pool and the detector. Links and associates[16] determined the attenuation distance (d) by measurement of the horizontal distance (d') from the computer-defined center of the left ventricle to a technetium marker placed on the chest wall overlying the center of the left ventricle in the 40° left anterior oblique projection. The actual depth of the center of the left ventricle in the chest during imaging in the 40° left anterior oblique projection is given by $d'/\sin 40°$ (see Fig. 12-3). This approach has been substantiated by others.[22-24] The distance of attenuation (d) has also been calculated by echocardiography[25] and from the left posterior oblique image of the radionuclide ventriculogram.[26] Verani and associates,[19] in a study of intra- and interobserver variability in radionuclide measurement of left ventricular volumes, found the determination of left ven-

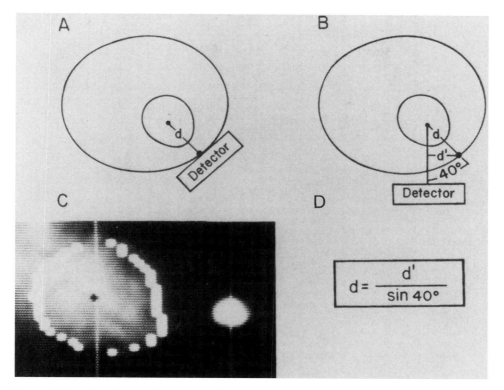

Figure 12-3 Calculation of the distance from the heart to the chest wall. Analysis of the anterior view. **A:** Depth of the center of the ventricle (d) along the left anterior oblique axis. **B:** Projection of d in the anterior view (d'). **C:** Measurement of d' as the horizontal distance from the computer-defined center of the ventricle to the technetium marker on the chest. **D:** Calculation of d from d'. (From Links et al,[16] reprinted with permission of the American Heart Association, Inc.)

tricular depth to be the main factor responsible for volume measurement variability.

Attenuation coefficient Links and associates[16] proposed that heart, lung, and chest wall attenuation could be approximated using the attenuation coefficient in water for the major technetium-99m (^{99m}Tc) energy photopeak (i.e., 0.15 cm^{-1}). Use of the linear attenuation coefficient of water for these measurements assumes the absence of Compton scatter and fails to take into account the large amount of air present in the chest, which may lower the average attenuation of photons from the heart. Chest wall attenuation studies using calculations from transmission computed tomography,[27] radionuclide sources in the esophagus,[28,29] and phantom studies[30,31] have demonstrated that chest wall attenuation in cardiac blood-pool imaging is considerably less than the attenuation coefficient for water. In these studies, an attenuation coefficient for cardiac blood-pool imaging in the range of 0.12 to 0.13 cm^{-1} has generally been demonstrated.

An attenuation coefficient for use in the measurement of ventricular volumes has been estimated by counting the activity of a ^{99m}Tc solution placed in the balloon of

a flotation catheter and measured in air compared with the activity detected with the balloon inside a cardiac chamber.[32] In 10 adult male patients, this yielded an attenuation coefficient of 0.12 cm^{-1}. Regardless of the method used, the attenuation coefficient will change constantly with respiration and cardiac motion. It is not currently clear whether these various limitations to the correction of emitted counts for tissue attenuation will alter computed left ventricular volumes to a clinically important extent. For most clinical applications, an error of 15 percent in the measurement of left ventricular volume is not likely to have an effect on patient management.

An alternative approach to the use of an assumed attenuation correction of observed activity from the region of the ventricle is to measure a *transmission factor.* One such approach relates the count rate of a capsule containing ^{99m}Tc measured in air to the capsule count rate in a retrocardiac location in the esophagus.[29] This method is illustrated in Fig. 12-4.

Some newer tomographic cameras directly obtain a three-dimensional attenuation map computed from simultaneously acquired transmission images (using external activity sources). The attenuation map is then directly

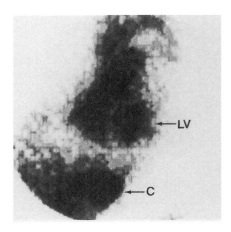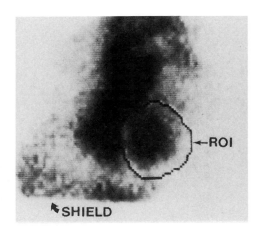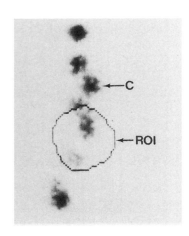

Figure 12-4 A capsule (C), containing a 1- to 2-mCi dose of ^{99m}Tc-sulfur colloid is attached to a sewing thread and the count rate in air is determined with a scintillation camera. The capsule is then swallowed by the patient. The intensity of the activity from the capsule dims when it reaches the level of the left ventricle (*right panel*). Without moving the patient, the patient's red blood cells are labeled in vivo with ^{99m}Tc pertechnetate (*left panel*), and a region of interest (ROI) is manually drawn surrounding the left ventricle (LV) (*central panel*). The capsule count rate from the esophagus compared with the capsule count rate in air is determined, enabling the calculation of a transmission factor for the capsule. This transmission factor is then used to adjust count rates from the left ventricle compared with venous blood activity measured in air in order to account for effects of tissue attenuation. (From Maurer et al,[29] reprinted with permission of the American Heart Association, Inc.)

employed as the basis for a more complete three-dimensional attenuation correction, as compared with the previously cited methods.

Self-attenuation As discussed earlier in this chapter, measurement of the intravascular volume of an organ is based on the premise that the volume is proportional to the radioactivity emitted from the organ. This does not imply that tracer activity from different locations within the cardiac blood pool is detected equally by an external counter. A point source within the heart farther from the gamma detector will be shielded by more blood-pool contents than a point source within the blood pool closer to the detector. This self-attenuation phenomenon[33] may become particularly important in a patient with coronary artery disease, in whom different segments of the left ventricle may contract to varying degrees. Schneider et al[34] studied the effects of simulated regional contraction abnormalities by using radionuclide techniques in a heart model. Regional contraction abnormality located in the anterior region of the blood pool (and with minimal self-attenuation effect) produced underestimation of the actual left ventricular ejection fraction. Regional contraction abnormality located in the posterior region of the blood pool (with maximal self-attenuation effect) produced overestimation of the actual left ventricular ejection fraction. When left ventricular ejection fractions were calculated from absolute left ventricular volumes measured by radionuclide methods, the correlation with actual left ventricular ejection fraction, as determined by contrast angiography, improved substantially. This may have resulted from correction for attenuation (in-

cluding the distance of blood-pool activity from the gamma detector) during the measurement of absolute ventricular volumes.

MEASUREMENT OF ACTIVITY DENSITY IN BLOOD

Many, but not all, radionuclide techniques for measuring ventricular volumes require the withdrawal of a blood sample from the patient for the purpose of counting blood radioactivity. Blood is withdrawn during the process of counting activity emitted from the ventricle. Activity in the blood sample is subsequently counted on the same detector used to image the heart. The blood may be counted on a flat Petri dish to minimize self-attenuation. A correction is made for physical decay of the tracer from the time of blood withdrawal to the time of counting.

If the concentration of activity in the blood sample will be related to more than one measurement of activity emitted from a ventricular chamber (e.g., serial volume measurements in a patient before and after drug intervention), then the stability of the tracer must be carefully monitored. Burns and associates[17] observed a mean in vivo half-time of ^{99m}Tc-labeled red blood cells (RBCs) of 4.1 h, but there was considerable interpatient and intrapatient variability.

The concentration of radioactive tracer in the blood pool may change with varying imaging conditions in addition to any alteration associated with changing ventricular volumes. Konstam and associates[35] observed an increase in blood activity concentration with exercise after in vivo RBC labeling with ^{99m}Tc. This increase was related to an increase in RBC count with exercise[35] and appears to result from splenic contraction with release of erythrocytes.[36] In contrast, Vatterott and associates, using the modified in vivo RBC labeling method of Callahan et al (see Chap. 11), found a rise in blood hematocrit value with exercise but no change in left ventricular blood radioactivity.[37]

Specific Implementations of Nongeometric Techniques

RELATIVE VOLUMES

Changes in ventricular size on serial assessments may be quantitated using relative volume measurements. For example, activity from the left ventricle may be compared before and after drug intervention. From Eq. (3), it is apparent that the count rate from the left ventricle for each measurement must be corrected for the time per frame and the number of cardiac cycles acquired. Patient positioning[38] and the approach to outlining the left ventricle and selecting a background region to correct for background activity must be consistent. The same detector system is used and tissue attenuation is assumed to be constant. Because no measurement of absolute volume is made, no blood sample is needed. However, a correction must be made for the physical decay of the tracer between serial measurements. The relative change in left ventricular volume may be expressed as the change in background- and decay-corrected left ventricular counts between serial assessments expressed as a percentage of initial counts.

NONGEOMETRIC VOLUMES FROM REGRESSION EQUATIONS

Early nongeometric methods for the estimation of left ventricular volumes compared the count rate over the left ventricle to the count rate from a blood sample withdrawn from the patient but made no direct attempt to correct the counted activity for tissue attenuation.[39,40] The resultant estimates were then fitted to volume measurements from contrast ventriculography using linear regression equations. However, for increased left ventricular volumes, the relationship between left ventricular counts and volumes is not linear, probably as a result of self-attenuation effects.[41] Furthermore, these early methods[39,40,42,43] assume that tissue attenuation is the same in all patients. Difficulty with volume estimates in very thin or very obese patients would be expected. A standard error of 28 ml in the measurement of left ventricular diastolic volume (mean diastolic volume, 189 ml) is not uncommon[43] and represents a 15 percent measurement error.

NONGEOMETRIC VOLUME MEASUREMENTS WITH CORRECTION FOR TISSUE ATTENUATION

In 1982, Links and associates[16] proposed a method for left ventricular volume measurement that provided a correction for tissue attenuation of emitted radioactivity for each individual patient. As discussed in an earlier section, this method assumed that the tissue attenuation coefficient (μ) for ^{99m}Tc in the cardiac blood pools was equivalent to the attenuation coefficient for water. The depth of the heart in the chest (d) was calculated geometrically (Fig. 12-3). The calculation of left ventricular volume could then be summarized by the following equation:

$$\text{vol}_{LV} = \frac{(\text{count rate from LV})e^{\mu d}}{\text{count rate/ml blood sample}} \qquad (4)$$

This approach has been substantiated by others.[22-24,44] Parrish and associates[45] have used a similar approach to measure left and right ventricular volumes in children. A high correlation of left ventricular volume measurements from nongeometric radionuclide methods with those from contrast ventriculography was found in children ($r = 0.94$, $p < 0.05$), but the standard error of the estimate was 25 ml, with the mean absolute error between radionuclide and cineangiographic volumes being 20 to 34 percent.

An alternative approach to the correction of left ventricular counts for tissue attenuation has been proposed by Harpen and associates.[46] Left ventricular attenuation is determined by analysis of the dynamics of the bolus of ^{99m}Tc-labeled RBCs observed during the first pass through the left ventricle before the beginning of data acquisition of the equilibrium blood-pool scan. If the total injected activity is measured in air (by counting the activity in the injection syringe placed on the face of the gamma camera) and again as it passes through the left ventricle attenuated by body tissues, the ratio of these two measurements (the transmission factor) can be used to correct for tissue attenuation of counts from the left ventricle during the equilibrium blood-pool study.

An approach to the measurement of left ventricular volumes that has been proposed by Nichols and associates[47] requires no geometric assumptions and avoids the problem of radiation attenuation correction. This method is based on the observation that the pixel within the left ventricle containing the most counts at diastole, as seen in the left anterior oblique projection, should correspond to the deepest region of the left ventricle (Fig. 12-5). If a first-pass study is obtained in the right anterior oblique projection (90° away from the left anterior oblique projection subsequently used for equilibrium imaging), then the widest portion of the ventricle (L) on the first-pass image will generally correspond to the depth of the pixel with the greatest activity on the left anterior oblique image. The maximum depth of the ventricle on

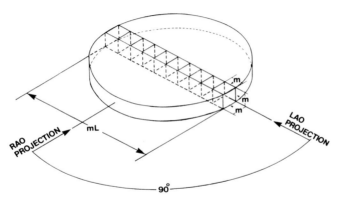

Figure 12-5 The depth of the pixel from the left ventricle that contains the highest count rate, as viewed from the left anterior oblique (LAO) projection is measured as the length of the corresponding column of voxels viewed on the right anterior oblique (RAO) projection, 90° away. Each voxel has a volume of m^3, so that the deepest pixel corresponds to a column of L voxels having a total volume of Lm^3. (From Nichols et al,[47] reprinted with permission of the American Heart Association, Inc.)

an ungated first-pass image will represent the depth at end diastole measured in units of pixels. The depth of the left ventricle (L) is converted to mL in centimeters, where m is a magnification factor relating 64 pixels on the computer image to a span of 18 cm in both the X and Y directions. The deepest column of blood in the left ventricle, as seen on the left anterior oblique view corresponding to the pixel with maximum diastolic counts (M), will have a volume of Lm^3 (Fig. 12-5). With complete mixing of the tracer in blood, the observed count rate per volume from the blood contained in the deepest pixel is

$$C = M/Lm^3 \qquad (5)$$

where M (following background correction) = the maximum count rate per pixel from the left ventricle, and Lm^3 = the maximum volume of a left ventricular pixel on the left anterior oblique view.

The volume of the left ventricle (vol_{LV}) at end diastole is

$$\text{diastolic } vol_{LV} = D/C = DLm^3/M \qquad (6)$$

where D = the observed total count rate from the ventricle at end diastole, with background correction.

Measurement of ventricular volume by this method compared favorably with actual volumes from a phantom and with clinical measurements obtained by ther-

modilution techniques in patients (Fig. 12-6). Nichols and associates[47] observed that the major source of error for this method is the measurement of ventricular depth from the first-pass study. Errors on the order of 10 percent would be expected for the average range of human end-diastolic volumes. Nevertheless, the approach is easily implemented, highly automated, and likely to be accurate as long as the first-pass acquisition is orthogonal to the subsequent acquisition angle for the blood-pool image. In fact, on cameras equipped with 90° dual-head geometry, this might be the method of choice.

Recently, Massardo and associates[48] have presented a similar method in which left ventricular volume is related to the ratio of total left ventricular region-of-interest counts to the count average of the "hottest" four-pixel region in the left ventricle as assessed on the left anterior oblique projection. Not only does this method eliminate the need for attenuation correction and peripheral blood sampling, but it also requires no measurement of the length of the long axis of the left ventricle. The same method can be applied to first-pass radionuclide angiography.[49]

Yen and associates[50] have taken a more elaborate approach and devised a conjugate counting technique that uses both an external reference and a patient blood sample. Figure 12-7 shows the series of images that must be acquired. This scheme explicitly measures and corrects for both body attenuation and self-attenuation, and may be the most theoretically accurate approach in the literature.

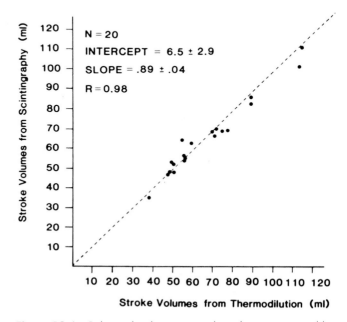

Figure 12-6 Relationship between stroke volumes measured by the scintigraphic method and thermodilution measurements. (From Nichols et al,[47] reprinted with permission of the American Heart Association, Inc.)

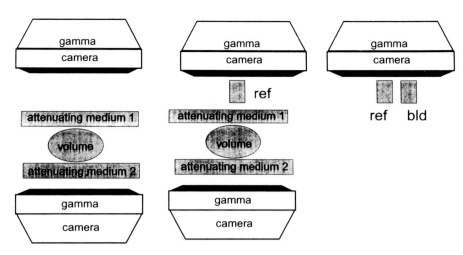

Figure 12-7 Schematic diagram of the series of three conjugate-view acquisitions required to quantitate left-ventricular "volume". The attenuating media 1 and 2 schematically represent overlying and underlying attenuating tissues in the patient's body. The "ref" (reference) source and "bld" (blood) sample are of equal geometry and volume but need not be the same activity. (From Yen et al,[50] A count-based radionuclide method for volume quantitation using conjugate imaging and an external reference source: Theoretical consideration and phantom study. *J Nucl Med* 35:644, 1994, reprinted with permission.)

LEFT VENTRICULAR VOLUMES FROM BLOOD-POOL TOMOGRAPHY

Tomographic gated blood-pool images have been used to generate absolute left ventricular volumes without attenuation correction, background correction, or geometric assumptions.[51-53] Plane projections are collected over a 180° or 360° arc around the patient. Tomographic blood-pool slices are created by filtered backprojection and oriented perpendicular to the cardiac axes (Fig. 12-8). Left ventricular blood-pool activity is isolated from surrounding structures on serial short-axis tomograms.[51] Left ventricular volume is determined based on the methods of Tauxe and associates.[54] The length of one pixel on the tomographic image is determined from a radioactive source of known length. The volume of a three-dimensional pixel or voxel can then be determined. For a tomographic slice with a depth of one pixel, the number of voxels within the left ventricular region times the volume per voxel will give the actual volume of the slice. From phantom studies, a threshold of 45 percent of the maximum counts per pixel in the reconstructed image has been used to define the borders of the left ventricle in some studies.[51,54] The sum of the volumes of the left ventricular slices in the tomographic sections yields the total left ventricular volume. Correlation coefficients relating tomographic radionuclide volumes to angiographic volumes have been in the range of $r = 0.81$ to 0.97, with a standard error of the estimate ranging from 13 to 27 cm³.[51-53]

Alternate approaches to the calculation of left ventricular volumes from blood-pool tomograms have been suggested that incorporate counts-based methods.[55-57] In one method,[55] tomographic slices that are one pixel thick are generated through the left ventricle, and ventricular counts are outlined with hand-drawn regions of interest.

Short Axis   Four Chamber   RAO Long Axis

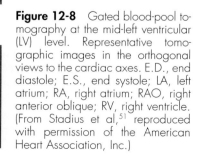

Figure 12-8 Gated blood-pool tomography at the mid-left ventricular (LV) level. Representative tomographic images in the orthogonal views to the cardiac axes. E.D., end diastole; E.S., end systole; LA, left atrium; RA, right atrium; RAO, right anterior oblique; RV, right ventricle. (From Stadius et al,[51] reproduced with permission of the American Heart Association, Inc.)

It is assumed that the distribution of radiotracer activity is homogeneous within the ventricular chamber, and that a similar homogeneous distribution of activity is present in each one-pixel-thick tomographic slice comprising the total left ventricular volume. The average count per pixel in the left ventricle, K, is determined by placing a 5×5-pixel rectangular region of interest centrally in each slice. The average number of counts per pixel in the rectangular region is determined for each tomographic slice through the left ventricle. These values are then averaged for all the left ventricular tomographic slices, yielding the value of K. For each tomographic slice, the total number of counts in the hand-drawn left ventricular region of interest is divided by K, yielding the total number of *contributing pixels* in each slice. The total number of contributing pixels in all of the tomographic slices encompassing the left ventricle can then be summed. The volume corresponding to each pixel can be determined, as described above, and multiplied by the total number of contributing pixels to yield the left ventricular volume at any selected time during the cardiac cycle. The potential advantage of this approach is that pixels at the edges of the left ventricle, which may be only partly contained in the left ventricular contour, will be weighted less heavily in the volume calculation compared with pixels located centrally in the left ventricular cavity. Again with blood-pool tomography, the inclusion of transmission-emission capability would allow for a full three-dimensional attenuation compensation. This should eliminate most artifactual distortions in left ventricular volume-rendered shape and hence improve subsequent volume calculations, whether geometric or count based.

Precautions for Left Ventricular Volume Determination

Numerous technical factors can substantially alter radionuclide measurements of left ventricular volume. Common to the various methods for calculation of left ventricular volume is a major dependence on accurate identification of the left ventricular outline.[58-60] Geometric methods will suffer most from left ventricular boundary variability, because a small error in measuring a linear dimension compounds itself to the third power when corresponding volumes are calculated. For instance, a 20 percent increase in boundary linear dimension of the ellipsoidal axes will result in over a 70 percent increase in left ventricular volume. Object scatter interference will also cause variability in left ventricular volume results.[59,60] The degree of such object scatter interference will depend on the camera spatial resolution, on the energy discrimination window setting, and on patient size. The inclusion of object-scattered events within the left ventricular boundary will affect counts-based methods in direct proportion to that interference. Geometric methods will likely be less sensitive to this source of error as they are only affected indirectly via the left ventricular boundary blurring and threshold level changes that result from this interference.

In general, counts-based methods provide more accurate estimates of left ventricular volume compared with geometric methods.[11,58] When geometric methods are used, tomographic approaches appear to provide better estimates of left ventricular volumes compared with planar methods.[58] Regardless of the method selected, validation of radionuclide left ventricular volumes against measurement from contrast ventriculography or phantom studies is needed to assure accurate results for the volumetric method in an individual laboratory. It should not be assumed that published accuracy measurements for a particular left ventricular volume methodology can be universally ported over to other institutional imaging systems without local validation.

Measurement of Cardiac Output by Radionuclide Methods

Systolic left ventricular performance is determined by heart rate, contractility, and loading conditions. However, the end result of systolic left ventricular performance—forward cardiac output—is also altered directly or indirectly by additional factors, including valvular regurgitation, intracardiac shunting, cardiac arrhythmias, right ventricular function, and pericardial dynamics. Reproducible noninvasive measurements of forward cardiac output can provide valuable insight into baseline hemodynamics and the consequences of pharmacologic agents and other interventions.

Forward cardiac output may be estimated from the measurement of absolute left ventricular volumes by multiplying stroke volume by heart rate. Cardiac outputs measured in this manner, both at rest and during exercise, have been validated in comparison to cardiac outputs measured by the Fick method.[61] However, when left-sided valvular regurgitation or intracardiac shunting is present, a correction is needed to separate forward cardiac output from regurgitant or shunt flow. Although potential methods for this correction are available (see Chap. 24), the accuracy of such correction is unclear. The presence of biventricular regurgitant lesions or bidirectional shunting makes the accurate assessment of forward cardiac output from equilibrium left ventricular volume measurements even more problematic. Major cardiac arrhythmias (e.g., atrial fibrillation) make accurate calculation of forward cardiac output from equilibrium left ventricular volumes impossible by current methods.

Noninvasive measurement of cardiac output can also

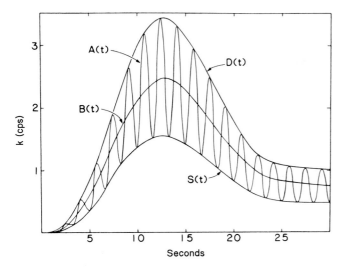

Figure 12-9 A left ventricular time–activity curve is shown. A(t), instantaneous; B(t), average; D(t), diastolic; S(t), systolic. (From Harpen et al,[46] reprinted with permission of the American Heart Association, Inc.)

be accomplished by first-pass radionuclide methods using indicator-dilution principles.[62-66] If a known quantity (*I*) of radioactive tracer is injected into a constantly flowing stream and the concentration of tracer can be determined by sampling as all of the tracer passes a point downstream, then the total flow (*F*) can be calculated as follows:

$$F = \frac{I}{\int_0^\infty c(t)\, dt} \qquad (7)$$

where *c* is the concentration of tracer in blood and *t* is time. Intravascular concentrations cannot be directly measured by an external counter. However, count rates can be detected in a volume of interest, and concentration and count rate are related.

It is assumed that

$$\frac{\int_0^\infty c(t)\, dt}{\int_0^\infty q(t)\, dt} = \frac{C_{eq}}{Q_{eq}} \qquad (8)$$

where C_{eq} = the blood concentration of tracer after complete equilibration in the vascular space, *q* = the mean height of the tracer curve during the bolus passage as recorded externally [e.g., the same as B(t) in Fig. 12-9], and Q_{eq} = the height of the tracer curve after complete equilibration. Therefore,

$$F = \frac{I}{\int_0^\infty q(t)\, dt \times C_{eq}/Q_{eq}}$$

or   (9)

$$F = \frac{Q_{eq}}{\int_0^\infty q(t)\, dt} \times \frac{I}{C_{eq}}$$

The quantity of radiotracer (*I*) divided by the equilibrium concentration of the radiotracer (C_{eq}) equals the distribution volume (V_d) of the tracer. The area (*A*) under the externally recorded passage of the tracer bolus is represented by $\int_0^\infty q(t)\, dt$. Blood flow is determined as

$$F = \frac{Q_{eq}}{A} \times V_d \qquad (10)$$

The height of the tracer curve after complete equilibration (Q_{eq}) may be obtained as the detected activity from a background-corrected left ventricular region of interest.[64] The area (*A*) under the averaged first-pass time–activity curve represents the total externally recorded counts from the passage of the tracer bolus. An averaged first-pass time–activity curve is shown in Fig. 12-9. Calculation of the area under the curve is facilitated by fitting the downslope of the curve with a gamma variate function, as shown in Fig. 12-10. The latter maneuver removes distortion of the downslope of the curve resulting from recirculation of the tracer. The distribution volume (V_d) is determined by dividing the known tracer dose (*I*) by the specific radioactivity of the equilibrated tracer in a blood sample (C_{eq}), drawn during external recording of the background-corrected activity curve.

Cardiac output determined by this method of exter-

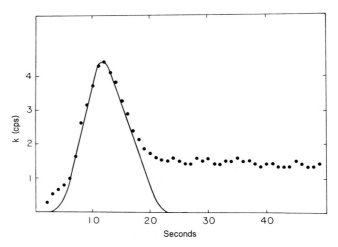

Figure 12-10 Gamma-variate extrapolation of first-pass time–activity curve. (From Harpen et al,[46] reprinted with permission of the American Heart Association, Inc.)

nal counting has shown excellent correlation ($r = 0.978$, standard error of the estimate 0.36, $p < 0.001$), compared with conventional invasive methods.[64] The first-pass method offers the advantage of measuring forward cardiac flow, which is especially important in patients with valvular regurgitation. The first-pass method allows calculation of cardiac output in spite of cardiac arrhythmias. In four patients with atrial fibrillation, Kelbaek and associates[64] found excellent agreement between first-pass radionuclide measurement of cardiac output and invasive cardiac outputs by the Fick method.

Nevertheless, a number of potential sources of error must be kept in mind in using the first-pass radionuclide method for determining cardiac output. The use of Eq. (7) requires certain assumptions, including (1) complete mixing of tracer between the injection and sampling sites, (2) complete initial injection of the tracer, and (3) complete assessment of the tracer at the sampling site until all tracer has flowed past without contamination by recycling tracer.[66] Satisfaction of these assumptions requires a bolus injection that is of good quality and adequate distance from injection site to sampling site to permit complete mixing of tracer and blood. Prolonged injection can produce recirculation of the tracer before the initial bolus leaves the field of view of the detector. This increases the area (A) under the first-pass curve, resulting in underestimation of cardiac output. Complete assessment of the first-pass of tracer at the sampling site requires a correction for recirculation by fitting the flow curve with a gamma variate or similar curve-fitting function. A prolonged bolus tends to contaminate the downslope of the time–activity curve, making curve fitting difficult.

Assumptions from Eq. (8) regarding the relationship of tracer concentration and observed tracer counts require that the transmission of counts be constant during the first-pass bolus and during equilibrium counting. This condition cannot be met completely, and some concern has been raised[67] as to the clinical significance of differences in background activity, scattered activity, and chest wall activity during the first-pass bolus and during equilibrium counting. Also, the radiopharmaceutical must remain entirely in the intravascular space during both first-pass and equilibrium counting. Diffusion of tracer out of the intravascular space probably occurs to a small extent following in vivo labeling of red blood cells, resulting in underestimation of equilibrium counts (Q_{eq}) and of cardiac output. Further pitfalls in the method can result from dead-time count losses when an older scintillation camera is being used and with improper region-of-interest selection.[68]

Left Ventricular Volumes and Cardiac Output: An Overview

Substantial progress had been made since nongeometric approaches to the measurement of left ventricular volumes by radionuclide ventriculography were first detailed in 1979. Problems of tissue attenuation, tissue cross talk and background-activity correction, and the need for peripheral blood sampling have been dealt with by a variety of new planar and tomographic methods of absolute volume estimation. As discussed earlier in this chapter, measurement of left ventricular end-diastolic volume enables study of the effects of ventricular preload on left ventricular contractility. Measurement of end-systolic volume enables assessment of ventricular contractility independent of preload variation. Therefore, measurement of absolute left ventricular volume is most likely to be clinically helpful in abnormal ventricular loading conditions, including valvular heart disease. Measurements of left ventricular volumes and of forward cardiac output are of fundamental importance in assessing changes in cardiac performance in response to drugs in the failing ventricle, and this is discussed in Chap. 17. It has been shown that some patients with coronary artery disease may be distinguished from normal subjects by the response of the left ventricular end-systolic volume to stress. An abnormal response of the left ventricular end-systolic volume to exercise may be observed in some patients with coronary artery disease even when the ejection-fraction response to exercise is normal.[69] Many of the principles for measurement of absolute left ventricular volumes can also be applied, potentially, to the measurement of absolute right ventricular volumes.[70] Approaches to the measurement of right ventricular volumes are made more difficult by the variable shape of the right ventricle and the lack of a simple, widely employed "gold standard" for measurement of right ventricular volumes. As radionuclide measurement of absolute ventricular volumes and forward cardiac output becomes more widely available, new applications will likely be found.

RADIONUCLIDE PRESSURE–VOLUME RELATIONS

Rationale

Left ventricular contractility may be assessed from isovolumic or ejection-phase indices or from analysis of ventricular function curves. Isovolumic-phase indices including peak dP/dt and maximum $(dP/dt)/P$ have proved useful in separating groups of patients with normal and depressed myocardial contractility. There has, however, been sufficient overlap of these values in normal subjects and patients with depressed myocardial contractility to limit the usefulness of these and other isovolumic indices in individual patients.[71]

Ejection-phase indices, including ejection fraction and ejection rate, have proven more clinically useful than isovolumic indices. As left ventricular dilation occurs, ejection-phase indices generally remain normal in the absence of heart failure. In left ventricular pressure overload, compensatory ventricular hypertrophy occurs, maintaining normal wall stress and normal ejection-phase indices. When cardiac failure from volume and/or pressure overload occurs, ejection-phase indices may become abnormal, reflecting depressed myocardial contractility or abnormal loading conditions.

Left ventricular contractility may be examined independently of loading conditions from ventricular end-systolic pressure–volume relations. The volume of the left ventricle at end systole is not dependent on the initial ventricular volume or preload,[3] but it is dependent on alteration of afterload. Afterload can be defined as the force acting on the fibers in the ventricular wall after the onset of shortening. Left ventricular afterload is determined by a number of variables, including the elasticity of the aorta and large arteries, tone of the systemic arterioles, viscosity of the blood, presence of aortic stenosis, and size and thickness of the left ventricle.

If the left ventricular end-systolic pressure and end-systolic volume are determined at different levels of afterload, the slope of the end-systolic pressure–volume relation may be calculated and used as an index of contractility that is relatively independent of loading conditions[72] (Fig. 12-1). Grossman and associates[73] found abnormality of the slope of the end-systolic pressure–volume relation to reflect clinically important impairment of contractile function in patients with cardiomyopathy. Support for this approach comes from animal studies[74–77] and from studies in humans[78–82] (see Fig. 12-11). Patients with high end-systolic afterload may develop a large end-systolic volume with minimal or no impairment of myocardial contractility. When afterload returns to normal, end-systolic left ventricular volume may then also normalize without a change in the contractile state of the left ventricle. Figure 12-1 illustrates how the contractile state of the left ventricle, as reflected in the slope of the end-systolic pressure–volume line, may remain constant when a change in left ventricular end-systolic volume results from a corresponding change in afterload. Carabello and Spann[83] have suggested that the presence of high end-systolic afterload may explain the relatively favorable prognosis observed in some patients presenting with aortic regurgitation and a large left ventricular end-systolic dimension. The left ventricular end-systolic volume may therefore provide a better index of ventricular contractility if it is related to the level of end-systolic afterload.

A number of potential limitations of end-systolic pressure–volume relationships in patients have been described. One limitation arises from the impracticality and potential danger of determining the slope of the end-systolic pressure–volume relation in patients. Changes in loading conditions may not be well tolerated in some patients. Furthermore, to assess left ventricular contractility by measuring multiple points on the end-systolic

pressure–volume curve, reflex changes in contractility must be avoided as afterload is changed. This requires the use of additional drugs that could have adverse effects in patients with impaired cardiac function. These problems with the measurement of multiple points on the end-systolic pressure–volume curve led to the consideration of a single point from the curve as a measure of ventricular inotropy. Since the X intercept of the end-systolic pressure–volume relation is usually not through zero volume and the X intercept may vary with changes in inotropy, an end-systolic pressure–volume ratio does not produce the same information regarding ventricular contractility as does the slope of the line relating end-systolic pressure to end-systolic volume.

A second limitation of the end-systolic pressure–volume relationship relates to the assumption that end-systolic pressure is an accurate measure of end-systolic afterload. Afterload relates not only to the pressure opposing ejection but also to the distribution of pressure over the surface to which the force is applied. By the Laplace relation, stress equals pressure times chamber radius divided by twice the wall thickness. Therefore, the effects of varied levels of ventricular afterload may be better related to end-systolic volume if ventricular wall thickness as well as pressure is taken into account by measuring left ventricular end-systolic stress. It has been suggested that the contractile state of the ventricle may be more effectively approximated by the relation-

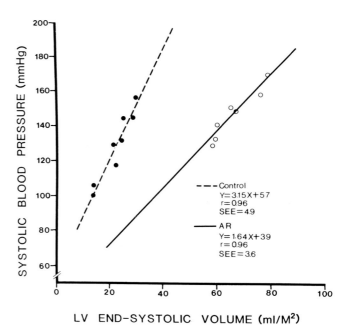

Figure 12-11 Systolic blood pressure–left ventricular end-systolic volume relationship at various levels of systolic blood pressure in control subjects (*solid circles*) and in asymptomatic patients with aortic regurgitation and a normal resting left ventricular ejection fraction (*open circles*). Note the differences in the slopes of the systolic blood pressure–left ventricular systolic volume relationship. (From Shen et al,[78] reproduced with permission of the American Heart Association, Inc.)

ship of end-systolic volume to the left ventricular end-systolic stress rather than to the pressure measurement.

The left ventricular end-systolic pressure–volume relationship may have other theoretical limitations as an index of myocardial contractility. Observed nonlinearity of the end-systolic pressure–volume relationship may limit its accurate characterization with a simple slope and volume intercept.[84] In the range of physiologic interventions in humans, this nonlinearity may be of limited importance.[85,86] Nevertheless, additional theoretical concerns have been expressed regarding dependence of the end-systolic pressure–volume relationship on left ventricular chamber size[86-89] and shape,[90] on left ventricular afterload,[91] on elevated left ventricular diastolic pressure,[92] and on left ventricular chamber stiffness.[93]

Noninvasive Approaches to Measurement of the End-Systolic Pressure–Volume Relationship

Assessment of ventricular contractility by a noninvasive measurement of the end-systolic pressure–volume relationship would offer many advantages for clinical work. The risk to the patient of contrast angiography would be avoided as well as any effects of the contrast material on ventricular contractility. Serial measurements could be made without limitation by a total contrast dose, and the effects of arrhythmias could be avoided. Furthermore, geometric assumptions inherent in the calculations of left ventricular volumes might be avoided.

NONINVASIVE MEASUREMENT OF END-SYSTOLIC VOLUME

Echocardiography has been used to estimate end-systolic volume. However, echocardiographic volume measurements require geometric assumptions that may result in limited accuracy when regional wall motion abnormality or ventricular dilation is present. In addition, delineation of ventricular chamber margins may be difficult in regions adjacent to papillary muscles. Echocardiography is technically limited in some patients, and the calculation of ventricular volumes is less automated than with radionuclide approaches.

Radionuclide measurement of left ventricular end-systolic volume has been discussed earlier in this chapter. It requires no geometric assumptions and can sample large numbers of cardiac cycles; arrhythmia can be rejected, contrast material can be avoided, and serial measurements can be performed. For these reasons, the use of radionuclide measurements of left ventricular end-systolic volume in the determination of end-systolic pressure–volume relationships appears to be an acceptable noninvasive alternative to angiographic volumes. Kronenberg and associates demonstrated that small changes in left ventricular end-systolic volume can be accurately

detected by radionuclide ventriculography. Radionuclide measurements of left ventricular end-systolic volumes and of the slope of the left ventricular end-systolic pressure–volume relationship correlated well with measurements obtained by contrast ventriculography in dogs.[94]

NONINVASIVE MEASUREMENT OF SYSTOLIC PRESSURE OR STRESS

In a study of normal subjects, Marsh and associates[95] confirmed a linear relationship of left ventricular end-systolic pressure and end-systolic dimension. Similarly, a linear relationship was demonstrated between the peak systolic blood pressure and end-systolic dimension. Although the slopes of the two relationships are not identical, the use of a relationship between peak systolic pressure and systolic length[95] or volume[96-98] appears to be a potentially useful measure of ventricular contractility that is independent of loading conditions. The importance of this observation is that peak systolic blood pressure may be recorded noninvasively by use of a sphygmomanometer. Unfortunately, not all authors have found the slope of the relationship between peak systolic blood pressure and end-systolic dimension to reliably reflect ventricular contractility,[81] and relatively few data are available to confirm that the noninvasive peak systolic blood pressure may be used in place of the end-systolic pressure from catheterization in patients with large stroke volumes and pulse pressures.[73] Marsh and colleagues have provided a noninvasive approach to the measurement of end-systolic pressure from the carotid pulse tracing,[95] but further confirmation is needed for this approach to the noninvasive measurement of the end-systolic pressure–volume relationship.

Left ventricular end-systolic stress determination requires measurement of left ventricular wall thickness, which may be accomplished noninvasively by echocardiography. Substitution of end-systolic stress for end-systolic pressure offers some potential advantages in the assessment of ventricular contractility. In a dilated ventricle, the effects of altered afterload may relate more to increased volume than increased pressure. Furthermore, ventricular wall thickness will influence the effect of end-systolic pressure on myocardial contractility.

SUBSTITUTION OF THE LEFT VENTRICULAR END-SYSTOLIC PRESSURE–VOLUME RATIO FOR THE SLOPE OF THE END-SYSTOLIC PRESSURE–VOLUME RELATIONSHIP

A further consideration in the assessment of ventricular contractility is the need for serial measurements under conditions of varying afterload to measure the slope of the end-systolic pressure–volume relationship.[99] This has been accomplished in patients through the administration of drugs such as methoxamine or nitroprusside, which alter afterload while presumably not substantially altering myocardial contractility[100] or by preload reduction by transient occlusion of the inferior vena cava.[85] Clinical applications of end-systolic pressure–volume relationships would be greatly facilitated if the risk and inconvenience to patients of repeated pressure–volume assessment under varying loading conditions could be obviated.

Sagawa and associates[101] described the end-systolic pressure–volume ratio as a new index of ventricular contractility. Nivatpumin and associates[102] constructed pressure–volume loops (Fig. 12-1) with micromanometer-tipped angiographic catheters in 35 patients. The ratio of peak systolic left ventricular pressure to end-systolic volume was obtained and found to reflect values for the peak ratio of left ventricular pressure to volume. This is not, however, the end-systolic pressure–volume ratio that was described by Sagawa et al as a measure of contractility.[101]

In patients undergoing cardiac catheterization for evaluation of chest pain, McKay and associates[96] found that a simple ratio of peak systolic left ventricular pressure to minimum systolic volume reasonably approximated the slope, E_{max}, of the isochronic pressure–volume line with maximum time-varying elastance. El-Tobgi and associates[103] evaluated systolic pressure–volume relationships in seven patients with normal coronary arteriograms and contrast ventriculograms, in five patients with a greater than 75 percent coronary artery stenosis and no evidence of previous myocardial infarction, and in eight patients with documented myocardial infarction and segmental akinesia by left ventriculography. The slope of the left ventricular end-systolic pressure–volume line was compared with the left ventricular end-systolic volume, the peak systolic pressure–volume ratio (at one point), and the volume axis intercept, V_0, for detection of left ventricular dysfunction. The slope of the left ventricular end-systolic pressure–volume relationship was the only one of these indices that could differentiate reliably between normal and impaired ventricles, whereas the peak systolic pressure–volume ratio did not (Fig. 12-12).

Role of the Left Ventricular End-Systolic Pressure–Volume Relationship

In patients with abnormal left ventricular loading conditions (e.g., valvular heart disease), assessment of ventricular contractility independent of preload and afterload is important in the understanding of disease pathophysiology and natural history. It is reasonable to expect that such an assessment will aid in the timing of treatment such as surgical valve replacement. A substantial literature confirms that the slope of the left ventricular end-

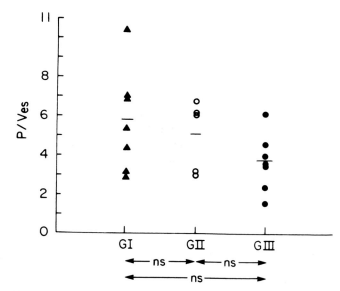

Figure 12-12 The ratio of peak left ventricular systolic pressure to end-systolic volume, P/V_{es} (mmHg/ml/m²), did not distinguish among the three groups of patients investigated. *Black triangles* represent subjects with normal coronary arteries (group I), *open circles* represent patients with coronary artery disease associated with normal left ventricular function (group II), and *black circles* represent patients with impaired left ventricular function (group III). (From El-Tobgi et al,[103] reprinted with permission from the American College of Cardiology, *Journal of the American College of Cardiology*, 3, 781, 1984.)

systolic pressure–volume relationship is useful in the assessment of ventricular contractility independent of loading conditions. Several studies suggest that the left ventricular end-systolic pressure–volume (or stress–volume) relationship may prove useful in determining the timing of valve replacement in regurgitant valvular heart disease,[104] verifying the importance of this index as a research tool. However, the slope of the left ventricular end-systolic pressure–volume relationship has not entered into general clinical use and is unlikely to do so unless it can be demonstrated that this index can provide conclusive information regarding the timing of valve replacement that is not available by other, less invasive means. The invasiveness of measuring the slope of the left ventricular end-systolic pressure–volume relationship, with its associated risk and inconvenience for the patient, makes the test unsuitable for serial measurements in conditions such as aortic regurgitation, which may have a lengthy natural history.

Attempts to assess ventricular contractility noninvasively from the slope of the peak systolic (or end-systolic) pressure/end-systolic volume relationship by using sphygmomanometry, carotid pulse tracings, radionuclide volume measurements, and echocardiographic measurements may make this index more clinically accessible and practical. Further verification is needed to determine whether noninvasive measurement of these indices can aid in making clinical decisions.

Less clear is the role of a simple systolic pressure–volume ratio for the assessment of ventricular contractility and guiding of therapy. The conflicting results[105,106] of available studies assessing the peak systolic (or end-systolic) pressure/end-systolic volume ratio as an index of ventricular contractility suggest that this measurement cannot be used interchangeably with the slope of the end-systolic pressure–volume relationship. The ratio of noninvasive peak systolic pressure to end-systolic volume does not appear to be ready for clinical use at the time of writing.

In addition to valvular heart disease, assessment of the slope of the left ventricular end-systolic pressure–volume relationship holds promise for clinical application in other conditions characterized by abnormal ventricular loading conditions. The effect of drug therapy on myocardial contractility in patients with heart failure is an important area that can be studied by the noninvasive end-systolic pressure–volume relationship. Pressure–volume indices have also been evaluated at rest and with exercise or atrial pacing in patients with coronary artery disease,[107–110] but no clinical advantage compared with the rest and exercise ejection fraction has been demonstrated.[111] The role of the systolic pressure–volume relationship in patients with coronary artery disease remains to be defined.

PRESSURE–VOLUME LOOPS IN THE ASSESSMENT OF LEFT VENTRICULAR PROPERTIES

Complete left ventricular pressure–volume loops of the type shown in Fig. 12-1 contain considerable information about left ventricular dynamics beyond that conveyed by the slope of the end-systolic pressure–volume line. When left ventricular pressure is measured, serial corresponding measurement of left ventricular volume throughout the cardiac cycle may be accurately obtained from equilibrium radionuclide ventriculography,[98] or from first-pass radionuclide angiocardiography,[112] permitting generation of pressure–volume loops. Complete pressure–volume loops not only provide characterization of pump performance with reasonable separation of ventricular properties from loading factors but also display systolic and diastolic ventricular properties in common terms and therefore help to clarify their interrelationships. Furthermore, pressure–volume loops provide a description of coupling between ventricle and vasculature, enabling predictions of stroke-volume and stroke-work responses to various loading interventions.[85,113]

Other Invasive and Noninvasive Approaches to Assessment of Left Ventricular Contractility

Efforts have continued to develop new load-independent indices to characterize the contractile state (and changes in the contractile state) of the left ventricle. In addition to independence of afterload or preload, an index of ventricular contractility should be unaltered by changes in the diastolic properties of the ventricle.[92,93] To be clinically applicable, an index of contractility should be reproducible, obtainable without significant risk to the patient, linear in its response to inotropic changes over an applicable clinical range, and, preferably, noninvasive.

In addition to the slope of the end-systolic pressure–volume relationship, several newer indices of left ventricular contractility have been proposed. The relationship between the maximal rate of left ventricular pressure development (dP/dt_{max}) and end-diastolic volume was found to be more sensitive to changes in the contractile state of the left ventricle compared with the slope of the end-systolic pressure–volume relation in dogs.[114] However, this invasively derived parameter has been less reproducible compared with the end-systolic pressure–volume slope in both animal models[114] and in humans[115] and was not a linear relation in some animal[116] and human studies.[115] A second invasive index of left ventricular contractility is the preload recruitable stroke work. This relationship of left ventricular stroke work and left ventricular end-diastolic volume has been found to be reproducible and appears to be linear over a broad range of left ventricular volumes.[114,115,117] The preload recruitable stroke volume has been less sensitive to changes in left ventricular contractility compared with the end-systolic pressure–volume relation in the range of interventions observed in some animal studies,[114] but this was not the case in other animal studies[117] and in humans.[115] As with the end-systolic pressure–volume relation, the preload recruitable stroke work depends on left ventricular size. Therefore, both indices may be more reliable for measuring serial changes in contractility in a single subject rather than as comparative indices of contractility in different patients.

Because of the coupling between the heart and the arterial system, contractility may also be assessed in relation to its adequacy compared with the load against which cardiac work is generated. Therefore, the end-systolic pressure–volume relation or end-systolic elastance (E_{es}) has been reexamined in the context of arterial elastance (E_a). Here, E_a is calculated as the relation of end-systolic left ventricular pressure to left ventricular stroke volume. In this framework, normal subjects with a left ventricular ejection fraction greater than or equal to 60 percent and ventricular elastance nearly twice as large as arterial elastance were observed to have maximal mechanical efficiency (defined as the ratio of stroke work to myocardial oxygen consumption per beat).[118] In patients with moderate heart failure and a left ventricular ejection fraction of 40 to 59 percent, left ventricular elastance was approximately equal to arterial elastance, thereby affording maximal stroke volume for a given end-diastolic volume. In patients with severe heart failure and a left ventricular ejection fraction of less than 40 percent, ventricular elastance was less than half of arterial elastance, resulting in increased left ventricular potential energy and decreased work efficiency. Thus, in the normal heart, ventriculoarterial coupling is set to provide high left ventricular work efficiency, in moderate left ventricular dysfunction ventriculoarterial coupling is matched to maintain stroke work at the expense of mechanical efficiency; and, in severe heart failure, both stroke work and work efficiency are depressed.[118] The relation of E_{es} to E_a has been derived through invasive studies. The potential for valid approximation of this index of cardiac function by noninvasive means is currently unclear.

The mean velocity of circumferential fiber shortening (Vcf) is an echocardiographic index that has been used to estimate left ventricular contractility noninvasively. Vcf is obtained as the difference between the left ventricular internal diameter in diastole minus the internal diameter in systole, divided by the internal diameter in diastole multiplied by the left ventricular ejection time. The left ventricular ejection time is obtained from noninvasive carotid pulse tracings[95,119] and corrected to a heart rate of 60 beats/min by dividing by the square root of the electrocardiographic R-R interval. Because Vcf is dependent on afterload, the latter has been incorporated by examining the left ventricular end-systolic wall stress to velocity of fiber shortening relation.[120] However, the relation upon which this index is based is not defined by parallel straight lines across contractile states, so single beat measurements may reflect this nonlinearity rather than abnormalities in contractility.[121]

Left ventricular peak power has been proposed as an index of left ventricular contractility.[122-127] Ventricular power is the instantaneous product of pressure and flow and is analogous to the area under a force-shortening velocity curve for isolated muscle.[124] Peak left ventricular power has been validated invasively as an index of left ventricular contractility by using micromanometer catheters to measure instantaneous left ventricular pressure and a conductance catheter to measure the rate of left ventricular volume change (dV/dt or flow). Peak ventricular power is dependent on preload, but this preload dependence can be obviated by dividing peak ventricular power (PWR_{pk}) by the square of end-diastolic volume (EDV). In a study of 24 patients with a dilated cardiomyopathy, Sharir and associates[124] showed that PWR_{pk}/EDV^2 was not altered significantly by either reducing preload by 30 percent using balloon occlusion of the inferior vena cava or by reducing afterload impedance by 50 percent by a bolus injection of nitroglycerin. In response to changes in contractility induced by intravenous dobutamine, verapamil, or esmolol, changes in PWR_{pk}/EDV^2 correlated closely with changes in the end-systolic pressure–volume relation ($r = 0.91$, $p < 0.001$).

Preload-adjusted peak power offers the substantial advantage that it can be measured at a single steady-state condition and does not appear to require multiple measurements from variably loaded cardiac cycles as has been requisite for most other indices.[121,124] In addition, peak left ventricular power can be measured noninvasively at rest and with exercise by radionuclide ventriculography and a computerized sphygmomanometric device.[126] Noninvasive measurement of PWR_{pk} has been validated by demonstrating a substantial increase in PWR_{pk}/EDV^2 with dobutamine infusion but no change with an infusion of nitroprusside regardless of the similar rise in left ventricular ejection fraction with both agents.[124] Confirmation of these promising findings by other investigators is needed.

ESTIMATION OF LEFT VENTRICULAR FILLING PRESSURE FROM PULMONARY ACTIVITY ON THE RADIONUCLIDE VENTRICULOGRAM

When the left heart fails, pulmonary blood volume increases. In the absence of mitral valve disease, changes in pulmonary blood volume can be used as an indicator of left ventricular filling pressure. Pulmonary blood volume may be estimated noninvasively by radionuclide techniques.[128] Lindsey and Guyton[129] used a scintillation probe to document increasing pulmonary blood volume related to left heart failure following constriction of the aorta in dogs. Nichols and associates[130] used cyclotron-generated carbon 11 (^{11}C) to label the blood with ^{11}C carboxyhemoglobin. Pulmonary blood volume was then monitored with a multicrystal positron camera at rest and during exercise. In patients with multivessel angiographic coronary artery disease and angina pectoris with ischemic ST-segment depression during exercise, pulmonary and cardiac blood volume increased with exercise. For patients with normal coronary arteries or single-vessel disease who did not develop angina pectoris or ischemic electrocardiographic changes with exercise, regional pulmonary blood volume remained unchanged with exercise and cardiac volume decreased. The authors concluded that an ischemic response to exercise testing was associated with a transient rise in pulmonary and cardiac blood volume related to exercise-induced left ventricular dysfunction. The exercise-induced increase in pulmonary blood volume with left ventricular dys-

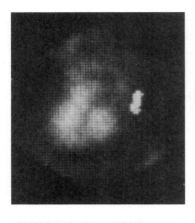

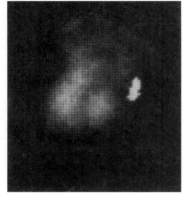

Rest

Exercise

Figure 12-13 End-diastolic frames from radionuclide ventriculograms in the left anterior oblique projection at rest and during exercise. Regions of interest have been drawn over the left lung field. The ratio of pulmonary blood volume during exercise as compared with that at rest was 1.16 in this patient presenting with substantial coronary artery disease. The exercise-induced increase in pulmonary activity is not apparent from visual comparison of the images obtained at rest and during exercise. (From Okada et al,[132] reproduced with permission.)

function may correspond to the interstitial edema observed on a chest radiogram in patients with left ventricular dysfunction following myocardial infarction.[131]

Assessment of pulmonary blood volume as an indicator of left ventricular filling pressure has been extended to radionuclide ventriculography.[132–137] Okada et al[132,133] used radionuclide ventriculography at rest and during supine exercise to assess pulmonary blood volume changes in 54 patients with indications for coronary arteriography. A ratio of exercise-to-rest left lung counts was generated from hand-drawn regions of interest (Fig. 12-13). In most patients with multiple-vessel coronary artery disease or with single-vessel coronary disease involving the left coronary artery, the exercise-to-rest pulmonary blood volume ratio was greater than 1.0 (Fig. 12-14). In patients with normal coronary arteries, the ratio was less than 1.0. In patients with single-vessel right

coronary artery disease, the exercise-to-rest pulmonary blood volume ratio was less than or equal to 1.0 in most cases. The authors postulated that exercise-induced ischemia in patients with single-vessel right coronary artery disease resulted in diminished pulmonary blood volume from right ventricular dysfunction.[132]

Okada and associates then compared exercise-induced changes in the pulmonary capillary wedge pressure with exercise-induced changes in the radionuclide pulmonary blood volume.[133] Nine subjects with a normal cardiac catheterization showed no increase in mean pulmonary capillary wedge pressure with exercise and had a normal pulmonary blood volume ratio. Thirteen patients with coronary artery disease, 15 patients with valvular heart disease, and 3 patients with cardiomyopathy showed an exercise-induced increase in pulmonary capil-

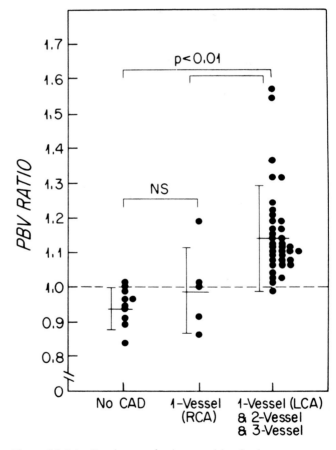

Figure 12-14 Distribution of pulmonary blood volume exercise–rest ratios (PBV ratio) according to extent of coronary artery disease. No CAD indicates no substantial coronary artery disease; 1-vessel (RCA): disease involving only the right coronary artery; 1-vessel (LCA): disease involving one of the two major branches of the left coronary artery; 2-vessel: stenosis in two of the three major coronary arteries; 3-vessel: stenosis in all three major coronary arteries. *Long horizontal bars* represent means, and *short horizontal bars* represent ±SD. (From Okada et al,[132] reproduced with permission.)

lary wedge pressure and had an abnormal pulmonary blood volume ratio (Fig. 12-15). Two patients with mitral stenosis had normal or near normal pulmonary blood volume ratios in response to exercise, although the pulmonary capillary wedge pressure rose with exercise. The authors suggested that in mitral stenosis the pulmonary blood volume is already increased at rest and relatively little further increase occurs with exercise. The authors concluded that the pulmonary blood volume ratio measured by exercise radionuclide ventriculography can be used to estimate noninvasively exercise-induced changes in left ventricular filling pressure (Fig. 12-16).

Left ventricular dysfunction also produces a progressive redistribution of pulmonary blood flow to the lung apices relative to the lung bases. Using regions of interest drawn over the apex and base of the right lung on resting radionuclide ventriculograms, Bateman and associates[134] demonstrated a significant correlation of the ratio of apex-to-base lung activity with the level of pulmonary capillary wedge pressure. Directional changes in pulmonary capillary wedge pressure following therapeutic in-

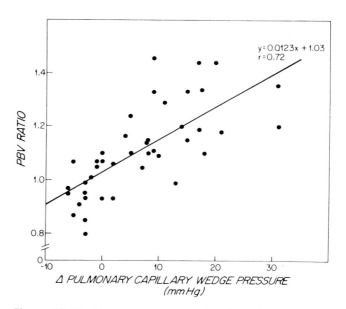

Figure 12-16 Linear regression analysis for pulmonary blood volume (PBV) ratio versus exercise-induced changes in pulmonary capillary wedge pressure. (From Okada et al,[133] reproduced with permission of the American Heart Association, Inc.)

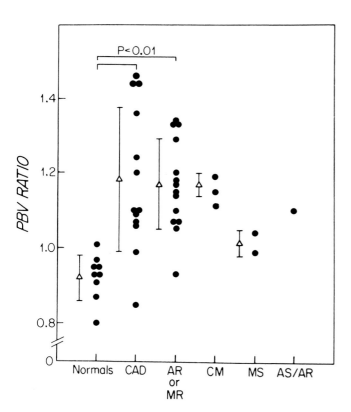

Figure 12-15 Distribution of pulmonary blood volume (PBV) ratios according to the diagnosis after cardiac catheterization. CAD, coronary artery disease; AR, aortic regurgitation; MR, mitral regurgitation; CM, cardiomyopathy; MS, mitral stenosis; AS/AR, combined aortic stenosis and AR. (From Okada et al,[133] reproduced with permission of the American Heart Association, Inc.)

terventions were reflected by changes in the apex-to-base lung perfusion ratio.

SUMMARY

Although widely used, the ventricular ejection fraction is influenced by ventricular preload and afterload as well as by myocardial contractility. This presents practical limitations in the evaluation of cardiac performance in patients with volume or pressure overload or underload states. Noninvasive measurement of diastolic and systolic ventricular volumes by radionuclide ventriculography enables assessment of ventricular preload or of contraction independent of preload. Combination of radionuclide volume measurement at end systole with end-systolic ventricular pressure measurement enables investigation of the end-systolic pressure–volume slope, which is a measure of ventricular contractility that is relatively independent of loading conditions. Ventricular preload is also indirectly assessed by measuring the pulmonary capillary wedge pressure. Assessment of pulmonary blood-pool activity can provide indirect measures of pulmonary capillary wedge pressure. Advances in the radionuclide measurement of ventricular volumes have resulted in increasing accuracy and ease of volume measurement. As ventricular volume measurement becomes a more routine part of the radionuclide ventriculogram study, the continued evolution of these measurements from a research tool to a clinical tool can be expected.

REFERENCES

1. Starling EH: *Linacre Lecture on the Law of the Heart (1915)*. London, Longmans, Green, 1918.
2. Ross J Jr: Afterload mismatch in aortic and mitral valve disease: Implications for surgical therapy. *J Am Coll Cardiol* 5:811, 1985.
3. Mitchell JH, Wildenthal K: Problems in measurement of myocardial contractility. *Proc R Soc Med* 65:542, 1972.
4. Sagawa K, Suga H, Shoukas AA, et al: End-systolic pressure/volume ratio: A new index of ventricular contractility. *Am J Cardiol* 40:748, 1977.
5. Nivatpumin T, Katz S, Scheuer J: Peak left ventricular systolic pressure/end-systolic volume ratio: A sensitive detector of left ventricular disease. *Am J Cardiol* 43:969, 1979.
6. Watkins J, Slutsky R, Tubau J, et al: Scintigraphic study of relation between left ventricular peak systolic pressure and end-systolic volume in patients with coronary artery disease and normal subjects. *Br Heart J* 48:39, 1982.
7. Kennedy JW, Trenholme SE, Kasser IS: Left ventricular volume and mass from single-plane cineangiocardiogram: A comparison of anteroposterior and right anterior oblique methods. *Am Heart J* 80:343, 1970.
8. Dodge HT, Sandler H, Ballew DW, et al: The use of biplane angiocardiography for the measurement of left ventricular volume in man. *Am Heart J* 60:762, 1960.
9. Mullins CB, Mason DT, Ashburn WL, et al: Determination of ventricular volume by radioisotope-angiography. *Am J Cardiol* 24:72, 1969.
10. Boucher CA, Bingham JB, Osbakken MD, et al: Early changes in left ventricular size and function after correction of left ventricular volume overload. *Am J Cardiol* 47:991, 1981.
11. Massie BM, Kramer BL, Gertz EW, et al: Radionuclide measurement of left ventricular volume: Comparison of geometric and counts-based methods. *Circulation* 65:725, 1982.
12. Seldin DW, Esser PD, Nichols AB, et al: Left ventricular volume determined from scintigraphy and digital angiography by a semi-automated geometric method. *Radiology* 149:809, 1983.
13. Uren RF, Newman HN, Hutton BF, et al: Geometric determination of left ventricular volume from gated blood-pool studies using a slant-hole collimator. *Radiology* 147:541, 1983.
14. Faber TL, Akers MS, Peshock RM, et al: Three-dimensional motion and perfusion quantification in gated single-photon emission computed tomograms. *J Nucl Med* 32:2311, 1991.
15. Corbett JR: Tomographic radionuclide ventriculography: Opportunity ignored? *J Nucl Cardiol* 1:567, 1994 (editorial).
16. Links JM, Becker LC, Shindledecker JG, et al: Measurement of absolute left ventricular volume from gated blood pool studies. *Circulation* 65:82, 1982.
17. Burns RJ, Druck MN, Woodward DS, et al: Repeatability of estimates of left-ventricular volume from blood-pool counts: Concise communication. *J Nucl Med* 24:775, 1983.
18. Fearnow EC III, Stanfield JA, Jaszczak RJ, et al: Factors affecting ventricular volumes determined by a count-based equilibrium method. *J Nucl Med* 26:1042, 1985.
19. Verani MS, Gaeta J, LeBlanc AD, et al: Validation of left ventricular volume measurements by radionuclide angiography. *J Nucl Med* 26:1394, 1985.
20. Seiderer M, Bohn I, Buell U, et al: Influence of background and absorption correction on nuclear quantification of left ventricular end-diastolic volume. *Br J Radiol* 56:183, 1983.
21. Herbst CP, Van Aswegen A, Kleynhans PHT, et al: Radionuclide determination of absolute LV volumes: Interstudy, interobserver and intraobserver variances. *Nucl Med Biol* 13:43, 1986.
22. Starling MR, Dell'Italia LJ, Nusynowitz ML, et al: Estimates of left-ventricular volumes by equilibrium radionuclide angiography: Importance of attenuation correction. *J Nucl Med* 25:14, 1984.
23. Starling MR, Dell'Italia LJ, Walsh RA, et al: Accurate estimates of absolute left ventricular volumes from equilibrium radionuclide angiographic count data using a simple geometric attenuation correction. *J Am Coll Cardiol* 3:789, 1984.
24. Petru MA, Sorensen SG, Chaudhuri TK, et al: Attenuation correction of equilibrium radionuclide angiography for noninvasive quantitation of cardiac output and ventricular volumes. *Am Heart J* 107:1221, 1984.
25. Thomsen JH, Patel AK, Rowe BR, et al: Estimation of absolute left ventricular volume from gated radionuclide ventriculograms: A method using phase image assisted automated edge detection and two-dimensional echocardiography. *Chest* 84:6, 1983.
26. Rabinovitch MA, Kalff V, Koral K, et al: Count-based left ventricular volume determination utilizing a left posterior oblique view for attenuation correction. *Radiology* 150:813, 1984.
27. Nickoloff EL, Perman WH, Esser PD, et al: Left ventricular volume: Physical basis for attenuation corrections in radionuclide determinations. *Radiology* 152:511, 1984.
28. Fearnow EC, Jaszczak RJ, Harris CC, et al: Esophageal source measurement of ^{99m}Tc attenuation coefficients for use in left ventricular volume determinations. *Radiology* 157:517, 1985.
29. Maurer AH, Siegel JA, Denenberg BS, et al: Absolute left ventricular volume from gated blood pool imaging with use of esophageal transmission measurement. *Am J Cardiol* 51:853, 1983.
30. Siegal JA, Wu RA, Maurer AH: The buildup factor: Effect of scatter on absolute volume determination. *J Nucl Med* 26:390, 1985.
31. Harris CC, Greer KL, Jaszczak RJ, et al: ^{99m}Tc attenuation coefficients in water-filled phantoms determined with gamma cameras. *Med Phys* 11:681, 1984.
32. Keller AM, Simon TR, Smitherman TC, et al: Direct

determination of the attenuation coefficient for radionuclide volume measurements. *J Nucl Med* 28:102, 1987.

33. Yeh EL, Yeh YS: Theoretical error in radionuclide ejection fraction study due to photon attenuation. *Eur J Nucl Med* 6:69, 1981.

34. Schneider RM, Jaszczak RJ, Coleman RE, et al: Disproportionate effects of regional hypokinesis on radionuclide ejection fraction: Compensation using attenuation-corrected ventricular volumes. *J Nucl Med* 25:747, 1984.

35. Konstam MA, Tu'meh S, Wynne J, et al: Effect of exercise on erythrocyte count and blood activity concentration after technetium-99m in vivo red blood cell labeling. *Circulation* 66:638, 1982.

36. Sandler MP, Kronenberg MW, Forman MB, et al: Dynamic fluctuations in blood and spleen radioactivity: Splenic contraction and relation to clinical radionuclide volume calculations. *J Am Coll Cardiol* 3:1205, 1984.

37. Vatterott PJ, Gibbons RJ, Hu DCK, et al: Assessment of left ventricular volume changes during exercise radionuclide angiography in coronary artery disease. *Am J Cardiol* 61:912, 1988.

38. Nelson TR, Slutsky RA, Verba JW: Effect of patient imaging angle on apparent cardiac volumes and the potential impact on measurement of valvular regurgitant fractions. *Invest Radiol* 18:406, 1983.

39. Slutsky R, Karliner J, Ricci D, et al: Left ventricular volumes by gated radionuclide angiography: A new method. *Circulation* 60:556, 1979.

40. Dehmer GJ, Lewis SE, Hillis LD, et al: Nongeometric determination of left ventricular volumes from equilibrium blood pool scans. *Am J Cardiol* 45:293, 1980.

41. Bacharach SL, Green MV, Borer JS, et al: ECG-gated scintillation probe measurement of left ventricular function. *J Nucl Med* 18:1176, 1977.

42. Konstam MA, Wynne J, Holman BL, et al: Use of equilibrium (gated) radionuclide ventriculography to quantitate left ventricular output in patients with and without left-sided valvular regurgitation. *Circulation* 64:578, 1981.

43. Clements IP, Brown ML, Smith HC: Radionuclide measurement of left ventricular volume. *Mayo Clin Proc* 56:733, 1981.

44. Wijns W, Melin JA, Decoster PM, et al: Radionuclide absolute left ventricular volumes during upright exercise: Validation in normal subjects by simultaneous hemodynamic measurements. *Eur J Nucl Med* 10:111, 1985.

45. Parrish MD, Graham TP Jr, Born ML, et al: Radionuclide ventriculography for assessment of absolute right and left ventricular volumes in children. *Circulation* 66:811, 1982.

46. Harpen MD, Dubuisson RL, Head GB III, et al: Determination of left-ventricular volume from first-pass kinetics of labeled red cells. *J Nucl Med* 24:98, 1983.

47. Nichols K, Adatepe MH, Isaacs GH, et al: A new scintigraphic method for determining left ventricular volumes. *Circulation* 70:672, 1984.

48. Massardo T, Gal RA, Grenier RP, et al: Left ventricular volume calculation using a count-based ratio method applied to multigated radionuclide angiography. *J Nucl Med* 31:450, 1990.

49. Gal RA, Grenier RP, Port SC, et al: Left ventricular volume calculation using a count-based ratio method applied to first-pass radionuclide angiography. *J Nucl Med* 33:2124, 1992.

50. Yen C-K, Lim AD, Lull RJ: A count-based radionuclide method for volume quantitation using conjugate imaging and an external reference source: Theoretical consideration and phantom study. *J Nucl Med* 35:644, 1994.

51. Stadius ML, Williams DL, Harp G, et al: Left ventricular volume determination using single-photon emission computed tomography. *Am J Cardiol* 55:1185, 1985.

52. Corbett JR, Jansen DE, Lewis SE, et al: Tomographic gated blood pool radionuclide ventriculography: Analysis of wall motion and left ventricular volumes in patients with coronary artery disease. *J Am Coll Cardiol* 6:349, 1985.

53. Bunker SR, Schmidt WP, Hartshorne MF, et al: Left ventricular volumes from single photon emission computed tomography (SPECT). *Circulation* 70(suppl II):II-448, 1984 (abstr).

54. Tauxe WN, Soussaline F, Todd-Pokropek A, et al: Determination of organ volume by single-photon emission tomography. *J Nucl Med* 23:984, 1982.

55. Bunker SR, Hartshorne MF, Schmidt WP, et al: Left ventricular volume determination from single-photon emission computed tomography. *Am J Roentgenol* 144:295, 1985.

56. Caputo GR, Graham MM, Brust KD, et al: Measurement of left ventricular volume using single-photon emission computed tomography. *Am J Cardiol* 56:781, 1985.

57. Gill JB, Moore RH, Miller DD, et al: Multigated blood pool tomography: Measurement of left ventricular volume and assessment of regional wall motion. *Circulation* 72(suppl III):III-136, 1985 (abstr).

58. Levy WC, Cerqueira MD, Matsuoka DT, et al: Four radionuclide methods for left ventricular volume determination: Comparison of a manual and an automated technique. *J Nucl Med* 33:763, 1992.

59. Levy WC, Jacobson AF, Cerqueira MD, et al: Radionuclide cardiac volumes: Effects of region of interest selection and correction for Compton scatter using a buildup factor. *J Nucl Med* 33:1642, 1992.

60. Jang S, Jaszczak RJ, Li J, et al: Cardiac ejection fraction and volume measurements using dynamic cardiac phantoms and radionuclide imaging. *IEEE Trans Nucl Sci* 41:2845, 1994.

61. Melin JA, Wijns W, Robert A, et al: Validation of radionuclide cardiac output measurements during exercise. *J Nucl Med* 26:1386, 1985.

62. MacIntyre WJ, Pritchard WH, Moir TW: The determination of cardiac output by the dilution method without arterial sampling. I. Analytical concepts. *Circulation* 18:1139, 1958.

63. Pritchard WH, MacIntyre WJ, Moir TW: The determination of cardiac output by the dilution method without arterial sampling. II. Validation of precordial recording. *Circulation* 18:1147, 1958.

64. Kelbaek H, Hartling OJ, Skagen K, et al: First-pass radionuclide determination of cardiac output: An improved gamma camera method. *J Nucl Med* 28:1330, 1987.

65. Harpen MD, Dubuisson RL, Head GB III, et al: Radionuclide determination of cardiac outputs and indices. *Eur J Nucl Med* 9:73, 1984.

66. Glass EC: Cardiac output and transit times, in Gelfand MJ, Thomas SR (eds): *Effective Use of Computers in Nuclear Medicine*. New York, McGraw-Hill, 1988, pp 228–247.

67. Glass EC: First-pass radionuclide determination of cardiac output: An improved gamma camera method. *J Nucl Med* 29:1154, 1988 (letter).

68. Glass EC, Rahimian J, Hines HH: Effect of region of interest selection on first-pass radionuclide cardiac output determination. *J Nucl Med* 27:1282, 1986.

69. Jones RH, McEwan P, Newman GE, et al: Accuracy of diagnosis of coronary artery disease by radionuclide measurement of left ventricular function during rest and exercise. *Circulation* 64:586, 1981.

70. Dell'Italia LJ, Starling MR, Walsh RA, et al: Validation of attenuation-corrected equilibrium radionuclide angiographic determinations of right ventricular volume: Comparison with cast-validated biplane cineventriculography. *Circulation* 72:317, 1985.

71. Peterson KL, Skloven D, Ludbrook P, et al: Comparison of isovolumic and ejection phase indices of myocardial performance in man. *Circulation* 49:1088, 1974.

72. Kass DA, Maughan WL, Guo ZM, et al: Comparative influence of load versus inotropic states on indexes of ventricular contractility: Experimental and theoretical analysis based on pressure–volume relationships. *Circulation* 76:1422, 1987.

73. Grossman W, Braunwald E, Mann T, et al: Contractile state of the left ventricle in man as evaluated from end-systolic pressure–volume relations. *Circulation* 56:845, 1977.

74. Suga H, Sagawa K, Shoukas AA: Load independence of the instantaneous pressure–volume ratio of the canine left ventricle and effects of epinephrine and heart rate on the ratio. *Circ Res* 32:314, 1973.

75. Suga H, Sagawa K, Kostiuk DP: Controls of ventricular contractility assessed by pressure–volume ratio, E_{max}. *Cardiovasc Res* 10:582, 1976.

76. Suga H, Sagawa K: Instantaneous pressure–volume relationships and their ratio in the excised, supported canine left ventricle. *Circ Res* 35:117, 1974.

77. Mahler F, Covell JW, Ross J Jr: Systolic pressure–diameter relations in the normal conscious dog. *Cardiovasc Res* 9:447, 1975.

78. Shen WF, Roubin GS, Choong CYP, et al: Evaluation of relationship between myocardial contractile state and left ventricular function in patients with aortic regurgitation. *Circulation* 71:31, 1985.

79. Magorien DJ, Shaffer P, Bush CA, et al: Assessment of left ventricular pressure–volume relations using gated radionuclide angiography, echocardiography and micromanometer pressure recordings: A new method for serial measurements of systolic and diastolic function in man. *Circulation* 67:844, 1983.

80. Iskandrian AS, Hakki AH, Bemis CE, et al: Left ventricular end-systolic pressure–volume relation: A combined radionuclide and hemodynamic study. *Am J Cardiol* 51:1057, 1983.

81. Borow KM, Neumann A, Wynne J: Sensitivity of end-systolic pressure–dimension and pressure–volume rela-

tions to the inotropic state in humans. *Circulation* 65:988, 1982.

82. Borow KM, Green LH, Grossman W, et al: Left ventricular end-systolic stress-shortening and stress-length relations in humans: Normal values and sensitivity to inotropic state. *Am J Cardiol* 50:1301, 1982.

83. Carabello BA, Spann JF: The uses and limitations of end-systolic indexes of left ventricular function. *Circulation* 69:1058, 1984.

84. Mirsky I, Tajima T, Peterson KL: The development of the entire end-systolic pressure–volume and ejection fraction–afterload relations: A new concept of systolic myocardial stiffness. *Circulation* 76:343, 1987.

85. Kass DA, Maughan WL: From "E_{max} to pressure–volume relations: A broader view. *Circulation* 77:1203, 1988.

86. Hsia HH, Starling MR: Is standardization of left ventricular chamber elastance necessary? *Circulation* 81:1826, 1990.

87. Suga H, Hisano R, Goto Y, et al: Normalization of end-systolic pressure–volume relation and E of different sized hearts. *Jpn Circ J* 48:136, 1984.

88. Foult J-M, Loiseau A, Nitenberg A: Size dependence of the end-systolic stress/volume ratio in humans: Implications for the evaluation of myocardial contractile performance in pressure and volume overload. *J Am Coll Cardiol* 16:124, 1990.

89. Nakano K, Sugawara M, Ishihara K, et al: Myocardial stiffness derived from end-systolic wall stress and logarithm of reciprocal of wall thickness: Contractility index independent of ventricular size. *Circulation* 82:1352, 1990.

90. Hanson DE, Cahill PD, DeCampli WM, et al: Valvular-ventricular interaction: Importance of the mitral apparatus in canine left ventricular systolic performance. *Circulation* 73:1310, 1986.

91. Maughan WL, Sunagawa K, Burkhoff D, et al: Effect of arterial impedance changes on the end-systolic pressure–volume relation. *Circ Res* 54:595, 1984.

92. Zile MR, Izzi G, Gaasch WH: Left ventricular diastolic dysfunction limits use of maximum systolic elastance as an index of contractile function. *Circulation* 83:674, 1991.

93. Aroney CN, Herrmann HC, Semigran MJ, et al: Linearity of the left ventricular end-systolic pressure–volume relation in patients with severe heart failure. *J Am Coll Cardiol* 14:127, 1989.

94. Kronenberg MW, Parrish MD, Jenkins DW Jr, et al: Accuracy of radionuclide ventriculography for estimation of left ventricular volume changes and end-systolic pressure–volume relations. *J Am Coll Cardiol* 6:1064, 1985.

95. Marsh JD, Green LH, Wynne J, et al: Left ventricular end-systolic pressure–dimension and stress–length relations in normal human subjects. *Am J Cardiol* 44:1311, 1979.

96. McKay RG, Aroesty JM, Heller GV, et al: Assessment of the end-systolic pressure–volume relationship in human beings with the use of a time-varying elastance model. *Circulation* 74:97, 1986.

97. Kono A, Maughan WL, Sunagawa K, et al: The use of left ventricular end-ejection pressure and peak pressure

in the estimation of the end-systolic pressure–volume relationship. *Circulation* 70:1057, 1984.

98. Starling MR, Gross MD, Walsh RA, et al: Assessment of the radionuclide angiographic left ventricular maximum time-varying elastance calculation in man. *J Nucl Med* 29:1368, 1988.

99. Carabello BA: Ratio of end-systolic stress to end-systolic volume: Is it a useful clinical tool? *J Am Coll Cardiol* 14:496, 1989 (editorial).

100. Freeman GL, Little WC, O'Rourke RA, et al: The effect of vasoactive agents on the left ventricular end-systolic pressure–volume relation in closed-chest dogs. *Circulation* 74:1107, 1986.

101. Sagawa K, Suga H, Shoukas AA, et al: End-systolic pressure/volume ratio: A new index of ventricular contractility. *Am J Cardiol* 40:748, 1977.

102. Nivatpumin T, Katz S, Scheuer J: Peak left ventricular systolic pressure/end-systolic volume ratio: A sensitive detector of left ventricular disease. *Am J Cardiol* 43:969, 1979.

103. El-Tobgi S, Fouad FM, Kramer JR, et al: Left ventricular function in coronary artery disease: Evaluation of slope of end-systolic pressure–volume line (E_{max}) and ratio of peak systolic pressure to end-systolic volume (P/V_{es}). *J Am Coll Cardiol* 3:781, 1984.

104. Carabello BA, Nolan SP, McGuire LB: Assessment of preoperative left ventricular function in patients with mitral regurgitation: Value of the end-systolic wall stress–end-systolic volume ratio. *Circulation* 64:1212, 1981.

105. Borow KM, Green LH, Mann T, et al: End-systolic volume as a predictor of postoperative left ventricular performance in volume overload from valvular regurgitation. *Am J Med* 68:655, 1980.

106. Pirwitz MJ, Lange RA, Willard JE, et al: Use of the left ventricular peak systolic pressure/end-systolic volume ratio to predict symptomatic improvement with valve replacement in patients with aortic regurgitation and enlarged end-systolic volume. *J Am Coll Cardiol* 24:1672, 1994.

107. Slutsky R, Karliner J, Gerber K, et al: Peak systolic blood pressure/end-systolic volume ratio: Assessment at rest and during exercise in normal subjects and patients with coronary heart disease. *Am J Cardiol* 46:813, 1980.

108. Dehmer GJ, Lewis SE, Hillis LD, et al: Exercise-induced alterations in left ventricular volumes and the pressure–volume relationship: A sensitive indicator of left ventricular dysfunction in patients with coronary artery disease. *Circulation* 63:1008, 1981.

109. Kalischer AL, Johnson LL, Johnson YE, et al: Effects of propranolol and timolol on left ventricular volumes during exercise in patients with coronary artery disease. *J Am Coll Cardiol* 3:210, 1984.

110. Pouleur H, Rousseau MF, Van Eyll C, et al: Assessment of left ventricular contractility from late systolic stress–volume relations. *Circulation* 65:1204, 1982.

111. Gibbons RJ, Clements IP, Zinsmeister AR, et al: Exercise response of the systolic pressure to end-systolic volume ratio in patients with coronary artery disease. *J Am Coll Cardiol* 10:33, 1987.

112. Purut CM, Sell TL, Jones RH: A new method to determine left ventricular pressure–volume loops in the clinical setting. *J Nucl Med* 29:1492, 1988.

113. Katz AM: Influence of altered inotropy and lusitropy on ventricular pressure–volume loops. *J Am Coll Cardiol* 11:438, 1988.

114. Little WC, Cheng C-P, Mumma M, et al: Comparison of measures of left ventricular contractile performance derived from pressure–volume loops in conscious dogs. *Circulation* 80:1378, 1989.

115. Feneley MP, Skelton TN, Kisslo KB, et al: Comparison of preload recruitable stroke work, end-systolic pressure–volume and dP/dt_{max}–end-diastolic volume relations as indexes of left ventricular contractile performance in patients undergoing routine cardiac catheterization. *J Am Coll Cardiol* 19:1522, 1992.

116. Van der Velde ET, Burkhoff D, Steendijk P, et al: Nonlinearity and load sensitivity of end-systolic pressure–volume relation of canine left ventricle in vivo. *Circulation* 83:315, 1991.

117. Rahko PS: Comparative efficacy of three indexes of left ventricular performance derived from pressure–volume loops in heart failure induced by tachypacing. *J Am Coll Cardiol* 23:209, 1994.

118. Sasayama S, Asanoi H: Coupling between the heart and arterial system in heart failure. *Am J Med* 90:5B, 1991.

119. Stefadouros MA, Dougherty MS, Grossman W, et al: Determination of systemic vascular resistance by a noninvasive technique. *Circulation* 47:101, 1973.

120. Colan SD, Borow KM, Neumann A: Left ventricular end-systolic wall stress–velocity of fiber shortening relation: A load-independent index of myocardial contractility. *J Am Coll Cardiol* 4:715, 1984.

121. Banerjee A, Brook MM, Klautz RJM, et al: Nonlinearity of the left ventricular end-systolic wall stress–velocity of fiber shortening relation in young pigs: A potential pitfall in its use as a single-beat index of contractility. *J Am Coll Cardiol* 23:514, 1994.

122. Stein PD, Sabbah HN: Ventricular performance measured during ejection: Studies in patients of the rate of change of ventricular power. *Am Heart J* 91:599, 1976.

123. Stein PD, Sabbah HN: Rate of change of ventricular power: An indicator of ventricular performance during ejection. *Am Heart J* 91:219, 1976.

124. Sharir T, Feldman MD, Haber H, et al: Ventricular systolic assessment in patients with dilated cardiomyopathy by preload-adjusted maximal power: Validation and noninvasive application. *Circulation* 89:2045, 1994.

125. Marmor A, Jain D, Cohen LS, et al: Left ventricular peak power during exercise: A noninvasive approach for assessment of contractile reserve. *J Nucl Med* 34:1877, 1993.

126. Marmor A, Sharir T, Shlomo IB, et al: Radionuclide ventriculography and central aorta pressure change in noninvasive assessment of myocardial performance. *J Nucl Med* 30:1657, 1989.

127. Marmor A, Jain D, Zaret B: Beyond ejection fraction. *J Nucl Cardiol* 1:477, 1994.

128. Weissler AM, McCraw BH, Warren JV: Pulmonary blood volume determined by a radioactive tracer technique. *J Appl Physiol* 14:531, 1959.

129. Lindsey AW, Guyton AC: Continuous recording of pulmonary blood volume: Pulmonary pressure and volume changes. *Am J Physiol* 197:959, 1959.

130. Nichols AB, Strauss HW, Moore RH, et al: Acute changes in cardiopulmonary blood volume during upright exercise stress testing in patients with coronary heart disease. *Circulation* 60:520, 1979.

131. Battler A, Karliner JS, Higgins CB, et al: The initial chest x-ray in acute myocardial infarction: Prediction of early and late mortality and survival. *Circulation* 61:1004, 1980.

132. Okada RD, Pohost GM, Kirshenbaum HD, et al: Radionuclide-determined change in pulmonary blood volume with exercise. *N Engl J Med* 301:569, 1979.

133. Okada RD, Osbakken MD, Boucher CA, et al: Pulmonary blood volume ratio response to exercise: A noninvasive determination of exercise-induced changes in pulmonary capillary wedge pressure. *Circulation* 65: 126, 1982.

134. Bateman TM, Gray RJ, Czer LSC, et al: Regional distribution of pulmonary blood volume: An index of pulmonary capillary wedge pressure determined from blood pool scintigraphy. *Am J Cardiol* 51:1404, 1983.

135. Tubau J, Slutsky RA, Gerber KH, et al: Pulmonary blood volume: Relationship to changes in left ventricular end-diastolic pressure during atrial pacing. *Am Heart J* 105:940, 1983.

136. Slutsky R: Pulmonary blood volume: The response to afterload in normal subjects and patients with previous myocardial infarction. *Invest Radiol* 17:241, 1982.

137. Liu P, Kiess MC, Strauss HW, et al: Comparison of ejection fraction and pulmonary blood volume ratio as markers of left ventricular function change after coronary angioplasty. *J Am Coll Cardiol* 8:511, 1986.

Functional Imaging and Phase Analysis of Blood-Pool Scintigrams

Elias H. Botvinick
Michael W. Dae
J. William O'Connell

Scintigraphic methods can well evaluate cardiac structure, perfusion, and function. Primary advantages of the scintigraphic method include its noninvasive nature, its ability to analyze pathophysiologic markers, its quantitative nature, and its amenability to computer analysis. A good example of these features is equilibrium blood-pool scintigraphy[1,2] which accurately and reproducibly determines regional and global ventricular function and also provides the basic data for determination and display of many regional functional parameters.

FUNCTIONAL OR PARAMETRIC IMAGES

Since background-corrected cardiac blood-pool counts are proportional to volume, regional counts and their serial alterations can yield information relating to regional stroke volume, ejection fraction, and ventricular filling rates (Fig. 13-1). Simple mathematical manipulations of the equilibrium time–activity curve can derive parameters characterizing the degree and sequence of chamber emptying.[3] When the equilibrium study is reconstructed as an image that spatially displays one of these derived parameters, a parametric (mathematic) or functional (physiologic) image is produced. These are powerful tools that can uniquely and rapidly display in a condensed, easily interpretable form, the regional distribution of often complex but clinically useful functional measurements.[4]

STROKE–VOLUME AND EJECTION FRACTION IMAGES

The stroke–volume (SV) image[5] is a parametric image that codes, in relative gray shades or in colors, the regional volume ejected with each cycle (Fig. 13-1). It represents the pixel-by-pixel difference between background-corrected end-diastolic (ED) and end-systolic (ES) counts and is obtained by subtracting the ES from the ED image. Unlike the amplitude image, the SV image recognizes signs and sets to zero (or black) pixels where SV is negative, where ES counts exceed ED counts. Thus, atrial regions and regions of apparent paradoxical motion are not visualized. The SV image provides an objective map of regional ventricular emptying.

Similarly, the ejection fraction (EF) image[6] codes the regional EF by dividing (pixel by pixel) the SV count value by the background-corrected ED count value (Fig. 13-1). The EF image can be an important supplement to other functional data, since global ventricular performance and EF may not reflect or localize regional dysfunction. It provides added accurate, objective detection of regional dysfunction, beyond the qualitative impression of the dynamic display. The converse of the SV image, the paradox image, reveals the difference between ES and ED images, accentuating atrial and dyskinetic segments[7] (Fig. 13-1).

Both SV and EF images can provide objective quantitative evidence of relative regional ventricular function in a single best septal projection owing to the dependence of scintigraphic data on counts rather than geometry.

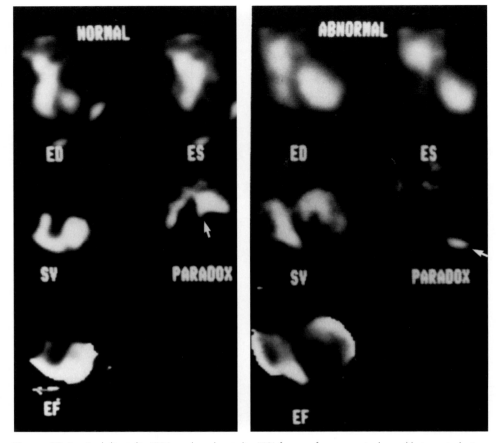

Figure 13-1 End-diastolic (ED) and end-systolic (ES) frames from a gated equilibrium study in a patient with normal ventricular function (*left*) and a patient with a left ventricular aneurysm (*right*). EF, ejection fraction image (intensity parallels ejection fraction); paradox, paradox image (intensity relates to increased volume in systole); SV, stroke–volume image (*right arrow* indicates dyskinesis in the left ventricle).

FIRST FOURIER HARMONIC TRANSFORMATION: AMPLITUDE AND PHASE IMAGES

Definition

The phase image is a computer-derived parametric image assembled from an analysis of the time–activity curve in each pixel location of the blood-pool scintigram.[8–10] Here, each curve is fitted with its first harmonic Fourier transform, equivalent to a symmetric cosine curve. Such a curve undergoes one complete sequence during each cardiac cycle from the onset of the electrocardiographic (ECG) R wave, or 0°, to the following R wave, or 360°. If ventricular contraction began immediately with the R wave and the time–activity curve was completely symmetric, it would mirror a cosine curve that began at the R wave and ended with the subsequent R wave. Because it remains symmetric with the periodicity of a cosine curve, regardless of its time of onset, the fitted curve, unlike the asymmetric raw-data curve, can be characterized by two features: its amplitude or height, and the phase angle, representing the angular location of its time of onset in the cardiac cycle.

With reference to the ventricles, the phase angle is expressed in degrees from 0° to 360° over the R-to-R interval (Fig. 13-2). Each pixel so characterized can be gray scale or color coded with reference to phase angle to present a functional image of such data—the phase image. The phase angle may be viewed as a relative measure of the timing of the loss of regional counts, chamber emptying, or contraction. To the extent that contraction follows conduction, display of phase-angle progression portrays the pattern of inter- and intraventricular conduction, and parallels the sequence of ventricular emptying or contraction.

Method of Derivation

The amplitude and phase images are parametric images derived by fitting this first Fourier harmonic to the time–

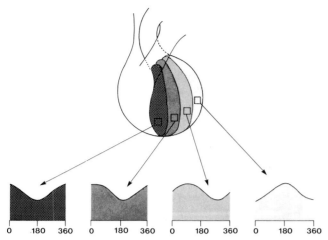

Figure 13-2 Diagrammatic sketch of the right and left ventricles and great vessels in the best septal left anterior oblique projections. The left ventricle has been divided into four regions characterized by varying time of contraction onset and phase angle. Pixels in the darkest region near the septum begin contraction at the electro-cardiographic R wave with a phase angle of 0°. Contiguous segments with progressively lighter gray shades are related to progressively delayed contraction and more delayed phase angles. Moving from the septum toward the lateral left ventricular wall, pixels in progressive segments demonstrate contraction onset one-eighth, one-quarter, and one-half of the way through the car-diac cycle with related phase angles of 45°, 90°, and 180°. Below the cardiac diagram are the first harmonic Fourier transforms related to each of the ventricular contraction segments. In this sketch, the fitted curves are expected to reproduce the timing of the raw volume (time–activity) curve without displacement, and electromechanical delay is assumed to be negligible. However, subsequent patient data will be influenced by other curve fit error and conduction delay. For this reason, for patient studies, the gray scale and left histogram margin is rotated to avoid a black–white interface in otherwise normal ventricular regions of interest. (From Frais et al,[8] reproduced with permission of the American Heart Association, Inc.)

activity curve on a pixel-by-pixel basis. The resultant fitted curve is of the form:

$$f(t) = A_o + A_1 \cos(t - w)$$

where t takes values between 0 and 360° and $f(t)$ is the fitted function

$$\sum_{k=1}^{N} f(k)/N$$

where
N = number of study frames
A_1 = first harmonic amplitude
A_o = mean time–activity curve value
w = first harmonic phase, the angular delay of the cosine maximum

The amplitude is an approximate proportionate mea-sure of stroke counts or SV. Phase angle is influenced by initial curve symmetry, here a measure of the symme-try of the time–activity curve, and describes the relative position of the peak of the fitted curve with respect to the gating trigger, generally the ECG R wave. Phase and amplitude are periodic functions, but can be applied with first-pass, blood-pool methods.[9]

Phase Image Analysis and Display

Blood-pool data for phase image analysis are best ac-quired with a narrow-beat-length window set by frame or list mode to provide technically optimal curves. For-ward–backward compilation may be employed to elimi-nate irregular terminal frame data drop-off in list mode acquisition. Images are acquired in a 64 × 64 matrix and interpolated to 128 × 128.

The phase image may be displayed and analyzed in steps. Each pixel in each projection of the phase images is initially coded in 256 shades of gray or 64 colors. Pixels with the fitted first harmonic demonstrating the same phase angle, with simultaneous count reduction or contraction onset, demonstrate the same gray shade or color. This display is reviewed visually to provide an overview of phase relations in preparation for the quanti-tative assessment that follows.

Next, the borders of each ventricle are outlined on the phase image (Fig. 13-3) and phase histograms of each ventricle or atrium are constructed from data in these respective regions, in the best septal left anterior oblique projection. The histogram relates phase angle, on the abscissa, to the number of pixels at any given phase angle on the ordinate. From these histograms, the mean phase angle and standard deviation of phase for each region of interest may be calculated. For the ventri-cles, the standard deviation of phase angle can be practi-cally related to the duration of contraction: the greater this duration, the less synchronous the ventricular con-traction. Movable cursors placed on the histogram may then be used to select a range of phase angles (as small as 2.8°). Pixels in the designated range of phase angles are coded white and, by selective, serial, progressive movement of the cursor window to higher phase angles, the progressive pattern of ventricular "contraction" is mapped (Fig. 13-4). An amplitude threshold may be applied outside the region of interest in an effort to suppress background. In each study, regions of earliest and latest phase angle in each ventricle are those that appeared first and last as the movable cursors are ad-vanced across the phase range in small increments. The sequential phase progression may be displayed in a dy-namic (16-frame) movie version of the gray-scale-coded image. In addition, amplitude and phase data may be combined in a single image with the display color coded

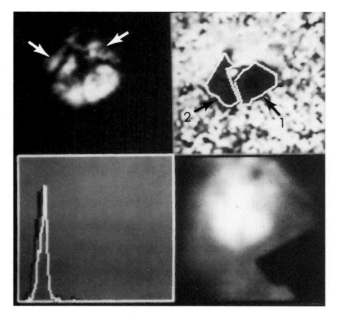

Figure 13-3 Normal amplitude (*top left*) and phase (*top right*) images in a patient with normal contraction and conduction. The composite blood-pool image (*bottom right*) guides identification of left (*arrow 1*) and right (*arrow 2*) ventricular regions of interest while the phase histograms generated from right (*black*) and left (*white*) ventricular regions are shown at *bottom left*. Homogeneous *dark gray* coloration in ventricular regions indicates early, coordinate contraction. Note the position of the histograms, early and nearly superimposed, consistent with early symmetric ventricular contraction, and the atrial region (*arrows, top left*) out of phase with the ventricles. The histograms shown here, and many throughout this presentation, are normalized to peak values within the respective region of interest. (From Dae et al,[10] reproduced with permission.)

for phase angle and intensity coded for amplitude. However, when assessing serial phase angle, or the site of earliest phase angle, separate phase images must be generated.

Normal Amplitude and Phase Image

The amplitude image in a normal subject presents, in relative intensities, the regional amplitude of blood-pool ejection from the cardiac chambers. If regional emptying is everywhere simultaneous and the proper frames are chosen, it will resemble the SV image. When the timing of regional systole does not parallel that of global systole, the amplitude distribution will better estimate true regional emptying independent of time constraints.

Amplitude depends on the ability of the fitted curve to reflect the full excursion of the regional time–activity curve. To the extent that this is not true, the parameter will err. Regions of reduced ventricular amplitude correspond to contraction abnormalities assessed on a count basis.

The sequence of phase variation in normal subjects shows an orderly progression across both ventricles with minor irregularities.[11] The site of the earliest left and right ventricular phase angle is always in the proximal septum but is also often noted at the left ventricular base, in the inferoapical region, and in the distal septum in some patients. The sequence of phase variation spreads concentrically in an inferoapical and lateral direction through the left ventricle (Fig. 13-4). In the normal subject, the phase image reveals a homogeneous ventricular pattern of a dark gray shade, corresponding to early phase angle without regions of gross phase delay.[12] The phase histogram of each ventricle approximates a narrow Gaussian distribution. The phase angle of the right ventricle is frequently earlier than that of the left ventricle. Overall, these results are consistent with the known temporal relationship between right and left ventricular conduction and contraction[13] and parallel the documented pattern of myocardial activation.

PHASE ANALYSIS FOR THE ASSESSMENT OF CONTRACTION ABNORMALITIES

Numerous authors have noted an increased phase angle in regions with contraction abnormalities. In early work,[14] akinetic and dyskinetic segments demonstrated impressive phase delay compared with normals. However, hypokinetic segments were often related to a less impressive phase angle. Subsequently, phase angle, standard deviation of phase angle, and phase histogram skewness have all been related to abnormal contraction.[12,13,15–19]

Phase analysis may be particularly helpful in the evaluation of ventricular aneurysms.[20,21] Akinetic or apparently dyskinetic segments may be detected in an otherwise normal ventricle, and a characteristic discrete secondary histogram peak is often present[20] (Fig. 13-5). The region of phase abnormalities can be superimposed on the ED frame to determine the percentage of ED volume involved in the aneurysm. This parameter correlates well with the percentage of akinetic segments measured angiographically. This pattern is well differentiated from that of ventricles with generalized contraction abnormalities that reveal even greater mean phase angle (Fig. 13-6).

ATRIAL PHASE ANALYSIS

While the atrial time–activity curve is not as simple, as predictable, or as easily extracted from the blood-pool

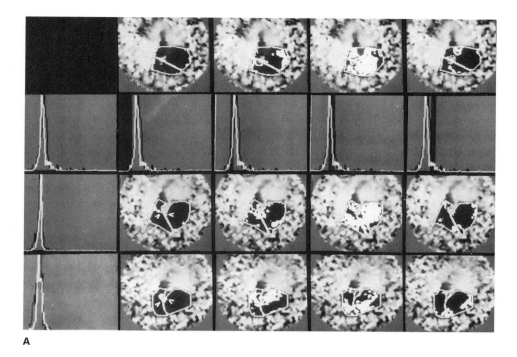

A

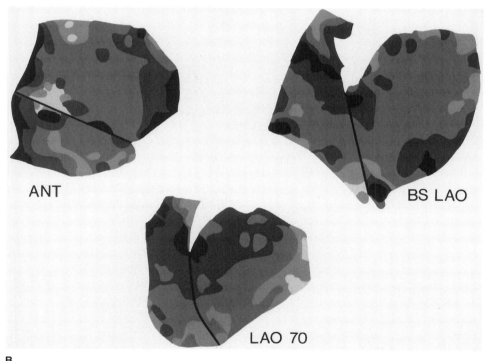

B

Figure 13-4 **A:** (*Top row*) Sequential phase images performed in the anterior projection in a normal patient. Here, both ventricles appear as homogeneous *dark gray* shades. The atria appear in *light* shades superior and to the left of the ventricles while the background is a random "salt and pepper" pattern and the ventricular histograms (*row 2*) are nearly superimposed. Similar findings are noted in relation to "best septal" (*row 3*) and 70° left anterior oblique (*bottom row*) projections. In each case, serial samplings of regional phase angles demonstrate earliest septal phase angle and symmetric biventricular phase progression. **B:** Diagrammatic representations of the same phase images, where regions of earliest phase angle are shown in *black*.

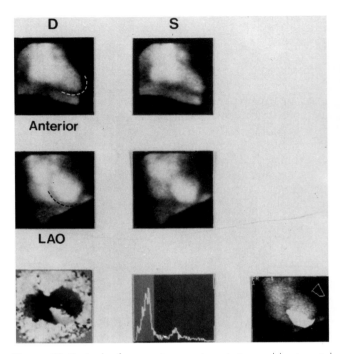

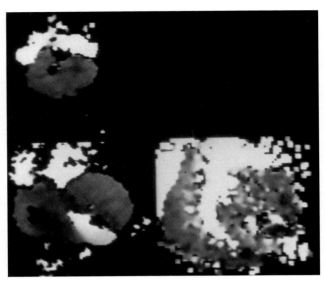

Figure 13-5   In the four *top* images in anterior and best septal left anterior oblique (LAO) projections are the diastolic (D) and systolic (S) frames from the equilibrium blood-pool scintigram in a patient with a well-defined apicoseptal aneurysm. The akinetic regions have been highlighted with a *dotted line* on the diastolic image in each projection. The *bottom row* shows the phase image generated from the left anterior oblique projection in this patient (*left*) and the phase histogram generated from the left ventricular region of interest in this same phase image (*middle*). Examination of the phase image reveals the left ventricle to be divided into two sharply defined components, a larger, more proximal region (*dark gray*) corresponding to an early phase angle component, and an apical region (*light gray*) corresponding to the location of dyskinesia in this projection. The phase histogram in this patient, with a segmental contraction abnormality, reveals two peaks and was divided at that phase angle equal to the normal left ventricular mean value plus 2 standard deviations. In the *right panel* of the *bottom row*, pixels corresponding to phase angles beyond this cutoff have been highlighted in *white* and superimposed on the end-diastolic frame. From such an analysis, the percentage of the end-diastolic volume involved in the severe segmental contraction abnormality or aneurysm can be simply and objectively calculated. (From Frais et al,[20] reprinted with permission from the American College of Cardiology, *Journal of the American College of Cardiology*, 4:987, 1984.)

Figure 13-6   Enhanced phase images in a normal patient (*top left*) and in patients with segmental (*bottom left*) and generalized (*bottom right*) contraction abnormalities. Note the nearly random phase distribution in the patient with generalized contraction abnormalities. (From Frais et al,[20] reprinted with permission from the American College of Cardiology, *Journal of the American College of Cardiology*, 4:987, 1984.)

image as the ventricular curve, atrial amplitude and phase can be characterized. Normal phase images demonstrate extreme phase delay of atrial regions similar to that observed in paradoxical ventricular segments. This is not unexpected, owing to the temporal opposition of atrial and ventricular emptying patterns (Figs. 13-3 to 13-6). Earlier atrial phase can be seen when the atrium is paced and triggering occurs from the atrial pacemaker spike. In such cases, regional phase angles are altered, yet the sequence appears to be preserved. Phase image documentation of ventricular–atrial conduction in the presence of ventricular pacing has been demonstrated,[22] and bypass pathways are well seen by phase image analysis when conduction occurs antegrade down the bypass pathway or with atrial pacing.

PHASE ANALYSIS OF VENTRICULAR CONDUCTION ABNORMALITIES

There seems to be a relatively good relationship between the phase angle and the timing of onset of ventricular systole. The phase angle has been correlated with the onset and sequence of regional emptying. This is a very difficult parameter to measure by other imaging modalities, because other methods, even angiography, do not have the ability to view the global ventricular contraction pattern and objectively discern the earliest and sequential contraction sites. Echocardiography, for example, has a limited sampling window, is observer dependent, and lacks the application of computerized methods to extract sequential wall-motion data objectively and readily,[23] yet it has been applied to the identification of contraction patterns in preexcitation with atrioventricular connections.[24] By comparison, the radionuclide gated blood-pool method is well suited to assess sequential wall motion over the cardiac chambers and is characterized by ease of digitization and computer analysis and by its ability to evaluate all of the central blood pool simultaneously.

Owing to the insufficiency of other methods, corroboration of the scintigraphic method has come from correlations of phase maps with expected contraction patterns based on known patterns of electrical activation. Conversely, since evidence suggests that excitation and contraction are generally linked,[25] the scintigraphic phase map has been used to assess patterns of electrophysiologic activation and conduction and has been extensively correlated with surface ECG and electrophysiologic data.

PHASE CHARACTERIZATION OF THE CONDUCTION SEQUENCE: VALIDATION IN ANIMAL MODELS

We evaluated 12 activation sequences during atrial and right and left ventricular pacing in four normal dogs.[26] For each sequence, phase maps generated in multiple projections were compared with epicardial maps obtained from a roving bipolar electrode after thoracotomy. In total, 34 sites were recorded and referenced to two intracardiac and two surface electrograms for each sequence. Pacing catheters were kept stationary during phase and epicardial mapping. In 11 of 12 sequences, epicardial breakthrough and the site of earliest contraction and phase angle occurred in the same region. Sequences were comparable in direction, speed of spread,

and location of terminal activity. Regions with synchronous excitation were comparable in distribution to regions with homogeneous contraction. The study demonstrated the close correlation between phase sequences and activation patterns in normal hearts. It supported the potential of the method as a noninvasive tool to delineate the spatial sequence of altered excitation in terms of a functional parameter.

PHASE ASSESSMENT OF THE ACTIVATION SITE AND CONDUCTION SEQUENCE: VALIDATION IN HUMANS

We compared the patterns of phase distribution and sequential phase changes over both right and left ventricles in 16 patients with normal electrical activation to those of eight patients with an artificial ventricular pacemaker and four patients with normal contraction and accessory atrioventricular connections[11] (Fig. 13-7). In each of the eight patients with a ventricular pacemaker, the site of earliest activation on phase imaging corresponded to the position of the pacing electrode as seen on the patient's radiograph and sequential phase changes spread from the initial focus through both ventricles. In those patients experiencing preexcitation, the site of earliest phase angle corresponded exactly to the site of the bypass tract determined by endocardial mapping in posterior, left paraseptal, left lateral, and right lateral locations. Dynamic changes were also seen.[14]

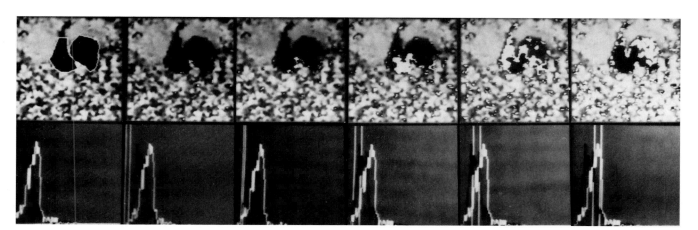

Figure 13-7 Sequential phase images and associated ventricular histograms in a patient with a right ventricular endocardial pacemaker. In contrast to the pattern in normal patients, the right ventricle, particularly at its apical and septal segments, is represented by a *darker gray* shade than that of the left ventricle. The sites of earliest phase angle are localized to the right ventricular apex and distal septum. Owing to the pacemaker effect on the septum, the phase histograms of each ventricle have a simultaneous onset. However, the left ventricular histogram demonstrates delayed upstroke and peak compared with that of the right ventricle, owing to delayed left ventricular activation. The sequence of phase changes demonstrates initial right ventricular apical and septal changes. The subsequent phase sequence involves the right ventricular body with later involvement of the right ventricular base and left ventricle. (From Botvinick et al,[11] reproduced with permission of the American Heart Association, Inc.)

Similarly, Turner and co-workers,[27] using least squares phase analysis, demonstrated that the sequence of inward ventricular movement paralleled the sequence of depolarization in 14 patients with pacemakers and in three with ventricular tachycardia. Further, the duration of spread of contraction onset or standard deviation of phase angle related well to the QRS duration. Bashore et al[28] later supported these findings and demonstrated the sensitivity of the method when phase image patterns accurately localized all of 35 right and 21 of 25 left ventricular pacing and premature contraction sites, regardless of the presence of wall-motion or contraction abnormalities. Sites as close as 1.5 cm were identified, whereas the surface ECG was both insensitive and nonspecific.

APPLICATIONS OF THE PHASE IMAGE IN CONDUCTION DISORDERS

Bundle Branch Block

In bundle branch block (BBB), the site of earliest phase angle is septal or paraseptal, similar to that noted in normal patients and consistent with the normal conduction pattern proximal to bundle branch bifurcation. Ventricular phase histograms are Gaussian, but that of the affected side always follows that of the contralateral ventricle.[8,29–31] The mean phase angles of the right ventricle in patients with right BBB and of the left ventricle in those with left BBB are delayed compared with that in patients with normal conduction. Machac and co-workers[31] demonstrated similar asynchrony and phase difference in artificial ventricular pacemaker rhythms and showed that the method permitted assessment of asynchrony within as well as between the ventricles (Fig. 13-7).

Left Anterior Fascicular Block

Left anterior fascicular block may be difficult to diagnose accurately from the surface ECG, particularly when an inferior myocardial infarction pattern is present. Dae et al[32] analyzed phase images in the 70° left anterior oblique projection in 13 patients with ECG evidence of left anterior fascicular block. In seven of the 13 patients, phase images confirmed the presence of anterior wall contraction delay. However, only two of these seven patients had narrow phase histograms and normal anterior wall amplitude consistent with an isolated conduction defect. The other five patients had broad histograms with reduced anterior wall amplitude consistent with anterior myocardial infarction. In the remaining six patients, anterior wall contraction preceded inferior wall contrac-

tion, a finding not consistent with left anterior fascicular block. This included four patients with a broad phase histogram and reduced inferior wall amplitude consistent with inferior infarction. Two other patients with ECG evidence of left anterior fascicular block had normal image activation sequences and normal amplitude maps. It appears that the phase image sequence, phase histogram, and phase amplitude image can be combined to clarify surface ECG findings attributed to left anterior fascicular block.

PHASE ANALYSIS IN PREEXCITATION WITH ATRIOVENTRICULAR CONNECTIONS

Phase image analysis has been applied successfully to identification of the preexcitation pathway and characterization of the conduction pattern in patients with preexcitation syndromes. In an initial examination,[12] the site of earliest ventricular phase angle correlated closely with the location of the bypass pathway, documented in an electrophysiologic study of 17 patients preexcited at rest (Fig. 13-8). The focus could be localized at times in some patients not obviously preexcited on the surface electrocardiogram. Sequential phase changes in 10 studies suggested *fusion* of normal septal and lateral bypass fronts.

Subsequently, we have studied more than 40 patients during preexcitation with excellent ability to identify the site of the pathway. There were only seven patients for whom image and electrophysiologic assessment grossly disagreed. These discrepancies not infrequently occurred in patients with two pathways: one identified on electrophysiologic testing, and the other seen on the phase image. On occasion, ambiguities at catheter study were clarified by image evaluation, whereas, in other cases, differences were related to a lack of preexcitation at image evaluation. In some cases, full endocardial mapping was unsuccessful. A difficult task for the imaging method is the specific resolution and differentiation of septal and paraseptal pathways.[33] Problems also arise owing to the difficulties related to triangulation in this nonselective imaging method. However, these can generally be overcome with primary reliance on the phase pattern in the best septal projection for right–left localization and utilization of anterior and 70° left anterior oblique projections for localization in the anterior–posterior plane. Recent work suggests the advantage of single photon emission computed tomography blood-pool imaging with superimposed phase mapping.[34,35] The method appears to be especially useful, not to diagnose the condition, but to clarify ambiguities at electrophysiologic study and provide increased security and accuracy of localization in patients who are to undergo catheter

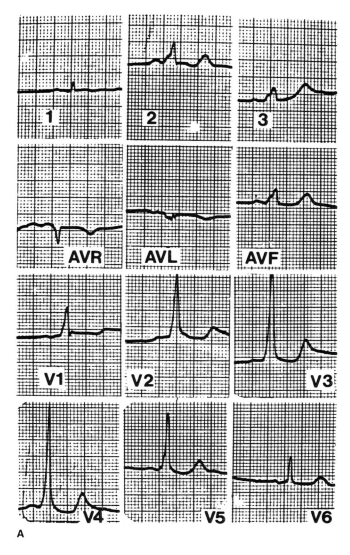

Figure 13-8 **A:** Surface 12-lead electrocardiogram in a patient with a left atrioventricular connection (preexcitation). Although a clear delta wave is apparent, the location of the delta wave is more consistent with a left posterior rather than a left lateral pathway. **B:** Anterior projection—phase image and right (*black*) and left (*white*) ventricular histograms in this same patient. Serial sampling of the spatial distribution of phase angle reveals the site of earliest phase angle at the high lateral left ventricular base.

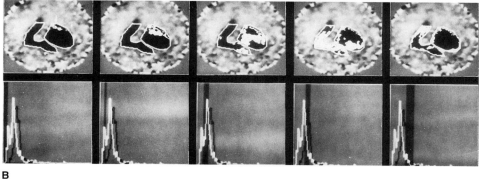

ablation or surgical resection of bypass pathways.[36,37] Phase imaging can identify the focus of preexcitation prior to invasive evaluation, indicate by its location the feasibility of catheter ablation, and potentially shorten the invasive mapping procedure.[38] Owing to its ability to map the pathway only when conducting antegrade, difficulties should be expected when seeking to apply the phase method to the localization of accessory pathways that appear to conduct only in the retrograde direction.

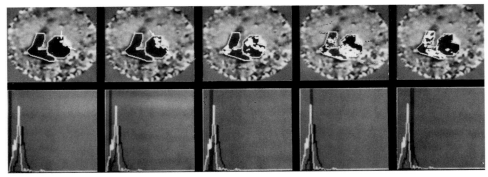

C

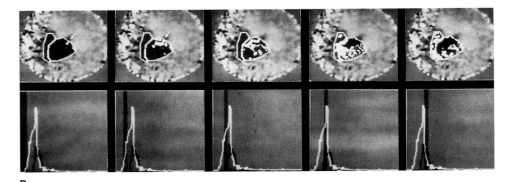

D

**WPW
Left Bypass**

Ant.

BS-LAO

LAO-70°

E

Figure 13-8 (*Continued*) C: Phase image and ventricular histograms in same patient in the best septal left anterior oblique projection. D: Sequential phase sampling indicates a left lateral basal focus as confirmed by the same analysis in the 70° left anterior oblique projection. Note the early occurrence of the left ventricular histogram (*white*). E: Diagrammatic sketches of sequential phase angles in anterior (Ant.), best septal (BS), and 70° left anterior oblique (LAO) projections. Earliest phase angle is shown in *black*. The changes summarize those illustrated above in the actual phase images and show the site of earliest phase angle in each projection to be located at the lateral left ventricular base.

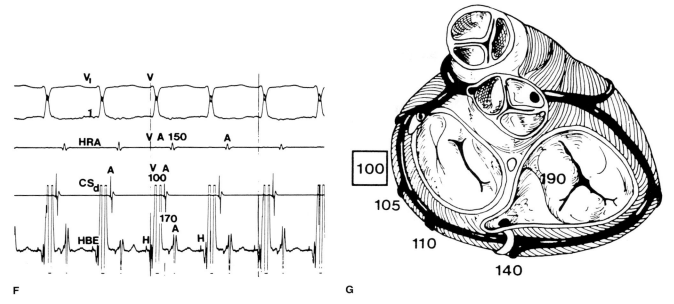

Figure 13-8 (Continued) F: Simultaneous surface leads V₁ and 1, together with recordings from the high right atrium (HRA), distal coronary sinus (CS_d), low atrial septum, and the His bundle electrocardiogram (HBE), are shown during orthodromic atrioventricular reentrant tachycardia. The sequence of retrograde atrial activation can be determined by noting the ventricular (V)–atrial (A) conduction time. During tachycardia, the atrial electrogram recorded from the distal coronary sinus preceded all other recorded atrial positions, confirming the presence of a left lateral atrioventricular accessory pathway. VA conduction times are noted. **G:** Diagrammatic cross section of the heart at the level of the atrioventricular groove in the same patient. Indicated are representative regional VA conduction times actually mapped at electrophysiologic study. The shortest interval, 100 ms, corresponds to the lateral left ventricular location determined above. (From Botvinick et al,[12] reprinted with permission from the American College of Cardiology, *Journal of the American College of Cardiology*, 3:799, 1984.)

EFFECTS OF ATRIAL PACING

The effects of atrial pacing on phase image evaluation were assessed in 11 patients with left or right lateral accessory atrioventricular connections and normal ventricular function[39] (Fig. 13-9). In six patients with minimal preexcitation at rest, ventricular phase patterns were normal. The site of earliest phase angle occurred at the site of the bypass pathway in the remaining patients. With atrial pacing, phase analysis was abnormal in all patients. Earliest phase angle always occurred at the site of the bypass pathway and that of the preexcited ventricle greatly preceded the earliest phase angle of the contralateral ventricle. Pacing made image abnormalities more obvious as preexcitation was augmented. The latter was again supported by the observation that atrial pacing moved the site of latest phase angle, the site of fusion, away from the bypass and brought a widening of the QRS complex. These findings were confirmed by a shortening of the H-Q interval in all patients during atrial pacing at electrophysiologic study.

PREEXCITATION VIA NODOVENTRICULAR AND FASCICULOVENTRICULAR CONNECTIONS

Accessory nodoventricular and fasciculoventricular connections may also present with ECG abnormalities including a delta wave resulting from preexcitation combined with a normal P-R interval. Nodoventricular pathways have been documented to play a significant role in sustained reentrant tachycardias and may add to the ambiguities of electrophysiologic and phase analysis.

Scintigraphic patterns were recorded in 11 patients during preexcitation by Mahaim pathways[40,41]—six nodoventricular and five fasciculoventricular confirmed on electrophysiologic study (Fig. 13-10). Their patterns paralleled the known activation sequence in 10 of 11 patients and could be differentiated from those in normal subjects, those with septal accessory atrioventricular connections with symmetric right and left ventricular phase variation, and from lateral right and left ventricular accessory atrioventricular pathways, with earliest phase angle in the lateral basal aspect of the affected

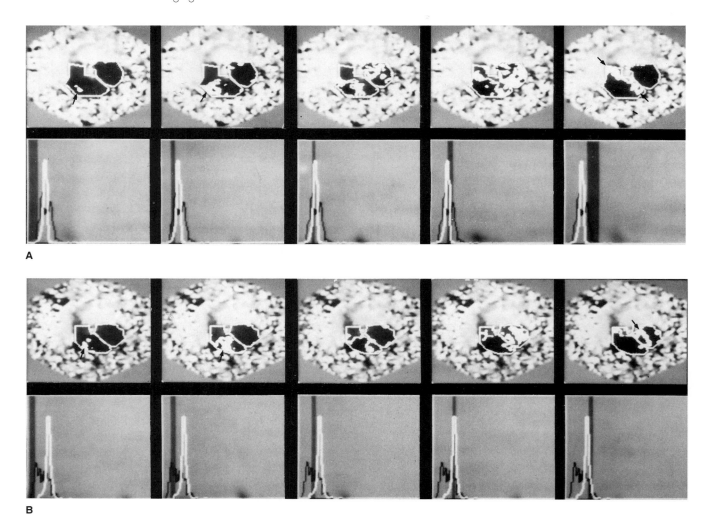

A

B

Figure 13-9 **A:** Phase image and phase histograms (right, *black*; left, *white*) with progressive phase sampling, in a patient with right bypass pathway, evaluated at rest in the best septal left anterior oblique projection. The site of earliest phase angle is seen localized to the anterior and lateral aspect of the right ventricle (*arrows, left panels*). However, the left ventricular changes are seen relatively early, and the regions of greatest phase angle, representing the last ventricular regions to demonstrate contraction onset, are localized to paraseptal and right basal areas in this projection (*arrow, right panel*). **B:** Corresponding findings in the same patient during rapid atrial pacing at a rate of 140 beats/min. Owing to the shorter refractory period of the accessory pathway, the patient is now maximally preexcited and the right ventricular phase histogram greatly precedes that of the left ventricle, as do right ventricular phase angles. Again, the site of earliest phase angle appears in the anterior and lateral right ventricular region (*black arrows, left panels*). With atrial pacing, however, left ventricular phase angles are relatively delayed, and left ventricular changes occur after right ventricular changes are nearly complete.

ventricle. But these patterns did not differ from those in right or left BBB without preexcitation. The strength of the imaging method was well demonstrated in two patients with both left lateral accessory atrioventricular and fasciculoventricular pathways. Their respective phase images showed alterations in the typical phase patterns associated first with the left lateral pathway and, after surgery, the pattern of right-sided phase delay consistent with the fasciculoventricular pathway.

PHASE ANALYSIS IN VENTRICULAR TACHYCARDIA

Recent work has documented the importance of sudden arrhythmic death, and much effort has been directed at its diagnosis, characterization, suppression, and cure. In particular, ventricular stimulation studies performed for diagnostic and therapeutic assessment may be conveniently combined with endocardial mapping procedures.

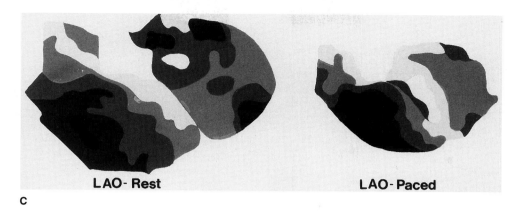

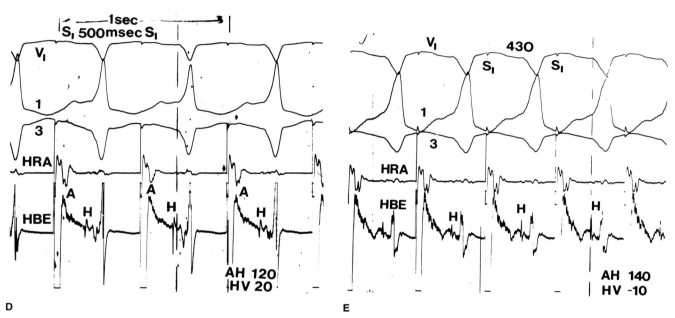

Figure 13-9 (Continued) C: Sketches of sequential phase changes in the best septal left anterior oblique projection at rest (*left*) and with atrial pacing (*right*). **D and E:** Electrophysiologic records obtained during atrial pacing at 120 (D) and 140 (E) beats/min. Each figure demonstrates simultaneous surface leads V_1, 1, and 3, as well as recordings from the high right atrium (HRA), low atrial septum, and the His bundle electrocardiogram (HBE). An increase in atrial pacing rate produced augmentation of conduction through the right-sided bypass pathway. Such predominance of conduction through the bypass pathway is reflected by a progressive widening of the QRS complex and increased prematurity of ventricular activation (V) as the HV interval moves from 20 to −10. Ventricular activation actually preceded His bundle activation at the more rapid pacing rate. (From Botvinick et al,[12] reprinted with permission from the American College of Cardiology, *Journal of the American College of Cardiology*, 3:799, 1984.)

The latter are increasingly important for differentiating among multiple foci and accurately localizing the focus. Such localization offers the best possibilities for catheter ablation while facilitating epicardial mapping at surgery, which will enable precise resection of the ectopic focus and the best opportunity of cure. Blood-pool imaging with phase mapping promises to provide an accurate noninvasive tool for the localization of these foci, aiding often complex, arduous, and sometimes ambiguous electrophysiologic evaluation while providing quantitative evaluation of ventricular size and function.

While patient stability is a requirement for such image analysis, so too is it required for catheter assessment. Owing to the statistical advantage of the parametric method, accurate maps of the ventricular tachycardia focus have been made with less than 1 min of acquisition time. Studies have been performed at the bedside or in the catheterization laboratory during tachycardia induction. While multiple projections are helpful for localization, the best septal, 70° left anterior oblique, and anterior are obtained in that priority, and even a single projection can aid localization of the focus.

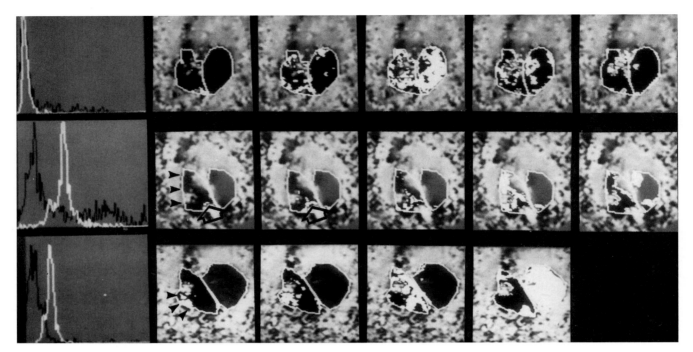

Figure 13-10 Phase analysis in Mahaim pathways—phase image comparison. In the *left panel of each row* are phase histograms for left (*white*) and right (*black*) ventricular regions of interest, obtained in the best septal left anterior oblique projection from the related phase image at right. Phase histograms and images are shown from a patient with normal conduction (*top*), a patient with documented nodoventricular bypass pathway (*middle*), and a patient with a right atrioventricular pathway (*bottom*). The pattern of phase progression in the patient with a nodoventricular connection has onset relatively low in the septum and progresses toward the right ventricle with late left ventricular activation. This pattern also differs from the conventional pattern in septal preexcitation, where the site of earliest phase angle is high in the base of the septum with near simultaneous phase progression through both ventricles. (From Bhandari et al,[40] reprinted with permission from the American College of Cardiology, *Journal of the American College of Cardiology*, 4:611, 1984.)

Swiryn and co-workers[42] first studied six patients with clinical ventricular tachycardia during sinus rhythm and during spontaneous or induced sustained ventricular tachycardia. Their phase map correlated with QRS morphology and axis in most but (not unexpectedly) not all tachycardias. The site of earliest phase angle usually demonstrated the tachycardia origin to lie at the border of a severe contraction abnormality.

We initially studied 25 patients during ventricular tachycardia, with 28 different foci.[43] Each underwent electrophysiologic study but, owing to difficulties encountered and patient intolerance, only 18 foci were successfully mapped. Several of these had to be studied sequentially to obtain the full body of electrophysiologic data. The phase image localized six right ventricular, 10 septal, and 12 left ventricular foci,[11] which corresponded to the same or adjacent endocardial sites in 14 and matched ECG findings in 10 others, including two patients with multiple foci. Again, the image foci often corresponded to the borders of discrete contraction abnormalities.

The surface ECG is limited in its capability to localize the electrical origin of ventricular tachycardia. Furthermore, the same focus of ventricular tachycardia can produce divergent ECG patterns as the conduction pathway is altered. Multiple foci of ventricular tachycardia present an additional problem, and scintigraphic study has been extremely useful in drawing attention to ventricular tachycardia foci not observed or only suspected after electrophysiologic assessment. Phase analysis of the ventricular tachycardia focus has been used to differentiate between a single focus with multiple conduction pathways and multiple foci.[44] This and a subsequent study demonstrate the apparent relationship between the ventricular tachycardia focus and ventricular function.[45]

We compared the blood-pool scintigram obtained at rest in sinus rhythm to that acquired sequentially during ventricular tachycardia in 11 patients who tolerated the rhythm and in eight who demonstrated hemodynamic deterioration. Those who were intolerant to the rhythm revealed a higher mean ventricular tachycardia rate and a greater relative fall in ED volume, SV, and cardiac output compared with the tolerant group. Intolerance appeared to relate to greater dysynchrony in wall motion and resulted in a lower ventricular tachycardia ejection fraction.

The scintigraphic method may be of value in confirming foci in the presence of insecure or incomplete electrophysiologic mapping. Phase localization could shorten the time of performing mapping in the catheterization laboratory or epicardial mapping in the operating room. When surgical incision or catheter ablation is contemplated, confirmation of ECG and electrophysiologic localizing data from a totally independent source, based on a totally independent mechanism, may be a useful measurement.

SUMMARY

Parametric images provide a useful, objective guide to the evaluation of regional contraction abnormalities and may be particularly valuable in serial function assessment. Phase analysis has been used successfully to clarify ambiguous surface ECG patterns, including delineation of anterior and inferior myocardial infarction patterns in the presence of left anterior fascicular block. Phase analysis is capable of mapping ventricular preexcitation foci and offers promise in the localization of foci responsible for ventricular tachycardia.

REFERENCES

1. Ashburn WL, Schelbert HR, Verba JW: Left ventricular ejection fraction: A review of several radionuclide angiographic approaches using the scintillation camera. *Prog Cardiovasc Dis* 20:267, 1978.
2. Botvinick EH, Glazer HB, Shosa DW: What is the reliability and the utility of scintigraphic methods for the assessment of ventricular function? in Rahimtoola SH (ed): *Controversies in Coronary Artery Disease*. Philadelphia, Davis, 1982.
3. Champeney DC: *Fourier Transforms and Their Physical Applications*. New York, Academic Press, 1973, p 8.
4. Goris ML: Functional or parametric images. *J Nucl Med* 23:360, 1982.
5. Gandsman EJ, North DL, Shulman RS, et al: Measurement of the ventricular stroke volume ratio by gated radionuclide angiography. *Radiology* 138:161, 1981.
6. Maddox DE, Holman BL, Wynne J, et al: Ejection fraction image: A noninvasive index of regional left ventricular wall motion. *Am J Cardiol* 41:1230, 1978.
7. Holman BL, Wynne J, Idoine J, et al: The paradox image: Noninvasive index of regional left ventricular dyskinesis. *J Nucl Med* 20:P661, 1979 (abstr).
8. Frais MA, Botvinick EH, Shosa DW, et al: Phase image

characterization of ventricular contraction in left and right bundle branch block. *Am J Cardiol* 50:95, 1982.
9. Walton S, Ell PJ, Jarritt PH, Swanton RH: Phase analysis of the first pass radionuclide angiocardiogram. *Br Heart J* 48:441, 1982.
10. Dae MW, Engelstad BL, Botvinick EH: Parametric imaging in cardiovascular medicine. *Cardiovasc Rev Rep* 6:16, 1985.
11. Botvinick EH, Frais MA, Shosa DW, et al: An accurate means of detecting and characterizing abnormal patterns of ventricular activation by phase image analysis. *Am J Cardiol* 50:289, 1982.
12. Botvinick E, Frais M, O'Connell W, et al: Phase image evaluation of patients with ventricular pre-excitation syndromes. *J Am Coll Cardiol* 3:799, 1984.
13. Clayton PD, Bulawa WF, Klausner SC, et al: The characteristic sequence for the onset of contraction in the normal human left ventricle. *Circulation* 59:671, 1979.
14. Botvinick E, Dunn R, Frais M, et al: The phase image: Its relationship to patterns of contraction and conduction. *Circulation* 65:551, 1982.
15. Turner DA, Shima MA, Ruggie N, et al: Coronary artery disease: Detection by phase analysis of rest/exercise radionuclide angiocardiograms. *Radiology* 148:539, 1983.
16. Mancini GBJ, Peck WW, Slutsky RA: Analysis of phase-angle histograms from equilibrium radionuclide studies: Correlation with semiquantitative grading of wall motion. *Am J Cardiol* 55:535, 1985.
17. Norris SL, Slutsky RA, Gerber KH, et al: Sensitivity and specificity of nuclear phase analysis versus ejection fraction in coronary artery disease. *Am J Cardiol* 53:1547, 1984.
18. Ratib O, Henze E, Schon H, et al: Phase analysis of radionuclide ventriculograms for the detection of coronary artery disease. *Am Heart J* 104:1, 1982.
19. Schwaiger M, Ratib O, Henze E, et al: Limitations of quantitative phase analysis of radionuclide angiograms for detecting coronary artery disease in patients with impaired left ventricular function. *Am Heart J* 108:942, 1984.
20. Frais M, Botvinick E, Shosa D, et al: Phase image characterization of localized and generalized left ventricular contraction abnormalities. *J Am Coll Cardiol* 4:987, 1984.
21. Jones L Jr, Weber PM, Schurr DA: Phase imaging of the left ventricular ECG-gated equilibrium blood pool radionuclide scan as a noninvasive method for detecting aneurysms. *Circulation* 62(suppl III):III-229, 1980 (abstr).
22. Rabinovitch MA, Stewart J, Chan W, et al: Scintigraphic demonstration of ventriculo-atrial conduction in the ventricular pacemaker syndrome. *J Nucl Med* 23:795, 1982.
23. DeMaria AN, Mason DT: Echocardiographic evaluation of disturbances of cardiac rhythm and conduction. *Chest* 71:439, 1977 (editorial).
24. DeMaria AN, Vera Z, Neumann A, et al: Alterations in ventricular contraction pattern in the Wolff–Parkinson–White syndrome—detection by echocardiography. *Circulation* 53:249, 1976.
25. Wyndham CR, Meeran MK, Smith T, et al: Epicardial activation of the intact human heart without conduction defect. *Circulation* 59:161, 1979.
26. Dae M, Davis J, Botvinick E, et al: Comparison of scintigraphic phase maps to epicardial activation maps in dogs. *J Nucl Med* 26:P57, 1985 (abstr).

27. Turner DA, Von Behren PL, Ruggie NT, et al: Noninvasive identification of initial site of abnormal ventricular activation by least-square phase analysis of radionuclide cineangiograms. *Circulation* 65:1511, 1982.

28. Bashore TM, Stine RA, Shaffer PB, et al: The noninvasive localization of ventricular pacing sites by radionuclide phase imaging. *Circulation* 70:681, 1984.

29. Links JM, Douglass KH, Wagner HN Jr: Patterns of ventricular emptying by Fourier analysis of gated blood-pool studies. *J Nucl Med* 21:978, 1980.

30. Swiryn S, Pavel D, Byrom E, et al: Sequential regional phase mapping of radionuclide gated biventriculograms in patients with left bundle branch block. *Am Heart J* 102:1000, 1981.

31. Machac J, Horowitz SF, Miceli K, et al: Quantification of cardiac conduction abnormalities using segmental vector Fourier analysis of radionuclide gated blood pool scans. *J Am Coll Cardiol* 2:1099, 1983.

32. Dae M, Wen YM, Botvinick E, et al: ECG left anterior fascicular block reveals diverse patterns on scintigraphic phase analysis. *Am Heart J* 117:861, 1989.

33. Oeff M, Scheinman MM, Abbott JA, et al: Phase image triangulation of accessory pathways in patients undergoing catheter ablation of posteroseptal pathways. *PACE* 14:1072, 1991.

34. Nakajima K, Bunko H, Tada A, et al: Nuclear tomographic phase analysis: Localization of accessory conduction pathway in patients with Wolff–Parkinson–White syndrome. *Am Heart J* 109:809, 1985.

35. Lucas JR, O'Connell JW, Lee RJ, et al: First harmonic (Fourier) analysis of gated SPECT blood pool scintigrams provides refined assessment of the site of initial activation of accessory pathways in patients with the Wolff–Parkinson–White syndrome. *J Nucl Med* 34:151P, 1993.

36. Nakajima K, Bunko H, Tada A, et al: Phase analysis in the Wolff–Parkinson–White syndrome with surgically proven accessory conduction pathways: Concise communication. *J Nucl Med* 25:7, 1984.

37. Dae M, Botvinick E, Schechtmann M, et al: Correlation of scintigraphic phase maps with intraoperative epicardial/endocardial maps and surgical results in patients with activation disturbances. *Circulation* 70(suppl II):II-371, 1984 (abstr).

38. Chan WWC, Kalff V, Dick M II, et al: Topography of preemptying ventricular segments in patients with Wolff–Parkinson–White syndrome using scintigraphic phase mapping and esophageal pacing. *Circulation* 67:1139, 1983.

39. Botvinick E, Dae MW, Scheinman M, et al: Augmented pre-excitation assessed by scintigraphic phase analysis during atrial pacing. *J Nucl Med* 26:P58, 1985 (abstr).

40. Bhandari A, Morady F, Shen EN, et al: Catheter-induced His bundle ablation in a patient with reentrant tachycardia associated with a nodoventricular tract. *J Am Coll Cardiol* 4:611, 1984.

41. Schechtmann N, Botvinick E, Dae M, et al: The scintigraphic characteristics of ventricular pre-excitation through Mahaim fibers with the use of phase analysis. *J Am Coll Cardiol* 13:882, 1989.

42. Swiryn S, Pavel D, Byrom E, et al: Sequential regional phase mapping of radionuclide gated biventriculograms in patients with sustained ventricular tachycardia: Close correlation with electrophysiologic characteristics. *Am Heart J* 103:319, 1982.

43. Botvinick E, Scheinman M, Morady F, et al: The scintigraphic assessment of sequential changes in ventricular volume, function and contraction pattern during ventricular tachycardia. *J Am Coll Cardiol* 1:711, 1983 (abstr).

44. Botvinick E, Schechtmann N, Dae M, et al: Scintigraphy provides a thorough evaluation of "electrical" and mechanical events during ventricular tachycardia. *J Am Coll Cardiol* 7:235A, 1986 (abstr).

45. Munoz L, Chin M, Krishnan R, et al: Scintigraphic phase analysis provides insight into the consequences of ventricular tachycardia. *J Nucl Med* 33:994, 1992 (abstr).

Measurement of Right Ventricular Function

Barry L. Zaret
Frans J. Th. Wackers

The ability to assess the function of the right ventricle accurately, reproducibly, and repeatedly has developed largely as a result of the advent of nuclear cardiologic techniques. Through the use of time–activity-curve analysis—the basis of radionuclide functional assessment—we have evaluated the physiologic complexities of the right ventricular chamber in a variety of relevant clinical circumstances. In contrast, evaluation of the right ventricle by conventional methodologies has been and will continue to be fraught with difficulty. This chamber has an unusual geometric shape, namely, that of a truncated pyramid, and it does not conform readily to configurations suitable for straightforward geometric analysis or modeling. In addition, the cross-sectional shape of the right ventricle is that of a crescent. In disease states associated with right ventricular enlargement, this crescentic configuration is lost, but this change in shape will not readily be appreciated from a mere analysis of the contours of conventional anterior and lateral images. Furthermore, the right ventricular wall is relatively thin and heavily trabeculated, which makes definition of the endocardial outlines on contrast angiograms quite difficult. As stated above, many of these difficulties are obviated by employing radioisotopic time–activity-curve analysis, thereby rendering inoperative geometric analytic considerations.

This chapter reviews radionuclide techniques for evaluating right ventricular function. Measurement parameters are defined and physiologic determinants are discussed. The clinical relevance of these measurements, particularly with respect to coronary artery disease

and chronic obstructive pulmonary disease, is emphasized.

TECHNIQUES

Three basic radionuclide techniques have been employed to evaluate the right ventricle: the conventional first-pass radionuclide angiocardiogram, the gated first-pass radionuclide angiocardiogram, and the equilibrium radionuclide angiocardiogram. All three studies generally employ technetium 99m (^{99m}Tc) as the primary radionuclide. However, a variety of short-lived tracers, usually generator produced, have also been employed.

First-pass radionuclide angiocardiograms are best obtained with a computerized multicrystal scintillation camera or the newer digital single-crystal cameras, which have special high count rate capabilities. For the first-pass study, it is optimal to use such instrumentation to alleviate problems associated with low count rate statistics and inadequate dead-time correction, which result in substantial data loss and inaccuracy. Conventional scintillation cameras are not configured to provide accurate and reliable first-pass data. (The technical details of first-pass study performance are presented in Chap. 10.)

Studies are obtained after the peripheral venous injection of the radioactive tracer. The injection site should not be distal to the antecubital fossa. Despite the fact that optimal anatomic separation of right atrium and

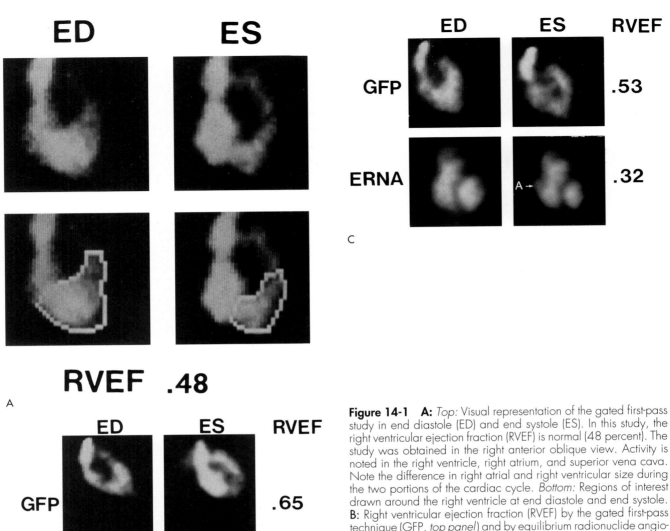

Figure 14-1 **A:** *Top:* Visual representation of the gated first-pass study in end diastole (ED) and end systole (ES). In this study, the right ventricular ejection fraction (RVEF) is normal (48 percent). The study was obtained in the right anterior oblique view. Activity is noted in the right ventricle, right atrium, and superior vena cava. Note the difference in right atrial and right ventricular size during the two portions of the cardiac cycle. *Bottom:* Regions of interest drawn around the right ventricle at end diastole and end systole. **B:** Right ventricular ejection fraction (RVEF) by the gated first-pass technique (GFP, *top panel*) and by equilibrium radionuclide angiocardiography (ERNA, *bottom panel*). RVEF is normal by both techniques, although higher by gated first-pass technique. During right ventricular systole, the right atrium (A, *arrow*) is well separated from the right ventricle, allowing a reasonably accurate assessment of RVEF by the equilibrium method. **C:** Right ventricular ejection fraction (RVEF) by the gated first-pass method (GFP, *top panel*) and by equilibrium radionuclide angiocardiography (ERNA, *bottom panel*). Although RVEF is normal by GFP (0.53), RVEF is calculated to be abnormal by ERNA (0.32). It can be appreciated that the right atrium (A, *arrow*) is not well separated from the right ventricle during right ventricular systole, resulting in an erroneously low calculation of RVEF.

right ventricle is achieved in the right anterior oblique view, the anterior position is employed for these first-pass studies. Acquiring in the anterior position will allow the most efficient analysis of both right and left ventricular functions with this technique. In the right anterior oblique position, the left ventricle is placed further away from the detector because of the overlap of the two ventricular chambers. Hence, left ventricular count data are somewhat attenuated and detected less efficiently.

This will detract from the reliability of analysis of the left heart phase, which usually is an important part of the total study. If one is only interested in the right ventricle, however, the right anterior oblique position is probably preferable.

Data analysis using the first-pass technique is relatively straightforward and has been reported previously.[1] Regions of interest are determined for both the right ventricle and background zones. A time–activity curve based on two to four beats is obtained, and right ventricular ejection fraction is derived from the average value of the data from each beat. Alternatively, the data from several beats can be summed, providing a composite time–activity curve. Recently, Johnson et al compared right ventricular ejection fraction by first-pass techniques with measurements by magnetic resonance imaging. An excellent correlation was noted when a two-region-of-interest processing method was employed.[2]

The gated first-pass technique provides a viable option for performing first-pass studies while utilizing conventional single-crystal gamma cameras[3] (Fig. 14-1). This is particularly relevant since this type of instrumentation is routinely available if nuclear studies are performed. The gated first-pass technique involves a conventional bolus injection of radioactivity, with acquisition of data in a multigated frame mode in concert with the R wave of the electrocardiogram (ECG). In this manner, data are summed during the bolus passage through the right heart, using the ECG as a synchronizing signal. In so doing, problems associated with accurate recognition of maxima and minima and with reliability of the data are overcome. Data acquisition is terminated when the radioactivity clearly has entered the lung field.

With both gated first-pass and conventional first-pass techniques, one must be concerned about streaming of the radioactive bolus. This can result in inadequate mixing and consequent inaccuracies in time–activity-curve analysis. By using the gated first-pass technique, one obtains a better visual analysis of right ventricular regional wall motion than with the conventional first pass obtained on a multicrystal camera.

The third general approach involves utilization of the equilibrium radionuclide angiocardiographic study. This technique provides the best means of qualitatively evaluating right ventricular regional contraction patterns. Since activity is present throughout the blood pool, studies are obtained in the left anterior oblique position. It is necessary to employ the left anterior oblique view because this is the only position in which right and left ventricles are adequately separated. In the left anterior oblique position, however, there is substantial right atrial–right ventricular overlap and, unfortunately, the right atrium is superimposed on the right ventricle with respect to the detector. Therefore, there will be a significant right atrial contribution to the right ventricular time–activity curve. Because of its anterior position with respect to the detector, this right atrial contamination can result in substantial error. Generally, right ventricular ejection fraction determined by the equilibrium technique will underestimate that measured by either first-pass approach. This problem has been dealt with to some extent through the use of a special caudally tilted slant-hole collimator.[4] Because of the problems stated above, it is the authors' preference to perform right ventricular quantitative analyses of ejection fraction with either the conventional first-pass or gated

first-pass techniques. These problems may be of even greater magnitude when studies are done during exercise rather than in the resting state.

The potential availability of other radionuclides may have a significant impact on right ventricular measurements, particularly by the first-pass technique. Two new generator-produced radioisotopes have been employed in first-pass studies involving right and left ventricles. These radioactive tracers have quite short physical half-lives compared with ^{99m}Tc (6 h). They are the osmium–iridium system, with iridium 191m having a physical half-life of 4.9 s;[5] and the mercury–gold system, with gold 195m having a half-life of 30.5 s.[6] Because of the extremely short half-life of these radioisotopes, repeated studies can be done using the first-pass technique, thereby providing multiple measurements suitable for evaluation of rapidly changing physiologic states and therapeutic effects. At present, neither system is available for commercial use. In addition, the ^{99m}Tc-labeled perfusion agents may be injected as a bolus, thereby enabling first-pass measurement of right ventricular function during a perfusion imaging study either at rest or during stress.

Another radioisotopic approach involves the use of gaseous radioactive tracers that are excreted via the lung. Krypton 81m, with a half-life of 13 s,[7,8] as well as xenon 133,[9] have been employed. Since the radioactivity is eliminated in the lungs, one can administer a continuous infusion that will result in steady-state blood-pool activity only in the right-sided cardiac structures. This allows for high count rate studies. Krypton has its major energy at 190 keV; therefore, it is an excellent agent for imaging with the conventional scintillation camera.

MEASUREMENT PARAMETERS

Clearly, the most common parameter of right ventricular function measured routinely over the past decade has been right ventricular ejection fraction. Reasonable correlations have been demonstrated between measurements of right ventricular ejection fraction obtained by the various techniques. The lower limit of normal for right ventricular ejection fraction ranges from 40 to 45 percent (Fig. 14-2). Right ventricular ejection fraction is particularly dependent on the afterload faced by the right ventricle. Reasonable correlations between right ventricular ejection fraction and either pulmonary artery systolic pressure or pulmonary vascular resistance have been demonstrated by a number of investigators[10–12] (Fig. 14-3). A less dramatic but nevertheless significant relationship also exists between right ventricular ejection fraction and preload as assessed by right atrial pressure and right ventricular end-diastolic volume.[10] The marked afterload dependence of right ventricular ejection frac-

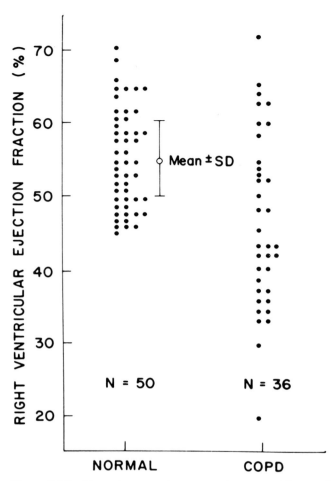

Figure 14-2 The right ventricular ejection fraction in 50 normal adult subjects and 36 patients with chronic obstructive pulmonary disease (COPD). Data were obtained with a computerized multi-crystal scintillation camera. The normal range for this study by this technique is from 45 to 65 percent. In patients with chronic obstructive pulmonary disease, the right ventricular ejection fraction ranged from 19 to 71 percent and was abnormal (less than 45 percent) in 19. (From Berger et al,[1] reproduced with permission.)

highly specific (100 percent). Based on these data, it would seem that the finding of right ventricular ejection fraction of 40 percent or less, at least in patients with chronic obstructive pulmonary disease, is reasonable evidence for the presence of pulmonary hypertension. This particular assessment is recommended in patients with chronic obstructive pulmonary disease.

In addition to right ventricular ejection fraction, right ventricular volumes and pressure–volume relations also can be assessed. Ventricular volumes can be measured directly from the nuclear data. Dell'Italia et al demonstrated good correlation between attenuation-corrected equilibrium radionuclide angiocardiographic determinations of right ventricular volume and biplane cineventriculography that had been validated by postmortem cast studies.[14] Right ventricular volumes may also be derived if cardiac output is determined by an independent modality, such as thermodilution. Stroke volume and ejection fraction then are used to calculate end-systolic and end-diastolic volumes. This approach has been employed in a number of studies, including reports by Brent et al,[10,15,16] Konstam et al,[17,18] and Mahler et al.[19,20] Volume measurements take on an independent importance in study of the failing ventricle, where changes in volume may be a more sensitive index of therapeutic efficacy than ejection fraction.

Because of the load dependence of right ventricular ejection fraction, it is important to define additional modalities for assessment of intrinsic contractility of this chamber. The same principles of ventricular systolic pressure–volume relations used to evaluate contractility of the left ventricle can also be applied to the right ventricle.[10,17] End-systolic or peak-systolic pressure–volume

tion can be used in a positive sense to aid in the diagnosis of pulmonary hypertension.[12] Brent et al demonstrated that the assessment of right ventricular ejection fraction at rest was helpful in distinguishing patients with resting pulmonary artery hypertension occurring in chronic obstructive pulmonary disease.[13] In a group of 30 patients with combined radionuclide and hemodynamic measurements, the value of right ventricular ejection fraction at rest could predict the presence of pulmonary hypertension, defined as a mean pulmonary artery pressure of greater than 20 mmHg (Fig. 14-4). Using a right ventricular ejection fraction of less than 45 percent was highly sensitive (100 percent) but less specific (55 percent), whereas a right ventricular ejection fraction of 40 percent or less was somewhat less sensitive (75 percent) but

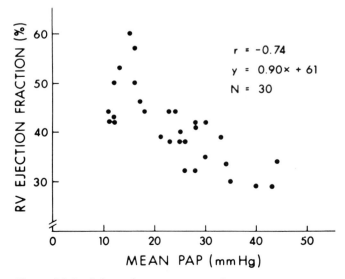

Figure 14-3 Relation between mean pulmonary artery pressure (PAP) and right ventricular (RV) ejection fraction. (From Brent et al,[13] reproduced with permission.)

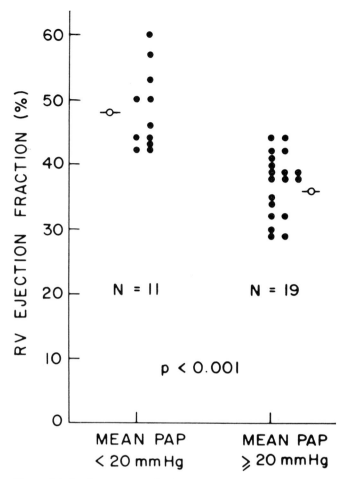

Figure 14-4 Comparison of right ventricular (RV) ejection fraction in patients with and in those without pulmonary artery hypertension. PAP, pulmonary artery pressure. (From Brent et al,[13] reproduced with permission.)

a complicated protocol including pulmonary artery catheterization and the administration of vasoactive drugs.

STUDIES IN CORONARY ARTERY DISEASE

A number of studies have demonstrated the frequent occurrence of right ventricular dysfunction in the course of acute myocardial infarction. These studies have employed both the first-pass and equilibrium techniques. The majority have emphasized the occurrence of right ventricular dysfunction, with or without other evidence of myocardial necrosis, as being predominantly a phenomenon associated with inferior wall myocardial infarction. This was initially demonstrated by Reduto et al[21] and Tobinick et al[22] and has since been confirmed by others.[23] Abnormal right ventricular ejection fraction may be noted in as many as approximately 50 percent of patients with inferior wall myocardial infarction. However, this frequency appears to have been reduced dramatically in patients treated with thrombolytic therapy. In the Thrombosis in Myocardial Infarction Phase II (TIMI II) study, only 5 percent of patients with inferior infarction manifested right ventricular regional dysfunction on equilibrium studies.[24] Abnormal right ventricular ejection fraction also has been associated with a characteristic ECG abnormality consisting of ST-segment elevation in lead V_{4R}.[25] Right ventricular dysfunction has also been a frequent concomitant of high-degree atrioventricular block in patients with inferior myocardial infarction.[26] A right ventricular ejection fraction of less than 35 percent is clearly associated with significant hemodynamic consequences.[27] As stated previously, right ventricular ejection fraction is an extremely load-dependent parameter. Therefore, one might expect that the presence of regional wall-motion abnormalities of right ventricular contraction would provide a more specific indicator of right ventricular infarction. This does indeed appear to be the case, based on the data of Starling et al[23] and Cabin et al.[28]

Although right ventricular infarction is traditionally associated with inferior infarction, right ventricular infarction and necrosis may also be concomitants of anterior wall infarction. Cabin et al demonstrated this in a series of 13 necropsy patients, most of whom also had coincident radionuclide ventricular function studies.[28,29] All patients with anterior wall infarction and concomitant right ventricular infarction had sustained extremely large degrees of left ventricular damage (average left ventricular ejection fraction = 15 percent), had right ventricular necrosis located anteriorly rather than posteriorly, and inevitably had involvement of the interventricular septum. Clinically, right ventricular infarction was not suspected in any of these patients despite evi-

data are obtained under varying afterload conditions and these points are connected (Fig. 14-5). A minimum of three points is required. The slope of the systolic pressure–volume relation is a reflection of the intrinsic contractility of the chamber and has been deemed E_{max}. This parameter provides a more load-independent index of ventricular performance. To generate an appropriate number of points, right ventricular afterload alteration should be undertaken. Infusions of nitroglycerin and nitroprusside, either alone or in combination, have been employed to alter pulmonary artery pressures. Whether the use of pressure–volume relations will provide clinically relevant data suitable for patient evaluation currently remains unclear. A number of studies have indicated the potential physiologic value of these measurements. Their clinical meaningfulness requires further definition and demonstration of efficacy, independent of that obtainable with resting ejection fraction or ventricular volumes alone. Clearly, measurement of E_{max} involves

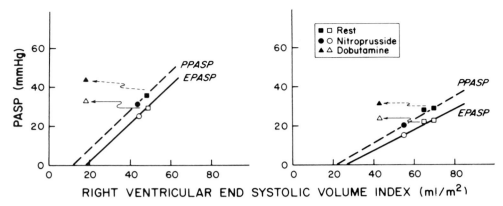

Figure 14-5 Systolic pressure–volume relations in two patients receiving dobutamine. Pulmonary artery systolic pressure (PASP) is plotted against right ventricular end-systolic volume index. The *dashed lines* refer to data derived using peak pulmonary artery systolic pressure (PPASP), and the *solid lines* refer to data obtained with pulmonary arterial end-systolic pressure (EPASP). Administration of dobutamine, an inotropic agent, results in a shift of the systolic pressure–volume relation to the left, corresponding to an increased contractile state. (From Brent et al,[10] reproduced with permission.)

dence of right ventricular dysfunction on radionuclide studies. This phenomenon merits further clinical attention, since patients with associated right ventricular infarction may have the hemodynamics of right ventricular infarction totally obscured by that of major left ventricular dysfunction. Despite left ventricular dysfunction, these patients may require increased intravascular volume to augment right ventricular forward output and place a severely compromised left ventricle in a more optimal hemodynamic status.

The presence of significant infarction-related right ventricular dysfunction raises the question of whether monitoring right ventricular function may be important in assessing thrombolytic therapy in the infarct patient. This was assessed by Schuler et al in a group of 19 patients with proximal right coronary obstruction and acute inferior wall myocardial infarction.[30] In the 12 patients in whom recanalization of the infarct artery was achieved, there was statistically significant early improvement in right ventricular ejection fraction (30 ± 9 percent to 39 ± 7 percent), with further improvement noted at 4 weeks (43 ± 5 percent). In contrast, in those patients without recanalization, right ventricular ejection fraction remained unchanged. However, a conflicting set of data on this question was reported by Verani et al, who evaluated 30 patients with inferior wall myocardial infarction, 19 of whom had right ventricular dysfunction on admission.[31] They noted an improvement in right ventricular ejection fraction in patients who had achieved successful recanalization. However, comparable improvement was noted both in control patients who did not receive therapy and in patients in whom recanalization was not achieved. The investigators concluded that right ventricular dysfunction following inferior wall infarction is often transient and tends to improve irrespective of thrombolytic therapy. Questions remain con-

cerning whether infarct-related right ventricular dysfunction occurs on an ischemic or a necrotic myocardial basis. Further natural history studies concerning the temporal sequence of change following various types of infarction are also necessary. Nevertheless, at this time, one can conclude that right ventricular assessment in appropriately selected acute-infarct patients can add significantly to overall evaluation and can define those in whom aggressive therapy with volume loading should be undertaken.

Right ventricular performance has also been assessed during exercise in patients with coronary artery disease. Data from our laboratory suggest that the major determinant of right ventricular dysfunction during exercise is the concomitant occurrence of left ventricular dysfunction.[32] This would suggest that left ventricular diastolic abnormality leading to elevated pulmonary artery pressure and increased right ventricular afterload stress is the major pathophysiologic mechanism involved. In our series, abnormalities occurred independently of the presence or absence of proximal right coronary artery stenosis. However, this is an area in which some controversy exists. In a recent study during right coronary angioplasty, it was noted that right ventricular ejection fraction fell and right ventricular wall-motion abnormalities developed during transient right coronary occlusion.[33] This, however, is a dramatic representation of ischemia and is not necessarily comparable to exercise-induced ischemia.

CHRONIC OBSTRUCTIVE PULMONARY DISEASE

Since the right ventricle sustains the major hemodynamic burden in chronic obstructive pulmonary disease, it is not surprising that a substantial effort has focused on evaluating right ventricular performance in this condition. Right ventricular failure carries an extremely poor prognostic impact in patients with chronic obstructive pulmonary disease. Development of pulmonary artery hypertension and subsequent right ventricular failure are associated with a 73 percent mortality within 4 years.[34] Indeed, cor pulmonale is a major cause of death in patients with chronic obstructive pulmonary disease. An assessment of right ventricular function at rest should be routine in patients with significant chronic obstructive pulmonary disease. In the initial series of Berger et al, all patients with cor pulmonale were identified by virtue of abnormal right ventricular ejection fraction (Fig. 14-6).[1] As stated above, abnormal right ventricular ejection fraction can also be used to identify those patients with chronic obstructive pulmonary disease who already manifest pulmonary hypertension. Identification prior to presentation with clinical heart failure can lead to appropriate interventions designed both to augment right ventricular performance and decrease right ventricular afterload. Right ventricular performance can be used to assess the efficacy of vasodilator therapy in patients with pulmonary hypertension and right ventricular dysfunction. Brent et al demonstrated the efficacy of this approach in a comparative assessment of nitroglycerin, hydralazine, and nitroprusside.[15] In that study, the primary arterial vasodilator hydralazine had the greatest effect with respect to both lowering pulmonary vascular resistance and improving right ventricular function (Fig. 14-7). This improvement was associated with a substantial increment in forward cardiac output and oxygen delivery. Similar observations have been made with terbutaline in this patient group.[16] Studies in the pulmonary disease group need not be limited to conventional disease types such as chronic bronchitis and emphysema. Additional studies have been performed in young adults with cystic fibrosis. In this group, additional relevant hemodynamic-clinical-radionuclide correlations have also been made.[35,36] In these patients, identification of right ventricular dysfunction prior to hemodynamic decompensation may also be of particular clinical relevance.

Exercise studies assessing right ventricular responses to physical stress have also been performed in pulmonary patients. These studies are of interest from both the clinical and physiologic standpoints. In patients with lung disease, it is clinically important to distinguish cardiac from respiratory causes of dyspnea, since underlying occult left ventricular dysfunction, either intrinsic or from another disease state, can also be present. Furthermore, the role of right ventricular dysfunction, either primary or secondary, in contributing to exercise intolerance should be defined. A different protocol must be employed to assess exercise ventricular performance in pulmonary patients.[37] A conventional graded, symptom-limited exercise test is not appropriate, since under such conditions

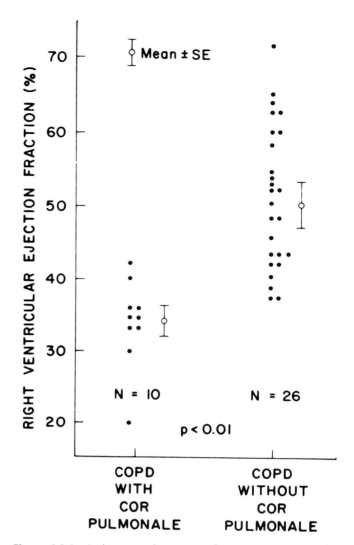

Figure 14-6 Right ventricular ejection fraction in patients with chronic obstructive pulmonary disease (COPD) with or without cor pulmonale. All patients with cor pulmonale demonstrate an abnormal right ventricular ejection fraction. It is of interest to note that nine additional patients without cor pulmonale also demonstrate depressed right ventricular ejection fraction. (From Berger et al,[1] reproduced with permission.)

respiratory disease patients may become markedly hypoxemic and acidemic. For this reason, exercise should involve a steady-state, submaximal response at approximately 50 to 60 percent of the effort required to produce maximal oxygen consumption. This level of exercise is selected because it is considered to be significantly below the anaerobic threshold in these patients and represents a functional level appropriate for their physical activity.

Using this exercise protocol, Matthay et al evaluated a group of patients with chronic obstructive pulmonary disease.[37] In this study, the majority of patients manifested an abnormal right ventricular response to exercise. The incidence of abnormality could be related directly

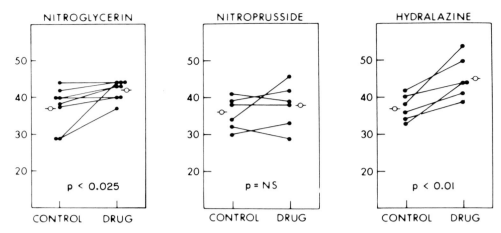

Figure 14-7 Right ventricular ejection fraction at control and after administration of nitroglycerin, nitroprusside, and hydralazine. Both nitroglycerin and hydralazine result in an increase in right ventricular ejection fraction, whereas nitroprusside does not. However, the increase in right ventricular ejection fraction noted with nitroglycerin is relatively modest. (From Brent et al,[15] reproduced with permission.)

to the functional severity of the underlying pulmonary disease. Abnormal right ventricular responses to exercise were noted in all patients with severe pulmonary disease. This response was evaluated further by Mahler et al in a combined hemodynamic and radionuclide study of 12 patients with chronic obstructive pulmonary disease, studied during upright exercise, in whom pulmonary artery pressures, right ventricular hemodynamics, cardiac output, and pleural pressure (measured with an esophageal balloon) were compared.[19] During steady-state upright exercise, it was noted that pulmonary artery pressure and pulmonary vascular resistance rose inordinately high and were associated with failure to augment right ventricular ejection fraction. In addition, right ventricular end-diastolic volumes increased, whereas right ventricular end-systolic volumes did not change. These data, as well as the data of Morrison et al,[38] show clearly that exercise performance in these patients with chronic obstructive pulmonary disease can be limited by right ventricular dysfunction in addition to respiratory impairment.

Right ventricular studies are also of value in assessing patients with acute respiratory distress syndrome[39] and patients receiving therapy with positive end-expiratory pressure (PEEP). In particular, PEEP, which may be associated with significant changes in intrathoracic pressures, would be expected to affect right ventricular function substantially. Schulman et al noted that the right ventricular response to PEEP was determined to a major extent by the degree of baseline right ventricular dysfunction.[40] Furthermore, on the basis of ventricular interaction, the extent of right ventricular impairment and dilatation were major influences on altered left ventricular diastolic function during PEEP.[41]

CONGESTIVE HEART FAILURE AND CARDIOMYOPATHY

Assessment of right ventricular performance may be of significant value in defining the composite hemodynamic status of patients with congestive heart failure. Konstam et al evaluated right ventricular ejection fraction, right ventricular volumes, and right ventricular pressure–volume relations in patients with heart failure.[18] They noted a significant negative correlation between right ventricular end-systolic pressure–volume slope and end-systolic volume. Their data also indicated that greatest improvement in right ventricular systolic emptying with vasodilators can be expected in those with the largest right ventricular end-systolic volume at baseline. Thus, estimation of right ventricular end-systolic volume by radionuclide techniques may be useful in identifying those patients most likely to benefit from appropriate vasodilator therapy.

Baker et al evaluated the relationship between resting right ventricular ejection fraction and exercise capacity in patients with chronic severe congestive heart failure.[42] They noted that there was an excellent correlation between right ventricular ejection fraction at rest and overall exercise capacity as measured by maximal oxygen consumption. In contrast, there was no correlation between left ventricular ejection fraction and this parameter of overall exercise performance. The same lack of correlation between left ventricular ejection fraction and exercise performance in heart failure had been noted previously.[43] The correlation between right ventricular ejection fraction and maximal oxygen consumption was somewhat stronger in patients with coronary disease than in those with dilated cardiomyopathy. It will require further study to define the underlying mechanism for these observations. The results may indicate the primary importance of the right ventricle with respect to overall cardiac function. Alternatively, this may indicate that right ventricular ejection fraction reflects the overall systolic and diastolic function of the left ventricle in addition to providing insights on primary right ventricular function. Since the right ventricle is markedly dependent on afterload conditions, abnormal left ventricular diastolic function in heart failure patients may be reflected more in right ventricular than left ventricular systolic measurements. In addition, important ventricular interactions are based on sharing of the interventricular septum and effects mediated via the pericardium. Whatever the underlying mechanism, it is clear that appropriate assessment of right ventricular function is an important aspect of the comprehensive assessment of patients with congestive heart failure. A recent long-term follow-up study of cardiomyopathy patients showed that, for comparable degrees of left ventricular dysfunction, those with associated right ventricular dysfunction had a poorer prognosis.[44]

From a diagnostic standpoint, preserved right heart function in the presence of left ventricular dysfunction in heart failure suggests coronary artery disease, hypertension, or aortic valve disease as the likely culprits, whereas marked biventricular dysfunction suggests primary myocardial disease or far-advanced disease of any etiology. In the setting of cardiomyopathy, however, the presence of tricuspid regurgitation must be considered, since this lesion may alter traditional physiologic relationships.[45]

CONGENITAL HEART DISEASE

Assessment of right ventricular performance can be of clinical significance in several congenital processes that primarily affect the right heart. Conditions such as tetralogy of Fallot, atrial septal defect, and pulmonic stenosis are but a few.[46,47] Right ventricular performance can be evaluated under conditions of rest and exercise. Depending on the condition, abnormal right ventricular performance may reflect either afterload stress or intrinsic myocardial dysfunction.

VALVULAR HEART DISEASE

Assessment of right ventricular function is of prime importance in disease of the mitral valve, particularly in the presence of elevated pulmonary artery pressures. The clinical recognition of right ventricular dysfunction and its potential impact on the postoperative status of patients undergoing mitral valve replacement requires definition.[48] In this instance, the primary determinant of right ventricular function appears to be afterload stress.[11] However, if the condition is sufficiently severe and of sufficient duration, then intrinsic right ventricular failure can develop with an associated fall in right ventricular function.[49-51] Preoperative assessment of right ventricular ejection fraction may play an important role in predicting surgical outcome in the treatment of regurgitant lesions.[52,53]

SEPTIC SHOCK

Kimchi et al demonstrated that right ventricular performance may be abnormal in patients with septic shock.[54] In a series of 25 patients with septic shock, depressed right ventricular ejection fraction was present in 13. This was seen in patients with both elevated and normal or low cardiac outputs. The presence of right ventricular dysfunction was not directly attributable to the presence of acute respiratory failure. In eight of the 13 patients, abnormal right ventricular function was accompanied by left ventricular dysfunction, while, in five patients, impairment occurred in the presence of normal left ventricular performance. In this clinical circumstance, there was no correlation between abnormal right ventricular afterload and depressed right ventricular ejection fraction. These data suggest that right ventricular dysfunction may be an important pathophysiologic mechanism in some patients with septic shock. Parker et al noted concomitant responses in right and left ventricular ejection fractions in both survivors and fatalities of septic shock, suggesting a more diffuse cardiac dysfunction.[55] Clearly, this parameter should be monitored in this patient subgroup.

CONCLUSION

Over the past decade, measurement of right ventricular performance by radionuclide techniques has become an accepted modality for the clinical evaluation of a variety of patients. Evaluation of right ventricular performance makes it possible to characterize many patients with both known and unsuspected dysfunction of this cardiac chamber. It is recommended that right ventricular performance be assessed routinely in patients with pulmonary disease, acute and chronic coronary disease, and congestive heart failure as well as in other clinical subsets in whom right ventricular dysfunction may play an important role in the overall clinical presentation. While echocardiography is now used frequently for evaluating left ventricular function, the precision and reproducibility inherent in radionuclide techniques for assessing the right ventricle suggest strongly that nuclear approaches should retain primacy in this arena. Further comparative echo–nuclear studies assessing the right ventricle would be of definite value.

REFERENCES

1. Berger HJ, Matthay RA, Loke J, et al: Assessment of cardiac performance with quantitative radionuclide angiocardiography: Right ventricular ejection fraction with reference to findings in chronic obstructive pulmonary disease. *Am J Cardiol* 41:897, 1978.

2. Johnson LL, Lawson MA, Blackwell GG, et al: Optimizing the method to calculate right ventricular ejection fraction from first-pass data acquired with a multicrystal camera. *J Nucl Cardiol* 2:372, 1995.

3. Morrison DA, Turgeon J, Ovitt T: Right ventricular ejection fraction measurement: Contrast ventriculography versus gated blood pool and gated first-pass radionuclide methods. *Am J Cardiol* 54:651, 1984.

4. Konstam MA, Kahn PC, Curran BH, et al: Equilibrium (gated) radionuclide ejection fraction measurement in the pressure or volume overloaded right ventricle: Comparison of three methods. *Chest* 86:681, 1984.

5. Treves S, Cheng C, Samuel A, et al: Iridium-191 angiocardiography for the detection and quantitation of left-to-right shunting. *J Nucl Med* 21:1151, 1980.

6. Wackers FJ, Giles RW, Hoffer PB, et al: Gold-195m, a new generator-produced short-lived radionuclide for sequential assessment of ventricular performance by first pass radionuclide angiocardiography. *Am J Cardiol* 50:89, 1982.

7. Horn M, Witztum K, Neveu C, et al: Krypton-81m imaging of the right ventricle. *J Nucl Med* 26:33, 1985.

8. Nienaber CA, Spielmann RP, Wasmus G, et al: Clinical use of ultrashort-lived radionuclide krypton-81m for noninvasive analysis of right ventricular performance in normal subjects and patients with right ventricular dysfunction. *J Am Coll Cardiol* 5:687, 1985.

9. Dahlstrom JA: Radionuclide assessment of right ventricular ejection fraction: A comparison of first pass studies with ¹³³Xe and ⁹⁹ᵐTc. *Clin Physiol* 2:205, 1982.

10. Brent BN, Berger HJ, Matthay RA, et al: Physiologic correlates of right ventricular ejection fraction in chronic obstructive pulmonary disease: A combined radionuclide and hemodynamic study. *Am J Cardiol* 50:255, 1982.

11. Cohen M, Horowitz SF, Machac J, et al: Response of the right ventricle to exercise in isolated mitral stenosis. *Am J Cardiol* 55:1054, 1985.

12. Schulman DS: Assessment of the right ventricle with radionuclide techniques. *J Nucl Cardiol* 3:253, 1996.

13. Brent BN, Mahler D, Matthay RA, et al: Noninvasive diagnosis of pulmonary arterial hypertension in chronic obstructive pulmonary disease: Right ventricular ejection fraction at rest. *Am J Cardiol* 53:1349, 1984.

14. Dell'Italia LJ, Starling MR, Walsh RA, et al: Validation of attenuation-corrected equilibrium radionuclide angiographic determinations of right ventricular volume: Comparison with cast-validated biplane cineventriculography. *Circulation* 72:317, 1985.

15. Brent BN, Berger HJ, Matthay RA, et al: Contrasting acute effects of vasodilators (nitroglycerin, nitroprusside, and hydralazine) on right ventricular performance in patients with chronic obstructive pulmonary disease and pulmonary hypertension: A combined radionuclide–hemodynamic study. *Am J Cardiol* 51:1682, 1983.

16. Brent BN, Mahler D, Berger HJ, et al: Augmentation of right ventricular performance in chronic obstructive pulmonary disease by terbutaline: A combined radionuclide and hemodynamic study. *Am J Cardiol* 50:313, 1982.

17. Konstam MA, Salem DN, Isner JM, et al: Vasodilator effect on right ventricular function in congestive heart failure and pulmonary hypertension: End-systolic pressure–volume relation. *Am J Cardiol* 54:132, 1984.

18. Konstam MA, Cohen SR, Salem DN, et al: Comparison of left and right ventricular end-systolic pressure–volume relations in congestive heart failure. *J Am Coll Cardiol* 5:1326, 1985.

19. Mahler DA, Brent BN, Loke J, et al: Right ventricular performance and central circulatory hemodynamics during upright exercise in patients with chronic obstructive pulmonary disease. *Am Rev Respir Dis* 130:722, 1984.

20. Mahler DA, Matthay RA, Snyder PE, et al: Volumetric responses of right and left ventricles during upright exercise in normal subjects. *J Appl Physiol* 58:1818, 1985.

21. Reduto LA, Berger HJ, Cohen LS, et al: Sequential radionuclide assessment of left and right ventricular performance after acute transmural myocardial infarction. *Ann Intern Med* 89:441, 1978.

22. Tobinick E, Schelbert HR, Henning H, et al: Right ventricular ejection fraction in patients with acute inferior and anterior myocardial infarction assessed by radionuclide angiography. *Circulation* 57:1078, 1978.

23. Starling MR, Dell'Italia LJ, Chaudhuri TK, et al: First transit and equilibrium radionuclide angiography in patients with inferior transmural myocardial infarction: Criteria for the diagnosis of associated hemodynamically significant right ventricular infarction. *J Am Coll Cardiol* 4:923, 1984.

24. Berger PB, Ruocco NA, Ryan TJ, et al: Frequency and significance of right ventricular dysfunction during inferior wall left ventricular myocardial infarction treated with thrombolytic therapy: Results from the thrombolysis in myocardial infarction (TIMI) II trial. *Am J Cardiol* 71:1148, 1993.

25. Braat SH, Brugada P, DeZwaan C, et al: Right and left ventricular ejection fraction in acute inferior wall infarction with or without ST segment elevation in lead V₄R. *J Am Coll Cardiol* 4:940, 1984.

26. Braat SH, DeZwaan C, Brugada P, et al: Right ventricular involvement with acute inferior wall myocardial infarction

identifies high risk of developing atrioventricular nodal conduction disturbances. *Am Heart J* 107:1183, 1984.

27. Dell'Italia LJ, Starling MR, Crawford MH, et al: Right ventricular infarction: Identification by hemodynamic measurements before and after volume loading and correlation with noninvasive techniques. *J Am Coll Cardiol* 4:931, 1984.

28. Cabin HS, Clubb KS, Wackers FJ: Regional right ventricular dysfunction: An excellent predictor of right ventricular necrosis with anterior as well as inferior myocardial infarction. *Circulation* 72(suppl III):III-413, 1985 (abstr).

29. Cabin HS, Clubb KS, Wackers FJ, et al: Right ventricular myocardial infarction with anterior wall left ventricular infarction: An autopsy study. *Am Heart J* 113:16, 1987.

30. Schuler G, Hofmann M, Schwarz F, et al: Effect of successful thrombolytic therapy on right ventricular function in acute inferior wall myocardial infarction. *Am J Cardiol* 54:951, 1984.

31. Verani MS, Tortoledo FE, Batty JW, et al: Effect of coronary artery recanalization on right ventricular function in patients with acute myocardial infarction. *J Am Coll Cardiol* 5:1029, 1985.

32. Berger HJ, Johnstone DE, Sands JM, et al: Response of right ventricular ejection fraction to upright bicycle exercise in coronary artery disease. *Circulation* 60:1292, 1979.

33. Verani MS, Guidry GW, Mahmarian JJ, et al: Effects of acute, transient coronary occlusion on right ventricular function in humans. *J Am Coll Cardiol* 20:1490, 1992.

34. Renzetti AD Jr, McClement JH, Litt BD: The Veterans Administration Cooperative Study of Pulmonary Function: Mortality in relation to respiratory function in chronic obstructive pulmonary disease. *Am J Med* 41:115, 1966.

35. Matthay RA, Berger HJ, Loke J, et al: Right and left ventricular performance in ambulatory young adults with cystic fibrosis. *Br Heart J* 43:474, 1980.

36. Canny GJ, de Souza ME, Gilday DL, et al: Radionuclide assessment of cardiac performance in cystic fibrosis: Reproducibility and effect of theophylline on cardiac function. *Am Rev Respir Dis* 130, 822, 1984.

37. Matthay RA, Berger HJ, Davies RA, et al: Right and left ventricular exercise performance in chronic obstructive pulmonary disease: Radionuclide assessment. *Ann Intern Med* 93:234, 1980.

38. Morrison DA, Adcock K, Collins CM, et al: Right ventricular dysfunction and the exercise limitation of chronic obstructive pulmonary disease. *J Am Coll Cardiol* 9:1219, 1987.

39. Sibbald WJ, Driedger AA, Myers ML, et al: Biventricular function in the adult respiratory distress syndrome: Hemodynamic and radionuclide assessment, with special emphasis on right ventricular function. *Chest* 84:126, 1983.

40. Schulman D, Biondi J, Matthay R, et al: The effect of positive end-expiratory pressure on right ventricular performance: Importance of baseline right ventricular function. *Am J Med* 84:57, 1988.

41. Schulman D, Biondi J, Matthay R, et al: Differing responses in right and left ventricular filling, loading and volumes during positive end-expiratory pressure. *Am J Cardiol* 64:772, 1989.

42. Baker BJ, Wilen MM, Boyd CM, et al: Relation of right ventricular ejection fraction to exercise capacity in chronic left ventricular failure. *Am J Cardiol* 54:596, 1984.

43. Franciosa JA, Park M, Levine TB: Lack of correlation between exercise capacity and indexes of resting left ventricular performance in heart failure. *Am J Cardiol* 47:33, 1981.

44. Lewis JF, Webber JD, Sutton LL, et al: Discordance in degree of right and left ventricular dilation in patients with dilated cardiomyopathy. *J Am Coll Cardiol* 21:649, 1993.

45. Schulman DS, Grandis DJ, Flores AR: Relationship between hemodynamics and right ventricular function in patients with cardiomyopathy: Important role of tricuspid regurgitation. *Chest* 107:14, 1995.

46. Reduto LA, Berger HJ, Johnstone DE, et al: Radionuclide assessment of right and left ventricular exercise reserve after total correction of tetralogy of Fallot. *Am J Cardiol* 45:1013, 1980.

47. Konstam MA, Idoine J, Wynne J, et al: Right ventricular function in adults with pulmonary hypertension with and without atrial septal defect. *Am J Cardiol* 51:1144, 1983.

48. Morise AP, Goodwin C: Exercise radionuclide angiography in patients with mitral stenosis: Value of right ventricular response. *Am Heart J* 112:509, 1986.

49. Iskandrian AS, Hakki A-H, Ren J-F, et al: Correlation among right ventricular preload, afterload and ejection fraction in mitral valve disease: Radionuclide, echocardiographic and hemodynamic evaluation. *J Am Coll Cardiol* 3:1403, 1984.

50. Morrison DA, Lancaster L, Henry R, et al: Right ventricular function at rest and during exercise in aortic and mitral valve disease. *J Am Coll Cardiol* 5:21, 1985.

51. Winzelberg GG, Boucher CA, Pohost GM, et al: Right ventricular function in aortic and mitral valve disease: Relation of gated first-pass radionuclide angiography to clinical and hemodynamic findings. *Chest* 79:520, 1981.

52. Hochreiter C, Niles N, Devereux RB, et al: Mitral regurgitation: Relationship of noninvasive descriptors of right and left ventricular performance to clinical and hemodynamic findings and to prognosis in medically and surgically treated patients. *Circulation* 73:900, 1986.

53. Borer JS, Wencker D, Hochreiter C: Management decisions in valvular heart disease: The role of radionuclide based assessment of ventricular function and performance. *J Nucl Cardiol* 3:72, 1996.

54. Kimchi A, Ellrodt AG, Berman DS, et al: Right ventricular performance in septic shock: A combined radionuclide and hemodynamic study. *J Am Coll Cardiol* 4:945, 1984.

55. Parker MM, McCarthy KE, Ognibene FP, Parillo JE: Right ventricular dysfunction and dilation, similar to left ventricular changes, characterize the cardiac depression of septic shock in humans. *Chest* 97:126, 1990.

Left Ventricular Diastolic Function

Daniel J. Lenihan
Thomas M. Bashore

It is widely understood and appreciated that overall left ventricular systolic function has a major impact on the management and prognosis of patients with heart disease. It is also becoming increasingly clear that left ventricular diastolic function is important and may be a harbinger of subsequent abnormal systolic function. Symptoms of congestive heart failure resulting from pulmonary venous congestion may, in fact, be largely a result of abnormal diastolic function and impaired active myocardial relaxation in addition to, or in lieu of, contractile abnormalities.[1] Extensive clinical and basic investigations have attempted to describe left ventricular diastolic filling characteristics in a meaningful way with the hope of finding therapeutic options to improve symptoms and/or prognosis in patients with diastolic heart failure.

Radionuclide ventriculography, a widely available and easily reproducible noninvasive clinical tool, has been used in a variety of clinical disease states to describe left ventricular diastolic filling using a time–activity curve reflective of ventricular volume throughout a cardiac cycle. This technique has added great insight into the pathophysiology of left ventricular diastolic filling both in normal patients and in those with important cardiac disease.[2]

This chapter first describes the physiologic determinants of normal diastolic filling and attempts to describe the complex interplay of factors that can dramatically affect left ventricular relaxation and filling. Subsequently, diagnostic techniques, including radionuclide ventriculography, that are typically used to examine di-astole are described, and specific advantages and disadvantages are highlighted. Lastly, clinical studies as well as basic investigations are overviewed to illustrate important aspects of left ventricular diastolic function that can be assessed noninvasively by radionuclide ventriculographic techniques with an emphasis on the management of important cardiac disease.

NORMAL LEFT VENTRICULAR FILLING: PHYSIOLOGIC DETERMINANTS

A tremendous interest in myocardial function at the cellular level coupled with precise physiologic measurements of the characteristics of left ventricular pressure and volume has led to a rapidly expanding appreciation of the major determinants of left ventricular diastolic filling. To understand what aspects of left ventricular diastolic filling can be measured and how therapeutic choices affect these measurements, one must be cognizant of the normal sequence of left ventricular relaxation and resultant filling as well as the cellular, hormonal, architectural, hemodynamic, and extrinsic interactions that affect each of these normal cardiac events.

Cellular Interactions in Diastole

Molecular biological techniques have broadened the understanding of myocardial aberrations at the myocyte

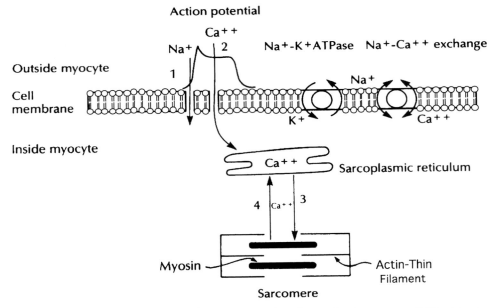

Figure 15-1   A schematic diagram of calcium (Ca^{++}) handling within the myocyte. (1) The initiation of an action potential with sodium (Na$^+$) influx across the cell membrane. (2) The action potential produces Ca^{2+} influx into the myocyte. This in turn stimulates a large release of Ca^{2+} (3) into the cytosol, which then interacts with contractile and regulatory proteins of the myofilament and allows cross-bridge attachments to occur. Calcium is then resequestered (4) by the sarcoplasmic reticulum calcium ATPase. (From Walsh,[106] reproduced with permission.)

and genetic level that are responsible for the pathogenesis of clinically apparent heart disease. From a variety of investigations, it is apparent that calcium plays a critical role in cellular events governing contraction and relaxation; the efficiency of the cellular calcium-handling mechanisms is an important determinant of myocardial relaxation and resultant left ventricular filling.

An overview of myocardial calcium handling at the myocyte level illustrates this point (Fig. 15-1). The process begins with an action potential that initiates contraction and allows the entry of a relatively small amount of calcium through the cell membrane.[1] This calcium influx, in turn, triggers the release of a large amount of calcium into the cytosol from the sarcoplasmic reticulum. The resultant high intracellular ionized calcium level allows actin–myosin cross-bridges to form, mediated by a conformational change in the myofilaments in the presence of adequate adenosine triphosphate (ATP), and contraction ensues. Myocardial relaxation must follow for the cycle to be perpetuated. Returning the intracellular calcium level to its original low concentration (10^{-7} mmol) is of paramount importance. This process of resequestration of calcium into the sarcoplasmic reticulum primarily occurs by a powerful ATP-requiring calcium pump, sarcoplasmic reticular calcium ATPase (SR Ca^{2+} ATPase). Other less important mechanisms reestablishing calcium homeostasis include the sarcolemmal sodium–calcium exchanger and sarcolemmal calcium

pumps.[3] Both contraction and relaxation are active, energy-requiring processes maintaining effective myocardial cell function.

The exact role that calcium homeostasis plays in myocardial disease processes in humans, particularly regarding abnormal left ventricular diastolic filling, remains unclear. In patients with heart failure due to systolic dysfunction, it appears that the resequestration of calcium may be impaired.[4] In patients with hypertrophic cardiomyopathy, the ability of the cell to maintain calcium homeostasis is, likewise, dysfunctional.[5] To emphasize the role of calcium handling in myocardial relaxation, an animal investigation (using hypoxia as a stress) documented a direct relationship between a rising end-diastolic pressure and a rising intracellular calcium level.[6] The exact mechanism leading to abnormal calcium homeostasis is likely multifactorial, however, and further studies will undoubtedly provide important new insights.[3]

Other investigations have examined the role of ATP in cardiac systolic and diastolic performance. The level of ATP content in human myocardial biopsy samples correlated fairly well with hemodynamic measures of left ventricular contractility and less well with parameters of left ventricular relaxation.[7] In animal models of hypoxia[8] and ischemia,[9] though, the ATP content has not correlated with alterations in myocardial diastolic distensibility. These data taken together suggest that ATP content, per se, may not play a critical role in diastolic performance, but ATP synthesis and utilization could be altered without any change in the absolute ATP content.

Hormonal Influences on Diastole

Activation of the neurohumoral system in congestive heart failure due to systolic dysfunction is widely understood and appreciated.[10,11] The roles that activation of the catecholamine response, the renin–angiotensin system, and the arginine–vasopressin system play in the pathophysiology of congestive heart failure are rapidly being delineated.[12] On the other hand, the effects of hormonal alterations on diastolic function are not well known, especially in the absence of systolic dysfunction.

The sympathetic system is a potent effector of left ventricular contraction and relaxation.[13] In normal humans, beta-adrenergic stimulation not only increases the force of contraction[14] but also improves active relaxation resulting in ventricular suction that augments early left ventricular diastolic filling.[15] The improvement in active left ventricular relaxation that occurs with beta-adrenergic stimulation may be more prominent than the improvement in contractile function.[16] The underlying cellular events that produce an improved rate of relaxation with beta-adrenergic stimulation are mediated by an increase in cAMP-dependent phosphorylation of phospholamban, the major regulatory protein of the SR Ca^{2+} ATPase,[17-19] resulting in increased calcium transport within the myocyte. The caveat remains that, while beta-adrenergic stimulation may improve diastolic filling, high circulating levels of endogenous beta-adrenergic agonists, epinephrine and norepinephrine, are clearly associated with increased mortality.[10,11] The exact roles that beta-adrenergic receptors and cAMP-mediated changes in myocyte calcium handling play in human heart failure and myocardial relaxation remain unknown. Beta-adrenergic blockers paradoxically improve myocardial contraction and relaxation in symptomatic patients with depressed contractility.[20] Alterations in a specific subtype of beta-adrenergic receptors might be primarily responsible for the contractile and/or lusitropic response to sympathetic stimulation.[21-24]

The renin–angiotensin system has an equally important impact on diastolic filling, at least indirectly. Angiotensin II is a potent vasoconstrictor. As a peripheral vasoconstrictor, angiotensin II may also raise left ventricular afterload and stimulate aldosterone secretion, which, in turn, promotes sodium retention. These effects markedly influence the loading conditions on the left ventricle and can impair diastolic filling. Angiotensin-converting enzyme inhibition improves diastolic filling in animal experiments[25] and, by this mechanism, may be responsible for the mortality reduction observed in

people with heart failure.[10] Animal investigations suggest that local angiotensin II production in hypertrophied myocardial cells may directly impair myocardial relaxation,[26] but this has yet to be demonstrated in humans.

Architectural/Structural Factors Affecting Diastole

The classic representation of the myocardium is to consider it in terms of layers of discrete muscle bundles. In this traditional view,[27] the left ventricle is wrapped in an outer spiral muscle bundle that winds clockwise from the base of the heart to the apex, where it then spirals in counterclockwise fashion inwardly back to the base. Sandwiched between these two spiral layers is a thick muscle band of circumferential fibers that surround the left ventricular cavity, forming the midwall everywhere except at the apex. The apex is thus much thinner than the rest of the ventricle.

This classic description of discrete muscle bundles has recently been challenged by several investigators.[28,29] In these studies, there appears to be a gradual transition of fiber orientation rather than discrete bundles, with a predominance of the circumferentially oriented fibers at the base of the heart and a gradual decrease in favor of the spiral fibers as the apex is approached. This alignment results in circumferential shortening being greater than longitudinal shortening during ventricular contraction. The spiral continuum also creates rotational motion during systole and results in less endocardial fiber shortening or lengthening compared with the epicardial fibers during systole and diastole. Anatomically and functionally, the ventricular septum appears to be more a part of the left ventricle than the right ventricle. The composite shape of the left ventricle that results from this complex muscular orientation has a significant effect on resultant wall forces. This geometry may even affect systolic wall forces differently than diastolic wall forces.[30]

The forces exerted on the ventricular walls are frequently expressed in terms of wall stress. In general, wall stress calculations are modifications of Laplace's law wherein stress is directly proportional to pressure and ventricular radius and is inversely related to wall thickness:

$$\text{stress} \; \alpha \; \frac{\text{pressure} \times \text{radius}}{\text{wall thickness}}$$

When one considers the fiber orientation within the ventricle and the heart's variable wall thickness, it becomes evident that the wall stress at the thinner left ventricular apex is greater than at the midchamber circumference. This may be an adaptive mechanism that results in the short axis dilating more than the long axis during volume overload, for instance. In this manner, the ventricle's normal ellipsoid shape may be transformed into a spherical shape when the need arises for the ventricle to contain more volume.[31] At any rate, the shape and variability in wall thickness results in heterogeneous stress throughout different areas of the left ventricle, and this would be expected to affect global as well as segmental filling patterns. There are, thus, anatomic reasons to expect heterogenous relaxation of the left ventricle, even in the normal state.

Other anatomic factors would also be expected to contribute to the diastolic filling pattern observed. The muscle fibers are supported by an extensive collagen network[32] that binds both large groups of muscle cells as well as individual myocytes to each other. In addition, there is a unique arrangement of collagen connecting with the adjacent capillaries that tends to hold these vessels open during ventricular systole. This extensive collagen network contributes greatly to the viscoelastic behavior of the myocardium and likely affects both systolic and diastolic performance.[33] Because the coronaries fill primarily in diastole, the impact of the blood surging into the coronary bed[34] and the resultant total coronary blood volume[35] may also influence the early diastolic properties of the myocardium, and these influences may contribute to the filling pattern observed in the ventricle.

Not only does the left ventricular architecture itself influence ventricular filling, but this rather heterogeneous structure is also influenced by the atria, the cardiac valves, the right ventricle, the pericardium, and the pleural pressure. In certain circumstances, any or all of these adjacent structures can directly or indirectly limit or restrain left ventricular filling. These anatomic/structural considerations are important to keep in mind when considering the factors that may lead to an observable alteration in the shape of the left ventricular volume curve and to the subsequent determination of both the early and late filling rates from this curve.

Principal Hemodynamic Determinants of Left Ventricular Diastolic Filling

Traditionally, diastole is defined from the time of aortic valve closure to the initiation of contraction (systole) and mitral valve closure. During this time frame, diastole can be divided into four phases: (1) *isovolumic relaxation* (from aortic valve closure to the opening of the mitral valve), (2) *rapid early mitral inflow* in which the majority of ventricular filling occurs, (3) *diastasis* (the plateau phase), and (4) *atrial systole* (atrial contribution to left ventricular filling) (Fig. 15-2).

In this traditional view, the ventricular volume curve reaches end ejection just prior to the period of isovolumic relaxation. The volume curve then remains flat, with no

Phases of Ventricular Filling

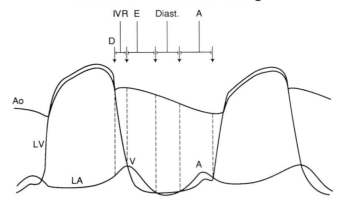

Figure 15-2 Schematic diagram of the phases of ventricular filling: Simultaneous aortic (Ao), left ventricular (LV), and left atrium (LA) pressures. V, "V" wave of LA pressure; A, "A" wave of LA pressure; D, dicrotic notch of Ao pressure signifying Ao valve closure; IVR, isovolumic relaxation period; E, early rapid filling of the left ventricle when the LA pressure exceeds LV pressure; Diast, diastasis or plateau phase of filling with little change in ventricular volume or pressure. The A-wave portion of LV filling corresponds to the A wave of LA pressure and atrial systole.

volume change until mitral valve opening. The onset of the rapid early mitral inflow then coincides with mitral valve opening at the point when left ventricular pressure falls below left atrial pressure. The time of minimum left ventricular volume represented on the volume curve is, in the strictest sense, neither end systole nor end ejection but rather represents ventricular volume just prior to mitral valve opening (Fig. 15-3).

Some data[35,36] suggest that considerable changes in the shape of the left ventricular cavity occur during "isovolumic" relaxation. Contrast angiographic studies have noted an apparent increase in left ventricular volume,[36,37] as well as considerable asynchrony of relaxation during this brief interval.[38] Abnormal outward movement in one area has been noted to be accompanied by inward movement in another; however, whether there is truly an increase in volume during the "isovolumic" phase remains controversial.[38]

The left ventricular pressure decay during the time of isovolumic relaxation has also been extensively studied. The left ventricular peak negative dP/dt has been found to occur at about the time of aortic valve closure. As a result, peak negative dP/dt has been used as a marker for the onset of isovolumic relaxation. The left ventricular pressure decline from aortic valve closure until mitral valve opening is exponential, and the time course of the pressure decay during this period has been used as an expression of active left ventricular relaxation (often referred to as *tau*).[39]

Once the mitral valve has opened and the ventricle begins filling, the early left ventricular pressure continues to decline despite the rapid inflow of blood—a phenome-

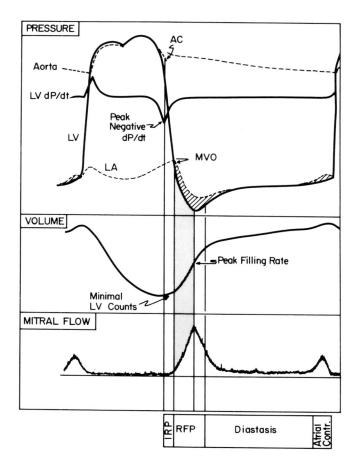

Figure 15-3 The aortic, left ventricular (LV), and left atrial (LA) pressures (*top panel*), the left ventricular volume curve (*center panel*), and mitral flow (*bottom panel*). The isovolumic relaxation period (IRP) occurs from aortic closure (AC) to mitral valve opening (MVO). Peak filling from the ventricular volume curve occurs at a point near minimal LV pressure when the LA–LV gradient is maximal. The ventricle has usually refilled about halfway by the time of peak filling. RFP, rapid filling period; Atrial Contr, atrial contraction period.

non that has led to the concept of left ventricular suction.[15] In fact, by the time of minimum left ventricular pressure, about 40 to 60 percent of the filling of the normal left ventricle may have occurred.[40,41] In humans and in animal models, this concept has been confirmed and may exert a significant effect on early diastolic filling.[15,42] Physiologic principles dictate that early mitral filling is determined by the pressure gradient between the left atrium and the left ventricle (or atrioventricular gradient), and this motive force has a profound effect on noninvasive or invasive determinations of left ventricular filling. Many factors influence the magnitude and timing of the atrioventricular gradient, including the isovolumic relaxation rate, loading conditions, and ventricular volume.[43] Thus, any intervention or change in clinical status of a patient that significantly affects the atrioventricular gradient or factors that determine its magnitude may

have an important impact on left ventricular diastolic filling characteristics.

Although a substantial portion of left ventricular diastolic filling depends on active relaxation and early left ventricular filling may be most influenced by active processes, passive left ventricular filling that occurs during the period of diastasis and with atrial contraction exerts an important effect on any measured parameter of diastole. Just as the onset of active relaxation is a gradual and regionally heterogeneous event, the end of active relaxation and the end of rapid filling are also gradual and heterogeneous events. The gradual shift from the rapid filling to the passive filling phase eventually results in the middiastolic loss of any gradient between the left atrium and the left ventricle, and middiastolic transmitral flow approaches zero. Atrial contraction then imparts additional momentum to the blood as the final surge of ventricular filling occurs. Mitral flow continues for up to 25 ms after the atrioventricular pressure crossover so that the reversal of the pressure gradient does not precisely coincide with flow cessation or to the precise moment of mitral valve closure.[44] From this discussion, it is clear that changes in heart rate from one study to the next, even in the same patient, would have a profound effect on diastolic filling characteristics.

The late filling that occurs during atrial contraction usually is responsible for up to 20 percent of left ventricular filling in a normal heart. Clinically, it has been widely observed that atrial contraction may be more important in patients with diastolic filling abnormalities, such as left ventricular hypertrophy due to aortic stenosis, and in this instance atrial contraction may be responsible for a much larger proportion of left ventricular filling.[45]

The importance of the passive filling characteristics of the left ventricle in the determination of global left ventricular function is unsettled. Rankin et al[40] have pointed out that, compared with the entire diastolic filling period, the period of rapid ventricular filling is quite short—so brief, in fact, that if there were no rapid filling phase, the heart might still be able to fill adequately prior to the next systole. This suggests that passive filling mechanisms may assume a greater role if rapid filling is impeded for any reason.

The passive filling of the left ventricle is often described in terms of the exponential left ventricular diastolic pressure–volume relationship (Fig. 15-4). The chamber stiffness is then defined as the change in pressure relative to a change in volume during this period, with its reciprocal ($\Delta V/\Delta P$) termed *chamber compliance*. In the poorly compliant left ventricle, a change in volume (ΔV) will result in larger change in pressure (ΔP) than would be observed in the normal ventricle.

Though the left ventricle volume and pressure are exponentially related in diastole, some authors[44] have argued that the *rate of mitral flow* during later diastole is actually linearly related to the change in pressure (ΔP)

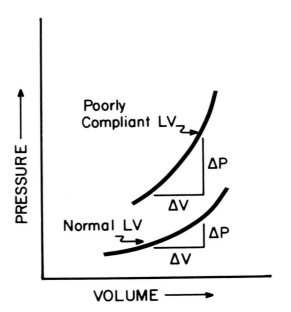

Figure 15-4 The diastolic pressure–volume relationship during diastasis. A normal pressure–volume relationship is contrasted with that of a poorly compliant left ventricle (LV). For a specific volume change (ΔV) in the normal LV, the poorly compliant LV develops a greater change in pressure (ΔP).

alone. If this is true, changes in volume (mitral flow) during later diastole would not be a function of both volume and pressure ($\Delta V/\Delta P$) but would require only an appropriate change in pressure to fill the ventricle adequately.

The effect of reduced left ventricular compliance on the radionuclide volume curve during the passive filling phase has not been systematically studied. In addition, while the measure of atrial contribution to late ventricular filling might provide interesting data regarding the marriage of atrial and ventricular hemodynamics, radionuclide angiography is generally unreliable for evaluating the tail end of the diastolic volume curve, and it is unlikely that useful data will emerge from its analysis.

Extrinsic Factors Affecting Diastole

The pericardium exerts an important restraining effect on left ventricular filling especially as ventricular volume increases. Since the pericardium surrounds all four cardiac chambers, any change in volume or systemic loading conditions will affect all of the chambers. This fact has led to the confirmation of a phenomenon in humans known as ventricular interdependence in which parallel changes in ventricular pressure and volume occur with acutely altered loading conditions in both the right and left ventricles.[46] Additionally, the atria may be more profoundly affected by pericardial restraint due to a reduced wall thickness compared with the ventricles. Therefore,

any given change in volume or load may result in a more pronounced corresponding pressure change in the atria than in the ventricles.[47] In patients with congestive heart failure or elevated intracardiac pressures,[48-50] the restraining effect of the pericardium appears to exert a critical influence on left ventricular filling and may play a primary role in determining exercise capacity. The classic example that illustrates the effect that the pericardium can have on left ventricular diastolic filling occurs with pericardial constriction. In patients with pericardial constriction that had not been operated on and who had hemodynamic confirmation of elevated and equalized filling pressures, the peak filling rate was increased when compared with that of normals, as were the first-third and first-half filling fractions. When the pericardium was removed, these same patients had identical diastolic filling indices as the control subjects.[49] Even in less prominent examples, the pericardium exerts an important influence on left ventricular filling.[50]

TECHNIQUES USED TO ASSESS DIASTOLIC FILLING

As interest in diastolic mechanisms of cardiac disease has risen, so has the enthusiasm to develop a reliable method of measuring diastolic filling characteristics. Available techniques to assess diastole include invasive measurements during cardiac catheterization as well as noninvasive assessment of left ventricular filling using Doppler echocardiography or radionuclide ventriculography.

Cardiac Catheterization

The ability to directly measure intracardiac pressures and oxygenation and to define the extent of epicardial coronary artery disease is unique to cardiac catheterization. Cardiac catheterization remains the single most precise and powerful tool used to assist in the clinical management of patients with cardiac disease and the examination of left ventricular diastolic filling is no exception.

Typically "diastolic dysfunction" or *diastolic heart failure* is defined as elevated left ventricular diastolic pressures and resultant pulmonary venous congestion in the presence of normal systolic function.[51] Diastolic heart failure can be identified most directly by a routine right and left heart catheterization (Fig. 15-5). However, to assess accurately the relative contribution of the many determinants previously mentioned that affect left ventricular diastolic filling and to define precisely the mechanisms in diastolic heart failure, high-fidelity micro-

Pressure Waveforms in Normal and Abnormal Left Ventricular Diastolic Filling

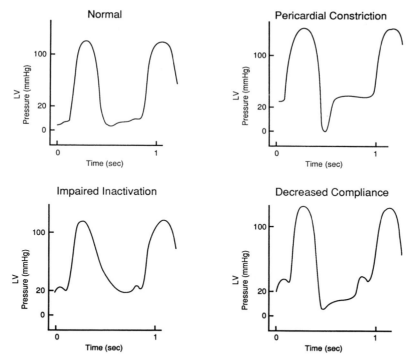

Figure 15-5 Pressure waveforms in normal and abnormal left ventricular (LV) diastolic filling that can be typically seen during cardiac catheterization. *Top left:* Normal pressure waveform. *Top right:* LV pressure waveform in pericardial constriction. A "dip and plateau" pattern is seen due to rapid early filling that is prematurely halted due to right and left ventricular interdependence in conjunction with LV maximal volume restriction due to the pericardium. *Bottom left:* LV pressure waveform in a patient with impaired inactivation. Notice that the LV pressure drop after systole is not as rapid and the LV pressure decline is occurring longer into diastole. *Bottom right:* LV pressure waveform in a patient with decreased compliance showing a large "A" wave at end diastole.

manometers and capacitance catheters with a greater frequency response are required.

The most common measurements performed during scientific investigations using cardiac catheterization to describe left ventricular relaxation and filling include (1) *loading conditions*, in particular, the left atrioventricular pressure gradient; (2) *left ventricular active relaxation*, as assessed by the time constant of isovolumic relaxation (tau); (3) *chamber characteristics*, using pressure–volume relations to estimate chamber compliance and myocardial elasticity; and (4) precise determinations of pressure by using high-fidelity micromanometers that enable the recording of the change in pressure over time, *dP/dt*. Peak positive *dP/dt* is a rough indicator of contractility, whereas peak negative *dP/dt* is a similarly gross indicator of relaxation. All of these measurements obtained during catheterization have limitations in accurately describing left ventricular diastolic function depending on the specific hemodynamic conditions in which they are obtained.[52] The invasive nature of cardiac catheterization limits the ability to measure repetitively diastolic filling in an individual after a pharmacologic or mechanical intervention.

Echocardiography

Left ventricular structure and function are routinely examined by echocardiography. Pulsed and continuous-wave Doppler echocardiographic measurements of mitral valve flow are widely available and frequently used to assess diastolic function noninvasively.[53] A variety of pulsed Doppler measurements are typically performed that include (1) *"E" wave*, peak early transmitral filling velocity; (2) *A wave*, peak late (or atrial) transmitral filling velocity; (3) *E-wave–A-wave ratio*, a ratio comparing the peak velocities; (4) *rate of deceleration of flow*, expressed as either time from peak filling velocity to baseline (deceleration time) or as pressure half-time; and (5) *velocity–time integral*, the area recorded by flow velocity over time (Fig. 15-6). Recent investigations have used continuous-wave Doppler interrogation of mitral regurgitation signals to describe diastolic filling characteristics in patients. The rate of decay of velocity from these signals has been correlated with peak negative *dP/dt*[54] and the time constant of isovolumic relaxation,[55] although these Doppler measurements are only semiquantitative because of important limitations of this technique.

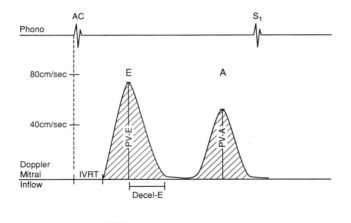

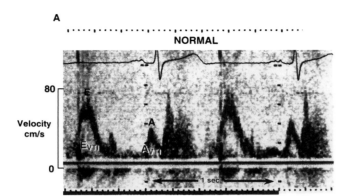

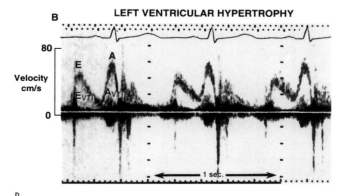

Figure 15-6 **A:** A diagram of typical measurements obtained from pulsed Doppler recordings. E, E wave; A, A wave; PV-E, peak velocity of E wave; PV-A, peak velocity of A wave; IVRT, isovolumic relaxation time; Decel-E, E velocity deceleration time; AC, aortic valve closure; S_1, S_1 heart sound at the initiation of systole. The *shaded area* is the velocity–time integral. **B:** Pulsed Doppler measurements in a normal patient and one with left ventricular hypertrophy. Note that the normal ratio of peak early (E) to late (A) transmitral velocity is reversed in the patient with hypertensive heart disease. (From Hoit and Walsh,[107] reproduced in modified form with permission.)

Extensive clinical investigation of Doppler-derived filling indices has been performed. However, because of the multifactorial nature of the parameters defined by this noninvasive tool[56,57] and issues related to reproducibility,[58] management decisions based on these measurements must be placed in the clinical context of each individual patient. Due to these shortcomings, it remains difficult to clearly define "normal" vs "abnormal" diastolic filling for a wide variety of patients.

Radionuclide Ventriculography

Radionuclide ventriculography is also widely available, and measurement of left ventricular diastolic function can be easily assessed, provided certain technical concerns are addressed.[2] Data obtained by radionuclide ventriculography, such as the left ventricular ejection fraction, are directly related to prognosis,[59] but, as with echocardiography, measurements of left ventricular diastolic function by radionuclide ventriculography have not been validated as predictors of outcome.

To describe ventricular diastolic filling accurately, a more complete time–activity curve is required than is typically used to calculate the left ventricular ejection fraction. Variability in the heart rate, and subsequently in diastolic time, makes it difficult to record events in late diastole, in particular, atrial systole. To obviate this problem, data must be collected into multiple R-R interval time windows (prospective bad-beat rejection) or by list-mode acquisition. Secondly, statistical variability of each data point on the time–activity curve due to attenuation or other factors can be large and must be fit mathematically with a Fourier harmonic or polynomial curve to obtain clinically useful data. Based on these requirements, first-pass methods are limited to assess left ventricular diastolic filling.

A variety of diastolic filling indices have been described using radionuclide ventriculography. These are the most common (Fig. 15-7): (1) *Left ventricular peak filling rate.* This is the maximum first derivative from the left ventricular volume curve and is typically normalized to either left ventricular diastolic volume or stroke volume. (2) *Time to peak filling rate.* The time from end systole to the time of peak filling rate. (3) *Filling fraction.* By using the stroke volume, a percentage of filling that has occurred can be calculated at different time points in diastole such as the first third (⅓ FF), the first half (½ FF), and the first two-thirds (⅔ FF). In addition, all of these same radionuclide ventriculographic indices can be similarly calculated by regional methods using the left anterior oblique projection to describe septal, apical, and lateral segmental diastolic filling of the left ventricle.[60]

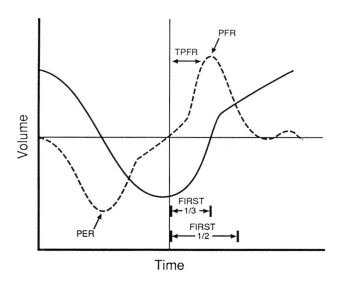
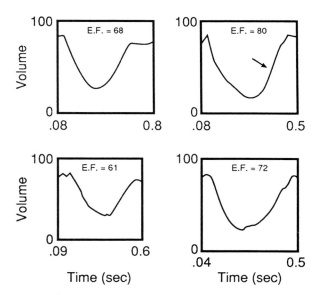

Figure 15-7 Diagram (*left*) and left ventricular time–volume curves from patients (*right*) as obtained during radionuclide ventriculography. The diagram illustrates typical measurements obtained from the volume (*solid*) curve and the first derivative (*dashed*) curve. PER, peak ejection rate; PFR, peak filling rate; TPFR, time to peak filling rate; First ⅓, first-third filling fraction; First ½, first-half filling fraction. See the text for details. The actual patient time–volume curves (*right*) illustrate early diastolic filling abnormalities in constrictive pericarditis. The *top left curve* is from a normal subject, the *top right curve* is from a patient with constrictive pericarditis, the *bottom left curve* is from the same patient after pericardiectomy, the *bottom right curve* is from a patient with restrictive cardiomyopathy, and the *arrow* indicates a rapid rate of diastolic filling in constrictive pericarditis (*top right*) that normalizes after surgery (*bottom left*). (From Gerson et al,[49] reproduced in modified form with permission.)

Radionuclide ventriculography is a very powerful noninvasive tool that is widely used to define left ventricular systolic function and with certain important technical adjustments can measure left ventricular diastolic filling accurately and reproducibly. Many indices of diastolic filling by radionuclide ventriculography correlate with accepted invasive parameters of diastolic filling[61,62] and with indices measured from Doppler echocardiography.[63] Nevertheless, limitations regarding the multifactorial determination inherent in noninvasive parameters of left ventricular filling using either radionuclide ventriculography or Doppler echocardiography prevent establishment of "normal" or "abnormal" filling indices for a wide spectrum of patients (Table 15-1).

Table 15-1   Factors Important in Determinations of Left Ventricular Filling

Loading conditions
Heart rate
Pericardial restraint
Active relaxation (time constant of isovolumic relaxation)
Chamber compliance
Myocardial elasticity
Asynchronous contraction/relaxation
Coronary blood flow

CLINICAL STUDIES ASSESSING LEFT VENTRICULAR DIASTOLIC FUNCTION

A wide variety of clinical investigations using radionuclide ventriculography or other techniques have described left ventricular diastolic filling in normal and diseased states.[64–67] It is clear that diastolic function is impaired when systolic function is depressed, and multiple studies have indicated that this direct relation is valid.[67,68] For purposes of clarity, the subsequent discussion focuses only on those studies with normal or near-normal left ventricular function in which diastolic heart failure or "dysfunction" is the predominant abnormality.

Several common conditions, such as long-standing hypertension resulting in left ventricular hypertrophy, coronary artery disease, or hypertrophic cardiomyopathy, are known to impair left ventricular diastolic filling.[69] Treatment directed at improving these conditions has resulted in variable improvement in diastolic filling indices obtained by radionuclide ventriculography or other invasive and noninvasive techniques. This section focuses primarily on clinical investigations using radionuclide angiographic methods; however, other techniques that have added significant insight into the pathophysiology of left ventricular diastolic filling may be highlighted.

Hypertension

The human heart responds to long-standing systemic hypertension by increasing wall thickness, thus normalizing wall stress and maintaining compensated left ventricular performance. If hypertension is left untreated, progressive left ventricular hypertrophy and ultimately congestive heart failure ensue.[70]

To reduce morbidity and mortality resulting from long-standing hypertension, an extensive array of medications has been developed over the years.[71] Many of these medications not only reduce blood pressure but also may regress the left ventricular hypertrophy that develops. As discussed previously, loading conditions on the left ventricle as well as the degree of hypertrophy are important determinants of myocardial relaxation and resultant diastolic filling. For example, radionuclide ventriculographic studies have demonstrated that the peak filling rate in hypertensive patients is lower than in matched normal controls,[72] indicating impaired diastolic filling. In addition, several studies indicate that the diastolic filling impairment in hypertensive heart disease may be related to the degree of hypertrophy,[65,73,74] although this has been a controversial point.[75] Other parameters of diastolic filling such as the time to peak filling rate (*prolonged*) and the first-third filling fraction (*reduced*) may be abnormal, further supporting the diagnosis of impaired left ventricular diastolic filling in hypertensive patients. From a clinical standpoint, significant variability in these indices exists,[76] however. Additionally, the limitations in exercise capacity frequently seen in patients with diastolic dysfunction appear to be related to the degree of hypertrophy and the inability of the heart to augment end-diastolic volume.[65]

Antihypertensive agents, in particular, calcium channel antagonists, beta-adrenergic blockers, or angiotensin-converting enzyme inhibitors, have all shown promise in reducing left ventricular hypertrophy and possibly improving diastolic filling.[75,77-79] The difficulty remains in documenting a clear improvement in left ventricular diastolic filling[77] or regression of hypertrophy with treatment, because of the variability of the techniques used.[80] In addition, a recent investigation of a group of predominantly hypertensive patients with diastolic dysfunction indicated that the peak filling rate appears to be most sensitive to loading conditions.[43] Antihypertensive agents profoundly affect loading conditions on the left ventricle, and this may explain the normalization of noninvasive indices with pharmacotherapy as opposed to a true improvement in left ventricular filling. This hypothesis was substantiated in humans during intravenous administra-

tion of verapamil.[81] In this study, patients with a reduced early peak filling rate, as assessed by Doppler echocardiography, had normalization of the E/A wave ratio during verapamil administration that was accompanied by worsening of active relaxation and an increase in left ventricular end-diastolic pressure. Furthermore, no study has clearly shown a reduction in cardiovascular morbidity or mortality related to an improvement in noninvasively determined diastolic filling or regression of hypertrophy. The important clinical parameter to monitor remains the systemic blood pressure in determining efficacy of therapy.

Coronary Artery Disease

Ischemic heart disease, in particular, acute ischemia, is known to impair left ventricular systolic and diastolic function.[82-84] The peak filling rate measured during radionuclide ventriculography may indicate important coronary disease, either symptomatic or silent.[85-87]

In many of these studies,[82,84-87] the peak filling rate was depressed despite a normal global ejection fraction, implicating diastolic dysfunction as the etiology of the depressed peak filling rate. Once the underlying coronary disease was treated with medication[88] or percutaneous transluminal angioplasty,[89] the peak filling rate improved, both globally and by regional analysis.[60] These investigations are the most compelling in providing evidence that a low peak filling rate may indicate diastolic dysfunction in coronary disease and that effective therapy for ischemia will improve left ventricular diastolic performance.

As discussed in the previous section, the peak filling rate by radionuclide ventriculography (or, for that matter, the E/A wave ratio by Doppler echocardiography) cannot be relied on as an indicator of effective therapy. When these studies of diastolic ventricular function in patients with coronary disease[88,89] are examined closely, other differences between the treated and control groups could explain a depressed peak filling rate compared with control and subsequent improvement in peak filling rate during therapy. For instance, in these investigations,[88,89] loading conditions before and after the intervention are not reported and significant differences in heart rate[88] were seen. Nonetheless, good evidence suggests that diastolic function is impaired with ischemia and treatment directed at improving ischemia will likely improve diastolic performance.

Hypertrophic Cardiomyopathy

Left ventricular hypertrophy, as detected by physical exam or noninvasive testing, is most commonly associated with hypertension or aortic stenosis; however, certain individuals have no inciting clinical etiology that explains left ventricular hypertrophy.[90,90a] These patients typically have first-degree relatives with similar structural myocardial abnormalities and, as a result, genetic analysis of these families has uncovered missense mutations in the beta cardiac myosin heavy-chain gene that may be an important marker for risk of sudden death.[91] This patient population with hypertrophic cardiomyopathy may have significant activity-limiting symptoms as a result of diastolic heart failure. Extensive clinical investigation using radionuclide ventriculography has described variable improvement in left ventricular diastolic filling during therapy for this condition.

As a result of significant myocardial hypertrophy, relaxation and diastolic filling are markedly impaired in many patients with hypertrophic cardiomyopathy. Several studies have examined the effects of calcium channel antagonists in this condition. Verapamil administration has been shown to shorten isovolumic relaxation period,[92] increase the peak filling rate, decrease the time to peak filling rate, and improve exercise tolerance in a majority of patients with hypertrophic cardiomyopathy even after 1 year of therapy.[93] Additionally, verapamil therapy may reduce the risk of hemodynamic decompensation caused by atrial fibrillation[94] and may make regional relaxation more synchronous.[95] Other calcium channel antagonists, such as diltiazem[96] and nifedipine,[97,98] have been investigated using echocardiographic and invasive measurements of left ventricular diastolic filling, and diastolic function apparently improved with these medications. All of these investigations have potentially important limitations in protocol design, resulting from alterations in load and heart rate during pharmacotherapy, that may explain the observed changes in filling indices. The most powerful clinical evidence of improvement in diastolic filling with pharmacotherapy for hypertrophic cardiomyopathy is the observed difference in exercise capacity.[93]

Aortic Stenosis

Significant aortic stenosis classically results in left ventricular hypertrophy by the same basic pathophysiology as that seen in hypertension. The major clinical difference between these two conditions is that aortic stenosis is a structural defect that can usually be corrected by aortic valve replacement. Following valve replacement, hypertrophy may regress and diastolic filling indices may also improve.[99] Interestingly, the myocardial thickening and interstitial fibrosis that resulted from prolonged outflow obstruction may not regress even years after adequate valve replacement.[100]

With respect to diastolic filling in patients who have significant aortic stenosis, radionuclide angiographic di-astolic filling indices can provide insight into those patients who may develop symptoms from important valvular stenosis. A recent study suggests that the time to peak filling rate may be surprisingly short or "supranormal" in these patients.[101]

Aging

The aging process of a normal human heart appears to involve at least some evidence of impaired diastolic filling as a result of decreased left ventricular distensibility.[102] Indices of diastolic filling appear to decrease over time,[103] and elderly patients may have severe congestive heart failure despite normal left ventricular systolic function.[104] Recent radionuclide ventriculographic data suggest that verapamil may improve the age-related impairment in diastolic filling,[105] but further confirmation is needed.

CONCLUSIONS

Diastolic function has become an important concept to understand in the clinical management of cardiac disease. The process of left ventricular diastolic filling is complex and involves many major determinants that can be affected singularly or in combination in disease states. Diastolic heart failure or diastolic dysfunction can be diagnosed by a variety of widely available tests, and certainly radionuclide ventriculographic techniques can be used effectively to establish the diagnosis.

Extensive clinical investigation using radionuclide ventriculography–derived indices of left ventricular diastolic filling has added tremendous insight into the characteristics of diastolic function in disease states. Therapy directed at improving symptoms in patients who have conditions known to impair diastolic function may be accompanied by improved left ventricular filling indices. There are still important limitations of radionuclide ventriculographic indices of left ventricular filling that should be accounted for when any individual patient is being assessed for impaired diastolic function. Future research must address the prognosis related to abnormal left ventricular filling indices and the influence that treatment has on patient outcomes.

REFERENCES

1. Grossman W: Diastolic dysfunction in congestive heart failure. *N Engl J Med* 325:1557, 1991.
2. Bonow RO: Radionuclide angiographic evaluation of left

ventricular diastolic function. *Circulation* 84(suppl I):I-208, 1991.

3. Morgan JP: Abnormal intracellular modulation of calcium as a major cause of cardiac contractile dysfunction. *N Engl J Med* 325:625, 1991.

4. Gwathmey JK, Copelas L, MacKinnon R, et al: Abnormal intracellular calcium handling in myocardium from patients with end-stage heart failure. *Circ Res* 61:70, 1987.

5. Gwathmey JK, Warren SE, Briggs GM, et al: Diastolic dysfunction in hypertrophic cardiomyopathy: Effect on active force generation during systole. *J Clin Invest* 87:1023, 1991.

6. Kihara Y, Grossman W, Morgan JP: Direct measurement of changes in intracellular calcium transients during hypoxia, ischemia, and reperfusion of the intact mammalian heart. *Circ Res* 65:1029, 1989.

7. Bashore TM, Magorien DJ, Letterio J, et al: Histologic and biochemical correlates of left ventricular chamber dynamics in man. *J Am Coll Cardiol* 9:734, 1987.

8. Wexler LF, Lorell BH, Momomura S-I, et al: Enhanced sensitivity to hypoxia-induced diastolic dysfunction in pressure-overload left ventricular hypertrophy in the rat: Role of high-energy phosphate depletion. *Circ Res* 62:766, 1988.

9. Momomura S-I, Ingwall JS, Parker A, et al: The relationships of high energy phosphates, tissue pH, and regional blood flow to diastolic distensibility in the ischemic dog myocardium. *Circ Res* 57:822, 1985.

10. Swedberg K, Eneroth P, Kjekshus J, et al: Hormones regulating cardiovascular function in patients with severe congestive heart failure and their relation to mortality. *Circulation* 82:1730, 1990.

11. Francis GS, Benedict C, Johnstone DE, et al: Comparison of neuroendocrine activation in patients with left ventricular dysfunction with and without congestive heart failure: A substudy of the studies of left ventricular dysfunction (SOLVD). *Circulation* 82:1724, 1990.

12. Parmley WW: Pathophysiology and current therapy of congestive heart failure. *J Am Coll Cardiol* 13:771, 1989.

13. Walsh RA: Sympathetic control of diastolic function in congestive heart failure. *Circulation* 82(suppl I):I-52, 1990.

14. Parker JD, Landzberg JS, Bittl JA, et al: Effects of β-adrenergic stimulation with dobutamine on isovolumic relaxation in the normal and failing human left ventricle. *Circulation* 84:1040, 1991.

15. Udelson JE, Bacharach SL, Cannon RO III, et al: Minimum left ventricular pressure during β-adrenergic stimulation in human subjects: Evidence for elastic recoil and diastolic "suction" in the normal heart. *Circulation* 82:1174, 1990.

16. Little WC, Rassi A Jr, Freeman GL: Comparison of effects of dobutamine and ouabain on left ventricular contraction and relaxation in closed-chest dogs. *J Clin Invest* 80:613, 1987.

17. Lindemann JP, Jones LR, Hathaway DR, et al: β-Adrenergic stimulation of phospholamban phosphorylation and Ca^{2+}-ATPase activity in guinea pig ventricles. *J Biol Chem* 258:464, 1983.

18. Luo W, Grupp IL, Harrer J, et al: Targeted ablation of the phospholamban gene is associated with markedly enhanced myocardial contractility and loss of β-agonist stimulation. *Circ Res* 75:401, 1994.

19. Vittone L, Grassi A, Chiappe L, et al: Relaxing effect of pharmacologic interventions increasing cAMP in rat heart. *Am J Physiol* 240:H441, 1981.

20. Eichhorn EJ, Bedotto JB, Malloy CR, et al: Effect of β-adrenergic blockade on myocardial function and energetics in congestive heart failure: Improvements in hemodynamic, contractile, and diastolic performance with bucindolol. *Circulation* 82:473, 1990.

21. Bristow MR, Ginsburg R, Minobe W, et al: Decreased catecholamine sensitivity and β-adrenergic-receptor density in failing human hearts. *N Engl J Med* 307:205, 1982.

22. Fowler MB, Laser JA, Hopkins GL, et al: Assessment of the β-adrenergic receptor pathway in the intact failing human heart: Progressive receptor down-regulation and subsensitivity to agonist response. *Circulation* 74:1290, 1986.

23. Motomura S, Zerkowski HR, Daul A, et al: On the physiologic role of beta-2 adrenoceptors in the human heart: In vitro and in vivo studies. *Am Heart J* 119:608, 1990.

24. Schafers RF, Adler S, Daul A, et al: Positive inotropic effects of the beta₂-adrenoceptor agonist terbutaline in the human heart: Effects of long-term beta₁-adrenoceptor antagonist treatment. *J Am Coll Cardiol* 23:1224, 1994.

25. Eberli FR, Apstein CS, Ngoy S, et al: Exacerbation of left ventricular ischemic diastolic dysfunction by pressure-overload hypertrophy: Modification by specific inhibition of cardiac angiotensin converting enzyme. *Circ Res* 70:931, 1992.

26. Schunkert H, Dzau VJ, Tang SS, et al: Increased rat cardiac angiotensin converting enzyme activity and mRNA expression in pressure overload left ventricular hypertrophy: Effects on coronary resistance, contractility, and relaxation. *J Clin Invest* 86:1913, 1990.

27. Robb JS, Robb RC: The normal heart: Anatomy and physiology of the structural units. *Am Heart J* 23:455, 1942.

28. Streeter DD, Sponitz HM, Patel DJ, et al: Fiber orientation in the canine left ventricle during diastole and systole. *Circ Res* 24:339, 1969.

29. Pearlman ES, Weber KT, Janicki JE, et al: Muscle fiber orientation and collagen content in the hypertrophied human heart. *Lab Invest* 46:158, 1982.

30. Rankin JS: The chamber dynamics of the intact left ventricle, in Baan J, Arntzenius AC, Yellin EL (eds): *Cardiac Dynamics*. The Hague, Martinus Nijhoff, 1980, pp 95–106.

31. Fischl SJ, Gorlin R, Herman MV: Cardiac shape and function in aortic valve disease: Physiologic and clinical implications. *Am J Cardiol* 39:170, 1977.

32. Caulfield JB, Borg TK: The collagen network of the heart. *Lab Invest* 40:364, 1979.

33. Weber KT, Janicki JS, Hunter WC, et al: The contractile behavior of the heart and its functional coupling to the circulation. *Prog Cardiovasc Dis* 24:375, 1982.

34. Brutsaert DL, Housman PR, Goethals MA: Dual control

of relaxation: Its role in the ventricular function in the mammalian heart. *Circ Res* 47:637, 1980.

35. Salisburg PF, Cross CE, Rieben PA: Influence of coronary artery pressure on myocardial elasticity. *Circ Res* 7: 794, 1980.

36. Ruttley MS, Adams DF, Cohn PF, et al: Shape and volume changes during "isovolumetric relaxation" in normal and asynergic ventricles. *Circulation* 50:306, 1974.

37. Gibson DG, Prewitt TA, Brown DJ: Analysis of left ventricular wall movement during isovolumic relaxation and its relation to coronary artery disease. *Br Heart J* 38:1010, 1976.

38. Gaash WH, Blaustein AS, Bing OHL: Asynchronous (segmental early) relaxation of the left ventricle. *J Am Coll Cardiol* 5:891, 1985.

39. Weiss JL, Frederiksen JW, Weisfeldt ML: Hemodynamic determinants of the time-course of fall in canine left ventricular pressure. *J Clin Invest* 58:751, 1976.

40. Rankin JS, Arentzen CE, Ring WS, et al: The diastolic mechanical properties of the intact left ventricle. *Fed Proc* 39:141, 1980.

41. Alderman EL, Glantz SA: Acute hemodynamic interventions shift the diastolic pressure–volume curve in man. *Circulation* 54:662, 1976.

42. Bahler RC, Martin P: Effects of loading conditions and inotropic state on rapid filling phase of left ventricle. *Am J Physiol* 248:H523, 1985.

43. Lenihan DJ, Gerson MC, Dorn GW II, et al: Effects of changes in atrioventricular gradient and isovolumic relaxation rates on radionuclide diastolic filling in man. *J Am Coll Cardiol* 25:358A, 1995 (abstr).

44. Laniado S, Yellin EL: Simultaneous recording of mitral valve echocardiogram and transmitral flow, in Kalmanson D (ed): *The Mitral Valve: A Pluridisciplinary Approach.* Acton, MA, Publishing Sciences Group, 1976, pp 156–172.

45. Sheikh K, Bashore TM, Kitzman DW, et al: Doppler left ventricular diastolic filling abnormalities in aortic stenosis and their relation to hemodynamic parameters. *Am J Cardiol* 63:1360, 1989.

46. Dell'Italia LJ, Walsh RA: Right ventricular diastolic pressure–volume relations and regional dimensions during acute alterations in loading conditions. *Circulation* 77:1276, 1988.

47. Hoit BD, Shao Y, Gabel M, et al: Influence of pericardium on left atrial compliance and pulmonary venous flow. *Am J Physiol* 264:H1781, 1993.

48. Carroll JD, Lang RM, Neumann AL, et al: The differential effects of positive inotropic and vasodilator therapy on diastolic properties in patients with congestive cardiomyopathy. *Circulation* 74:815, 1986.

49. Gerson MC, Colthar MS, Fowler NO: Differentiation of constrictive pericarditis and restrictive cardiomyopathy by radionuclide ventriculography. *Am Heart J* 118: 114, 1989.

50. Reynertson SI, Konstadt SN, Louie EK, et al: Alterations in transesophageal pulsed Doppler indexes of filling of the left ventricle after pericardiotomy. *J Am Coll Cardiol* 18:1655, 1991.

51. Dougherty AH, Naccarelli GV, Gray EL, et al: Congestive heart failure with normal systolic function. *Am J Cardiol* 54:778, 1984.

52. Walsh RA: Evaluation of ventricular diastolic function using invasive techniques. *Am J Card Imaging* 4:1, 1990.

53. DeMaria AN, Wisenbaugh TW, Smith MD, et al: Doppler echocardiographic evaluation of diastolic dysfunction. *Circulation* 84(suppl I):I-288, 1991.

54. Chen C, Rodriquez L, Guerrero JL, et al: Noninvasive estimation of the instantaneous first derivative of left ventricular pressure using continuous-wave Doppler echocardiography. *Circulation* 83:2101, 1991.

55. Nishimura RA, Schwartz RS, Tajik AJ, et al: Noninvasive measurement of rate of left ventricular relaxation by Doppler echocardiography: Validation with simultaneous cardiac catheterization. *Circulation* 88:146, 1993.

56. Choong CY, Herrmann HC, Weyman AE, et al: Preload dependence of Doppler-derived indexes of left ventricular diastolic function in humans. *J Am Coll Cardiol* 10:800, 1987.

57. Appleton CP, Hatle LK, Popp RL: Relation of transmitral flow velocity patterns to left ventricular diastolic function: New insights from a combined hemodynamic and Doppler echocardiographic study. *J Am Coll Cardiol* 12:426, 1988.

58. Fast JH, Van Dam I, Heringa A, et al: Limits of reproducibility of mitral pulsed Doppler spectra. *Am J Cardiol* 61:891, 1988.

59. Gradman A, Deedwania P, Cody R, et al: Predictors of total mortality and sudden death in mild to moderate heart failure. *J Am Coll Cardiol* 14:564, 1989.

60. Bonow RO, Vitale DF, Bacharach SL, et al: Asynchronous left ventricular regional function and impaired global diastolic filling in patients with coronary artery disease: Reversal after coronary angioplasty. *Circulation* 71:297, 1985.

61. Magorien DJ, Shaffer P, Bush CA, et al: Assessment of left ventricular pressure–volume relations using gated radionuclide angiography, echocardiography and micromanometer pressure recordings: A new method for serial measurements of systolic and diastolic function in man. *Circulation* 67: 844, 1983.

62. Magorien DJ, Shaffer P, Bush C, et al: Hemodynamic correlates for timing intervals, ejection rate and filling rate derived from the radionuclide angiographic volume curve. *Am J Cardiol* 53:567, 1984.

63. Spirito P, Maron BJ, Bonow RO: Noninvasive assessment of left ventricular diastolic function: Comparative analysis of Doppler echocardiographic and radionuclide angiographic techniques. *J Am Coll Cardiol* 7:518, 1986.

64. Bianco JA, Filiberti AW, Baker SP, et al: Ejection fraction and heart rate correlate with diastolic peak filling rate at rest and during exercise. *Chest* 88:107, 1985.

65. Cuocolo A, Sax FL, Brush JE, et al: Left ventricular hypertrophy and impaired diastolic filling in essential hypertension: Diastolic mechanisms for systolic dysfunction during exercise. *Circulation* 81:978, 1990.

66. Kass DA, Wolff MR, Ting C-T, et al: Diastolic compliance of hypertrophied ventricle is not acutely altered by pharmacologic agents influencing active processes. *Ann Intern Med* 119:466, 1993.

67. Grossman W, McLaurin LP, Rolett EL: Alterations in

left ventricular relaxation and diastolic compliance in congestive cardiomyopathy. *Cardiovasc Res* 13:514, 1979.

68. Miura T, Miyazaki S, Guth BD, et al: Heart rate and force-frequency effects on diastolic function of the left ventricle in exercising dogs. *Circulation* 89:2361, 1994.

69. Lenihan DJ, Gerson MC, Hoit BD, et al: Mechanisms, diagnosis, and treatment of diastolic heart failure. *Am Heart J* 130:153, 1995.

70. Frohlich ED, Apstein C, Chobanian AV, et al: The heart in hypertension. *N Engl J Med* 327:998, 1992.

71. The Fifth Report of the Joint National Committee on Detection, Evaluation, and Treatment of High Blood Pressure (JNC V). *Arch Intern Med* 153:154, 1993 (special article).

72. Inouye I, Massie B, Loge D, et al: Abnormal left ventricular filling: An early finding in mild to moderate systemic hypertension. *Am J Cardiol* 53:120, 1984.

73. Fouad FM, Slominski JM, Tarazi RC: Left ventricular diastolic function in hypertension: Relation to left ventricular mass and systolic function. *J Am Coll Cardiol* 3:1500, 1984.

74. Iriarte M, Murga N, Sagastagoitia D, et al: Congestive heart failure from left ventricular diastolic dysfunction in systemic hypertension. *Am J Cardiol* 71:308, 1993.

75. Shahi M, Thom S, Poulter N, et al: Regression of hypertensive left ventricular hypertrophy and left ventricular diastolic function. *Lancet* 336:458, 1990.

76. Little WC, Downes TR: Clinical evaluation of left ventricular diastolic performance. *Prog Cardiovasc Dis* 32:273, 1990.

77. Inouye IK, Massie BM, Loge D, et al: Failure of antihypertensive therapy with diuretic, beta-blocking and calcium channel-blocking drugs to consistently reverse left ventricular diastolic filling abnormalities. *Am J Cardiol* 53:1583, 1984.

78. Habib GB, Mann DL, Zoghbi WA: Normalization of cardiac structure and function after regression of cardiac hypertrophy. *Am Heart J* 128:333, 1994.

79. Schulman SP, Weiss JL, Becker LC, et al: The effects of antihypertensive therapy on left ventricular mass in elderly patients. *N Engl J Med* 322:1350, 1990.

80. Gottdiener JS, Livengood SV, Meyer PS, et al: Should echocardiography be performed to assess effects of antihypertensive therapy? Test–retest reliability of echocardiography for measurement of left ventricular mass and function. *J Am Coll Cardiol* 25:424, 1995.

81. Nishimura RA, Schwartz RS, Holmes DR Jr, et al: Failure of calcium channel blockers to improve ventricular relaxation in humans. *J Am Coll Cardiol* 21:182, 1993.

82. Bertrand ME, Lablanche JM, Fourrier JL, et al: Left ventricular systolic and diastolic function during acute coronary artery balloon occlusion in humans. *J Am Coll Cardiol* 12:341, 1988.

83. Applegate RJ, Walsh RA, O'Rourke RA: Comparative effects of pacing-induced and flow-limited ischemia on left ventricular function. *Circulation* 81:1380, 1990.

84. Bowman LK, Cleman MW, Cabin HS, et al: Dynamics of early and late left ventricular filling determined by Doppler two-dimensional echocardiography during percutaneous transluminal coronary angioplasty. *Am J Cardiol* 61:541, 1988.

85. Bonow RO, Bacharach SL, Green MV, et al: Impaired left ventricular diastolic filling in patients with coronary artery disease: Assessment with radionuclide angiography. *Circulation* 64:315, 1981.

86. Reduto LA, Wickemeyer WJ, Young JB, et al: Left ventricular diastolic performance at rest and during exercise in patients with coronary artery disease: Assessment with first-pass radionuclide angiography. *Circulation* 63: 1228, 1981.

87. Polak JF, Kemper AJ, Bianco JA, et al: Resting early peak diastolic filling rate: A sensitive index of myocardial dysfunction in patients with coronary artery disease. *J Nucl Med* 23:471, 1982.

88. Bonow RO, Leon MB, Rosing DR, et al: Effects of verapamil and propranolol on left ventricular systolic function and diastolic filling in patients with coronary artery disease: Radionuclide angiographic studies at rest and during exercise. *Circulation* 65:1337, 1981.

89. Bonow RO, Kent KM, Rosing DR, et al: Improved left ventricular diastolic filling in patients with coronary artery disease after percutaneous transluminal coronary angioplasty. *Circulation* 66:1159, 1982.

90. Maron BJ, Bonow RO, Cannon RO III, et al: Hypertrophic cardiomyopathy: Interrelations of clinical manifestations, pathophysiology, and therapy [First of two parts]. *N Engl J Med* 316:780, 1987.

90a. Maron BJ, Bonow RO, Cannon RO III, et al: Hypertrophic cardiomyopathy: Interrelations of clinical manifestations, pathophysiology, and therapy [Second of two parts]. *N Engl J Med* 316:844, 1987.

91. Watkins H, Rosenzweig A, Hwang D-S, et al: Characteristics and prognostic implications of myosin missense mutations in familial hypertrophic cardiomyopathy. *N Engl J Med* 326:1108, 1992.

92. Betocchi S, Bonow RO, Bacharach SL, et al: Isovolumic relaxation period in hypertrophic cardiomyopathy: Assessment by radionuclide angiography. *J Am Coll Cardiol* 7:74, 1986.

93. Bonow RO, Dilsizian V, Rosing DR, et al: Verapamil-induced improvement in left ventricular diastolic filling and increased exercise tolerance in patients with hypertrophic cardiomyopathy: Short- and long-term effects. *Circulation* 72:853, 1985.

94. Bonow RO, Frederick TM, Bacharach SL, et al: Atrial systole and left ventricular filling in hypertrophic cardiomyopathy: Effect of verapamil. *Am J Cardiol* 51:1386, 1983.

95. Bonow RO, Vitale DF, Maron BJ, et al: Regional left ventricular asynchrony and impaired global left ventricular filling in hypertrophic cardiomyopathy: Effect of verapamil. *J Am Coll Cardiol* 9:1108, 1987.

96. Iwase M, Sotobata I, Takagi S, et al: Effects of diltiazem on left ventricular diastolic behavior in patients with hypertrophic cardiomyopathy: Evaluation with exercise pulsed Doppler echocardiography. *J Am Coll Cardiol* 9:1099, 1987.

97. Paulus WJ, Lorell BH, Craig WE, et al: Comparison of the effects of nitroprusside and nifedipine on diastolic

properties in patients with hypertrophic cardiomyopathy: Altered left ventricular loading or improved muscle inactivation? *J Am Coll Cardiol* 2:879, 1983.

98. Lorell BH, Paulus WJ, Grossman W, et al: Modification of abnormal left ventricular diastolic properties by nifedipine in patients with hypertrophic cardiomyopathy. *Circulation* 65:499, 1982.

99. Murakami T, Hess OM, Gage JE, et al: Diastolic filling dynamics in patients with aortic stenosis. *Circulation* 73:1162, 1986.

100. Krayenbuehl HP, Hess OM, Monrad ES, et al: Left ventricular myocardial structure in aortic valve disease before, intermediate, and late after aortic valve replacement. *Circulation* 79:744, 1989.

101. Archer SL, Mike DK, Hetland MB, et al: Usefulness of mean aortic valve gradient and left ventricular diastolic filling pattern for distinguishing symptomatic from asymptomatic patients. *Am J Cardiol* 73:275, 1994.

102. Gerstenblith G, Frederiksen J, Yin FCP, et al: Echocardiographic assessment of a normal adult aging population. *Circulation* 56:273, 1977.

103. Iwase M, Nagata K, Izawa H, et al: Age-related changes in left and right ventricular filling velocity profiles and their relationship in normal subjects. *Am Heart J* 126:419, 1993.

104. Topol EJ, Traill TA, Fortuin NJ: Hypertensive hypertrophic cardiomyopathy of the elderly. *N Engl J Med* 312:277, 1985.

105. Arrighi JA, Dilsizian V, Perrone-Filardi P, et al: Improvement of the age-related impairment in left ventricular diastolic filling with verapamil in the normal human heart. *Circulation* 90:213, 1994.

106. Walsh RA: Advances in our understanding of congestive heart failure. *Focus Opinion Intern Med* 1(5):3, 1994.

107. Hoit BD, Walsh RA: Diastolic function in hypertensive heart disease, in Gaasch WH, LeWinter MM (eds): *Left Ventricular Diastolic Dysfunction and Heart Failure.* Philadelphia, Lea & Febiger, 1993, pp 354–372.

Ambulatory Left Ventricular Function Monitoring

Diwakar Jain
Barry L. Zaret

The ability to monitor various physiologic parameters continuously during routine physical activities has contributed significantly to our understanding of several complex physiologic and pathologic phenomena. Electrocardiographic (ECG) and blood pressure monitoring are used routinely for the evaluation of ambulatory patients with coronary artery disease and hypertension.[1-4] In comparison with these well-established techniques, continuous left ventricular function monitoring is a relatively recent development. In the relatively short period of time since its introduction, several studies have shown the potential of this technique for understanding several complex pathophysiologic issues associated with a number of cardiovascular disorders. In this chapter, we describe the technical aspects of continuous ambulatory left ventricular function monitoring, the results of various studies carried out using this technique in different patient populations, and the future developments and applications of this technique.

INSTRUMENTATION

Left ventricular function at rest and during exercise can be evaluated using a number of techniques, such as radionuclide imaging, contrast ventriculography, and echocardiography. To date, however, continuous ambulatory left ventricular function monitoring can be carried out only by the radionuclide technique, which employs a miniature radiation detector that is positioned on the chest over the left ventricular blood pool, after stable blood-pool labeling with technetium 99m.[5] The detector used in this device is a nonimaging, high-sensitivity detector that continuously acquires counts from the left ventricular blood pool. Changes in these counts represent cyclic changes in left ventricular blood volume. The counts are recorded on a suitable recording medium. A time–activity curve is generated from these counts from which a number of indices of systolic and diastolic function of the left ventricle such as ejection fraction, relative cardiac output, peak ejection rate, and peak filling rate can be derived. Of these indices, global left ventricular ejection fraction is by far the most commonly used index of left ventricular function. These techniques have technical constraints imposed by the physical half-life of the radiotracer used, difficulties in adequately separating the left ventricular blood pool from contiguous cardiac and extracardiac structures, scatter and background activity, tissue attenuation, and statistical noise associated with the use of radioisotopes. These considerations must be taken into account while using these techniques.

Earlier attempts to monitor left ventricular function continuously were made in the early 1980s by using the nuclear stethoscope, which consisted of a single photomultiplier tube with a lead collimator mounted on a movable arm and interfaced to a computer for recording and analyzing the data acquired by the photomultiplier tube.[6,7] However, this equipment was bulky and difficult to use for prolonged periods. Moreover, the equipment could be used only in patients who were either lying down or sitting up in a chair. Due to these limitations, this instrument is no longer in use and has largely been replaced by newer devices: c-VEST™ and Cardioscint, which are described next.

c-VEST™

This was initially described by Wilson et al in 1983.[8] This miniaturized device is portable and can be used in ambulatory patients. It has undergone several technical improvements since initial introduction. In its present form, the device is comprised of a nonimaging detector and a semirigid plastic vestlike garment with a bracket to hold the detector on the chest, two ECG channels, and a recording device that is a modified Holter monitor to record the scintigraphic and ECG data for several hours on an ordinary magnetic tape.[9–11] The nuclear data are in the form of sequential gamma counts, obtained 32 times per second. The tape is read off-line using a dedicated minicomputer.

The nonimaging detector used in this device is a 5.5-cm-diameter sodium iodide crystal equipped with a parallel-hole collimator. The detector weighs about 1.5 lb. Another smaller cadmium telluride detector is used to monitor background activity over the lung field. The plastic garment that is used to mount the device on the chest weighs 1.5 lb. The associated electronics and the recorder are placed in a lightweight shoulder-strap bag (weighing about 4.5 lb) that is carried by the patient (Fig. 16-1). Thus, monitoring can be carried out under ambulatory conditions.

The principle used for data generation and analysis is similar to that for classic gamma-camera equilibrium radionuclide angiocardiography. The blood pool is labeled with technetium 99m in a standard manner. Baseline gamma-camera equilibrium radionuclide angiocardiographic imaging is carried out in the left anterior oblique view to visualize the left ventricle and assess left ventricular ejection fraction. This also helps in positioning the detector over the left ventricle. A positioning target with several lead markers that fits into the bracket for the miniature detector is employed to determine the optimal position and angulation of the bracket (Fig. 16-2). After appropriate positioning, the device continuously monitors left ventricular time activity and a two-channel ECG. Patients can be monitored for periods from 2 to 6 h. For longer monitoring periods, repeat blood-pool labeling with additional injections of radioisotope is necessary.

The radionuclide data are summed for 15 to 60 s and displayed in graphic form (Fig. 16-3). A number of indices are derived from the summed data to evaluate quantitatively systolic and diastolic left ventricular function. Of these, left ventricular ejection fraction is the

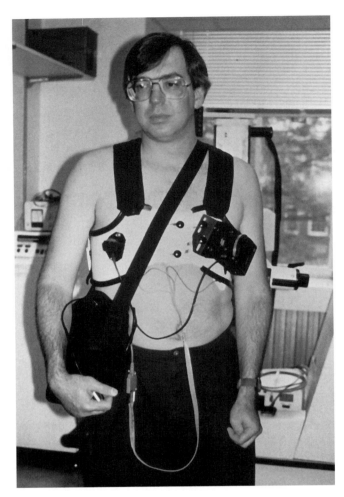

Figure 16-1 A subject wearing the c-VEST. The detector is housed in a bracket in the plastic vestlike garment. The shoulder-strap bag contains the electronics. (From Zaret and Jain,[10] reproduced with permission.)

most widely used and relatively easily obtained index of left ventricular function. Left ventricular ejection fraction measured by this technique correlates well with conventional gamma-camera left ventricular ejection fraction obtained at rest and during treadmill exercise.[12,13] A fall of 0.05 ejection-fraction units or more lasting more than 1 to 2 min is considered abnormal. This assessment is based on variability data and the range of responses noted in normal subjects.

Cardioscint

This device has a smaller and lighter detector that is 48 mm in diameter and 39 mm in height and weighs only 0.14 kg. Instead of a photomultiplier tube, this instrument contains cesium iodide scintillation crystal (14 × 14 × 8 mm) equipped with a 1-cm-long converging collimator. The crystal is optically coupled to a photodi-

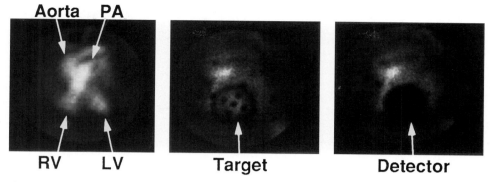

Figure 16-2 Static imaging in the left anterior oblique position demonstrating c-VEST positioning. *Left:* A static blood-pool image in the left anterior oblique view. PA, pulmonary artery; RV, right ventricle; LV, left ventricle. *Middle:* The static image with the positioning target over the left ventricular blood pool. *Right:* The positioning target has been replaced by the detector.

ode. The nuclear data and ECG are interfaced to a micro-computer for on-line analysis. The data can be displayed in either real time in beat-to-beat mode or can be averaged over 10 to 300 s. The detector can be positioned either under gamma-camera control or blindly using a blind positioning algorithm similar to that used by nuclear stethoscope. Background can be determined automatically or manually. Left ventricular ejection fraction obtained with this device at rest or during atrial pacing correlates well with gamma-camera-derived ejection fraction.[14,15] This device can be used only in recumbent patients and is thus useful only for studies in coronary care and intensive care units. An important limitation is the lack of a reliable system to hold the device in a constant position over an extended period of time. From a practical standpoint, this has severely limited its utilization.

Validation Studies

A number of studies have correlated the results obtained by using miniature detectors with those derived from conventional gamma cameras. The c-VEST detector has also been used to track left ventricular function under conditions when rapid left ventricular function changes are expected. Kayden et al employed the c-VEST detector in the cardiac catheterization laboratory to study left ventricular ejection-fraction changes during angioplasty of the left anterior descending coronary artery in patients with preserved resting left ventricular function.[16] A total of 18 inflations were studied in 12 patients. The mean duration of each balloon inflation was 70 ± 16 s. Ejection fraction changed from 53 ± 8 percent at baseline to 28 ± 11 percent at peak inflation. An absolute fall of 10 percent or more in ejection fraction was observed

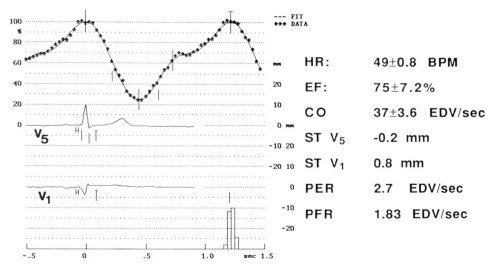

HR:	49±0.8 BPM
EF:	75±7.2%
CO	37±3.6 EDV/sec
ST V₅	-0.2 mm
ST V₁	0.8 mm
PER	2.7 EDV/sec
PFR	1.83 EDV/sec

Figure 16-3 Summed time–activity curve from the data obtained over 30 s along with a two-channel electrocardiogram and a list of the derived parameters. (From Zaret and Jain,[10] reproduced with permission.)

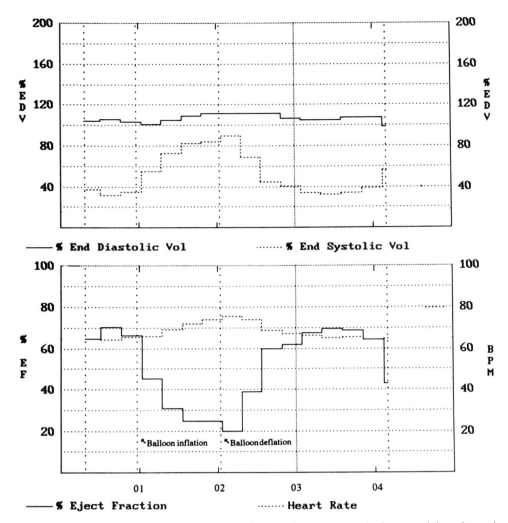

Figure 16-4 Trend of left ventricular ejection fraction, heart rate, and relative end-diastolic and end-systolic volumes during coronary angioplasty. The data have been averaged over 15 s. Note a marked reduction in the ejection fraction and an increase in the end-systolic volume with the inflation of balloon. (From Kayden et al,[16] reproduced with permission.)

in 17 of 18 inflations. The changes in ejection fraction were associated with a minimal but significant increase in end-diastolic volume (4 ± 3 percent) and a major increase in end-systolic volume (69 ± 43 percent). Interestingly, chest pain occurred in only 10 of 18 inflations, and ischemic ST-segment changes were observed in only seven inflations. The fall in ejection fraction was noted within 15 s of balloon inflation and generally antedated the chest pain. This indicates the greater sensitivity of changes in left ventricular function for detecting myocardial ischemia in comparison with symptoms of chest pain or ST depression. Furthermore, profound reduction in left ventricular ejection fraction frequently occurred unaccompanied by symptoms or ST-segment changes. These observations are of importance in studies of silent ischemia, as is described in a later section of this chapter. Figure 16-4 shows the data trend from a patient during

angioplasty of the left anterior descending coronary artery.

Tamaki et al studied the effect of routine activities such as standing, walking, eating, and mental stress on left ventricular function in 18 normal subjects by using the c-VEST.[17] The authors observed that left ventricular ejection fraction (in percent units) increases by 3 ± 4 percent with standing alone, 10 ± 5 percent with walking, 18 ± 9 percent with stair climbing, and 2 ± 3 percent during eating. Exposure to a cold environment resulted in a decrease of 5 ± 4 percent. During graded upright bicycle and treadmill exercise, marked increases in the left ventricular ejection fraction and end-diastolic volume were accompanied by a marked decrease in end-systolic volume. Interestingly, most of the changes in ejection fraction and volumes occurred in the early part of exercise, with no further change in the later part of exercise, whereas heart rate, systolic blood pressure, and double product continued to rise progressively throughout the exercise. Bairy et al studied the effect of several routine activities and mental stress on left ventricular ejection fraction in 18 normal subjects[18] and found similar results with walking and stair climbing. In their study, 14 of the 18 subjects showed a fall in ejection fraction with cold pressor testing. Four of 18 subjects showed a fall in ejection fraction in response to laboratory-induced mental stress. Mortelmans et al studied the effect of standing, walking, climbing stairs, intravenous isosorbide dinitrate, Trendelenburg position, and inflation of cuffs around the thighs on left ventricular volumes and ejection fraction in normal healthy subjects.[19] With standing, there was no change in ejection fraction but, with walking and stair climbing, ejection fraction increased by 7 percent and 21 percent, respectively. Trendelenburg increased left ventricular end-diastolic volume by 3 percent, while administration of isosorbide dinitrate and inflation of cuffs around thighs decreased it by 6 percent and 2 percent, respectively.

Imbriaco et al studied the repeatability of c-VEST–determined left ventricular function changes in response to different stimuli in patients with coronary artery disease by performing two separate c-VEST studies 5 days apart.[20] Left ventricular function was monitored at rest, during change of position from supine to upright, during sustained isometric exercise (handgrip), and after administration of sublingual nitroglycerin. Significant changes in the heart rate, left ventricular ejection fraction, end-diastolic volume, end-systolic volume, stroke volume, and cardiac output occurred with these stimuli. However, the magnitude of these changes was similar between the two c-VEST studies. These results demonstrate good reproducibility for measuring left ventricular function responses to different stimuli.

STUDIES IN MYOCARDIAL INFARCTION

Several studies have demonstrated that ambulatory monitoring of left ventricular function can provide relevant information in patients with acute myocardial infarction.[21-24] Breisblatt et al performed ambulatory monitoring of left ventricular function during routine activities, exercise, and mental stress in 35 patients with acute myocardial infarction who did not receive thrombolytic therapy.[21] Observed in 23 patients were 56 episodes of transient left ventricular dysfunction. Of these episodes, 22 occurred during exercise and 13 during mental stress: 75 percent were silent and only 39 percent were associated with ST-segment change. A correlation was observed between the presence of reversible perfusion abnormalities recorded during a separately obtained stress

thallium-201 study and the occurrence of transient left ventricular dysfunction during exercise or mental stress.

Kayden et al performed ambulatory left ventricular function monitoring in acute myocardial infarction patients receiving thrombolytic therapy.[22] The patients were monitored over a period of 187 ± 56 min. Transient left ventricular dysfunction, as defined by 5 percent unit or greater fall in ejection fraction lasting 1 min or longer, was observed in 12 of 33 patients during routine ambulation. Only two episodes in one patient were accompanied by chest pain or ECG changes. Clinical follow-up over 19 ± 5 months demonstrated a highly significant relationship between the occurrence of silent left ventricular dysfunction during the prehospital discharge monitoring period and subsequent cardiac events. Of the 11 patients with cardiac events (death, myocardial infarction, or unstable angina requiring urgent intervention), eight had left ventricular dysfunction during routine monitoring. Likewise, eight (75 percent) of 12 patients with an abnormality on c-VEST monitoring had a cardiac event compared with only three (14 percent) of 21 with no abnormality over a mean follow-up period of 19 months ($p < 0.01$). Clinical variables including the results of exercise radionuclide angiocardiography and myocardial perfusion imaging did not predict cardiac events in this study.

This study highlights the potential role of ambulatory monitoring in the risk stratification of patients following acute myocardial infarction in the thrombolytic era. Since exercise studies with perfusion imaging or ventricular function analysis may not provide the optimal prognostic information in patients with acute myocardial infarction treated with thrombolytic agents, the results of ambulatory function studies take on further significance.[25-27] The exact mechanism by which ambulatory monitoring of left ventricular function is predictive of subsequent cardiac events in patients with acute myocardial infarction treated with thrombolytic agents is largely speculative. Spontaneous episodes of left ventricular dysfunction may reflect the instability of the atherosclerotic plaque, luminal thrombosis, or abnormal coronary vasomotion. There is a need for further large-scale studies to evaluate the role of predischarge ambulatory monitoring of left ventricular function for risk stratification of patients with acute myocardial infarction receiving thrombolytic therapy.

In another study, ambulatory monitoring of left ventricular function was carried out in 17 patients admitted with unstable angina or non-Q-wave myocardial infarction on an average of 3 ± 2 days after hospital admission.[23] Patients were monitored in either the coronary care unit or in the step-down care unit for 145 ± 45 min. Of 17 patients, 11 (68 percent) manifested 23 episodes of spontaneous transient left ventricular dysfunction. These episodes occurred in the absence of ECG changes in all but two instances. Only one patient experienced chest pain. Most episodes (57 percent) were no-

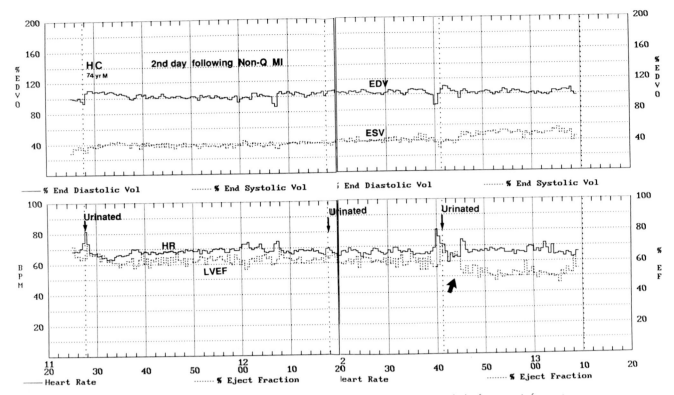

Figure 16-5   Data trend from a patient with recent non-Q-wave myocardial infarction. Left ventricular function was monitored for nearly 2 h. *Top:* Relative end-diastolic (EDV) and end-systolic (ESV) volumes. *Bottom:* Heart rate (HR) (*solid line*) and left ventricular ejection fraction (LVEF) (*dotted line*) trends. Note an asymptomatic episode of fall in left ventricular ejection fraction (*arrow*) that was not accompanied by any sustained change in heart rate. This episode occurred nearly 15 min after urination. There is no change in end-diastolic volume, but there is an increase in end-systolic volume. (From Zaret et al,[9] reproduced with permission.)

ticed during routine activities or at rest. Several episodes were associated with eating (4 percent) or urination/defecation (22 percent). The episodes lasted 8.7 ± 12 min, and the fall in ejection fraction averaged 8 ± 15 percent units. Figure 16-5 shows the data trend from a patient with non-Q-wave myocardial infarction showing spontaneous episodes of left ventricular dysfunction. Similar results have been reported by Yang et al.[24]

STUDIES IN STABLE CORONARY ARTERY DISEASE

Tamaki and colleagues performed c-VEST monitoring in 39 ambulatory patients with coronary artery disease for an average period of 2.6 h.[12] Thirty-six episodes of a transient fall in left ventricular ejection fraction were observed in 16 patients. Two-thirds of the episodes were not accompanied by any symptoms, and ECG abnormalities were noted in only 11 episodes. In 10 of the 12 symptomatic episodes, ventricular dysfunction occurred 30 to 90 s prior to the onset of symptoms. Sheldahl et

al found similar results when monitoring patients with coronary artery disease under a variety of circumstances, including snow shoveling and physical exercise in a hot environment.[28,29]

Vassiliadis et al studied the occurrence of left ventricular dysfunction during routine daily activities in patients with coronary artery disease.[30] Transient left ventricular dysfunction was common during activities such as walking, urinating, or eating and was not associated with any symptoms or ST depression. This transient left ventricular dysfunction was more common in patients with abnormal ejection-fraction response to exercise on a separately performed rest–exercise gated blood-pool imaging, compared with patients who showed a normal ejection-fraction response with exercise.

Mohiuddin et al monitored left ventricular function with the c-VEST during exercise in 27 patients with stable coronary artery disease to determine the temporal sequence of events during ischemic episodes.[31] Seventeen episodes of exercise-induced left ventricular ejection-fraction abnormalities were observed in 17 patients, of which eight (47 percent) were electrocardiographically silent and 12 (71 percent) were silent symptomatically.

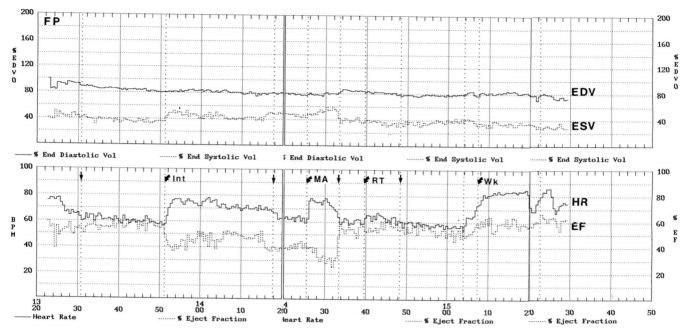

Figure 16-6 Trended data for left ventricular ejection fraction (LVEF), heart rate (HR), and relative end-diastolic volume (EDV) and end-systolic volume (ESV) over 2¼ h in a patient undergoing a mental stress protocol. *Curved arrows* indicate the start of specific interventions, and *vertical arrows* indicate the end of an intervention and start of relaxation. After an initial period of stabilization, the patient underwent a structured interview (Int). Note a marked decrease in ejection fraction, associated with a slight increase in heart rate. Mental arithmetic (MA) resulted in a further fall in ejection fraction with no change in heart rate. A neutral task (RT) did not result in any change in ejection fraction. With walking (WK), there is a marked increase in heart rate but no change in ejection fraction.

Exercise-induced ischemia occurred in a temporal sequence of first ejection-fraction abnormalities, then ST depressions, and finally symptoms. After discontinuation of exercise, ejection fraction recovered sooner than symptoms or ST abnormalities. Thus, c-VEST monitoring may be helpful in detecting ischemic episodes in coronary artery disease that remain electrocardiographically or symptomatically silent. c-VEST monitoring may be helpful in understanding the pathophysiology of the cascade of changes associated with exercise stress-induced myocardial ischemia.

Continuous left ventricular function monitoring has been used to study changes in left ventricular function at rest and during exercise following pharmacotherapy.[13] Left ventricular function was evaluated at rest and during exercise without any drug, and again after administration of nitroglycerin or nifedipine in patients with coronary disease and in normal subjects. In patients with coronary artery disease, abnormal left ventricular ejection-fraction responses were observed during the control exercise period. However, ejection fraction increased during exercise after administration of nitroglycerin or nifedipine. In normal subjects, resting and exercise ejection fraction remained unchanged between control and posttreatment studies.

Taki et al studied left ventricular function at rest and

during supine ergometer exercise before and 4 weeks after coronary artery bypass grafting in patients with coronary artery disease.[32] Only 13 percent of patients had a normal left ventricular ejection-fraction response to exercise prior to surgery, whereas 60 percent had a normal ejection-fraction response to exercise following coronary artery surgery. The mean ejection-fraction change from rest to peak exercise improved from -6.4 ± 8.8 percent to 5.0 ± 7.4 percent after surgery for the entire group.

STUDIES DURING MENTAL STRESS

We recently performed continuous left ventricular function monitoring in a group of 30 patients with chronic stable coronary artery disease and myocardial ischemia previously documented on stress thallium imaging.[33] Patients were monitored for a period of 2 to 3 h. They underwent mental stress with serial mental arithmetic and a structured interview as well as low-level physical exercise during the monitoring. In addition, their psychological profile was evaluated for type-A behavior, traits of anger, hostility, anxiety, somatization, and depression. During mental arithmetic, half of the 30 patients (group I) developed a significant drop in left ventricular ejection fraction and the remaining 15 (group II) showed no significant drop in ejection fraction. Figure 16-6 shows the data trend in a patient with mental stress-induced drop in left ventricular ejection fraction. The average drop in ejection fraction with mental stress was 14 ± 8 percent units in group I. None of these episodes of fall in ejection fraction was accompanied by chest pain or ST-segment depression. Both groups were comparable with respect to demographic variables, extent of perfusion abnormalities on stress thallium imaging, and medications. Both groups showed a marked increase in systolic blood pressure, a moderate increase in diastolic blood pressure, and a slight increase in heart rate with mental stress. In contrast, the two groups differed significantly with respect to psychological profiles. Group I patients had higher scores for type-A behavior, anger, and hostility when compared with group II patients.

This study highlights the role of behavioral and psychological factors in provoking silent left ventricular dysfunction in patients with coronary artery disease. Furthermore, this form of left ventricular dysfunction is not accompanied by chest pain or ST-segment depression. In a follow-up study, group I patients had a higher frequency of cardiac events over a period of 1 year.[34] Of the total of 12 events (reinfarction, unstable angina requiring admission to the hospital, and revascularization), nine occurred in group I patients and only three occurred in group II patients. Thus, patients with mental stress-induced left ventricular dysfunction had a higher incidence of cardiac events: nine (60 percent) versus three (20 percent) of 15 ($p = 0.025$). Similar findings were noted at 2-year follow-up. Figure 16-7 shows the event-free survival curves in both groups of patients. This study shows the prognostic importance of mental stress-induced left ventricular dysfunction in patients with coronary artery disease. This observation requires further evaluation in larger patient populations. In another study, mental stress-induced left ventricular dysfunction was associated with greater prevalence of silent myocardial ischemia on Holter monitoring.[35,36]

The issue of reproducibility of mental stress-induced left ventricular dysfunction was investigated in a recent study where a cohort of patients with coronary artery disease underwent a battery of mental stress tasks (mental arithmetic, anger recall, and color stroop) during continuous left ventricular function monitoring on two different occasions 4 to 8 weeks apart, with no change in medication in the interim.[37] Overall, left ventricular function response to mental stress was highly reproducible. Of the various mental stress tasks, response to anger recall was most reproducible.

The effect of routine antianginal medication on men-

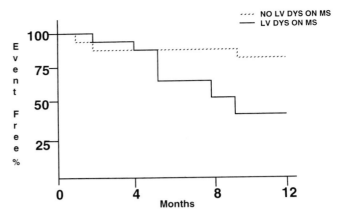

Figure 16-7 Cardiac event-free survival rate in two groups of patients with chronic stable angina. One group of patients had left ventricular dysfunction (Dys) in response to mental stress (MS), and the other group had no left ventricular dysfunction in response to mental stress. A significantly greater proportion of patients with mental stress-induced left ventricular dysfunction developed cardiac events over 1 year. (From Jain et al,[34] reproduced with permission.)

tal stress-induced left ventricular dysfunction was studied recently in patients with chronic stable angina who underwent ambulatory left ventricular function monitoring and treadmill exercise testing twice: on a calcium channel antagonist and on placebo.[38] Treatment with the calcium channel antagonist improved ischemic indices on the treadmill exercise test but did not affect mental stress-induced left ventricular dysfunction. Thus, there may be discordance between the effects of antianginal medications on exercise-induced versus mental stress-induced myocardial ischemia in patients with coronary artery disease. This observation is particularly important because, traditionally, treatment of coronary artery disease is guided by the improvement in symptoms and exercise-induced ischemia.

To understand the mechanism of mental stress-induced left ventricular dysfunction, a pilot study was performed in patients undergoing endoscopic transthoracic sympathectomy because of severe coronary artery disease and intractable angina pectoris.[39] Endoscopic transthoracic sympathectomy is a recently developed, less traumatic surgical approach for cervical and thoracic sympathectomy. This procedure was initially used for the treatment of hyperhidrosis but is currently being used in patients with severe intractable angina who are not suitable for revascularization treatment. A small group of patients with severe coronary artery disease underwent ambulatory left ventricular function monitoring with mental stress testing before and after endoscopic transthoracic sympathectomy. Of the four patients with mental stress-induced left ventricular dysfunction in the baseline study, only one developed left ventricular dysfunction with mental stress after endoscopic transthoracic sympathectomy. This study indicates the role of cardiac sympathetic nervous system in mental stress-induced left ventricular dysfunction.

STUDIES IN HYPERTENSION

Breisblatt et al monitored left ventricular function during exercise, mental stress, and routine activities in 31 patients with hypertension.[40] Patients with left ventricular hypertrophy showed episodes of fall in left ventricular ejection fraction during exercise and mental stress as well as during routine daily activities. These episodes of fall in ejection fraction were associated with an increase in blood pressure. This study shows that a fall in left ventricular ejection fraction is relatively common during daily activities in hypertensive patients with left ventricular hypertrophy. Whether this is purely an afterload-related phenomenon or is due to left ventricular dysfunction is not known. The prognostic significance of this finding and its relationship to antihypertensive treatment are not known.

STUDIES IN CARDIAC TRANSPLANTATION

Following successful cardiac transplantation, most patients continue to have subnormal exercise capacity despite normal left ventricular function. The exact etiology of this limitation of exercise capacity is not known. To address this issue, we studied 11 patients who had undergone cardiac transplantation 24 ± 17 months earlier as therapy for end-stage heart failure due to cardiomyopathy or coronary artery disease.[41] Patients were monitored during level walking at a brisk pace for 7 to 10 min, which resulted in symptoms of shortness of breath and tiredness. There was a marked increase in left ventricular ejection fraction (16 ± 5 percent units) that was accompanied by a marked increase in relative end-diastolic volume (+8.1 ± 7.0 percent) and a marked reduction in relative end-systolic volume (−12 ± 6 percent). Cardiac output increased 1.8-fold. Changes in left ventricular volumes and cardiac output were maximal within the first 3 to 4 min and then remained at a plateau. In contrast, increase in heart rate was more gradual, with a maximum increase of 20 ± 7 beats/min seen close to the end of walking. From these data, it was hypothesized that the increase in cardiac output with exercise is attained as a result of an increase in left ventricular end-diastolic volume and stroke volume without an appropriate increase in heart rate. This may be responsible for limited effort tolerance in cardiac transplant patients. Thus, the limitation of effort capacity in this patient population may be related to inadequate heart rate response rather than to myocardial dysfunction or altered ventricular function reserve. This study also highlights the potentially useful role of ambulatory monitoring of left ventricular function for obtaining important physiologic information.

STUDIES IN PARKINSON'S DISEASE

Nappi et al studied left ventricular function and blood pressure in patients with Parkinson's disease with and without a history of postural hypotension, with the patients in supine and then assuming an upright position.[42] In patients with postural hypotension, change in posture from the supine to the upright position induced a significant fall in end-diastolic volume, end-systolic volume, stroke volume, left ventricular ejection fraction, and cardiac output along with a reduction in peripheral vascular resistance. In patients without postural hypotension, ejection fraction increased upon changing posture from the supine to the upright position with no changes in stroke volume, cardiac output, or peripheral vascular resistance. Therefore, abnormalities in the regulation of peripheral vascular tone during postural change result in marked changes in parameters of cardiac function in patients with Parkinson's disease and postural hypotension.

STUDIES IN PATIENTS UNDERGOING HEMODIALYSIS

Singh et al performed continuous left ventricular function monitoring in patients with chronic renal failure during hemodialysis.[43] Asymptomatic episodes of ejection-fraction fall were observed commonly. These episodes were associated with a rise in end-systolic volume, while heart rate, blood pressure, and end-diastolic volume remained unchanged. ST-segment depression was observed only rarely during these episodes, but perfusion abnormalities were common when sestamibi was injected either during or after the dialysis. These data indicate that spontaneous changes in left ventricular function and perfusion are common in patients with chronic renal failure during hemodialysis but are rarely associated with chest pain or ST-segment depression. The therapeutic and prognostic implications of this observation, however, are not clear at this stage.

STUDIES IN SYNDROME X

Taki et al studied left ventricular function during exercise and recovery in patients with angina pectoris, ST-segment depression during exercise, and angiographically normal coronary arteries (syndrome X) and in patients with atypical chest pain without ST-segment depression during exercise and normal coronary arteries.[44] Left ventricular ejection-fraction response to exercise was impaired in patients with syndrome X but not in patients with atypical chest pain and no ST depression on exercise. The magnitude of ejection-fraction overshoot upon stopping exercise was lower, with the time to ejection-fraction overshoot longer in patients with syndrome X.

STUDIES IN HYPERTROPHIC CARDIOMYOPATHY

Functional response to exercise in patients with nonobstructive hypertrophic cardiomyopathy was studied using continuous left ventricular function monitoring.[45] Patients who were unable to increase left ventricular ejection fraction on exercise had impaired exercise capacity and a higher ejection fraction at rest, compared with patients who had normal ejection fraction at rest that increased further with exercise. Septal wall thickness and the septum-to-posterior wall-thickness ratio were not predictive of the impairment in exercise capacity in this patient population.

STUDIES IN SLEEP APNEA

Using continuous monitoring of left ventricular function and pulmonary arterial pressure, Garpestad et al investigated cardiac function in patients with sleep apnea during the cycles of obstruction and resumption of ventilation.[46] Repetitive oscillations of systemic arterial pressure were observed in association with changes in respiration and sleep state. Recovery from apnea was associated with an abrupt decrease in left ventricular stroke volume. Although heart rate increased with recovery, this was not sufficient to compensate for the observed decrease in stroke volume so that cardiac output fell. Recovery was also associated with a significant increase in pulmonary artery pressure. Abrupt decreases in left ventricular stroke volume and cardiac output at apnea termination occurring coincident with the nadir of oxygen saturation may contribute to compromised tissue oxygen delivery in patients with sleep apnea.

FUTURE DIRECTIONS

Ambulatory left ventricular function monitoring appears to provide important diagnostic as well as prognostic information in a wide spectrum of patients with coronary artery disease as well as several other cardiac and noncardiac disorders. Ambulatory left ventricular function monitoring has added a new dimension to the concept of silent myocardial ischemia. This technique may provide a unique opportunity for studying the hemodynamic correlates of coronary vascular reactivity and spontaneous changes in coronary arterial tone. These coronary vascular characteristics may form the basis for some of the adverse cardiovascular events observed in patients with stable coronary artery disease and in acute coronary syndromes treated with thrombolytic therapy. Currently, detection of exercise-induced ischemia constitutes an important basis for predicting ischemic cardiac events, for risk stratification, and for guiding treatment in patients with coronary artery disease. In real life, however, the majority of adverse cardiac events occur during routine daily activities and not during exercise stress.[47] The exact trigger for these adverse events in not known. A test modality based on the detection of abnormalities occurring at rest or during routine activities appears appealing for risk stratification of patients with coronary artery disease. Preliminary studies in patients with stable coronary artery disease or following thrombolysis support this notion. However, further studies involving larger numbers of patients are needed to substantiate these results.

This technique has also helped in understanding the interaction between behavioral profile and mental stress-induced changes in cardiac function in patients with coronary artery disease. Mental stress is now recognized as an important provocateur of silent left ventricular dysfunction. Mental stress-induced left ventricular dysfunction appears to be an important adverse prognostic sign in patients with chronic stable angina. Current data indicate that mental stress testing should be considered in the comprehensive evaluation of patients with coronary artery disease.

Further miniaturization of the detector and supporting electronics used for ambulatory left ventricular function monitoring are under way, and these technical refinements would make this technique more user friendly and widely acceptable. Future developments also include the capability for on-line processing of data with a real-time display of measurements of left ventricular function.

This would facilitate a simultaneous assessment of hemodynamic, biochemical, and metabolic accompaniments of silent left ventricular dysfunction.

The foregoing clinical investigations strongly suggest that ambulatory monitoring of left ventricular function will continue to play an important investigative and clinical role in cardiology.

REFERENCES

1. Deanfield JE, Selwyn AP, Chierchia S, et al: Myocardial ischemia during daily life in patients with stable angina: Its relation to symptoms and heart rate change. *Lancet* 1:753, 1983.
2. Miller-Craig MW, Bishop CN, Raftery EB: Circadian variation of blood pressure. *Lancet* 1:795, 1978.
3. Gottlieb SO, Gottlieb SH, Achuff SC, et al: Silent ischemia on Holter monitoring predicts mortality in high risk postinfarction patients. *JAMA* 259:1030, 1988.
4. Deedwania PC, Carabjal EV: Silent myocardial ischemia: A clinical perspective. *Arch Intern Med* 151:2373, 1991.
5. Callahan RJ, Froelich JW, McKusick KA, et al: A modified method for the in vivo labeling of red blood cells with Tc-99m: Concise communication. *J Nucl Med* 23:315, 1982.
6. Wagner HN Jr, Wake R, Nickoloff E, Natarajan TK: The nuclear stethoscope: A simple device for the generation of left ventricular volume curves. *Am J Cardiol* 38:747, 1976.
7. Berger HJ, Zaret BL: Beat-to-beat left ventricular performance assessed from equilibrium cardiac blood pool using a computerized nuclear probe. *Circulation* 67:133, 1981.
8. Wilson RA, Sullivan PJ, Moore RH, et al: An ambulatory ventricular function monitor: Validation and preliminary clinical results. *Am J Cardiol* 52:601, 1983.
9. Zaret BL, Wackers FJ: Nuclear cardiology [Second of two parts]. *N Engl J Med* 329:855, 1993.
10. Zaret BL, Jain D: Continuous monitoring of left ventricular function with miniaturized nonimaging detectors, in Zaret BL, Beller GA (eds): *Nuclear Cardiology: State of the Art and Future Directions.* St Louis, CV Mosby, 1993, pp 137–145,
11. Cohn PF: Myocardial dysfunction in silent myocardial ischemia as demonstrated by ambulatory radionuclide left ventricular function studies. *Cardiol Clin* 10:473, 1992.
12. Tamaki N, Yasuda T, Moore R, et al: Continuous monitoring of left ventricular function by an ambulatory radionuclide detector in patients with coronary artery disease. *J Am Coll Cardiol* 12:669, 1988.
13. Mohiuddin IH, Kambara H, Ohkusa T, et al: Clinical evaluation of cardiac function by ambulatory ventricular scintigraphic monitoring (VEST): Validation and study of the effects of nitroglycerin and nifedipine in patients with

and without coronary artery disease. *Am Heart J* 123:386, 1992.
14. Broadhurst P, Cashman P, Raftery EB, Lahiri A: Clinical validation of a miniature nuclear probe system for continuous on-line monitoring of cardiac function and ST-segment. *J Nucl Med* 32:37, 1991.
15. Jain D, Allam AH, Wackers FJ, Zaret BL: Validation of a new non-imaging miniature probe for serial on-line left ventricular ejection fraction. *J Nucl Med* 32(suppl):1038, 1991 (abstr).
16. Kayden DA, Remetz MS, Cabin HS, et al: Validation of continuous radionuclide left ventricular function monitoring in detecting silent myocardial ischemia during balloon angioplasty of the left anterior descending artery. *Am J Cardiol* 67:1339, 1991.
17. Tamaki N, Gill JB, Moore RH, et al: Cardiac response to daily activities and exercise in normal subjects assessed by an ambulatory ventricular function monitor. *Am J Cardiol* 59:1164, 1987.
18. Bairy N, Yang LD, Berman DS, Rozanski A: Comparison of physiological ejection fraction response to activities of daily living: Implications for clinical testing. *J Am Coll Cardiol* 16:847, 1990.
19. Mortelmans L, Cabrera EZ, Dorny N, et al: Left ventricular function changes during pharmacological and physiological interventions and routine activities monitored in healthy volunteers by a portable radionuclide probe (VEST). *Int J Card Imaging* 7:79, 1991.
20. Imbriaco M, Cuocolo A, Pace L, et al: Repeatability of hemodynamic responses to cardiac stimulations by ambulatory monitoring of left ventricular function. *J Nucl Biol Med* 37:238, 1993.
21. Breisblatt W, Weiland FL, McLain JR, et al: Usefulness of ambulatory radionuclide monitoring of left ventricular function early after acute myocardial infarction for predicting residual myocardial ischemia. *Am J Cardiol* 62:1005, 1988.
22. Kayden D, Wackers FJTh, Zaret BL: Silent left ventricular dysfunction during routine activity after thrombolytic therapy for acute myocardial infarction. *J Am Coll Cardiol* 15:1500, 1990.
23. Jain D, Vita NA, Wackers FJTh, Zaret BL: Transient silent left ventricular dysfunction in non-Q wave myocardial infarction and unstable angina. *J Nucl Med* 32(suppl):938, 1991 (abstr).
24. Yang L, Freeman MR, Hsia T, Armstrong PW: Episodes of ejection fraction fall frequently occur at rest in patients with coronary artery disease. *J Nucl Med* 32:1038, 1991 (abstr).
25. Tilkemeier PL, Guiney TE, LaRaia PJ, Boucher CA: Prognostic value of predischarge low-level exercise thallium testing after thrombolytic treatment of acute myocardial infarction. *Am J Cardiol* 66:1203, 1990.
26. Haber HL, Beller GA, Watson DD, Gimple LW: Exercise thallium-201 scintigraphy after thrombolytic therapy with or without angioplasty for acute myocardial infarction. *Am J Cardiol* 71:1257, 1993.
27. Jain D, Wackers FJTh, Zaret BL: Radionuclide Imaging in the thrombolytic era, in Becker R (ed): *Modern Era of Coronary Thrombolysis*, 1st ed. Norwell, MA, Kluwer, 1994, pp 195–218.

28. Sheldahl LM, Wilke NA, Dougherty S, et al: Response to snow shoveling in men with and without ischemic heart disease. *J Am Coll Cardiol* 17:94A, 1991.

29. Sheldahl LM, Wilke NA, Dougherty S, Tristani FE: Cardiac response to combined moderate heat and exercise in men with coronary artery disease. *Am J Cardiol* 70:186, 1992.

30. Vassiliadis IV, Machac J, Sharma S, et al: Detection of silent left ventricular dysfunction during daily activities in coronary artery disease patients by the nuclear VEST. *J Nucl Biol Med* 37:198, 1993.

31. Mohiuddin IH, Tamaki N, Kambara H, et al: Detection of exercise-induced silent ischemia and the sequence of ischemic events in coronary artery disease by radionuclide ambulatory ventricular function monitoring. *Jpn Circ J* 58:689, 1994.

32. Taki J, Muramori A, Nakajima K, Bunko H, et al: Cardiac response to exercise before and after coronary artery bypass grafting: Evaluation by continuous ventricular function monitor [in Japanese]. *Kaku Igaku* 28:1313, 1991.

33. Burg MM, Jain D, Soufer R, et al: Role of behavioral and psychological factors in mental stress-induced silent left ventricular dysfunction in coronary artery disease. *J Am Coll Cardiol* 22:440, 1993.

34. Jain D, Burg MM, Soufer RS, Zaret BL: Prognostic significance of mental stress induced left ventricular dysfunction in patients with coronary artery disease. *Am J Cardiol* 76:31, 1995.

35. Legault SE, Langer A, Armstrong PW, Freeman MR: Usefulness of ischemic response to mental stress in predicting silent myocardial ischemia during ambulatory monitoring. *Am J Cardiol* 75:1007, 1995.

36. Legault SE, Freeman MR, Langer A, Armstrong PW: The pathophysiology and time course of silent myocardial ischemia during mental-stress: Clinical, anatomic and physiologic correlates. *Br Heart J* 73:242, 1995.

37. Jain D, Burg M, Soufer R, et al: Day to day reproducibility of mental stress induced LV dysfunction. *J Am Coll Cardiol* 27(Suppl):240A, 1996 (abstr).

38. Jain D, Burg M, Soufer R, et al: Discordant effects of amlodipine on exercise-induced vs mental stress induced myocardial ischemia in patients with angina. *J Nucl Med* 37:59P, 1996 (abstr).

39. Lomsky M, Jain D, Claes G, et al: Endoscopic transthoracic sympathicotomy protects against mental stress induced LV dysfunction in patients with severe angina: Pilot study results. *Circulation* 92:I-677, 1995.

40. Breisblatt WM, Wolf CJ, McElhinny B, et al: Comparison of ambulatory left ventricular ejection fraction and blood pressure in systemic hypertension in patients with and without increased left ventricular mass. *Am J Cardiol* 67:597, 1991.

41. Jain D, Lee FA, Revkin J, et al: Reduced exercise capacity in patients following cardiac transplantation: Excellent ventricular function—A primary Starling effect but inadequate heart rate response during exercise. *J Nucl Med* 33:939, 1992 (abstr).

42. Nappi A, Cuocolo A, Iazzetta N, et al: Ambulatory monitoring of left ventricular function in patients with Parkinson's disease and postural hypotension. *Eur J Nucl Med* 21:1312, 1994.

43. Singh N, Langer A, Freeman MR, Goldstein MB: Myocardial alterations during hemodialysis: Insights from new noninvasive technology. *Am J Nephrol* 14:173, 1994.

44. Taki J, Nakajima K, Muramori A, et al: Left ventricular dysfunction during exercise in patients with angina pectoris and angiographically normal coronary arteries (syndrome X). *Eur J Nucl Med* 21:98, 1994.

45. Taki J, Nakajima K, Shimizu M, et al: Left ventricular functional reserve in nonobstructive hypertrophic cardiomyopathy: Evaluation by continuous left ventricular function monitoring. *J Nucl Med* 35:1937, 1994.

46. Garpestad E, Katayama H, Parker JA, et al: Stroke volume and cardiac output decrease at termination of obstructive apneas. *J Appl Physiol* 73:1743, 1992.

47. Mittleman MA, Maclure M, Tofler GH, et al: Triggering of acute myocardial infarction by heavy physical exertion: Protection against triggering by regular exercise. *N Engl J Med* 329:1677, 1993.

Response of Left Ventricular Function to Drug Intervention

Ajit R. Bhagwat
Michael W. Farrar

Direct assessment of the response of left ventricular function to drug interventions was limited in the past to invasive techniques such as right and left heart catheterization. The advent of reliable echocardiographic and radionuclide techniques over the past two decades has broadened the ability to evaluate left ventricular function. Although these tests do not replace invasive techniques, they often provide additional information when studying left ventricular function and supplant invasive procedures for the purposes of many drug studies and in many clinical situations. The general availability, extremely low risk, good reproducibility, and relative low cost (as compared with the overall costs of cardiac catheterization) have made noninvasive study of left ventricular function in response to drug intervention particularly attractive.

This chapter reviews the use and value of radionuclide ventriculography in the evaluation of changes in left ventricular function related to drug interventions. Studies utilizing this technique for the evaluation of doxorubicin cardiotoxicity, therapy of congestive heart failure and ischemic heart disease, and response of the left ventricle to specific drugs are reviewed and, when possible, compared with other available techniques. Guidelines are generated for the clinician as to the general use, advantages, and disadvantages of these techniques in specific patient care circumstances.

ACCURACY OF SERIAL MEASUREMENTS

The serial variability of radionuclide ventriculography must be known before data involving drug intervention can be interpreted accurately. At least two studies from Yale University have evaluated the serial variability of radionuclide ventriculograms. In the first study,[1] three first-pass quantitative radionuclide ventriculograms separated by an average of 4.3 days were performed in 20 patients. Left ventricular ejection fraction, normalized mean ejection rate, and regional wall motion were assessed with each radionuclide ventriculogram. Ejection fraction and ejection rate did not differ significantly in individuals on any of the three radionuclide ventriculograms, with a mean difference of sequential ejection fraction measurements of 4.4 ± 3.6 percent (absolute change) and of sequential ejection rates of 0.56 ± 0.47 s^{-1}. Fluctuations in heart rate or blood pressure did not account for variations in measurement. Patients with normal left ventricular function had greater variability in ejection rate than those with abnormal function. Of 20 patients, 19 showed constant regional wall-motion analysis.

In the second study,[2] 83 patients with various types of stable heart disease underwent assessment of left ventricular ejection fraction by radionuclide ventriculography utilizing multiple gated blood-pool imaging. Ejection fraction was determined twice in 70 patients: on the same day at intervals separated by 1 to 2 h in 41 patients and 1 to 5 days apart in 29 patients. The baseline ejection fraction ranged widely in these patients (18 to 91 percent) and was normal in 37 patients. There was no significant difference in mean serial variability of the absolute left ventricular ejection fraction performed on the same or separate days (3.3 ± 3.1 percent versus 4.3 ± 3.1 percent, respectively). However, the mean variability of absolute left ventricular ejection fraction was significantly greater in normal patients than in abnormal patients (5.4 ± 4.4 percent versus 2.1 ± 2.0 percent, respectively, $p < 0.01$). A serial change in left ventricular ejection fraction of 5 percent or more was more common in normal patients [19 (51 percent) of 37] than in abnormal patients [4 (12 percent) of 33]. One patient with an abnormal baseline ejection fraction had a 10 percent or more absolute change in ejection fraction on repeat testing, whereas six patients with a normal baseline ejection fraction exhibited the same phenomenon. When relative, rather than absolute, changes in ejection fraction were considered, there was no significant difference among those patients with normal and abnormal ejection fractions (8.0 ± 7.2 percent versus 6.6 ± 6.3 percent, respectively). As shown in other studies, ejection fraction by gated studies correlated well with data from first-pass radionuclide ventriculograms ($r = 0.94$) and from contrast angiography ($r = 0.84$). Intra- and interobserver variabilities of absolute ejection-fraction measurement were minimal and not different for patients with normal versus abnormal left ventricular function.

As can be seen, radionuclide ventriculography enables accurate serial assessment of left ventricular function with a high degree of reproducibility. As pointed out by these authors, however, it is particularly important to consider the baseline ejection fraction when assessing response to drug intervention. An absolute change in left ventricular ejection fraction of 10 percent or more in normal patients is necessary in order to attribute the change to a nonrandom physiologic alteration, whereas a change of 5 percent or more in an abnormal ventricle is significant.[2] This can be explained by considering that a normal left ventricle has intact functional reserve and can increase pump function by responding to a variety of stimuli. In contrast, the abnormal ventricle is less prone to manifest spontaneous fluctuations in ejection fraction or other indices of left ventricular function, since it has less functional reserve and is presumably functioning at close to maximum effort.*

Mechanism of Serial Changes

While measurement of left ventricular ejection fraction by radionuclide ventriculography is helpful in assessing the response of the left ventricle to a drug intervention, it does not necessarily reflect the mechanism of action of the drug. An increase in left ventricular ejection fraction or cardiac index with a lowering of left ventricular filling pressure may result from altered loading conditions rather than an inotropic effect.[3] The identification of the predominant hemodynamic effect and usefulness of a drug in human subjects is often complex and frequently requires evaluation of various hemodynamic, radionuclide (ejection fraction and ventricular volumes), and clinical parameters. Coupling these with exercise testing is particularly useful in assessing the effect of drug intervention. In addition, short- and long-term results of drug intervention must be evaluated separately.

MONITORING OF DOXORUBICIN CARDIOTOXICITY

Doxorubicin hydrochloride (adriamycin), an anthracycline antibiotic, is extremely useful in the treatment of many neoplastic diseases.[4] However, a cumulative dose-related cardiomyopathy develops in some patients, limiting further use of the drug and effective treatment of the tumor.[5-8] Various methods, including serial radionuclide ventriculography, have been proposed to monitor cardiotoxicity and enable certain patients to continue therapy safely without developing cardiomyopathy.[6] The value of serial radionuclide ventriculograms and other methods in following therapy are discussed below. However, it is important initially to review some basic aspects of the natural history of doxorubicin cardiotoxicity in order to understand the rationale behind the various methods of monitoring therapy.

Types and Frequency of Cardiotoxicity

Cardiotoxicity of doxorubicin may be acute or chronic.[6,8] Transient left ventricular dysfunction occurring within a few hours of drug administration, generally in patients with limited cardiac reserve, has been reported, although the mechanism is poorly defined.[8]

The dose-related cumulative toxicity of doxorubicin, resulting in cardiomyopathy, is well known.[5-8] The incidence and probably the severity of cardiomyopathy vary with the schedule of administration[6,9] and the presence of various risk factors, the most important of which is total prior drug dosage.[6,7,10] While the frequency of cardiomyopathy has ranged from 0.4 to 9 percent in all patients receiving the drug,[6] more meaningful data are obtained when considering total cumulative drug dosage. Von Hoff et al[7] have outlined the probability of developing congestive heart failure (cardiomyopathy) with varying total drug dosage, as shown in Fig. 17-1. Of 3941 retrospectively reviewed patients receiving doxorubicin, only 88 (2.2 percent) developed congestive heart failure. The risk of congestive heart failure correlated directly with total cumulative dose and increased

---

*Unless stated otherwise, a percentage change in ejection fraction shall indicate an absolute rather than a relative change (for example, a change in ejection fraction by 5 percent would represent a change from 55 to 60 percent, *not* 55 to 57.75 percent).

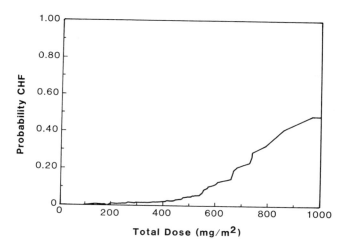

Figure 17-1 Cumulative probability of developing congestive heart failure (CHF) versus total cumulative dose of doxorubicin. (From Von Hoff et al,[7] reproduced with permission.)

to 3.5 percent of patients given 400 mg/m², 7 percent given 550 mg/m², and 15 percent given 700 mg/m². As the total dose of doxorubicin increases above 700 mg/m², the incidence of congestive heart failure continues to rise linearly. Thus, as quoted in many studies,[6,11–13] clinical congestive heart failure may occur in up to one-third of patients receiving high doses of doxorubicin. The incidence of subclinical cardiac toxicity is higher as measured by multiple invasive and noninvasive techniques.[14] This has led to the recommendation that doxorubicin therapy be empirically stopped when the total cumulative dose has reached 550 mg/m².[6] However, it is clear that patients show marked individual sensitivity to doxorubicin, with congestive heart failure occurring in some patients at doses much less than this, yet with other patients safely receiving over 1000 mg/m².[6,7,12,15] This individual variability has produced the interest in developing effective techniques to identify and monitor those patients at higher risk of developing cardiomyopathy.

SCHEDULE OF DOSE ADMINISTRATION

The schedule of drug administration also plays an important role in the development of doxorubicin cardiomyopathy.[7,9] As seen in Fig. 17-2, the incidence of congestive heart failure with cumulative drug doses greater than 550 mg/m² is less in patients receiving a smaller dose of doxorubicin on a weekly schedule (0.8 percent) compared with patients either receiving a single larger dose every 3 weeks (2.9 percent) ($p = 0.0001$) or for 3 sequential days every 3 weeks (2.4 percent) ($p = 0.06$).[7,16] Legha et al[9] compared standard doxorubicin administration every 3 weeks with prolonged infusion of drug (over 48 or 96 h) every 3 weeks and found less cardiotoxicity as measured by endomyocardial biopsy in the prolonged

continuous infusion group. Of 21 patients receiving the prolonged infusion, only two were forced to discontinue therapy because of abnormal biopsy findings. Of the 30 patients receiving standard treatment, 14 developed abnormal biopsy results precluding further drug therapy. Patients in the prolonged infusion group received a higher mean total dosage of doxorubicin (600 mg/m²) than the standard therapy group (465 mg/m²) ($p = 0.002$), and 13 patients in the prolonged infusion group were able to receive greater than 550 mg/m², as compared with only four in the standard therapy group. Only one patient, however, in the entire study developed congestive heart failure (standard therapy group, total cumulative dose, 540 mg/m²). Clinical antineoplastic activity was the same with both regimens.

Despite the promising effects of weekly administration or prolonged continuous infusion of doxorubicin in preventing cardiotoxicity, the every-3-weeks dosage schedule remains the most commonly used in clinical oncology.[17] The weekly schedule causes difficulty with overlapping myelosuppression from preceding courses, limiting its applicability.[9] The clinical significance of the prolonged infusion method in prevention of cardiotoxicity has not yet been confirmed by other studies. It is likely that the prolonged continuous infusion and other methods of doxorubicin administration may decrease cardiotoxicity due to exposure of the heart to lower peak blood levels of the drug.[6,9]

PREVIOUS CARDIOVASCULAR DISEASE

Preexisting cardiac disease (coronary, valvular, or myocardial disease or long-standing hypertension, defined as a diastolic blood pressure greater than 100 mmHg obtained at least 5 years prior to therapy) has also been

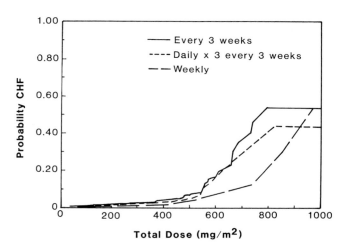

Figure 17-2 Cumulative probability of developing congestive heart failure (CHF) versus total cumulative doxorubicin dose at different dosage schedules (daily × 3 every weeks indicates administration of drug daily on 3 sequential days every 3 weeks). (From Von Hoff et al,[7] reproduced with permission.)

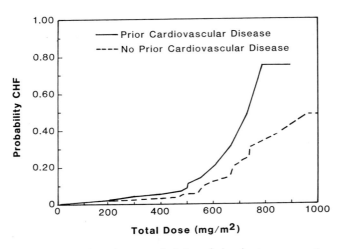

Figure 17-3 Cumulative probability of developing congestive heart failure (CHF) versus total cumulative doxorubicin dose in patients with and without prior cardiovascular disease. (From Von Hoff et al,[7] reproduced with permission.)

reported as a significant risk factor for development of doxorubicin cardiomyopathy.[7,15,18] The basis for this can be understood by considering that morphologic myocardial degeneration precedes evidence of functional abnormalities, and that once a critical level of morphologic damage is reached from any cause, myocardial function deteriorates rapidly and overt congestive heart failure occurs.[12,19,20] It is tempting to speculate that the already diseased heart requires less additional morphologic alteration in order to deteriorate functionally. However, studies examining the importance of prior cardiovascular disease as a risk factor for doxorubicin cardiotoxicity are somewhat conflicting. Von Hoff et al[7] examined this variable in their review of risk factors and found a trend toward a higher incidence of doxorubicin cardiotoxicity in those patients with underlying hypertension and/or prior cardiac disease (Fig. 17-3). However, only 475 of 3941 patients evaluated by Von Hoff et al had definite underlying hypertension and/or cardiac disease, and the trend did not reach statistical significance ($p = 0.08$). Morgan et al[15] noted that four of 11 patients with previous cardiac disease required discontinuation of doxorubicin therapy due to decreases in left ventricular ejection fraction by radionuclide ventriculography, while only two of 74 patients without previous cardiac disease required discontinuation of therapy. However, two of the four patients with cardiac disease also received concurrent chest irradiation, while none of the 74 patients without cardiac disease received this therapy.

As can be seen, the importance of underlying hypertension or preexisting cardiovascular disease is less well defined as a risk factor for doxorubicin cardiotoxicity than are other factors, such as total drug dose.[6,10] In fact, Choi et al[21] were able to administer doxorubicin safely to patients with an abnormal baseline resting left ventricular ejection fraction (less than 55 percent) by monitoring serial radionuclide ventriculograms. Of 45 patients with an abnormal baseline resting left ventricular ejection fraction (mean ejection fraction, 46 ± 6 percent; range, 30 to 54 percent), 39 had no known antecedent heart disease and 16 had received prior chest radiation therapy. Twenty-nine patients received doxorubicin and were studied serially with radionuclide ventriculograms. After a mean dose of doxorubicin of 313 ± 144 mg/m² (range, 120 to 600 mg/m²), the left ventricular ejection fraction was unchanged (47 ± 9 percent). Of 12 patients receiving at least 350 mg/m², the ejection fraction was slightly but significantly changed (48 ± 4 percent versus 43 ± 8 percent, $p < 0.05$). Only one patient developed congestive heart failure (total dose, 460 mg/m²). While these results are encouraging, it should be pointed out that these were relatively low cumulative doses of doxorubicin (at 350 mg/m², the probability of developing congestive heart failure is less than 3.5 percent)[7] in a small number of patients.

MEDIASTINAL IRRADIATION

Mediastinal radiation therapy is an important risk factor in doxorubicin cardiotoxicity.[6,10,11,15,17,20,22,23] Alexander et al,[11] using multivariate regression analysis in 55 patients receiving doxorubicin, were able to show that high-dose mediastinal radiation (6000 rad or greater) was the only independent risk factor besides total cumulative doxorubicin dose to contribute to a decline in ejection fraction measured by radionuclide ventriculography. Bristow et al[20] noted more severe abnormalities of endomyocardial biopsy specimens in patients with previous mediastinal radiation therapy who were receiving doxorubicin.

OTHER RISK FACTORS

Concurrent administration of other cytotoxic agents—cyclophosphamide in particular, but also actinomycin D, mitomycin C, and dacarbazine—has also been reported to increase the risk of developing doxorubicin cardiomyopathy.[6] However, most studies have not been able to show that concurrent therapy with cyclophosphamide or other cytotoxic agents has a significant effect on doxorubicin cardiotoxicity.[7,11,13,15,20]

Advanced age has been reported to be a risk factor for doxorubicin cardiomyopathy.[6] Von Hoff et al[7] noted a generally increasing risk with more advanced age, independent of total drug dose or schedule of administration (Fig. 17-4; $p = 0.0027$ when comparing all age groups). As noted with other risk factors, the differences do not begin to achieve significance until a total cumulative dose of approximately 500 to 600 mg/m² is administered. Bristow et al[20] noted an increased incidence of congestive heart failure in patients 70 years of age or older who were treated with doxorubicin. Alexander et al[11] were unable to show a correlation of doxorubicin cardiotoxic-

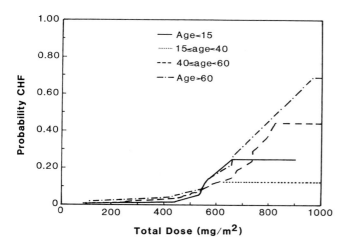

Figure 17-4 Cumulative probability of developing congestive heart failure (CHF) versus total cumulative doxorubicin dose in different age groups. (From Von Hoff et al,[7] reproduced with permission.)

ity with age but point out that their definition of advanced age was only 60 years or older, since only three patients in their series exceeded the age of 70. However, doxorubicin therapy should probably be administered more cautiously in patients who are elderly.

NATURAL HISTORY

Mortality related to congestive heart failure caused by doxorubicin has traditionally been reported to be high, on the order of approximately 50 to 60 percent.[7,20] The onset of congestive heart failure may be insidious, with sinus tachycardia as the earliest finding, or it may be abrupt, presenting as acute pulmonary edema precipitated by intravenous hydration in preparation for chemotherapy.[6,10] Typical signs and symptoms of congestive heart failure, such as dyspnea, nonproductive cough, increased jugular venous pressure, gallop rhythm, pedal edema, hepatomegaly, cardiomegaly, and pleural effusion are common.[6,7] Von Hoff et al[7] noted the onset of congestive heart failure at any time between 0 and 231 days following the last dose of doxorubicin, with a mean interval of 33 days. Cardiotoxicity proven by endomyocardial biopsy has been reported 7 years after completion of doxorubicin therapy.[24] In the 88 patients with doxorubicin-induced congestive heart failure reported by Von Hoff et al,[7] death occurred within 70 days of diagnosis of congestive heart failure in 63 patients, with heart failure felt to be responsible for 38 deaths. Twenty-five patients died secondary to tumor progression, and congestive heart failure remained unresolved but stable in 12, partially resolved in eight, and completely resolved in five.

Once cardiac dysfunction and congestive heart failure ensue, they are not always progressive.[7,11,13,20,25] Alex-

ander et al[11] noted that, in 11 of 55 patients with moderate or severe doxorubicin cardiotoxicity as measured by radionuclide ventriculography (see below), the left ventricular ejection fraction remained stable or improved slightly (+4 percent, $p < 0.005$, in the six patients with moderate toxicity) following discontinuation of doxorubicin. In the patients with severe toxicity and overt congestive heart failure, complete resolution of heart failure occurred in two patients, partial improvement in two, and death secondary to heart failure in one.

Ritchie et al[13] reported that four of eight patients with depression of ejection fraction by radionuclide ventriculography (less than 45 percent) and/or congestive heart failure improved over 2 to 6 months following discontinuation of doxorubicin therapy, often with dramatic changes in ejection fraction. Improvements in left ventricular ejection fraction from 17 to 65 percent, 37 to 61 percent, 26 to 57 percent, and 26 to 43 percent were noted. Bristow et al[20] noted progression of toxicity by endomyocardial biopsy in only one of 33 patients following cessation of doxorubicin therapy.

Schwartz et al[26] noted that 40 of 46 patients in whom clinical congestive heart failure developed as a result of doxorubicin cardiotoxicity improved significantly with standard treatment of congestive heart failure with digitalis, diuretics, and afterload-reducing agents and discontinuation of doxorubicin. Only one patient died as a result of congestive heart failure and only 14 (30 percent) of the 46 had any evidence of congestive heart failure at the time of their most recent follow-up exam after completion of therapy. No cases of worsening of congestive heart failure occurred during the follow-up period. Of the total of 1487 patients evaluated in the study, only three developed congestive heart failure late after completion of therapy. Thus, this study suggests that the natural history of clinical congestive heart failure secondary to doxorubicin cardiotoxicity is not as bad as initially thought and that most patients improve with appropriate therapy.

The long-term effects of doxorubicin on myocardial function were studied by Lipshultz et al,[27] who assessed the cardiac status of 115 children who had been treated for acute lymphoblastic leukemia with doxorubicin 1 to 15 years earlier and in whom the disease was in continuous remission. They found that 57 percent of the patients had abnormalities of left ventricular afterload (measured as end-systolic wall stress) or contractility (measured as the stress–velocity index). The cumulative dose of doxorubicin was the most significant predictor of abnormal cardiac function ($p < 0.002$). Of patients who received one dose of doxorubicin, 17 percent had slightly elevated age-adjusted afterload and none had decreased contractility. In contrast, 65 percent of patients who received at least 228 mg/m² of doxorubicin had increased afterload (59 percent of the patients), decreased contractility (23 percent), or both. Increased afterload was due to reduced ventricular wall thickness, not to hypertension or ventricular dilatation. In multivariate analysis restricted to patients who received at least 228 mg/m^2 of doxorubicin, the only significant predictive factor was a higher cumulative dose ($p = 0.01$), which predicted decreased contractility, and an age of less than 4 years at treatment ($p = 0.003$), which predicted increased afterload. Afterload increased progressively in 24 of 34 patients evaluated serially. Eleven patients had congestive heart failure within 1 year of treatment with doxorubicin; five of them had recurrent heart failure 3.7 to 10.3 years after completing doxorubicin treatment, and two required heart transplantation. No patient had late congestive heart failure as a new event. The authors hypothesized that the loss of myocytes during doxorubicin treatment in childhood might result in inadequate left ventricular mass and clinically important heart disease in later years.

HISTOLOGY

A brief discussion of the histology of doxorubicin cardiotoxicity is necessary because of the use of endomyocardial biopsy in monitoring therapy. The histologic findings are nonspecific and may be seen with other cardiomyopathies.[6] They are easily distinguishable, however, from lesions resulting from arterial occlusion or radiation therapy.[10] Focal damage, scattered throughout the heart, is initially seen, but diffuse involvement occurs as a larger cumulative dose of doxorubicin is used.[10] Myofibrillar loss and cytoplasmic vacuolization are characteristic.[22] Fibrosis is less frequent but may occur, and an inflammatory response is absent.[22] Evaluation by electron microscopy shows myocyte vacuolization and dilated mitochondria.[6] Histologic changes have been reported to occur in almost all patients treated with a cumulative doxorubicin dose of 240 mg/m^2,[22] although evidence of histologic changes has been noted with doses as low as 45 mg/m^2,[20] and severe histologic toxicity with only 100 mg/m^2.[5] Histologic evidence of cardiotoxicity may be seen within the first 24 h to several days following doxorubicin administration.[13]

While severe histologic toxicity may be seen by light microscopy, more subtle changes require electron-microscopic evaluation.[22] In fact, use of electron microscopy with light microscopy versus light microscopy alone may partially explain some of the discrepancies between studies regarding the sensitivity and value of histologic changes in monitoring doxorubicin cardiotoxicity.[28] Necropsy studies of histologic findings may report poor correlations between histologic toxicity and clinical toxicity, since electron microscopy cannot be routinely performed (specimens must be immediately preserved for electron microscopy in order to prevent postmortem artifact).[5,28–30] Most studies utilizing endomyocardial biopsy for evaluation of doxorubicin cardiotoxicity employ routine evaluation of specimens by electron microscopy.[12,16,18–20,22,28,29]

Methods for Early Detection of Doxorubicin Cardiotoxicity

To continue therapy with doxorubicin and avoid cardiotoxicity in a patient whose tumor is responding to the drug, various methods have been proposed to monitor patients and enable early detection of cardiotoxicity. Noninvasive methods such as serial physical examinations, chest x-rays, cardiac enzymes (no study has examined the usefulness of isoenzyme measurements), electrocardiograms (ECGs), M-mode echocardiograms, systolic time intervals, technetium-pyrophosphate scans, and QRS–Korotkoff measurements have been disappointing and are not felt to have sufficient predictive accuracy to justify their use for this purpose.[6,10,31–35] Until recently, radionuclide ventriculography was the only noninvasive method that had been used with good predictive accuracy in detection and monitoring of doxorubicin cardiotoxicity. In recent years, however, the role of other noninvasive techniques—including Doppler echocardiography, dobutamine echocardiography, and iodine-123 (^{123}I)–metaiodobenzylguanidine (MIBG) scintigraphy,[36–39] indium-111–labeled antimyosin antibody imaging, and magnetic resonance spectroscopy—in the detection of early doxorubicin-induced cardiotoxicity has been studied with encouraging results. Invasive methods such as endomyocardial biopsy, in conjunction with right heart catheterization, are also important in guiding doxorubicin therapy so as to avoid cardiotoxicity.[19,20,22,29,40] Radionuclide ventriculography coupled with endomyocardial biopsy has been proposed as an important method for following the condition of these patients.[12,41]

RADIONUCLIDE VENTRICULOGRAPHY

Perhaps the most widely known study using radionuclide ventriculography for this purpose was performed by Alexander and associates.[11] In this investigation, 55 patients receiving doxorubicin therapy were prospectively studied with serial first-pass radionuclide ventriculograms. Cardiotoxicity was divided into mild, moderate, or severe and defined as follows: Patients with severe toxicity developed congestive heart failure with a decrease in left ventricular ejection fraction to less than 30 percent. Moderate toxicity was defined as no congestive heart failure, with an absolute decrease in left ventricular ejection fraction by at least 15 percent to a final value of 45 percent or less. Patients with mild toxicity did not have congestive heart failure but demonstrated a 10 percent or more reduction in left ventricular ejection fraction while not fulfilling criteria of moderate toxicity. First-pass radionuclide ventriculograms were obtained several hours before a doxorubicin dose in order to avoid confusion with acute toxicity. Two to 12 studies per patient were obtained, and 23 patients had baseline radionuclide ventriculography prior to doxorubicin therapy. The 32 patients without a baseline study all had at least three radionuclide ventriculograms after initiation of doxorubicin. Normal left ventricular ejection fraction was defined as 50 percent or greater. Baseline mean left ventricular ejection fraction was similar in all four patient groups. Only three patients in this study had known antecedent heart disease, and only four had an abnormal baseline left ventricular ejection fraction.

Patients were divided into four groups, depending on total cumulative doxorubicin dose. Twenty group I patients received less than 350 mg/m^2. Eight patients received 350 to 449 mg/m^2 and made up group II. Group III patients, eight in total, received 450 to 549 mg/m^2, and 19 group IV patients received 550 mg/m^2 or more. In group I patients, no cardiotoxicity was noted, and mean left ventricular ejection fraction following doxorubicin therapy was unchanged from baseline (60 versus 61 percent, respectively). In group II patients, the mean ejection fraction following therapy was 53 percent versus a mean baseline value of 60 percent ($p < 0.01$). Group III patients had a mean decrease in left ventricular ejection fraction from 62 to 50 percent ($p < 0.01$), and group IV patients from 62 to 47 percent ($p < 0.01$). Five patients developed severe cardiotoxicity (one in group III and four in group IV) and had received cumulative doxorubicin doses ranging from 490 to 715 mg/m^2. All of these patients had moderate cardiotoxicity, as defined above, prior to developing congestive heart failure, and they had a further decrease in ejection fraction in response to continued doxorubicin. Moderate toxicity was present at a mean of 90 mg/m^2 less than the mean doxorubicin dose associated with severe toxicity. Moderate toxicity developed in six other patients, in all of whom doxorubicin was discontinued. None of these six patients developed congestive heart failure or a further decline in ejection fraction (mean follow-up, 2.5 months; range, 1 to 4 months). Mild toxicity developed in 11 patients (three in group II, four in group III, and four in group IV). Four continued therapy with doxorubicin, three died of noncardiac causes, and doxorubicin was discontinued in four. No patient with mild toxicity developed congestive heart failure (mean follow-up, 3 months; range, 2 to 5 months).

A number of conclusions were derived from this study. While there was a weak overall correlation between absolute decline in left ventricular ejection fraction and cumulative dose toxicity as measured by radionuclide ventriculography did not occur with a cumulative dose of less than 350 mg/m^2. Moderate toxicity was predictive of congestive heart failure and signaled the need to discontinue doxorubicin. Mild toxicity required only careful observation during continued doxorubicin therapy.

The Yale group has reported their experience in a larger number of patients treated with doxorubicin.[42] Of 1115 patients monitored with serial radionuclide ventriculography, 54 with baseline normal left ventricular function developed cardiotoxicity. Of these 54 patients, 33 received more than 450 mg/m^2 of doxorubicin, while 21 received smaller doses (mean dose, 309 $\pm$ 132 mg/m^2 in these 21). Only three patients developed congestive heart failure (all received 550 mg/m^2 or more) and all had evidence of moderate cardiotoxicity prior to developing heart failure.

In another report by the Yale group,[26] congestive heart failure developed in 46 (16 percent) of 282 patients at high risk for doxorubicin cardiotoxicity. These high-risk patients were defined as those that received 450 mg/m^2 or more of doxorubicin therapy, those that sustained a fall in absolute left ventricular ejection fraction by 10 percent or more to a value of 50 percent or less, or those with a baseline left ventricular ejection fraction of less than 50 percent. Patients developing congestive heart failure showed greater reductions in left ventricular ejection fraction (23 $\pm$ 14 percent) than those without congestive heart failure (12 $\pm$ 10 percent, $p < 0.001$). Of 46 patients, 40 (87 percent) showed improvement in their congestive heart failure with routine treatment and only one (2 percent) had worsening of heart failure despite treatment (this patient was also the only patient in the series whose death was attributed to the heart failure).

The Yale group has recommended the following method of monitoring patients for doxorubicin cardiotoxicity.[26] Baseline radionuclide ventriculography is obtained prior to administration of 100 mg/m^2 of doxorubicin. Each study is obtained at least 3 weeks after the last dose of drug. If the left ventricular ejection fraction is normal (greater than or equal to 50 percent), then a second study is obtained after 250 to 300 mg/m^2. If the patient has risk factors for development of doxorubicin cardiotoxicity (known cardiovascular disease, radiation therapy to the thorax, abnormal ECG, or concomitant cyclophosphamide therapy), then the next radionuclide ventriculogram is obtained after a dose of 400 mg/m^2. In the absence of these risk factors, the study is delayed until a cumulative dose of 450 mg/m^2 is reached. Subsequent studies are obtained prior to each dose. Doxorubicin is stopped if an absolute decrease in left ventricular ejection fraction of 10 percent or more occurs, associated with a drop in left ventricular ejection fraction to 50 percent or less. If the baseline left ventricular ejection fraction is 30 percent or less, doxorubicin is contraindicated. If the left ventricular ejection fraction is between 30 and 50 percent, radionuclide ventriculography is obtained prior to each dose and doxorubicin is stopped if there is a fall in absolute units by 10 percent or more or left ventricular ejection fraction falls to less than 30 percent.

In 70 high-risk patients in the course of whose treatment these guidelines were strictly adhered to, only two (2.9 percent) developed congestive heart failure, which was mild and easily treated in both. In contrast, of 212 high-risk patients for whom these recommendations were not closely followed, 44 (20.8 percent) developed congestive heart failure secondary to doxorubicin. The difference in incidence of congestive heart failure between the two groups is statistically significant ($p < 0.001$). In addition, 25 of the 44 patients in the second group had heart failure that was judged to be moderate to severe.

Using these criteria, one-third of patients with baseline left ventricular ejection fraction of less than 50 percent were able to receive high-dose therapy safely, and all patients with abnormal baseline left ventricular ejection fractions in whom the monitoring recommendations were adhered to remained free of congestive heart failure. Thus, the investigators concluded that strict adherence to these guidelines reduced both the incidence and severity of doxorubicin-induced congestive heart failure. It should be noted, however, that the efficacy of these guidelines was evaluated in high-risk patients only. As is discussed later in this section, it is not clear whether applying these guidelines to a population at low risk of developing doxorubicin cardiotoxicity will significantly reduce the incidence of congestive heart failure and be cost-effective, as the incidence of congestive heart failure is minimal regardless of monitoring.[18]

Ritchie, Singer, and colleagues, from the University of Washington, have also evaluated the use of serial radionuclide ventriculograms to monitor doxorubicin therapy.[13,43,44] Thirty-six patients from a Veterans Administration hospital population were evaluated prospectively with radionuclide ventriculograms.[13] In this study, however, patients were treated with either doxorubicin or daunorubicin, another anthracycline antibiotic chemically similar to doxorubicin and also with significant cardiotoxicity.[6] Radionuclide ventriculograms were obtained just prior to drug administration. In eight patients, additional radionuclide measurement of left ventricular ejection fraction was made at 5 min, 1 h, and 4 h following drug administration. Twelve patients were studied 24 h after drug administration. Of these, seven had repeat ejection fractions at 1 week following drug administration. The left ventricular ejection fraction obtained immediately prior to drug administration (mean, 60 ± 2 percent) did not change significantly at 5 min (62 ± 3 percent), 1 h (61 ± 2 percent), or 4 h (66 ± 2 percent) ($p > 0.05$). No single patient had an ejection fraction change of more than 10 percent. Mean ejection fraction at 24 h (60 ± 5 percent) and 1 week (64 ± 3 percent) also did not significantly differ from

baseline (63 ± 2 percent) ($p > 0.05$). Eight patients had significant depression of left ventricular ejection fraction (less than 45 percent), with total cumulative drug dosages of 280 to 600 mg/m^2 (seven patients received more than 380 mg/m^2). No patient receiving less than 280 mg/m^2 developed depression of the left ventricular ejection fraction. Congestive heart failure occurred in four patients, all of whom had depression of the left ventricular ejection fraction. Seven patients who died had necropsy examination of the heart. In this group, only the single patient with depression of the ejection fraction exhibited histologic evidence of cardiotoxicity, yet all but one of the patients had received at least 400 mg/m^2 of drug. However, histologic evaluation was limited to necropsy data only, excluding more sensitive detection of histologic toxicity by electron microscopy.[5,28] Furthermore, it may not be appropriate to extrapolate data from patients receiving daunorubicin for use in the care of patients receiving doxorubicin, since congestive heart failure secondary to daunorubicin may occur at higher total cumulative drug doses than with doxorubicin.[6,45,46] Nevertheless, the authors were able to conclude that serial radionuclide ventriculography just prior to drug administration was useful in guiding therapy, whereas ejection-fraction determinations shortly following drug therapy were not helpful or necessary.

Morgan et al[15] evaluated the use of radionuclide ventriculography to detect and monitor doxorubicin cardiotoxicity in 98 patients, with 91 receiving at least 200 mg/m^2 of the drug. The other seven patients received 100 to 200 mg/m^2 but had risk factors for doxorubicin cardiotoxicity, including cardiovascular disease and/or mediastinal radiation therapy. Of all patients, 32 had risk factors (including 11 patients who received a total cumulative dose greater than 550 mg/m^2) and 66 had no risk factors. First-pass radionuclide ventriculograms were obtained in patients prior to each doxorubicin dose except in 14 patients in whom the study was obtained prior to every second dose. Serial evaluation in 10 patients was not started until the total dose reached at least 250 mg/m^2 (all subsequently underwent at least three studies). Criteria to discontinue doxorubicin therapy included a left ventricular ejection fraction of less than 40 percent in patients with risk factors or less than 35 percent in patients without risk factors or a decrease in ejection fraction of 14 percent or more over three successive studies. Sixty-two patients exhibited no significant change in ejection fraction (defined as initial ejection fraction minus final ejection fraction of 7 percent or less), 11 showed an initial drop in ejection fraction of 8 to 14 percent but with no later change in ejection fraction, and 25 demonstrated a progressive, dose-related decline in ejection fraction. Of these last 25 patients, 14 were in the group with risk factors and 11 in the group without. Thus, 14 (43.75 percent) of 32 risk-factor patients and 11 (16.7 percent) of 66 no-risk-factor patients devel-

e declines in ejection fraction (p =
atients receiving less than 550 mg/m²
 the difference was still statistically sig-
19, chi-squared test). However, criteria
)xorubicin therapy, as outlined above,
ıny patient without risk factors, while
h risk factors required discontinuation
se eight, one received 730 mg/m², an-
, and six less than 550 mg/m² (120
If the eight patients, three developed
ıilure.

ıncluded that all patients undergoing
py should have baseline radionuclide
 long with determination of risk fac-
ı cardiotoxicity. In patients with risk
ıl baseline left ventricular ejection
nt), ejection fraction should be deter-
lose of doxorubicin. In patients with-
dionuclide ventriculography should
e each dose after a cumulative dose
ched. By using these guidelines and
 above for discontinuation of ther-
:hat doxorubicin cardiotoxicity may
ﾞnificant number of patients.

ıtriculography has also been used
characterization of left ventricular
ʲ and after doxorubicin therapy. In
 of 12 patients, Lee and associates
 fall in both rapid and slow ventric-
 following treatment with 193 ±
ıbicin.[47] Evidence of diastolic im-
 the presence of a left ventricular
ter than or equal to 55 percent.
 have been made using Doppler
hus, in patients receiving doxoru-
ırs that noninvasive evidence of
ar dysfunction may precede sys-
ʲsfunction. However, the signifi-
ıstolic left ventricular dysfunction
 treatment is currently unknown.
ıe of writing to indicate whether
;gestive of subclinical left ventric-
on have any useful role for the
eart failure or for determining
;e.

PHY

ies on the role of Doppler echo-
tection of doxorubicin-induced
ı reported by Lee et al[47] and
 showed that diastolic left ven-
ıncluding isovolumetric relax-
 filling velocities, and ratio of
ies, showed significant changes
ʲxorubicin who had preserved

left ventricular systolic function. It was suggested on the basis of these studies that monitoring of the left ventricular diastolic indexes may be useful in early detection of doxorubicin-induced cardiotoxicity. Stoddard et al,[49] in their prospective study of 26 patients, used Doppler indexes of diastolic filling to predict doxorubicin-induced systolic dysfunction. They observed that prolongation of the isovolumetric relaxation time almost always preceded reduction in systolic function. A more than 37 percent increase in isovolumetric relaxation time was 78 percent sensitive and 88 percent specific for predicting the ultimate development of doxorubicin-induced systolic dysfunction. The indexes of diastolic filling remained impaired and isovolumetric relaxation time prolonged 3 months after the last doxorubicin dose. It was concluded that doxorubicin-induced systolic dysfunction could be reliably predicted by prolongation of Doppler-derived isovolumetric relaxation time.

DOBUTAMINE ECHOCARDIOGRAPHY

Dobutamine echocardiography is a well-established technique for the diagnosis of cardiac dysfunction in patients with coronary artery disease. Klewer et al[50] applied this technique in an attempt to unmask latent left ventricular dysfunction in children and young adults previously treated with doxorubicin and compared it with normal controls. They observed that end-systolic left ventricular free-wall dimension and percent left ventricular free-wall thickening were decreased in doxorubicin-treated patients at rest compared with values in control subjects, but dobutamine infusion magnified these differences. In particular, shortening fraction and end-systolic left ventricular wall stress were abnormal only during inotropic stimulation in their asymptomatic doxorubicin-treated group. Percent left ventricular posterior wall thickening and end-systolic left ventricular wall stress appeared to be more sensitive than shortening fraction for differentiating individual doxorubicin-treated patients from control subjects during moderate inotropic stimulation with dobutamine. Prospective studies are needed to establish the utility of dobutamine echocardiography in predicting left ventricular systolic dysfunction in oncology patients.

IODINE-123–MIBG SCINTIGRAPHY

Vacuolar destruction of cardiac neurons has been reported in a rat model of doxorubicin-induced cardiotoxicity.[36] Damage to intrinsic cardiac neurons, induced by daunorubicin (a drug closely related to doxorubicin) has also been reported.[37] Doxorubicin is an anthracycline antibiotic that blocks ribonucleic acid (RNA) synthesis and also inhibits deoxyribonucleic acid (DNA) synthesis. Neurons are rich in RNA and depend on it for normal function. It is likely that cessation of RNA synthesis as a result of doxorubicin administration results in severe neuronal damage. Recently, radiolabeled MIBG, an analog of the adrenergic neurotransmitter norepinephrine (NE), has been developed. Changes in myocardial MIBG accumulation are reported to reflect cardiac adrenergic neuron integrity and function.[38,39,51] Therefore, it has been speculated that dose-dependent impairment of cardiac adrenergic neuron activity occurs in doxorubicin-induced cardiomyopathy and may be a new indicator for the detection of doxorubicin cardiomyopathy. To test this hypothesis, Wakasugi et al[52] assessed alterations in myocardial MIBG accumulation in a rat model of doxorubicin-induced cardiomyopathy. The degree of vacuolar degeneration of myocardial cells was analyzed in relation to the duration and the dose of doxorubicin. It was observed that MIBG accumulation in the myocardium decreased and its washout increased in a doxorubicin dose-dependent manner. It was concluded that the appearance of impaired cardiac adrenergic neuron activity in the presence of slight myocardial impairment (scattered or focal vacuolar degeneration) indicates that MIBG scintigraphy may be a useful method for detection of doxorubicin-induced cardiomyopathy. Valdes Olmos et al[53] reported a study in six patients in whom they could demonstrate a good correlation between decrease in left ventricular function and faster myocardial ^{123}I-MIBG washout rate. Ono and Takahashi[54] performed ^{123}I-MIBG scintigraphy in 19 patients treated with doxorubicin. Low uptake into and rapid washout from the myocardium, especially in the lateral and inferior segments, were noted in patients with cardiotoxicity and the effect was dose dependent. These abnormal areas corresponded to areas of decreased glucose metabolism observed by positron emission tomography. Left ventricular ejection fractions were normal. Hence, it was concluded that ^{123}I-MIBG scintigraphy may be a useful measure in detecting cardiotoxicity related to doxorubicin in an early stage.

INDIUM-111–ANTIMYOSIN ANTIBODY STUDIES

Indium-111–antimyosin antibody studies enable noninvasive detection of myocardial damage in vivo. This antibody binds to intracellular myosin only when sarcolemmal disruption occurs and the cell is irreversibly damaged. It has been shown that the morphologic damage in the myocytes present in doxorubicin cardiotoxicity can be detected by antimyosin scans,[55] that intensity of antimyosin uptake relates to the cumulative dose of doxorubicin,[56] and that antimyosin uptake precedes ejection-fraction deterioration.[56] Carrio et al,[57] in a recent study, compared the utility of the antimyosin scan and the MIBG scan in predicting doxorubicin cardiotoxicity at intermediate (240 to 300 mg/m^2) and maximal (420 to 500 mg/m^2) cumulative doses of doxorubicin. While both the antimyosin scan and the MIBG scan were supe-

Table 17-1   Biopsy Grading System for Doxorubicin Cardiotoxicity

Grade 0	No change from normal.
Grade 1	Minimal numbers of cells (<5% of total number of cells per block) with early change (early myofibrillar loss and/or distended sarcoplasmic reticulum).
Grade 2A (midway between 1 and 2)	Small groups of cells involved (5–15% of total number), some of which have definite change (marked myofibrillar loss and/or cytoplasmic vacuolization).
Grade 2	Groups of cells (16–25% of total number), some of which have definite change (marked myofibrillar loss and/or cytoplasmic vacuolization).
Grade 2B (midway between 2 and 3)	Groups of cells involved (26–35%), some of which have definite change (marked myofibrillar loss and/or cytoplasmic vacuolization).
Grade 3	Diffuse cell damage (>35% of total number of cells) with marked change (total loss of contractile elements, loss of organelles, and mitochondrial and nuclear degeneration).

From Bristow et al,[18] adapted with permission.

rior to radionuclide ventriculography in predicting the risk of significant functional impairment, at intermediate cumulative doses the antimyosin scan was superior to the MIBG scan in this study. The authors found that patients with more intense antimyosin uptake present at intermediate doxorubicin doses tended to be those with more severe functional impairment at maximal cumulative doses.

ENDOMYOCARDIAL BIOPSY

Endomyocardial biopsy has also been reported as a sensitive and specific method for detecting and monitoring doxorubicin cardiotoxicity.[6,10] Histologic changes are graded according to the scale in Table 17-1. Both light and electron microscopy are used, and histologic toxicity is based on the prevalence and severity of myocardial cellular damage.[18] Bristow et al[20] reported endomyocardial biopsy findings in 33 patients receiving doxorubicin therapy (mean cumulative dose, 368 mg/m^2; range, 45 to 545 mg/m^2). Seven patients also had repeat biopsies. Right heart catheterization for hemodynamic measurement was performed at the time of biopsy in 38 of 40 instances.

In 34 of the 39 biopsy samples obtained following doxorubicin therapy, histologic changes of toxicity were present. When cumulative doses greater than 240 mg/m^2 were considered, histologic changes were seen in 27 of 29 patients. Histologic changes were seen in one patient with a total dose of only 45 mg/m^2, whereas one patient with a cumulative dose of 400 mg/m^2 had a normal biopsy. The lowest dose with severe histologic changes (grade 3) was 272 mg/m^2. Seven patients in

(21 percent) developed congestive heart fail... ...umented by cardiac catheterization): five developed heart failure during therapy, while one patient developed heart failure 1 week after discontinuation of doxorubicin and a second patient developed heart failure 23 months after doxorubicin therapy. Five of the seven patients showed severe histologic changes (grade 3) on biopsy and a significantly greater degree of myocyte damage when compared with dose-matched controls. Congestive heart failure occurred at doses of 330 to 545 mg/m^2. In 14 patients approaching standard dose limitation (550 mg/m^2 cumulative dose) and in whom continued doxorubicin therapy was indicated, the authors used endomyocardial biopsy and right heart catheterization to determine whether further doxorubicin could safely be given. Seven patients had the drug discontinued; of these, one developed congestive heart failure a week later and ultimately died of this. Seven patients safely continued therapy without developing heart failure.

Bristow et al[18] have been able to predict the occurrence of congestive heart failure in patients receiving doxorubicin therapy by using a combination of biopsy score and catheterization score to stratify risk. The biopsy grading system in Table 17-1 is used to assess histologic toxicity. Catheterization score is as listed in Table 17-2 and incorporates both resting and exercise hemodynamics. Patients are then categorized as to the risk of developing congestive heart failure at the time of study or within an additional 100 mg/m^2 dose limit, as noted in Table 17-3. The risk subsets in Table 17-3 are based on biopsy and hemodynamic data and not on clinical risk factors. Of 35 no-risk or low-risk subset patients prospectively studied, none developed congestive heart failure as therapy with doxorubicin continued. Eight of 33 moderate-risk and high-risk subset patients, however, developed congestive heart failure (only one received further doxorubicin) when prospectively evaluated following study.

Limitations of endomyocardial biopsy   Critics of the use of endomyocardial biopsy for monitoring doxorubicin cardiotoxicity point out that other studies that examine the relationship of histologic changes with clinical cardiotoxicity have not demonstrated the correlation to be very good.[5,30] Isner et al[5] retrospectively reviewed necropsy findings from 64 patients who received either doxorubicin or daunorubicin. Total drug dosages ranged from 85 to 900 mg/m^2. Of 20 patients with documented clinical cardiotoxicity (defined as impaired left ventricular systolic performance as assessed by hemodynamic, echocardiographic, or clinical parameters), seven (35 percent) showed no histologic evidence of toxicity. Of 44 patients without clinical evidence of cardiotoxicity, 23 had histologic toxicity (mild in 15 and severe in four). The authors thus reported a sensitivity of histologic toxicity of 65 percent, a specificity of histologic toxicity of

48 percent, and a predictive accuracy of histologic toxicity of only 36 percent. The authors concluded that this predictive accuracy was not significantly different from random variation in toxicity and that endomyocardial biopsy was an unreliable method for the detection of doxorubicin cardiotoxicity. It should be pointed out,

Table 17-2   Catheterization Grading System[a]

Grade	Abnormality
0	Normal (not meeting criteria for grade 1–3 abnormality).
1	Mild abnormality, any of the following: (a) Hemodynamics at rest: Right ventricular end-diastolic pressure (RVEDP) > 8 but < 12 mmHg or mean right atrial pressure ($\overline{RA}$) > 7 but < 10 mmHg, left ventricular end-diastolic pressure (LVEDP) ≥ 12 but ≤ 15 mmHg or mean pulmonary wedge pressure ($\overline{PW}$) > 10 but < 15 mmHg, cardiac index (CI) < 2.5 but ≥ 2.2 liters/min/m^2 with A-V O$_2$ difference > 5 vol%. (b) Exercise hemodynamics: RVEDP > 5 but < 9 mmHg above pressure at rest, PW > 5 but < 11 mmHg above pressure at rest, exercise factor (change in cardiac output ÷ change in O$_2$ consumption) ≥ 4 but < 6.
2	Moderate abnormality, any of the following: (a) Two or more of the above. (b) Pressure at rest: $\overline{PW}$ ≥ 15 but < 20 mmHg, LVEDP ≥ 15 but < 20 mmHg, RVEDP ≥ 12 but < 17 mmHg or RA > 10 but ≤ 15, CI < 2.2 but ≥ 1.8 with A-V O$_2$ difference > 5 vol%. (c) Exercise hemodynamics: RVEDP ≥ 9 mmHg above pressure at rest, $\overline{PW}$ ≥ 10 mmHg above pressure at rest, exercise factor < 4.
3	Severe abnormality, any of the following: (a) Two or more moderate abnormalities. (b) Hemodynamics at rest: $\overline{PW}$ or LVEDP ≥ 20 mmHg, RVEDP ≥ 18 or RA ≥ 16 mmHg, CI < 1.8 liters/min/m^2 with A-V O$_2$ difference > 5 vol%.

[a] Hemodynamic grading system based on right heart catheterization for doxorubicin cardiotoxicity.
From Bristow et al,[18] reproduced with permission.

Table 17-3   Risk Subsets in Patients Receiving Doxorubicin (Probability of Developing Overt Heart Failure in Next 100 mg/m^2)

Risk	Biopsy Score	Catheter-ization Score	Actual No. Developing CHF Within 100 mg/m^{2a}
No	≤ 2A	< 1	0/42
Low (< 10%)	2	≤ 1	1/31
	≤ 2A	2	
Moderate (10–25%)	2	2	2/16
	2B	≤ 1	
	2B	2	
	3	—	
High (> 25%)	≥ 1	3	14/31

[a] Total number of patients with symptomatic congestive heart failure (CHF) at the time of study or within 10 mg/m^2 additional time limit, over total number of patients studied.
From Bristow et al,[18] reproduced with permission.

however, that the study by Isner et al[5] reported only light-microscopy findings, since evaluation was limited to necropsy. Furthermore, it is important to note that Bristow and colleagues have not advocated endomyocardial biopsy *alone* to assess doxorubicin cardiotoxicity but use this technique in conjunction with other invasive and noninvasive techniques.[20] Nevertheless, in another paper by Bristow et al,[19] four of 50 patients with biopsy scores of only 1 showed moderate or severe hemodynamic abnormalities at right heart catheterization. Interestingly, one of these patients had received mediastinal radiation therapy, and the authors point out a potential problem in evaluating histologic toxicity in patients receiving this form of treatment. The technique of giving mediastinal irradiation at their institution involves delivery of approximately 3000 rad to the right ventricle but only 1500 rad to the left ventricle. Since endomyocardial biopsy specimens are obtained from the right ventricle, potentiation of histologic changes of doxorubicin cardiotoxicity by radiation therapy may be greater than functional changes of cardiac performance, since measured functional changes are primarily related to the left ventricle. Although the authors state that this disparity must be considered in using endomyocardial biopsy for dose limitation of doxorubicin therapy, no specific guidelines have been established.

It has also been suggested that endomyocardial biopsy specimens may not represent the histology of the heart as a whole.[6] However, samples are routinely obtained from different sites at the time of biopsy and have shown excellent correlation of histologic findings when compared with each other.[19]

Finally, it is important to consider the expense and the complication rate of endomyocardial biopsy. Bristow and associates routinely perform endomyocardial biopsy and right heart catheterization as an outpatient procedure in most patients.[12,20] Complications of endomyocardial biopsy include arrhythmias and myocardial perforation.[58] The risk is low in experienced hands, however, and the complication rate is less than that of routine cardiac catheterization.[58] The incidence of complications in over 4000 patients undergoing endomyocardial biopsy at Stanford University was less than 1 percent.[58] Only four patients developed cardiac tamponade and none required thoracotomy. Four patients developed arrhythmias (atrial fibrillation in three and sustained ventricular arrhythmias in one) as a result of the procedure.

USE OF RADIONUCLIDE VENTRICULOGRAPHY WITH ENDOMYOCARDIAL BIOPSY

Radionuclide ventriculography has also been used in conjunction with endomyocardial biopsy in order to assess doxorubicin cardiotoxicity.[12,41] Druck et al[41] studied 33 patients receiving doxorubicin therapy (total doses ranging from 144 to 954 mg/m²; mean, 452 mg/m²) with 27 patients having both radionuclide ventriculograms and endomyocardial biopsies. In this report, nine patients with abnormal biopsy findings had normal radionuclide ventriculograms. Eighteen patients, all of whom also had abnormal biopsy findings, had abnormal radionuclide ventriculograms. Of these 18 patients, five are included with normal resting studies but an abnormal ejection-fraction response to exercise. Significant abnormalities on endomyocardial biopsy were noted in all patients with a resting left ventricular ejection fraction of 45 percent or less. These authors concluded that radionuclide ventriculography correlated well with endomyocardial biopsy results and allowed radionuclide ventriculography to be reliably used in detecting early doxorubicin cardiotoxicity and in management of further therapy. The authors stated that exercise radionuclide ventriculography is indicated when the rest study is normal but not when the rest ejection fraction is abnormal. It was also felt that doxorubicin therapy should be stopped in any patient with a resting left ventricular ejection fraction of less than 45 percent, exclusive of other cardiac disease. Finally, it was pointed out that endomyocardial biopsy was useful in separating doxorubicin cardiotoxicity from other possible causes of abnormal radionuclide ventriculograms. However, these conclusions are based on retrospective data analysis; results of prospective evaluation using these criteria are not available. In addition, the method of biopsy grading and level of exercise were not described in this report.

McKillop et al,[12] from Stanford University, have also reported the use of radionuclide ventriculography in conjunction with endomyocardial biopsy to assess doxorubicin cardiotoxicity. Thirty-seven patients already receiving doxorubicin therapy underwent study including rest and exercise gated radionuclide ventriculography, endomyocardial biopsy, and right heart catheterization. Cumulative doxorubicin dose ranged from 100 to 636 mg/m² at the time of study (mean dose, 412 mg/m²). Five patients underwent two sets of studies, and in five patients exercise studies could not be performed (three with abnormal and two with normal resting left ventricular ejection fractions). A normal resting left ventricular ejection fraction was defined as greater than 45 percent. Failure to increase the left ventricular ejection fraction by 5 percent or more from the resting value during maximum exercise was considered an abnormal exercise response. Histologic changes on endomyocardial biopsy specimens were graded according to criteria listed in Table 17-1, and catheterization scores assigned were based on criteria listed in Table 17-2. Patients were stratified into no-, low-, moderate-, or high-risk subsets for development of congestive heart failure, as outlined in Table 17-3, for data analysis. The authors observed that in 19 patients at moderate or high risk of congestive heart failure, only 10 had an abnormal resting left ventricular ejection fraction (seven of 12 in the high-risk group only).

Abnormal resting left ventricular ejection fraction was noted in one of seven no-risk patients and four of 13 low-risk patients. Thus, an abnormal resting left ventricular ejection fraction had only a 53 percent sensitivity and 75 percent specificity for detecting patients at moderate or high risk of developing congestive heart failure secondary to doxorubicin, using biopsy and hemodynamic findings as a "gold standard." The corresponding sensitivity of the resting radionuclide ventriculogram for predicting the occurrence of clinical heart failure was not established. The authors concluded that a single resting radionuclide ventriculogram lacked sufficient sensitivity as a screening technique to detect patients at risk of developing congestive heart failure upon further treatment with doxorubicin.

Addition of an exercise radionuclide ventriculogram correctly detected seven of nine moderate-risk or high-risk patients with a normal resting study but also yielded seven false-positive studies (no-risk or low-risk patients). Thus, sensitivity increased markedly (to 89 percent), but specificity dropped sharply (to 41 percent). Sensitivity in high-risk patients increased to 100 percent. The two false-negative studies in patients with moderate or high risk of congestive heart failure correlated with normal hemodynamics at catheterization but moderate risk by biopsy. Of the 13 false-positive resting and exercise radionuclide ventriculograms, 12 occurred in patients without identifiable heart disease. It was speculated that the decrease in specificity of the exercise study resulted from the detection of minor nonspecific abnormalities not immediately related to the risk of developing cardiotoxicity in these patients with false-positive results.

A previous study by these authors addressed the issue of cost-benefit considerations in monitoring patients for doxorubicin cardiotoxicity.[18] In this study, patients were divided into those with risk factors (previous mediastinal irradiation, previous heart disease and/or long-standing hypertension, age greater than 70 years, and total dose of doxorubicin 550 mg/m² or more) and those without risk factors as well as those monitored for cardiotoxicity (the majority by endomyocardial biopsy and right heart catheterization) and those not monitored. Results are as noted in Table 17-4. As can be seen, the incidence of congestive heart failure was negligible in patients without risk factors regardless of the presence or absence of cardiac monitoring. In patients with risk factors, the incidence of congestive heart failure and resultant mortality was higher than in nonmonitored patients, although the difference did not achieve statistical significance. Nevertheless, the authors felt that this trend would have become statistically significant if the size of the patient sample had been larger. It is important to note that symptoms of congestive heart failure, as assessed by the New York Heart Association class, were less in monitored than in unmonitored risk-factor patients ($p = 0.034$).

Based on the observations of the above studies, these investigators from Stanford University have suggested the following guidelines in monitoring patients for doxorubicin cardiotoxicity.[12] Patients without risk factors should be treated until an empiric dose limit is attained (the authors suggest 450 mg/m²). If further doxorubicin therapy is contemplated, rest and exercise radionuclide ventriculograms are then obtained. If the exercise left ventricular ejection fraction response is normal, this test is serially repeated after each 100 mg/m² of additional doxorubicin (or every other dose). If the exercise study is abnormal but the resting ejection fraction is normal, a resting radionuclide ventriculogram is obtained after each 50 to 60 mg/m² of doxorubicin. If both the initial resting and exercise radionuclide ventriculograms are abnormal at 450 mg/m² and a baseline value is not available, endomyocardial biopsy and right heart catheterization are performed. These invasive studies are also performed if the subsequent studies show deterioration of resting or exercise ejection fractions (decline of resting value by 10 percent or exercise ejection-fraction response converting from normal to abnormal).

In patients with risk factors for development of doxorubicin cardiotoxicity, resting and exercise radionuclide ventriculograms are obtained prior to receipt of the third dose of doxorubicin. If the exercise ejection-fraction response is normal, this is followed serially after each additional 100 mg/m² of drug. If results of the exercise test are abnormal, resting ejection fraction is followed serially after each 100 mg/m² dose until a total dose of 350 mg/m² is achieved, after which the test is repeated after each additional 50 mg/m². Endomyocardial biopsy and right heart catheterization are not performed in patients with risk factors if the initial resting and exercise radionuclide ventriculograms are abnormal, but they are performed if deterioration in either occurs (as noted above). Doxorubicin is stopped if the endomyocardial biopsy and the right heart catheterization show that the patient is at moderate or high risk as listed in Table 17-3. By using this method of following serial resting and exercise radionuclide ventriculograms, few false negatives will be encountered and prior baseline studies are not necessary, since the test is so sensitive. Because of the limited specificity of the radionuclide test in this setting, endomyocardial biopsy and right heart catheterization are used to verify the presence of increased risk of cardiotoxicity, since at least half of patients with abnormal radionuclide test results can safely receive at least 100 mg/m² of additional doxorubicin, guided by endomyocardial biopsy and hemodynamic data.

Although the authors note that a single resting radionuclide ventriculogram lacks the sensitivity to be used as a screening test, it should be noted that this may not apply to the test when followed serially.[11,18] It should also be pointed out that exercise studies may frequently not be feasible in patients receiving doxorubicin, since

Table 17-4 Efficacy of Monitoring Patients for Doxorubicin Cardiotoxicity

Group	Number Responding to DXR	Number Developing CHF	CHF Incidence	Number Dead of CHF
I. All patients				
No monitoring	126	12	0.10	6
Monitored	80	3	0.04	0
II. No risk factors				
No monitoring	68	2	0.03	1
Monitored	31	0	0.00	0
III. Risk factors				
No monitoring	58	10	0.17	5
Monitored	49	3	0.06	0

Probability for CHF (Fisher exact, two-tailed): group IA vs. IB, $p = 0.14$; group IIIA vs. IIIB, $p = 0.107$.
Probability for mortality incidence (Fisher exact, two-tailed): group IA vs. IB, $p = 0.102$; group IIIA vs. IIIB, $p = 0.087$.
DXR, doxorubicin; CHF, congestive heart failure.
From Bristow et al,[18] reproduced with permission.

these patients are often debilitated and quite ill. Also, the addition of the exercise study might simply make the radionuclide test too sensitive, necessitating invasive procedures in these patients, half of whom do not have important cardiotoxicity. Furthermore, many institutions do not have pathologists experienced in interpreting results of endomyocardial biopsy or personnel with the capability of performing this procedure with an acceptably low morbidity. Therefore, the availability of this method of monitoring patients is limited.

Cost must also be considered. Since no study has shown that regional wall-motion abnormalities or other parameters measured by radionuclide ventriculography (such as absolute left ventricular volumes) add additional information to the left ventricular ejection fraction alone in serial monitoring of patients treated with doxorubicin, a limited radionuclide ventriculogram using one or two views only with measurement of left ventricular ejection fraction, or measurement of ejection fraction with a non-imaging probe,[59] should be considered to minimize cost. While it is difficult to compare costs of one regimen with another for monitoring doxorubicin therapy because of the individual variability with which patients respond to doxorubicin and the variation in test costs from one institution to another, addition of the costs of exercise testing and invasive studies is significant. Furthermore, once rest and exercise radionuclide ventriculograms become abnormal in the Stanford regimen but endomyocardial biopsy and right heart catheterization demonstrate safety in administering an additional 100 mg/m² of doxorubicin (seen in 50 percent of patients because of the low specificity of rest and exercise radionuclide ventriculography), these invasive studies must again be repeated in order to administer therapy safely beyond the additional 100 mg/m², further increasing the cost.

The method outlined by Bristow et al[18] may be particularly useful in the patient who has already received a significant dose of doxorubicin (450 mg/m² or more) and in whom a baseline measurement of left ventricular function is not available. Furthermore, the method may also be particularly helpful in patients with underlying heart disease or where other factors may confound the use of serial measurements of the left ventricular ejection fraction (e.g., large variations in hematocrit or in intravascular volume).

Summary

Much controversy exists in the literature regarding the use of various techniques for early detection and monitoring of doxorubicin cardiotoxicity. However, a number of important conclusions can be drawn from the studies reviewed.

From a cost–benefit standpoint, it is simply not reasonable at present to monitor routinely all patients receiving doxorubicin for evidence of cardiotoxicity, as the overall incidence of congestive heart failure is low and only a small subgroup of patients will benefit from monitoring. However, it would be unfortunate to stop therapy empirically at a dose of 550 mg/m² or lower in the patient who is responding well to doxorubicin and has no evidence of clinical cardiotoxicity. While no technique of monitoring cardiotoxicity is perfect, the methods proposed by the Yale group[26] and by the investigators at Stanford University[12] appear to be clinically sound and suggest that many patients can be safely treated with doxorubicin at doses greater than 550 mg/m². The method using serial resting radionuclide ventriculograms[26] has virtually no morbidity, relatively low cost, and acceptable sensitivity and specificity for following patients at high risk of cardiac toxicity. The invasive method outlined by the Stanford group[12] is more precise but has the disadvantages of greater expense and some potential morbidity.

The following guidelines are proposed for monitoring patients for doxorubicin cardiotoxicity. All patients should be assessed for the presence of risk factors predisposing them to doxorubicin cardiotoxicity. These should include prior or concurrent mediastinal radiation therapy, underlying cardiovascular disease (including long-standing hypertension), and age 70 years or greater. In general, only patients with risk factors or those expected to receive high-dose therapy (more than 550 mg/m²) need be monitored. In patients without risk factors, the likelihood of receiving more than 550 mg/m² can usually be assessed early in the course of treatment. Since most regimens employ doses of 50 to 70 mg/m² of doxorubicin every 3 to 4 weeks,[17] a decision regarding institution of monitoring can generally be made prior to a total dose of 250 to 350 mg/m², since a switch to another chemotherapy agent would generally be made if the patient is not responding by this time. Thus, a baseline radionuclide ventriculogram could be obtained after the third dose of drug in a low-risk patient who is responding to treatment and likely to benefit from high doses of doxorubicin (such as a patient with small cell carcinoma of the lung[60]). Patients showing an unexpectedly favorable response to treatment where the tumor response to therapy was unpredictable prior to starting doxorubicin and where high-dose therapy might continue would also fall into this category. The occasional patient who is not likely to survive continued therapy but continues to receive doxorubicin for palliation or other reasons would not be a candidate for monitoring. In the patient without risk factors where high-dose therapy is likely, repeat radionuclide ventriculography would be obtained at 450 mg/m² and then prior to each successive dose. Doxorubicin would be discontinued if the current Yale criteria were met.[26]

In patients with risk factors (excluding prior receipt of 550 mg/m² of doxorubicin), a baseline radionuclide ventriculogram should be obtained prior to starting doxorubicin therapy. If the left ventricular ejection fraction is greater than 50 percent, a repeat study should be obtained after reaching a total of 250 to 350 mg/m² of drug and then prior to each additional doxorubicin dose. Doxorubicin is discontinued if the left ventricular ejection fraction declines by 10 percent or more to a value of 50 percent or less. If the baseline ejection fraction is less than 30 percent, doxorubicin should not be given. It may be preferable to use the endomyocardial biopsy method, as outlined by the Stanford group,[12] for patients with a baseline left ventricular ejection fraction of less than 50 percent. If desired, however, serial radionuclide ventriculography alone can be utilized, employing the Yale method.[26] In this group of patients, radionuclide ventriculograms should be obtained prior to each dose of doxorubicin. Doxorubicin is discontinued if the left ventricular ejection fraction falls to less than 30 percent or decreases by an absolute value of 10 percent or more.

The method of monitoring cardiotoxicity outlined by the Stanford group[12] appears advantageous in the following circumstances. Patients who have already received a significant dose of doxorubicin (450 mg/m² without baseline cardiac evaluation or patients receiving at least 350 mg/m² remotely) should have resting and exercise radionuclide ventriculography and be followed in the manner previously outlined by these authors.[12] Patients with extreme fluctuations in left ventricular ejection fraction, but not meeting definite criteria for discontinuation by the Yale group,[26] should also undergo exercise radionuclide ventriculography; if the results are abnormal, endomyocardial biopsy and right heart catheterization should be performed, since this method determines cardiotoxicity more precisely. Patients who have symptoms of congestive heart failure but for whom the diagnosis of congestive heart failure is uncertain—particularly if the resting left ventricular ejection fraction is abnormal but definite criteria for discontinuation of doxorubicin are not met—should have endomyocardial biopsy and right heart catheterization. As previously noted, patients with baseline left ventricular ejection fractions below 40 percent are also probably best monitored by endomyocardial biopsy and hemodynamic measurement. Finally, patients meeting criteria for discontinuation of doxorubicin, as outlined by the Yale group,[26] but in whom continued therapy with doxorubicin is deemed imperative, should have endomyocardial biopsy and right heart catheterization. In all of these patients, criteria for discontinuation of doxorubicin therapy are based on biopsy and catheterization data (moderate-risk or high-risk patients in Table 17-3). In addition, if exercise radionuclide ventriculography is indicated but the patient is unable to exercise adequately, endomyocardial biopsy and right heart catheterization are performed.

These guidelines should enable clinicians to guide doxorubicin therapy safely and in a rational and cost-effective manner. It is realized that an occasional patient may not fit well into these categories and, as in all of clinical medicine, sound clinical judgment alone will best determine the risks and benefits of continuing therapy.

Future Developments

Although it is possible to reduce the incidence of severe cardiomyopathy by careful monitoring, some cardiac damage remains inevitable for patients receiving anthracyclines. Since cardiotoxicity appears to be mediated by a different mechanism than the antitumor effect,[61] there has been a continuing search both for less cardiotoxic anthracyclines and for agents that might be given concurrently to block cardiotoxicity. So far, there has been little success with the former approach, but some blocking agents have shown promise. Although the use of antioxidant agents has proved disappointing, the bispiperazindione compound known as ICRF-187 seems to offer more hope.[62] ICRF-187 appears to prevent the formation of intramyocardial iron ions by chelation of anthracycline without interfering with antimitotic activity elsewhere. Significant cardioprotection has been demonstrated in animal models,[63] adult studies,[64,65] and more recently in a small number of children.[66]

There is increasing interest in the role of afterload-reducing agents, both for the support of the failing ventricle and in preservation of residual myocardial function. Many clinicians are now considering the use of angiotensin-converting enzyme inhibitors in patients who have previously received anthracyclines, although as yet few data are available from clinical trials.[67] Again, careful assessment of left ventricular function both before institution of therapy and once treatment is established will be crucial. Measurement of diastolic as well as systolic function may be particularly relevant here to detect patients with more restrictive and noncompliant ventricles, in whom vasodilatation may be detrimental.[68,69]

THERAPY OF CONGESTIVE HEART FAILURE: EVALUATION BY RADIONUCLIDE VENTRICULOGRAPHY

Evaluation of the response of the failing left ventricle to drug interventions is difficult. Ventricular performance is influenced by multiple factors—including the contractile state of the ventricle, heart rate, preload, and afterload[70]—and mechanisms of action of pharmacologic agents are frequently complex, affecting more than one variable.[3] For these reasons, multiple techniques are often necessary to demonstrate a response to drug intervention. Radionuclide ventriculography is one technique that has been employed to measure this response.[70] However, measurement of the left ventricular ejection fraction alone has limitations in the evaluation of patients with severe congestive heart failure.[70-74] Addition of other parameters measured by radionuclide ventriculography, such as left ventricular volumes, stroke volume, cardiac output, and exercise ejection-fraction response, has been proposed to improve the usefulness of the technique in evaluating therapy of congestive heart failure.[75-77] However, limitations still exist.[74]

While there are conflicting data in the literature concerning the value of radionuclide ventriculography in the assessment of the therapy of congestive heart failure, the clinical response of an individual patient to a drug remains the most important goal to the clinician and investigator in determining the usefulness of any given therapy for congestive heart failure or any other condition. However, addition of radionuclide modalities, as well as other invasive and noninvasive techniques, may add important information as to the mechanisms involved and the quantitation of the actual response to

therapy, particularly when large groups of patients are studied.[2,3,70,72]

Limitations of Ejection Fraction Measurement

Simple measurement of the radionuclide left ventricular ejection fraction alone is an insensitive determinant of the response of the severely dilated and depressed left ventricle to a drug intervention in an individual patient.[70-74] As stated earlier, at least a 5 percent absolute change in left ventricular ejection fraction is required in order to attribute the response to a nonrandom physiologic alteration.[2] However, a relatively large change in stroke volume of the severely dilated and depressed left ventricle must occur before a significant (more than 5 percent) absolute change in left ventricular ejection fraction occurs.[72,74] For example, in a patient with a left ventricular end-diastolic volume of 300 ml and left ventricular ejection fraction of 15 percent, a 33 percent improvement in stroke volume resulting from vasodilator therapy would increase stroke volume from 45 to 60 ml. In this patient, measured ejection fraction would increase from 15 to only 20 percent, a barely significant change.[72] If end-diastolic volume were 400 ml and ejection fraction 15 percent, the same 15-ml increase in stroke volume would change the value from 60 to 75 ml, with ejection fraction increasing from 15 to only 18.75 percent, a change that could not be definitely attributed to the drug intervention.[2] Thus, the improvement in left ventricular function may be obscured by the small but expected serial variability in radionuclide ejection-fraction measurements in the patient with a massively increased end-diastolic volume.[72,74]

Other factors probably also contribute to the limitations of radionuclide ejection-fraction measurement in the evaluation of the heart failure patient. Mitral regurgitation, frequently present in these patients, results in a total stroke volume, as measured by radionuclide ventriculography, that exceeds actual forward stroke volume.[74] While forward stroke volume may be increased by a vasodilator agent, total stroke volume may show relatively less improvement because of the reduction of regurgitant fraction.[72,74] Also, changes in heart rate related to drug intervention may substantially alter the regurgitant fraction. These various changes in total stroke volume, forward stroke volume, and regurgitant fraction may produce a variable response of the ejection fraction to a drug intervention. In addition, differential effects of a vasodilator drug on mitral regurgitation may play a role. While an agent that predominantly reduces left ventricular afterload may result in improved ejection-fraction measurements, concomitant preload reduction may decrease mitral valve orifice area and eliminate the low impedance outlet of mitral regurgitation, resulting in reduction of measured global ejection fraction.[74] Direct alteration of left ventricular compliance by a drug with additional vasodilator actions may also alter ventricular filling, resulting in ambiguous ejection-fraction changes.[72,74]

Specific Studies Examining Ejection-Fraction Measurements in Response to Drug Therapy

Specific studies examining the left ventricular ejection-fraction responses to specific drug interventions are detailed in Table 17-5. Most of the studies have shown an improvement in mean left ventricular ejection fraction following therapy. However, left ventricular ejection-fraction responses varied substantially among individual patients, and improvement in ejection fraction, when noted, was frequently not of demonstrable physiologic significance. When compared with hemodynamic changes, radionuclide ejection-fraction responses have correlated poorly with clinical improvement in patients following drug therapy. In the study by Goldberg et al,[72] patients responding to hydralazine as demonstrated by invasive hemodynamic measurement could not be separated from those not responding on the basis of the change in radionuclide ejection fraction after drug administration, either at rest or during exercise. In this study, there were no statistically significant correlations between changes in ejection fraction and changes in invasively measured hemodynamic variables following hydralazine therapy. The authors concluded that ejection-fraction response to hydralazine could not accurately be used to predict the hemodynamic response to drug therapy in severe congestive heart failure. Other authors have also reported poor correlations between radionuclide ejection-fraction responses and both clinical and hemodynamic improvement with pharmacologic treatment of congestive heart failure.[85,86] Haq et al[73] specifically compared noninvasive techniques, including radionuclide ejection fraction, with hemodynamic responses to various vasodilator agents and combinations in patients with congestive heart failure. These investigators concluded that radionuclide ventriculography was of little value in predicting the hemodynamic response to a drug in an individual patient with a left ventricular ejection fraction of 30 percent or less.

Value of Ventricular Volumes and Cardiac Output Determined by Radionuclide Ventriculography in Assessing Drug Response

Because of the limitations of the radionuclide left ventricular ejection fraction in assessing response to drug intervention in patients with congestive heart failure, radionuclide measurements of ventricular volumes, stroke volume, and cardiac output have been advocated in order to improve the value of radionuclide ventriculography

for this purpose.[75,76,87] Determination of left ventricular volumes from gated radionuclide ventriculograms has been well described, and values have shown an excellent correlation with those measured by contrast ventriculography.[88,89] Direct measurement of cardiac output by radionuclide ventriculography can be accomplished by determination of left ventricular end-diastolic volume and subsequent determination of stroke volume by multiplying left ventricular ejection fraction by left ventricular end-diastolic volume; cardiac output is equal to calculated stroke volume × heart rate.[90] Scintigraphic cardiac output and stroke volume measurements have been shown to have an excellent correlation with thermodilution values in patients without intracardiac shunts or valvular regurgitation.[90]

A technically less demanding approach to the measurement of drug-induced changes in ventricular volumes and cardiac output involves the determination of relative ventricular volumes. Following correction for background activity, left ventricular counts are proportional to left ventricular volumes. Changes in background-corrected stroke counts (end-diastolic counts minus end-systolic counts) are proportional to changes in stroke volume. Further, changes in background-corrected stroke counts times heart rate are proportional to changes in cardiac output.[76] Use of this technique, however, does not allow for comparison of data between different subjects, owing to differences for each subject of attenuation, scatter, radioisotope dosage, and timing of study. While count–volume relationships are linear for a given subject, counts represent relative rather than absolute manifestations of volume change and changes are most accurately graded as a percentage change from baseline. When this technique was compared with a percentage change from baseline of Fick cardiac outputs in normal subjects, correlations were excellent.[76]

Although reduction in left ventricular volume in the patient with congestive heart failure may indicate a beneficial effect of drug intervention, it does not necessarily indicate the mechanism of action of the drug.[3] In addition, while this may be of value in documenting drug response in a group of patients, it is probably of less practical value to the clinician in treating an individual patient than is a measured change in ejection fraction or cardiac output. Perhaps the most important benefit of measuring changes in left ventricular volume in patients with congestive heart failure lies in the ability to measure changes in cardiac output by utilizing this technique.

Specific Studies Evaluating Left Ventricular Volume and Cardiac Output Responses to Drug Intervention

Specific studies examining the value of radionuclide ventricular volume and cardiac output measurements to as-

Table 17-5 Specific Studies Examining Ejection-Fraction Measurements in Response to Drug Therapy

Reference	Drug	Radionuclide Parameters	Patients Studied	Findings and Conclusions
Colucci et al[78]	Prazosin (up to 24 mg/day) vs. placebo; oral	Resting LVEF	22 patients with severe CHF → 10 treated with prazosin (baseline mean LVEF, 24.8 ± 2.2%). Similar baseline LVEF in placebo group.	LVEF improved after 2 months of prazosin to 32.1 ± 2.9%[b] (5% absolute change in 3 patients). LVEF fell to pretreatment levels 48 h after prazosin withdrawal in 6 patients; returned to long-term treatment levels after a single dose. One patient in placebo group improved LVEF from 13 to 18% after switched to prazosin but remained in severe CHF. Prazosin patients improved treadmill exercise duration and functional class. Clinical evidence of attenuation after 2 months, although still improved over baseline.
Rude et al[3]	Amrinone, pirbuterol, prazosin, all oral	Resting LVEF	34 patients with refractory CHF; 1–2 days of therapy.	9 patients treated with amrinone → LVEF improved from 20 ± 3% to 31 ± 5%;[b] 12 patients treated with pirbuterol → LVEF improved from 20 ± 3% to 26 ± 4%;[b] 13 patients treated with prazosin → LVEF improved from 18 ± 3% to 23 ± 4%.[b]
LeJemtel et al[79]	Amrinone, oral	Resting LVEF	5 patients with severe left ventricular dysfunction.	LVEF improved from 14 ± 8% to 21 ± 8%.[b] All showed > 5% absolute increase in LVEF (average 7%).
Awan et al[80]	Captopril, oral	Resting LVEF	9 patients with CHF (baseline mean LVEF, 23 ± 2%).	LVEF improved to 28 ± 2% after 1 week of therapy.[b] LVEF improved by 5% or more (absolute change) in only 4 patients and decreased in 1 patient.
Dzau et al[81]	Captopril, oral	Resting LVEF	7 patients with severe left ventricular dysfunction (baseline mean LVEF, 12 ± 3%).	LVEF improved to 26 ± 7% after 4.6 ± 1.6 months of therapy.[b]
Arnold et al[82]	Digoxin, oral	Resting LVEF	10 patients with chronic CHF.	LVEF fell from 41 ± 14% to 30 ± 14% after withdrawal of chronic digoxin therapy.[b] Significant worsening of CI and PCWP also occurred.
Goldberg et al[72]	Hydralazine (50–100 mg q 6 h), oral	Rest and exercise LVEF	9 patients with severe CHF (baseline mean LVEF, 21 ± 6%).	LVEF improved to 26 ± 7% after 48 h of therapy;[b] however, only 5 patients showed 5% or more absolute increase in LVEF. Exercise LVEF improved from 21 ± 8% to 24 ± 9%;[a] only 2 patients had 5% or more absolute increase in exercise LVEF from baseline exercise value and LVEF fell in 3. Of 9 patients, 6 responded hemodynamically to hydralazine (20% or more reduction in systemic vascular resistance). No significant correlation between changes in LVEF and hemodynamic changes.
Massie et al[83,84]	Captopril, oral	Resting LVEF	15 patients with CHF (baseline mean LVEF, 20 ± 6%).	LVEF increased to 25 ± 6% after 3 months[b] and to 30 ± 12% in 12 patients after mean therapy of 22 months.[b] Six patients did not show a 5% or more absolute increase in LVEF; 6 patients showed greater than 10% absolute increase in LVEF. Poor correlation between hemodynamic measurements and changes in clinical class, exercise tolerance, heart size, and LVEF.
Haq et al[73]	Nitrates, prazosin, hydralazine, hydralazine and nitrates; all oral	Resting LVEF	12 patients with refractory CHF (mean baseline LVEF, 19.2 ± 7.6%). Drug doses titrated to lowest PCWP with maximum CO.	LVEF not significantly changed with therapy (18.1 ± 7.5%); 5% or greater absolute change in LVEF in 50% of patients → only 2 had increase in LVEF by 5%. PCWP decreased from 29 ± 3 mmHg to 20 ± 4 mmHg ($p < 0.001$) (decreased significantly in all but 3 patients). CI increased from 2.0 ± 0.02 liters/min to 2.7 ± 0.2 liters/min ($p < 0.01$) (improved significantly in all but 2 patients).
Feldman et al[71]	Vesnarinone (60 mg/day oral)	Resting LVEF	239 patients with CHF (LVEF ≤ 30%).	No significant change in LVEF after 6 weeks. Functional class did not improve. However, significant improvement in quality of life and mortality noted at 6 weeks.

CHF, congestive heart failure; CI, cardiac index; CO, cardiac output; LVEF, left ventricular ejection fraction; PCWP, pulmonary capillary wedge pressure.
[a] Statistically significant improvement, but not physiologically significant.
[b] Statistically and physiologically significant improvement (>5% absolute change in LVEF).

sess the effects of drug intervention are detailed in Table 17-6. Again, the data reveal conflicting results regarding the utility of these measurements. Massie et al[87] noted that changes in left ventricular ejection fraction resulting from a single dose of oral captopril were almost entirely due to reduction in left ventricular end-diastolic volume, and that captopril reduced ventricular volume and filling pressure with a less significant effect on cardiac output. The authors concluded that there was good agreement between radionuclide and hemodynamic findings and that radionuclide ventriculograms may be a valuable method of following patients when volumes are also determined.

Hindman et al[91] found no significant change in radionuclide ejection fraction or ventricular volumes at rest or during exercise with hydralazine therapy despite significant improvement in invasively monitored parameters such as pulmonary capillary wedge pressure and cardiac output. The authors concluded that the hemodynamic improvement noted, without improvement in ventricular volumes or ejection fraction, may reflect an alteration in left ventricular compliance with the drug or reflect insensitivity of the radionuclide technique in patients with severely dilated ventricles and depressed left ventricular function.

Firth et al[74] noted that changes in cardiac index produced by nitroprusside infusion bore no relation to absolute changes in left ventricular ejection fraction, end-diastolic volume index, end-systolic volume index, or cardiac index by radionuclide ventriculography. While there was a fair correlation between change in pulmonary capillary wedge pressure and change in left ventricular end-diastolic volume in this study, the correlation was too loose to allow good predictive accuracy of using end-diastolic volume to monitor hemodynamic change. Furthermore, nitroprusside produced a considerably greater percentage change in invasively measured variables than in those determined by radionuclide study.

Use of Exercise Radionuclide Ventriculography

Exercise radionuclide ventriculography did not yield additional meaningful information when compared with rest studies of the response of the failing left ventricle to drug intervention.[72,87,91] Several studies, however, have noted the absence of change of resting ejection fraction with drug therapy but improvement in radionuclide values during exercise after drug administration.[76,93,94] These studies are detailed in Table 17-7. Murray et al[93] and Firth et al[94] studied the effects of digitalis on ventricular function and concluded that benefit may be manifest only during dynamic exercise. In the study by Firth et al,[94] the effect was apparent only in those patients with well-preserved left ventricular function at rest.

Goldman et al[77] noted an improvement in left ventricular function during exercise following prazosin therapy, but they saw no improvement at rest. The authors noted that, in the patient with less severe congestive heart failure, sympathetic vasomotor activity at rest may be normal. During exercise, however, an exaggerated sympathetic discharge may inhibit the normal decrease in systemic vascular resistance. It was postulated, therefore, that prazosin would not improve resting left ventricular function but enables appropriate vasodilatation during exercise and subsequent improvement in left ventricular function.

Summary

As can be seen, there are wide discrepancies in the medical literature concerning the value of radionuclide techniques in assessing drug therapy in patients with congestive heart failure. Multiple factors probably account for this lack of agreement. Timing of studies following drug intervention, route of administration of the drug, and differential short- and long-term effects of individual drugs may play a role. Variance of medication dosage may also be important. Evaluation of drugs with multiple mechanisms of action may be difficult. Different effects of the drugs in patients with different types of underlying cardiac disease may also be a significant factor. Finally, differences in the severity of congestive heart failure, size of left ventricular end-diastolic volume, and presence or absence of valvular regurgitation have an important effect on the various reported results.

Nevertheless, some conclusions can be derived regarding the value of radionuclide ventriculography in assessing the response of the left ventricle to drug intervention. Radionuclide ventriculography by itself is a valid technique in evaluating drug response and effects in groups of patients without severe left ventricular dysfunction and without valvular regurgitation in formal pharmacologic studies. Additional measurement of left ventricular absolute volumes may help separate drug effects that alter the inotropic state of the myocardium compared with drug effects that alter the ejection fraction by producing changes in ventricular loading conditions. The left ventricular end-diastolic volume may be used to assess changes in left ventricular preload in response to drug treatment. The left ventricular end-systolic volume may produce an index of left ventricular function that is independent of ventricular preload. Furthermore, determination of left ventricular volumes in addition to the left ventricular ejection fraction allows for accurate determination of left ventricular stroke volume and cardiac output, potentially eliminating the need for invasive hemodynamic monitoring in patients without severe left ventricular dysfunction and without valvular regurgitation.

Table 17-6 Specific Studies Evaluating Left Ventricular Volume and Cardiac Output Responses to Drug Intervention

Reference	Drug	Radionuclide Parameters	Patients Studied	Findings and Conclusions
Massie et al[87]	Captopril (25 mg), oral	Rest and exercise LVEF and ventricular volumes	14 patients with CHF (9 with secondary MR; baseline mean LVEF, $19 \pm 6\%$).	Radionuclide findings compared with rest and exercise invasively measured hemodynamic changes. LVEF increased to $22 \pm 5\%$ after single drug dose.[a] LVEDV decreased from 388 ± 81 ml to 350 ± 77 ml ($p < 0.01$). LVEDP decreased from 24 ± 10 mmHg to 17 ± 9 mmHg ($p < 0.001$). Stroke volume did not change significantly, by either radionuclide or invasive measurement. CI measured only invasively and not significantly changed. Changes at exercise similar to those at rest.
Ritchie et al[75]	Sublingual nitroglycerin	Resting LVEF, relative ventricular volumes and COs	23 patients with wide spectrum of cardiac disease (baseline LVEF range, 10–20% to 60–70%; 8 of 26 studies with baseline LVEF $\geq 50\%$). Patients with MR excluded.	Mean LVEF increased by $15.6 \pm 2.2\%$ ($p < 0.001$) (increased in 18 of 26; unchanged in 8). Relative cardiac output increased in 9 of 26 and decreased in 3; increased by mean of $5.3 \pm 3.8\%$ (NS). LVEDV decreased by $10.7 \pm 2.1\%$ ($p < 0.001$). LVESV decreased by $18.5 \pm 2.6\%$ ($p < 0.001$).
Hindman et al[91]	Hydralazine (50–75 mg q 6 h), oral	Rest and exercise LVEF and ventricular volumes	12 patients with CAD (4 with CHF); 10 had secondary MR; 9 studied by radionuclide testing. Baseline mean LVEF, 23%; range, 12–31%.	No significant change in LVEF or LVEDV (mean baseline value 263 ± 83 ml) after either 48 h or 1 month of therapy, despite significant improvement, reduction in PCWP or improvement in CO at rest or with exercise. Radionuclide LVEF or ventricular volumes with exercise also showed no significant improvement.
Poliner et al[92]	Prazosin, oral	Resting LVEF, ventricular volumes, and CO	7 patients with severe CHF (mean baseline LVEF, $14 \pm 4\%$).	LVEF increased to $27 \pm 5\%$ after 48 h of therapy.[b] Significant improvement in invasively measured PCWP and PAP. LVEDV unchanged (mean baseline, 212 ± 33 ml). LVESV decreased from 175 ± 17 ml to 152 ± 9 ml ($p < 0.05$) and radionuclide CO increased from 3.1 to 5.8 liters/min (no p value). Authors suggested increased contractility as major mechanism of improvement.
Firth et al[74]	Nitroprusside infusion	Resting LVEF, LVEDVI, LVESVI, and CI	12 patients with severe CHF (mean baseline LVEF, $19 \pm 5\%$).	LVEF increased to $23 \pm 5\%$ during peak infusion.[a] LVEF increased by <5% absolute change in 11 of 12. LVEDVI decreased from 185 ± 61 ml/m² to 152 ± 55 ml/m² ($p < 0.001$) and LVESVI decreased from 150 ± 51 to 120 ± 45 ml/m² ($p < 0.001$). Radionuclide CI did not change significantly (baseline, 3.13 ± 1.02 liters/min/m²; 2.89 ± 0.99 liters/min/m² during peak infusion). Thermodilution CI increased from 2.06 ± 0.41 liters/min/m² to 2.91 ± 0.62 liters/min/m² ($p < 0.005$). PCWP also decreased significantly.
Loeb et al[92a]	Dopamine (IV)	CO, CI, and PCWP	27 patients with severe CHF	CI increased from 1.8 to 2.5 liters/min/m² but PCWP increased from 24 to 30 mmHg.
Liang et al[92b]	Dobutamine (continuous IV infusion for 72 h)	Maximal exercise time, NYHA class, LVEF, and CO	15 patients with dilated cardiomyopathy (NYHA class III or IV)	Significant increase in maximal exercise time, LVEF, and CO, and improved NYHA class as compared with placebo.

CAD, coronary artery disease; CHF, congestive heart failure; CO, cardiac output; IV, intravenous; LVEDP, left ventricular end-diastolic pressure; LVEDV, left ventricular end-diastolic volume; LVEDVI, left ventricular end-diastolic volume index; LVESV, left ventricular end-systolic volume; LVESVI, left ventricular end-systolic volume index; MR, mitral regurgitation; PAP, pulmonary artery pressure; PCWP, pulmonary capillary wedge pressure; q6h, every 6 h.
[a] Statistically significant improvement but not physiologically significant.
[b] Statistically and physiologically significant improvement (>5% absolute change in LVEF).

Table 17-7   Specific Studies Examining Addition of Exercise Ejection-Fraction Response for Evaluation of Left Ventricular Response to Drug Therapy

Reference	Drug	Radionuclide Parameters	Patients Studied	Findings and Conclusions
Murray et al[93]	Intravenous ouabain, chronic oral digoxin	Rest and exercise LVEF	10 patients with CHF and in sinus rhythm (mean baseline LVEF, 32 ± 3%).	LVEF did not change significantly after ouabain (31 ± 2%) or 6 weeks of digoxin therapy (36 ± 4%). Invasively measured hemodynamic parameters did not change either. Mean baseline exercise LVEF (29 ± 2%) did increase after ouabain (36 ± 3%)[b] but not with digoxin (34 ± 4%). SVI increased significantly after both ouabain and digoxin. CI increased after drug therapy but not to a significant degree.
Goldman et al[77]	Prazosin (8–20 mg/day), oral	Rest and exercise LVEF	15 patients with CHF (mean baseline LVEF, 36 ± 14%).	LVEF not significantly changed after 7–12 weeks of therapy (37 ± 14%). Only 3 patients showed absolute change of 5% or more in rest LVEF. With exercise, LVEF increased from 34 ± 14% to 42 ± 17%[b] and 9 patients showed ≥5% absolute increase. Exercise duration and total work capacity also improved significantly with therapy but correlated to only a fair degree with changes in LVEF.
Firth et al[94]	Digoxin, oral	Rest and exercise LVEF, ventricular volumes, stroke volume, and CI	14 patients with ischemic heart disease (8 with LVEF < 50% and 6 with LVEF > 50%). Baseline mean LVEF of 33% in 8 patients with abnormal LVEFs; 68% in patients with normal LVEFs.	For both groups and all patients as a whole, resting and exercise LVEF, SVI, and CI did not change significantly following drug therapy. LVEF responses varied widely for all patients. In patients with baseline abnormal LVEFs, LVEDV and LVESV increased with exercise and were unaffected by digoxin.

CI, cardiac index; LVEDV, left ventricular end-diastolic volume; LVEF, left ventricular ejection fraction; LVESV, left ventricular end-systolic volume; SVI, stroke volume index.
[a] Statistically significant improvement but not physiologically significant (no examples in this table).
[b] Statistically and physiologically significant improvement (>5% absolute change in LVEF).

However, the need for monitoring the effects of inotropic or vasodilator drug interventions in clinical patient care exists primarily in patients with severe left ventricular dysfunction. In these patients, the validity of radionuclide ventriculography by itself for evaluating a drug effect in an individual patient is less reliable, as responses may be variable and routine use of the test for this purpose in clinical situations is not advocated. Clinically important improvement in left ventricular function related to drug treatment that may be measurable by invasive monitoring may not be demonstrated by radionuclide ventriculography in individual patients. However, the technique may be used in conjunction with other methods such as hemodynamic invasive monitoring or exercise testing for the study of drug effects in groups of patients, since changes which may not be physiologically significant for an individual patient may be significant for the group as a whole.

Additional measurements from the radionuclide ventriculogram such as the regurgitant index might improve characterization of drug-induced improvement in forward cardiac output by allowing for such confounding factors as mitral regurgitation. However, regurgitant index has been found to be of limited value when used in patients with significant left ventricular dysfunction[95,96] or with concomitant tricuspid regurgitation.[97] To measure small changes in forward cardiac output in patients with a dilated left ventricle and severe left ventricular dysfunction, it must be possible to determine accurately what percentage of total stroke volume contributes to forward ejection.

EVALUATION OF DRUG INTERVENTIONS IN ISCHEMIC HEART DISEASES

Radionuclide ventriculography, by assessment of global and segmental left ventricular function, has been valuable in establishing the usefulness and safety of various drugs in patients with ischemic heart disease.[98–107] Determining the safety of administering an antianginal agent with significant myocardial depressant activity to a patient with myocardial ischemia is a commonly encountered clinical problem.[108] Radionuclide techniques have also been used in assessing the safety of drug withdrawal in these patients[109] as well as determining the mechanisms of protection from ischemia exerted by anti-anginal medications.[110-113]

Results of these studies have important implications in the practical treatment of patients with ischemic heart disease. The assessment of myocardial viability and prediction of changes in left ventricular performance in response to pharmacologic therapy or surgical revascularization are important.[70] In addition, the drugs themselves may affect the validity of radionuclide ventriculographic tests used to determine the presence or absence of coronary artery disease. These issues are addressed in the next section.

Evaluation of Nitrate Therapy by Radionuclide Ventriculography

Borer et al[99] studied the effect of sublingual nitroglycerin on global and regional left ventricular function at rest and during exercise in 47 patients with coronary artery disease and 25 patients without heart disease. Gated radionuclide ventriculograms revealed resting segmental wall-motion abnormalities in 17 patients with coronary artery disease, with new segmental abnormalities appearing in 40 of the 47 patients during exercise. In seven of the 17 patients with resting segmental abnormalities, no difference in wall motion was noted during exercise. All 47 coronary artery disease patients exhibited abnormal ejection-fraction responses to exercise (less than 5 percent absolute increase in ejection fraction from rest to exercise), with a reduction of left ventricular ejection fraction in 42 cases. Following administration of nitroglycerin, resting left ventricular ejection fraction in the patients with coronary artery disease increased from a mean of 45 to 50 percent ($p < 0.02$). Nitroglycerin increased the left ventricular ejection fraction attained during exercise from a mean value of 36 to 48 percent ($p < 0.001$). While this value improved in all patients with coronary artery disease except one, the degree of improvement varied and was not of clear physiologic significance in some patients, particularly those with baseline exercise-ejection fractions of 20 percent or less. In some patients, exercise ejection-fraction response became normal following pretreatment with nitroglycerin. In all 47 patients, segmental wall-motion abnormalities during exercise improved following nitroglycerin pretreatment and normalized in some patients. In normal subjects, resting ejection fraction increased from a mean value of 58 to 71 percent ($p < 0.01$) following nitroglycerin pretreatment, although exercise ejection fraction was unchanged by nitroglycerin. No normal subject manifested regional wall-motion abnormalities. The authors concluded that prophylactic nitroglycerin improved regional left ventricular function and ejection fraction during exercise in patients with coronary artery disease.

Rozanski et al[100] used a combination of thallium myocardial perfusion imaging and radionuclide ventriculography to study the effects of nitroglycerin on myocardial ischemia in 17 patients with resting segmental wall-motion abnormalities. Radionuclide ventriculography was performed at rest, before, and after a sufficient nitroglycerin dose to lower the systolic blood pressure 10 mmHg or raise the heart rate by at least 10 beats per minute. Of 49 segmental wall-motion abnormalities at rest, 22 improved after nitroglycerin while 27 failed to change. The presence or absence of thallium redistribution following exercise thallium testing (without nitroglycerin) correctly predicted the wall-motion response to nitroglycerin in 39 of the 49 segments. Thallium redistribution images were normal in 21 of 22 segments improving with nitroglycerin, and abnormal in 18 of 27 segments not showing improvement ($p < 0.001$). The authors concluded that postexercise and redistribution thallium myocardial imaging predicts the response of segmental wall-motion abnormalities to nitroglycerin and, therefore, that nitroglycerin may help to assess the potential reversibility of ischemia in resting areas of abnormal wall motion.

Hellman et al[101] compared response of radionuclide left ventricular ejection fraction with nitroglycerin administration to change in left ventricular ejection fraction following coronary artery bypass graft surgery in 12 patients. Preoperative resting mean left ventricular ejection fraction rose from 30 to 36 percent following administration of nitroglycerin ($p < 0.01$) and rose to 38 percent following surgery ($p < 0.05$). In nine patients, ejection fraction increased after nitroglycerin administration. Six of these nine also manifested an increase in ejection fraction following surgery. Fifty-four resting segmental wall-motion abnormalities were present preoperatively. Of 40 hypokinetic segments, 17 improved after surgery, 13 of these having improved in response to nitroglycerin. Of seven akinetic segments, two improved after surgery and both improved in response to nitroglycerin. No other akinetic segments had responded to nitroglycerin. None of the seven dyskinetic segments improved following nitroglycerin administration or surgery. Thus, the authors concluded that the radionuclide ventriculogram response to nitroglycerin is useful for predicting regional wall-motion and global left ventricular responses to coronary artery bypass graft surgery.

In patients with unstable angina pectoris, Breisblatt et al[114] used a nonimaging radionuclide probe together with invasive hemodynamic monitoring to evaluate the mechanism of action of and dosage response to intravenous nitroglycerin. Assessment of peak systolic pressure–end-systolic volume relations suggested altered loading rather than augmented contractility as the principal hemodynamic mechanism of action of intravenous nitroglycerin in these patients.

Evaluation of Beta-Blocker Therapy by Radionuclide Ventriculography

NORMAL SUBJECTS

Marshall et al[113] evaluated the effects of maximally tolerated doses of oral propranolol on resting, exercise, and postexercise left ventricular function by radionuclide ventriculography in seven normal subjects. At rest, propranolol did not significantly change mean left ventricular ejection fraction (baseline, 63 ± 5 percent, and 65 ± 5 percent after propranolol; mean dose, 434 ± 99 mg/day). At 160 mg/day of propranolol, decrements in mean left ventricular ejection fraction with exercise and increases in mean left ventricular end-diastolic volume with exercise were noted, but neither change was statistically significant, and mean exercise ejection-fraction response remained normal (5 percent or greater absolute increase in ejection fraction with exercise). At peak propranolol dosage, however, mean left ventricular ejection fraction with exercise was significantly less than control (67 ± 5 percent versus 73 ± 5 percent, respectively; $p < 0.02$), and mean exercise ejection-fraction response was abnormal (only 2 percent absolute increase from rest value). At peak propranolol dosage, the exercise left ventricular end-diastolic volume was significantly greater than at rest ($p < 0.05$). Postexercise changes were not significantly different from control.

EFFECT OF PROPRANOLOL ON RESTING LEFT VENTRICULAR EJECTION FRACTION IN PATIENTS WITH CORONARY ARTERY DISEASE

Marshall et al[102] also studied the effects of propranolol on resting global and regional left ventricular function as assessed by radionuclide ventriculography in 22 stable patients with coronary artery disease. Propranolol was given in doses titrated to maximal clinical improvement or tolerance. Mean peak dose was 165 ± 13 mg/day (range, 80 to 240 mg/day). Baseline mean left ventricular ejection fraction was 63 ± 3 percent, 63 ± 3 percent at intermediate dosage levels, and 64 ± 3 percent at peak dosage ($p > 0.05$ for all comparisons). Although individual variation was noted, no significant trends in ejection-fraction measurement were encountered, including three patients with baseline ejection fractions of less than 50 percent and four patients with a history of congestive heart failure. No changes in regional wall-motion abnormalities were noted in the six patients in whom these were present at rest.

Reduto et al[109] used radionuclide ventriculography to assess the effect of propranolol withdrawal on resting left ventricular function in 18 stable patients with coronary artery disease scheduled to undergo coronary artery bypass graft surgery. Baseline mean left ventricular ejection fraction while on a mean dose of propranolol of 224 ± 9 mg/day (range, 160 to 640 mg/day) was 59.1

$\pm$ 2.4 percent. Following complete propranolol withdrawal, mean ejection fraction was 59.2 ± 2.5 percent ($p > 0.05$). Five patients had abnormal baseline ejection fractions (range, 43 to 48 percent) and no change was noted in these patients, as well, following drug withdrawal. The largest increase in ejection fraction noted was 8 percent and the largest decrease was 10 percent. No significant change was noted in resting regional wall-motion abnormalities following propranolol withdrawal.

While these studies suggest that oral propranolol has minimal effects on global or regional left ventricular function at rest (despite substantial improvement in angina pectoris and reduction of resting heart rate), it should be noted that the majority of the patients studied had normal left ventricular ejection fractions at rest.

Rainwater et al[106] noted variation in the effect of oral propranolol on resting left ventricular function in 30 patients with coronary artery disease related to the presence or absence of previous myocardial infarction. Left ventricular ejection fraction was measured by a nonimaging scintillation probe following intravenous injection of technetium 99m. Of the 30 patients, 15 studied had sustained a previous myocardial infarction. In the 15 patients without prior infarction, resting left ventricular ejection fraction was 53 ± 1 percent (normal in all patients). In the 15 patients with prior infarction, resting ejection fraction was 40 ± 1 percent (abnormal in all 15 patients). Following 1 week of oral propranolol therapy (40 mg every 6 h), resting ejection fraction was unchanged in the patients without previous infarction (52 ± 1 percent), but it decreased significantly in the group with prior infarction (36 ± 1 percent, $p < 0.05$).

EFFECT OF PROPRANOLOL ON EXERCISE LEFT VENTRICULAR EJECTION-FRACTION RESPONSE IN PATIENTS WITH CORONARY ARTERY DISEASE

Marshall et al[113] evaluated the effects of oral propranolol on exercise left ventricular ejection-fraction response in 18 stable patients with coronary artery disease: 17 had normal baseline left ventricular ejection fractions at rest and six had resting regional wall-motion abnormalities. Before propranolol therapy, 14 of the 18 patients showed an abnormal exercise ejection-fraction response (less than 5 percent absolute increase in ejection fraction). Propranolol improved exercise ventricular function in 10 but failed to produce significant improvement in four. Among these patients as a group, at peak propranolol dosage (mean dose, 162 ± 47 mg/day; range, 80 to 240 mg/day), exercise ejection fraction increased from 48 ± 11 percent to 58 ± 8 percent ($p < 0.01$). In the four patients with normal baseline exercise ejection-fraction responses, propranolol produced a small but insignificant decrease in exercise ejection fraction. No significant changes in left ventricular end-diastolic volume during exercise were noted after propranolol therapy in the 18 patients. Twenty-six segmental wall-motion abnormalities were present in response to exercise prior to propranolol therapy, and propranolol improved exercise performance in 21 of these areas ($p < 0.005$). In the 14 patients with an abnormal exercise ejection-fraction response, left ventricular ejection fraction 5 min after exercise was also significantly greater than the control value (63 ± 4 percent versus 55 ± 7 percent, $p < 0.005$). The postexercise values were not significantly changed in the other four patients with normal exercise ejection-fraction response. The authors concluded that, in patients with coronary artery disease and an abnormal exercise ejection-fraction response, clinically effective antianginal doses of propranolol improved exercise and postexercise regional and global left ventricular performance. However, propranolol had no significant effect on exercise left ventricular performance in patients with coronary artery disease and a baseline normal response to exercise.

Rainwater et al[106] evaluated the effects of propranolol in 30 patients with coronary artery disease and an abnormal baseline exercise ejection-fraction response. Following 1 week of oral propranolol therapy (40 mg every 6 h), exercise left ventricular ejection fraction improved in the 15 patients without previous myocardial infarction (45 ± 1 percent after propranolol versus 37 ± 2 percent before propranolol, $p < 0.01$) and in the 15 patients with a previous myocardial infarction (36 ± 1 percent after propranolol versus 30 ± 1 percent before propranolol, $p < 0.05$). Ten of the patients without previous infarction and seven with prior infarction had a 5 percent absolute increase over baseline exercise ejection fraction following propranolol therapy. Based on these and other[105–115] trials, it is concluded that high-dose propranolol prevents exercise-induced left ventricular dysfunction and that for the diagnosis of coronary artery disease exercise radionuclide ventriculography should not be performed while the patient is on high-dose beta-blocker therapy.

Evaluation of Calcium Channel Blocker Therapy by Radionuclide Ventriculography

Petru et al[107] evaluated the effects of high-dose diltiazem on exercise left ventricular performance in eight patients with coronary artery disease. All patients were evaluated after 1 week of diltiazem therapy (360 mg/day) and 1 week of placebo. Resting mean left ventricular ejection fraction on placebo was 53 ± 2 percent, with mean exercise ejection fraction 48 ± 2 percent. Resting left ventricular ejection fraction improved to 64 ± 2 percent on diltiazem ($p < 0.005$), and exercise ejection fraction improved to 62 ± 6 percent ($p < 0.005$). Treadmill exercise duration also improved ($p < 0.01$).

Chew et al[108] used radionuclide ventriculography in conjunction with hemodynamic invasive monitoring to evaluate the safety of administering intravenous verapamil to patients with ischemic heart disease. Fifteen patients had stable coronary artery disease with normal or moderately reduced baseline left ventricular ejection fraction (mean, 56 ± 10 percent; range, 42 to 69 percent), and seven had acute uncomplicated myocardial infarction (mean baseline ejection fraction, 49 ± 16 percent; range, 29 to 67 percent). Three additional patients (two with stable coronary artery disease and one with acute myocardial infarction) had severe left ventricular dysfunction (ejection fractions of 20 percent, 22 percent, and 35 percent) with elevated pulmonary capillary wedge pressures (20 mmHg or greater). Patients were given a verapamil bolus intravenously (0.145 mg/kg; mean dose, 17 ± 3 mg) followed by an infusion of 0.005 mg/kg/min (mean duration, 21 ± 5 min). Hemodynamic measurements and repeat radionuclide ventriculography were obtained after 5 to 10 min of drug infusion. In the patients with stable coronary artery disease and uncomplicated myocardial infarction, left ventricular ejection fractions were unchanged following the drug (56 ± 9 percent predrug and 50 ± 15 percent postdrug). Heart rate also remained unchanged, but significant reductions in mean arterial pressure and systemic vascular resistance occurred, coupled with significant increases in cardiac index and stroke volume index. Pulmonary capillary wedge pressure increased slightly but significantly ($p < 0.01$), while left ventricular stroke work index fell significantly ($p < 0.01$). In the three patients with preexisting severe left ventricular dysfunction, administration of verapamil was associated with a marked drop in mean arterial pressure and stroke volume index with an abrupt increase in pulmonary capillary wedge pressure, resulting in clinical evidence of congestive heart failure. Left ventricular ejection fraction fell from 20 to 17 percent in one patient but this measurement was not repeated in the other two. While no precise guidelines were available, it was concluded that verapamil could safely be given in the face of mild to moderate left ventricular dysfunction because the intrinsic depressant property of the drug was almost completely offset by the potent vasodilatation produced. In patients with severe underlying left ventricular dysfunction and elevation of the pulmonary capillary wedge pressure, clinical worsening of heart failure may occur secondary to the myocardial depressant effects of the drug.

Evaluation of Multiple Antianginal Agents by Radionuclide Ventriculography

Pfisterer et al[116] compared the effects of nitroglycerin, nifedipine, and metoprolol in patients with coronary artery disease affecting the left anterior descending coronary artery only, as assessed by hemodynamic invasive monitoring and radionuclide ventriculography. Nine patients had angina and exercise-induced ischemia and seven patients had previous anterior transmural myocardial infarction and no ischemic changes by thallium perfusion imaging. In the nine patients with ischemia only, baseline mean left ventricular ejection fraction was 64.7 ± 6.6 percent and fell to 56.7 ± 12.2 percent with exercise. In the seven patients with prior infarction, baseline mean left ventricular ejection fraction was 41.9 ± 12.7 percent and remained unchanged after exercise (42.7 ± 17.8 percent). Worsening of regional wall-motion abnormalities occurred in the patients with ischemia during exercise, but little change was noted in the patients with previous infarction. In the 16 patients overall, left ventricular ejection fraction during exercise increased following nitroglycerin (0.8 mg sublingually; ejection fraction, 58.2 ± 16.5 percent; control, 50.6 ± 16.1 percent; $p < 0.001$) and following nifedipine (5 ng/kg/min intravenously; ejection fraction, 57.9 ± 14.0 percent; $p < 0.01$). Cardiac index and systemic vascular resistance were unchanged after nitroglycerin, but both improved significantly with nifedipine ($p < 0.001$). Only nitroglycerin significantly reduced left ventricular end-diastolic volume ($p = 0.001$), whereas both drugs improved pulmonary capillary wedge pressure. Finally, regional wall motion improved to similar degrees following administration of both drugs. Following metoprolol (0.15 mg/kg intravenously), however, exercise left ventricular ejection fraction (52.5 ± 11.3 percent) was not significantly changed from control, while regional wall motion improved, but to a lesser degree than with nitroglycerin or nifedipine. Cardiac index was significantly less than control ($p < 0.001$) and pulmonary capillary wedge pressure greater than control ($p < 0.02$). Left ventricular end-diastolic volume was unchanged. The authors concluded that all three agents improved regional myocardial performance despite widely differing mechanisms of action of the drugs, thereby providing rationale for combined use of these agents in patients with ischemic heart disease.

Nesto et al[117] evaluated the effects of nifedipine on patients with ischemic heart disease who were already on stable doses of propranolol and nitrates. Rest and exercise radionuclide ventriculograms were performed on 16 patients on baseline therapy (heart rate less than 60 beats per minute and systolic blood pressure greater than 110 mmHg) and after 7 days of nifedipine (80 to 120 mg/day). Mean left ventricular ejection fraction fell from 61 to 46 percent during exercise ($p < 0.01$), and 27 regions developed hypokinesis while on baseline therapy. Resting ejection fraction decreased to 54 percent with the addition of nifedipine ($p < 0.005$), but exercise ejection fraction did not fall significantly (53 percent), and only 14 hypokinetic segments were noted ($p < 0.05$). The

time to onset of angina during exercise also increased significantly. Thus, while nifedipine depressed resting ejection fraction, global and regional left ventricular performance during exercise was improved.

Evaluation of Coronary Artery Spasm by Radionuclide Techniques

Myocardial thallium perfusion imaging in conjunction with the administration of ergonovine or methacholine has been shown to be a valuable method for the diagnosis of coronary artery spasm.[118] Buda et al[119] evaluated 28 patients with atypical chest pain by thallium myocardial perfusion imaging at rest, following exercise, and after ergonovine administration (0.05 to 0.25 mg intravenously). Sixteen of these patients developed coronary artery spasm following administration of ergonovine, documented by chest pain, ECG changes, and myocardial perfusion defects. Coronary artery spasm was also confirmed by angiography in 15 of the 16 patients. Seven patients had significant fixed obstructive coronary disease (50 percent or greater luminal narrowing of at least one major coronary artery) with superimposed spasm, while eight had no significant coronary artery disease. Exercise thallium testing was abnormal in seven of eight patients with fixed coronary stenoses and normal in seven of eight without significant stenoses. Thus, it was concluded that thallium myocardial perfusion imaging could detect coronary artery spasm induced by ergonovine, and exercise thallium testing could differentiate patients with normal coronary arteries and spasm from those with spasm superimposed on fixed coronary artery lesions.

DiCarlo et al[120] used thallium myocardial perfusion imaging following the administration of intravenous ergonovine to detect coronary artery spasm in patients with atypical chest pain: 26 patients with normal coronary arteries or angiographically insignificant lesions were studied. Thallium was injected following infusion of maximal ergonovine dosage (0.20 mg) or onset of chest pain. Four patients developed chest pain associated with ischemic ST-segment changes or reversible myocardial perfusion defects (two with both, one with ECG changes only, and one with perfusion defect only). Nine additional patients developed chest pain but without either ECG or myocardial perfusion changes. Thirteen patients did not experience chest pain with ergonovine administration, although two developed reversible thallium perfusion defects. The four patients with chest pain and abnormal thallium images and/or ECG changes were restudied after institution of nitrates or calcium antagonists. None of the four patients manifested ECG abnormalities or thallium perfusion defects. All four became asymptomatic or have had marked reduction of chest

Table 17-8 Radionuclide Ventriculographic Assessment of the Response of Ventricular Function to Various Drugs

Drug	Reference	Method	Patients Studied	Radionuclide Findings	Comments
Disopyramide (oral)	Gottdiener et al[128]	Rest and exercise RNV	22 patients with normal LV function; 12 patients with LV dysfunction.	No change in rest or exercise LVEF in either group with 150 mg PO q 6 h. Decrease in LVEF at rest and exercise in patients with LV dysfunction following 300 mg PO.[a]	Use loading dose with caution in patients with LV dysfunction.
Disopyramide (oral)	Kowey et al[129]	Rest RNV	7 patients with normal LV function; 9 patients with LV dysfunction.	All 9 patients with LV dysfunction had a decrease in LVEF after 300 mg PO;[a] decrease in LVEF in only 1 with normal LV function.	Patients with LV dysfunction particularly susceptible to negative inotropic effect.
Disopyramide procainamide quinidine (oral)	Wisenberg et al[130]	Rest and exercise RNV	17 patients with baseline LVEF of >40%.	No statistically significant difference in LVEF following drug therapy with any agent, but downward trend in LVEF, especially with disopyramide; 1 patient with baseline LVEF of 22% developed pulmonary edema with disopyramide and was excluded from further study.	Caution should be used when administering any of the agents to patients with LV dysfunction.
Quinidine, procainamide (oral)	Smitherman et al[131]	Rest RNV	8 patients with ischemic heart disease.	No change in LVEF with either agent but baseline LVEF not specified.	No significant deleterious effect in patients with ischemic heart disease.
Amiodarone (oral)	Sugrue et al[132]	Rest RNV	30 patients with hypertrophic cardiomyopathy and chronic oral amiodarone.	No change in rest LVEF; peak ejection rate decreased at 1 month, returned to normal at 6 months. Five patients had > 6% absolute increase in LVEF; 6 patients > 6% absolute decrease in LVEF.	No change in radionuclide indices of LV function with chronic therapy.
Mexiletine (oral)	Stein et al[133]	Rest RNV	10 patients with LV dysfunction (mean LVEF 28%).	No change in LVEF after 48 h of therapy. No change in RVEF with therapy.	No effect on LV function in patients with preexisting LV dysfunction.
Imipramine, doxepin (oral)	Veith et al[134]	Rest and exercise RNV	24 patients with varying heart disease (9 with abnormal LVEFs).	No change in LVEF with chronic therapy. No change in LVEF in patients with LV dysfunction. No worsening of arrhythmias or heart block.	Can be used safely in patients with heart disease (not adequately tested in patients with severe LV dysfunction).
Nitroprusside (infusion)	Shah et al[135]	Rest RNV	16 patients with acute myocardial infarction.	Improved LVEF with infusion;[a] regional wall motion improved in 18/67 abnormal segments, worsened in 1. Improved pulmonary capillary wedge pressure; cardiac index unchanged.	Improved global and regional LV performance in acute myocardial infarction.

pain with chronic drug therapy. On the other hand, seven of the nine patients with chest pain in response to ergonovine but no ECG or thallium perfusion changes have continued to have chest pain that has been unchanged despite medical therapy.

Johnson et al[121] evaluated the effects of verapamil and nifedipine on global left ventricular function in 10 patients with documented coronary artery spasm. Eight patients had normal coronary arteries, while two patients also had significant obstructive coronary artery disease. Rest and exercise radionuclide ventriculography was performed during placebo therapy, following 2 months of verapamil therapy (400 ± 80 mg/day), and following 2 months of nifedipine therapy (82 ± 31 mg/day). Baseline resting left ventricular ejection fraction ranged from 26 to 80 percent, with a mean of 61 percent on placebo, 65 percent on verapamil, and 60 percent on nifedipine (differences not significant). Exercise ejection fraction rose to 69 percent on placebo, 71 percent on verapamil, and 71 percent on nifedipine ($p < 0.05$ when

Table 17-8 (Continued)

Drug	Reference	Method	Patients Studied	Radionuclide Findings	Comments
Digoxin (oral)	Rainwater et al[136]	Rest and exercise RNV and thallium imaging	9 patients with ischemic heart disease.	Resting LVEF improved;[b] exercise LVEF unchanged. Improvement or worsening of myocardial perfusion imaging correlated with improvement or worsening of LVEF.	Change in LVEF with digoxin in ischemic heart disease predicts change in perfusion imaging.
Aminophylline (infusion)	Matthay et al[137]	Rest RNV	15 patients with COPD; 5 normal patients.	Improved RVEF and LVEF in both groups with drug infusion.[a]	Acute improvement in biventricular function, unrelated to degree of pulmonary compromise.
Terbutaline (subcutaneous)	Hooper et al[138]	Rest RNV	11 patients with severe COPD.	Improved RVEF and LVEF following 0.25 mg subcutaneously.[a] Left ventricular end-diastolic volume decreased. Insignificant increase in cardiac output.	May be beneficial in COPD patients because of hemodynamic effects.
Oxygen	Olvey et al[139]	Rest and exercise RNV	18 patients with severe COPD and normal LV function.	Resting RVEF and LVEF unchanged with oxygen. RVEF[a] and LVEF[b] improved with oxygen during exercise.	Right ventricular reserve abnormal in most patients with COPD and improved with oxygen during exercise.
Glucose-insulin-potassium infusion	Whitlow et al[140]	Rest RNV	28 patients with acute myocardial infarction (13 infusion, 15 placebo).	LVEF improved in infusion group.[a] Regional wall motion and left ventricular end-systolic and end-diastolic volumes also improved. All parameters worsened in control group.	Improved global and regional left ventricular function in acute myocardial infarction.
Angiotensin (infusion)	Bianco et al[141]	Rest RNV	6 normal patients; 10 patients with ischemic heart disease.	Hypertensive response with decreased LVEF[a] in both groups. Effect varied among patients.	Angiotensin infusion test not helpful in separating normal patients from patients with ischemic heart disease.
Captopril (oral)	Blaufox et al[142]	Rest and exercise RNV	16 patients with essential hypertension.	Abnormal exercise LVEF response with hypertension; normalized following captopril therapy.	Abnormal LVEF response to exercise present in hypertension, which may be normalized with therapy.
Anesthesia induction	Giles et al[143]	Nuclear probe	18 patients during induction for CABG surgery.	LVEF decreased in all patients by 1 min after intubation.[a] Recovered in 15/18 by 5 min.	Profound LV depression occurs during anesthesia induction, highlighting need for close LV monitoring.

CABG, coronary artery bypass graft; COPD, chronic obstructive pulmonary disease; LV, left ventricle; LVEF, left ventricular ejection fraction; PO, oral; RNV, radionuclide ventriculogram; RVEF, right ventricular ejection fraction; q 6 h, every 6 h.
[a] Statistically and physiologically significant improvement (e.g., > 5% absolute change in LVEF).
[b] Statistically significant improvement but not physiologically significant.

compared with rest). Left ventricular end-diastolic volume index increased significantly from rest to exercise with verapamil but not with placebo or nifedipine. All patients, including two with abnormal baseline ejection fractions (26 and 46 percent), showed no change or had a slight improvement in ejection fraction with exercise while on nifedipine and verapamil. The authors concluded that, in patients with coronary artery spasm, left ventricular performance at rest and during exercise was not significantly altered by verapamil or nifedipine.

Summary

Exercise radionuclide ventriculography has been widely used for the noninvasive detection of coronary artery disease. If an absolute increase in left ventricular ejection fraction from rest to peak exercise of less than 5 percent is regarded as an abnormal response, the test has a sensitivity of approximately 90 percent when used for this purpose.[122–124] However, therapy with antianginal agents may affect the validity of the test in screening an individual patient for coronary artery disease. Patients with undiagnosed chest pain and treated with maximal doses of beta blockers may have an abnormal exercise ejection-fraction response despite having normal coronary arteries. Although intermediate doses of beta blockers (160 mg/day) did not have a statistically significant effect on test results, the patients studied have consisted almost entirely of young, healthy adults with completely normal cardiac function. The effect of intermediate doses of beta blockers on the left ventricular ejection-fraction response to exercise in older patients has not been clearly established and may also importantly alter diagnostic accuracy of coronary disease detection by radionuclide ventriculography. For the detection of coronary artery disease, however, it is probably best to use methods other than exercise radionuclide ventriculography when the patient is on high-dose beta-blocker therapy.

Although nitroglycerin has been noted to produce a normal exercise ejection-fraction response in some patients with coronary artery disease and a previously abnormal response, the effect of long-acting nitrates on diagnostic test accuracy has not been extensively studied. Nevertheless, it is probably prudent to avoid using exercise radionuclide ventriculography for determining the presence or absence of coronary artery disease in the patient already on high-dose nitrate therapy. Similar considerations may apply to diagnostic testing with radionuclide ventriculography in patients receiving calcium channel blockers.

Analysis of segmental wall-motion abnormalities, an integral part of exercise radionuclide ventriculography, should aid in the diagnostic accuracy of the test when used for detection of coronary artery disease. As shown in the studies reviewed, however, antianginal medications may also normalize segmental wall motion during exercise and thus alter test results.

From the data reviewed, there is little question that radionuclide ventriculography is a valuable tool for assessing the usefulness of drug therapy in ischemic heart disease and for assessing the mechanisms of protection from ischemia by the drugs. The safety of drug administration is also well assessed by this technique. As in the evaluation of the therapy of congestive heart failure, however, the ejection fraction alone is inadequate in many cases. Assessment of regional wall motion and measurement of left ventricular volumes provide data not available from measurement of the global left ventricular ejection fraction.

An interesting application of radionuclide techniques is for the evaluation of myocardial segment viability with radionuclide ventriculography before and after nitroglycerin or with thallium myocardial perfusion imaging in order to predict the response of left ventricular function to coronary artery bypass graft surgery. While this is certainly not necessary in the average patient undergoing revascularization surgery, it may give the clinician addi-

tional important information in the patient with "borderline" left ventricular function being considered for this therapy.

The use of thallium perfusion imaging in conjunction with ergonovine administration for the diagnosis of coronary artery spasm outside of the cardiac catheterization laboratory is attractive, since it may eliminate the need for repeat cardiac catheterization in many of these patients. While provocative testing with ergonovine in the setting of the coronary care unit has been safely performed in several centers,[120] serious complications, including myocardial infarction, have been reported.[125] In addition, coronary artery spasm, both spontaneous and ergonovine-induced, has been noted to be unresponsive to sublingual and intravenous nitroglycerin in some patients, with death resulting.[126,127] Intracoronary nitroglycerin was necessary to reverse the spasm in other patients.[126,127] Thus, at present, the method of using thallium perfusion imaging with ergonovine testing outside of the cardiac catheterization laboratory should be regarded as experimental and should not be routinely advocated for the diagnosis of coronary artery spasm.

MISCELLANEOUS DRUG EFFECTS

A variety of pharmaceutical agents have been studied in various patient groups and clinical situations by radionuclide techniques to evaluate the effects on left ventricular function. It is beyond the scope of this chapter to review these studies extensively. Table 17-8 outlines some of these drug studies that have been performed.

SUMMARY

This chapter has reviewed the use of radionuclide techniques in the evaluation of the response of left ventricular function to drug interventions. It is hoped that this chapter will aid the clinician in developing practical criteria for the use of these radionuclide techniques in the evaluation of individual patient therapy and in the meaningful interpretation of drug studies involving radionuclide testing that appear in the literature.

REFERENCES

1. Marshall RC, Berger HJ, Reduto LA, et al: Variability in sequential measures of left ventricular performance

assessed with radionuclide angiocardiography. *Am J Cardiol* 41:531, 1978.

2. Wackers FJT, Berger HJ, Johnstone DE, et al: Multiple gated cardiac blood pool imaging for left ventricular ejection fraction: Validation of the technique and assessment of variability. *Am J Cardiol* 43:1159, 1979.

3. Rude RE, Grossman W, Colucci WS, et al: Problems in assessment of new pharmacologic agents for the heart failure patient. *Am Heart J* 102:584, 1981.

4. Blum RM, Carter SK: Adriamycin: A new anticancer drug with significant clinical activity. *Ann Intern Med* 80:249, 1974.

5. Isner JM, Ferrans VJ, Cohen SR, et al: Clinical and morphologic cardiac findings after anthracycline chemotherapy. *Am J Cardiol* 51:1167, 1983.

6. Von Hoff DD, Rozencweig M, Piccart M: The cardiotoxicity of anticancer agents. *Semin Oncol* 9:23, 1982.

7. Von Hoff DD, Layard MW, Basa P, et al: Risk factors for doxorubicin-induced congestive heart failure. *Ann Intern Med* 91:710, 1979.

8. Bristow MR, Billingham ME, Mason JW, et al: Clinical spectrum of anthracycline antibiotic cardiotoxicity. *Cancer Treat Rep* 62:873, 1978.

9. Legha SS, Benjamin RS, Mackay B, et al: Reduction of doxorubicin cardiotoxicity by prolonged continuous intravenous infusion. *Ann Intern Med* 96:133, 1982.

10. Henderson IC, Frei E III: Adriamycin cardiotoxicity. *Am Heart J* 99:671, 1980.

11. Alexander J, Dainiak N, Berger HJ, et al: Serial assessment of doxorubicin cardiotoxicity with quantitative radionuclide angiocardiography. *N Engl J Med* 300:278, 1979.

12. McKillop JH, Bristow MR, Goris ML, et al: Sensitivity and specificity of radionuclide ejection fractions in doxorubicin cardiotoxicity. *Am Heart J* 106:1048, 1983.

13. Ritchie JL, Singer JW, Thorning D, et al: Anthracycline cardiotoxicity: Clinical and pathologic outcomes assessed by radionuclide ejection fraction. *Cancer* 46:1109, 1980.

14. Palmeri ST, Bonow RO, Myers CE, et al: Prospective evaluation of doxorubicin cardiotoxicity by rest and exercise radionuclide angiography. *Am J Cardiol* 58:607, 1986.

15. Morgan GW, McIlveen BM, Freedman A, et al: Radionuclide ejection fraction in doxorubicin cardiotoxicity. *Cancer Treat Rep* 65:629, 1981.

16. Torti FM, Bristow MR, Howes AE, et al: Reduced cardiotoxicity of doxorubicin delivered on a weekly schedule: Assessment by endomyocardial biopsy. *Ann Intern Med* 99:745, 1983.

17. Di Marco A: Anthracycline antibiotics, in Holland JF, Frei E (eds): *Cancer Medicine.* Philadelphia, Lea and Febiger, 1982, p 900.

18. Bristow MR, Lopez MB, Mason JW, et al: Efficacy and cost of cardiac monitoring in patients receiving doxorubicin. *Cancer* 50:32, 1982.

19. Bristow MR, Mason JW, Billingham ME, et al: Dose–effect and structure–function relationships in doxorubicin cardiomyopathy. *Am Heart J* 102:709, 1981.

20. Bristow MR, Mason JW, Billingham ME, et al: Doxorubicin cardiomyopathy: Evaluation by phonocardiography, endomyocardial biopsy, and cardiac catheterization. *Ann Intern Med* 88:168, 1978.

21. Choi BW, Berger HJ, Schwartz PE, et al: Serial radionuclide assessment of doxorubicin cardiotoxicity in cancer patients with abnormal baseline resting left ventricular performance. *Am Heart J* 106:638, 1983.

22. Billingham ME, Mason JW, Bristow MR, et al: Anthracycline cardiomyopathy monitored by morphologic changes. *Cancer Treat Rep* 62:865, 1978.

23. Donaldson SS, Glick JM, Wilbur JR: Adriamycin activating a recall phenomenon after radiation therapy. *Ann Intern Med* 81:407, 1974.

24. Freter CE, Lee TC, Billingham ME, et al: Doxorubicin cardiac toxicity manifesting seven years after treatment: Case report and review. *Am J Med* 80:483, 1986.

25. Gottdiener JS, Mathisen DJ, Borer JS, et al: Doxorubicin cardiotoxicity: Assessment of late left ventricular dysfunction by radionuclide cineangiography. *Ann Intern Med* 94:430, 1981.

26. Schwartz RG, McKenzie WB, Alexander J, et al: Congestive heart failure and left ventricular dysfunction complicating doxorubicin therapy: Seven-year experience using serial radionuclide angiocardiography. *Am J Med* 82:1109, 1987.

27. Lipshultz SE, Colan SD, Gelber RD, et al: Late cardiac effects of doxorubicin therapy for acute lymphoblastic leukemia in childhood. *N Engl J Med* 324:808, 1991.

28. Bristow MR, Billingham ME, Mason JW: Adriamycin cardiotoxicity. *Am J Cardiol* 53:263, 1984 (letter).

29. Mason JW, Bristow MR, Billingham ME, et al: Invasive and noninvasive methods of assessing adriamycin cardiotoxic effects in man: Superiority of histopathologic assessment using endomyocardial biopsy. *Cancer Treat Rep* 62:857, 1978.

30. Isner JM: Adriamycin cardiotoxicity: Reply. *Am J Cardiol* 53:263, 1984 (letter).

31. Fulkerson PK, Talley R, Kleinman D, et al: Noninvasive profile in the prospective monitoring of adriamycin cardiomyopathy. *Cancer Treat Rep* 62:881, 1978.

32. Gorton SJ, Wilson GA, Sutherland R, et al: The predictive value of myocardial radioisotope scanning in animals treated with doxorubicin. *J Nucl Med* 21:518, 1980.

33. Chacko AK, Gordon DH, Bennett JM, et al: Myocardial imaging with Tc-99m pyrophosphate in patients on adriamycin treatment for neoplasia. *J Nucl Med* 18:680, 1977.

34. Henderson IC, Sloss LJ, Jaffe N, et al: Serial studies of cardiac function in patients receiving adriamycin. *Cancer Treat Rep* 62:923, 1978.

35. Ewy GA, Jones SE, Friedman MJ, et al: Noninvasive cardiac evaluation of patients receiving adriamycin. *Cancer Treat Rep* 62:915, 1978.

36. Mettler FP, Young DM, Ward JM: Adriamycin-induced cardiotoxicity (cardiomyopathy and congestive heart failure) in rats. *Cancer Res* 37:2705, 1977.

37. Smith B: Damage to the intrinsic cardiac neurones by rubidomycin (daunorubicin). *Br Heart J* 31:607, 1969.

38. Sisson JC, Shapiro B, Meyers L, et al: Metaiodobenzylguanidine to map scintigraphically the adrenergic nervous system in man. *J Nucl Med* 28:1625, 1987.

39. Sisson JC, Wieland DM, Sherman P, et al: Metaiodoben-

zylguanidine as an index of the adrenergic nervous system integrity and function. *J Nucl Med* 28:1620, 1987.

40. Friedman MA, Bozdech MJ, Billingham ME, et al: Doxorubicin cardiotoxicity: Serial endomyocardial biopsies and systolic time intervals. *JAMA* 240:1603, 1978.

41. Druck M, Bar-Shlomo BZ, Gulenchyn K, et al: Radionuclide angiography and endomyocardial biopsy in the assessment of doxorubicin cardiotoxicity. *Am J Cardiol* 47:401, 1981 (abstr).

42. Schwartz RG, McKenzie WB, Sager PT, et al: Utility of monitoring doxorubicin cardiotoxicity with resting first pass radionuclide angiocardiography for prevention of irreversible congestive heart failure: A seven year experience in 1115 patients. *J Am Coll Cardiol* 5:452, 1985 (abstr).

43. Singer JW, Narahara KA, Ritchie JL, et al: Time- and dose-dependent changes in ejection fraction determined by radionuclide angiography after anthracycline therapy. *Cancer Treat Rep* 62:945, 1978.

44. Kennedy JW, Sorensen SG, Ritchie JL, et al: Radionuclide angiography for the evaluation of anthracycline therapy. *Cancer Treat Rep* 62:941, 1978.

45. Von Hoff DD, Rozencweig M, Layard M, et al: Daunomycin-induced cardiotoxicity in children and adults: A review of 110 cases. *Am J Med* 62:200, 1977.

46. Wiernik PH, Schimpff SC, Schiffer CA, et al: Randomized clinical comparison of daunorubicin (NSC 82151) alone with a combination of daunorubicin, cytosine arabinoside (NSC 63878), 6-thioguanine (NSC 752) and pyrimethamine (NSC 3061) for the treatment of acute nonlymphocytic leukemia. *Cancer Treat Rep* 60:41, 1976.

47. Lee BH, Goodenday LS, Muswick GJ, et al: Alterations in left ventricular diastolic function with doxorubicin therapy. *J Am Coll Cardiol* 9:184, 1987.

48. Marchandise B, Schroeder E, Bosly A, et al: Early detection of doxorubicin cardiotoxicity: Interest of Doppler echocardiographic analysis of left ventricular filling dynamics. *Am Heart J* 118:92, 1989.

49. Stoddard MF, Seeger J, Liddell NE, et al: Prolongation of isovolumetric relaxation time as assessed by Doppler echocardiography predicts doxorubicin-induced systolic dysfunction in humans. *J Am Coll Cardiol* 20:62, 1992.

50. Klewer SE, Goldberg SJ, Donnerstein RL, et al: Dobutamine stress echocardiography: A sensitive indicator of diminished myocardial function in asymptomatic doxorubicin-treated long-term survivors of childhood cancer. *J Am Coll Cardiol* 19:394, 1992.

51. Wieland DM, Wu J-L, Brown LE, et al: Radiolabeled adrenergic neuron-blocking agents: adrenomedullary imaging with [131I]iodobenzylguanidine. *J Nucl Med* 21:349, 1980.

52. Wakasugi S, Wada A, Hasegawa Y, et al: Detection of abnormal cardiac adrenergic neuron activity in adriamycin-induced cardiomyopathy with iodine-125–metaiodobenzylguanidine. *J Nucl Med* 33:208, 1992.

53. Valdes Olmos RA, ten Bokkel Huinink WW, Greve JC, et al: I-123 MIBG and serial radionuclide angiocardiography in doxorubicin-related cardiotoxicity. *Clin Nucl Med* 17:163, 1992.

54. Ono M, Takahashi T: ^{123}I-MIBG scintigraphy in cardiotoxicity related to antineoplastic agents. *Jpn J Nucl Med* 31:451, 1994.

55. Estorch M, Carrio I, Berna L, et al: Indium-111–antimyosin scintigraphy after doxorubicin therapy in patients with advanced breast cancer. *J Nucl Med* 31:1965, 1990.

56. Carrio I, Estorch M, Berna L, et al: Assessment of anthracycline-induced myocardial damage by quantitative indium 111 myosin-specific monoclonal antibody studies. *Eur J Nucl Med* 18:806, 1991.

57. Carrio I, Estorch M, Berna L, et al: Indium-111–antimyosin and iodine-123–MIBG studies in early assessment of doxorubicin cardiotoxicity. *J Nucl Med* 36:2044, 1995.

58. Fowles RE, Mason JW: Endomyocardial biopsy. *Ann Intern Med* 97:885, 1982.

59. Strashun AM, Goldsmith SJ, Horowitz SF: Gated blood pool scintigraphic monitoring of doxorubicin cardiomyopathy: Comparison of camera and computerized probe results in 101 patients. *J Am Coll Cardiol* 8:1082, 1986.

60. Sarna GP, Holmes EC, Zbigniew P, et al: Lung cancer, in Haskell CM (ed): *Cancer Treatment*. Philadelphia, WB Saunders, 1985, pp 205–206.

61. Young RC, Ozols RF, Myers CE: The anthracycline antineoplastic drugs. *N Engl J Med* 305:139, 1981.

62. Myers CE, McGuire WP, Liss RH, et al: Adriamycin: The role of lipid peroxidation in cardiac toxicity and tumor response. *Science* 197:165, 1977.

63. Wang G, Finch MD, Trevan D, et al: Reduction of daunomycin toxicity by Razoxane. *Br J Cancer* 43:871, 1981.

64. Speyer JL, Green MD, Kramer E, et al: Protective effect of the bispiperazinedione ICRF-187 against doxorubicin-induced cardiac toxicity in women with advanced breast cancer. *N Engl J Med* 319:745,1988.

65. Speyer JL, Greer MD, Zelenieuch-Jagnotte A, et al: ICRF permits longer treatment with doxorubicin in women with breast cancer. *J Clin Oncol* 10:117, 1992.

66. Bu'Lock FA, Gabriel HM, Oakhill A, et al: Cardioprotection by ICRF187 against high dose anthracycline toxicity in children with malignant disease. *Br Heart J* 70:185, 1993.

67. Lipshultz SE, Colan SD, Mone SM, et al: Afterload reduction therapy in long term survivors of childhood cancer treated with doxorubicin. *Circulation* 84:II-659, 1991 (abstract).

68. Mortensen SA, Olsen HS, Baandrup U: Chronic anthracycline cardiotoxicity: Haemodynamic and histopathological manifestations suggesting a restrictive endomyocardial disease. *Br Heart J* 55:274, 1986.

69. Bu'Lock FA, Mott MG, Oakhill A, et al: Left ventricular diastolic function after anthracycline chemotherapy in childhood: Relation with systolic function, symptoms and pathophysiology. *Br Heart J* 73:340, 1995.

70. Steingart RM, Wexler JP, Blaufox MD: Pharmacologic intervention in cardiovascular nuclear medicine procedures. *Semin Nucl Med* 9:80, 1981.

71. Feldman AM, Bristow MR, Parmley WW, et al: Effects of vesnarinone on morbidity and mortality in patients with heart failure. *N Engl J Med* 329:149, 1993.

72. Goldberg MJ, Franklin BA, Rubenfire M, et al: Hydralazine therapy in severe chronic heart failure: Inability of

radionuclide left ventricular ejection fraction measurement to predict the hemodynamic response. *J Am Coll Cardiol* 2:887, 1983.

73. Haq A, Rakowski H, Baigrie R, et al: Vasodilator therapy in refractory congestive heart failure: A comparative analysis of hemodynamic and noninvasive studies. *Am J Cardiol* 49:439, 1982.

74. Firth BG, Dehmer GJ, Markham RV Jr, et al: Assessment of vasodilator therapy in patients with severe congestive heart failure: Limitations of measurements of left ventricular ejection fraction and volumes. *Am J Cardiol* 50:954, 1982.

75. Ritchie JL, Sorensen SG, Kennedy JW, et al: Radionuclide angiography: Noninvasive assessment of hemodynamic changes after administration of nitroglycerin. *Am J Cardiol* 43:278, 1979.

76. Sorensen SG, Ritchie JL, Caldwell JH, et al: Serial exercise radionuclide angiography: Validation of count-derived changes in cardiac output and quantitation of maximal exercise ventricular volume change after nitroglycerin and propranolol in normal men. *Circulation* 61:600, 1980.

77. Goldman SA, Johnson LL, Escala E, et al: Improved exercise ejection fraction with long-term prazosin therapy in patients with heart failure. *Am J Med* 68:36, 1980.

78. Colucci WS, Wynne J, Holman BL, et al: Long-term therapy of heart failure with prazosin: A randomized double blind trial. *Am J Cardiol* 45:337, 1980.

79. LeJemtel TH, Keung E, Ribner HS, et al: Sustained beneficial effects of oral amrinone on cardiac and renal function in patients with severe congestive heart failure. *Am J Cardiol* 45:123, 1980.

80. Awan NA, Evenson MK, Needham KE, et al: Efficacy of oral angiotensin-converting enzyme inhibition with captopril therapy in severe chronic normotensive congestive heart failure. *Am Heart J* 101:22, 1981.

81. Dzau VJ, Colucci WS, Williams GH, et al: Sustained effectiveness of converting-enzyme inhibition in patients with severe congestive heart failure. *N Engl J Med* 302:1373, 1980.

82. Arnold SB, Byrd RC, Meister W, et al: Long-term digitalis therapy improves left ventricular function in heart failure. *N Engl J Med* 303:1443, 1980.

83. Massie BM, Kramer BL, Topic N: Lack of relationship between the short-term hemodynamic effects of captopril and subsequent clinical responses. *Circulation* 69:1135, 1984.

84. Massie BM, Kramer BL, Topic N: Long-term captopril therapy for chronic congestive heart failure. *Am J Cardiol* 53:1316, 1984.

85. Levine TB, Franciosa JA, Cohn JN: Acute and long-term response to an oral converting-enzyme inhibitor, captopril, in congestive heart failure. *Circulation* 62:35, 1980.

86. Fouad FM, Tarazi RC, Bravo EL, et al: Long-term control of congestive heart failure with captopril. *Am J Cardiol* 49:1489, 1982.

87. Massie B, Kramer BL, Topic N, et al: Hemodynamic and radionuclide effects of acute captopril therapy for heart failure: Changes in left and right ventricular volumes and function at rest and during exercise. *Circulation* 65:1374, 1982.

88. Dehmer GJ, Lewis SE, Hillis LD, et al: Nongeometric determination of left ventricular volumes from equilibrium gated blood pool scans. *Am J Cardiol* 45:293, 1980.

89. Links JM, Becker LC, Shindledecker JG, et al: Measurement of absolute left ventricular volume from gated blood pool studies. *Circulation* 65:82, 1982.

90. Dehmer GJ, Firth BG, Lewis SE, et al: Direct measurement of cardiac output by gated equilibrium blood pool scintigraphy: Validation of scintigraphic volume measurements by a nongeometric technique. *Am J Cardiol* 47:1061, 1981.

91. Hindman MC, Slosky DA, Peter RH, et al: Rest and exercise hemodynamic effects of oral hydralazine in patients with coronary artery disease and left ventricular dysfunction. *Circulation* 61:751, 1980.

92. Poliner L, Twieg D, Parkey R, et al: Radionuclide angiographic and hemodynamic assessment of prazosin in patients with medically refractory heart failure. *Am J Cardiol* 43:403, 1979 (abstr).

92a. Loeb HS, Ostrenga JP, Gaul W, et al: Beneficial effects of dopamine combined with intravenous nitroglycerin on hemodynamics in patients with severe left ventricular failure. *Circulation* 68:813, 1983.

92b. Liang C-S, Sherman LG, Doherty JU, et al: Sustained improvement of cardiac function in patients with congestive heart failure after short-term infusion of dobutamine. *Circulation* 69:113, 1984.

93. Murray RG, Tweddel AC, Bastian BC, et al: The clinical value of digitalis therapy in cardiac failure. *Circulation* 62(suppl III):III-232, 1980 (abstr).

94. Firth BG, Dehmer GJ, Corbett JR, et al: Effect of chronic oral digoxin therapy on ventricular function at rest and peak exercise in patients with ischemic heart disease: Assessment with equilibrium gated blood pool imaging. *Am J Cardiol* 46:481, 1980.

95. Lam W, Pavel D, Byrom E, et al: Radionuclide regurgitant index: Value and limitations. *Am J Cardiol* 47:292, 1981.

96. Nicod P, Corbett JR, Firth BG, et al: Radionuclide techniques for valvular regurgitant index: Comparison in patients with normal and depressed ventricular function. *J Nucl Med* 23:763, 1982.

97. Rigo P, Alderson PO, Robertson RM, et al: Measurement of aortic and mitral regurgitation by gated cardiac blood pool scans. *Circulation* 60:306, 1979.

98. Salel AF, Berman DS, DeNardo GL, et al: Radionuclide assessment of nitroglycerin influence on abnormal left ventricular segmental contraction in patients with coronary heart disease. *Circulation* 53:975, 1976.

99. Borer JS, Bacharach SL, Green MV, et al: Effect of nitroglycerin on exercise-induced abnormalities of left ventricular regional function and ejection fraction in coronary artery disease: Assessment by radionuclide cineangiography in symptomatic and asymptomatic patients. *Circulation* 57:314, 1978.

100. Rozanski A, Berman D, Levy R, et al: Thallium-201 redistribution scintigraphy predicts the response to left ventricular asynergic segments to nitroglycerin administration. *Am J Cardiol* 47:484, 1981 (abstr).

101. Hellman C, Carpenter J, Blau F, et al: Myocardial viability: Assessment with first pass radionuclide angiography

following nitroglycerin. *J Nucl Med* 19:705, 1978 (abstr).

102. Marshall RC, Berger HJ, Reduto LA, et al: Assessment of cardiac performance with quantitative radionuclide angiocardiography: Effects of oral propranolol on global and regional left ventricular function in coronary artery disease. *Circulation* 58:808, 1978.

103. Wisenberg G, Marshall R, Schelbert H, et al: The effect of oral propranolol on left ventricular function at rest and during exercise in normals and in patients with coronary artery disease as determined by radionuclide angiography. *J Nucl Med* 20:639, 1979 (abstr).

104. Marshall R, Wisenberg G, Schelbert H, et al: Radionuclide evaluation of the effect of oral propranolol on left ventricular function during exercise in patients with coronary artery disease. *Am J Cardiol* 43:398, 1979 (abstr).

105. Berger H, Lachman A, Sands M, et al: Exercise left ventricular performance during high dose oral propranolol in coronary artery disease. *Circulation* 62(suppl III):III-202, 1980 (abstr).

106. Rainwater J, Steele P, Kirch D, et al: Effect of propranolol on myocardial perfusion images and exercise ejection fraction in men with coronary artery disease. *Circulation* 65:77, 1982.

107. Petru MA, Crawford MH, Sorensen SG, et al: Improvement of exercise left ventricular performance by high dose diltiazem in patients with angina due to fixed coronary artery disease. *Clin Res* 29:815A, 1981 (abstr).

108. Chew CYC, Hecht HS, Collett JT, et al: Influence of severity of ventricular dysfunction on hemodynamic responses to intravenously administered verapamil in ischemic heart disease. *Am J Cardiol* 47:917, 1981.

109. Reduto LA, Berger HJ, Geha A, et al: Radionuclide assessment of ventricular performance during propranolol withdrawal prior to aortocoronary bypass surgery. *Am Heart J* 96:714, 1978.

110. Slutsky R, Curtis G, Battler A, et al: Effect of sublingual nitroglycerin on left ventricular function at rest and during spontaneous angina pectoris: Assessment with a radionuclide approach. *Am J Cardiol* 44:1365, 1979.

111. McEwan MP, Berman ND, Morch JE, et al: Effect of intravenous and intracoronary nitroglycerin on left ventricular wall motion and perfusion in patients with coronary artery disease. *Am J Cardiol* 47:102, 1981.

112. Port S, Cobb FR, Jones RH: Effects of propranolol on left ventricular function in normal men. *Circulation* 61:358, 1980.

113. Marshall RC, Wisenberg G, Schelbert HR, et al: Effect of oral propranolol on rest, exercise and postexercise left ventricular performance in normal subjects and patients with coronary artery disease. *Circulation* 63:572, 1981.

114. Breisblatt WM, Vita NA, Armuchastegui M, et al: Usefulness of serial radionuclide monitoring during graded nitroglycerin infusion for unstable angina pectoris for determining left ventricular function and individualized therapeutic dose. *Am J Cardiol* 61:685, 1988.

115. Brown EJ, Wynne J, Holman BL, et al: Beneficial effect of beta-adrenergic blockade on regional left ventricular wall motion determined by radionuclide regional ejection fraction imaging. *Circulation* 62(suppl III):III-78, 1980 (abstr).

116. Pfisterer M, Glaus L, Burkart F: Comparative effects of nitroglycerin, nifedipine and metoprolol on regional left ventricular function in patients with one-vessel coronary disease. *Circulation* 67:291, 1983.

117. Nesto RW, White HD, Ganz P, et al: Addition of nifedipine to maximum beta-blocker and nitrate therapy: Divergent effects on global and regional left ventricular performance at rest and exercise. *Circulation* 70(suppl II):II-43, 1984 (abstr).

118. Gerson MC, Noble RJ, Wann LS, et al: Noninvasive documentation of Prinzmetal's angina. *Am J Cardiol* 43:329, 1979.

119. Buda AJ, Doherty PW, Goris ML, et al: The value of exercise thallium-201 myocardial perfusion imaging in differentiating subgroups of patients with coronary artery spasm. *Circulation* 57–58(suppl II):II-135, 1978 (abstr).

120. DiCarlo LA, Botvinick EH, Canhasi BS, et al: Value of noninvasive assessment of patients with atypical chest pain and suspected coronary spasm using ergonovine infusion and thallium-201 scintigraphy. *Am J Cardiol* 54:744, 1984.

121. Johnson SM, Mauritson DR, Corbett J, et al: Effects of verapamil and nifedipine on left ventricular function at rest and during exercise in patients with Prinzmetal's variant angina pectoris. *Am J Cardiol* 47:1289, 1981.

122. Borer JS, Bacharach SL, Green MV, et al: Real-time radionuclide cineangiography in the non-invasive evaluation of global and regional left ventricular function at rest and during exercise in patients with coronary artery disease. *N Engl J Med* 296:839, 1977.

123. Berger HJ, Reduto LA, Johnstone DE, et al: Global and regional left ventricular response to bicycle exercise in coronary artery disease: Assessment by quantitative radionuclide angiocardiography. *Am J Med* 66:13, 1979.

124. Caldwell JH, Hamilton GW, Sorenson SG, et al: The detection of coronary artery disease with radionuclide techniques: A comparison of rest–exercise thallium imaging and ejection fraction response. *Circulation* 61:610, 1980.

125. Waters DD, Theroux P, Szlachcic J, et al: Ergonovine testing in a coronary care unit. *Am J Cardiol* 46:922, 1980.

126. Buxton A, Goldberg S, Hirshfeld JW, et al: Refractory ergonovine-induced coronary vasospasm: Importance of intracoronary nitroglycerin. *Am J Cardiol* 46:329, 1980.

127. Buxton AE, Goldberg S, Harken A, et al: Coronary-artery spasm immediately after myocardial revascularization: Recognition and management. *N Engl J Med* 304:1249, 1981.

128. Gottdiener JS, DiBianco R, Fletcher RD, et al: Effects of disopryamide on left ventricular function: Assessment by radionuclide cineangiography. *Circulation* 62(suppl III):III- 147, 1980 (abstr).

129. Kowey P, Friedman P, Podrid P, et al: Use of radionuclide ventriculography for assessment of changes in myocar-

dial performance induced by disopryamide phosphate. *Circulation* 62(suppl III):III-231, 1980 (abstr).

130. Wisenberg G, Zawadowski AG, Gebhardt VA, et al: Effects on ventricular function of disopyramide, procainamide and quinidine as determined by radionuclide angiography. *Am J Cardiol* 53:1292, 1984.

131. Smitherman TC, Gottlich CM, Narahara KA, et al: Myocardial contractility in patients with ischemic heart disease during long-term administration of quinidine and procainamide. *Chest* 76:552, 1979.

132. Sugrue DD, Dickie S, Myers MJ, et al: Effect of amiodarone on left ventricular ejection and filling in hypertrophic cardiomyopathy as assessed by radionuclide angiography. *Am J Cardiol* 54:1054, 1984.

133. Stein J, Podrid P, Lown B: Effects of oral mexilitine on left and right ventricular function. *Am J Cardiol* 54:575, 1984.

134. Veith RC, Raskind MA, Caldwell JH, et al: Cardiovascular effects of tricyclic antidepressants in depressed patients with chronic heart disease. *N Engl J Med* 306:954, 1982.

135. Shah PK, Berman D, Pichler M, et al: Improved global and regional ventricular performance with nitroprusside in acute myocardial infarction. *J Nucl Med* 20:640, 1979 (abstr).

136. Rainwater JO, Jensen DP, Vogel RA, et al: Effects of chronic digitalis administration on exercise ventricular performance and myocardial perfusion images in coronary disease. *Am J Cardiol* 43:433, 1979 (abstr).

137. Matthay RA, Berger HJ, Loke J, et al: Effects of aminophylline upon right and left ventricular performance in chronic obstructive pulmonary disease. *Am J Med* 65:903, 1978.

138. Hooper W, Slutsky R, Kocienski D, et al: The effect of terbutaline on right and left ventricular function and size in obstructive lung disease. *Am J Cardiol* 47:491, 1981 (abstr).

139. Olvey SK, Reduto LA, Deaton WJ, et al: First pass radionuclide assessment of right and left ventricular performance in chronic hypoxic lung disease: Effect of oxygen upon exercise reserve. *Clin Res* 27:192A, 1979 (abstr).

140. Whitlow PL, Rogers WJ, Smith LR, et al: Enhancement of left ventricular function by glucose–insulin–potassium infusion in acute myocardial infarction. *Am J Cardiol* 49:811, 1982.

141. Bianco JA, Laskey WK, Makey DG, et al: Angiotensin infusion effects on left ventricular function: Assessment in normal subjects and in patients with coronary disease. *Chest* 77:172, 1980.

142. Blaufox MD, Wexler JP, Sherman RA, et al: Left ventricular ejection fraction and its response to therapy in essential hypertension. *Nephron* 28:112, 1981.

143. Giles R, Berger H, Barash P, et al: Profound alterations in left ventricular performance during anesthesia induction for coronary surgery detected with the computerized nuclear probe. *Circulation* 62(suppl III):III-146, 1980 (abstr).

CLINICAL APPLICATIONS

Selection of Noninvasive Tests in the Emergency Room and in the Coronary Care Unit

Myron C. Gerson
Daniel J. Lenihan

Management of patients with acute myocardial infarction has changed dramatically over the past two decades. Previously, the approach to the patient with acute myocardial infarction was largely supportive. Coronary care units (CCUs) provided an environment in which arrhythmic and hemodynamic complications of acute myocardial infarction could be identified, monitored, and treated. Treatment of the patient with acute myocardial infarction has now evolved from a supportive role to a role of acute intervention, designed to restore coronary artery blood flow and preserve jeopardized myocardium. Patients in the early hours of a myocardial infarction have been approached with thrombolytic drugs, acute percutaneous transluminal coronary angioplasty (PTCA), and, in some cases, emergent coronary artery bypass surgery. Based on evidence that nearly 90 percent of acute myocardial infarctions are related to intracoronary thrombosis,[1] large cooperative studies have documented that restoration of vessel patency during the initial hours of myocardial infarction can reduce mortality[2-5] as well as the extent of left ventricular dysfunction after myocardial infarction.[6-8]

This new emphasis in the treatment of acute myocardial infarction has created many challenges for the field of nuclear cardiology. Nuclear cardiology procedures are needed that can accurately predict whether a patient presenting to the emergency room with chest pain has a noncardiac source of symptoms, appropriate for outpatient evaluation, or whether an acute ischemic syndrome is present and requires prompt inpatient evaluation. Patients who have evidence of evolving myocardial in-

farction would likely benefit from a rapid noninvasive test that can accurately determine whether the infarct-associated artery is patent or occluded and whether substantial residual viable myocardium is present.[9] This may be particularly important following thrombolytic therapy when emergent angiography and intervention may be considerably more risky.[10]

This chapter examines the role of cardiac nuclear medicine in the thrombolytic era. The traditional roles for radionuclide studies in the patient with acute myocardial infarction are also examined in terms of infarct identification, sizing, localization, detection of complications, and assessment of prognosis. The role of nuclear cardiology is examined in a context of other noninvasive tests including electrocardiography, cardiac enzyme measurement, and echocardiography.

ELECTROCARDIOGRAPHY IN ASSESSMENT OF ACUTE MYOCARDIAL INFARCTION

The electrocardiogram (ECG) is an inexpensive and readily available tool for the early diagnosis of acute myocardial infarction.[11-23] In a study of 3697 patients presenting with at least 30 min of chest pain, Rude et al[11] showed that new pathologic Q waves or ST-segment elevation provided good prediction of enzymatic myocardial necrosis, whereas left bundle branch block or depression of the ST segment did not. The diagnostic correlation between occlusion of the left anterior descending (LAD) coronary artery and ECG changes in the anterior precordial leads has been reported to be 90 percent.[18] In the instance of right coronary artery occlusion, diagnostic ECG changes have been detected in leads III and aVF in 70 to 90 percent of patients.[18-20] Proximal occlusion of the right coronary artery is also associated with right ventricular myocardial infarction, which is suggested when there is ST-segment elevation in lead V_{4R} or V_1.[21-23] Occlusion of the circumflex coronary artery is the most electrocardiographically silent of the occlusions in the coronary system; diagnostic ECG changes in the lateral leads were seen in approximately 50 percent of the patients.[18,19] Conversely, the ECG may falsely suggest the presence of acute myocardial infarction with a "pseudoinfarction" pattern in patients with left ventricular hypertrophy, left bundle branch block, Wolff-Parkinson-White syndrome, pulmonary embolus, intracranial hemorrhage, or hyperkalemia.[17]

Numerous investigators have evaluated the clinical significance and prognosis of infarct type when classified into Q-wave versus non-Q-wave infarction. Correlation between the presence or absence of pathologic Q waves on the ECG with the transmural or nontransmural extent of infarction has been poor.[24-26] In most studies, the short-term mortality in patients with non-Q-wave myocardial infarction has been about half that observed in patients with Q-wave infarction.[27] This finding appears to reflect the lower peak total creatine kinase (CK), higher left ventricular ejection fraction (LVEF), and smaller infarct size in patients with non-Q-wave, compared to Q-wave, infarction. However, patients with non-Q-wave myocardial infarction often have more residual jeopardized myocardium than patients with Q-wave infarction, leading to a higher reinfarction rate in the former group. Among patients with infarction Q waves, those with anterior myocardial infarction have a higher mortality than those with an inferior infarction in the majority of series.

PLASMA ENZYMES IN THE DIAGNOSIS OF MYOCARDIAL INFARCTION

Measurement of cardiac enzymes in the serum is fundamental to the diagnosis of acute myocardial infarction. In patients treated with thrombolytic therapy, cardiac enzyme levels can often confirm that successful myocardial reperfusion has occurred. Traditional serologic markers of cardiac enzyme release include CK, aspartate transaminase, and lactic dehydrogenase. The isoenzymes and subforms of CK provide sensitive and specific markers for acute myocardial infarction and for successful myocardial reperfusion.

The isoenzymes of CK are found in three major organ systems—CK-MM is predominantly found in mature skeletal muscle, CK-BB in brain tissue, and CK-MB in cardiac muscle. The CK-MB isoenzyme constitutes approximately 15 to 20 percent of cytosolic CK in mature human myocardium. The remaining 80 percent is CK-MM. Isoenzyme CK-MB is present in small quantities in tissues other than myocardium including small intestine, uterus, prostate, tongue, and diaphragm. Therefore, a patient with trauma or a surgical procedure that involves one of these organs may have release of CK-MB into the serum, thus possibly causing misdiagnosis of a myocardial infarction.[28] The patient who presents with acute cerebral ischemic or hemorrhagic stroke may also present diagnostic difficulties. The differentiating point between CK-MB released at the time of a stroke and that of acute myocardial infarction is the timing of the rise and fall of cardiac enzymes. In stroke, there is a slow and progressive rise in CK-MB until the fourth to sixth day,[29,30] whereas in acute myocardial infarction the peak CK value usually occurs between 18 and 24 h after onset of symptoms with a relatively rapid decline. Other factors that may alter CK time release patterns in acute myocardial infarction include reperfusion following thrombolysis, which causes accelerated washout, and renal failure, which may cause persistently elevated CK levels.

The use of CK-MB for the diagnosis of acute myocardial infarction provides a sensitive and specific marker.[31,32] However, blood levels of CK-MB often remain in the normal range for the first 8 to 10 h following onset of acute myocardial infarction.[33,34] The use of CK isoforms has shown promise in the early diagnosis of myocardial infarction and in the prediction of reperfusion following thrombolytic therapy.[33,35-42]

Both CK-MM and CK-MB exist in tissue and plasma isoforms. Release of CK-MB isoforms into the circulation is believed to be more specific for myocardial necrosis than is release of CK-MM isoforms, but both isoforms may be released with either cardiac or skeletal muscle injury. The CK-MB isoforms in the plasma are equally divided between CK-MB$_2$ (the tissue form) and CK-MB$_1$ (the plasma form) and amount to only 0.5 to 1.0 IU/liter of each form under baseline conditions in normal individuals.[33] Relatively small increments in the CK isoform MB$_2$ appearing in the plasma may lead to detection of acute myocardial infarction. A ratio of CK-MB$_2$ to CK-MB$_1$ of 1.5 or greater in the plasma has been reported to provide reliable diagnosis of acute myocardial infarction, increasing from a sensitivity within 2 h of onset of symptoms of 12 percent to 59 percent at 2 to 4 h and 92 percent at 4 to 6 h.[37] Although it has been stated that CK isoforms provide significantly more rapid diagnosis of acute myocardial infarction than by conventional measurement of CK-MB enzyme activity curves,[37] comparison of CK isoform diagnosis to direct measurement of CK-MB mass by immunodiffusion (rather than CK-MB enzymatic activity) has provided comparable early diagnosis of acute myocardial infarction in some studies.[39]

Enzymes other than CK have proved helpful in establishing the diagnosis of acute myocardial infarction. Lactic dehydrogenase begins to elevate approximately 10 h after onset of clinical symptoms and peaks at 24 to 48 h. Lactic dehydrogenase and its isoenzymes are occasionally useful late in the presentation of acute myocardial infarction, at a time when CK levels may have already returned to baseline.

For ruling out acute myocardial infarction in the emergency room, one group of authors[36] found a measurement of plasma myoglobin, obtained between 3 and 6 h following onset of chest pain, to have a negative predictive value for acute myocardial infarction of 89 percent. Myoglobin was significantly more sensitive for identification of myocardial infarction in the 3- to 6-h post-onset time frame compared to measurement of CK-MB mass or troponin T. However, others found no similar advantage with a plasma myoglobin assay.[39] The absence of myoglobin in the plasma at 6 h following the onset of chest pain may help to exclude acute myocardial infarction, but the presence of myoglobin is nonspecific and may reflect skeletal muscle injury.

Troponin consists of three cardiac-specific components that regulate the interaction of actin and myosin during the cardiac cycle. Troponin T and troponin I plasma measurements can provide accurate diagnosis of acute myocardial infarction, but current assay methods have not provided any clear advantage for early infarct detection compared to assessment of CK-MB mass, CK isoforms, or plasma myoglobin.[36,39]

In summary, measurements of CK-MB mass, myoglobin, CK isoforms, and troponin T and I can all provide accurate diagnosis of acute myocardial infarction. None is diagnostic with sufficient rapidity to influence the decision in most patients to start thrombolytic drug therapy. All provide sufficient diagnostic accuracy by 6 to 8 h after onset of chest pain for use in excluding a diagnosis of acute myocardial infarction in the emergency room, but no single cardiac enzyme method has been shown to perform best in this setting. For purposes of evaluating noninvasive imaging modalities in the diagnosis of acute myocardial infarction, measurement of CK-MB provides a practical "gold standard." Pathologic correlation, although more definitive, favors the generation of study series with relatively large and complicated infarcts.

ECHOCARDIOGRAPHY IN ASSESSMENT OF ACUTE MYOCARDIAL INFARCTION

Echocardiography provides a convenient method for rapidly evaluating the patient with acute cardiac symptoms in the emergency room, the cardiac catheterization laboratory, or the CCU. Two-dimensional echocardiography provides not only detection and quantification of regional wall-motion abnormalities but also assessment of cardiac chamber size, global ventricular function, cardiac valvular structure, pericardial visualization, and assessment of regional wall motion in complications of acute myocardial infarction. Doppler echocardiography and color flow imaging provide assessments of regurgitant valvular abnormalities, cardiac shunts, and elevated pulmonary artery pressure, which may develop as complications of myocardial infarction.

One of the principal echocardiographic methods for detecting myocardial ischemia is by demonstrating wall motion abnormalities in the ischemic segment.[43-59] The occurrence of such abnormalities almost immediately after the onset of myocardial ischemia was first described by Tennant and Wiggers in 1935.[43] More recently, PTCA has allowed clinical documentation of reversible regional myocardial dysfunction in response to sudden coronary artery occlusion.[60,61] In patients who undergo acute coronary artery occlusion in the setting of PTCA, Labovitz et al[60] have documented a sequence of ischemic manifestations consisting of left ventricular diastolic impairment followed by systolic impairment and then angina. The ECG changes suggestive of ischemia preceded systolic wall-motion abnormality in the study of Labovitz, but in numerous other studies systolic regional wall-motion abnormality has preceded ECG changes.[61]

In evaluating the left ventricle for findings that may be secondary to ischemia, wall-thickening abnormalities may also be noted.[62-67] However, there continues to be no consensus on the use of endocardial wall motion versus wall thickening as the most appropriate echocardiographic index of ischemic dysfunction. Regardless of whether impaired regional wall motion or abnormal myocardial thickening is considered, two-dimensional echocardiography will generally overestimate myocardial infarct size.[68-72] This may result from the "tethering" effect of infarcted myocardial walls on motion of normally perfused adjacent myocardium.[68] More frequently, echocardiographic overestimation of infarct size results from adjacent severely hypokinetic or akinetic segments containing viable ("stunned") myocardium.

Echocardiography may be used to assist in the initial diagnosis of acute myocardial infarction. Heger et al[49] evaluated 44 patients who were admitted to the hospital with acute Q-wave myocardial infarction. Complete echocardiographic studies were performed on 37 of these patients within 48 h of admission. Segmental wall-motion abnormalities were identified in each of the 37 patients and correlation to location of ECG findings was excellent.

Patients with typical chest pain and Q-wave myocardial infarction on ECG rarely present diagnostic difficulty. It is the patient who presents with non-Q-wave myocardial infarction, left bundle branch block, or paced rhythm for whom an accurate echocardiographic diagnosis of myocardial infarction would be most helpful.[56,73-76] To confirm or exclude acute myocardial infarction, Loh et al[56] evaluated 30 patients with an acute chest pain syndrome but no ST-segment elevation or Q waves on the initial ECG. Using the presence of severe hypokinesis as the criterion for an abnormal echocardiographic study, 10 of 12 patients (83 percent) with subsequent enzymatic documentation of acute non-Q-wave myocardial infarction and 18 of 18 patients (100 percent) without acute myocardial infarction were correctly identified. Arvan and Varat[76] studied 50 patients with acute chest pain and a possible acute non-Q-wave myocardial infarction. The presence or absence of non-Q-wave myocardial infarction was subsequently established by serial measurement of CK-MB fraction. The sensitivity and specificity of the two-dimensional echocardiogram for identifying a non-Q-wave myocardial infarction were 66 percent and 91 percent, respectively. Therefore, the diagnosis of myocardial infarction by two-dimensional echocardiography appears to be less accurate for non-Q-wave than for Q-wave myocardial infarction.

Overall, the echocardiogram provides many advantages in the examination of the patient with chest pain. These include rapid availability, brief imaging time, relatively low cost, excellent visualization of regional myocardial contraction, and potential for quantitation of global and regional left ventricular function. As discussed later in this chapter, echocardiography is the procedure of choice for detection of many of the complications of acute myocardial infarction and also provides useful prognostic information. The principal limitation of echocardiography in acute myocardial infarction relates to its inability to determine whether left ventricular dysfunction is related to acute myocardial necrosis, old myocardial necrosis, myocardial ischemia, or "stunned myocardium."

RADIONUCLIDE STUDIES IN ACUTE MYOCARDIAL INFARCTION

Technetium Pyrophosphate Infarct-Avid Imaging

Infarct-avid imaging with technetium 99m (^{99m}Tc) pyrophosphate is based on the observation that calcium is deposited in irreversibly damaged myocardial cells.[77] The ^{99m}Tc pyrophosphate is taken up by bone and, under certain pathologic conditions, by myocardial structures containing crystalline or amorphous calcium phosphate. In acute myocardial infarction, ^{99m}Tc pyrophosphate uptake may be present 12 to 24 h postinfarction, but more

BLOOD POOL   3 HOUR DELAY

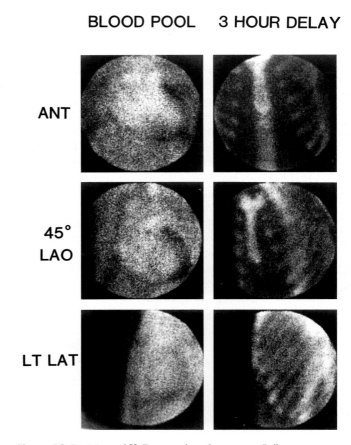

Figure 18-1 Normal ^{99m}Tc pyrophosphate scan. Following intravenous ^{99m}Tc- pyrophosphate injection, the right and left ventricular blood pools are demonstrated in multiple projections. The appearance of the ventricular blood pools can be used to guide localization of pyrophosphate activity in the heart on delayed images. Three hours following tracer injection, the osseous structures of the thorax are clearly visualized without evidence of ^{99m}Tc pyrophosphate activity in the myocardium. ANT, anterior; LAO, left anterior oblique; LT LAT, left lateral.

intense myocardial activity is usually observed at 24 to 72 h (Figs. 18-1 and 18-2). Presumably, this relates to delayed time to calcium deposition in damaged myocardium and delayed time to development of sufficient myocardial blood flow to deliver the tracer to the infarct region. Pyrophosphate delivery is greatest to damaged myocardial regions with a reduction of coronary blood flow to 20 to 40 percent of that in normal regions. Pyrophosphate accumulation in the central necrotic zone may be minimal.[79-82] Using tomographic imaging to measure ^{99m}Tc pyrophosphate activity in dogs following coronary artery ligation, good correlation of scintigraphic infarct size and anatomic infarct weight has been observed ($r = 0.98$).[83] However, the correlation was weaker ($r = 0.81$) for infarcts involving less than 10 g of myocardium. It has been reported that as little as 1 g of myocardial necrosis in an animal model may be detectable as ^{99m}Tc pyrophosphate myocardial activity when imaged by single photon emission computed tomography (SPECT).[83-85]

More controversial has been the uptake of ^{99m}Tc pyrophosphate in ischemic but noninfarcted myocardium. In an early report, Willerson et al[86] found evidence of ^{99m}Tc pyrophosphate activity in 7 of 101 patients presenting with chest pain but in whom myocardial infarction was subsequently ruled out. All 7 patients had unstable angina. Uptake of ^{99m}Tc pyrophosphate was diffuse rather than focal in distribution and was mild in intensity. Several groups of investigators have demonstrated in animal models that ^{99m}Tc pyrophosphate is accumulated in myocardial segments subjected to severe ischemia followed by reperfusion.[87-89] In a resultant setting of "stunned myocardium," focal accumulation of ^{99m}Tc pyrophosphate was two to four times greater than tracer activity in nonischemic zones. Nevertheless, tracer activity was significantly less in stunned myocardium compared to the 14- to 17-fold increase in ^{99m}Tc pyrophosphate activity observed in infarcted myocardium. This may account for identification of diffuse, mild ^{99m}Tc pyrophosphate activity in some patients with unstable angina,[86,90] whereas focal uptake of tracer in the absence of myocardial infarction has been noted only infrequently in humans.[91]

Following ^{99m}Tc pyrophosphate injection, cardiac imaging is delayed at least 3 h to allow clearance of the tracer from the cardiac blood pool. Images are collected in multiple planar projections or using SPECT with or without subtraction of blood pool activity.[92] Normal planar ^{99m}Tc pyrophosphate cardiac images (see Fig. 18-1) clearly delineate the bony structures of the thorax, with no tracer activity in the region of the myocardium. Abnormal pyrophosphate activity in the area of the heart may be focal (see Fig. 18-2) and localizable to a myocardial region or may be diffuse throughout the ventricular myocardium. The latter pattern of diffuse myocardial

activity must be differentiated from residual tracer activity in the cardiac blood pools. The intensity of myocardial tracer activity is graded as minimal (1+), definite but less than bony uptake (2+), equal to bony uptake (3+), or greater than bony uptake (4+), with specification of a focal or diffuse pattern.

Wynne and Holman[93] tabulated the results from 22 reported series consisting of 935 patients having, in most cases, historical, ECG, and enzymatic criteria for myocardial infarction. They found an overall sensitivity of the ^{99m}Tc pyrophosphate scan of 93 percent. A high level of diagnostic sensitivity is dependent on optimal timing of pyrophosphate imaging—usually 2 to 5 days following the onset of infarction. Therefore, in patients presenting late following onset of acute myocardial infarction, at a time when serum levels of cardiac enzymes may have already returned to baseline, ^{99m}Tc pyrophosphate may be particularly helpful for identification of acute myocardial infarction.[94]

The sensitivity of ^{99m}Tc pyrophosphate imaging is greater in myocardial infarcts associated with pathologic Q waves, compared to non-Q-wave infarcts.[95-98] This probably reflects the larger size of Q-wave infarcts, because infarcts involving less than 3 g of myocardium are frequently not detected by planar pyrophosphate imaging methods. The calculated sensitivity also varies depending on the diagnostic criteria used for the radionuclide diagnosis of infarction. Focal myocardial ^{99m}Tc pyrophosphate activity localized to one or more myocardial segments is fairly specific for myocardial infarction. If the diffuse pattern of ^{99m}Tc pyrophosphate activity in the region of the heart is accepted as a criterion for acute myocardial infarction, additional infarcts will be detected, but numerous conditions other than acute myocardial infarction may also produce abnormality.

The reported sensitivity of the ^{99m}Tc pyrophosphate scan for detection of acute non-Q-wave myocardial in-

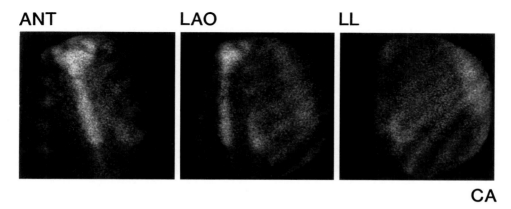

Figure 18-2 Technetium 99m pyrophosphate images obtained 2 days following onset of chest pain in a man with enzymatic documentation of acute myocardial infarction. Abnormal focal pyrophosphate uptake is present in the apex, anterior, and septal walls of the left ventricle. (From Gerson,[78] reproduced with permission.)

ANT   LAO   LL

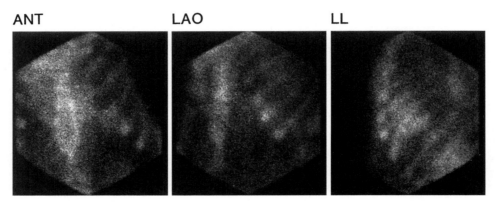

Figure 18-3 Accumulation of ^{99m}Tc pyrophosphate in skeletal muscle following direct-current cardioversion. Activity located along the upper left parasternal area on the anterior view and the lateral chest wall on the left lateral view corresponds to the location of the cardioversion paddles. The absence of abnormal tracer accumulation in the region of the heart on the left anterior oblique view aids in making the correct diagnosis from the scintigrams. The CK-MB fraction and ECG changes of acute myocardial infarction were absent. (From Gerson,[78] reproduced with permission.)

farction has varied widely.[95-98] An early report[99] documented focal ^{99m}Tc pyrophosphate uptake in 6 patients and 2+ diffuse uptake in 11 patients from a group of 17 individuals with non-Q-wave myocardial infarction. A different series[97] noted focal or diffuse ^{99m}Tc pyrophosphate uptake in just 52 percent of 31 patients who had non-Q-wave acute myocardial infarction by ECG and CK-MB fraction criteria. Detection of many patients with non-Q-wave myocardial infarction has required acceptance of diffuse ^{99m}Tc pyrophosphate uptake as clinically useful evidence of acute myocardial infarction.[96]

Wynne and Holman[93] compiled a specificity for the ^{99m}Tc pyrophosphate scan in acute myocardial infarction of 83 percent among 1334 patients. Focal ^{99m}Tc pyrophosphate activity usually corresponds to acute myocardial infarction but may be observed in areas of old myocardial infarction.[100-103] After acute myocardial infarction, most areas of ^{99m}Tc pyrophosphate activity can be expected to resolve within 1 month.[104] Technetium pyrophosphate activity in an area of old myocardial scar would be expected to change little on a follow-up study several weeks later. Several other conditions have been reported to produce or simulate focal ^{99m}Tc pyrophosphate activity in the region of the myocardium, including valvular calcification,[105] fibrosis surrounding prosthetic valves,[106] electrical cardioversion[107-111] (Fig. 18-3), cardiac contusion,[112,113] high voltage electrical injury,[114] or invasion of the myocardium by metastatic tumor.[115] Focal uptake of ^{99m}Tc pyrophosphate has been observed with acute pericarditis,[116] although accompanying myocarditis may be responsible for ^{99m}Tc pyrophosphate activity in some of these cases.

Specificity of the diffuse pattern of ^{99m}Tc pyrophosphate activity in the region of the heart appears to be low. Prasquier et al[117] observed diffuse ^{99m}Tc pyrophosphate

uptake of 2+ or greater intensity in the region of the heart in 70 of 483 (14.4 percent) patients during routine bone scans. However, exclusion of the diffuse pattern as a criterion for myocardial infarction will lower the sensitivity of planar ^{99m}Tc pyrophosphate studies to approximately 66 percent.[118]

Infarct-Avid Imaging with Labeled Antimyosin Antibodies

Radiolabeled antimyosin monoclonal antibodies and their Fab fragments are highly specific markers of myocardial necrosis,[119-125] and may more accurately delineate infarct size[126,127] compared to ^{99m}Tc pyrophosphate scanning.[88,128] When introduced into the extracellular space, radiolabeled antimyosin antibodies can enter through the interrupted cell membrane of an irreversibly damaged myocyte and attach to myosin molecules. Because myosin heavy chains are relatively insoluble in extracellular fluid, they remain inside the irreversibly damaged myocyte and are available for antimyosin binding. The high concentration of myosin in the heart results in extensive availability for interaction with antimyosin antibodies in irreversibly damaged myocardium.

Antimyosin antibodies have been produced by fusing immunized mouse spleen cells with myeloma cells to form a hybridoma capable of producing monoclonal antimyosin. To improve blood pool clearance and the ratio of target to nontarget activity, the antibodies are split into Fab fragments by papain digestion. The resultant Fab fragment is then complexed to the chelating agent diethylene triamine pentaacetic acid (DTPA),[119] which facilitates binding to 2 mCi of indium 111 (^{111}In). Following intravenous injection of ^{111}In antimyosin, there is an initial blood pool phase. At 16 to 48 h following injection, imaging can be performed with a medium energy collimator, accumulating 1 million counts per view in multiple planar projections. Alternatively, images may be acquired in a tomographic format.

Appropriate application of ^{111}In antimyosin as an infarct-avid tracer requires documentation that the tracer is taken up into necrotic myocytes only. This documentation has been provided by electron microscopy studies in which microspheres coated with antibodies specific for myosin were observed to attach in large numbers to irreversibly damaged myocytes with a disrupted cell membrane. Few or no antimyosin-coated microspheres adhered to myocardial cells with intact cell membranes.[120] In a canine model, Khaw et al[121] showed that regions of myocardial infarction defined by triphenyl–tetrazolium chloride staining corresponded to the region of myosin antibody fragment uptake. Coronary occlusion without histochemical or histologic evidence for infarction did not lead to the accumulation of antimyosin antibody fragments.

Myocardial distribution of ^{111}In antimyosin and ^{99m}Tc pyrophosphate has been compared in animal models of acute myocardial infarction with or without coronary reperfusion. The results of these studies have at times been conflicting.[123,125] Beller et al[122] compared myocardial uptake of iodine 125 (^{125}I)-labeled antimyosin fragments and ^{99m}Tc pyrophosphate in dogs with ligation of the LAD coronary artery. Maximal uptake of labeled antimyosin fragments was located in the subendocardial region of the center of the infarct, where regional myocardial flow measured by microspheres was most severely impaired (1 to 10 percent of normal). In contrast, ^{99m}Tc pyrophosphate was concentrated in the subepicardium in samples taken from the periphery of the myocardial infarct, where flow was 31 to 50 percent of normal. In a canine reperfused myocardial infarct model, Khaw et al[123] showed that intravenous ^{99m}Tc pyrophosphate overestimated myocardial infarct size as established by triphenyl–tetrazolium chloride staining but ^{111}In antimyosin fragment imaging did not. These findings confirm reports by Bianco et al[88] and Gerber and Higgins,[128] who observed uptake of ^{99m}Tc pyrophosphate into myocardium that was determined to be noninfarcted by triphenyl–tetrazolium chloride staining. Thus, it appears that labeled antimyosin fragments may offer an advantage compared to ^{99m}Tc pyrophosphate for imaging of acute myocardial infarction, because antimyosin may be taken up more specifically by irreversibly damaged myocytes and because antimyosin distribution correlates more closely with the distribution of necrotic myocardial cells in the infarct region.[129]

Several studies have examined the accuracy of ^{111}In antimyosin imaging for detection of acute myocardial infarction in humans.[130-134] The sensitivity of ^{111}In antimyosin imaging for detection of acute Q-wave myocardial infarction in 372 patients presenting with prolonged chest pain was 95 percent. More limited experience with this technique is available in patients with non-Q-wave myocardial infarction. Among 72 such patients, the sensitivity of ^{111}In antimyosin for infarct detection was 86 percent.[131,132,134] Antimyosin imaging in patients with stable chest pain and no evidence of acute myocardial infarction is also limited, but among 48 such patients, the reported specificity was 92 percent.[132,134] However, in the preliminary report of a multicenter trial of antimyosin imaging, Berger et al[132] noted that 21 of 44 patients with unstable angina (48 percent) had focal uptake of ^{111}In antimyosin that was indistinguishable from that in acute myocardial infarction. Interpretation of the results of that large multicenter trial is made difficult by the fact that in 30 percent of patients entered into the study, no conclusive determination could be made from the clinical data concerning the presence or absence of myocardial necrosis.

Available studies suggest that acute myocardial necrosis may be readily detected with antimyosin imaging in either anterior or inferoposterior myocardial infarction (Figs. 18-4 and 18-5). However, ^{111}In antimyosin uptake has generally been more faint on planar images in inferior compared to anterior infarcts. Antimyosin uptake is thought to be relatively specific for acute as opposed to remote myocardial necrosis. In one study, the heart-to-lung ratio of ^{111}In antimyosin uptake decreased from 1.93 ± 0.51 at 24 h to 1.77 ± 0.025 between 4 and 15 days, to 1.54 ± 0.12 between 50 and 100 days, and to 1.42 ± 0.16 between 125 and 270 days following onset of acute myocardial infarction. The corresponding ratio in controls was 1.24 ± 0.11.[135] Abnormal antimyosin uptake could be documented up to 154 days postinfarction. In data from Tamaki et al,[136] 7 of 11 patients with antimyosin imaging 2 weeks to 9 months following acute myocardial infarction had focal antimyosin uptake in the region of prior myocardial infarction. Yamada et al[137] observed ^{111}In antimyosin activity in 71 percent of 14 patients studied 1.5 months to 1 year following acute myocardial infarction. Qualitative antimyosin uptake in acute myocardial infarction in humans does not appear to depend strongly on the presence or absence of a patent infarct-related artery. Uptake of ^{111}In antimyosin has been documented in acute myocardial infarcts in humans when the associated coronary artery is persistently occluded, when the artery becomes patent following thrombolysis, or when the infarct-associated artery opens spontaneously.[131] Nevertheless, canine studies of ^{111}In antimyosin uptake in experimental acute myocardial infarction have suggested that measures of quantitative tracer uptake may be dependent on the level of residual myocardial blood flow to the infarct zone.[138,139]

Imaging with radiolabeled antimyosin has shown substantial promise for detection of ongoing cell necrosis

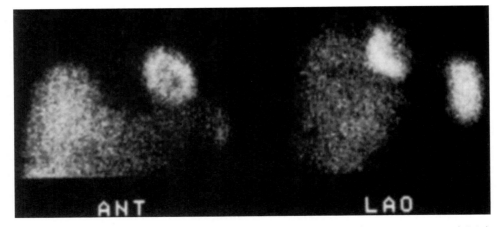

Figure 18-4   Anterior (*left*) and 45° left anterior oblique (LAO) (*right*) images acquired 26 h following injection of ^{111}In antimyosin in a patient with an acute anteroseptal myocardial infarction and successful reperfusion therapy. (From Khaw et al,[131] Acute myocardial infarct imaging with indium-111 labeled monoclonal antimyosin Fab, reprinted with permission from the *Journal of Nuclear Medicine* 28:1671, 1987.)

in patients with myocarditis,[140–146] including those with underlying systemic disorders including systemic lupus erythematosus,[147] polymyositis,[148] sarcoidosis,[149] Lyme disease,[150] Churg-Strauss vasculitis,[151] acute rheumatic fever,[152] and pheochromocytoma[153]; those with myocardial toxicity induced by drugs including doxorubicin[154–156]; and tricyclic antidepressants[157]; in cardiomyopathy[158–163]; and in rejection of a cardiac transplant.[140,164–171] Although these represent potentially important clinical roles for radiolabeled antimyosin, these observations also suggest that antimyosin imaging will not be specific for acute myocardial necrosis related to

coronary artery occlusion in patients with other ongoing processes—including hypertrophic cardiomyopathy,[159,172,173] myocarditis,[140–142,174] and dilated cardiomyopathy[158]—that could result in myocyte necrosis.

More recent advances in the development of antimyosin tracers have included the use of smaller monoclonal antibody fragments, antibodies with altered molecular charge designed to improve tracer distribution in target and nontarget tissues,[175–177] and antibodies labeled with ^{99m}Tc.[178–181] Because antimyosin antibody is a potentially immunogenic protein, removal of the immunogenic portions of the molecule is desirable even though allergic

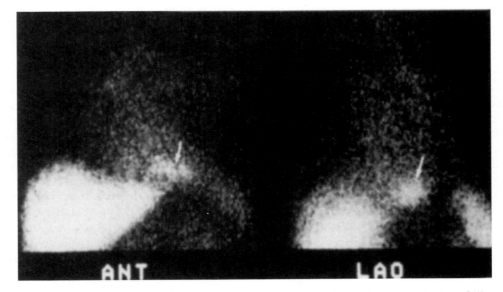

Figure 18-5   Anterior (*left*) and 45° LAO (*right*) images acquired 25 h following injection of ^{111}In antimyosin in a patient with an acute inferior myocardial infarction (*arrows*) and successful reperfusion therapy. (From Khaw et al,[131] Acute myocardial infarct imaging with indium-111 labeled monoclonal antimyosin Fab, reprinted with permission from the *Journal of Nuclear Medicine* 28:1671, 1987.)

reactions to antimyosin have not been described in available series to date.[130,131,133,134] Replacement of ^{111}In antimyosin with [99mTc] antimyosin is potentially advantageous for numerous reasons.

1. [99mTc] is less expensive than [111]In.
2. [99mTc] antimyosin has been reported to clear from the cardiac blood pools more rapidly than ^{111}In antimyosin, permitting earlier cardiac imaging following injection.[178,179]
3. The shorter physical half-life of [99mTc] (6 h) compared to the half-life of [111]In (67 h) permits administration of a larger amount of tracer activity, improving counting statistics.
4. The 140-keV energy of [99mTc] is ideally suited for imaging on a conventional gamma camera, whereas the higher energy emissions of ^{111}In are poorly absorbed by the thin sodium iodide crystal used in gamma cameras.
5. As is the case with ^{111}In antimyosin, the initial blood pool phase following [99mTc] antimyosin injection can be used to generate radionuclide ventriculograms for measurement of left ventricular function.

GLUCARIC ACID

A practical limitation of infarct-avid imaging with ^{111}In antimyosin is the requirement to wait 1-2 days following tracer injection for blood pool clearance before acquiring clinically useful images. An infarct-avid tracer that may be rapidly imaged after injection would have potential utility for identification of acutely infarcted versus viable myocardium in the emergency room. Technetium 99m glucaric acid has been suggested as such a tracer.[182–184]

Several [99mTc] complexes containing carbohydrate ligands have been used as infarct-avid agents, including [99mTc] glucoheptonate, [99mTc] gluconate, and [99mTc] glucaric acid (or glucarate). Technetium 99m glucaric acid, a 6-carbon dicarboxylic acid, shows rapid blood pool clearance with urinary excretion. Bone uptake is limited. In a canine model, Orlandi et al[182] demonstrated [99mTc] glucaric acid uptake in areas of triphenyl–tetrazolium chloride documented myocardial infarction after 90 min of coronary artery occlusion followed by 3 h of reperfusion. Uptake of [99mTc] glucaric acid was not observed in regions of myocardial ischemia without evidence of myocardial infarction in canines, but others have reported [99mTc] glucaric acid uptake in myocardial ischemia in the absence of myocardial infarction in a swine model.[185] The specific utility of [99mTc] glucaric acid for early identification of infarcted myocardium will require extensive additional validation in animal models and in humans.

Thallium 201 Myocardial Perfusion Imaging (Figs. 18-6 and 18-7)

The sensitivity of ^{201}Tl scintigraphy for detection of acute myocardial infarction depends on the timing of imaging. Wackers et al[186] detected evidence of myocardial hypoperfusion in 94 percent of patients with acute myocardial infarction when imaging with ^{201}Tl was performed within 24 h following the onset of chest pain. Thallium 201 images acquired more than 24 h following the onset of symptoms were abnormal in 72 percent of patients with ECG and enzymatic evidence of acute myocardial infarction. When imaging was performed more than 24 h following the onset of chest pain, only 52 percent of patients having a nontransmural myocardial infarction were detected. Patients with resting myocardial perfusion defects apparent within 24 h following the onset of chest pain may have normalization of the ^{201}Tl images when rescanned at a later time. This may represent resolution of reversible ischemia in a region surrounding a small myocardial infarction.

Although a properly timed ^{201}Tl myocardial perfusion scan appears to be highly sensitive for detection of acute myocardial infarction, it is also relatively nonspecific. Approximately one-half to three-quarters of patients with an old myocardial infarction will have a persistent thallium perfusion defect.[188,189] Furthermore, resting ^{201}Tl perfusion defects are not specific for the presence of irreversibly damaged myocardium. Reversible resting myocardial ischemia can produce resting ^{201}Tl defects in patients with unstable angina pectoris,[190,191] stable angina pectoris,[191] or even silent myocardial ischemia.[190,191]

Separation of reversible resting myocardial ischemia from myocardial scar is possible in some cases by the use of rest and delayed redistribution images.[192] Regions of severe myocardial ischemia may exhibit delayed uptake of ^{201}Tl into the myocardium (Fig. 18-8). Three to 4 h later, improved or uniform myocardial perfusion may be present, suggesting that myocardial scar is absent. Since at least 5 g of myocardium must be hypoperfused to permit detection by planar imaging,[193] small infarcts located in an ischemic zone may not be identified as infarcts by the rest–redistribution technique. Nevertheless, the practical clinical implication of a myocardial region containing an initial thallium defect that is improved or no longer present on repeat imaging 3 h later is illustrated by the subsequent response of such a region to surgical revascularization. Berger et al[191] found that 37 of 48 myocardial segments containing an initial resting ^{201}Tl defect with evidence of thallium redistribution 3 h later reverted toward normal initial thallium uptake postoperatively. Contrast angiographic assessment showed that myocardial regions containing persistent resting ^{201}Tl defects were more likely to have akinetic or dyskinetic wall motion than regions with thallium redistribution, which were more often normal or, at most, hypokinetic.[191]

ANT   LAO   LL

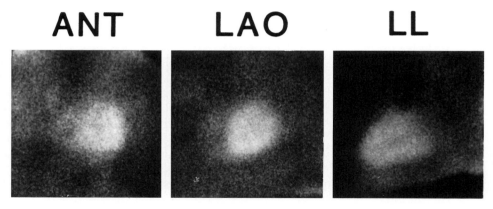

Figure 18-6   Normal ^{201}Tl myocardial perfusion in a patient with no evidence of myocardial infarction. Left image, anterior; center, left anterior oblique; right, left lateral. (From Gerson,[187] reproduced with permission.)

Lomboy et al[194] have used rest and 4-h redistribution planar ^{201}Tl images to study 31 patients 2 ± 1 days following a Q-wave myocardial infarction. Patients with evidence of viable myocardium, defined by the presence of a less than 50 percent reduction in maximal ^{201}Tl activity or by an increase in counts by 15 percent or greater on delayed images (representing redistribution) were compared to patients with no evidence of viable myocardium. Patients with viable myocardium were significantly more likely to have a patent infarct-related artery at angiography, had smaller infarcts by enzymatic criteria, and had higher levels of LVEF by radionuclide measurement at 3 ± 2 days postinfarction. At late follow-up 64 ± 95 days postinfarction, LVEF improved in patients with viable myocardium from 57 ± 13 percent to 66 ± 10 percent ($p < 0.05$) but deteriorated in patients with no initial evidence of viable myocardium from 53 ± 10 percent to 46 ± 8 percent ($p < 0.05$). Although a rest–redistribution ^{201}Tl scan performed 2 ± 1 days following the onset of acute myocardial infarction provided statistically

significant prognostic information, the information was not available until after decisions regarding reperfusion therapy had already been made.

Regions of diminished ^{201}Tl myocardial activity may also be observed in the absence of atherosclerotic CAD. Resting ^{201}Tl myocardial perfusion defects may be observed in the presence of coronary artery spasm,[195] sarcoidosis, metastatic carcinoma,[196] aortic stenosis,[197] and, occasionally, in cardiomyopathy.[198,199] Abnormal resting (or exercise) ^{201}Tl myocardial perfusion in patients with normal coronary arteries and either mitral valve prolapse[200–203] or hypertrophic cardiomyopathy[204,205] appears to be uncommon.

Technetium 99m Sestamibi Myocardial Perfusion Imaging

Technetium 99m sestamibi provides a distinct alternative to ^{201}Tl for the study of relative myocardial blood flow

ANT   45° LAO   70° LAO

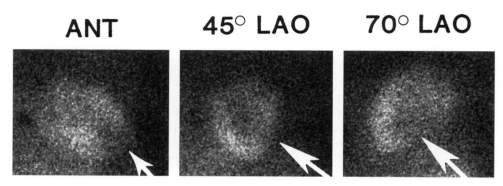

Figure 18-7   Inferoposterior, inferolateral (*large arrows*), and inferoapical (*small arrow*) hypoperfusion at rest in a 46-year-old man with acute myocardial infarction. Left image, anterior; center, 45° left anterior oblique; right, 70° left anterior oblique. (From Gerson,[187] reproduced with permission.)

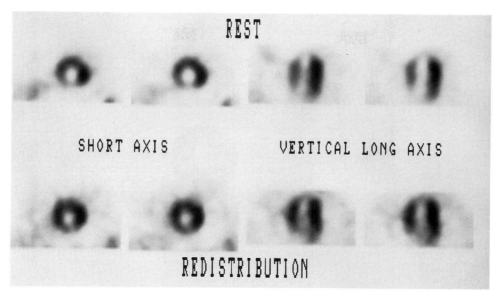

Figure 18-8 Demonstration of severe resting myocardial ischemia by rest and redistribution imaging following injection of [201]Tl. After injection of ^{201}Tl with the patient at rest and free of anginal symptoms there is evidence of anteroseptal, apical, and inferior wall hypoperfusion. Three hours later, improved tracer distribution is observed in each of the ischemic myocardial segments.

distribution in acute myocardial infarction. The kinetics and imaging properties of ^{99m}Tc sestamibi have been reviewed in detail in Chap. 1. Technetium 99m sestamibi provides improved physical imaging properties compared to ^{201}Tl because its 140-keV photopeak is better suited to imaging with a conventional gamma camera, and it is less attenuated by overlying soft tissue. The 6-h physical half-life of ^{99m}Tc results in improved organ dosimetry compared to ^{201}Tl and allows administration of larger tracer doses. The principal clinical difference between the two tracers is the lack of clinically important redistribution of ^{99m}Tc sestamibi.[206] This property permits a number of potentially important applications in the patient with acute myocardial infarction.

In canine models of permanent coronary artery occlusion and of 2-h coronary occlusion followed by reperfusion, Verani et al[207] showed a good correlation of ^{99m}Tc sestamibi infarct size, measured from planar myocardial images 48 h postocclusion, in comparison to anatomic infarct size by triphenyl–tetrazolium chloride staining ($r = 0.85$). Infarct size from planar ^{99m}Tc sestamibi images tended to overestimate anatomic infarct size. When tomographic imaging of ^{99m}Tc sestamibi myocardial activity was compared to anatomic infarct size in the same canine models, an excellent correlation was obtained ($r = 0.95$), without overestimation of infarct size. Accurate estimation of myocardial infarct size by ^{99m}Tc sestamibi has also been reported in humans. In 14 patients studied 5 days after acute myocardial infarction, Santoro et al[208] compared tomographic ^{99m}Tc sestamibi estimates of myocardial infarct size to the amount of necrotic tissue estimated from CK-MB curves and found a good correlation ($r =$

$0.91, p < 0.001$). Similarly, Gibbons et al[209] found a good correlation of tomographic ^{99m}Tc sestamibi infarct size measured 6 to 14 days after myocardial infarction and radionuclide LVEF obtained 1 day later ($r = -0.82, p < 0.01$). In contrast, ECG Q waves showed little relation to ^{99m}Tc sestamibi infarct size or to a radionuclide LVEF obtained before hospital discharge.[210]

Of particular importance is the potential use of serial ^{99m}Tc sestamibi images to identify the extent of myocardium at risk and the effect of treatment in acute myocardial infarction. This principle is illustrated in Fig. 18-9. When a patient presents to the emergency room with chest pain, ECG evidence of evolving myocardial infarction, and indications for thrombolysis, administration of the thrombolytic drug should not be delayed for cardiac imaging. It would, however, be useful to be able to document the extent of myocardium at risk for infarction at the time of presentation. If ^{99m}Tc sestamibi is made available in the emergency room for prompt administration when the patient with an evolving myocardial infarction is about to receive thrombolytic therapy, then the lack of myocardial redistribution of sestamibi can be used to advantage. Cardiac imaging can be delayed for several hours, until the patient is clinically stable, following the injection of ^{99m}Tc sestamibi. Because sestamibi does not redistribute, the distribution of sestamibi on the myocardial images will correspond to the distribution of myocardial blood flow before reperfusion therapy. A second dose of ^{99m}Tc sestamibi can then be administered hours or days later to document myocardial tracer distribution subsequent to reperfusion therapy. If in the comparison of images from prethrombo-

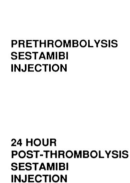

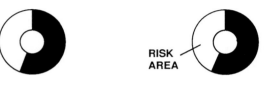

PRETHROMBOLYSIS SESTAMIBI INJECTION

RISK AREA

24 HOUR POST-THROMBOLYSIS SESTAMIBI INJECTION

LARGE FIXED DEFECT (WHITE)

DEFECT RESOLUTION

IMPLICATION:

EITHER: 1) MYOCARDIAL NECROSIS, 2) STUNNED MYOCARDIUM, OR 3) ?? RESTING ISCHEMIA (PERSISTENT OCCLUSION)

MYOCARDIAL SALVAGE (OR INITIAL CORONARY SPASM WITH RESOLUTION)

Figure 18-9 Diagrammatic representation of short-axis myocardial tomograms obtained from ^{99m}Tc sestamibi injections before (*top*) and after (*bottom*) coronary artery thrombolysis. **Right**: Resolution of the prethrombolysis sestamibi defect after repeat injection of sestamibi postthrombolysis. Defect resolution on serial images suggests myocardial salvage of the risk area. **Left**: The fixed defect on prethrombolysis and postthrombolysis images suggests that myocardial necrosis or stunned myocardium (or both) is present. Resting myocardial ischemia resulting from a persistent coronary artery occlusion is probably a less likely etiology for a persistent defect of this severity.

lytic to postthrombolytic sestamibi injection, the size of the perfusion defect is unchanged, the implication is that reperfusion has not been successful. This might result from failure of the thrombolytic agent (or acute angioplasty procedure) to reestablish vessel patency. It might also result if myocardial infarction has been completed before patency of the infarct-related vessel is restored. Alternatively, defects associated with prethrombolytic and postthrombolytic injection of sestamibi that correspond in size and location could relate to old myocardial infarction or to postischemic dysfunction ("stunned myocardium").[211,212] Concordant sestamibi defects from tracer injections before and several days after reperfusion therapy appear to correspond to regions of myocardial necrosis related to failed reperfusion therapy rather than postischemic myocardial dysfunction or persistent ischemia in most cases from available animal or clinical studies.[207–209,213]

When the ^{99m}Tc sestamibi defect resulting from tracer injection prior to reperfusion therapy is larger than the defect size associated with a repeat injection of sestamibi following reperfusion therapy, the reduction in perfusion defect size appears to correspond to salvaged myocardium.[208,209] In the setting of acute myocardial infarction, a decrease in the size of the sestamibi defect over time (usually associated with tracer injections before and then following reperfusion therapy) has correlated with restored patency of the infarct-related artery and has predicted late recovery of myocardial function.[208] The presence of extensive myocardium at risk, as identified by serial ^{99m}Tc sestamibi studies, may identify a subgroup of patients with acute myocardial infarction who may benefit most from revascularization therapy.

Dual Isotope Imaging with ^{111}In Antimyosin and ^{201}Tl or ^{99m}Tc Sestamibi

Several groups of investigators have noted the substantial clinical potential of combined imaging with an infarct-avid tracer and a tracer of myocardial perfusion in patients with acute myocardial infarction. Johnson et al[214] administered 2 mCi ^{111}In antimyosin to 42 patients within 48 h of onset of chest pain. At approximately 48 h following antimyosin injection, each patient received approximately 2 mCi ^{201}Tl. Simultaneously, dual-isotope SPECT acquisition was performed, with one energy window set for the 70-keV photopeak of ^{201}Tl and one set for the 247-keV photopeak of ^{111}In. Indium antimyosin uptake and thallium 201 defects that corresponded in size and location were classified as "matches" (Fig. 18-10). The implication of a match was that all underperfused myocardium was necrotic. Multivessel CAD was absent in 5 of the 6 patients with matched defects who went on to angiography. None of the 14 patients with matched defects went on to have a recurrent ischemic coronary event in the hospital and none of the 14 had evidence of residual ischemia on a predischarge low level stress test.

In comparison, patients with antimyosin uptake and a larger thallium defect were considered to have a "mismatch." The implication of a mismatch was that not all underperfused myocardium was recently and irreversibly damaged. Of 23 patients with mismatches studied by Johnson et al,[214] 9 had a previous myocardial infarction. Seventeen of the 23 patients with mismatched thallium and antimyosin activity underwent coronary arteriography during or immediately following initial hospitalization. Fifteen of the 17 patients had multivessel CAD. Of the 23 patients with a mismatch, 16 developed evidence of recurrent ischemia ($p < 0.01$ versus patients with matched activity) including recurrent chest pain in 10, myocardial infarct extension in 3, ischemic pulmonary edema in 1, and stress test evidence of residual ischemia in 6. The authors concluded that myocardium identified by a thallium defect but no antimyosin uptake (a mismatch) represents either old myocardial scar, ischemia consisting of myocardium with reduced blood flow supply, or slowly recovering ("stunned") myocardium. Eleven of the 23 patients with mismatches also had thallium 4-h redistribution scans. In 4 of these 11 patients, thallium redistribution was detected in the same region as the thallium/antimyosin mismatch, suggesting the presence of viable myocardium. Verification that viable myocardium is responsible for a specific myocardial region of thallium/antimyosin mismatch might be better accomplished through the addition of thallium reinjection, but these data are not available at the time of writing.

Occasionally, "overlap" of ^{201}Tl activity (uptake) and ^{111}In antimyosin activity may be noted, despite the favorable spatial resolution of SPECT imaging. This uptake pattern appears to correspond to islands of viable myocardium within the infarct territory or to nontransmural infarction. A similar "overlap pattern" has been described with dual isotope imaging with ^{111}In antimyosin and ^{99m}Tc sestamibi in a porcine model of nontransmural myocardial infarction.[215] Although the overlap pattern suggests the presence of residual myocardial ischemia, this finding does not appear to be predictive of in-hospital cardiac complications.[180]

Radionuclide Ventriculography

The myocardium is not directly visualized by radionuclide ventriculography. Therefore, the presence of acute myocardial infarction can only be inferred from radionu-

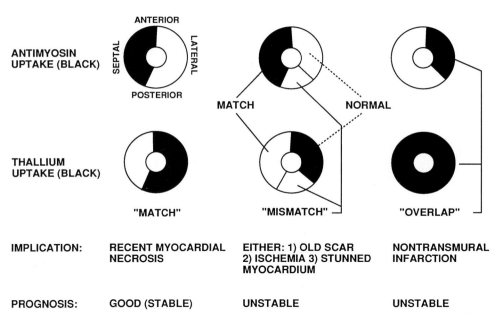

Figure 18-10 Diagrammatic representation of short-axis myocardial tomograms illustrating findings from dual-isotope myocardial imaging with ^{111}In antimyosin and [201]Tl. **Left**: Concordant area of anteroseptal ^{111}In antimyosin uptake (*dark area*) and anteroseptal ^{201}Tl perfusion defect (*light area*—lack of uptake). These concordant areas constitute a "match" and are consistent with recent myocardial necrosis. Because all hypoperfused myocardium is already necrotic, a stable clinical course is likely. **Center**: An anteroseptal match is again present. However, there is also a posterior wall "mismatch," involving diminished posterior wall perfusion by ^{201}Tl imaging in the absence of posterior wall necrosis by ^{111}In antimyosin imaging. If the mismatch corresponds to old myocardial necrosis, then the patient has an extensive combination of old posterior and acute anteroseptal myocardial infarction. Alternatively, the posterior wall mismatch may correspond to residual myocardial ischemia or to stunned myocardium. The combination of acute anteroseptal myocardial infarction and posterior wall ischemia or stunning would likely portend an unstable clinical course. **Right**: The anteroseptal and posterior walls have normal ^{111}In antimyosin and ^{201}Tl scintigraphic findings. However, there is abnormal uptake of ^{111}In antimyosin in the lateral myocardial wall and maintained ^{201}Tl uptake in the same segment. This suggests the coexistence of myocardial scar and viable muscle in the lateral wall, perhaps related to nontransmural myocardial infarction. This "overlap" pattern may correspond to increased risk for an unstable clinical course.

clide evidence of regional and global abnormalities of ventricular function arising in a clinical context suggesting infarction. Global disturbances of left ventricular function may, however, be observed in a wide variety of cardiac disorders. Regional myocardial dysfunction is visualized by radionuclide ventriculography in the vast majority of patients with acute myocardial infarction,[216,217] but it may also result from healed myocardial infarction or myocardial ischemia. Regional left ventricular wall-motion abnormality may also be visualized in noncoronary heart disease, including valvular cardiac disorders[218] and cardiomyopathy.

As is discussed later in this chapter in the section on prognosis, the resting LVEF is a powerful predictor of in-hospital and late cardiac events following acute myocardial infarction. Also the change in global and regional left ventricular function during hospitalization for acute myocardial infarction is a powerful predictor of subsequent cardiac events.[219]

RELATIVE ROLES OF ECG, ENZYMATIC, AND IMAGING TECHNIQUES FOR DETECTION OF ACUTE MYOCARDIAL INFARCTION

Imaging tests are not generally needed to diagnose the presence of acute Q-wave myocardial infarction except when supportive evolutionary ECG and enzymatic changes are absent or unavailable. Detection of non-Q-wave acute myocardial infarction in the absence of typical abnormalities of the CK-MB fraction is often difficult. When cardiac enzymatic changes are equivocal, focal abnormal myocardial activity on an infarct-avid scan provides useful confirmation that acute myocardial infarction is present (high specificity). However, many patients with non-Q-wave acute myocardial infarction will not be identified by ^{99m}Tc pyrophosphate imaging and up to one-sixth of non-Q-wave infarctions will not be detectable by ^{111}In antimyosin imaging.[132,134] In non-Q-wave myocardial infarction, abnormal myocardial perfusion is ordinarily detectable by ^{201}Tl scintigraphy, but the likelihood of detection begins to decrease as early as 6 h following the onset of symptoms.

Evaluation of the Patient Presenting to the Emergency Department with Chest Pain

The presence of ST-segment elevation greater than 1 mm on the resting ECG identifies a group of patients with chest pain having a very high likelihood of acute myocardial infarction.[220] Conversely, patients who present to the emergency department with sharp or stabbing chest pain that has a positional component, or that is reproduced by chest wall palpation, and in whom the resting ECG is normal, have a very low likelihood that an acute ischemic cardiac syndrome is present. Most patients in this latter group require no acute cardiac therapy and do not require hospitalization.[221-224] The majority of patients who present to an emergency department for evaluation of chest pain have symptoms and ECG findings that fall between these two extremes, and rapid cardiac diagnosis is often difficult.

CLINICAL AND ECG PREDICTORS

Lee et al[223] prospectively validated a multivariable algorithm (Fig. 18-11) designed to identify patients presenting to the emergency department with chest pain in whom the risk of myocardial infarction was sufficiently small that 12 h of observation in the emergency department was satisfactory to exclude the presence of myocardial infarction. The algorithm was applied in a validation study of 2684 patients. On the basis of the algorithm, 957 patients (36 percent) were classified as low risk for acute myocardial infarction. Of the 957 low-risk patients, 771 patients (81 percent) did not have abnormal cardiac enzymes or recurrent chest pain during 12 h of observation and were candidates for discharge from the emergency department. Follow-up of these 771 patients showed that 4 had a nonfatal myocardial infarction (0.5 percent) and 5 patients died from complications of ischemic heart disease 3 days or more after presentation (0.6 percent). Within 3 days following presentation, an additional 8 patients (1.0 percent) in the low-risk group eligible for early discharge from the emergency department underwent cardiac catheterization and this was followed by coronary artery revascularization. Among the 1727 patients at high risk based on the algorithm in Fig. 18-11, 739 patients (43 percent) had an acute myocardial infarction and 491 (28 percent) had a final diagnosis of unstable angina. The algorithm in Fig. 18-11 provides good separation of patients into high-risk and low-risk groups, but 331 of the patients who were assigned to the low-risk group had a final diagnosis of either acute myocardial infarction or unstable angina. Only 186 initially "low-risk" patients were subsequently identified in the emergency department as requiring hospital admission. Thus, at least 145 of the 771 patients who were identified for early discharge from the emergency room (19 percent) had an acute coronary syndrome as the final diagnosis. Although the protocol based on clinical and ECG data provided substantial risk stratification for patients presenting to the emergency department with chest pain, it is unclear that a protocol for early discharge of low-risk patients from the emergency department would be widely applied if one-fifth of the "low-risk" patients have important CAD.

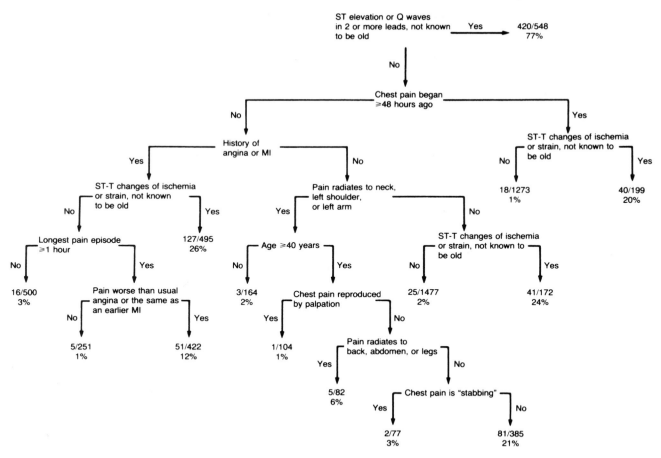

Figure 18-11 Algorithm for prediction of risk of acute myocardial infarction based on clinical and ECG data acquired in the emergency room. Based on the algorithm, patients presenting to the emergency department with chest pain are classified into low risk (< 7 percent) or high risk (> 7 percent) subgroups for acute myocardial infarction. (From Lee et al,[223] reproduced with permission.)

Newer cardiac enzyme determinations, with assessment of CK isoforms, troponin T, and serum myoglobin all offer considerable promise for speeding the diagnosis of acute myocardial infarction.[225,226] Yet, before a patient can be discharged from the emergency department, assurance is also needed that the patient does not have unstable angina, with its associated cardiac risks. Furthermore, a diagnostic test would be useful in the evaluation of patients with chest pain in the emergency department if that test could distinguish those patients requiring further diagnostic evaluation for CAD from patients with noncoronary artery-related chest pain.

TREADMILL ECG IN THE EMERGENCY DEPARTMENT

Treadmill ECG, echocardiography, and myocardial perfusion imaging have each been applied in the emergency department setting. Treadmill ECG has been found to be safe in selected low-risk patients presenting to the emergency department with chest pain and having a normal resting ECG.[227-229] In this setting, patients with

exercise-induced ST-segment depression have been found to have a low[227] to moderate[229] likelihood that angiographic CAD is present. Conversely, low-risk patients with no exercise-induced ST-segment depression have been discharged rapidly from the emergency department or from the hospital, and cardiac events have been rare at 6 months of follow-up in these small studies.[227-229] It should be emphasized that these low-risk patients with normal resting ECG would be expected to have few cardiac events on short-term follow-up based on the classification of Lee et al,[223] with or without further risk stratification using exercise ECG. The diagnostic and prognostic value of treadmill exercise testing for patients entering the emergency department with chest pain might be more valuable clinically in patients with a moderate risk that an acute ischemic event is present. However, the usefulness of treadmill exercise testing may be reduced in this group because baseline ECG abnormalities are more commonly present. Also, the safety of treadmill ECG in moderate-risk patients presenting with chest pain is currently unknown.

ECHOCARDIOGRAPHY IN THE EMERGENCY DEPARTMENT

Echocardiography may be an appropriate test for further determining cardiac diagnosis and prognosis in patients presenting to the emergency department with chest pain and an intermediate clinical likelihood that an acute ischemic syndrome is present. In contrast to the treadmill ECG, echocardiography should also be of value in patients with ST-segment depression or T wave abnormalities on the resting ECG. Use of echocardiography in this setting is based on the observation that approximately 83 to 100 percent of patients with acute myocardial infarction and a technically adequate two-dimensional echocardiogram have visible regional wall-motion abnormalities.[49,56,230,231] Resting two-dimensional echocardiography provides definite advantages in terms of portability, speed of examination, and moderate cost. It also has a number of disadvantages, including subjectivity of interpretation, technically inadequate images in 5 to 10 percent of patients, lack of precise quantitation of regional left ventricular function, in particular subtle regional abnormalities, and, most importantly, inability to distinguish acute from old myocardial infarction.[232,233]

Sabia et al[232] conducted a prospective study of 180 patients presenting to the emergency room with symptoms suggestive of acute myocardial infarction. Patients with less than a 30-min duration of pain or with symptoms readily explained by musculoskeletal abnormalities, local trauma, or pulmonary pathology were excluded. Two-dimensional echocardiography performed in the emergency department was technically adequate in 169 of 180 patients (94 percent). Based on conventional clinical and ECG criteria, and without knowledge of the echocardiographic findings, 140 study patients were admitted to the hospital and 40 patients were not admitted. Follow-up cardiac enzyme determinations were made on all study patients to determine the presence or absence of acute myocardial infarction. Greater than or equal to 1 mm of ST-segment elevation was present in just 9 of the 30 patients who evolved an acute myocardial infarction. Pathologic Q waves were present equally in patients with and without an acute myocardial infarction. An echocardiographic regional wall-motion abnormality was present in 27 of the 29 patients with a technically adequate echocardiogram. Of the 140 patients without an acute myocardial infarction who had a technically adequate echocardiogram, 58 had no regional or global left ventricular wall-motion abnormality (41 percent), 22 had diffuse left ventricular dysfunction without a regional wall-motion abnormality (16 percent), and 60 had a regional wall-motion abnormality (43 percent). Thirteen patients with acute myocardial infarction had a complication in the hospital consisting of cardiogenic shock, life-threatening arrhythmias, or postinfarction angina; each patient had a resting regional wall-motion abnormality on echocardiography in the emergency department. This study suggests that echocardiographic evaluation of left ventricular regional wall motion in the emergency department provides significantly better prediction of acute myocardial infarction compared to clinical and ECG findings. A normal echocardiogram potentially identifies a subgroup of those patients presenting with at least 30 min of chest pain who are at low risk for evolving an acute myocardial infarction or associated complications. Conversely, a left ventricular regional or global wall-motion abnormality on the emergency department echocardiogram was identified in 59 percent of study patients who did not evolve a myocardial infarction. Echocardiography could not be used to differentiate acute myocardial infarction from unstable angina or old myocardial infarction.

THALLIUM 201 MYOCARDIAL PERFUSION IMAGING IN THE EMERGENCY DEPARTMENT

Myocardial perfusion imaging provides an alternative method for identifying patients in the emergency room with an acute ischemic syndrome requiring hospital admission.[234,235] In an early study, Wackers et al[234] studied prospectively 203 patients with possible acute myocardial infarction by performing ^{201}Tl myocardial scintigraphy within 10 h after the last episode of chest pain. Of 203 patients, 49 had positive, 47 had questionable, and 107 had normal ^{201}Tl scans. Patients with unstable angina and a normal ^{201}Tl scan were unlikely to progress to myocardial infarction or other major cardiac complications. An abnormal or equivocal ^{201}Tl scan result identified a high-risk subgroup of 96 patients including 41 patients who subsequently evolved a myocardial infarction (43 percent) and 20 patients with unstable angina that was otherwise uncomplicated (21 percent). In large part, because of its inability to identify specifically old myocardial infarction, at least one-third of these patients who presented to the emergency department with chest pain and were at moderate clinical risk would have been admitted to the hospital based on results of ^{201}Tl imaging but would not have had a final diagnosis of acute myocardial infarction or unstable angina.

TECHNETIUM 99m SESTAMIBI IMAGING IN THE EMERGENCY DEPARTMENT

Compared to ^{201}Tl, ^{99m}Tc sestamibi permits imaging with a larger administered activity, resulting in superior counting statistics and provides images with less soft-tissue attenuation artifact. Perhaps the most important characteristic of ^{99m}Tc sestamibi for imaging patients presenting to the emergency department with chest pain is its lack of tracer redistribution. When injected during an episode of myocardial ischemia, ^{99m}Tc sestamibi will demonstrate evidence of hypoperfusion even if imaging is delayed. This is in contrast to ^{201}Tl, which may show tracer redistribution, obscuring any evidence of ischemia if imaging does not immediately follow tracer injection.

Bilodeau et al[236] studied 45 patients with ^{99m}Tc sestamibi injection in the emergency room or coronary care unit and tomographic imaging during and up to 4 h after chest pain. All patients were admitted to the hospital with a diagnosis of unstable angina and had no prior history of myocardial infarction. Tomographic ^{99m}Tc sestamibi studies following tracer injection during pain were abnormal in 25 of 26 patients with a 50 percent or greater luminal diameter stenosis by angiography. The 12-lead ECG obtained at the time of tracer injection had a diagnostic sensitivity of only 35 percent for detection of angiographic disease. In the pain-free state, radionuclide imaging and ECG recording had sensitivities of 65 percent and 38 percent, respectively. Specificity for tomographic sestamibi imaging was 79 percent during chest pain and 84 percent in the pain-free state, whereas for the 12-lead ECG specificities were 74 percent both with and without chest pain. This early study established the ability of rest ^{99m}Tc sestamibi imaging to accurately identify the presence or absence of CAD and was particularly sensitive following tracer injection during chest pain.

This approach was examined further by Varetto et al[237] who used rest ^{99m}Tc sestamibi imaging to study 64 patients presenting to the emergency department with chest pain and a nondiagnostic resting ECG. The patients were then followed for 11 ± 3 months for evidence of major cardiac events, including death, myocardial infarction, and coronary artery revascularization. Thirty patients had a perfusion defect by resting ^{99m}Tc sestamibi imaging, including 13 patients with subsequent enzymatic evidence of myocardial infarction, 14 patients with subsequent evidence of CAD by coronary arteriography or exercise myocardial perfusion imaging, and 3 patients with probable false-positive ^{99m}Tc sestamibi scans. None of the patients with a normal rest ^{99m}Tc sestamibi scan following injection in the emergency department was diagnosed as having CAD disease on follow-up. At 18 months of follow-up, five revascularization procedures and one death occurred in the group of patients with a perfusion defect. No cardiac events occurred in the patients without a resting ^{99m}Tc sestamibi defect. The authors noted that of the 14 patients without myocardial infarction but with subsequent evidence of CAD, 11 were pain free at the time of ^{99m}Tc sestamibi administration. In these patients, remission of chest pain occurred 2 to 8 h before tracer injection.

These results have been confirmed by Hilton et al[238] and others.[239] In a study of 102 emergency room patients[238] with typical angina and a normal or nondiagnostic 12-lead ECG, ^{99m}Tc sestamibi was injected during chest pain and the patients were followed for in-hospital cardiac complications (i.e., cardiac death, nonfatal myo-

cardial infarction, or need for immediate coronary intervention). Multivariable regression analysis identified an abnormal perfusion image as the only independent predictor of adverse cardiac events. Of 70 patients with a normal perfusion scan, only 1 had a cardiac event (recurrent angina leading to angiography and coronary bypass surgery) during follow-up of at least 90 days. In comparison, 12 of 17 patients (71 percent) with an abnormal ^{99m}Tc sestamibi scan and 2 of 15 patients with an equivocal scan (13 percent) had cardiac events ($p = 0.0004$ versus patients with a normal scan) including 12 patients with myocardial infarction and 1 with cardiac death. An abnormal or equivocal ^{99m}Tc sestamibi scan provided a sensitivity of 94 percent and specificity of 83 percent in the prediction of adverse cardiac events. Initial myocardial perfusion imaging with ^{99m}Tc sestamibi distinguished between most (85 percent) patients with very low or very high risk for short-term cardiac events (< 2 percent and > 70 percent, respectively) and was significantly more accurate than standard clinical and ECG variables.

Thus, ^{99m}Tc sestamibi, when injected during chest pain in the emergency department or early following resolution of prolonged chest pain, provides accurate prediction of adverse cardiac events and appears to be a useful tool for triage of patients with chest pain in the emergency department. Following ^{99m}Tc sestamibi injection, its lack of redistribution permits stabilization of the patient with antianginal drug therapy before imaging without apparent loss of diagnostic accuracy. Initial data suggest that in patients presenting to the emergency department with chest pain, a nondiagnostic ECG, and negative cardiac enzymes, ^{99m}Tc sestamibi imaging at rest is more accurate for exclusion of myocardial ischemia than is resting echocardiography,[240] but additional studies are needed.

LOCALIZATION OF ACUTE MYOCARDIAL INFARCTION

In patients with healed myocardial infarction, the 12-lead ECG can distinguish infarcts involving the anterior wall from those involving the posterior left ventricular wall, but more precise ECG localization of myocardial infarction has been limited in accuracy.[241-243] In 23 patients with fatal acute myocardial infarction, Wackers et al[244] considered five anatomic infarct locations (septal, anterior, inferior, lateral, and posterior). They found good agreement of the scintigraphic location of myocardial infarct by ^{201}Tl imaging with the postmortem infarct location in 91 percent of patients. Agreement between the ECG infarct location and the infarct location at postmortem examination occurred in only 70 percent of patients. Thus, in Wackers' study, ^{201}Tl scintigraphy provided more precise anatomic location of acute myocardial infarct compared to the ECG. Myocardial perfusion scintigraphy may prove particularly helpful in localizing myocardial infarcts in patients with left bundle branch block or with non-Q-wave infarction. Thallium tomography provides improved spatial resolution compared to planar imaging and can be expected to further improve infarct localization. The rest–redistribution thallium scintigram can help differentiate regions of acute myocardial infarction from resting myocardial ischemia,[192] but it does not separate acute from old regions of infarction.

Localization of acute myocardial infarction by ^{99m}Tc pyrophosphate imaging has been reported to agree closely with the anatomic location at autopsy.[95] Fewer data exist concerning the accuracy of acute myocardial infarct localization by ^{99m}Tc pyrophosphate in patients with smaller nonfatal infarcts. Concordant ECG and ^{111}In antimyosin acute infarct localization was reported by Johnson et al[130] in 43 of 44 patients. Correlation of ^{111}In antimyosin acute infarct location with autopsy data is limited.[245]

Radionuclide ventriculography and echocardiography[72] can provide accurate localization of left ventricular regional dysfunction but cannot delineate the cause of dysfunction except in some cases, through an intervention such as nitrate administration.[246] The latter approach may reverse dysfunction caused by myocardial ischemia.

RIGHT VENTRICULAR INFARCTION

Right ventricular myocardial infarction frequently complicates inferoposterior myocardial infarction. Right ventricular impairment has been observed in up to 45 percent of patients with inferior myocardial infarction[247-249] and is particularly likely to occur with right coronary artery occlusion when preexisting right ventricular hypertrophy is present.[250-252] Limited right ventricular infarction can also occur with isolated occlusion of the LAD coronary artery, but anterior descending artery occlusion does not result in infarction of sufficient right ventricular myocardium to produce right ventricular hemodynamic impairment.[253,254]

Right ventricular infarction is suggested clinically by neck vein distension and hypotension with no pulmonary congestion in patients with inferoposterior infarcts. Diagnosis of right ventricular infarction is important clinically because it often identifies patients with acute myocardial infarction and hypotension who will have a favorable response to volume loading, and because it identifies a high-risk subgroup of patients with an inferoposterior myocardial infarction.[255-258]

Accumulation of ^{99m}Tc pyrophosphate in the region

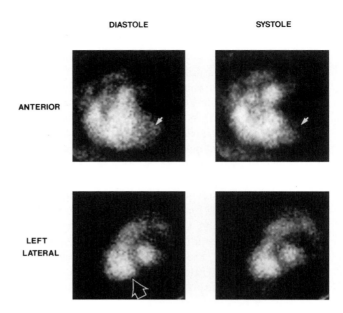

DIASTOLE   SYSTOLE

ANTERIOR

LEFT LATERAL

Figure 18-12 Resting radionuclide ventriculogram in a patient with right ventricular myocardial infarction. On the anterior images, vigorous contraction of the left ventricle is shown by the small arrows. The right ventricle (*large arrow*) is enlarged and hypocontractile.

of the right ventricular myocardium has been described in 33 to 37.5 percent of patients with clinical, ECG, and enzymatic evidence of acute inferior myocardial infarction.[259,260] Pyrophosphate activity in the right ventricular myocardium is located anteriorly and medially to activity located in the infarcted inferior left ventricular wall. It may appear to extend to the sternum on anterior and left anterior oblique images. The presence of ^{99m}Tc pyrophosphate activity in the right ventricular myocardium is thought to be specific for the presence of right ventricular myocardial necrosis.

Radionuclide ventriculography has also demonstrated right ventricular abnormalities in patients with hemodynamic evidence of right ventricular infarction[259] (Fig. 18-12). Segmental akinesis of the right ventricular free wall and an increased ratio of right ventricular to left ventricular chamber area have been described.[259] A lower right ventricular ejection fraction has been observed in patients with inferior compared to anterior myocardial infarction,[257] and these findings have been associated with ^{99m}Tc pyrophosphate activity in the right ventricle, suggesting right ventricular infarction.[261]

Radionuclide identification of right ventricular abnormality can identify a spectrum of pathology associated with inferior myocardial infarction. Cohn et al[262] described a clinical syndrome of right ventricular infarction consisting of ECG evidence of inferior myocardial infarction, distended neck veins, hypotension, and heart block. However, patients with right ventricular infarction by autopsy examination may not have hemodynamic evidence of right ventricular infarction during life.[263] Rigo et al[264] described a patient with inferior myocardial infarction not complicated by cardiogenic shock who had marked right ventricular dilatation without abnormality of right or left ventricular filling pressures. Following volume loading, the right ventricular filling pressure increased to 13 mmHg, suggesting right ventricular dysfunction. This observation has been confirmed by others,[134] suggesting that radionuclide ventriculography or ^{99m}Tc pyrophosphate imaging may detect evidence of right ventricular abnormality in patients with inferior myocardial infarction without measurable right ventricular dysfunction by baseline invasive hemodynamic monitoring. A further aspect of the spectrum of right ventricular involvement in inferior myocardial infarction has been suggested by Baigrie et al.[265] Of 37 consecutive patients who consented to invasive hemodynamic monitoring and who also had ECG evidence of transmural acute inferior myocardial infarction, 29 had hemodynamic evidence consistent with right ventricular infarction. In that study, hemodynamic evidence of right ventricular infarction consisted of either disproportionate elevation of the right compared to the left ventricular filling pressure or a right ventricular stroke–work index less than 5 g · m/m^2. However, ^{99m}Tc pyrophosphate images confirmed the presence of acute right ventricular myocardial infarction in only 5 patients. In acute inferior myocardial infarction, it appears that measurable hemodynamic dysfunction of the right ventricle may result from ischemia without right ventricular infarction. This is supported by sequential radionuclide ventriculographic studies demonstrating initial right ventricular dysfunction and a return to normal function by the third day following acute inferior wall infarction.[257] Therefore, in acute inferior wall infarction there appears to be a spectrum of right ventricular involvement, which includes (1) severe clinical and hemodynamic right ventricular infarction, (2) measurable hemodynamic impairment related to limited right ventricular infarction without the clinical syndrome of severe right ventricular infarction, (3) noninvasive evidence of right ventricular infarction without hemodynamic evidence of infarction until after a volume load is administered, and (4) ischemic dysfunction of the right ventricle without right ventricular infarction.

Echocardiographically, patients with right ventricular myocardial infarction often exhibit akinesis or dyskinesis of the inferior and posterior segments of the left ventricle and abnormal ventricular septal motion. Paradoxical ventricular septal motion is a common finding, which may be due to acute right ventricular volume overload or to injury of the inferior portion of the ventricular septum. Patients with right ventricular myocardial infarction have a very high incidence of right ventricular enlargement and right ventricular lateral and inferior segment akinesis or dyskinesis.[266]

Experimentally, the ventricular septum contributes both to right ventricular and left ventricular[267,268] performance, and production of isolated ventricular septal ischemia can cause right ventricular dysfunction.[269] Destruction of the right ventricular free wall does not compromise resting right ventricular function, suggesting that the intact ventricular septum may maintain right ventricular performance following free right ventricular wall injury.[270] Mikell et al[271] showed that patients with right ventricular infarction and abnormal septal systolic thickening on echocardiography had significantly higher right ventricular filling pressures (19 ± 3 mmHg versus 12 ± 5 mmHg, $p = 0.04$) and right ventricular dimensions in diastole (32 ± 8 mm versus 20 ± 3 mm, $p = 0.02$) compared to patients with normal septal thickening.

Although noninvasive imaging has been of help in revealing a spectrum of right ventricular infarction, its clinical role remains to be clarified. In the hypotensive patient with acute inferior myocardial infarction, invasive hemodynamic monitoring can both provide diagnostic confirmation of right ventricular dysfunction and guide therapy. Assessment of ECG lead V_{4R} for evidence of ST-segment elevation provides powerful prognostic information in patients with inferior myocardial infarction,[258] and no added benefit from myocardial imaging has been established.

COMPLICATIONS OF ACUTE MYOCARDIAL INFARCTION

Because of its high resolution, versatility, and portability, echocardiography is the principal noninvasive imaging modality for detection of complications early in acute myocardial infarction. Radionuclide imaging techniques can provide a more quantitative assessment of left ventricular function and extent of hypoperfusion in acute myocardial infarction and can provide powerful prognostic information. When radionuclide imaging is performed in the setting of acute myocardial infarction, the reader must be prepared to detect evidence of complications of myocardial infarction.

Left Ventricular Aneurysm

Left ventricular aneurysm has been reported to be present in 17.5 percent of patients with myocardial infarction who come to autopsy.[272] A true left ventricular aneurysm consists of a localized convex protrusion of the entire thickness of the left ventricular wall, with the mouth of the aneurysm usually at least as large as the maximal diameter of the aneurysm and the wall of the aneurysm consisting of fibrotic left ventricular myocardium.[273] Protrusion is present in both systole and diastole. Ventricular aneurysms may be akinetic or dyskinetic, but because they contain few if any normal myocardial fibers, they are not usually hypokinetic. In contrast, a dyskinetic left ventricular segment that bulges during systole but contributes to normal ventricular shape during diastole often contains a mixture of viable muscle and fibrosis.[274] Although true left ventricular aneurysms related to CAD frequently cause left heart failure, they seldom undergo expansion or rupture.[275] Left ventricular aneurysm may be suspected from the presence of pathologic Q waves and associated persistent ST-segment elevation on the ECG.[276,277]

Technetium-99m-pyrophosphate activity has been observed in left ventricular aneurysms, but it is not clinically helpful because this finding is more suggestive of acute myocardial infarction.[278,279] Distortion of the left ventricular contour correctly suggesting the presence of left ventricular aneurysm has been observed on ^{201}Tl scintigrams, but the latter technique has poor sensitivity for the detection of aneurysms.[280]

Radionuclide ventriculography is reported to be highly sensitive (approximately 96 percent) and specific (approximately 98 percent) for detecting the presence of left ventricular aneurysm compared to findings from contrast ventriculography[281-284] and from cardiac surgery.[282] The radionuclide technique permits separation of left ventricular aneurysm (Fig. 18-13) from general-ized left ventricular hypokinesis in most cases.[281,283] It has proved accurate for localization of ventricular aneurysm,[282] for assessment of the extent of the ventricle involved by the aneurysm,[281,285] and for assessment of the noninvolved segments.[286-288]

By two-dimensional echocardiography, a left ventricular aneurysm can be identified by the presence of a clearly defined, localized interruption in the diastolic configuration of the left ventricle.[276,289-291] Visser et al,[289] studying 422 patients prospectively, found that two-dimensional echocardiography detected left ventricular aneurysm with a sensitivity of 93 percent and specificity of 94 percent.

Left Ventricular Pseudoaneurysm

Pseudoaneurysm is much less common than true aneurysm and results from a rupture of the myocardium that is contained by the pericardium. Thus, parietal pericardium and clot are in direct contact with left ventricular intracavitary blood, with no myocardial elements in the pseudoaneurysm. Characteristically, pseudoaneurysms have narrow necks. Detection of pseudoaneurysms is important because of their propensity to fatal rupture[275] and their amenability to surgical repair.

Equilibrium (Fig. 18-14) and first-pass (Fig. 18-15) radionuclide ventriculography have been used to identify left ventricular pseudoaneurysms.[292-300] Pseudoaneurysm

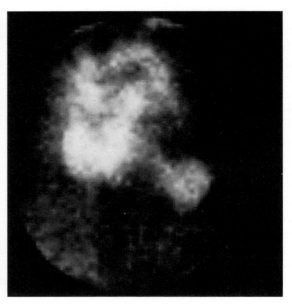

DIASTOLE **SYSTOLE**

Figure 18-13 Left ventricular aneurysm imaged in the anterior projection. A mural thrombus is suggested by the squared-off shape of the left ventricular apex and was confirmed by two-dimensional echocardiography.

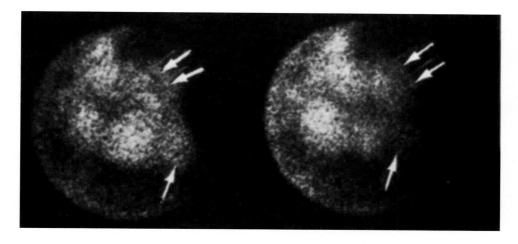

30°RAO

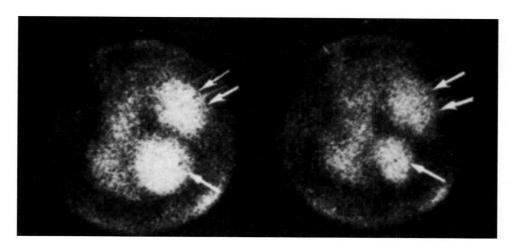

45°LAO

Figure 18-14 Gated cardiac blood pool scan, with end-diastolic images on the left and end-systolic images on the right. The false aneurysm is indicated by double arrows and the main left ventricular cavity by a single arrow. The interventricular septum and the right ventricle are well visualized in the 45° left anterior oblique (LAO) scintigrams, as is the apparent separation between the left ventricle and the false aneurysm. In the 30° right anterior oblique (RAO) views, the anterolateral wall and the apex appear akinetic. (From Sweet et al,[294] by permission.)

is typically identified on radionuclide ventriculography by the presence of a "discrete paraventricular chamber" connected to the main ventricular blood pool by a narrow neck.[293] Identification may be further confirmed by filling of the pseudoaneurysm after the main left ventricular cavity on a first-pass study[294] and by paradoxic bulging of the pseudoaneurysm during systole. Definitive diagnosis of pseudoaneurysm requires identification of a narrow neck. Several authors[294] have encountered difficulty identifying the narrow neck between the left ven-

tricular cavity and the pseudoaneurysm cavity using radionuclide imaging.

The combination of two-dimensional echocardiography with Doppler echocardiography has proved helpful in the diagnosis of left ventricular pseudoaneurysm.[297,301-311] Characteristics of pseudoaneurysm by two-dimensional echocardiography include (1) a sharp discontinuity of the endocardial image at the site of the pseudoaneurysm communication with the left ventricular cavity; (2) a saccular or globular contour of the pseu-

45°LAO   30°RAO

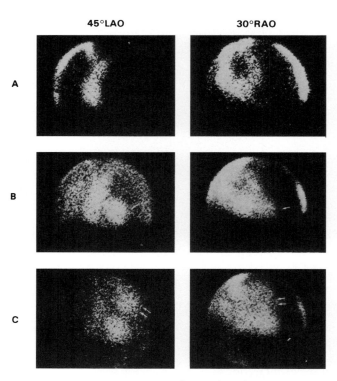

Figure 18-15 Representative 5-s frames from first-pass isotopic angiocardiograms performed in the 45° left anterior oblique (LAO) and 30° right anterior oblique (RAO) projections. Time 0 is defined as the appearance of the isotope in the superior vena cava. In frame A (0 to 5 s), the isotope has passed through the superior vena cava, the right atrium, and the right ventricle and into the proximal pulmonary artery. By frame B (10 to 15 s), the left ventricle (*single arrow*) has been visualized but the false aneurysm is not seen. Frame C (25 to 30 s) shows the false aneurysm (*double arrows*) fully visualized by delayed filling, presumably from the left ventricle. (From Sweet et al,[294] by permission.)

doaneurysm chamber; and (3) the presence of a relatively narrow orifice in comparison with the diameter of the body of the pseudoaneurysm.[301] Color Doppler echocardiography can provide physiologic correlation to the anatomic evidence of left ventricular pseudoaneurysm from two-dimensional echocardiography. A turbulent jet of flow into the pseudoaneurysm during systole and reversal of flow during diastole may be demonstrated by color Doppler imaging. Although the sensitivity and specificity have not been established in a large series, it appears that echocardiography provides the most accurate and convenient modality for noninvasive detection of pseudoaneurysm of the left ventricle.

Ventricular Septal Rupture and Mitral Regurgitation

Prompt detection of ventricular septal rupture is clinically important because surgical repair often produces

a more favorable outcome than medical management.[312–314] Two-dimensional echocardiography has proved successful in visualizing defects in the septum after acute inferior myocardial infarction.[315-319] The combination of two-dimensional echocardiography with Doppler echocardiography appears to provide the noninvasive diagnostic procedure of choice for detection of ventricular septal rupture in myocardial infarction at this time.[315,316,320-322] In particular, color Doppler flow imaging appears to provide a rapid and accurate method for detection of acute ventricular septal rupture and differentiation of this complication from acute mitral regurgitation in acute myocardial infarction.[315]

Detection and differentiation of ventricular septal rupture and mitral regurgitation complicating acute myocardial infarction have received relatively little attention in the nuclear cardiology literature. Gustafson et al[323] investigated systolic murmurs arising early in the course of acute myocardial infarction in 5 patients. Evaluation for the presence of left-to-right intracardiac shunting was accomplished by radioisotope injection into a central vein, followed by gamma camera detection and computer analysis of pulmonary blood flow curves. (Methods for radioisotope detection of intracardiac shunts are described in detail in Chap. 27.) Three patients had evidence of early pulmonary recirculation of the tracer, suggesting the presence of a left-to-right shunt. Ventricular septal rupture was confirmed at autopsy in each case. Two patients with no radioisotope evidence of a shunt were presumed to have mitral regurgitation as the cause of the murmur and recovered. The stroke–volume ratio by radionuclide ventriculogram (see Chap. 24) might theoretically prove helpful for detecting the presence of ventricular septal rupture or acute mitral regurgitation, but few data are available that describe this application. The clinical consequences of significant acute mitral regurgitation or ventricular septal defect complicating myocardial infarction are usually profound and the stroke count ratio may underestimate the acute hemodynamic burden, as a result of a lack of time for adaptation to acute volume overload. It would not be expected that the hemodynamic severity of acute valvular regurgitation or an acute shunt could be accurately assessed by comparing the resultant radionuclide stroke–volume ratio to values reported in patients with chronic valvular regurgitation or shunt lesions in whom gradual adaptation to volume overload of the left ventricle was possible.

Pericardial Effusion

Whereas almost all patients with acute transmural myocardial infarction who come to autopsy have evidence of a localized fibrinous pericarditis overlying the site of infarction, only about 10 to 15 percent of patients with acute myocardial infarction have signs or symptoms of pericardial effusion.[324] Echocardiography is the procedure of choice for detecting pericardial effusion and for quantitating its size.[325,326] Although definitive hemodynamic diagnosis of pericardial tamponade is made from invasive measurement of ventricular pressures, the diagnosis may be strongly suspected from echocardiography. In a patient with jugular venous distension and hypotension, echocardiographic evidence of substantial pericardial effusion with diastolic compression of the right atrium and right ventricle strongly suggests a diagnosis of pericardial tamponade.

The presence of pericardial effusion may sometimes be suggested by the presence of a halo (low photon density) surrounding the heart on a radionuclide ventriculogram. The features of pericardial effusion detected from radionuclide ventriculography are illustrated in Fig. 11-29.

RELATIONSHIP OF NONINVASIVE CARDIAC IMAGING TO ACUTE INTERVENTION IN MYOCARDIAL INFARCTION

Imaging Prior to Thrombolysis

Early interventions in acute myocardial infarction with intravenous thrombolysis, percutaneous transluminal coronary angioplasty, or urgent coronary artery bypass surgery can reestablish blood flow to the distribution of the occluded coronary artery. Numerous studies document that the earlier that patency (or revascularization) of the infarct-related artery is provided, the greater will be the degree of myocardial salvage and the likelihood of the patient's survival.[2,327] Therefore, thrombolysis should not be delayed to perform noninvasive imaging unless the indication for thrombolysis is in doubt. For example, if clinical features are present that suggest the patient's chest pain and ECG findings may be related to pericarditis rather than acute myocardial infarction, then imaging by two-dimensional echocardiography would be advisable before considering administration of a thrombolytic drug. If uncertainty exists as to whether the patient has chest pain related to acute myocardial infarction or to acute aortic dissection, then thrombolysis would be withheld until the aorta could be studied, usually by contrast aortography or transesophageal echocardiography.

Although timely administration of thrombolytic drugs has been clearly documented to improve left ventricular function and survival in patients with acute myocardial infarction, only a minority of patients presenting to the hospital with acute myocardial infarction are actually treated with thrombolytic therapy.[328] At the time of writing, thrombolytic drug administration is generally considered appropriate when a patient (1) presents within 6 h of onset of symptoms with more than 30 min of ongoing ischemic chest pain, (2) has ST-segment elevation consistent with myocardial injury, and (3) has no contraindication to thrombolytic therapy. However, these current guidelines probably apply to only about 25 percent of patients with acute myocardial infarction.[329]

Although ST-segment elevation on the ECG has proved valuable for identification of patients with acute myocardial infarction who are likely to benefit from thrombolytic treatment, it is not clear that this ECG assessment is the optimal identifier. It has been suggested that the size of the risk area of a persistently occluded coronary artery is inversely related to the LVEF measured 3 days postinfarction and is an important predictor of cardiac death in these patients.[330] In 27 patients without prior evidence of myocardial infarction, Feiring et al[330] administered, immediately prior to intracoronary streptokinase, intracoronary ^{99m}Tc-macroaggregated albumin to determine myocardial risk area in acute myocardial infarction. The myocardial risk area could not be predicted from the sum of ST-segment elevation, acute angiographic LVEF, cardiac index, left ventricular end-diastolic pressure, or the location of coronary artery occlusion within the occluded vessel. These findings suggest that accurate noninvasive assessment of myocardial risk area could prove valuable in aiding in the selection of patients for thrombolytic treatment.

At present, no noninvasive test can accurately measure the extent of the risk area in acute myocardial infarction and provide that measurement prior to and without delaying thrombolysis. Two-dimensional echocardiography can verify the presence of segmental left ventricular wall-motion abnormality in a patient with prolonged chest pain who is being considered for acute thrombolysis.[74] However, two-dimensional echocardiography cannot differentiate necrotic myocardium, old myocardial scar, and myocardial ischemia. Also, two-dimensional echocardiography is likely to overestimate the size of the risk area. Administration of ^{99m}Tc sestamibi immediately prior to thrombolysis, with imaging after thrombolysis, provides a potential approach to the assessment of risk area without delaying thrombolysis. However, ^{99m}Tc sestamibi imaging has not been shown to be helpful in guiding selection of patients for thrombolytic therapy.

Imaging within 24 h after Thrombolysis

An ideal noninvasive test performed soon following administration of a thrombolytic drug would (1) establish whether patency of the infarct-related artery has been restored, (2) demonstrate the size and location of the necrotic zone and remaining myocardial risk area, and (3) accurately define prognosis. Numerous noninvasive imaging tests have been examined in the early postthrombolytic state. The strength and limitations of selected noninvasive tests early following administration of a thrombolytic drug will be considered in this section.

Although two-dimensional echocardiography holds substantial promise for estimating the combined myocardial ischemic and necrotic area and for assessing prognosis in acute myocardial infarction,[74,331] the role of echocardiography in documenting myocardial reperfusion in response to thrombolytic therapy in acute myocardial infarction is limited. Regional wall-motion abnormalities that are observed prior to thrombolytic therapy and that resolve after thrombolytic therapy suggest reperfusion, but if stunned myocardium is present, there may be a lack of early improvement of regional wall motion abnormalities.[332,333] Charuzi et al[333] noted improvement of left ventricular function 10 days after thrombolysis, but not on an immediate postthrombolytic echocardiographic study. Topol et al[332] evaluated the functional recovery of 20 patients with acute myocardial infarction who received recombinant tissue-type plasminogen activator. There was no improvement in contraction of the reperfused infarct zone during the first 24 h following thrombolysis. Function of the reperfused infarct zone showed improvement 10 days after coronary thrombolysis. It appears that two-dimensional echocardiography can be used to identify myocardial salvage several days following thrombolysis but is currently unable to identify accurately patients in the initial 24 h following thrombolytic therapy who require a further revascularization procedure.

The proposed use of ^{99m}Tc pyrophosphate imaging to identify coronary artery patency following acute thrombolytic therapy is based on observations concerning the time after infarction when pyrophosphate uptake begins to occur. In acute myocardial infarction without thrombolytic treatment, pyrophosphate uptake is seldom observed within 12 h following onset of myocardial infarction.[334] Acute myocardial infarction followed by restoration of coronary artery flow produced pyrophosphate uptake in the infarction zone within 4.5 h in dogs.[335] Subsequently, Wheelan et al[336] reported findings from pyrophosphate imaging 7 $\pm$ 2 h following onset of chest pain and 3 h following streptokinase administration in 14 patients with acute myocardial infarction. Eight of 11 patients who came to angiography 15 days later had a patent infarct-related vessel, and each of these patients had intense, early pyrophosphate uptake. Two of three patients with a persistent coronary artery occlusion following acute infarction did not have early pyrophosphate uptake. Identification of successful reperfusion in response to thrombolytic therapy from early ^{99m}Tc-pyro-

phosphate uptake has been substantially less successful in more recent studies[337] with Manyari et al[338] reporting early pyrophosphate uptake to be 60 percent sensitive and 50 percent specific for detection of successful reperfusion. Therefore, it remains to be established whether ^{99m}Tc pyrophosphate imaging has any useful role for demonstrating patency of the infarct-related artery early following thrombolysis. Use of ^{111}In antimyosin in a similar role remains to be reported but is not likely to be clinically useful because of delayed clearance of the antibody from the central circulation.[339,340]

The imaging characteristics of ^{201}Tl in relation to coronary artery occlusion and reperfusion have been extensively studied in laboratory animals and in humans.[341] In the absence of substantial collateral circulation, ^{201}Tl injection in the setting of coronary artery occlusion will demonstrate a perfusion defect. If ^{201}Tl is injected during coronary artery occlusion, initial images will document the extent of ischemia. If thallium imaging is repeated (without further thallium injection) following restoration of vessel patency by thrombolytic therapy, thallium redistribution compared to the initial images will demonstrate regions of salvaged myocardium.[342,343] Absence of ^{201}Tl redistribution following successful reperfusion suggests that myocardial necrosis has occurred.[344] In comparison, if ^{201}Tl is injected soon after reperfusion by a thrombolytic drug, thallium activity in the infarct zone will reflect hyperemic myocardial blood flow more than tissue viability.[345,346] As a result, normal or even increased thallium activity may be observed in the myocardial region supplied by the previously occluded vessel even though myocardial necrosis has occurred. Conversely, if ^{201}Tl is injected soon after reperfusion by thrombolytic drugs and a ^{201}Tl defect is present, then myocardial necrosis is likely to be present. An alternative approach to ^{201}Tl myocardial imaging in patients undergoing thrombolytic treatment is to inject two separate thallium doses, one prior to thrombolysis and one at least 24 h after therapy. With this approach, improvement in size of thallium defect on serial images will predict patency of the infarct-related artery and improvement in regional myocardial function. A clinical limitation of these approaches is that if thallium is injected before thrombolysis, then thallium imaging will delay administration of the thrombolytic drug, with a delay in time to vessel patency and a decrease in clinical benefit in terms of myocardial salvage and survival advantage. If ^{201}Tl is administered early after thrombolysis, it will reflect coronary blood flow rather than tissue survival. For these reasons, routine thallium imaging on the day of thrombolytic treatment has not become popular.

Technetium 99m myocardial imaging agents such as sestamibi offer a potential advantage compared to ^{201}Tl in that clinically important redistribution of the tracer following injection is absent. Technetium-99m-sestamibi can be injected immediately prior to thrombolysis, and the prethrombolysis tracer distribution may be recorded by imaging after thrombolysis when the patient is clinically stable. Injection of ^{99m}Tc sestamibi within hours following thrombolysis in an animal model is associated with tracer distribution in direct relation to myocardial blood flow in regions with viable but hypocontractile (i.e., stunned) myocardium.[207,347-349] Although myocardial blood flow is restored and ^{99m}Tc sestamibi uptake is related to myocardial blood flow, scintigraphic images of the reperfused myocardial segment may still reveal an apparent perfusion defect. Sinusas et al[350] have shown that this may be a consequence of altered left ventricular geometry. These authors demonstrated that reperfused regions of stunned myocardium contained perfusion defects that were largest at end-systole. In end-systole normal myocardial segments thicken maximally and appear brightest. Postischemic stunned myocardial segments do not thicken normally and may actually thin during systole. Because the thickness of the ischemic left ventricular wall is less than twice the full width half maximum point spread function of the imaging system, the ischemic wall is not fully detected and a perfusion defect is displayed. Thus, although myocardial blood flow is normal and ^{99m}Tc sestamibi activity is normal in the stunned myocardial segment, a defect will be present on the scintigraphic image as a result of the partial volume effect.[350] Over the next several days, if myocardial contraction gradually normalizes, the associated scintigraphic defect will also tend to normalize. In contrast, restoration of flow to infarcted myocardium is associated with reduced uptake of ^{99m}Tc sestamibi and the scintigraphic defect resulting from myocardial scar will not decrease over time.[207,347,348,350] As previously discussed, ^{99m}Tc sestamibi injection during coronary artery occlusion in humans can identify the resultant myocardial risk area; separate ^{99m}Tc sestamibi injection several days following successful thrombolysis reveals a scintigraphic defect that corresponds to myocardial infarct size, and the change in defect size between the two images identifies the extent of salvaged myocardium.[351,352] Thus, comparison of initial sestamibi images obtained prior to reflow with images acquired following a separate ^{99m}Tc sestamibi injection days to weeks later is predictive of patency of the infarct-related artery by demonstrating recovery of peri-infarction ischemic zones.[353]

Positron emission tomography (PET) offers great potential for differentiation of metabolically intact but hypocontractile myocardium from necrotic myocardium early following acute myocardial infarction. However, PET is costly and not widely available, particularly for imaging in or near the emergency room or CCU during the first day after myocardial infarction. Further development of noninvasive imaging is needed to provide information related to infarct artery patency, infarct size,

and risk area at an earlier time to assist in decisions concerning further coronary revascularization.

Summary of Clinical and Experimental Reperfusion Studies

Concisely summarizing the available literature regarding resting radionuclide imaging in severely ischemic but reperfused myocardium is difficult. The variety of clinical or experimental conditions in which each investigation was performed creates complexity in defining clear patterns of radionuclide uptake. This parallels the uncertain clinical criteria for determining effective reperfusion with thrombolytic therapy. Figure 18-16 illustrates common clinical and experimental radionuclide imaging characteristics for four different tracers during five different ischemic myocardial states. For purposes of clarity, each myocardial condition is considered separately although human myocardium after infarction may have several coexistent abnormalities.

Severe resting myocardial ischemia is exemplified by unstable angina pectoris, in which a thrombus suddenly produces severe but subtotal coronary artery stenosis. In this setting, ^{201}Tl imaging is effective in delineating severe reversible ischemia, when redistribution images are obtained in addition to initial rest images.[211,354] Resting ^{99m}Tc sestamibi,[236] ^{99m}Tc tetrofosmin, and ^{99m}Tc Q12 imaging are all likely to demonstrate perfusion defects in the presence of severe resting ischemia. Furthermore, PET imaging with ^{18}F fluorodeoxyglucose (FDG)[355] or ^{11}C acetate[356] is effective in detecting resting myocardial ischemia accurately. Similarly, all of the above radionuclide agents are capable of detecting myocardial infarction (or scar) with specific advantages and disadvantages of each method.[348,357-360] Thallium-201 and ^{18}F FDG imaging have proven to be particularly reliable clinically for differentiating viable from infarcted myocardium. Technetium-99m-labeled agents usually show reduced activity in the diseased zone. However, the pattern observed following ^{99m}Tc tracer injection at rest has not clearly separated severely ischemic from infarcted tissue as compared to observations from combined rest and redistribution ^{201}Tl images.[361-367]

In contrast, the phenomenon of stunned myocardium, or prolonged postischemic systolic dysfunction, has been less extensively investigated. Stunned myocardium has been simulated in experimental animal models of coronary artery occlusion followed by reperfusion. Increasingly, stunned myocardium is also being recognized in humans. For example, following acute coronary artery thrombosis and subsequent emergent percutaneous coronary angioplasty, hypocontractile regional left ventricular function often persists in the distribution of a now patent coronary artery with restored coronary

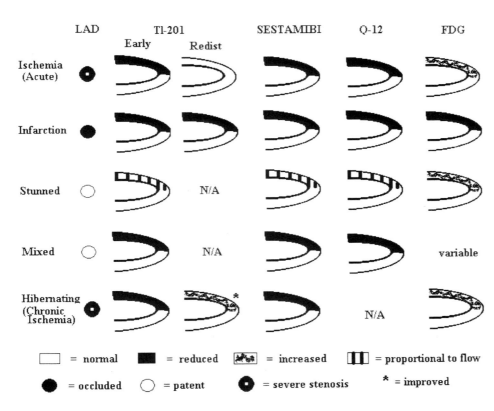

LAD   Tl-201   SESTAMIBI   Q-12   FDG
Early   Redist

Ischemia (Acute)

Infarction

Stunned   N/A

Mixed   N/A   variable

Hibernating (Chronic Ischemia)   *   N/A

☐ = normal   ■ = reduced   ▨ = increased   ▥ = proportional to flow

● = occluded   ○ = patent   ◉ = severe stenosis   * = improved

Figure 18-16 Comparative schematic images of radionuclide tracers in different ischemic myocardial conditions. See text for details. All images are analogous to a vertical long axis view on SPECT imaging with the anterior and apical segments represented as the area at risk. The shaded areas indicate perturbations in relative tracer activity during imaging. LAD, left anterior descending; ^{201}Tl, thallium; Q-12, [99m]Tc Q12; FDG, fluorodeoxyglucose imaging; N/A, not available; *, improved activity from baseline imaging when reinjection performed. The circular schema represent the status of the left anterior descending (LAD) coronary artery at the time of imaging.

blood flow. The available data suggest that radionuclide imaging indicates normal or reduced myocardial activity in the diseased zone corresponding to myocardial blood flow at the time of injection. Thallium-201, ^{99m}Tc sestamibi, [99m]Tc Q12, and ^{18}F FDG have all been investigated with appropriate models to detect myocardial stunning.[211,358,360,368,369]

Hibernating myocardium (i.e., severely ischemic and dysfunctional but viable myocardium) has also been investigated by ^{201}Tl and PET imaging.[370-374] To date, ^{99m}Tc sestamibi has been less useful clinically for this condition,[361] and ^{99m}Tc tetrofosmin and Q12 have not been studied adequately.

Clinically, it is common for a patient to have a mixture of myocardial infarction and stunned myocardium. The extent of infarction depends on several factors including duration of coronary occlusion, presence of collateral vessels, and adequacy of reperfusion. Wall-motion studies early after reperfusion do not accurately define the amount of salvaged myocardium. Radionuclide imaging in this instance is not well validated but may have clinical utility. In experimental animal models of mixed myocardial infarction and stunned myocardium, ^{201}Tl activity appears to be reduced[358] as does ^{99m}Tc sestamibi[351] and [99m]Tc Q12.[358,369] It appears from these data that the degree of reduction in activity with these agents in the risk zone correlates with severity of infarction. A similar infarction/reperfusion study using [18]F

FDG revealed increased FDG activity in the ischemic but viable border zone.[359]

Current standards of treatment for myocardial infarction do not include radionuclide imaging as a routine peri-infarction diagnostic test. Recent investigation suggests that radionuclide imaging, particularly with ^{99m}Tc-labeled compounds, may impart important clinical data on extent of infarction and degree of tissue viability.

PROGNOSTIC IMPLICATIONS OF NONINVASIVE IMAGING AT REST IN ACUTE MYOCARDIAL INFARCTION

The Prethrombolytic Era

In acute myocardial infarction, coronary artery occlusion results in a central zone of myocardial necrosis that is often surrounded by peri-infarction ischemia. In addition, the neurohumoral and mechanical responses to myocardial infarction often induce ischemia in the distributions of stenotic noninfarct-related arteries. As a result, assessment of regional myocardial blood flow or regional myocardial contraction can often provide insight into the extent of myocardium in jeopardy as well as the extent of myocardial necrosis. Measures of the combined extent of jeopardized and necrotic myocardium provide powerful prediction of both in-hospital and subsequent cardiac complications of acute myocardial infarction.[375] This and the next section consider the prognostic importance of clinical, ECG, and imaging data acquired at rest early in the hospital course of acute myocardial infarction. Subsequent diagnosis of residual CAD and assessment of prognosis following initial recovery from acute myocardial infarction require addition of a stress modality, and these topics are discussed in Chap. 19 and 23.

Detection of residual myocardial ischemia following acute myocardial infarction often results when the patient reports recurrent chest pain.[376,377] When recurrent chest pain in the hospital is associated with transient ischemic ST-segment depression, anatomically extensive CAD is usually present and the patient is at high risk for extension of the infarction zone.[377,378] Signs of clinical left heart failure also generally correspond to the presence of residual myocardial ischemia and portend a poor in-hospital outcome with medical therapy.[379] More recently it has been documented that silent myocardial ischemia after an initially uncomplicated myocardial infarction is also associated with increased risk for subsequent complications of myocardial infarction.[380]

In the prethrombolytic era, Holman et al[381] found that increasing intensity and extent of focal activity in the heart on a ^{99m}Tc pyrophosphate scan predicted an increasing incidence of in-hospital congestive heart failure and death. Patients found to have a large, intense area of focal pyrophosphate activity in the heart were also likely to develop recurrent myocardial infarction, unstable angina, or cardiac death following hospital discharge.[381] The measured area of pyrophosphate activity in acute myocardial infarction patients provided greater predictive value for postdischarge cardiac complications compared to the peak level of total CK.[381] The "doughnut sign" of extensive myocardial pyrophosphate activity surrounding a central, less-intense region of tracer activity carried a particularly unfavorable prognosis. Ahmad et al[382] followed 30 survivors of acute myocardial infarction for a mean of 28 months, including 8 patients with this sign. The 83 percent mortality in the group of patients with the doughnut sign was significantly greater than the 6 percent mortality associated with less extensive focal pyrophosphate activity.

The ^{111}In antimyosin scan has also been used to evaluate prognosis in patients with acute myocardial infarction before the wide use of thrombolytic therapy. In a preliminary report of 497 patients followed for up to 5 months after acute myocardial infarction, the Antimyosin Multicenter Trial Group observed that a high-risk antimyosin scan (defined when more than 50 percent of the myocardium demonstrated ^{111}In antimyosin uptake) was a more powerful predictor of cardiac death and

nonfatal reinfarction than conventional clinical, ECG, and enzymatic parameters.[383] Nevertheless, prediction of cardiac complications from either ^{111}In antimyosin or ^{99m}Tc pyrophosphate imaging alone is likely to be limited because these techniques provide no information regarding the extent of peri-infarction or distant ischemia. Combination of imaging with an infarct-avid tracer and with a myocardial perfusion tracer offers greater promise for assessment of prognosis in patients with acute myocardial infarction not treated with thrombolytic or early revascularization measures.

The ^{201}Tl myocardial perfusion scintigram has proved to be a useful predictor of in-hospital complications of acute myocardial infarction.[384,385] The size of the perfusion defect early in the course of acute myocardial infarction has provided an estimate of the total extent of hypoperfused myocardium, including both necrotic and ischemic muscle. Myocardial perfusion scintigraphy with ^{201}Tl was performed safely in the earliest stages of myocardial infarction where imaging instrumentation was available in the coronary care unit and provided that a ^{201}Tl dose was available when needed. Silverman et al[384] used ^{201}Tl scintigraphy to study hemodynamically stable patients within 15 h of onset of symptoms resulting from acute myocardial infarction. A high thallium defect score corresponding to at least a moderate reduction of activity involving 40 percent or more of the left ventricle identified a patient subgroup with a 46 percent in-hospital mortality. A lower ^{201}Tl defect score identified a patient subgroup with a 3 percent in-hospital mortality. Thallium 201 scintigraphy was a better predictor of in-hospital mortality than a variety of clinical indicators including age, sex, history of previous infarct, location of the acute infarct, and Killip[386] clinical class.

Myocardial perfusion imaging has also proven useful in prediction of late cardiac events following acute myocardial infarction. In a study of 42 patients with acute myocardial infarction not treated by acute revascularization and not complicated by pulmonary edema or cardiogenic shock, Silverman et al[384] obtained quantitative ^{201}Tl myocardial perfusion images within 15 h following the onset of symptoms. At least moderate reduction in ^{201}Tl activity involving 40 percent or more of the left ventricle identified 13 high-risk patients with a 92 percent mortality at 9 months of follow-up. For 29 patients with less than 40 percent of the left ventricle hypoperfused, the total mortality at follow-up was 7 percent. Combinations of clinical variables including age, gender, history of previous infarct, acute infarct location, peak CK, and clinical class at the time of admission lacked the prognostic power of either qualitative or quantitative ^{201}Tl scintigraphy.[384,385] In addition, the presence of lung thallium uptake on rest thallium images following admission to the hospital for acute myocardial infarction or unstable angina has been correlated with clinical heart failure and has been found to be predictive of increased risk for cardiac death over the subsequent 9 months.[387]

Dual-isotope ^{201}Tl myocardial perfusion and ^{111}In antimyosin infarct-avid imaging have been used in acute myocardial infarction for combined assessment of myocardial ischemia and necrosis and have provided good prediction of in-hospital cardiac complications.[214] "Matched" [201]Tl defects and ^{111}In antimyosin uptake suggested that all underperfused myocardium was necrotic. In patients with matched defects, no recurrent ischemic coronary events occurred during the hospital stay. "Mismatched" [201]Tl defects and ^{111}In antimyosin uptake suggested that myocardial ischemia (or old myocardial scar) was present outside the acute infarct zone. Among 23 patients with myocardial infarction within 48 h prior to the injection of dual tracer, a mismatch predicted recurrent angina or infarction, ischemic pulmonary edema, or stress test evidence of residual ischemia in 16 patients. Therefore, the ^{201}Tl and ^{111}In antimyosin dual-isotope scan can potentially identify and quantitate residual myocardial ischemia as well as myocardial necrosis. The principal drawbacks to this approach are the difficulty in separating old myocardial infarction from residual myocardial ischemia and the 24- to 48-h time delay from the beginning of myocardial infarction to the time of ^{111}In antimyosin imaging.

Echocardiographic assessment of in-hospital prognosis after acute myocardial infarction is based on estimation of global and regional impairment of left ventricular function.[74,331,388–394] In an early study,[49] echocardiographic studies were performed on 44 patients with acute myocardial infarction. Nine segments of the left ventricle were analyzed to develop a wall-motion index. Patients with uncomplicated myocardial infarction had a wall-motion index of 3.2 ± 2.4. This wall-motion index was significantly less than that of patients with pulmonary edema (9.7 ± 3.1) or with both pulmonary edema and hypotension (10.6 ± 4.8, $p < 0.001$). Subsequently, the early detection of high-risk patients with acute myocardial infarction by an echocardiographic wall-motion index was reported by Horowitz et al.[74] Technically adequate echocardiograms were obtained in 43 of 60 patients within 8 h of hospital admission. A wall-motion index was developed on the basis of echocardiographic evaluation of 12 left ventricular segments. A cardiac complication was defined as hypotension requiring pharmacologic agents for support, refractory pulmonary edema, third-degree heart block, ventricular fibrillation presenting at least 24 h after admission, or death. A wall-motion index of 8 or greater was found in 11 of 13 patients who suffered a cardiac complication and in 5 of 30 patients without a cardiac complication ($p < 0.05$, sensitivity 85 percent, specificity 83 percent). Thus, the wall-motion index allowed identification of patients with acute myocardial infarction who were at high risk for the development of in-hospital complications.

The LVEF by radionuclide ventriculography is a powerful predictor of cardiac complications in patients with acute myocardial infarction.[385,395–398] In a study from the prethrombolytic era by Shah et al,[395] death due to cardiac pump failure occurred in 6 of 11 patients (55 percent) with a LVEF of 30 percent or less measured within 24 h of the onset of symptoms of a first acute transmural myocardial infarction. In contrast, only 1 of 45 patients with a higher initial LVEF died in the hospital ($p < 0.001$). Assessment of regional myocardial contraction by radionuclide ventriculography has also been found predictive of early mortality in acute myocardial infarction.[385] In-hospital prognosis and clinical functional class have been related not only to regional myocardial function in the infarcted zone but also to regional function of noninfarcted areas.[399] These findings provide support for the concept that in-hospital prognosis in acute myocardial infarction is a function of both the extent of infarcted myocardium and the presence of ischemia in noninfarcted segments (e.g., ischemia at a distance). In the prethrombolytic era, assessment of global and regional left ventricular function by radionuclide ventriculography early in the course of acute myocardial infarction was also predictive of long-term cardiac prognosis. Becker et al[398] studied 91 consecutive patients admitted to the hospital with evident or strongly suspected acute myocardial infarction. Patients with pulmonary edema or shock were excluded. Radionuclide ventriculography and ^{201}Tl myocardial scintigraphy were performed within 15 h of the onset of symptoms. The patients were followed clinically for 6 months following acute myocardial infarction, and apparent cardiac death occurred in 12 patients (13 percent). Scintigraphic variables were more strongly associated with mortality than a variety of clinical variables, including Killip clinical class and peak serum CK. When 3 patients with noncardiac death were excluded, the presence of a left ventricular ejection fraction less than or equal to 35 percent identified a patient subgroup with a 60 percent mortality at 6 months. Patients with a presenting left ventricular ejection fraction greater than 35 percent had an 11 percent mortality in 6 months.

Ong et al[385] examined prospectively the prognostic value of radionuclide imaging performed within 24 h of the onset of symptoms of acute transmural myocardial infarction in patients not treated with a thrombolytic drug. Radionuclide ventriculography and ^{201}Tl scintigraphy were performed in 222 patients who were found to be in Killip class I or II on admission to the hospital. The total mortality rate after 90 days of follow-up was 13 percent. Based on previous studies by Killip and Kimball[386] and Norris et al,[400] five clinical variables were analyzed for prediction of prognosis: age, Killip class, infarct location, presence of pulmonary congestion on chest radiograph, and history of prior myocardial infarction. The peak serum CK level was also evaluated.

Based on criteria established in a preliminary study, three prospective radionuclide criteria were found to be univariately predictive of prognosis: LVEF less than 30 percent, abnormal contraction of more than 70 percent of left ventricular regions, and a quantitative thallium defect score greater than 32.0.[401] By stepwise logistic regression, LVEF provided the greatest improvement over the best clinical model for prediction of 90-day mortality. Although a LVEF less than 30 percent was the single variable predicting the greatest relative risk of mortality, an optimal predictive model included both LVEF and Killip class. This is in agreement with the findings of the Multicenter Postinfarction Research Group, who found independent predictive information concerning prognosis after acute myocardial infarction from clinical evidence of heart failure in the acute hospital phase and from evidence of depressed LVEF in the late hospital phase.[402] One explanation for these latter findings is that LVEF measured late in the course of myocardial infarction predicts the extent of myocardial scar, and clinical evidence of left heart failure early in the course of acute infarction identifies the presence of extensive reversible myocardial ischemia. In the study by Ong et al,[385] LVEF was measured within 24 h of onset of acute myocardial infarction and might be expected to identify both necrotic and extensive ischemic myocardium.

In addition to the resting LVEF measured within 24 h after the onset of acute myocardial infarction, the subsequent short-term change in LVEF has been observed to be a powerful predictor of early (1 month) and late (1 year) mortality.[219] In 138 patients with an initial LVEF less than 55 percent within 24 h after onset of acute myocardial infarction, LVEF was remeasured 7 to 14 days later. Patients with a 5 percent or greater increase in LVEF had a 4 percent early and 6 percent late mortality, whereas patients with a 5 percent or greater decrease in LVEF had a 56 percent early and 67 percent late mortality ($p < 0.01$ for both).

The presence of a left ventricular aneurysm, including a "distinct diastolic deformity" of the ventricle, by radionuclide ventriculography may also predict a high risk of death in the year following initial acute anterior myocardial infarction.[285] Whether the presence of a left ventricular aneurysm provides prognostic information in this setting—that is, independent of the LVEF—is less clear.[403]

Beyond the prognostic information provided by the LVEF, the frequency of premature ventricular beats has also been found to be an independent predictor of outcome after acute myocardial infarction.[404-406] Risk stratification strategies following acute myocardial infarction have been described, which combine assessment of the extent of infarcted and ischemic myocardium by measurement of LVEF or thallium defect size, with 24-h ambulatory ECG[407] or the signal-averaged ECG.[408]

Several studies have applied multivariable analysis to both clinical and imaging data in the assessment of in-hospital and late prognosis in acute myocardial infarction.[385,397,398,409] Patients who are initially free of infarct-related complications (Killip class I) or who have at most evidence of mild left heart failure (Killip class II) have been evaluated in most of these studies. Radionuclide LVEF,[385,397,398] radionuclide regional wall-motion assessment,[385,397] two-dimensional echocardiographic LVEF,[397] and extent of ^{201}Tl defect[385,398] have provided improved prediction of in-hospital complications of acute myocardial infarction compared to combinations of clinical variables[386,400] and compared to the peak level of serum CK.[385,398]

In patients with acute inferior myocardial infarction, the presence of greater than 1 mm of ST-segment depression in the anterior precordial ECG leads has been found univariately predictive of increased in-hospital mortality.[410] Radionuclide studies have demonstrated that in the majority of patients with inferior infarction and precordial ST-segment depression, these precordial changes represent reciprocal changes from an anatomically extensive inferior myocardial infarction with frequent involvement of posterolateral and inferoseptal segments.[401,411-415] When submitted to stepwise logistic regression analysis, precordial ST-segment depression in patients with inferior myocardial infarction has provided less prognostic information compared to the radionuclide LVEF measured within 48 h following hospital admission.[401]

The Thrombolytic Era

Once a diagnosis of acute myocardial infarction is established by clinical and ECG criteria, thrombolytic or other revascularization therapy should not be delayed to accomodate additional noninvasive testing.[416,417] Nevertheless, the extent of myocardium in jeopardy prior to revascularization therapy can be assessed by the injection of the nonredistributing myocardial perfusion tracer, ^{99m}Tc sestamibi,[207-209,212] prior to revascularization, and imaging can be delayed until the patient is stable following treatment. Repeat injection of ^{99m}Tc sestamibi 24 h or more following thrombolysis or revascularization and after subsidence of acute myocardial infarction demonstrates the extent of myocardial infarction.[207-209,212] When a revascularization procedure or successful coronary thrombolysis is carried out between these two ^{99m}Tc sestamibi injections, the difference in perfusion defect size between the two sestamibi studies represents the extent of salvaged myocardium.[207-209,212] Miller et al[418] studied 274 consecutive patients with ^{99m}Tc sestamibi injection on arrival at the hospital with acute myocardial infarction (to measure myocardium at risk prior to reperfusion therapy) and at hospital discharge (to measure final infarct size). The median defect size on tomographic imaging was 27 percent of the left ventricle at presentation to the hospital and 12 percent at hospital discharge, with a median estimate of salvaged myocardium of 9 percent of the left ventricle. During a median duration of follow-up of 12 months, there were seven cardiac deaths and one resuscitated out-of-hospital cardiac arrest. There was a significant association between infarct size (predischarge scan defect size) and cardiac mortality ($p < 0.003$). Two-year mortality was 7 percent for patients whose infarct size was 12 percent of the left ventricle or greater versus 0 percent for patients with an infarct size of less than 12 percent. There was also a significant relationship between initial myocardial risk area and cardiac mortality ($p = 0.009$). The estimate of the extent of salvaged myocardium was unrelated to cardiac mortality.[418] After successful reperfusion therapy, myocardial infarct size determined from hospital discharge ^{99m}Tc sestamibi images was inversely correlated with resting LVEF by radionuclide ventriculography 1 year later (20 patients, $r = -0.78$, $p < 0.0001$).[419] Although myocardial infarct size by noninvasive imaging continues to be an important predictor of late prognosis after acute myocardial infarction in the thrombolytic era, it may be less predictive of cardiac events than it was in the prethrombolytic era. This may be a result of the improving prognosis associated with acute myocardial infarction. In 1980, Silverman et al[384] reported a 92 percent mortality at 9 months of follow-up in 13 patients presenting with at least a moderate reduction in resting ^{201}Tl activity involving at least 40 percent of the left ventricle. In 1993, McCallister et al[420] followed 16 patients with an open infarct-related artery and an infarct size by ^{99m}Tc sestamibi imaging of 42 to 68 percent of the left ventricle, and reported only one death at 13 months of follow-up.

Late prognosis and improvement in regional left ventricular function have also been predicted by ^{111}In antimyosin imaging in patients treated with thrombolytic drugs for acute myocardial infarction.[421,422] Van Vlies et al[421] injected antimyosin into 21 patients within 24 h of presentation with acute myocardial infarction, and imaging was performed 24 h later. A ratio of ^{111}In antimyosin count density in the myocardial infarct zone to the count density in a left lung region was calculated. Patients with a low antimyosin count density ratio, reflecting limited myocardial necrosis, were most likely to show improvement in echocardiographic left ventricular regional wall motion from the time of admission to the time of hospital discharge. A count density ratio less than or equal to 1.95 was consistently associated with only mild left ventricular contractile dysfunction at the time of hospital discharge, even if left ventricular dysfunction on admission to the hospital was extensive. In patients hospitalized for acute myocardial infarction,

Maddahi and Di Carli[422] studied the relationship between the extent of ^{111}In antimyosin cardiac activity and subsequent cardiac death or nonfatal myocardial infarction over a mean of 5 months of follow-up. Death or infarction occurred in 25 percent of patients with antimyosin uptake in more than 10 myocardial segments, whereas similar cardiac events occurred in only 5 percent of patients with less extensive ^{111}In antimyosin activity ($p < 0.0001$).

Few reports have appeared in the thrombolytic era evaluating the prognostic implications of early ^{201}Tl imaging and radionuclide ventriculography. Early in the course of acute myocardial infarction, injection of ^{201}Tl immediately following thrombolysis results in tracer distribution that reflects hyperemic blood flow rather than tissue viability.[342] Left ventricular global and regional wall motion during the 24 h period following successful acute thrombolysis may remain reduced due to the presence of stunned myocardium. Consequently, the extent of myocardial infarction will be overestimated by imaging studies of left ventricular regional wall motion in the early postthrombolytic period. Numerous studies of left ventricular global and regional function following acute revascularization therapy for acute myocardial infarction have been performed 1 to 2 weeks postinfarction when postinfarction myocardial stunning is usually resolved.[423–427] In the Thrombolysis in Myocardial Infarction (TIMI) phase II study, resting radionuclide ventriculography was performed 1 to 2 weeks after intravenous thrombolytic treatment in 2567 patients.[423] Patients with a LVEF less than 30 percent had a 1-year mortality of 9.9 percent. Patients with LVEF greater than or equal to 50 percent had a 1-year mortality of 1.2 percent. The authors compared their data to that of the Multicenter Post-infarction Research Group (MPRG).[405] At any level of LVEF, mortality was lower in the TIMI II patients compared to the MPRG patients treated in the prethrombolytic era.[423] Although mortality was lower in the thrombolytic era, resting LVEF remained an important prognostic index.

Candell-Riera et al[424] evaluated prospectively the prognostic role of submaximal exercise testing, ^{201}Tl scintigraphy, rest and exercise radionuclide ventriculography, two-dimensional echocardiography, Holter monitoring, and cardiac catheterization in 115 patients with an uncomplicated first acute myocardial infarction. At 5 years of follow-up, any combination of a test detecting residual ischemia or functional capacity, or both (exercise testing or ^{201}Tl scintigraphy), together with a test assessing left ventricular function (echocardiography or radionuclide ventriculography) best predicted complications, including severe angina, New York Heart Association class III or IV heart failure, reinfarction, angioplasty, cardiac surgery, or death following an uncomplicated first myocardial infarction.[425] Coronary arteriography did not add prognostic information to the noninvasive studies.

Table 18-1   Uses of Radionuclide Testing in Diagnosis of Acute Myocardial Infarction

Indication	Test	Class
1. Right ventricular infarction	Rest RNA	IIa
	^{99m}Tc pyrophosphate	IIa
2. Infarction not diagnosed by standard means—early presentation with successful reperfusion	Rest myocardial perfusion imaging	IIb
	^{99m}Tc pyrophosphate	IIb
3. Infarction not diagnosed by standard means—late presentation	^{99m}Tc pyrophosphate	IIa
4. Routine diagnosis	Any technique	III

Class I, usually appropriate and considered useful; class II, acceptable but usefulness less well established; class IIa, weight of evidence in favor of usefulness; class IIb, can be helpful but not well established by evidence; class III, generally not appropriate; RNA, radionuclide angiography; Tc, technetium. From American College of Cardiology/American Heart Association Task Force,[434] reprinted with permission from the American College of Cardiology, *Journal of the American College of Cardiology*, 25:521, 1995.

Measurement of resting LVEF 7 to 14 days following acute myocardial infarction has also been found to be predictive of ventricular tachycardia and arrhythmic death.[426] In a study of 301 consecutive survivors of acute myocardial infarction, including 205 (68 percent) patients treated with a thrombolytic drug, McClements et al[426] found the resting LVEF to be more predictive than the signal-averaged ECG and the Holter monitor for arrhythmic events over 1 year of follow-up. These findings were extended by Hohnloser et al[428] who found a patent infarct-related artery to be the single best predictor of cardiac death, ventricular fibrillation, or ventricular tachycardia during the first year after acute myocardial infarction. The highest predictive accuracy for severe arrhythmic events was provided by the combination of patency of the infarct-related artery, radionuclide LVEF, and detection of late potentials. In the Survival and Ventricular Enlargement (SAVE) study, patency of the infarct-related artery and the left ventricular ejection

fraction each provided independent predictive information on multivariable analysis for survival over 3.5 years.[429]

Thus, in the thrombolytic era, assessment of risk area and infarct size by ^{99m}Tc sestamibi imaging and LVEF by radionuclide ventriculography can provide powerful prognostic data following acute myocardial infarction. These tests, carried out at rest relatively early after acute infarction, appear to provide predictive information similar to that obtained later after myocardial infarction when noninvasive imaging is combined with limited exercise or pharmacologic stress.[424,425]

Although it is clear that noninvasive imaging can provide prognostic information following acute myocardial infarction, it is not clear that routine noninvasive testing is necessary in this setting.[430,431] Myers et al[427] compared the prediction of cardiac outcome by the patient's own cardiologist to a second prediction that included noninvasive testing with an exercise ECG, a rest

Table 18-2   Uses of Radionuclide Testing in Risk Assessment, Prognosis, and Assessment of Therapy After Acute Myocardial Infarction

Indication	Test	Class
1. Rest RV/LV function	Rest RNA	I
2. Presence/extent of stress-induced ischemia	Stress myocardial perfusion imaging	I
	Stress RNA	IIa
3. Assessment of myocardial viability in patients with LV dysfunction in planning revascularization	Rest–redistribution ^{201}Tl imaging	I
	Stress–redistribution–reinjection ^{201}Tl imaging	I
	PET imaging with ^{18}F fluorodeoxyglucose[a]	I
	Dobutamine RNA	IIb
	Postexercise RNA	IIb
	Post-NTG RNA	IIb
4. Detection of infarct size	Rest myocardial perfusion imaging	IIa
5. Acute measurement of myocardium at risk	Rest ^{99m}Tc sestamibi perfusion imaging	IIa
6. Measurement of myocardial salvage	Sequential rest myocardial imaging with ^{99m}Tc sestamibi	IIa

LV (RV), left (right) ventricular; [a]The relative cost of positron emission computed tomography (PET), thallium (Tl)-201 or technetium (Tc)-99m agents and lesser availability of PET must be considered when selecting this technique. ^{18}F, fluorine-18; NTG, nitroglycerin; other abbreviations as in Table 18-1. Adapted from American College of Cardiology/American Heart Association Task Force,[434] reprinted with permission from the American College of Cardiology, *Journal of the American College of Cardiology*, 25:521, 1995.

radionuclide ventriculogram, and a 24-h Holter monitor. In 147 patients age 65 years or older, addition of the noninvasive test results did not significantly improve prediction of cardiovascular death or recurrent myocardial infarction compared to clinical variables alone.[427] As is the case in patients with suspected chronic CAD, noninvasive testing will provide the most useful prognostic information in patients with residual clinical uncertainty concerning the level of risk following acute myocardial infarction. Clinical data and diagnostic measures that are already available may provide sufficient risk stratification after myocardial infarction in some patients. For example, patients who develop congestive heart failure or recurrent angina following acute myocardial infarction are at high risk for subsequent cardiac events, and noninvasive tests will do little to alter their prognostic assessment.[432,433]

CONCLUSIONS

In most cases, acute myocardial infarction can be diagnosed accurately from the 12-lead ECG and serial measurements of cardiac enzymes. The diagnosis of acute myocardial infarction may remain unclear (1) if the infarction is not associated with Q waves on the ECG (e.g., when infarction is interrupted by successful reperfusion therapy), (2) if the patient presents late in the course of infarction when cardiac enzymes have already returned to normal, or (3) if infarction involves primarily the right ventricle. In these circumstances, radionuclide imaging is frequently of value (Table 18-1). Mechanical complications of acute myocardial infarction including acute mitral regurgitation, acquired ventricular septal defect, ventricular pseudoaneurysm, and cardiogenic shock can be rapidly and accurately assessed by echocardiography. Specific complications of acute myocardial infarction may at times be suggested by findings from radionuclide imaging.

In the thrombolytic era, radionuclide testing can provide other valuable information in the patient with acute myocardial infarction (Table 18-2). The LVEF can be quantitated by radionuclide ventriculography, and this provides a reliable predictor of in-hospital and late cardiac complications. Residual jeopardized myocardium can be estimated accurately by serial measurements of left ventricular perfusion before and after thrombolytic treatment with ^{99m}Tc sestamibi perfusion imaging. In patients with left ventricular dysfunction, myocardial viability can be assessed with ^{201}Tl myocardial perfusion imaging to guide the use of further revascularization. Both myocardial perfusion imaging and radionuclide measurement of left ventricular function continue to provide valuable prognostic data in the patient with acute myocardial infarction treated with thrombolytic or revascularization therapy.

REFERENCES

1. DeWood MA, Spores J, Notske RN, et al: Prevalence of total coronary occlusion during the early hours of transmural myocardial infarction. *N Engl J Med* 303: 897, 1980.
2. Gruppo Italiano per lo studio della streptochinasi nell 'infarto miocardico (GISSI): Effectiveness of intravenous thrombolytic treatment in acute myocardial infarction. *Lancet* 1:397, 1986.
3. Simoons ML, Serruys PW, van den Brand M, et al: Early thrombolysis in acute myocardial infarction: Limitation of infarct size and improved survival. *J Am Coll Cardiol* 7:717, 1986.
4. European Cooperative Study Group for Streptokinase Treatment in Acute Myocardial Infarction: Streptokinase in acute myocardial infarction. *N Engl J Med* 301: 797, 1979.
5. Kennedy JW, Ritchie JL, Davis KB, et al: The Western Washington randomized trial of intracoronary streptokinase in acute myocardial infarction: A 12-month follow-up report. *N Engl J Med* 312:1073, 1985.
6. The ISAM Study Group: A prospective trial of intravenous streptokinase in acute myocardial infarction (ISAM): Mortality, morbidity, and infarct size at 21 days. *N Engl J Med* 314:1465, 1986.
7. Raizner AE, Tortoledo FA, Verani MS, et al: Intracoronary thrombolytic therapy in acute myocardial infarction: A prospective, randomized, controlled trial. *Am J Cardiol* 55:301, 1985.
8. Ritchie JL, Cerqueira M, Maynard C, et al: Ventricular function and infarct size: The Western Washington intravenous streptokinase in myocardial infarction trial. *J Am Coll Cardiol* 11:689, 1988.
9. Braunwald E, Kloner RA: The stunned myocardium: Prolonged, postischemic ventricular dysfunction. *Circulation* 66:1146, 1982.
10. Williams DO, Braunwald E, Knatterud G, et al: One-year results of the thrombolysis in myocardial infarction investigation (TIMI) phase II trial. *Circulation* 85:533, 1992.
11. Rude RE, Poole WK, Muller JE, et al: Electrocardiographic and clinical criteria for recognition of acute myocardial infarction based on analysis of 3,697 patients. *Am J Cardiol* 52:936, 1983.
12. Zarling EJ, Sexton H, Milnor P Jr: Failure to diagnose acute myocardial infarction: The clinicopathologic experience at a large community hospital. *JAMA* 250: 1177, 1983.
13. Slater DK, Hlatky MA, Mark DB, et al: Outcome in suspected acute myocardial infarction with normal or minimally abnormal admission electrocardiographic findings. *Am J Cardiol* 60:766, 1987.
14. Boden WE, Kleiger RE, Gibson RS, et al: Favourable

long term prognosis in patients with non-Q wave acute myocardial infarction not associated with specific electrocardiographic changes. *Br Heart J* 61:396, 1989.

15. Brush JE Jr, Brand DA, Acampora D, et al: Use of the initial electrocardiogram to predict in-hospital complications of acute myocardial infarction. *N Engl J Med* 312:1137, 1985.

16. Lee TH, Rouan GW, Weisberg MC, et al: Clinical characteristics and natural history of patients with acute myocardial infarction sent home from the emergency room. *Am J Cardiol* 60:219, 1987.

17. Taussig AS: Misleading ECGs: Patterns of infarction. *J Cardiovasc Med* 9:1147, 1983.

18. Blanke H, Cohen M, Schlueter GU, et al: Electrocardiographic and coronary arteriographic correlations during acute myocardial infarction. *Am J Cardiol* 54:249, 1984.

19. Huey BL, Beller GA, Kaiser DL, Gibson RS: A comprehensive analysis of myocardial infarction due to left circumflex artery occlusion: Comparison with infarction due to right coronary artery and left anterior descending artery occlusion. *J Am Coll Cardiol* 12:1156, 1988.

20. Fuchs RM, Achuff SC, Grunwald L, et al: Electrocardiographic localization of coronary artery narrowings: Studies during myocardial ischemia and infarction in patients with one-vessel disease. *Circulation* 66:1168, 1982.

21. Erhardt LR, Sjogren A, Wahlberg I: Single right-sided precordial lead in the diagnosis of right ventricular involvement in inferior myocardial infarction. *Am Heart J* 91:571, 1976.

22. Croft CH, Nicod P, Corbett JR, et al: Detection of acute right ventricular infarction by right precordial electrocardiography. *Am J Cardiol* 50:421, 1982.

23. Chou TC, van der Bel-Kahn J, Allen J, et al: Electrocardiographic diagnosis of right ventricular infarction. *Am J Med* 70:1175, 1981.

24. Freifeld AG, Schuster EH, Bulkley BH: Nontransmural versus transmural myocardial infarction: A morphologic study. *Am J Med* 75:423, 1983.

25. Mirvis DM, Ingram L, Holly K, et al: Electrocardiographic effects of experimental nontransmural myocardial infarction. *Circulation* 71:1206, 1985.

26. Phibbs B: "Transmural" versus "subendocardial" myocardial infarction: An electrocardiographic myth. *J Am Coll Cardiol* 1:561, 1983.

27. Ferlinz J: Acute myocardial infarction: Does the lack of Q waves help or hinder? *J Am Coll Cardiol* 15:1208, 1990.

28. Feld RD, Witte DL: Presence of creatine kinase BB isoenzyme in some patients with prostatic carcinoma. *Clin Chem* 23:1930, 1977.

29. Norris JW, Hachinski VC, Myers MG, et al: Serum cardiac enzymes in stroke. *Stroke* 10:548, 1979.

30. Byer E, Ashman R, Toth LA: Electrocardiograms with large, upright T waves and long Q-T intervals. *Am Heart J* 33:796, 1947.

31. Grande P, Christiansen C, Pedersen A, Christensen MS: Optimal diagnosis in acute myocardial infarction: A cost-effectiveness study. *Circulation* 61:723, 1980.

32. Hackel DB, Reimer KA, Ideker RE, et al: Comparison of enzymatic and anatomic estimates of myocardial infarct size in man. *Circulation* 70:824, 1984.

33. Roberts R, Kleiman NS: Earlier diagnosis and treatment

of acute myocardial infarction necessitates the need for a "new diagnostic mind-set." *Circulation* 89:872, 1994.

34. Lee TH, Goldman L: Serum enzyme assays in the diagnosis of acute myocardial infarction. *Ann Intern Med* 105:221, 1986.

35. Jaffe AS, Serota H, Grace A, et al: Diagnostic changes in plasma creatine kinase isoforms early after the onset of acute myocardial infarction. *Circulation* 74:105, 1986.

36. de Winter RJ, Koster RW, Sturk A, Sanders GT: Value of myoglobin, troponin T, and CK-MB$_{mass}$ in ruling out an acute myocardial infarction in the emergency room. *Circulation* 92:3401, 1995.

37. Puleo PR, Guadagno PA, Roberts R, et al: Early diagnosis of acute myocardial infarction based on assay for subforms of creatine kinase-MB. *Circulation* 82:759, 1990.

38. Prager NA, Suzuki T, Jaffe AS, et al: Nature and time course of generation of isoforms of creatine kinase, MB fraction in vivo. *J Am Coll Cardiol* 20:414, 1992.

39. Mair J, Morandell D, Genser N, et al: Equivalent early sensitivities of myoglobin, creatine kinase MB mass, creatine kinase isoform ratios, and cardiac troponins I and T for acute myocardial infarction. *Clin Chem* 41:1266, 1995.

40. Shiesh S-C, Ting W-K, Jap T-S: Measurement of creatine kinase isoforms by agarose gel electrophoresis in the diagnosis of myocardial infarction. *Clin Biochem* 25:293, 1992.

41. Kanemitsu F, Okigaki T: Creatine kinase MB isoforms for early diagnosis and monitoring of acute myocardial infarction. *Clin Chim Acta* 206:191, 1992.

42. Chattington P, Clarke D, Neithercut WD: Creatine kinase isoform electrophoresis for the early confirmation of myocardial infarction detected by timed sequential CK slope analysis. *Postgrad Med J* 70:805, 1994.

43. Tennant R, Wiggers CJ: The effect of coronary occlusion on myocardial contraction. *Am J Physiol* 112: 351, 1935.

44. Corya BC, Rasmussen S, Knoebel SB, et al: Echocardiography in acute myocardial infarction. *Am J Cardiol* 36:1, 1975.

45. Kerber RE, Marcus ML, Wilson R, et al: Effects of acute coronary occlusion on the motion and perfusion of the normal and ischemic interventricular septum: An experimental echocardiographic study. *Circulation* 54:928, 1976.

46. Heikkila J, Nieminen M: Echoventriculographic detection, localization, and quantification of left ventricular asynergy in acute myocardial infarction. *Br Heart J* 37:46, 1975.

47. Feigenbaum H, Corya BC, Dillon JC, et al: Role of echocardiography in patients with coronary artery disease. *Am J Cardiol* 37:775, 1976.

48. Bloch A, Morard J, Mayor C, et al: Cross-sectional echocardiography in acute myocardial infarction. *Am J Cardiol* 43:387, 1979.

49. Heger JJ, Weyman AE, Wann LS, et al: Cross-sectional echocardiographic analysis of the extent of left ventricular asynergy in acute myocardial infarction. *Circulation* 61:1113, 1980.

50. Weyman AE, Franklin TD Jr, Hogen RD, et al: Impor-

tance of temporal heterogeneity in assessing the contraction abnormalities associated with acute myocardial ischemia. *Circulation* 70:102, 1984.

51. Kerber RE, Abboud FM: Echocardiographic detection of regional myocardial infarction: An experimental study. *Circulation* 47:997, 1973.

52. Kerber RE, Marcus ML, Ehrhardt J, et al: Correlation between echocardiographically demonstrated segmental dyskinesis and regional myocardial perfusion. *Circulation* 52:1097, 1975.

53. Jacobs JJ, Feigenbaum H, Corya BC, Phillips JF: Detection of left ventricular asynergy by echocardiography. *Circulation* 48:263, 1973.

54. Fogelman AM, Abbasi AS, Pearce ML, Kattus AA: Echocardiographic study of the abnormal motion of the posterior left ventricular wall during angina pectoris. *Circulation* 46:905, 1972.

55. Horowitz RS, Morganroth J, Parrotto C, et al: Immediate diagnosis of acute myocardial infarction by two-dimensional echocardiography. *Circulation* 65:323, 1982.

56. Loh IK, Charuzi Y, Beeder C, et al: Early diagnosis of nontransmural myocardial infarction by two-dimensional echocardiography. *Am Heart J* 104:963, 1982.

57. Gibson RS, Bishop HL, Stamm RB, et al: Value of early two dimensional echocardiography in patients with acute myocardial infarction. *Am J Cardiol* 49:1110, 1982.

58. Sasaki H, Charuzi Y, Beeder C, et al: Utility of echocardiography for the early assessment of patients with nondiagnostic chest pain. *Am Heart J* 112:494, 1986.

59. Sabia P, Abbott RD, Afrookteh A, et al: Importance of two-dimensional echocardiographic assessment of left ventricular systolic function in patients presenting to the emergency room with cardiac-related symptoms. *Circulation* 84:1615, 1991.

60. Labovitz AJ, Lewen MK, Kern M, et al: Evaluation of left ventricular systolic and diastolic dysfunction during transient myocardial ischemia produced by angioplasty. *J Am Coll Cardiol* 10:748, 1987.

61. Wohlgelernter D, Cleman M, Highman HA, et al: Regional myocardial dysfunction during coronary angioplasty: Evaluation by two-dimensional echocardiography and 12 lead electrocardiography. *J Am Coll Cardiol* 7:1245, 1986.

62. Komer RR, Edalji A, Hood WB: Effects of nitroglycerin on echocardiographic measurement of left ventricular wall thickness and regional myocardial performance during acute coronary ischemia. *Circulation* 59:926, 1979.

63. Kerber RE, Martins JB, Marcus ML: Effect of acute ischemia, nitroglycerin, and nitroprusside on regional myocardial thickening, stress, and perfusion. *Circulation* 60:121, 1979.

64. Gallagher KP, Kumada T, Koziol JA, et al: Significance of regional wall thickening abnormalities relative to transmural myocardial perfusion in anesthetized dogs. *Circulation* 62:1266, 1980.

65. Traill TA: Wall thickness changes considered as regional myocardial function in ischemic heart disease. *Herz* 5:275, 1980.

66. Pandian NG, Kieso RA, Kerber RE: Two dimensional echocardiography in experimental coronary stenosis: II. Relationship between systolic wall thinning and regional myocardial perfusion in severe coronary stenosis. *Circulation* 66:603, 1982.

67. Guth BD, White FC, Gallagher KP, Bloor CM: Decreased systolic wall thickening in myocardium adjacent to ischemic zones in conscious swine during brief coronary artery occlusion. *Am Heart J* 107:458, 1984.

68. Force T, Kemper A, Perkins L, et al: Overestimation of infarct size by quantitative two-dimensional echocardiography: The role of tethering and of analytic procedures. *Circulation* 73:1360, 1986.

69. Wyatt HL, Meerbaum S, Heng MK, et al: Experimental evaluation of the extent of myocardial dyssynergy and infarct size by two-dimensional echocardiography. *Circulation* 63:607, 1981.

70. Weiss JL, Bulkley BH, Hutchins GM, Mason SJ: Two-dimensional echocardiographic recognition of myocardial injury in man: Comparison with postmortem studies. *Circulation* 63:401, 1981.

71. Lieberman AN, Weiss JL, Jugdutt BI, et al: Two-dimensional echocardiography and infarct size: Relationship of regional wall motion and thickening to the extent of myocardial infarction in the dog. *Circulation* 63:739, 1981.

72. Meltzer R, Woythaler J, Buda A, et al: Two-dimensional echocardiographic quantification of infarct size alteration by pharmacologic agents. *Am J Cardiol* 43:387, 1979.

73. Nixon JV, Narahara KA, Smitherman TC: Estimation of myocardial involvement in patients with acute myocardial infarction by two-dimensional echocardiography. *Circulation* 62:1248, 1980.

74. Horowitz RS, Morganroth J: Immediate detection of early high-risk patients with acute myocardial infarction using two-dimensional echocardiographic evaluation of left ventricular regional wall motion abnormalities. *Am Heart J* 103:814, 1982.

75. Mahias-Narvarte H, Adams KF, Willis PW: Evolution of regional left ventricular wall motion abnormalities in acute Q and non-Q wave myocardial infarction. *Am Heart J* 113:1369, 1987.

76. Arvan S, Varat MA: Two-dimensional echocardiography versus surface electrocardiography for the diagnosis of acute non-Q wave myocardial infarction. *Am Heart J* 110:44, 1985.

77. Shen AC, Jennings RB: Myocardial calcium and magnesium in acute ischemic injury. *Am J Pathol* 67:417, 1972.

78. Gerson MC: Myocardial imaging in myocardial infarction: Technetium vs thallium. *Cardiovasc Clin* 13:223, 1983.

79. Willerson JT, Parkey RW, Bonte FJ, et al: Pathophysiologic considerations and clinicopathological correlates of technetium-99m stannous pyrophosphate myocardial scintigraphy. *Semin Nucl Med* 10:54, 1980.

80. Lewis M, Buja LM, Saffer S, et al: Experimental infarct sizing using computer processing and a three-dimensional model. *Science* 197:167, 1977.

81. Stokely EM, Buja LM, Lewis SE, et al: Measurement of acute myocardial infarcts in dogs with ^{99m}Tc-stannous pyrophosphate scintigrams. *J Nucl Med* 17:1, 1976.

82. Willerson JT, Parkey RW, Stokely EM, et al: Infarct sizing with technetium-99m stannous pyrophosphate scintigraphy in dogs and man: Relationship between scintigraphic and precordial mapping estimates of infarct size in patients. *Cardiovasc Res* 11:291, 1977.

83. Lewis SE, DeVous MD Sr, Corbett JR, et al: Measurement of infarct size in acute canine myocardial infarction by single-photon emission computed tomography with technetium-99m pyrophosphate. *Am J Cardiol* 54:193, 1984.

84. Corbett JR, Lewis SE, Wolfe CL, et al: Measurement of myocardial infarct size by technetium pyrophosphate single-photon tomography. *Am J Cardiol* 54: 1231, 1984.

85. Corbett JR, Lewis M, Willerson JT, et al: ^{99m}Tc-pyrophosphate imaging in patients with acute myocardial infarction: Comparison of planar imaging with single-photon tomography with and without blood pool overlay. *Circulation* 69:1120, 1984.

86. Willerson JT, Parkey RW, Bonte FJ, et al: Technetium stannous pyrophosphate myocardial scintigrams in patients with chest pain of varying etiology. *Circulation* 51:1046, 1975.

87. Okuda K, Nohara R, Fujita M, et al: Technetium-99m-pyrophosphate uptake as an indicator of myocardial injury without infarct. *J Nucl Med* 35:1366, 1994.

88. Bianco JA, Kemper AJ, Taylor A, et al: Technetium-99m(Sn^{2+})pyrophosphate in ischemic and infarcted dog myocardium in early stages of acute coronary occlusion: Histochemical and tissue-counting comparisons. *J Nucl Med* 24:485, 1983.

89. Nohara R, Kambara H, Okuda K, et al: Effect of diltiazem on stunned myocardium evaluated with ^{99m}Tc-pyrophosphate imaging in canine heart. *Jpn Circ J* 56:262, 1992.

90. Lessem J, Johansson BW, Nosslin B, Thorell J: Myocardial scintigraphy with ^{99m}Tc-pyrophosphate in patients with unstable angina pectoris. *Acta Med Scand* 203:491, 1978.

91. Abdulla AM, Canedo MI, Cortez BC, et al: Detection of unstable angina by ^{99m}technetium pyrophosphate myocardial scintigraphy. *Chest* 69:168, 1976.

92. Corbett JR, Lewis SE, Dehmer G, et al: Simultaneous display of gated technetium-99m stannous pyrophosphate and gated blood-pool scintigrams. *J Nucl Med* 22:671, 1981.

93. Wynne J, Holman BL: Acute myocardial infarct scintigraphy with infarct-avid radiotracers. *Med Clin North Am* 64:119, 1980.

94. Olson HG, Lyons KP, Butman S, et al: Validation of technetium-99m stannous pyrophosphate myocardial scintigraphy for diagnosing acute myocardial infarction more than 48 hours old when serum creatine kinase-MB has returned to normal. *Am J Cardiol* 52:245, 1983.

95. Poliner LR, Buja LM, Parkey RW, et al: Clinicopathologic findings in 52 patients studied by technetium-99m stannous pyrophosphate myocardial scintigraphy. *Circulation* 59:257, 1979.

96. Ahmad M, Dubiel JP, Logan KW, et al: Limited clinical diagnostic specificity of technetium-99m stannous pyrophosphate myocardial imaging in acute myocardial infarction. *Am J Cardiol* 39:50, 1977.

97. Massie BM, Botvinick EH, Werner JA, et al: Myocardial scintigraphy with technetium-99m stannous pyrophosphate: An insensitive test for nontransmural myocardial infarction. *Am J Cardiol* 43:186, 1979.

98. Rude RE, Rubin HS, Stone MJ, et al: Radioimmunoassay of serum creatine kinase B isoenzyme in the diagnosis of acute myocardial infarction. Correlation with technetium-99m stannous pyrophosphate myocardial scintigraphy. *Am J Med* 68:405, 1980.

99. Willerson JT, Parkey RW, Bonte FJ, et al: Acute subendocardial myocardial infarction in patients: Its detection by technetium-99m stannous pyrophosphate myocardial scintigrams. *Circulation* 51:436, 1975.

100. Olson HG, Lyons KP, Aronow WS, et al: Follow-up technetium-99m stannous pyrophosphate myocardial scintigrams after acute myocardial infarction. *Circulation* 56:181, 1977.

101. Wisneski JA, Rollo FD, Gertz EW: Correlation of ^{99m}Tc-pyrophosphate myocardial accumulation with left ventricular wall motion abnormalities. *Cardiology* 66:85, 1980.

102. Cowley MJ, Kawamura K, Karp RB, et al: Persistently positive ^{99m}Tc-polyphosphate myocardial scintigrams after acute infarction: Angiographic, histochemical and electron microscopic correlations. *Circulation* 53, 54(suppl II):II-218, 1976 (abstr).

103. Ahmad M, Dubiel JP, Verdon TA Jr, et al: Technetium 99m stannous pyrophosphate myocardial imaging in patients with and without left ventricular aneurysm. *Circulation* 53:833, 1976.

104. Krause T, Kasper W, Zeiher A, et al: Relation of technetium-99m pyrophosphate accumulation to time interval after onset of acute myocardial infarction as assessed by a tomographic acquisition technique. *Am J Cardiol* 68:1575, 1991.

105. Jengo JA, Mena I, Joe SH, et al: The significance of calcific valvular heart disease in Tc-99m pyrophosphate myocardial infarction scanning: Radiographic, scintigraphic, and pathological correlation. *J Nucl Med* 18:776, 1977.

106. Seo I, Donoghue G: Tc-99m-pyrophosphate accumulation on prosthetic valves. *Clin Nucl Med* 5:367, 1980.

107. Pugh BR, Buja LM, Parkey RW, et al: Cardioversion and "false positive" technetium-99m stannous pyrophosphate myocardial scintigrams. *Circulation* 54: 399, 1976.

108. Davison R, Spies SM, Przybylek J, et al: Technetium-99m stannous pyrophosphate myocardial scintigraphy after cardiopulmonary resuscitation with cardioversion. *Circulation* 60:292, 1979.

109. DiCola VC, Freedman GS, Downing SE, et al: Myocardial uptake of technetium-99m stannous pyrophosphate following direct current transthoracic countershock. *Circulation* 54:980, 1976.

110. Sonnenblick M, Gelmont D, Keren A, et al: Positive radionuclide myocardial infarction pattern after ventricular fibrillation and direct current countershock. *Chest* 71:673, 1977.

111. Cowley MJ, Mantle JA, Rogers WJ, et al: Technetium-99m stannous pyrophosphate myocardial scintigraphy:

Reliability and limitations in assessment of acute myocardial infarction. *Circulation* 56:192, 1977.

112. Brantigan CO, Burdick D, Hopemar AR, et al: Evaluation of technetium scanning for myocardial contusion. *J Trauma* 18:460, 1978.

113. Go RT, Doty DB, Chiu CL, et al: A new method of diagnosing myocardial contusion in man by radionuclide imaging. *Radiology* 116:107, 1975.

114. Datz FL, Lewis SE, Parkey RW, et al: Radionuclide evaluation of cardiac trauma. *Semin Nucl Med* 10:187, 1980.

115. Harford W, Weinberg MN, Buja LM, et al: Positive ^{99m}Tc-stannous pyrophosphate myocardial image in a patient with carcinoma of the lung. *Radiology* 122: 747, 1977.

116. Fleg JL, Siegel BA, Roberts R: Detection of pericarditis with ^{99m}Tc pyrophosphate images. *Am J Cardiol* 39: 273, 1977 (abstr).

117. Prasquier R, Taradash MR, Botvinick EH, et al: The specificity of the diffuse pattern of cardiac uptake in myocardial infarction imaging with technetium-99m stannous pyrophosphate. *Circulation* 55:61, 1977.

118. Lyons KP, Olson HG, Aronow WS: Pyrophosphate myocardial imaging. *Semin Nucl Med* 10:168, 1980.

119. Khaw BA, Fallon JT, Strauss HW, Haber E: Myocardial infarct imaging of antibodies to canine cardiac myosin with indium-111-diethylenetriamine pentaacetic acid. *Science* 209:295, 1980.

120. Khaw BA, Scott J, Fallon JT, et al: Myocardial injury: Quantitation by cell sorting initiated with antimyosin fluorescent spheres. *Science* 217:1050, 1982.

121. Khaw BA, Gold HK, Leinbach RC, et al: Early imaging of experimental myocardial infarction by intracoronary administration of ^{131}I-labeled anticardiac myosin (Fab′)$_2$ fragments. *Circulation* 58:1137, 1978.

122. Beller GA, Khaw BA, Haber E, Smith TW: Localization of radiolabeled cardiac myosin-specific antibody in myocardial infarcts: Comparison with technetium-99m stannous pyrophosphate. *Circulation* 55:74, 1977.

123. Khaw BA, Strauss HW, Moore R, et al: Myocardial damage delineated by indium-111 antimyosin Fab and technetium-99m pyrophosphate. *J Nucl Med* 28:76, 1987.

124. Meerdink DJ, Leppo JA: Transcapillary exchange of indium 111-labeled anticardiac myosin Fab and thallium 201 in isolated reperfused rabbit hearts. *J Nucl Cardiol* 1:236, 1994.

125. Takeda K, LaFrance ND, Weisman HF, et al: Comparison of indium-111 antimyosin antibody and technetium-99m pyrophosphate localization in reperfused and nonreperfused myocardial infarction. *J Am Coll Cardiol* 17:519, 1991.

126. Antunes ML, Seldin DW, Wall RM, Johnson LL: Measurement of acute Q-wave myocardial infarct size with single photon emission computed tomography imaging of indium-111 antimyosin. *Am J Cardiol* 63:777, 1989.

127. Johnson LL, Lerrick KS, Coromilas J, et al: Measurement of infarct size and percentage myocardium infarcted in a dog preparation with single photon-emission computed tomography, thallium-201, and indium-111-monoclonal antimyosin Fab. *Circulation* 76:181, 1987.

128. Gerber KH, Higgins CB: Quantitation of size of myocardial infarctions by computerized transmission tomography: Comparison with hot-spot and cold-spot radionuclide scans. *Invest Radiol* 18:238, 1983.

129. Khaw BA, Gold HK, Yasuda T, et al: Scintigraphic quantification of myocardial necrosis in patients after intravenous injection of myosin-specific antibody. *Circulation* 74:501, 1986.

130. Johnson LL, Seldin DW, Becker LC, et al: Antimyosin imaging in acute transmural myocardial infarctions: Results of a multicenter clinical trial. *J Am Coll Cardiol* 13:27, 1989.

131. Khaw BA, Yasuda T, Gold HK, et al: Acute myocardial infarct imaging with indium-111-labeled monoclonal antimyosin Fab. *J Nucl Med* 28:1671, 1987.

132. Berger H, Lahiri A, Leppo J, et al: Antimyosin imaging in patients with ischemic chest pain: Initial results of phase III multicenter trial. *J Nucl Med* 29:805, 1988 (abstr).

133. Braat SH, de Zwaan C, Teule J, et al: Value of indium-111 monoclonal antimyosin antibody for imaging in acute myocardial infarction. *Am J Cardiol* 60:725, 1987.

134. Volpini M, Giubbini R, Gei P, et al: Diagnosis of acute myocardial infarction by indium-111 antimyosin antibodies and correlation with the traditional techniques for the evaluation of extent and localization. *Am J Cardiol* 63:7, 1989.

135. Bhattacharya S, Liu X-J, Senior R, et al: ^{111}In antimyosin antibody uptake is related to the age of myocardial infarction. *Am Heart J* 122:1583, 1991.

136. Tamaki N, Yamada T, Matsumori A, et al: Indium-111-antimyosin antibody imaging for detecting different stages of myocardial infarction: Comparison with technetium-99m-pyrophosphate imaging. *J Nucl Med* 31: 136, 1990.

137. Yamada T, Tamaki N, Morishima S, et al: Time course of myocardial infarction evaluated by indium-111-antimyosin monoclonal antibody scintigraphy: Clinical implications and prognostic value. *J Nucl Med* 33:1501, 1992.

138. Mody FV, Buxton DB, Araujo LI, et al: Blood flow-dependent uptake of indium-111 monoclonal antimyosin antibody in canine acute myocardial infarction. *J Am Coll Cardiol* 21:233, 1993.

139. Merhi Y, Arsenault A, Carrier M, Latour J-G: Effect of reperfusion on ^{111}In-antimyosin monoclonal antibody uptake by salvaged and necrotic myocardium in the dog. *Cardiovascular Res* 27:1504, 1993.

140. Carrio I, Berna L, Ballester M, et al: Indium-111 antimyosin scintigraphy to assess myocardial damage in patients with suspected myocarditis and cardiac rejection. *J Nucl Med* 29:1893, 1988.

141. Yasuda T, Palacios IF, Dec GW, et al: Indium 111-monoclonal antimyosin antibody imaging in the diagnosis of acute myocarditis. *Circulation* 76:306, 1987.

142. Rezkalla S, Kloner RA, Khaw BA, et al: Detection of experimental myocarditis by monoclonal antimyosin antibody, Fab fragment. *Am Heart J* 117:391, 1989.

143. Lekakis J, Nanas J, Moustafellou A, et al: Antimyosin scintigraphy for detection of myocarditis. Scintigraphic follow-up. *Chest* 104:1427, 1993.

144. Matsuura H, Palacios IF, Dec GW, et al: Intraventricular conduction abnormalities in patients with clinically sus-

pected myocarditis are associated with myocardial necrosis. *Am Heart J* 127:1290, 1994.

145. Morguet AJ, Munz DL, Kreuzer H, Emrich D: Scintigraphic detection of inflammatory heart disease. *Eur J Nucl Med* 21:666, 1994.

146. Castell J, Fraile M, Garcia A, et al: Pericardial and myocardial localization of antimyosin in a case of acute myocarditis. *J Nucl Med* 35:469, 1994.

147. Morguet AJ, Sandrock D, Stille-Siegener M, Figulla HR: Indium-111-antimyosin Fab imaging to demonstrate myocardial involvement in systemic lupus erythematosus. *J Nucl Med* 36:1432, 1995.

148. Le Guludec D, Lhote F, Weinmann P, et al: New application of myocardial antimyosin scintigraphy: Diagnosis of myocardial disease in polymyositis. *Ann Rheum Dis* 52:235, 1993.

149. Knapp WH, Bentrup A, Ohlmeier H: Indium-111-labelled antimyosin antibody imaging in a patient with cardiac sarcoidosis. *Eur J Nucl Med* 20:80, 1993.

150. Bergler-Klein J, Sochor H, Stanek G, et al: Indium 111-monoclonal antimyosin antibody and magnetic resonance imaging in the diagnosis of acute lyme myopericarditis. *Arch Intern Med* 153:2696, 1993.

151. Krause T, Schumichen C, Beck A, et al: Scintigraphy using 111-indium-labeled antimyosin in Churg-Strauss vasculitis with myocardial involvement. *Nuklearmedizin* 29:177, 1990.

152. Malhotra A, Narula J, Yasuda T, et al: Indium-111-monoclonal antimyosin antibody imaging for diagnosis of rheumatic myocarditis. *J Nucl Med* 31:841, 1990 (abstr).

153. Case records of the Massachusetts General Hospital. *N Engl J Med* 318:970, 1988.

154. Carrio I, Lopez-Pousa A, Estorch M, et al: Detection of doxorubicin cardiotoxicity in patients with sarcomas by indium-111-antimyosin monoclonal antibody studies. *J Nucl Med* 34:1503, 1993.

155. Hiroe M, Ohta Y, Fujita N, et al: Myocardial uptake of ^{111}In monoclonal antimyosin Fab in detecting doxorubicin cardiotoxicity in rats. Morphological and hemodynamic findings. *Circulation* 86:1965, 1992.

156. Estorch M, Carrio I, Berna L, et al: Indium-111-antimyosin scintigraphy after doxorubicin therapy in patients with advanced breast cancer. *J Nucl Med* 31:1965, 1990.

157. Marti V, Ballester M, Udina C, et al: Evaluation of myocardial cell damage by In-111-monoclonal antimyosin antibodies in patients under chronic tricyclic antidepressant drug treatment. *Circulation* 91:1619, 1995.

158. Obrador D, Ballester M, Carrio I, Berna L, Pons-Llado G: High prevalence of myocardial monoclonal antimyosin antibody uptake in patients with chronic idiopathic dilated cardiomyopathy. *J Am Coll Cardiol* 13:1289, 1989.

159. Dec GW, Palacios I, Yasuda T, et al: Antimyosin antibody cardiac imaging: Its role in the diagnosis of myocarditis. *J Am Coll Cardiol* 16:97, 1990.

160. Obrador D, Ballester M, Carrio I, et al: Presence, evolving changes, and prognostic implications of myocardial damage detected in idiopathic and alcoholic dilated cardiomyopathy by ^{111}In monoclonal antimyosin antibodies. *Circulation* 89:2054, 1994.

161. Werner GS, Figulla HR, Munz DL, et al: Myocardial

162. Huguet M, Garcia A, Francino A, et al: Myocardial uptake of antimyosin antibody in idiopathic dilated cardiomyopathy and its relation to functional and morphological parameters. *Nucl Med Commun* 15:943, 1994.

163. Obrador D, Ballester M, Carrio I, et al: Active myocardial damage without attending inflammatory response in dilated cardiomyopathy. *J Am Coll Cardiol* 21:1667, 1993.

164. Frist W, Yasuda T, Segall G, et al: Noninvasive detection of human cardiac transplant rejection with indium-111 antimyosin (Fab) imaging. *Circulation* 76(suppl V):V-81, 1987.

165. Addonizio LJ, Michler RE, Marboe C, et al: Imaging of cardiac allograft rejection in dogs using indium-111 monoclonal antimyosin Fab. *J Am Coll Cardiol* 9:555, 1987.

166. Ballester-Rodes M, Carrio-Gasset I, Abadal-Berini L, et al: Patterns of evolution of myocyte damage after human heart transplantation detected by indium-111 monoclonal antimyosin. *Am J Cardiol* 62:623, 1988.

167. Ballester M, Obrador D, Carrio I, et al: Indium-111-monoclonal antimyosin antibody studies after the first year of heart transplantation. Identification of risk groups for developing rejection during long-term follow-up and clinical implications. *Circulation* 82:2100, 1990.

168. Johnson LL, Cannon PJ: Antimyosin imaging in cardiac transplant rejection. *Circulation* 84(suppl I):I-273, 1991.

169. Latre JM, Arizon JM, Jimenez-Heffernan A, et al: Noninvasive radioisotopic diagnosis of acute heart rejection. *J Heart Lung Transplant* 11:453, 1992.

170. Owunwanne A, Shihab-Eldeen A, Sadek S, et al: Is cyclosporine toxic to the heart? *J Heart Lung Transplant* 12:199, 1993.

171. Allen MD, Shoji Y, Fujimura Y, et al: Effect of cyclosporine on the uptake of monoclonal antibody to cardiac myosin. *J Heart Lung Transplant* 10:775, 1991.

172. Nishimura T, Nagata S, Uehara T, et al: Assessment of active myocardial damage dilated-phase in hypertrophic cardiomyopathy by using In-111-antimyosin Fab myocardial scintigraphy. *J Nucl Med* 32:1333, 1991.

173. Nakata T, Gotoh M, Yonekura S, et al: Myocardial accumulation of monoclonal antimyosin Fab in hypertrophic cardiomyopathy and postpartum cardiomyopathy. *J Nucl Med* 32:2291, 1991.

174. Lambert K, Isaac D, Hendel R: Myocarditis masquerading as ischemic heart disease: The diagnostic utility of antimyosin imaging. *Cardiology* 82:415, 1993.

175. Khaw BA, Narula J: Antibody imaging in the evaluation of cardiovascular diseases. *J Nucl Cardiol* 1:457, 1994.

176. Khaw BA, Klibanov A, O'Donnell SM, et al: Gamma imaging with negatively charge-modified monoclonal antibody: Modification with synthetic polymers. *J Nucl Med* 32:1742, 1991.

177. Narula J, Torchilin VP, Petrov A, et al: In vivo targeting of acute myocardial infarction with negative-charge, polymer-modified antimyosin antibody: Use of different cross-linkers. *J Nucl Cardiol* 2:26, 1995.

178. Senior R, Bhattacharya S, Manspeaker P, et al: [99mTc-]

antimyosin antibody imaging for the detection of acute myocardial infarction in human beings. *Am Heart J* 126:536, 1993.

179. Taillefer R, Boucher L, Lambert R, et al: Technetium-99m antimyosin antibody (3-48) myocardial imaging: Human biodistribution, safety and clinical results in detection of acute myocardial infarction. *Eur J Nucl Med* 22:453, 1995.

180. Schoeder H, Topp H, Friedrich M, et al: Thallium and indium antimyosin dual-isotope single-photon emission tomography in acute myocardial infarction to identify patients at further ischaemic risk. *Eur J Nucl Med* 21:415, 1994.

181. Pak KY, Nedelman MA, Kanke M, et al: An instant kit method for labeling antimyosin Fab' with technetium-99m: Evaluation in an experimental myocardial infarct model. *J Nucl Med* 33:144, 1992.

182. Orlandi C, Crane PD, Edwards DS, et al: Early scintigraphic detection of experimental myocardial infarction in dogs with technetium-99m-glucaric acid. *J Nucl Med* 32:263, 1991.

183. Ohtani H, Callahan RJ, Khaw BA, et al: Comparison of technetium-99m-glucarate and thallium-201 for the identification of acute myocardial infarction in rats. *J Nucl Med* 33:1988, 1992.

184. Yaoita H, Fischman AJ, Wilkinson R, et al: Distribution of deoxyglucose and technetium-99m-glucarate in the acutely ischemic myocardium. *J Nucl Med* 34:1303, 1993.

185. Johnson LL, Verdesca SA, Schofield L, et al: Technetium-99m glucarate uptake in a swine model of demand ischemia. *J Nucl Med* 37:50P, 1996 (abstr).

186. Wackers FJTh, Sokole EB, Samson G, et al: Value and limitations of thallium-201 scintigraphy in the acute phase of myocardial infarction. *N Engl J Med* 295:1, 1976.

187. Gerson MC: Applications of thallium-201 myocardial perfusion imaging in acute myocardial infarction. *Cardiovasc Rev Rep* 2:801, 1981.

188. Blood DK, McCarthy DM, Sciacca RR, et al: Comparison of single-dose and double-dose thallium-201 myocardial perfusion scintigraphy for the detection of coronary artery disease and prior myocardial infarction. *Circulation* 58:777, 1978.

189. Niess GS, Logic JR, Russell RO Jr, et al: Usefulness and limitations of thallium-201 myocardial scintigraphy in delineating location and size of prior myocardial infarction. *Circulation* 59:1010, 1979.

190. Wackers FJTh, Lie KI, Liem KL, et al: Thallium-201 scintigraphy in unstable angina pectoris. *Circulation* 57:738, 1978.

191. Berger BC, Watson DD, Burwell LR, et al: Redistribution of thallium at rest in patients with stable and unstable angina and the effect of coronary artery bypass surgery. *Circulation* 60:1114, 1979.

192. Gibson RS, Watson DD, Taylor GJ, et al: Prospective assessment of regional myocardial perfusion before and after coronary revascularization surgery by quantitative thallium-201 scintigraphy. *J Am Coll Cardiol* 1:804, 1983.

193. Mueller TM, Marcus ML, Ehrhardt JC, et al: Limitations of thallium-201 myocardial perfusion scintigrams. *Circulation* 54:640, 1976.

194. Lomboy CT, Schulman DS, Grill HP, et al: Rest-redistribution thallium-201 scintigraphy to determine myocardial viability early after myocardial infarction. *J Am Coll Cardiol* 25:210, 1995.

195. Parodi O, Uthurralt N, Severi S, et al: Transient reduction of regional myocardial perfusion during angina at rest with ST-segment depression or normalization of negative T waves. *Circulation* 63:1238, 1981.

196. Lubell DL, Goldfarb CR: Metastatic cardiac tumor demonstrated by ^{201}Tl scan. *Chest* 78:98, 1980.

197. Bailey IK, Come PC, Kelly DT, et al: Thallium-201 myocardial perfusion imaging in aortic valve stenosis. *Am J Cardiol* 40:889, 1977.

198. Bulkley BH, Hutchins GM, Bailey I, et al: Thallium 201 imaging and gated cardiac blood pool scans in patients with ischemic and idiopathic congestive cardiomyopathy. A clinical and pathologic study. *Circulation* 55:753, 1977.

199. Beer N, Kertsnuz Y, Collet H: Diagnosis of Chagas cardiomyopathy by thallium 201 perfusion imaging. *Am J Cardiol* 45:396, 1980 (abstr).

200. Massie B, Botvinick EH, Shames D, et al: Myocardial perfusion scintigraphy in patients with mitral valve prolapse: Its advantage over stress electrocardiography in diagnosing associated coronary artery disease and its implications for the etiology of chest pain. *Circulation* 57:19, 1978.

201. Klein GJ, Kostuk WJ, Boughner DR, et al: Stress myocardial imaging in mitral leaflet prolapse syndrome. *Am J Cardiol* 42:746, 1978.

202. Greenspan M, Iskandrian AS, Croll MN, et al: Exercise myocardial scintigraphy in patients with mitral valve prolapse. *Clin Res* 27:172A, 1979 (abstr).

203. Staniloff HM, Huckell VF, Morch JE, et al: Abnormal myocardial perfusion defects in patients with mitral valve prolapse and normal coronary arteries. *Am J Cardiol* 41:433, 1978 (abstr).

204. Rubin KA, Morrison J, Padnick MB, et al: Idiopathic hypertrophic subaortic stenosis: Evaluation of anginal symptoms with thallium-201 myocardial imaging. *Am J Cardiol* 44:1040, 1979.

205. Huckell VF, Staniloff HM, Feiglin DH, et al: The demonstration of segmental perfusion defects in hypertrophic cardiomyopathy imitating coronary artery disease. *Am J Cardiol* 41:438, 1978 (abstr).

206. Okada RD, Glover D, Gaffney T, Williams S: Myocardial kinetics of technetium-99m-hexakis-2-methoxy-2-methylpropyl-isonitrile. *Circulation* 77:491, 1988.

207. Verani MS, Jeroudi MO, Mahmarian JJ, et al: Quantification of myocardial infarction during coronary occlusion and myocardial salvage after reperfusion using cardiac imaging with technetium-99m hexakis 2-methoxyisobutyl isonitrile. *J Am Coll Cardiol* 12:1573, 1988.

208. Santoro GM, Bisi G, Sciagra R, et al: Single photon emission computed tomography with technetium-99m hexakis 2-methoxyisobutyl isonitrile in acute myocardial infarction before and after thrombolytic treatment: Assessment of salvaged myocardium and prediction of late functional recovery. *J Am Coll Cardiol* 15:301, 1990.

209. Gibbons RJ, Verani MS, Behrenbeck T, et al: Feasibility of tomographic ^{99m}Tc-hexakis-2-methoxy-2-methylpropyl-isonitrile imaging for the assessment of myocardial area at risk and the effect of treatment in acute myocardial infarction. *Circulation* 80:1277, 1989.

210. Christian TF, Clements IP, Behrenbeck T, et al: Limitations of the electrocardiogram in estimating infarction size after acute reperfusion therapy for myocardial infarction. *Ann Int Med* 114:264, 1991.

211. Sinusas AJ, Watson DD, Cannon JM Jr, Beller GA: Effect of ischemia and postischemic dysfunction on myocardial uptake of technetium-99m-labeled methoxyisobutyl isonitrile and thallium-201. *J Am Coll Cardiol* 14:1785, 1989.

212. Pellikka PA, Behrenbeck T, Verani MS, et al: Serial changes in myocardial perfusion using tomographic technetium-99m-hexakis-2-methoxy-2-methylpropylisonitrile imaging following reperfusion therapy of myocardial infarction. *J Nucl Med* 31:1269, 1990.

213. Canby RC, Silber S, Pohost GM: Relations of the myocardial imaging agents ^{99m}Tc-MIBI and ^{201}Tl to myocardial blood flow in a canine model of myocardial ischemic insult. *Circulation* 81:289, 1990.

214. Johnson LL, Seldin DW, Keller AM, et al: Dual isotope thallium and indium antimyosin SPECT imaging to identify acute infarct patients at further ischemic risk. *Circulation* 81:37, 1990.

215. Morguet AJ, Munz DL, Klein HH, et al: Myocardial distribution of indium-111-antimyosin Fab and technetium-99m-sestamibi in experimental nontransmural infarction. *J Nucl Med* 33:223, 1992.

216. Reduto LA, Berger HJ, Cohen LS, et al: Sequential radionuclide assessment of left and right ventricular performance after acute transmural myocardial infarction. *Ann Intern Med* 89:441, 1978.

217. Pichler M, Shah PK, Peter T, et al: Wall motion abnormalities and electrocardiographic changes in acute transmural myocardial infarction: Implications of reciprocal ST segment depression. *Am Heart J* 106:1003, 1983.

218. Osbakken MD, Bove AA, Spaan JF: Left ventricular regional wall motion and velocity of shortening in chronic mitral and aortic regurgitation. *Am J Cardiol* 47:1005, 1981.

219. Traina M, Rotolo A, Raineri M, et al: Prognostic significance of the evolution of left ventricular ejection fraction in patients with acute myocardial infarction not treated with thrombolytic therapy. *Eur Heart J* 14:1034, 1993.

220. Goldman L, Cook EF, Brand DA, et al: A computer protocol to predict myocardial infarction in emergency department patients with chest pain. *N Engl J Med* 318:797, 1988.

221. Lee TH, Cook EF, Weisberg M, et al: Acute chest pain in the emergency room. Identification and examination of low-risk patients. *Arch Intern Med* 145:65, 1985.

222. Rouan GW, Lee TH, Cook EF, et al: Clinical characteristics and outcome of acute myocardial infarction in patients with initially normal or nonspecific electrocardiograms (a report from the Multicenter Chest Pain Study). *Am J Cardiol* 64:1087, 1989.

223. Lee TH, Juarez G, Cook EF, et al: Ruling out acute myocardial infarction. A prospective multicenter validation of a 12-hour strategy for patients at low risk. *N Engl J Med* 324:1239, 1991.

224. Pozen MW, D'Agostino RB, Selker HP, et al: A predictive instrument to improve coronary-care-unit admission practices in acute ischemic heart disease. A prospective multicenter clinical trial. *N Engl J Med* 310:1273, 1984.

225. Puleo PR, Meyer D, Wathen C, et al: Use of a rapid assay of subforms of creatine kinase MB to diagnose or rule out acute myocardial infarction. *N Engl J Med* 331: 561, 1994.

226. Antman EM, Grudzien C, Sacks DB: Evaluation of a rapid bedside assay for detection of serum cardiac troponin T. *JAMA* 273:1279, 1995.

227. Tsakonis JS, Shesser R, Rosenthal R, et al: Safety of immediate treadmill testing in selected emergency department patients with chest pain: A preliminary report. *Am J Emerg Med* 9:557, 1991.

228. Kerns JR, Shaub TF, Fontanarosa PB: Emergency cardiac stress testing in the evaluation of emergency department patients with atypical chest pain. *Ann Emerg Med* 22:794, 1993.

229. Lewis WR, Amsterdam EA: Utility and safety of immediate exercise testing of low-risk patients admitted to the hospital for suspected acute myocardial infarction. *Am J Cardiol* 74:987, 1994.

230. Horowitz RS, Morganroth J, Parrotto C, et al: Immediate diagnosis of acute myocardial infarction by two-dimensional echocardiography. *Circulation* 65:323, 1982.

231. Visser CA, Lie KI, Kan G, et al: Detection and quantification of acute, isolated myocardial infarction by two dimensional echocardiography. *Am J Cardiol* 47:1020, 1981.

232. Sabia P, Afrookteh A, Touchstone DA, et al: Value of regional wall motion abnormality in the emergency room diagnosis of acute myocardial infarction. A prospective study using two-dimensional echocardiography. *Circulation* 84(suppl I):I-85, 1991.

233. Peels CH, Visser CA, Funke Kupper AJ, et al: Usefulness of two-dimensional echocardiography for immediate detection of myocardial ischemia in the emergency room. *Am J Cardiol* 65:687, 1990.

234. Wackers FJTh, Lie KI, Liem KL, et al: Potential value of thallium-201 scintigraphy as a means of selecting patients for the coronary care unit. *Br Heart J* 41:111, 1979.

235. Mace SE: Thallium myocardial scanning in the emergency department evaluation of chest pain. *Am J Emerg Med* 7:321, 1989.

236. Bilodeau L, Theroux P, Gregoire J, et al: Technetium-99m sestamibi tomography in patients with spontaneous chest pain: Correlations with clinical, electrocardiographic and angiographic findings. *J Am Coll Cardiol* 18:1684, 1991.

237. Varetto T, Cantalupi D, Altieri A, Orlandi C: Emergency room technetium-99m sestamibi imaging to rule out acute myocardial ischemic events in patients with nondiagnostic electrocardiograms. *J Am Coll Cardiol* 22: 1804, 1993.

238. Hilton TC, Thompson RC, Williams HJ, et al: Technetium-99m sestamibi myocardial perfusion imaging in the

emergency room evaluation of chest pain. *J Am Coll Cardiol* 23:1016, 1994.

239. Tatum JL, Ornato JP, Jesse RL, et al: A diagnostic strategy using Tc-99m sestamibi for evaluation of patients with chest pain in the emergency department. *Circulation* 90:I-367, 1994 (abstr).

240. Varetto T, Cantalupi D, Cerruti A, et al: Tc99m sestamibi and 2D-echo imaging for rule-out of acute ischemia in patients with chest pain and non-diagnostic ECG. *Circulation* 90:I-367, 1994 (abstr).

241. Sullivan W, Vlodaver Z, Tuna N, et al: Correlation of electrocardiographic and pathologic findings in healed myocardial infarction. *Am J Cardiol* 42:724, 1978.

242. Roberts WC, Gardin JM: Location of myocardial infarcts: A confusion of terms and definitions. *Am J Cardiol* 42:868, 1978.

243. Warner RA, Hill NE, Mookherjee S, Smulyan H: Diagnostic significance for coronary artery disease of abnormal Q waves in the "lateral" electrocardiographic leads. *Am J Cardiol* 58:431, 1986.

244. Wackers FJTh, Becker AE, Samson G, et al: Location and size of acute transmural myocardial infarction estimated from thallium-201 scintiscans: A clinicopathologic study. *Circulation* 56:72, 1977.

245. Budihna NV, Micinski M, Latific-Jasnic D, Cerar A: Indium-111-antimyosin uptake in acute and remote myocardial infarction: Comparison with pathohistologic findings. *J Nucl Med* 33:587, 1992.

246. Helfant RH, Pine R, Meister SG, et al: Nitroglycerin to unmask reversible asynergy. Correlation with post coronary bypass ventriculography. *Circulation* 50:108, 1974.

247. Isner JM, Roberts WC: Right ventricular infarction complicating left ventricular infarction secondary to coronary artery disease. *Am J Cardiol* 42:885, 1978.

248. Ratliff NB, Hackel DB: Combined right and left ventricular infarction: Pathogenesis and clinicopathologic correlations. *Am J Cardiol* 45:217, 1980.

249. Erhardt LR: Clinical and pathological observations in different types of acute myocardial infarction: A study of 84 patients deceased after treatment in a coronary care unit. *Acta Med Scand* 560(suppl):7, 1974.

250. Forman MB, Wilson BH, Sheller JR, et al: Right ventricular hypertrophy is an important determinant of right ventricular infarction complicating acute inferior left ventricular infarction. *J Am Coll Cardiol* 10:1180, 1987.

251. Kopelman HA, Forman MB, Wilson BH, et al: Right ventricular myocardial infarction in patients with chronic lung disease: Possible role of right ventricular hypertrophy. *J Am Coll Cardiol* 5:1302, 1985.

252. Kaul S, Hopkins JM, Shah PM: Chronic effects of myocardial infarction on right ventricular function: A noninvasive assessment. *J Am Coll Cardiol* 2:607, 1983.

253. Andersen HR, Falk E, Nielsen D: Right ventricular infarction: Frequency, size and topography in coronary heart disease: A prospective study comprising 107 consecutive autopsies from a coronary care unit. *J Am Coll Cardiol* 10:1223, 1987.

254. Cabin HS, Clubb KS, Wackers FJTh, Zaret BL: Right ventricular myocardial infarction with anterior wall left ventricular infarction: An autopsy study. *Am Heart J* 113:16, 1987.

255. Dell'Italia LJ, Lembo NJ, Starling MR, et al: Hemodynamically important right ventricular infarction: Follow-up evaluation of right ventricular systolic function at rest and during exercise with radionuclide ventriculography and respiratory gas exchange. *Circulation* 75:996, 1987.

256. Haines DE, Beller GA, Watson DD, et al: A prospective clinical, scintigraphic, angiographic and functional evaluation of patients after inferior myocardial infarction with and without right ventricular dysfunction. *J Am Coll Cardiol* 6:995, 1985.

257. Steele P, Kirch D, Ellis J, et al: Prompt return to normal of depressed right ventricular ejection fraction in acute inferior infarction. *Br Heart J* 39:1319, 1977.

258. Zehender M, Kasper W, Kauder E, et al: Right ventricular infarction as an independent predictor of prognosis after acute inferior myocardial infarction. *N Engl J Med* 328:981, 1993.

259. Sharpe DN, Botvinick EH, Shames DM, et al: The noninvasive diagnosis of right ventricular infarction. *Circulation* 57:483, 1978.

260. Wackers FJTh, Lie KI, Sokole EB, et al: Prevalence of right ventricular involvement in inferior wall infarction assessed with myocardial imaging with thallium-201 and technetium-99m pyrophosphate. *Am J Cardiol* 42:358, 1978.

261. Tobinick E, Schelbert HR, Henning H, et al: Right ventricular ejection fraction in patients with acute anterior and inferior myocardial infarction assessed by radionuclide angiography. *Circulation* 57:1078, 1978.

262. Cohn JN, Guiha NH, Broder MI, et al: Right ventricular infarction: Clinical and hemodynamic features. *Am J Cardiol* 33:209, 1974.

263. Lopez-Sendon J, Coma-Canella I, Gamallo C: Sensitivity and specificity of hemodynamic criteria in the diagnosis of acute right ventricular infarction. *Circulation* 64:515, 1981.

264. Rigo P, Murray M, Taylor DR, et al: Right ventricular dysfunction detected by gated scintiphotography in patients with acute inferior myocardial infarction. *Circulation* 52:268, 1975.

265. Baigrie RS, Haq A, Morgan CD, et al: The spectrum of right ventricular involvement in inferior wall myocardial infarction: A clinical, hemodynamic and noninvasive study. *J Am Coll Cardiol* 1:1396, 1983.

266. Jugdutt BI, Sussex BA, Sivaram CA, et al: Right ventricular infarction: Two-dimensional echocardiographic evaluation. *Am Heart J* 107:505, 1984.

267. Brooks H, Holland R, Al-Sadir J: Right ventricular performance during ischemia: An anatomic and hemodynamic analysis. *Am J Physiol* 233:H505, 1977.

268. Fixler DE, Monroe GA, Wheeler JM: Hemodynamic alterations during septal or right ventricular ischemia in dogs. *Am Heart J* 93:210, 1977.

269. Starr I, Jeffers WA, Meade RH: The absence of conspicuous increments in venous pressure after severe damage to the right ventricle of the dog with a discussion of the relation between clinical congestive failure and heart disease. *Am Heart J* 26:291, 1943.

270. Bakos ACP: The question of the function of the right

ventricular myocardium: An experimental study. *Circulation* 1:724, 1950.

271. Mikell FL, Asinger RW, Hodges M: Functional consequences of interventricular septal involvement in right ventricular infarction: Echocardiographic, clinical, and hemodynamic observations. *Am Heart J* 105:393, 1983.
272. Schlichter J, Hellerstein HK, Katz LN: Aneurysm of the heart: A correlative study of one hundred and two proved cases. *Medicine* 33:43, 1954.
273. Cabin HS, Roberts WC: True left ventricular aneurysm and healed myocardial infarction. Clinical and necropsy observations including quantification of degrees of coronary arterial narrowing. *Am J Cardiol* 46:754, 1980.
274. Gorlin R, Klein MD, Sullivan JM: Prospective correlative study of ventricular aneurysm: Mechanistic concept and clinical recognition. *Am J Med* 42:512, 1967.
275. Vlodaver Z, Coe JI, Edwards JE: True and false left ventricular aneurysms: Propensity for the latter to rupture. *Circulation* 51:567, 1975.
276. Weyman AE, Peskoe SM, Williams ES, et al: Detection of left ventricular aneurysms by cross-sectional echocardiography. *Circulation* 54:936, 1976.
277. Mills RM Jr, Young E, Gorlin R, et al: Natural history of S-T segment elevation after acute myocardial infarction. *Am J Cardiol* 35:609, 1975.
278. Kelly RJ, Cowan RJ, Maynard CD, et al: Localization of ^{99m}Tc-Sn-pyrophosphate in left ventricular aneurysms. *J Nucl Med* 18:342, 1977.
279. Ahmad M, Dubiel JP, Verdon TA Jr, et al: Technetium 99m stannous pyrophosphate myocardial imaging in patients with and without left ventricular aneurysm. *Circulation* 53:833, 1976.
280. Gerson MC, Varma DGK, Nishiyama H, et al: Evidence of left ventricular aneurysm by thallium-201 myocardial scintigraphy. *Clin Nucl Med* 8:133, 1983.
281. Rigo P, Murray M, Strauss HW, et al: Scintiphotographic evaluation of patients with suspected left ventricular aneurysm. *Circulation* 50:985, 1974.
282. Friedman ML, Cantor RE: Reliability of gated heart scintigrams for detection of left-ventricular aneurysm: Concise communication. *J Nucl Med* 20:720, 1979.
283. Dymond DS, Jarritt PH, Britton KE, et al: Detection of postinfarction left ventricular aneurysms by first pass radionuclide ventriculography using a multicrystal gamma camera. *Br Heart J* 41:68, 1979.
284. Hopkins GB, Kan MK, Salel AF: Scintigraphic assessment of left ventricular aneurysms. *JAMA* 240:2162, 1978.
285. Meizlish JL, Berger HJ, Plankey M, et al: Functional left ventricular aneurysm formation after acute anterior transmural myocardial infarction: Incidence, natural history, and prognostic implications. *N Engl J Med* 311:1001, 1984.
286. Winzelberg GG, Strauss HW, Bingham JB, et al: Scintigraphic evaluation of left ventricular aneurysm. *Am J Cardiol* 46:1138, 1980.
287. Stephens JD, Dymond DS, Spurrell RAJ: Radionuclide and hemodynamic assessment of left ventricular functional reserve in patients with left ventricular aneurysm and congestive cardiac failure: Response to exercise stress and isosorbide dinitrate. *Circulation* 61:536, 1980.
288. Dymond DS, Stephens J, Stone D, et al: Assessment of function of contractile segments in patients with left ventricular aneurysms by quantitative first pass radionuclide ventriculography. Haemodynamic correlation at rest and exercise. *Br Heart J* 43:125, 1980.
289. Visser CA, Kan G, David GK, et al: Echocardiographic-cineangiographic correlation in detecting left ventricular aneurysm: A prospective study of 422 patients. *Am J Cardiol* 50:337, 1982.
290. Baur HR, Daniel JA, Nelson RR: Detection of left ventricular aneurysm on two dimensional echocardiography. *Am J Cardiol* 50:191, 1982.
291. Barrett MJ, Charuzi Y, Corday E, et al: Ventricular aneurysm: Cross-sectional echocardiographic approach. *Am J Cardiol* 46:1133, 1980.
292. Botvinick EH, Shames D, Hutchinson JC, et al: Noninvasive diagnosis of a false left ventricular aneurysm with radioisotope gated cardiac blood pool imaging. *Am J Cardiol* 37:1089, 1976.
293. Winzelberg GG, Miller SW, Okada RD, et al: Scintigraphic assessment of false left ventricular aneurysms. *AJR Am J Roentgenol* 135:569, 1980.
294. Sweet SE, Sterling R, McCormick JR, et al: Left ventricular false aneurysm after coronary bypass surgery: Radionuclide diagnosis and surgical resection. *Am J Cardiol* 43:154, 1979.
295. Dymond DS, Elliott AT, Banim S: Detection of a false left ventricular aneurysm by first-pass radionuclide ventriculography. *J Nucl Med* 20:851, 1979.
296. Perkins PJ: Radioisotope diagnosis of false left ventricular aneurysm. *Am J Roentgenol* 132:117, 1979.
297. Katz RJ, Simpson A, DiBianco R, et al: Noninvasive diagnosis of left ventricular pseudoaneurysm: Role of two dimensional echocardiography and radionuclide gated pool imaging. *Am J Cardiol* 44:372, 1979.
298. Onik G, Recht L, Edwards JE, et al: False left-ventricular aneurysm: Diagnosis by noninvasive means. *J Nucl Med* 21:177, 1980.
299. Park CH, Levy HA, Savage M: The use of scintigraphic studies in mid-ventricular obstructive cardiomyopathy to rule out pseudoaneurysm. *Clin Nucl Med* 10:463, 1985.
300. Sabah I, Yoshikawa J, Kato H, et al: Noninvasive diagnosis of pseudoaneurysm of the left ventricle. *Jpn Heart J* 20:95, 1979.
301. Catherwood E, Mintz GS, Kotler MN, et al: Two-dimensional echocardiographic recognition of left ventricular pseudoaneurysm. *Circulation* 62:294, 1980.
302. Gatewood RP Jr, Nanda NC: Differentiation of left ventricular pseudoaneurysm from true aneurysm with two dimensional echocardiography. *Am J Cardiol* 46:869, 1980.
303. Ginsberg F, Rosenberg RJ, Sziklas JJ, Spencer RP: Varied appearance of cardiac pseudoaneurysms on blood pool images. *Clin Nucl Med* 12:430, 1987.
304. Roelandt JRTC, Sutherland GR, Yoshida K, Yoshikawa J: Improved diagnosis and characterization of left ventricular pseudoaneurysm by Doppler color flow imaging. *J Am Coll Cardiol* 12:807, 1988.
305. Natello GW, Nanda NC, Zachariah ZP: Color Doppler recognition of left ventricular pseudoaneurysm. *Am J Med* 85:432, 1988.
306. Bach M, Berger M, Hecht SR, Strain JE: Diagnosis of left

ventricular pseudoaneurysm using contrast and Doppler echocardiography. *Am Heart J* 118:854, 1989.

307. Tunick PA, Slater W, Kronzon I: The hemodynamics of left ventricular pseudoaneurysm: Color Doppler echocardiographic study. *Am Heart J* 117:1161, 1989.

308. Schwarz J, Hamad N, Hernandez G, et al: Doppler color-flow echocardiographic recognition of left ventricular pseudoaneurysm. *Am Heart J* 116:1353, 1988.

309. Smeal WE, Dianzumba SB, Joyner CR: Evaluation of pseudoaneurysm of the left ventricle by echocardiography and pulsed Doppler. *Am Heart J* 113:1508, 1987.

310. Olalla JJ, Vazquez de Prada JA, Duran RM, et al: Color Doppler diagnosis of left ventricular pseudoaneurysm. *Chest* 94:443, 1988.

311. Alam M, Rosman HS, Lewis JW, Brymer JF: Color Doppler features of left ventricular pseudoaneurysm. *Chest* 95:231, 1989.

312. Sanders RJ, Kern WH, Blount SG Jr: Perforation of the interventricular septum complicating myocardial infarction. *Am Heart J* 51:736, 1956.

313. Moore CA, Nygaard TW, Kaiser OL, et al: Postinfarction ventricular septal rupture: The importance of location of infarction and right ventricular function in determining survival. *Circulation* 74:45, 1986.

314. Montoya A, McKeever L, Scanlon, P, et al: Early repair of ventricular septal rupture. *Am J Cardiol* 45:345, 1980.

315. Harrison MR, MacPhail B, Gurley JC, et al: Usefulness of color Doppler flow imaging to distinguish ventricular septal defect from acute mitral regurgitation complicating acute myocardial infarction. *Am J Cardiol* 64:697, 1989.

316. Maurer G, Czer LSC, Shah PK, Chaux A: Assessment by Doppler color flow mapping of ventricular septal defect after acute myocardial infarction. *Am J Cardiol* 64:668, 1989.

317. Eisenberg PR, Barzilai B, Perez JE: Noninvasive detection by Doppler echocardiography of combined ventricular septal rupture and mitral regurgitation in acute myocardial infarction. *J Am Coll Cardiol* 4:617, 1984.

318. Farcot JC, Boisante L, Rigaud M, et al: Two dimensional echocardiographic visualization of ventricular septal rupture after acute anterior myocardial infarction. *Am J Cardiol* 45:370, 1980.

319. Drobac M, Gilbert B, Howard R, et al: Ventricular septal defect after myocardial infarction: Diagnosis by two-dimensional contrast echocardiography. *Circulation* 67:335, 1983.

320. Zachariah ZP, Hsiun MC, Nanda NC, Camarano GP: Diagnosis of rupture of the ventricular septum during acute myocardial infarction by Doppler color flow mapping. *Am J Cardiol* 59:162, 1987.

321. Miyatake K, Okamoto M, Kinoshita N, et al: Doppler echocardiographic features of ventricular septal rupture in myocardial infarction. *J Am Coll Cardiol* 5:182, 1985.

322. Stevenson JG, Kawabori I, Guntheroth WG: Differentiation of ventricular septal defects from mitral regurgitation by pulsed Doppler echocardiography. *Circulation* 56:14, 1977.

323. Gustafson A, Nordenfelt I, White T: Diagnosis of ventricular septal defect in acute myocardial infarction without cardiac catheterization. *Acta Med Scand* 198:471, 1975.

324. Lichstein EM, Liu HM, Gupta P: Pericarditis after acute myocardial infarction: Incidence of complications and significance of electrocardiogram on admission. *Am Heart J* 87:246, 1974.

325. Feigenbaum H, Waldhausen JA, Hyde LP: Ultrasound diagnosis of pericardial effusion. *JAMA* 191:711, 1965.

326. Riba AL, Morganroth J: Unsuspected substantial pericardial effusions detected by echocardiography. *JAMA* 236:2623, 1976.

327. Sheehan FH, Mathey DG, Schofer J, et al: Factors that determine recovery of left ventricular function after thrombolysis in patients with acute myocardial infarction. *Circulation* 71:1121, 1985.

328. Hospital Data Services, Inc, Division of Pharmaceutical Data Services Inc, US Hospital Drug and Diagnosis Audit Thrombolytic Market, Phoenix, AZ, 1988.

329. Grines CL, DeMaria AN: Optimal utilization of thrombolytic therapy for acute myocardial infarction: Concepts and controversies. *J Am Coll Cardiol* 16:223, 1990.

330. Feiring AJ, Johnson MR, Kioschos JM, et al: The importance of the determination of the myocardial area at risk in the evaluation of the outcome of acute myocardial infarction in patients. *Circulation* 75:980, 1987.

331. Gibson RS, Bishop HL, Stamm RB, et al: Value of early two dimensional echocardiography in patients with acute myocardial infarction. *Am J Cardiol* 49:1110, 1982.

332. Topol EJ, Weiss JL, Brinker JA, et al: Regional wall motion improvement after coronary thrombolysis with recombinant tissue plasminogen activator: Importance of coronary angioplasty. *J Am Coll Cardiol* 6:426, 1985.

333. Charuzi Y, Beeder C, Marshall LA, et al: Improvement in regional and global left ventricular function after intracoronary thrombolysis: Assessment with two-dimensional echocardiography. *Am J Cardiol* 53:662, 1984.

334. Parkey RW, Bonte FJ, Meyer SL, et al: A new method for radionuclide imaging of acute myocardial infarction in humans. *Circulation* 50:540, 1974.

335. Long R, Symes J, Allard J, et al: Differentiation between reperfusion and occlusion myocardial necrosis with technetium-99m pyrophosphate scans. *Am J Cardiol* 46:413, 1980.

336. Wheelan K, Wolfe C, Corbett J, et al: Early positive technetium-99m stannous pyrophosphate images as a marker of reperfusion after thrombolytic therapy for acute myocardial infarction. *Am J Cardiol* 56:252, 1985.

337. Kondo M, Takahashi M, Matsuda T, et al: Clinical significance of early myocardial 99mTc-pyrophosphate uptake in patients with acute myocardial infarction. *Am Heart J* 113:250, 1987.

338. Manyari DE, Thompson CR, Duff HJ, et al: Usefulness of early positive technetium-99m stannous pyrophosphate scan in predicting reperfusion after thrombolytic therapy for acute myocardial infarction. *Am J Cardiol* 61:16, 1988.

339. Leger J, Chevalier J, Larue C, et al: Imaging of myocardial infarction in dogs and humans using monoclonal anti-

bodies specific for human myosin heavy chains. *J Am Coll Cardiol* 18:473, 1991.

340. Narula J, Nicol PD, Southern JF, et al: Evaluation of myocardial infarct size before and after reperfusion: Dual-tracer imaging with radiolabeled antimyosin antibody. *J Nucl Med* 35:1076, 1994.

341. Beller GA: Role of myocardial perfusion imaging in evaluating thrombolytic therapy for acute myocardial infarction. *J Am Coll Cardiol* 9:661, 1987.

342. Granato JE, Watson DD, Flanagan TL, et al: Myocardial thallium-201 kinetics during coronary occlusion and reperfusion: Influence of method of reflow and timing of thallium-201 administration. *Circulation* 73:150, 1986.

343. Melin JA, Wijns W, Keyeux A, et al: Assessment of thallium-201 redistribution versus glucose uptake as predictors of viability after coronary occlusion and reperfusion. *Circulation* 77:927, 1988.

344. Granato JE, Watson DD, Flanagan TL, Beller GA: Myocardial thallium-201 kinetics and regional flow alterations with 3 hours of coronary occlusion and either rapid reperfusion through a totally patent vessel or slow reperfusion through a critical stenosis. *J Am Coll Cardiol* 9:109, 1987.

345. Okada RD, Pohost GM: The use of preintervention and postintervention thallium imaging for assessing the early and late effects of experimental coronary arterial reperfusion in dogs. *Circulation* 69:1153, 1984.

346. Forman R, Kirk ES: Thallium-201 accumulation during reperfusion of ischemic myocardium: Dependence on regional blood flow rather than viability. *Am J Cardiol* 54:659, 1984.

347. Okada RD, Glover DK, Nguyen KN, Johnson G III: Technetium-99m sestamibi kinetics in reperfused canine myocardium. *Eur J Nucl Med* 22:600, 1995.

348. Freeman I, Grunwald AM, Hoory S, Bodenheimer MM: Effect of coronary occlusion and myocardial viability on myocardial activity of technetium-99m-sestamibi. *J Nucl Med* 32:292, 1991.

349. Li Q-S, Frank TL, Franceschi D, et al: Technetium-99m methoxyisobutyl isonitrile (RP30) for quantification of myocardial ischemia and reperfusion in dogs. *J Nucl Med* 29:1539, 1988.

350. Sinusas AJ, Shi QX, Vitols PJ, et al: Impact of regional ventricular function, geometry, and dobutamine stress on quantitative ⁹⁹ᵐTc-sestamibi defect size. *Circulation* 88:2224, 1993.

351. Sinusas AJ, Trautman KA, Bergin JD, et al: Quantification of area at risk during coronary occlusion and degree of myocardial salvage after reperfusion with technetium-99m methoxyisobutyl isonitrile. *Circulation* 82:1424, 1990.

352. Wackers FJTh, Gibbons RJ, Verani MS, et al: Serial quantitative planar technetium-99m isonitrile imaging in acute myocardial infarction: Efficacy for noninvasive assessment of thrombolytic therapy. *J Am Coll Cardiol* 14:861, 1989.

353. St. Gibson W, Christian TF, Pellikka PA, et al: Serial tomographic imaging with technetium-99m-sestamibi for the assessment of infarct-related arterial patency following reperfusion therapy. *J Nucl Med* 33:2080, 1992.

354. Sinusas AJ, Bergin JD, Edwards NC, et al: Redistribution of ⁹⁹ᵐTc-sestamibi and ²⁰¹Tl in the presence of a severe coronary artery stenosis. *Circulation* 89:2332, 1994.

355. Kalff V, Schwaiger M, Nguyen N, et al: The relationship between myocardial blood flow and glucose uptake in ischemic canine myocardium determined with fluorine-18-deoxyglucose. *J Nucl Med* 33:1346, 1992.

356. Chan SY, Brunken RC, Phelps ME, Schelbert HR: Use of the metabolic tracer carbon-11-acetate for evaluation of regional myocardial perfusion. *J Nucl Med* 32:665, 1991.

357. Dilsizian V, Rocco TP, Freedman NMT, et al: Enhanced detection of ischemic but viable myocardium by the reinjection of thallium after stress-redistribution imaging. *N Engl J Med* 323:141, 1990.

358. Lenihan DJ, Gerson MC, Gabel M, et al: Influence of stunned but viable myocardium on Q12 and thallium uptake after reperfusion in canine myocardial infarction. *Circulation* 92(suppl I):I-789, 1995 (abstr).

359. Schwaiger M, Schelbert HR, Ellison D, et al: Sustained regional abnormalities in cardiac metabolism after transient ischemia in the chronic dog model. *J Am Coll Cardiol* 6:336, 1985.

360. Schwaiger M, Neese RA, Araujo L, et al: Sustained nonoxidative glucose utilization and depletion of glycogen in reperfused canine myocardium. *J Am Coll Cardiol* 13:745, 1989.

361. Cuocolo A, Pace L, Ricciardelli B, et al: Identification of viable myocardium in patients with chronic coronary artery disease: Comparison of thallium-201 scintigraphy with reinjection and technetium-99m-methoxyisobutyl isonitrile. *J Nucl Med* 33:505, 1992.

362. Altehoefer C, vom Dahl J, Messmer BJ, et al: Fate of the resting perfusion defect as assessed with technetium-99m methoxy-isobutyl-isonitrile single-photon emission computed tomography after successful revascularization in patients with healed myocardial infarction. *Am J Cardiol* 77:88, 1996.

363. Sawada SG, Allman KC, Muzik O, et al: Positron emission tomography detects evidence of viability in rest technetium-99m sestamibi defects. *J Am Coll Cardiol* 23:92, 1994.

364. Altehoefer C, Kaiser H-J, Dorr R, et al: Fluorine-18 deoxyglucose PET for assessment of viable myocardium in perfusion defects in ⁹⁹ᵐTc-MIBI SPET: A comparative study in patients with coronary artery disease. *Eur J Nucl Med* 19:334, 1992.

365. Soufer R, Dey HM, Ng CK, Zaret BL: Comparison of sestamibi single-photon emission computed tomography with positron emission tomography for estimating left ventricular myocardial viability. *Am J Cardiol* 75:1214, 1995.

366. Rocco TP, Dilsizian V, Strauss HW, Boucher CA: Technetium-99m isonitrile myocardial uptake at rest. II. Relation to clinical markers of potential viability. *J Am Coll Cardiol* 14:1678, 1989.

367. Matsunari I, Fujino S, Taki J, et al: Myocardial viability assessment with technetium-99m-tetrofosmin and thallium-201 reinjection in coronary artery disease. *J Nucl Med* 36:1961, 1995.

368. Moore CA, Cannon J, Watson DD, et al: Thallium 201

kinetics in stunned myocardium characterized by severe postischemic systolic dysfunction. *Circulation* 81:1622, 1990.

369. Okada RD, Nguyen KN, Lauinger M, et al: Effects of no flow and reperfusion on technetium-99m-Q12 kinetics. *J Nucl Med* 36:2103, 1995.

370. Ragosta M, Beller GA, Watson DD, et al: Quantitative planar rest–redistribution ^{201}Tl imaging in detection of myocardial viability and prediction of improvement in left ventricular function after coronary bypass surgery in patients with severely depressed left ventricular function. *Circulation* 87:1630, 1993.

371. Dilsizian V, Freedman NMT, Bacharach SL, et al: Regional thallium uptake in irreversible defects. Magnitude of change in thallium activity after reinjection distinguishes viable from nonviable myocardium. *Circulation* 85:627, 1992.

372. Dilsizian V, Perrone-Filardi P, Arrighi JA, et al: Concordance and discordance between stress-redistribution-reinjection and rest-redistribution thallium imaging for assessing viable myocardium. Comparison with metabolic activity by positron emission tomography. *Circulation* 88:941, 1993.

373. Gropler RJ, Geltman EM, Sampathkumaran K, et al: Functional recovery after coronary revascularization for chronic coronary artery disease is dependent on maintenance of oxidative metabolism. *J Am Coll Cardiol* 20:569, 1992.

374. Gropler RJ, Geltman EM, Sampathkumaran K, et al: Comparison of carbon-11-acetate with fluorine-18-fluorodeoxyglucose for delineating viable myocardium by positron emission tomography. *J Am Coll Cardiol* 22:1587, 1993.

375. Schuster EH, Bulkley BH: Ischemia at a distance after acute myocardial infarction: A cause of early postinfarction angina. *Circulation* 62:509, 1980.

376. Benhorin J, Andrews ML, Carleen ED, et al: Occurrence, characteristics and prognostic significance of early postacute myocardial infarction angina pectoris. *Am J Cardiol* 62:679, 1988.

377. Muller JE, Rude RE, Braunwald E, et al: Myocardial infarct extension: Occurrence, outcome, and risk factors in the multicenter investigation of limitation of infarct size. *Ann Intern Med* 108:1, 1988.

378. Bosch X, Theroux P, Waters DD, et al: Early postinfarction ischemia: Clinical, angiographic, and prognostic significance. *Circulation* 75:988, 1987.

379. Wiener RS, Moses HW, Richeson JF, Gatewood RP Jr: Hospital and long-term survival of patients with acute pulmonary edema associated with coronary artery disease. *Am J Cardiol* 60:33, 1987.

380. Ouyang P, Chandra NC, Gottlieb SO: Frequency and importance of silent myocardial ischemia identified with ambulatory electrocardiographic monitoring in the early in-hospital period after acute myocardial infarction. *Am J Cardiol* 65:267, 1990.

381. Holman BL, Chisholm RJ, Braunwald E: The prognostic implications of acute myocardial infarct scintigraphy with ^{99m}Tc-pyrophosphate. *Circulation* 57: 320, 1978.

382. Ahmad M, Logan KW, Martin RH: Doughnut pattern of technetium-99m pyrophosphate myocardial uptake in patients with acute myocardial infarction: A sign of poor long-term prognosis. *Am J Cardiol* 44:13, 1979.

383. Berger HJ, and the Antimyosin Multicenter Trial Group: Prognostic significance of the extent of antimyosin uptake in unstable ischemic heart disease: Early risk stratification. *Circulation* 78(suppl II):II-131, 1988.

384. Silverman KJ, Becker LC, Bulkley BH, et al: Value of early thallium-201 scintigraphy for predicting mortality in patients with acute myocardial infarction. *Circulation* 61:996, 1980.

385. Ong L, Green S, Reiser P, et al: Early prediction of mortality in patients with acute myocardial infarction: A prospective study of clinical and radionuclide risk factors. *Am J Cardiol* 57:33, 1986.

386. Killip T III, Kimball JT: Treatment of myocardial infarction in a coronary care unit: A two year experience with 250 patients. *Am J Cardiol* 20:457, 1967.

387. Jain D, Lahiri A, Raftery EB, Raval U: Clinical and prognostic significance of lung thallium uptake on rest imaging in acute myocardial infarction. *Am J Cardiol* 65:154, 1990.

388. Kan G, Visser CA, Lie KI, Durrer D: Early two-dimensional echocardiographic measurement of left ventricular ejection fraction in acute myocardial infarction. *Eur Heart J* 5:210, 1984.

389. Nishimura RA, Tajik AJ, Shub C, et al: Role of two-dimensional echocardiography in the prediction of in-hospital complications after acute myocardial infarction. *J Am Coll Cardiol* 4:1080, 1984.

390. Isaacsohn JL, Earle MG, Kemper AJ, Parisi AF: Postmyocardial infarction pain and infarct extension in the coronary care unit: Role of two-dimensional echocardiography. *J Am Coll Cardiol* 11:246, 1988.

391. Nishimura RA, Reeder GS, Miller FA Jr, et al: Prognostic value of predischarge 2-dimensional echocardiogram after acute myocardial infarction. *Am J Cardiol* 53:429, 1984.

392. Kloner RA, Parisi AF: Acute myocardial infarction: Diagnostic and prognostic applications of two-dimensional echocardiography. *Circulation* 75:521, 1987.

393. Berning J, Steensgaard-Hansen F: Early estimation of risk by echocardiographic determination of wall motion index in an unselected population with acute myocardial infarction. *Am J Cardiol* 65:567, 1990.

394. Van Reet RE, Quinones MA, Poliner LR, et al: Comparison of two-dimensional echocardiography with gated radionuclide ventriculography in the evaluation of global and regional left ventricular function in acute myocardial infarction. *J Am Coll Cardiol* 3:243, 1984.

395. Shah PK, Pichler M, Berman DS, et al: Left ventricular ejection fraction determined by radionuclide ventriculography in early stages of first transmural myocardial infarction: Relation to short-term prognosis. *Am J Cardiol* 45:542, 1980.

396. Dewhurst NG, Hannan WJ, Muir AL: Prognostic value of radionuclide ventriculography after myocardial infarction. *Q J Med* 49:479, 1981.

397. Abrams DS, Starling MR, Crawford MH, et al: Value of noninvasive techniques for predicting early complications in patients with clinical class II acute myocardial infarction. *J Am Coll Cardiol* 2:818, 1983.

398. Becker LC, Silverman KJ, Bulkley BH, et al: Comparison of early thallium-201 scintigraphy and gated blood pool imaging for predicting mortality in patients with acute myocardial infarction. *Circulation* 67:1272, 1983.

399. Wynne J, Sayres M, Maddox DE, et al: Regional left ventricular function in acute myocardial infarction: Evaluation with quantitative radionuclide ventriculography. *Am J Cardiol* 45:203, 1980.

400. Norris RM, Brandt PWT, Caughey DE, et al: A new coronary prognostic index. *Lancet* 1:274, 1969.

401. Ong L, Valdellon B, Coromilas J, et al: Precordial S-T segment depression in inferior myocardial infarction. Evaluation by quantitative thallium-201 scintigraphy and technetium-99m ventriculography. *Am J Cardiol* 51:734, 1983.

402. Greenberg H, McMaster P, Dwyer EM Jr, et al: Left ventricular dysfunction after acute myocardial infarction: Results of a prospective multicenter study. *J Am Coll Cardiol* 4:867, 1984.

403. Alexopoulos D, Horowitz SF, Macari-Hinson MM, et al: Left ventricular aneurysm and prognosis after first anterior wall acute myocardial infarction. *Am J Cardiol* 63:362, 1989.

404. Schulze RA Jr, Strauss HW, Pitt B: Sudden death in the year following myocardial infarction: Relation to ventricular premature contractions in the late hospital phase and left ventricular ejection fraction. *Am J Med* 62:192, 1977.

405. The Multicenter Postinfarction Research Group: Risk stratification and survival after myocardial infarction. *N Engl J Med* 309:331, 1983.

406. Bigger JT Jr, Fleiss JL, Kleiger R, et al: The relationships among ventricular arrhythmias, left ventricular dysfunction, and mortality in the 2 years after myocardial infarction. *Circulation* 69:250, 1984.

407. Hakki A-H, Nestico PF, Heo J, et al: Relative prognostic value of rest thallium-201 imaging, radionuclide ventriculography and 24 hour ambulatory electrocardiographic monitoring after acute myocardial infarction. *J Am Coll Cardiol* 10:25, 1987.

408. Gomes JA, Winters SL, Stewart D, et al: A new noninvasive index to predict sustained ventricular tachycardia and sudden death in the first year after myocardial infarction: Based on signal-averaged electrocardiogram, radionuclide ejection fraction and Holter monitoring. *J Am Coll Cardiol* 10:349, 1987.

409. Griffin BP, Shah PK, Diamond GA, et al: Incremental prognostic accuracy of clinical, radionuclide and hemodynamic data in acute myocardial infarction. *Am J Cardiol* 68:707, 1991.

410. Hlatky MA, Califf RM, Lee KL, et al: Prognostic significance of precordial ST-segment depression during inferior acute myocardial infarction. *Am J Cardiol* 55:325, 1985.

411. Goldberg HL, Borer JS, Jacobstein JG, et al: Anterior S-T segment depression in acute inferior myocardial infarction: Indicator of posterolateral infarction. *Am J Cardiol* 48:1009, 1981.

412. Lew AS, Weiss AT, Shah PK, et al: Precordial ST segment depression during acute inferior myocardial infarction: Early thallium-201 scintigraphic evidence of adjacent

posterolateral or inferoseptal involvement. *J Am Coll Cardiol* 5:203, 1985.

413. Boden WE, Bough EW, Korr KS, et al: Inferoseptal myocardial infarction: Another cause of precordial ST-segment depression in transmural inferior wall myocardial infarction? *Am J Cardiol* 54:1216, 1984.

414. Billadello JJ, Smith JL, Ludbrook PA, et al: Implications of "reciprocal" ST segment depression associated with acute myocardial infarction identified by positron tomography. *J Am Coll Cardiol* 2:616, 1983.

415. Gibson RS, Crampton RS, Watson DD, et al: Precordial ST-segment depression during acute inferior myocardial infarction: Clinical, scintigraphic and angiographic correlations. *Circulation* 66:732, 1982.

416. Franzosi MG, Mauri F, Pampallona S, et al: The GISSI study: Further analysis. *Circulation* 76(Suppl II):II-52, 1987.

417. O'Keefe JH Jr, Grines CL, DeWood MA, et al: Factors influencing myocardial salvage with primary angioplasty. *J Nucl Cardiol* 2:35, 1995.

418. Miller TD, Christian TF, Hopfenspirger MR, et al: Infarct size after acute myocardial infarction measured by quantitative tomographic ^{99m}Tc sestamibi imaging predicts subsequent mortality. *Circulation* 92:334, 1995.

419. Christian TF, Behrenbeck T, Gersh BJ, Gibbons RJ: Relation of left ventricular volume and function over one year after acute myocardial infarction to infarct size determined by technetium-99m sestamibi. *Am J Cardiol* 68:21, 1991.

420. McCallister BD Jr, Christian TF, Gersh BJ, Gibbons RJ: Prognosis of myocardial infarctions involving more than 40% of the left ventricle after acute reperfusion therapy. *Circulation* 88:1470, 1993.

421. Van Vlies B, Baas J, Visser CA, et al: Predictive value of indium-111 antimyosin uptake for improvement of left ventricular wall motion after thrombolysis in acute myocardial infarction. *Am J Cardiol* 64:167, 1989.

422. Maddahi J, DiCarli M: Antimyosin monoclonal antibody imaging to assess myocardial viability in the setting of thrombolysis. *Am J Cardiac Imaging* 7:45, 1993.

423. Zaret BL, Wackers FJTh, Terrin ML, et al: Value of radionuclide rest and exercise left ventricular ejection fraction in assessing survival of patients after thrombolytic therapy for acute myocardial infarction: Results of Thrombolysis in Myocardial Infarction (TIMI) phase II study. *J Am Coll Cardiol* 26:73, 1995.

424. Candell-Riera J, Permanyer-Miralda G, Castell J, et al: Uncomplicated first myocardial infarction: Strategy for comprehensive prognostic studies. *J Am Coll Cardiol* 18:1207, 1991.

425. Olona M, Candell-Riera J, Permanyer-Miralda G, et al: Strategies for prognostic assessment of uncomplicated first myocardial infarction: 5-year follow-up study. *J Am Coll Cardiol* 25:815, 1995.

426. McClements BM, Adgey AAJ: Value of signal-averaged electrocardiography, radionuclide ventriculography, Holter monitoring and clinical variables for prediction of arrhythmic events in survivors of acute myocardial infarction in the thrombolytic era. *J Am Coll Cardiol* 21:1419, 1993.

427. Myers MG, Baigrie RS, Charlat ML, Morgan CD: Are

routine non-invasive tests useful in prediction of outcome after myocardial infarction in elderly people? *Lancet* 342:1069, 1993.

428. Hohnloser SH, Franck P, Klingenheben T, et al: Open infarct artery, late potentials, and other prognostic factors in patients after acute myocardial infarction in the thrombolytic era. A prospective trial. *Circulation* 90: 1747, 1994.

429. Lamas GA, Flaker GC, Mitchell G, et al: Effect of infarct artery patency on prognosis after acute myocardial infarction. *Circulation* 92:1101, 1995.

430. Tibbits PA, Evaul JE, Goldstein RE, et al: Serial acquisition of data to predict one-year mortality rate after acute myocardial infarction. *Am J Cardiol* 60:451, 1987.

431. Work JW, Ferguson JG, Diamond GA: Limitations of a conventional logistic regression model based on left ventricular ejection fraction in predicting coronary events after myocardial infarction. *Am J Cardiol* 64:702, 1989.

432. Nicod P, Gilpin E, Dittrich H, et al: Influence on prognosis and morbidity of left ventricular ejection fraction with and without signs of left ventricular failure after acute myocardial infarction. *Am J Cardiol* 61:1165, 1988.

433. Dwyer EM Jr, Greenberg HM, Steinberg G, et al: Clinical characteristics and natural history of survivors of pulmonary congestion during acute myocardial infarction. *Am J Cardiol* 63:1423, 1989.

434. Report of the American College of Cardiology/American Heart Association Task Force on Assessment of Diagnostic and Therapeutic Cardiovascular Procedures (Committee on Radionuclide Imaging), Developed in Collaboration with the American Society of Nuclear Cardiology: Guidelines for clinical use of cardiac radionuclide imaging. *J Am Coll Cardiol* 25:521, 1995.

Postmyocardial Infarction Test Selection

Anthony P. Morise

As a concept, risk stratification following a myocardial infarction–the separation of patients into groups with differing levels of risk concerning future coronary events–has significant theoretical as well as practical appeal. Most would agree that, at least at the conceptual level, risk stratification is both desirable and necessary for the purposes of quality patient care, which in the current economic milieu must also consider cost. Risk stratification is a dynamic never-ending clinical process that commences at the initial presentation of the patient for medical care. However, where there is substantial disagreement pertains to the means or methods of risk stratification. These considerations are further complicated by the ever-evolving management of acute myocardial infarction, the continuously improving means to evaluate patients both invasively and noninvasively, and the constantly expanding knowledge of the biological and biochemical processes that contribute to the occurrence and natural history of coronary atherosclerosis.

This chapter reviews the literature dealing with risk stratification following a myocardial infarction. I acknowledge beforehand that any recommendations pursuant from this discussion are limited by what is available in the literature and that any position taken will likely have both advocates and detractors. Prior to my analysis, I discuss several fundamental concepts that have influenced my analytic approach.

FUNDAMENTAL CONCEPTS

Definition of Risk and Prognostic End Points

Risk is defined as the possibility of loss or harm, which in the context of a myocardial infarction means death

or nonfatal reinfarction. These so-called "hard" events are the putative end points of risk stratification. Other so-called "soft" events such as unstable angina, congestive heart failure, hospitalization, or revascularization do incur loss on the individual but are generally of a different quality and degree of reversibility, i.e., economic loss or loss of useful time versus loss of life or heart muscle. There is frequently bias inherent in these soft events, e.g., the diagnostic test results that are often used to make decisions regarding revascularization are the object of an investigation. These soft events are generally more plentiful than hard events and allow for a greater prevalence of total events in an analysis. Nevertheless, the hard events are the bottom line of any assessment of prognosis and this review places an emphasis on hard end points.

Other end points have been used as surrogates for death and reinfarction, e.g., extent of coronary disease, left ventricular ejection fraction, or infarct artery patency. While there is frequently a general statistical correlation between hard events and these surrogates, using them as end points for risk stratification studies is fraught with many problems, not the least of which is that a significant number of patients with unfavorable surrogate end points do not die or suffer reinfarction. This review does not consider these surrogate end points.

Determinants of Risk

An assumption of risk stratification is that what is found now, will predict the future. For a stress testing strategy, this usually implies that the presence of significant inducible ischemia predicts future events. For an angiography-based strategy, this usually implies that the presence of three-vessel/left main disease or lesion-specific characteristics predicts the future. If these factors play a large role in determining risk, then risk stratification employing these approaches should be successful. But if the atherosclerotic plaque and its stability are the basis for risk of death or reinfarction, do either of these technologies provide answers in this regard?

Incremental Value

The clinical value of any variable, be it a clinical descriptor such as diabetes or a diagnostic test result, can be best appreciated in the context of other already available data.[1,2] The difference in relative value is referred to as the incremental value. When a variable is shown to have a strong univariate relationship with prognosis, but no relationship when incorporated into a multivariable model, it may be stated to have no incremental value. This is generally due to the presence of redundant information in the variable of interest and some other variable. This redundancy of variables is referred to by statisticians as multicollinearity. A familiar scenario might consider the additional prognostic value of a test such as exercise testing over already available clinical data, e.g., age, gender, and symptoms. This assumes that there is already demonstrable clinical value for the clinical variables. To demonstrate significant incremental value, usually multivariable analytic methods are employed. For this reason, this review considers almost exclusively studies that employed multivariable approaches to determining variables that predict risk independent of other data.

Selection Bias

The selection and exclusion of patients for evaluation based on prior knowledge of clinical data or a test result is, in general, a process to be avoided in any evaluation of a diagnostic or prognostic strategy. If the risk of events is similar in the excluded and included groups, then the clinical value of the method under scrutiny will not be misrepresented. However, this usually is not the case. Nevertheless, in the postmyocardial infarction setting, it is often necessary to select groups of patients based on the presence or absence of predetermined predictors of risk. This is, however, not necessarily selection bias but part of the risk stratification process whereby as the high-risk patients declare themselves by manifesting complications of myocardial infarction, the larger group is "whittled down" to a smaller and presumably lower-risk group. In the context of postmyocardial infarction risk stratification, the patients with uncomplicated early in-

hospital courses might constitute such a "whittled down" group. Therefore, in evaluating studies, attention will be paid to how the initial study groups were determined, with particular emphasis on patient age and history of prior infarction.

Publication Bias

One factor that can be neither ignored nor effectively adjusted for is publication bias. This phenomenon occurs for at least three general reasons. First, negative study results are not submitted for review by investigators who did not find the expected outcome. This may be due to poor study design, a type II or beta statistical error relating to sample size, or bias of the investigators not to submit data that run counterintuitively to their preconceived expectations. Second, a particular journal's interests may or may not be served by the results of a particular study introducing a reporting bias. Third, a study may not be published because the results are negative and there is a lack of new insight into the problem investigated. In any review of this sort, the influence of publication bias is present but virtually impossible to adjust for effectively. Nevertheless, the reader should be aware that the data that were reviewed were what was available in the literature and that the literature in general is affected by publication bias.

Treatment Eras

Over the last 10 years, it has become obvious that as the treatment of acute myocardial infarction advances, we enter new eras where the standard of care changes dramatically. Such an era was ushered in with the evidence from clinical megatrials that thrombolytic therapy had a major impact on the prognosis of acute myocardial infarction. Thus, the terms *prethrombolytic era* and *thrombolytic era* were born. With the results of recently reported trials, we may be on the brink of yet another era: the *primary angioplasty era*. While defining eras is best left to historians, what is clear is that in the foreseeable future, there will be three inherently different groups of patients that will require different considerations for risk stratification: patients who receive as primary therapy either (1) thrombolytic therapy, (2) infarct vessel angioplasty, or (3) neither. The first two of these three groups will be expanding in size, with the latter group hopefully decreasing in size.

Given what was stated earlier, this analysis considers studies with respect to treatment era. For the purposes of this study, the prethrombolytic era will end in 1985. Unless thrombolytic status is clearly delineated in the methods section of a study, studies that enrolled patients prior to 1985 are considered as prethrombolytic era studies. Studies that enrolled patients after 1985 or that explicitly indicated that thrombolytic therapy was given are considered thrombolytic era studies. Studies that explicitly state that they dealt with angioplasty as initial therapy on presentation are considered primary angioplasty era studies.

NO REPERFUSION THERAPY

Clinical Variables

In the 1990s, patients may not receive reperfusion therapy, i.e., intravenous thrombolysis or primary angioplasty, for several reasons[3]: (1) they may appear for care at a time period too late for clinical benefit, e.g., more than 12 h after symptom onset; (2) they may have an equivocal electrocardiogram; (3) they may have a contraindication to reperfusion therapy; (4) they may refuse reperfusion therapy; or (5) the patient's physician may decide against reperfusion therapy for other reasons not outlined above. The frequency of reperfusion therapy not being given can vary greatly and may currently be as high as two-thirds of potential candidates.[3]

The analysis of this group begins with a consideration of studies published from the prethrombolytic era. Extrapolating this analysis to the thrombolytic era is not assumed, as prethrombolytic era patients are not necessarily the same as patients in the thrombolytic era who do not receive reperfusion therapy. In general, because of the favorable effect of reperfusion therapy on mortality, patients who do not receive it are at higher risk than those who do receive it.[3]

Table 19-1 lists 15 prethrombolytic postmyocardial infarction studies with multivariable analysis of clinical variables where patients were not excluded because they did not undergo noninvasive or invasive testing.[4-18] All of the studies represent populations of substantial size with only one study containing fewer than 500 patients. Several multicenter studies are represented: the Multicenter Postinfarction Research Group (MPIRG), the Multicenter Investigation of the Limitation of Infarct Size (MILIS), the Secondary Prevention Reinfarction Israeli Nifedipine Trial (SPRINT), and the Multicenter Diltiazem Postinfarction Trial (MDPT). In addition, the five studies denoted with an asterisk represent studies from the United States and Canada, with the core unit being in San Diego. The last study is a multicenter study from Belgium. Therefore, the 15 studies represent at least seven different groups of patients.

All studies except for two used mortality as a solitary end point. The other two utilized reinfarction as the end point.[9,11] In addition, the study by Kornowski et al[17] evaluated death and reinfarction separately. All studies except one[6] were prospective. The average frequency of women enrolled was 25 percent, indicating that conclusions drawn may not be immediately transferable to women. Most studies did not limit their enrollment to patients with ST-segment elevation, i.e., those destined in most cases to develop Q-wave infarctions. This is in distinction to most studies in the thrombolytic era, which by design enrolled patients preferentially with ST-segment elevation. Given that non-Q-wave infarctions are presently considered to be closer to unstable angina in terms of pathophysiology, evaluation, and treatment,[19] this review does not separately analyze data for non-Q-wave infarction. Nevertheless, the impact of non-Q-wave infarctions on the results of prethrombolytic studies could be considerable.

A review of Table 19-1 indicates that study designs were somewhat different, e.g., regarding age and prior infarction exclusions and the point in time when follow-

Table 19-1 Prethrombolytic Era: Studies with Clinical Variables

Ref	Sample Size	% Women	Age Limit	Prospective	FU Entry	Prior MI	Non-Q MI	Multicenter
4	940	19	<65	Yes	Disch	Yes	Yes	No
5	221	23	No	No	Adm	Yes	Yes	No*
6	818	32	No	Yes	Disch	Yes	Yes	Yes*
7	997	22	No	Yes	Disch	Yes	No	Yes*
8	1736	27	No	Yes	Disch	No	Yes	Yes*
9	3666	24	No	Yes	Disch	Yes	Yes	Yes*
10	866	22	<70	Yes	Adm	Yes	Yes	MPIRG
11	866	22	<70	Yes	Adm	Yes	Yes	MPIRG
12	779	22	<70	Yes	Adm	Yes	Yes	MPIRG
13	866	22	<70	Yes	Adm	Yes	Yes	MPIRG
14	2466	20	No	Yes	Hosp	Yes	Yes	MDPT
15	532	27	<76	Yes	Disch	No	Yes	MILIS
16	5839	26	No	Yes	Adm	Yes	No	SPRINT
17	3695	24	No	Yes	Disch	No	No	SPRINT
18	2312	27	No	Yes	Disch	Yes	Yes	Yes

Adm, at admission; Disc, at discharge; FU Entry, time of entry into follow-up; Hosp, in-hospital; MI, myocardial infarction. For multicenter abbreviations, see the text.
*Multicenter study with its base in San Diego, CA.

up commenced. For this reason, conclusions concerning predictor variables need to consider study design.

For all studies without age restrictions on enrollment, increasing age was found to be an independent predictor of mortality. These included the SPRINT, Belgium, MDPT, and San Diego–based studies.

Of the 12 mortality studies that did not exclude patients with prior myocardial infarctions, prior myocardial infarction was an independent predictor of mortality in nine. However, in the three studies where independence was not found,[10,11,13] radionuclide left ventricular ejection fraction was included in the analysis. Since prior myocardial infarction generally predicts reduced left ventricular function, the redundant information in these two variables may have canceled the predictive value of prior myocardial infarction.

All studies in Table 19-1 evaluated variables that were clinical descriptors of left ventricular dysfunction. Most commonly these were defined as rales on an early in-hospital physical examination. In addition, Killip class, pulmonary congestion on chest x-ray, an S3 gallop, diuretic use, and peak heart rate were evaluated in some. Of the 15 studies, 11 demonstrated independent predictability of clinical heart failure variables for death. Of the four that failed to show independence, one also included left ventricular ejection fraction[13] and the other three used reinfarction[9,11] and sudden cardiac death[15] rather than total cardiac mortality as end points.

Only four of the studies evaluated predischarge chest pain/angina pectoris. Two used death as the end point,[6,13] one used reinfarction,[11] and one used both.[17] With one exception, each study indicated that predischarge angina was an independent predictor of the respective end point. The study by Kornowski et al[17] failed to show that predischarge angina predicted death. Two other studies not included in Table 19-1 also shed some light on the prognostic significance of postinfarction angina. Both of these studies involved groups who underwent postinfarction coronary angiography. Galjee et al[20] evaluated 231 patients, with a first infarction 27 of whom developed early postinfarction angina. On multivariable analysis, early postinfarction angina as well as left ventricular ejection fraction were independent predictors of 1-year mortality. It was difficult, however, to determine what other clinical variables were included in the analysis. Taylor et al[21] evaluated 106 patients and found that, after multivariable analysis of clinical and angiographic data, postinfarction angina was a significant predictor of reinfarction but not of death.

Concerning several other commonly considered clinical descriptors, there was a mixed response. The presence of diabetes mellitus was independently predictive of mortality in five of six studies where it was evaluated.[9,12,16–18] Anterior wall infarction location was independently predictive in only three of 10 studies where it was considered. Given that anterior infarctions are usually larger

and associated with lower ejection fractions than are inferior infarctions, lack of independence probably reflects redundant prognostic information between anterior infarction location and heart failure variables. High-grade atrioventricular block was predictive in only two of five studies where it was considered. In nine studies that considered gender, none found that gender was an independent predictor of mortality. However, the study by Greenland et al,[16] which analyzed men and women separately, found that the predictors of hospital and 1-year mortality were different for men and women, with a greater emphasis on diabetes in women.

An additional study not included in Table 19-1 is the study by Feinberg et al.[22] This subset analysis of the SPRINT study analyzed 1841 patients with a first inferior myocardial infarction. Age, Killip class, and elevated blood sugar were independently associated with in-hospital mortality.

In summary, review of these studies identifies several preadmission clinical descriptors (advanced age, prior myocardial infarction, and diabetes mellitus) and in-hospital postinfarction complications (early heart failure and predischarge angina) as predictors of death and/or reinfarction.

Left Ventricular Ejection Fraction

As noted earlier, left ventricular ejection fraction was considered in several of the studies listed in Table 19-1. In each case, patients were not excluded from the study if they did not have ejection fraction data. Therefore, only a fraction of these groups had ejection-fraction data. Ejection fraction data were determined most often by radionuclide methods and occasionally by catheterization. The usual cut point evaluated as a discrete variable was a left ventricular ejection fraction of less than or equal to 40 percent. Of the nine studies in Table 19-1 that considered ejection fraction, six found independent predictability for ejection fraction when analyzed with clinical variables.[8,10,12–15]

In addition, six other prethrombolytic studies were found that considered ejection fraction, but excluded patients from consideration who did not have ejection-fraction data.[20,21,23–26] Three studies utilized predischarge radionuclide studies,[23,25,26] and three used invasive angiography.[20,21,24] Each study found that the left ventricular ejection fraction was an independent predictor of death. In the study by Fioretti et al,[26] ejection fraction was a predictor only in those patients ineligible for exercise testing.

In summary, the majority of studies found that left ventricular ejection fraction was an independent predictor of death in postinfarction patients studied in the prethrombolytic era.

Table 19-2 Prethrombolytic Era: Exercise-Testing Studies

Ref	Sample Size	% Women	Mean Days After MI	Follow-up (Years)	End Point	% Cardiac Mortality (Annual)	% No Exercise	No Exercise Mortality (Annual)
27	205	22	21	1	D	11.7	21	?
28	236	20	16	1	D	12.0	24	14
29	205	18	12	1	D	5.8	12	?
30	225	13	11	5	D	11.1	40	?
31	667	20	15	1	D	5.0	22	14
32	466	18	12	1	D + MI	7.0	68	15
33	72	5	13	1	D or MI	16.6	?	?
34	301	?	10	2.4	D or MI	4.3	46	10.2
35	245	15	Predischarge	10	D	2.2	52	?
36	300	16	13	1	D	7.0	26	27

D, death; MI, myocardial infarction.

Exercise Electrocardiography

Beginning in the late 1970s, the exercise test entered into the risk stratification equation with an exponential increase in the number of studies assessing its merits. Table 19-2 displays features of 10 such studies reported using patients from the prethrombolytic era.[27-36] These studies are noteworthy for the number of patients who actually underwent exercise testing. All but one have a sample size of over 200. The largest study, involving 667 patients, was by the MPIRG. As noted in Table 19-1, women represent a distinct minority of the patients in each study, with the average being even lower than noted in Table 19-1. All studied populations of patients with uncomplicated postinfarction courses who were evaluated with exercise electrocardiography at or shortly following the point of discharge from the hospital. All had a minimum follow-up time of 1 year, with one study having a follow-up duration of 10 years. Each study considered cardiac mortality as the principal end point, with reinfarction also considered in three studies. All used patients who had a mix of Q-wave and non-Q-wave infarctions. No study could be found that involved entirely Q-wave infarctions.

The percentage of all eligible patients who were exercised varied greatly. However, in each case where mortality data were available, the annual cardiac mortality rate for the group who did not receive an exercise test was significantly greater than for the group who received an exercise test.

Concerning potential predictor variables, one of the greatest difficulties centered on the lack of uniformity in both the use and the definition of these variables. The most consistent variable in terms of presence and definition (seven studies) was the presence or absence of exercise induced angina. In only two of those seven studies, however, was it found to be an independent predictor. All 10 studies considered ST-segment changes and systolic blood pressure responses, but the definitions varied widely. Abnormal systolic blood pressure response was an independent predictor in five of the 10 studies while

ST-segment change (either elevation or depression) was an independent predictor in only two of 10 studies. Exercise capacity also had a wide range of definition and was an independent predictor in five of nine studies where it was considered.

In summary, due to inconsistencies in the variables evaluated as well as other potential methodologic problems, no exercise test variable was consistently demonstrated to be an independent predictor of postinfarction death or reinfarction. Of those variables considered, exercise capacity and abnormal systolic blood pressure response were the most likely candidates for risk discriminators. Previously, Froelicher et al analyzed 25 prethrombolytic studies that evaluated the prognostic ability of exercise testing.[37] However, they did not limit their analysis to studies that used multivariable analysis. Similar to the present analysis, they concluded that exercise capacity and systolic blood pressure response were the only variables that predicted risk and that patients excluded from exercise testing have a higher mortality than those who undergo exercise testing.

Stress Imaging

Given the lack of convincing evidence that exercise-induced ischemia manifested as ST-segment depression reliably predicted death or reinfarction, other stress modalities were explored. However, although numerous studies from the prethrombolytic era evaluated noninvasive imaging in this setting, only a handful incorporated multivariable analysis, used hard end points, and evaluated patients within 3 weeks after infarction (Table 19-3).[38-42] This is surprising given the enthusiasm with which investigators attacked this question. The following discussion considers each study individually.

The study by Hung et al[38] compared the ability of exercise electrocardiography, planar thallium scintigraphy, and radionuclide ventriculography to discriminate hard events 1 year after infarction. Their study was prospective and involved only men. Using the Cox propor-

Table 19-3 Prethrombolytic Era: Noninvasive Imaging Studies

Ref	Stess	Imaging Modality	Sample Size	% Women	End Point
38	Exercise	Thallium + RNA	117	0	D + MI
39	Dipyridamole	Thallium	51	31	D + MI
40	Exercise	RNA	106	1	D or MI
41	Exercise	RNA	117	33	Hard + soft
42	Exercise	RNA	183	13	D

D, death; MI, myocardial infarction; RNA, radionuclide angiography.

tional hazards model, peak treadmill workload and the exercise-induced change in left ventricular ejection fraction were chosen as independent predictors. Large thallium-201 (^{201}Tl) total and reversible perfusion defect scores were univariately predictive of hard cardiac events but were not predictive by multivariable analysis.

The study by Leppo et al[39] prospectively evaluated the ability of predischarge intravenous dipyridamole–planar thallium scintigraphy to discriminate hard events over 19 months of follow-up (annual cardiac mortality, 10 percent). When clinical, resting ejection fraction, and thallium variables were subjected to stepwise logistic regression analysis, only the presence of any thallium redistribution was selected as a predictor ($p = 0.02$). Infarction location, ejection fraction, and the number of thallium defects were of marginal significance ($p = 0.1$ to 0.2). Given the small sample size, it is not clear whether a larger sample size would have demonstrated these other variables to be significant predictors. In another small study by Gimple et al[43] that did not employ multivariable analysis, predischarge dipyridamole thallium studies were performed on 40 patients. Within 6 months, one patient died and three had reinfarction. The authors found that redistribution of thallium outside of the infarct zone was a sensitive and specific predictor of events (hard plus soft). In a larger study employing predischarge exercise thallium scintigraphy where multivariable analysis was not used, Gibson et al[44] prospectively evaluated 140 patients. Among the 49 patients with a single fixed defect and normal lung uptake, there was one death (2 percent) and no reinfarctions over 15 months of follow-up. Among the remaining 91 patients with more abnormal thallium studies, there were six deaths (7 percent) and a hard-event rate of 16 percent.

The study by Morris et al[40] prospectively evaluated the ability of rest and exercise radionuclide angiography to discriminate death or reinfarction in a group of predominantly men over a 2-year follow-up period. These authors did not incorporate exercise test variables into their analysis. Using a Cox proportional hazards model on clinical and radionuclide data, they found that both rest and exercise ejection fraction were independent predictors of death. There was also significant incremental value, as indicated by the differences in chi-square values for the nuclear data over the clinical data. No variables,

however, were predictors of nonfatal reinfarction. Like the study by Morris et al, the study by Corbett et al[41] prospectively evaluated the ability of rest and exercise radionuclide angiography to discriminate cardiac events, which in this study included death, reinfarction, and medically refractory angina over a 6-month follow-up period. Using stepwise discriminant analysis of clinical, exercise, and scintigraphic variables, they found that exercise ejection fraction data were the only independent predictors of cardiac events. Finally, the study by Mazzotta et al[42] prospectively evaluated the ability of exercise testing and exercise radionuclide angiography to predict cardiac death. This study had the largest sample size and followed patients for a mean of 4 years. Using a Cox regression model, only exercise left ventricular ejection fraction was an independent predictor. Considering that the 4-year mortality was only 6 percent (1.5 percent annual mortality), it is remarkable that any variables were found to be predictors.

In summary, the dearth of studies in the prethrombolytic era that employed multivariable analysis makes it difficult to define adequately the prognostic value of postinfarction noninvasive stress imaging in the context of other known clinical variables. This is despite the apparent successes of exercise thallium testing in this capacity, which is based on studies that did not employ multivariable analysis.[44] Nevertheless, available studies do suggest that both perfusion and function variables have independent predictability for death following acute myocardial infarction.

Coronary Angiography

The top half of Table 19-4 lists six studies from the prethrombolytic era that considered angiographic variables using multivariable analysis with hard prognostic end points.[20,21,24,45–47] Only one[47] studied patients prior to discharge from the hospital and all had age exclusions to study entry. As noted in the previous tables, women are not well represented, with three studies exclusively involving men. Coronary angiographic variables were expressed in different ways: jeopardy or myocardial scores, number of diseased vessels or lesions, multivessel

Table 19-4 Coronary Angiography Studies

Ref	Sample Size	% Women	Age Limit	Prior MI	Uncomplicated
			Prethrombolytic Era		
21	106	26	<67	Yes	No
45	325	0	<60	No	Yes
24	605	0	<60	Yes	Yes
46	259	0	<61	Yes	Yes
47	303	6	<69	No	Yes
20	231	12	<65	No	No
			Thrombolytic Era		
58	553	17	<70	Yes	No
57	1043	20	<71	Yes	Yes
64	1043	20	<70	Yes	Yes
77	708	20	<76	Yes	No
78	245	18	<76	Yes	No

MI, myocardial infarction.

disease, or discrete stenosis severity. Irrespective of how they were expressed, significant independent predictability for death was found in four of the six studies. Two of the studies considered reinfarction and both found the angiographic variables to be predictive.

Incremental Value

As stated earlier, incremental value is the prognostic value of a variable over and above already available data, e.g., exercise test data over clinical data. Properly designed incremental studies should perform separate analyses of clinical data, clinical data plus stress test, and clinical data plus stress test plus angiographic variables to assess adequately the predictability of data at each stage of the risk stratification process. This reflects the sequential flow of clinical decision making that patients generally receive.

Two studies were found that provide both qualitative and quantitative incremental analyses. The study by Leroy et al[47] evaluated 303 patients with a first myocardial infarction. Their analysis suggested that angiography was an independent predictor of mortality, but did not provide incremental value if clinical plus exercise electrocardiographic data (that were not all independently significant taken alone) were forced into the model. They did find that exercise electrocardiography had statistically significant incremental value over clinical variables. However, the exercise test was not performed prior to discharge. In another incremental evaluation, Tibbits et al,[48] using the MPIRG database, found that exercise testing and ejection fraction added little to the prognostic ability of clinical variables.

It is the opinion of this reviewer that, while there are studies that demonstrate independent predictability of a number of clinically, noninvasively, and invasively derived data, there are an insufficient number of adequately designed studies in the prethrombolytic era to determine the incremental value of invasive and noninvasive testing in the risk stratification of postinfarction patients.

THROMBOLYTIC THERAPY

Clinical Variables

The analysis of this group begins with a consideration of studies that both enrolled patients in the thrombolytic trials and used multivariable analysis with hard end points. In Table 19-5 are listed 11 studies[49-59] from the thrombolytic era that represent nine study groups, including eight multicenter studies: Global Utilization of Streptokinase and Tissue Plasminogen Activator for Occluded Coronary Arteries (GUSTO-1), the European Cooperative Study Group (ECSG), the Thrombolysis in Myocardial Infarction study (TIMI-2), the Gruppo Italiano per lo Studio della Sopravvivenza nell'Infarto Miocardico (GISSI-2), the Western Washington Intravenous/Intracoronary Streptokinase Trial (WWIST), the APSAC Intervention Mortality Study (AIMS), International Joint Efficacy Comparison of Thrombolytics Trial (INJECT), and the Interuniversity Cardiology Institute of the Netherlands trial. Most of these studies involved a large sample size, with women representing only about 20 percent of the patients.

Analysis of these 11 studies revealed findings similar to what was noted in the prethrombolytic studies. Of the nine that included patients with prior myocardial infarction, all nine found this preadmission characteristic to be an independent predictor of death and/or reinfarction. Likewise, all studies found advancing age to be an independent predictor of death irrespective of whether there were age limitations to study enrollment. Clinical variables consistent with in-hospital left ventricular dysfunction were found to be independent predictors of death in the nine studies that considered mor-

Table 19-5 Thrombolytic Era: Studies with Clinical Variables

Ref	Sample Size	% Women	Age Limit	FU Time	Prior MI	End Point	Multicenter
49	41,021	25	No	1 m	Yes	D	GUSTO-1
50	1398	26	No	1 m	Yes	D	INJECT
51	2819	18	<76	6 w	Yes	D	TIMI-2
52	10,219	18	No	6 m	Yes	D	GISSI-2
53	9752	21	No	6 m	No	D	GISSI-2
54	8907	18	No	6 m	Yes	MI	GISSI-2
55	456	23	<70	1 y	No	MI	No
56	1258	18	<71	1 y	Yes	D	AIMS
57	1043	?	<71	2 y	Yes	D	ECSG
58	533	?	No	3 y	Yes	D	Yes
59	618	15	<76	5 y	Yes	D	WWIST

D, death; FU, mean follow-up duration; m, month; MI, myocardial infarction; w, weeks; y, years. *Multicenter study based in San Diego, CA. For other multicenter-study abbreviations, see the text.

tality. These heart failure variables, however, were not predictors of reinfarction.[54,55]

Diabetes mellitus was an independent predictor in only two of the eight studies where it was considered. However, in the two studies[49,51] where it was found to be a predictor (including the large GUSTO cohort), the end point was death within 6 weeks of infarction. In five of the other six studies (three from GISSI), the follow-up period was 6 months or greater. This suggests that diabetes mellitus is an independent predictor of very early postinfarction mortality.

Anterior infarction location was an independent predictor in five of 10 studies where it was considered in the analysis. On the other hand, a clinical variable that could be a surrogate of anterior infarction, i.e., the number of leads with ST-segment elevation, was found to be an independent predictor of death in two studies where it was considered. Both the TIMI-2 and GISSI-2 studies,[51,52] which had some of the most comprehensive multivariable analyses, had this finding. The large GUSTO cohort study did not report that this variable was analyzed.[49] In addition, a substudy of the INJECT trial[50] found that early ST-segment resolution was a strong independent predictor of improved 35-day mortality.

Concerning postinfarction angina, none of the studies in Table 19-5 considered it as a possible predictor except the GISSI-2 study.[52,54] For the entire group of 10,219 patients, postinfarction angina was a good univariate predictor but not an independent predictor of 6-month mortality or reinfarction. However, this variable was analyzed along with exercise test variables rather than separately with just the other clinical variables. The strongest variable for predicting death or reinfarction in GISSI-2 was the ineligibility for an exercise test irrespective of whether it was for cardiac or noncardiac reasons. In a prospective collaborative study involving patients participating in the GISSI-2 study,[60] the conditions of 453 patients who were less than 71 years of age and who underwent angiography after their first infarction were followed for 1 year. Of potential clinical and angiographic variables, early ischemia (transient, spontaneous

ST-segment depression or elevation with or without angina) was the only independent predictor of in-hospital cardiac events (essentially reinfarctions). It did not, however, predict events at 1 year.

Of the nine studies that considered gender, several found gender to be a univariate predictor of mortality, but none found it to be an independent predictor. None of the studies, however, analyzed men and women separately. Given what was found in the previously cited study by Greenland et al[16] (which analyzed men and women separately, thus yielding gender-specific differences in the clinical variables that predict mortality) and what has been published more recently,[61] a consensus conclusion concerning gender and risk of death following infarction is not possible.

In summary, it would appear that the same clinical variables that were important and independent predictors of death and reinfarction in the prethrombolytic era continue to be important predictors in the thrombolytic era.

Left Ventricular Ejection Fraction

The ECSG study[57] found that resting radionuclide left ventricular ejection fraction was an independent predictor of death even though the ejection fraction data were added into the model after the exercise test data. The TIMI-2 study[62] found a similar independent relationship as the ECSG study, but the only exercise variables included in the analysis were derived from the exercise ejection fraction. In addition, the study also noted that when the rest and exercise ejection fractions were both included in the analysis, exercise ejection fraction was not a predictor and added nothing to discrimination over and above the rest ejection fraction. The WWIST and Netherlands trials also found resting ejection fraction to be an independent predictor.[58,59]

Figure 19-1 compares the ejection fraction and mortality data for a prethrombolytic study (MPIRG)[10] with

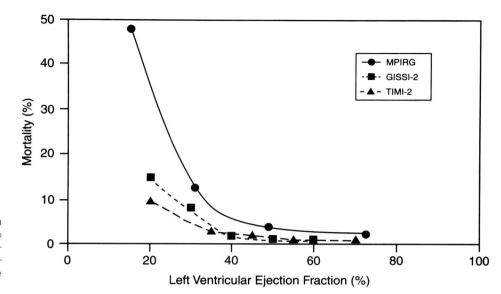

Figure 19-1 Compared are data from one prethrombolytic and two thrombolytic studies concerning mortality (y-axis) and left ventricular ejection fraction at rest (x-axis). See the text for discussion.

data from two thrombolytic studies (GISSI-2 and TIMI-2).[52,62] While there are significant differences between the studies and the analysis shown on the graph is not multivariable in nature, from a purely univariate perspective, the curves are qualitatively very similar, revealing an exponential increase in mortality as ejection fraction decreases. This suggests that, while quantitative evaluations of mortality between the two eras may indicate an improved mortality in the thrombolytic era, the correlation between ejection fraction and mortality has not changed from the prethrombolytic to the thrombolytic era.

Exercise Electrocardiography

Few studies in the thrombolytic era have considered exercise testing in a multivariable analysis in which clinical and exercise test variables were evaluated separately from imaging variables. Six studies (two from GISSI-2) adequately analyzed exercise electrocardiogram variables regarding death[52,57,63,64] or reinfarction.[54,55] In only one study[57] did exercise test variables show independent predictability. In this study, an inadequate systolic blood pressure response was predictive even after the inclusion of ejection fraction and angiographic variables into the analysis. In no study were ST-segment variables found to be predictive of death or reinfarction. However, in the two studies where the inability to perform exercise testing was considered as a variable, there was strong independent prediction concerning mortality.[52,57] The disappointing performance of exercise testing raises doubt as to the value of exercise as a provocative method

in the postinfarction patient who has received thrombolytic therapy.

Stress Imaging

Compared with the previous prethrombolytic analysis, more studies appear to be available that used multivariable analysis to assess the independent prognostic ability of stress imaging. The number of studies noted in Table 19-6, however, is still disappointingly small.[62,63,65–74] In fact, if those studies that considered hard and soft end points together (i.e., events) are removed, the number of remaining studies is very similar to that of Table 19-3. It would seem that many investigations have focused on subsetting patients by test responses rather than assessing the predictability of imaging data considered in the context of other clinical and imaging derived variables. Many of the studies utilized a mix of patients who received various interventional therapies including thrombolytic therapy. For several studies, it was not possible to determine whether any patients received thrombolytic therapy.[71,72] Of the three differing modalities represented in Table 19-6 (nuclear myocardial perfusion, radionuclide left ventricular function, and echocardiographic wall motion), each has one study that enrolled at least 900 patients and used death as a separate end point.

The first of these is a study reported by Krone et al[63] representing the Multicenter Myocardial Ischemia Research Group (the current metamorphosis of the MPIRG) population. These authors found that exercise test duration, ^{201}Tl ischemia, and the combination of these two variables were strong univariate predictors of

Table 19-6 Thrombolytic Era: Noninvasive Imaging Studies

Ref	Stress	Imaging Modality	Sample Size	End Point	Modality Predicts	Mortality Rate %	Positive Test (%)	End-point Rate (%) + Test	End-point Rate (%) − Test
63	Exercise	Planar thallium	936	D	Yes	1	13	10	4
				D + MI	Yes	1	13	6	0
65	Exercise	SPECT Thallium	210	D or MI	No	3	56–66	?	?
66	Dipyridamole	Planar thallium	50	Events	Yes	0	52	45	0
67	Dipyridamole	Planar thallium	71	D or MI	No	3	51	17	11
68	Adenosine	SPECT Thallium	92	D + MI	Yes	9	?	?	?
69	Exercise	SPECT Sestamibi	134	Events	Yes	3	?	?	?
70	Exercise	RNA	94	Events	Yes	3	31	26	2
62	Exercise	RNA	2567	D	No	2	16	5	1
71	Exercise	Echo	40	Events	Yes	8	43	35	0
72	Exercise	Echo	67	Events	Yes	4	30	50	12
73	Exercise	Echo	70	D or MI	Yes	21	39	48	14
74	Dipyridamole	Echo	925	D	Yes	4	44	7	2

D, death; Echo, two-dimensional echocardiography; MI, myocardial infarction; RNA, radionuclide angiogram; +, positive; −, negative

death and/or reinfarction. Following their multivariable analysis, however, they found that only the combination of myocardial ischemia demonstrated by ^{201}Tl imaging and failure to reach stage III of a modified Bruce treadmill protocol was independently predictive of death and/or reinfarction. However, they enrolled patients 1 to 2 months after acute coronary events with unstable angina and non-Q-wave infarctions in addition to patients with Q-wave infarctions. While myocardial ischemia by ^{201}Tl imaging was predictive of hard cardiac end points in this heterogeneous group of patients presenting with a variety of acute ischemic events, the study does not clarify the predictability of death or reinfarction by thallium testing in patients treated with a thrombolytic drug for an evolving Q-wave infarction. A similar study by Miller et al[75] enrolled 137 patients with acute ischemic events (31 infarctions) who were unable to exercise maximally. The patients were further evaluated with sestamibi SPECT imaging following dipyridamole infusion. The authors found that an abnormal sestamibi study was an independent predictor of death or reinfarction. However, the frequency of an abnormal sestamibi scan was very high (66 percent).

The second large cohort study was reported by Zaret et al[62] and represents the TIMI-2 population. These authors found that exercise left ventricular ejection fraction failed to be a predictor of death after the rest ejection fraction study had been considered.

The third large study by Picano et al[74] reported on 925 patients from the Echo Persantine Italian Cooperative (EPIC) trial and found that exercise wall-motion data were independently predictive of death. However, they studied a population in which only half of the patients received thrombolytic therapy and they did not analyze these patients separately.

A study reported by Miller et al[65] retrospectively evaluated a group of 210 patients with exercise thallium scintigraphy about 9 days after infarction. A subset of 131 of these patients who received thrombolytic therapy alone was analyzed separately. After 2 years, they were unable to find a survival difference between those patients that had high-risk scans and those that did not. In addition, no thallium variables were independently predictive of death in the postthrombolytic patients. An earlier study by Tilkemeier et al[76] that did not employ multivariable analysis also failed to show that exercise thallium perfusion variables predicted cardiac events following thrombolytic therapy.

Given the limited ability of exercise testing to discriminate patients at risk, several studies evaluated pharmacologic testing. Two studies found that dipyridamole or adenosine thallium studies could be safely performed 4 to 5 days after infarction.[66,68] Both found that pharmacologic thallium perfusion imaging variables predicted the respective end points evaluated. A third study was unable to show that dipyridamole–thallium results could predict death or reinfarction.[67] However, this study included patients who underwent angioplasty prior to thallium imaging. Finally, the EPIC study[74] evaluated dual dose dipyridamole echocardiography about 10 days after infarction and found that wall-motion changes predicted death.

For most of the studies in Table 19-6, the mortality rates were generally low, with only one study with a mortality rate greater than 10 percent.[73] In fact, the three largest cohorts had mortality rates of 1 to 4 percent. This observation is not unusual in the thrombolytic era.[3] While it may be possible to find a statistical association between a particular imaging modality and death in groups with such low mortality rates, it may be difficult to identify the precise patients at risk. For example, in those three large cohort studies in Table 19-6, the absolute difference in mortality rate between those with positive and negative imaging tests was narrow, ranging from 5 to 7 percent for positive tests to 0 to 1 percent for negative tests. While these differences are statistically significant, the group with positive tests is still a fairly low-risk group. The practical implication of this is that a significant percentage of those patients with positive tests will not be at high risk. If a test is associated with a high positive response rate, this could lead to statistically significant yet clinically inefficient stratification. On the other hand, those with negative results will have a very low risk of death.

Coronary Angiography

In the bottom half of Table 19-4 are listed five studies reported from the thrombolytic literature.[57,58,64,77,78] Compared with prethrombolytic studies, age restrictions, though present, were somewhat less restrictive, and the representation of women was better, though still only 20 percent at best. As with prethrombolytic studies, angiographic variables were independent predictors of death even when ejection fraction was included in the analysis.

Only a handful of studies assess specific coronary artery lesion characteristics and their prognostic implications. Ellis et al[79] evaluated 174 patients who had successful thrombolysis without angioplasty. Using multivariable analysis, these authors were unable to find any lesion-related variables that predicted recurrent ischemic events despite having an event rate of 23 percent. Davies et al[80] found that a plaque ulceration index determined by quantitative angiography after successful thrombolysis defined a high-risk subset of patients. However, their study did not utilize multivariable analysis. On the other hand, in another study where multivariable analysis was used, Wall et al[81] found that neither quantitative coronary angiographic dimensions nor qualitative coronary lesion morphology predicted early events.

A series of retrospective observational studies[82–85] consider the question of whether coronary angiography predicts the site of a subsequent myocardial infarction. Each study suggests that the angiographic appearance of a vessel does not reliably predict a subsequent total vessel occlusion with infarction. These studies do not disprove the prognostic value of angiographic data based on the extent of atherosclerosis. They do, however, indicate that coronary artery segments without hemodynamically significant lesions may be involved in a subsequent infarction. They also imply that sudden changes in plaques, e.g., rupture, are more likely operative as a mechanism of infarction than is gradual progression of existing stenoses.

Incremental Value

As was the case for data from the prethrombolytic era, few studies from the thrombolytic era provide data that are incremental by design and contain quantitative assessments of prognostic ability. The study by Arnold et al[57] evaluated 1043 patients with exercise testing, left ventricular ejection fraction, and angiography. The subsequent multivariable analysis was assessed using receiver operating characteristic (ROC) curve area analysis. The authors compared the curve areas for all clinical data, clinical data plus exercise testing, clinical data plus exercise testing plus ejection fraction, and all previous data plus angiography. They found that the respective ROC curve areas for these four incremental stages increased as follows: 0.70 ± 0.05, 0.73 ± 0.05, 0.75 ± 0.05, and 0.78 ± 0.04. Despite demonstrating a progressive increase in the discrimination of mortality, these increases were not statistically significant (as suggested by the overlapping standard errors). The study by Mahmarian et al[68] evaluated 92 patients with quantitative adenosine SPECT thallium imaging performed an average of 5 days after infarction in addition to coronary angiography (36 percent of patients received thrombolytic therapy). The authors performed incremental comparisons of clinical, clinical plus angiographic, and clinical plus scintigraphic variables by using a global chi-square test. They found that clinical plus scintigraphic variables had significantly higher chi-square values than either clinical variables alone or clinical plus angiographic variables.

Therefore, as noted earlier for the prethrombolytic era, there are an insufficient number of studies to assess adequately the incremental value of noninvasive and invasive testing in patients receiving thrombolytic therapy. However, none of the cited studies indicated that angiographic data had significant incremental value over clinical and noninvasive data.

EVALUATION OF STRATEGIES

The discussion to this point has dealt with studies that assessed the prognostic ability of clinical data, noninvasive testing, and angiography by using multivariable methods. The following discussion emphasizes those studies that considered strategies for postinfarction risk stratification.

Prethrombolytic Era

One of the earliest studies was by Debusk et al,[86] who considered 665 men stratified first by historical factors such as age, prior infarction or angina, and early postinfarction heart failure, angina, or ventricular arrhythmias. The 62 patients with two or more of these high-risk historical factors had a 6-month hard-event rate of 17.7 percent. The second stratification considered those in whom exercise testing was not performed (6-month hard-event rate, 6.4 percent). The third stratification considered the remaining patients who underwent exercise testing (6-month hard-event rate, 4.6 percent). Those patients that had negative exercise tests had a 6-month hard-event rate of 3.9 percent (positive test, 9.7 percent). Thus, this study provided the basis for believing that patients could be assigned to differing risk groups by the use of simple clinical and exercise variables.

Another study from the prethrombolytic era is that by Ross et al,[87] who proposed a strategy in which patients with prior infarction and those with early postinfarction heart failure and angina were recommended for coronary angiography. The next stratification point was exercise testing. Those with positive tests defined by ischemia or exercise capacity criteria were recommended for angiography. For those who did not undergo exercise testing, left ventricular ejection fraction was measured and, if it was between 0.20 and 0.44, coronary angiography was recommended. This scheme was developed in 1848 patients and applied to a separate set of 780 patients. The discharge to 1 year mortality rate for those identified in the first stage of stratification was 21 percent. The respective exercise test positive and negative mortality rates were 6 percent and 1 percent. The respective ejection fractions of greater than 44 percent and less than or equal to 44 percent mortality rates were 6 percent and 12 percent.

Therefore, there is justification for the consideration of a risk stratification strategy that does not require angiography for patients who do not undergo reperfusion therapy.

Thrombolytic Era

In 1993, the SWIFT (Should We Intervene Following Thrombolysis?) Trial Study group reported on a 1-year follow-up comparison of 800 patients randomized to one of two treatment strategies following thrombolysis:

early coronary angiography versus conservative care.[88] At 1 year, the respective death and reinfarction rates for the conservative care group were 5.0 percent and 12.9 percent and those for the early angiography group were 5.8 percent and 15.1 percent (all comparisons not different).

A similar evaluation was undertaken as part of the TIMI-2 study. Over 3300 patients were randomized to either conservative or invasive strategies. Similar annual death and reinfarction rates were noted at 1, 2, and 3 years after infarction for both strategies.[89,90] Analysis of subsets of TIMI-2 revealed no differences in outcome relating to age.[91] However, patients with prior myocardial infarction[89] fared better with the invasive strategy, and those diabetic patients with a first myocardial infarction fared better with the conservative strategy.[92] Given the retrospective nature of these subset analyses, these findings can be taken as only interesting hypotheses for future studies.

Olona and colleagues[93,94] evaluated 115 patients who had an uncomplicated first infarction. The authors performed predischarge exercise testing, exercise thallium scintigraphy, rest radionuclide ventriculography, rest echocardiography, and cardiac catheterization on all patients. Using multivariable methods, they compared the ability of various combinations of test strategies to predict cardiac complications that included both hard and soft end points. Their follow-up extended up to 5 years and resulted in two basic conclusions: (1) the combination of a test to detect residual ischemia and ventricular function provides significant prognostic information in uncomplicated patients with a first infarction, and (2) cardiac catheterization did not improve on the predictive power of the noninvasive tests. Their study, however, did not explore the possibility of whether noninvasive tests improve the predictive power of cardiac catheterization. Likewise, they failed to consider clinical variables such as age, diabetes, or infarction location in their analysis.

No randomized studies have addressed this controversial topic of routine predischarge coronary angiography following thrombolytic therapy for treatment of acute myocardial infarction. This was considered in nonrandomized groups in the TIMI-2 trial,[95] which compared 197 patients assigned to conservative management (i.e., tissue plasminogen activator, heparin, and aspirin only) and routine coronary angiography, with 1461 patients assigned to conservative management without routine angiography (unless there was spontaneous or induced ischemia). At the end of 1 year, there were no significant differences (or even suggestive trends) in death or reinfarction between the two groups.

Therefore, as with the prethrombolytic studies, there is a basis for applying risk stratification to patients who receive thrombolytic therapy, and this strategy does not require predischarge angiography in all patients.

PRIMARY ANGIOPLASTY

Data regarding risk stratification in patients treated with primary angioplasty for acute myocardial infarction are currently very limited. Most studies present comparisons of primary angioplasty with thrombolytic therapy.

DeBoer et al[96] evaluated 301 patients randomized to primary angioplasty or streptokinase therapy. Limiting their prognostic end points to in-hospital death or reinfarction, they found that age, Killip class on admission, prior myocardial infarction, and streptokinase therapy were independent predictors. However, while they did adjust the analysis for thrombolytic therapy, they did not analyze these variables along with the results of angiography, i.e., data already and automatically available. Stone et al[97] reported on 395 patients randomized to primary angioplasty or thrombolytic therapy with tissue plasminogen activator. They found that advanced age was the only baseline predictor of in-hospital death, and that this was true in both men and women. In a separate report dealing with the same group of patients, heart failure on admission to the hospital was a predictor of recurrent ischemia.[98] Mark et al[99] reported on 270 patients from the Primary Angioplasty Registry analyzing their data concerning the factors that related to baseline and 6-month costs. They found that age, anterior infarction, initial Killip class, the number of diseased vessels, recurrent ischemia, and heart failure were predictive of increased costs. Although this study did not address the hard end points, its results are consistent concerning the variables that were identified as important predictors of worse outcomes in other analyses and the analysis did include angiography results. Hopefully, future analyses of this database, when it has increased in size, will evaluate the data using death and reinfarction as end points.

Given that patients who receive primary angioplasty have undergone a procedure that provides prognostic information, i.e., coronary angiography, any analysis of risk stratification should be undertaken with the intent of determining whether clinical variables or noninvasive testing results add independent incremental information over that already available from the angiograms. This is essentially the reverse of what has been intended from the preprimary angioplasty analyses. Only the study by Mark et al[99] considered this type of analysis, but their study did not consider hard or soft end points.

CURRENT RECOMMENDATIONS

Despite the shortcomings of the available literature, it is appropriate that a clinical strategy be recommended based on what we do know about the postinfarction patient and the predictors of risk assessed in this literature review. There is a lack of compelling data that coronary angiography should be performed in all postmyocardial infarction patients. Therefore, clinical and test characteristics that place patients into high- and low-risk groups should be considered. In fact, given the absence of a significant volume of data to support routinely employing an invasive strategy, the proposed recommendations might well serve as a strategy to be tested in a future clinical trial.

Preadmission Historical Characteristics

Patients with prior myocardial infarction or diabetes should be considered at increased risk of death or reinfarction. Consideration for coronary angiography is recommended unless contraindications exist. While those of advanced age are clearly at increased risk, it is the judgment of this reviewer that advanced age does not mandate an invasive approach, particularly in light of the greater opportunity for complications in the elderly.

In-Hospital Characteristics

It would likewise seem reasonable that patients with postinfarction angina/ischemia or symptoms of or physical or radiographic findings suggestive of left ventricular failure be considered for coronary angiography. This would be irrespective of response to medical therapy or lack of persistence after initial observation. These recommendations concerning prehospital and in-hospital characteristics hold regardless of whether thrombolytic therapy is given.

Predischarge Testing

For those patients without the previously mentioned unfavorable preadmission or in-hospital characteristics, provocative testing should be considered. Given that exercise testing in both the prethrombolytic or the thrombolytic analyses was not a consistent predictor of risk and given the inability to perform exercise in a significant proportion of patients, some other stress provocation may be considered. Given the independent predictability of pharmacologic testing and the apparent safety of performing this early in the postinfarction course, dipyridamole myocardial perfusion imaging studies would be appropriate at 4 to 5 days after infarction. At this point in their course, many patients who will have complicated courses will have declared themselves and most questions over whether a patient can be stressed pharmacologically will become moot. I should caution the reader that while this approach seems reasonable from the available literature, it has not been subjected to larger clinical trials where issues of safety can be more appropriately explored. Along the same lines, given that dipyridamole echocardiography may require higher doses (to induce ischemic wall-motion abnormalities) than perfusion studies and the lack of data for the safe use of this higher dose in the early postinfarction period, it should be considered a secondary alternative to dipyridamole nuclear perfusion imaging studies. For whatever reason, those patients deemed as inappropriate for pharmacologic testing should be considered for angiography.

Given the lower mortality rates of uncomplicated postinfarction patients who received thrombolytic therapy, provocative testing that is positive may be less than effective in declaring risk due to the likely low predictive value of a positive test for death or reinfarction. However, those patients with studies suggesting low risk (a single fixed defect) should have an excellent prognosis. These low-risk patients do not need to undergo further predischarge exercise testing unless required for a precardiac rehabilitation evaluation.

Given the current emphasis on limiting cost and reducing hospital stay, it is difficult to see where assessments of left ventricular function (aside from clinical assessments) will fit in a schema such as that just outlined. While not supportable by the previous analysis, one might consider routine radionuclide angiography or echocardiography in those with an uncomplicated first anterior wall infarction. If the ejection is less than or equal to 40 percent, coronary angiography should be considered. If it is greater than 40 percent, pharmacologic stress testing should be considered.

Coronary Angiography

Recent studies suggest that the use of coronary angiography in postinfarction patients is increasing in the United States[100,101] and is significantly greater in the United States compared with Canada[102] despite a lack of difference in outcomes. The validity of this preference for invasive data is not supported by data from the TIMI-2 or SWIFT studies. It is likely that this trend is related to the (1) greater availability of angiography in the US compared with Canada, (2) the desire of US physicians to know the coronary anatomy (in particular the status of the infarct-related artery), and (3) the lack of any financial deterrent to the performance of routine coronary angiography. This state of affairs emphasizes the need for well-designed clinical trials to evaluate both the incremental value of coronary angiography as well as the value of routine coronary angiography with emphasis on the status of the infarct-related artery as well as on lesion characteristics.

Primary Angioplasty

Patients who receive this therapy and who experience no postinfarction complications should initially be stratified based on the angiographic results. No studies are presently available for clear guidance as to the need or value of exercise or pharmacologic stress testing. These studies should be performed selectively where questions of angiographic significance of residual coronary artery lesions arise. Again, these patients should receive a simple exercise electrocardiographic test (if able) as a precardiac rehabilitation evaluation.

FUTURE CHALLENGES

Data from studies cited in this review leave much to be desired concerning our state of knowledge of postinfarction risk stratification. Future endeavors in this area should concentrate on two principle areas: (1) well-designed prospective studies and (2) development of methods to assess and define the real predictor of risk for acute ischemic events: the unstable plaque.

Prognostic Studies

If a single conclusion can be drawn from the previous analysis, it is that the majority of prognostic postinfarction studies were either not well designed by current standards or failed to analyze their data adequately. Two recent surveys of studies that employed multivariable analysis to determine risk predictors are very enlightening in this regard.[103,104] One of these surveys specifically evaluated the postinfarction prognostic literature.[104] The authors of these articles outline specific methodologic guidelines that should be followed in order to allow for improved interpretation and reduced inconsistency of results. Future studies should all be judged based on these guidelines. Designers of studies and journal reviewers should take heed.

To summarize, studies should be prospective, properly sized to allow for hard-event analysis (with death alone analyzable), and randomized if comparing two or more strategies. Consideration should be given to allowing for analysis of data by gender, prior infarction and diabetic status, and specific reperfusion therapy (if given). Analysis should be multivariable and incremental at strategic stratification points, e.g., admission, early in-hospital, and predischarge. There should be quantitative measures of discrimination that can be compared at various incremental stages, e.g., ROC curve areas. Consideration for randomizing patients to routine angiography versus a defined conservative strategy should be given high priority in order to determine the incremental and relative values of each. The best of both diagnostic approaches should be employed with quantitative analysis wherever possible. Multicenter studies are encouraged perhaps as part of other megatrials, as a single center is unlikely to be able to accomplish the above, especially concerning adequate sample size.

Unstable Plaque Discrimination

Finally, the aspects of coronary pathology that truly define and determine risk need to be determined and quantified such that diagnostic strategies can be developed. We know that fibrous cap thickness,[105] plaque inflammation,[106] and undoubtedly other factors play some role in determining which plaques will rupture and when. Strategies designed to define these potential predictors need to be developed. Currently, intravascular ultrasound and magnetic resonance imaging hold promise in this regard, but other noninvasive approaches need to be explored. Perhaps when we have reached the summit of this quite formidable mountain, we will have the means by which to stratify patients that can be agreed on by all.

REFERENCES

1. Kaul S, Beller GA: Evaluation of the incremental value of a diagnostic test: a worthwhile exercise in this era of cost consciousness? *J Nucl Med* 33:1732, 1992.
2. Christian TF: The incremental value of noninvasive stress testing for the diagnosis of coronary artery disease. *ACC Curr J Rev* 3:60, 1994.
3. Anderson HV, Willerson JT: Thrombolysis in acute myocardial infarction. *N Engl J Med* 329:703, 1993.
4. Davis HT, DeCamilla J, Bayer LW, Moss AJ: Survivorship patterns in the posthospital phase of myocardial infarction. *Circulation* 60:1252, 1979.
5. Henning H, Gilpin EA, Covell JW, et al: Prognosis after acute myocardial infarction: A multivariate analysis of mortality and survival. *Circulation* 59:1124, 1979.
6. Madsen EB, Gilpin E, Henning H, et al: Prediction of late mortality after myocardial infarction from variables measured at different times during hospitalization. *Am J Cardiol* 53:47, 1984.
7. Maisel AS, Gilpin E, Hoit B, et al: Survival after hospital discharge in matched populations with inferior and anterior myocardial infarction. *J Am Coll Cardiol* 6:731, 1985.
8. Ahnve S, Gilpin E, Dittrich H, et al: First myocardial infarction: Age and ejection fraction identify a low risk group. *Am Heart J* 116:925, 1988.
9. Gilpin E, Ricou F, Dittrich H, et al: Factors associated with recurrent myocardial infarction within one year after acute myocardial infarction. *Am Heart J* 121:457, 1991.
10. Multicenter Postinfarction Research Group: Risk stratification and survival after myocardial infarction. *N Engl J Med* 309:331, 1983.
11. Dwyer EM, McMaster P, Greenberg H, and the Multicenter Postinfarction Research Group: Nonfatal cardiac events and recurrent infarction in the year after acute myocardial infarction. *J Am Coll Cardiol* 4:365, 1984.
12. Smith JW, Marcus FI, Serokman R, with the Multicenter Postinfarction Research Group: Prognosis of patients with diabetes mellitus after acute myocardial infarction. *Am J Cardiol* 54:718, 1984.
13. Benhorin J, Andrews ML, Carleen ED, Moss AJ, and the Multicenter Postinfarction Research Group: Occurrence, characteristics, and prognostic significance of early postacute myocardial infarction angina pectoris. *Am J Cardiol* 62:679, 1988.
14. Marcus FI, Friday K, McCans J, et al: Age-related prognosis after acute myocardial infarction (the Multicenter Diltiazem Postinfarction Trial). *Am J Cardiol* 65:559, 1990.
15. Mukharji J, Rude RE, Poole WK, et al, and the MILIS Study Group: Risk factors for sudden death after acute myocardial infarction: Two-year follow-up. *Am J Cardiol* 54:31, 1984.
16. Greenland P, Reicher-Ross H, Goldbourt U, Behar S, and the Israeli SPRINT Investigators: In-hospital and 1-year mortality in 1,524 women after myocardial infarction. *Circulation* 83:484, 1991.
17. Kornowski R, Goldbourt U, Zion M, et al, and the SPRINT Study Group: Predictors and long-term prognostic significance of recurrent infarction in the year after a first myocardial infarction. *Am J Cardiol* 72:883, 1993.
18. Pardaens J, Lesaffre E, Willems JL, DeGeest H: Multivariate survival analysis for the assessment of prognostic factors and risk categories after recovery from acute myocardial infarction: The Belgian situation. *Am J Epidemiol* 122:805, 1985.
19. TIMI IIIB Investigators: Effects of tissue plasminogen activator and a comparison of early invasive and conservative strategies in unstable angina and non-Q-wave myocardial infarction. *Circulation* 89:1545, 1994.
20. Galjee MA, Visser FC, DeCock CC, Van Eenige MJ: The prognostic value, clinical, and angiographic characteristics of patients with early postinfarction angina after a first myocardial infarction. *Am Heart J* 125:48, 1992.
21. Taylor GJ, Humphries JO, Mellits ED, et al: Predictors of clinical course, coronary anatomy and left ventricular function after recovery from acute myocardial infarction. *Circulation* 62:960, 1980.
22. Feinberg MS, Boyko V, Goldbourt U, et al, and the SPRINT Study Group: Early risk stratification of patients with a first inferior wall acute myocardial infarction. *Int J Cardiol* 48:31, 1995.
23. Ahnve S, Gilpin E, Henning H, et al: Limitations and advantages if the ejection fraction for defining high

risk after acute myocardial infarction. *Am J Cardiol* 58:872, 1986.

24. White HD, Norris RM, Brown MA, et al: Left ventricular end-systolic volume after recovery from myocardial infarction. *Circulation* 76:44, 1987.

25. Ong L, Green S, Reiser P, Morrison J: Early prediction of mortality in patients with acute myocardial infarction: A prospective study of clinical and radionuclide risk factors. *Am J Cardiol* 57:33, 1986.

26. Fioretti P, Brower RW, Simoons ML, et al. Relative value of clinical variables, bicycle ergometry, rest radionuclide ventriculography and 24 hour ambulatory electrocardiographic monitoring at discharge to predict 1 year survival after myocardial infarction. *J Am Coll Cardiol* 8:40, 1986.

27. Madsen EB, Rasmussen S, Svendsen TL: Multivariate long-term prognostic index from exercise ECG after acute myocardial infarction. *Eur J Cardiol* 11:435, 1980.

28. Weld FM, Chu K, Bigger JT, Rolnitzky LM: Risk stratification with low-level exercise testing 2 weeks after acute myocardial infarction. *Circulation* 64:306, 1981.

29. Williams WL, Nair RC, Higginson LAJ, et al: Comparison of clinical and treadmill variables for the prediction of outcome after myocardial infarction. *J Am Coll Cardiol* 4:477, 1984.

30. Waters DD, Bosch X, Bouchard A, et al: Comparison of clinical variables and variables derived from a limited predischarge exercise test as predictors of early and late mortality after myocardial infarction. *J Am Coll Cardiol* 5:1, 1985.

31. Krone RJ, Gillespie JA, Weld FM, et al, and the Multicenter Postinfarction Research Group: Low-level exercise testing after myocardial infarction: Usefulness in enhancing clinical risk stratification. *Circulation* 71:80, 1985.

32. Madsen EB, Gilpin E, Ahnve S, et al: Prediction of functional capacity and use of exercise testing for predicting risk after acute myocardial infarction. *Am J Cardiol* 56:839, 1985.

33. Starling MR, Crawford MH, Henry RL, et al: Prognostic value of electrocardiographic exercise testing and noninvasive assessment of left ventricular ejection fraction soon after acute myocardial infarction. *Am J Cardiol* 57:532, 1986.

34. Campbell S, A'Hern R, Quigley P, et al: Identification of patients at low risk of dying after acute myocardial infarction, by simple clinical and submaximal exercise test criteria. *Eur Heart J* 9:938, 1988.

35. Froelicher ES: Usefulness of exercise testing shortly after acute myocardial infarction for predicting 10-year mortality. *Am J Cardiol* 74:318, 1994.

36. Fioretti P, Brower RW, Simoons ML, et al: Prediction of mortality during the first year after acute myocardial infarction from clinical variables and stress test at hospital discharge. *Am J Cardiol* 55:1313, 1985.

37. Froelicher VF, Perdue S, Pewen W, Risch M: Application of meta-analysis using an electronic spread sheet to exercise testing in patients after myocardial infarction. *Am J Med* 83:1045, 1987.

38. Hung J, Goris ML, Nash E, et al: Comparative value of maximal treadmill testing, exercise thallium myocardial perfusion scintigraphy and exercise radionuclide ventriculography for distinguishing high- and low-risk patients soon after myocardial infarction. *Am J Cardiol* 53:1221, 1984.

39. Leppo JA, O'Brien J, Rothendler JA, et al: Dipyridamole–thallium-201 scintigraphy in the prediction of future cardiac events after acute myocardial infarction. *N Engl J Med* 310:1014, 1984.

40. Morris KG, Palmeri ST, Califf RM, et al: Value of radionuclide angiography for predicting specific cardiac events after acute myocardial infarction. *Am J Cardiol* 55:318, 1985.

41. Corbett JR, Nicod P, Lewis SE, et al: Prognostic value of submaximal exercise radionuclide ventriculography after myocardial infarction. *Am J Cardiol* 52:82A, 1983.

42. Mazzotta G, Camerini A, Scopinaro G, et al: Predicting severe ischemic events after uncomplicated myocardial infarction by exercise testing and rest and exercise radionuclide ventriculography. *J Nucl Cardiol* 1:246, 1994.

43. Gimple LW, Hutter AM, Guiney TE, Boucher CA: Prognostic utility of predischarge dipyridamole thallium imaging compared to predischarge submaximal exercise electrocardiography and maximal exercise thallium imaging after uncomplicated acute myocardial infarction. *Am J Cardiol* 64:1243, 1989.

44. Gibson RS, Watson DD, Craddock GB, et al: Prediction of cardiac events after uncomplicated myocardial infarction: A prospective study comparing predischarge exercise thallium-201 scintigraphy and coronary angiography. *Circulation* 68:321, 1983.

45. Norris RM, Barnaby PF, Brandt PWT, et al: Prognosis after recovery from first acute myocardial infarction: Determinants of reinfarction and sudden death. *Am J Cardiol* 53:408, 1984.

46. Sanz G, Castaner A, Betriu A, et al: Determinants of prognosis in survivors of myocardial infarction. *N Engl J Med* 306:1065, 1982.

47. Leroy F, Lablache J, McFadden EP, et al: Relative prognostic value of clinical, exercise, and angiographic data after a first myocardial infarction. *Coronary Artery Dis* 4:727, 1993.

48. Tibbits PA, Evaul JE, Goldstein RE, et al, and the Multicenter Postinfarction Research Group: Serial acquisition of data to predict one-year mortality rate after acute myocardial infarction. *Am J Cardiol* 60:451, 1987.

49. Lee KL, Woodlief LH, Topol EJ, et al, for the GUSTO-I Investigators: Predictors of 30-day mortality in the era of reperfusion for acute myocardial infarction. *Circulation* 91:1659, 1995.

50. Schroder R, Wegschieder K, Schroder K, et al, for the INJECT Trial Group: Extent of early ST segment elevation resolution: A strong predictor of outcome in patients with acute myocardial infarction and a sensitive measure to compare thrombolytic regimens. *J Am Coll Cardiol* 26:1657, 1995.

51. Murphy JF, Kahn MG, Krone RJ: Prethrombolytic versus thrombolytic era risk stratification of patients with acute myocardial infarction. *Am J Cardiol* 76:827, 1995.

52. Volpi A, DeVita C, Franzosi MG, et al, and the Ad Hoc Working Group of the Gruppo Italiano per lo Studio della Sopravvivenza nell'Infarto Miocardico (GISSI)-2 Data Base: Determinants of 6-month mortality in survi-

vors of myocardial infarction after thrombolysis. *Circulation* 88:416, 1993.

53. Maggioni AP, Maseri A, Fresco C, et al, on Behalf of the Investigators of the Gruppo Italiano per lo Studio della Sopravvivenza nell'Infarto Miocardico (GISSI-2): Age-related increase in mortality among patients with first myocardial infarctions treated with thrombolysis. *N Engl J Med* 329:1442, 1993.

54. Ad Hoc Working Group of GISSI-2 Data Base: Volpi A, DeVita C, Franzosi MG, et al: Predictors of nonfatal reinfarction in survivors of myocardial infarction after thrombolysis. *J Am Coll Cardiol* 24:608, 1994.

55. Rivers JT, White HD, Cross DB, et al: Reinfarction after thrombolytic therapy for acute myocardial infarction followed by conservative management: Incidence and effect of smoking. *J Am Coll Cardiol* 16:340, 1990.

56. AIMS Trial Study Group: Long-term effects if intravenous anistreplase in acute myocardial infarction: Final report of the AIMS study. *Lancet* 335:427, 1990.

57. Arnold AER, Simoons ML, Detry JR, et al: Prediction of mortality following hospital discharge after thrombolysis for acute myocardial infarction: Is there a need for coronary angiography? *Eur Heart J* 14:306, 1993.

58. Simoons ML, Vos J, Tijssen JGP, et al: Long-term benefit of early thrombolytic therapy in patients with acute myocardial infarction: 5 year follow-up of a trial conducted by the Interuniversity Cardiology Institute of the Netherlands. *J Am Coll Cardiol* 14:1609, 1989.

59. Cerquiera MD, Maynard C, Ritchie JL, et al: Long-term survival in 618 patients from the Western Washington Streptokinase in Myocardial Infarction Trials. *J Am Coll Cardiol* 20:1452, 1992.

60. Silva P, Galli M, Campolo L, for the IRES (Ischemia Residua) Study Group: Prognostic significance of early ischemia after acute myocardial infarction in low-risk patients. *Am J Cardiol* 71:1142, 1993.

61. Vaccarino V, Krumholz HM, Berkman LF, Horwitz RI: Sex differences in mortality after myocardial infarction. *Circulation* 91:1861, 1995.

62. Zaret BL, Wackers FJT, Terrin ML, et al, for the TIMI Study Group: Value of radionuclide angiography rest and exercise left ventricular ejection fraction in assessing survival of patients after thrombolytic therapy for acute myocardial infarction: Results of Thrombolysis in Myocardial Infarction (TIMI) Phase II Study. *J Am Coll Cardiol* 26:73, 1995.

63. Krone RJ, Gregory JJ, Freedland KE, et al, for the Multicenter Ischemia Research Group: Limited usefulness of exercise testing and thallium scintigraphy in evaluation of ambulatory patients several months after recovery from an acute coronary event: Implications for management of stable coronary heart disease. *J Am Coll Cardiol* 24:1274, 1994.

64. Lenderink T, Simoons ML, Van Es G, et al, for the European Cooperative Study Group: Benefit of thrombolytic therapy is sustained throughout five years and is related to TIMI perfusion grade 3 but not grade 2 flow at discharge. *Circulation* 92:1110, 1995.

65. Miller TD, Gersh BJ, Christian TF, et al: Limited prognostic value of thallium-201 exercise treadmill testing early after myocardial infarction in patients treated with thrombolysis. *Am Heart J* 130:259, 1995.

66. Brown KA, O'Meara J, Chamber CE, Plante DA: Ability of dt-201 imaging one to four days after acute myocardial infarction to predict in-hospital and late recurrent myocardial ischemic events. *Am J Cardiol* 65:160, 1990.

67. Hendel RC, Gore JM, Alpert JS, Leppo JA: Prognosis following interventional therapy for acute myocardial infarction: Utility of dipyridamole thallium scintigraphy. *Cardiology* 79:73, 1991.

68. Mahmarian JJ, Mahmarian AC, Marks GF, et al: Role of adenosine thallium-201 tomography for defining long-term risk in patients after acute myocardial infarction. *J Am Coll Cardiol* 25:1333, 1995.

69. Travin MI, Dessouki A, Cameron T, Heller GV: Use of exercise technetium-99m sestamibi SPECT imaging to detect residual ischemia and for risk stratification after acute myocardial infarction. *Am J Cardiol* 75:665, 1995.

70. Zhu W, Gibbons RJ, Bailey KR, Gersh BJ: Predischarge exercise radionuclide angiography in predicting multivessel coronary artery disease and subsequent cardiac events after thrombolytic therapy for acute myocardial infarction. *Am J Cardiol* 74:554, 1994.

71. Ryan T, Armstrong WF, O'Donnell JA, Feigenbaum H: Risk stratification after acute myocardial infarction by means of exercise two-dimensional ec. *Am Heart J* 114:1305, 1987.

72. Applegate RJ, Dell'Italia LJ, Crawford MH: Usefulness of two-dimensional echocardiography during low-level exercise testing early after uncomplicated acute myocardial infarction. *Am J Cardiol* 60:10, 1987.

73. Quintana M, Lindvall K, Ryden L, Brolund F: Prognostic value of predischarge exercise stress echocardiography after acute myocardial infarction. *Am J Cardiol* 76:1115, 1995.

74. Picano E, Landi P, Bolognese L, et al, for the EPIC Study Group: Prognostic value of dipyridamole echocardiography early after uncomplicated myocardial infarction: A large-scale, multicenter trial. *Am J Med* 95:608, 1993.

75. Miller DD, Stratmann HG, Shaw L, et al: Dipyridamole technetium 99m sestamibi myocardial tomography as an independent predictor of cardiac event-free survival after acute ischemic events. *J Nucl Cardiol* 1:172, 1994.

76. Tilkemeier PL, Guiney TE, LaRaia PJ, Boucher CA: Prognostic value of predischarge low-level exercise thallium testing after thrombolytic treatment of acute myocardial infarction. *Am J Cardiol* 66:1203, 1990.

77. Muller DWM, Topol EJ, Ellis SG, et al, and the Thrombolysis and Angioplasty in Myocardial Infarction (TAMI) Study Group: Multivessel coronary artery disease: A key predictor of short-term prognosis after reperfusion therapy for acute myocardial infarction. *Am Heart J* 121:1042, 1991.

78. Stadius ML, Davis K, Maynard C, et al: Risk stratification for 1 year survival based on characteristics identified in the early hours of acute myocardial infarction. *Circulation* 1986.74:703,

79. Ellis SG, Topol EJ, George BS, et al: Recurrent ischemia without warning: Analysis of risk factors for in-hospital ischemic events following successful thrombolysis with

intravenous tissue plasminogen activator. *Circulation* 80:1159, 1989.

80. Davies SW, Marchant B, Lyons JP, et al: Irregular coronary lesion morphology after thrombolysis predicts early clinical instability. *J Am Coll Cardiol* 18:669, 1991.

81. Wall TC, Mark DB, Califf RM, et al: Prediction of early recurrent myocardial ischemia and coronary reocclusion after successful thrombolysis: A qualitative and quantitative angiographic study. *Am J Cardiol* 63:423, 1989.

82. Little WC, Constantinescu M, Applegate RJ, et al: Can coronary angiography predict the site of a subsequent myocardial infarction in patients with mild-to-moderate coronary artery disease? *Circulation* 78:1157, 1988.

83. Ambrose JA, Tannenbaum MA, Alexopoulos D, et al: Angiographic progression of coronary artery disease and the development of myocardial infarction. *J Am Coll Cardiol* 12:56, 1988.

84. Nobuyoshi M, Tanaka M, Nosaka H, et al: Progression of coronary atherosclerosis: Is coronary spasm related to progression? *J Am Coll Cardiol* 18:904, 1991.

85. Giroud D, Li JM, Urban P, Meier B, Rutishauser W: Relation of the site of acute myocardial infarction to the most severe coronary arterial stenosis at prior angiography. *Am J Cardiol* 69:729, 1992.

86. DeBusk RF, Kraemer HC, Nash E, et al: Stepwise risk stratification soon after acute myocardial infarction. *Am J Cardiol* 52:1161, 1983.

87. Ross J, Gilpin E, Madsen EB, et al: A decision scheme for coronary angiography after acute myocardial infarction. *Circulation* 79:292, 1989.

88. SWIFT (Should We Intervene Following Thrombolysis?) Study Group: SWIFT trial of delayed elective intervention vs conservative treatment after thrombolysis with anistreplase in acute myocardial infarction. *BMJ* 302:555, 1991.

89. Williams DO, Braunwald E, Knatterud G, et al, and the TIMI Investigators: One-year results of the Thrombolysis in Myocardial Infarction (TIMI) Phase II Trial. *Circulation* 85:533, 1992.

90. Terrin ML, Williams DO, Kleiman NS, et al, for the TIMI II Investigators: Two- and three-year results of the thrombolysis in myocardial infarction (TIMI) phase II clinical trial. *J Am Coll Cardiol* 22:1763, 1993.

91. Aguirre FV, McMahon RP, Mueller HS, et al, for the TIMI II Investigators: Impact of age on clinical outcome and postlytic management strategies in patients treated with intravenous thrombolytic therapy. *Circulation* 90:78, 1994.

92. Mueller HS, Cohen LS, Braunwald E, et al, for the TIMI Investigators: Predictors of early morbidity and mortality after thrombolytic therapy of acute myocardial infarction. *Circulation* 85:1254, 1992.

93. Candell-Riera J, Permanyer-Miralda G, Castell J, et al: Uncomplicated first myocardial infarction: Strategy for comprehensive prognostic studies. *J Am Coll Cardiol* 18:1207, 1991.

94. Olona M, Candell-Riera J, Permanyer-Miralda G, et al: Strategies for prognostic assessment of uncomplicated first myocardial infarction: 5-year follow-up study. *J Am Coll Cardiol* 25:815, 1995.

95. Rogers WJ, Babb JD, Baim DS, et al, for the TIMI II Investigators: Selective versus routine predischarge coronary angiography after therapy with recombinant tissue-type plasminogen activator, heparin and aspirin for acute myocardial infarction. *J Am Coll Cardiol* 17:1007, 1991.

96. DeBoer MK, Hoorntje JCA, Ottervanger JP, et al: Immediate coronary angioplasty versus intravenous streptokinase in acute myocardial infarction: Left ventricular ejection fraction, hospital mortality and reinfarction. *J Am Coll Cardiol* 23:1004, 1994.

97. Stone GW, Grines CL, Browne KF, et al: Comparison of in-hospital outcome in men versus women treated by either thrombolytic therapy or primary coronary angioplasty for acute myocardial infarction. *Am J Cardiol* 75:987, 1995.

98. Stone GW, Grines CL, Browne KF, et al: Implications of recurrent ischemia after reperfusion therapy in acute myocardial infarction: A comparison of thrombolytic therapy and primary angioplasty. *J Am Coll Cardiol* 26:66, 1995.

99. Mark DB, O'Neill WW, Brodie B, et al: Baseline and 6-month costs of primary angioplasty therapy for acute myocardial infarction: Results from the primary angioplasty registry. *J Am Coll Cardiol* 26:688, 1995.

100. Nicod P, Gilpin EA, Dittrich H, et al: Trends in use of coronary angiography in subacute phase of myocardial infarction. *Circulation* 84:1004, 1991.

101. Every NR, Larson EB, Litwin PE, et al, for the Myocardial Infarction Triage and Intervention Project Investigators: The association between on-site cardiac catheterization facilities and the use of coronary angiography after acute myocardial infarction. *N Engl J Med* 329:546, 1993.

102. Rouleau JL, Moye LA, Pfeffer MA, et al, for the SAVE Investigators: A comparison of management patterns after acute myocardial infarction in Canada and the United States. *N Engl J Med* 328:779, 1993.

103. Concato J, Feinstein AR, Holford TR: The risk of determining risk with multivariable models. *Ann Intern Med* 118:201, 1993.

104. Marx BE, Feinstein AR: Methodologic sources of inconsistent prognoses for post-acute myocardial infarction. *Am J Med* 98:537, 1995.

105. Loree HM, Kamm RD, Stringfellow RG, Lee RT: Effects of fibrous cap thickness on peak circumferential stress in model atherosclerotic vessels. *Circ Res* 71:850, 1992.

106. Van der Wal AC, Becker AE, Van der Loos CM, Das PK: Site of intimal rupture or erosion of thrombosed coronary atherosclerotic plaques is characterized by an inflammatory process irrespective of the dominant plaque morphology. *Circulation* 89:36, 1994.

Test Accuracy, Test Selection, and Test Result Interpretation in Chronic Coronary Artery Disease

Myron C. Gerson

Numerous alternatives are available to the clinician assessing a patient for the presence or absence of coronary artery disease (CAD). When the possibility of CAD arises, approaches include coronary arteriography, exercise electrocardiography (ECG), myocardial perfusion scintigraphy, stress echocardiography, or exercise radionuclide ventriculography. Alternatively, the possibility of CAD may be so remote that no testing is necessary. This chapter and the chapter that follows review the relative accuracy of noninvasive tests for detection of CAD. The basis for test selection is discussed and the significance of test results considered. Selection of patients for revascularization procedures and noninvasive assessment of prognosis in CAD are considered in Chaps. 22 and 23.

MEASURES OF TEST ACCURACY

Selection of a Reference Standard

The coronary arteriogram is most commonly used as the reference or gold standard for measuring the accuracy of noninvasive tests used to detect CAD, but limitations of this approach must be kept in mind. Most studies using the coronary arteriogram as a gold standard have relied on subjective determinations of coronary artery narrowing. Unless a coronary artery stenosis is clearly delineated in multiple orthogonal projections, the per-

centage reduction in the vessel lumen cannot be accurately determined. Even when visualized in multiple views, eccentric or irregular lesions may remain difficult to assess accurately. Substantial interobserver variation in the estimation of coronary artery luminal stenosis has been reported.[1,2] To determine a percentage of luminal diameter reduction, it must be possible to measure the diameter of a corresponding normal coronary artery segment accurately. This approach has practical limitations in the evaluation of atherosclerotic CAD, which frequently involves the entire length of the coronary vessel.[3] This is likely to be one of the reasons why there is no consensus as to what percentage reduction in coronary artery luminal diameter constitutes a clinically important coronary artery stenosis. When multiple coronary stenoses occur in series in a vessel, determination of the clinical and hemodynamic importance of the lesions becomes even more difficult.[4] Additionally, coronary artery stenoses may assume greater importance in the presence of concomitant valvular heart disease.[5] Diseases such as hypertensive heart disease may also produce subendocardial ischemia in hypertrophied myocardium supplied by a "noncritical" coronary stenosis.[6]

Limitations of coronary arteriography as a gold standard for the assessment of CAD are listed in Table 20-1. These present limitations will likely be reduced in the future with quantitative approaches to the measurement of the coronary artery lumen size rather than subjective assessment of percentage stenosis.[7-9] Studies have shown that coronary blood flow is better estimated from lumen size than from percentage stenosis.[10]

Table 20-1   Limitations of Coronary Angiography as a "Gold Standard" for the Assessment of Coronary Disease

1. Technical limitations:
   Overlap of vessels
   Limited number of projections for viewing each vessel
   Interobserver variability in interpretation
   Invasive nature, finite morbidity and mortality

2. Physiologic limitations:
   Does not determine the physiologic significance of the anatomic lesion
   Comparison of "normal" and abnormal arterial segments in a disease that diffusely involves the vessel lumen
   Measurement of percentage stenosis instead of actual lumen size
   Effect of serial stenoses or stenoses of varying length on blood flow
   Angiography supplies little information regarding resistance to coronary blood flow
   Difficulty in assessment of the blood-flow contribution of coronary collaterals
   Difficulty in assessment of the effect of other forms of heart disease (e.g., aortic stenosis, aortic regurgitation) on coronary blood flow
   when a coronary stenosis is present
   (?) limited prognostic power
   May not detect transient reductions in coronary blood flow (or resultant myocardial damage) related to
       Coronary artery spasm
       Coronary thrombosis with recanalization
       Coronary embolization with recanalization

Advantages of coronary arteriography as a "gold standard" for coronary disease assessment
   Provides an individual reference standard for each patient
   Provides a readily available reference standard for quality control of noninvasive tests
   Provides good prediction of need for coronary bypass surgery particularly in patients with left main disease and some patients with triple-vessel disease
   Provides essential anatomic information for patients requiring coronary artery bypass surgery or percutaneous transluminal coronary angioplasty

A second limitation of the coronary arteriogram as a gold standard for demonstrating the presence or absence of important CAD is that the significance of coronary lesions is not clearly defined by anatomy alone. In one study, caliper measurements of the percentage of coronary stenosis were compared to a Doppler measurement of the reactive hyperemic response of coronary flow velocity following release after 20 s of coronary arterial occlusion at the time of coronary artery surgery.[11] The authors concluded that "the physiologic effects of the majority of coronary obstructions cannot be determined accurately by conventional angiographic approaches."[11] Other data[12] suggest that assessment of myocardial perfusion using thallium 201 (^{201}Tl) better predicts the physiologic importance of a coronary stenosis than does the angiographic percentage of stenosis. Furthermore, not all myocardial ischemia and scar can be causally related to a fixed anatomic coronary artery stenosis. Myocardial infarction resulting from coronary artery spasm, embolization, or thrombosis with subsequent recanalization may leave little or no evidence of abnormality by coronary arteriography[13] but may produce perfusion abnormality detectable by noninvasive testing. Reversible myocardial hypoperfusion related to coronary artery spasm may occur at rest or during exercise[14] in patients with no fixed coronary artery stenosis and may be documented by ECG or myocardial scintigraphy.[15] Myocardial hypoperfusion related to coronary spasm, embolism, or thrombosis, although uncommon in the overall population, might produce a clinically relevant percentage of positive noninvasive test results in a

population having a low prevalence of fixed coronary artery stenoses (e.g., middle-aged women with atypical chest pain).

Despite these limitations, the coronary arteriogram is a practical reference standard. For an individual hospital, it provides a useful standard for evaluating the performance of noninvasive tests locally. Also, invasive assessment of coronary anatomy in combination with the patient's history provides fundamental information for guiding treatment of CAD with coronary artery bypass surgery and percutaneous transluminal coronary angioplasty. Data are now available from long-term clinical outcome studies that can provide a more direct indication of the significance of findings from tests of cardiac physiology and function beyond the correlative information obtained from coronary arteriography.

A noninvasive test may perform a useful role by providing sufficient clinical data, beyond that available from the history and physical examination, to permit an accurate diagnosis, which, in turn, obviates the need for a more expensive or more hazardous test or intervention. For example, a normal exercise test may under certain circumstances obviate the need for cardiac catheterization. Alternatively, a noninvasive test may provide information that is not available from other sources, including coronary arteriography. An example is the use of an exercise ^{201}Tl myocardial scintigram to clarify the significance of an angiographic coronary artery stenosis that is of borderline anatomic importance and bears an unclear relationship to clinical symptoms. Noninvasive testing is also more suitable for serial testing than invasive testing.

Predictive Value of a Test Result

Prevalence, sensitivity, specificity, and predictive value are defined below:

$$Sensitivity = \frac{\text{no. patients with disease having positive test}}{\text{total no. patients with disease}}$$

$$= \frac{\text{true positives}}{\text{true positives} + \text{false negatives}}$$

$$Specificity = \frac{\text{no. patients without disease having negative test}}{\text{total no. patients without disease}}$$

$$= \frac{\text{true negatives}}{\text{true negatives} + \text{false positives}}$$

$$\frac{Predictive\ value}{\text{of positive test}} = \frac{\text{true positives}}{\text{true positives} + \text{false positives}}$$

Given a positive test result, the *predictive value* of a positive test is a statement of the probability that the disease tested for is present. However, the predictive value of a test result is highly dependent on the prevalence of disease in the population under study. If, for example, the exercise ECG has a sensitivity of 80 percent and a specificity of 75 percent, a positive test result in a group of 100 patients with typical angina (and, therefore, a 90 percent pretest prevalence of CAD) will correctly suggest the presence of CAD in 97 percent of cases. In 100 asymptomatic subjects (with an approximate 5 percent prevalence of CAD), a positive exercise test consisting of 1 mm of horizontal or downsloping ST-segment depression will identify 4 of 5 patients with CAD but will be falsely positive in an additional 24 patients without CAD. The predictive value of a positive test in the asymptomatic group will be 14 percent.[16] Most (but not all) studies of exercise testing in asymptomatic patients confirm that a large proportion of positive exercise tests in a low-prevalence population is falsely positive.[17,18]

Sensitivity, Specificity, and Selection Biases

The sensitivity and specificity of a test are independent of the prevalence of disease in the population tested.[19] Test sensitivity and specificity may, however, be altered by biases introduced in the process of selecting patients and tests. An example of an apparent increase in test sensitivity related to "pretest bias"[20] might occur if 100 patients underwent thallium myocardial scintigraphy prior to coronary angiography but each patient had historical and ECG documentation of previous transmural myocardial infarction. The severity of myocardial hypoperfusion is usually greater in a patient with myocardial scar compared to a patient with similar coronary anatomy without myocardial scar, so the likelihood of visualizing an area of abnormal rest or exercise thallium myocardial perfusion is increased in patients with prior myocardial infarction.

An apparent decline over time in the specificity of the exercise radionuclide ventriculogram for the detection of CAD has been reported.[20] This does not represent a change in the accuracy of the radionuclide ventriculogram but represents a change over time in the criteria used to select patients for testing. If the result of a noninvasive test, whether it be exercise ECG, stress scintigraphy, or stress echocardiography, is used to determine if the patient will or will not proceed to coronary arteriography, then the apparent specificity of that noninvasive test in comparison to arteriography will decrease. The cause for this finding is posttest selection bias and is illustrated in Fig. 20-1. If 100 patients were referred for exercise myocardial perfusion imaging and all patients went on to coronary arteriography, it might be found that 70 patients had arteriographic disease and 30 did not. This might occur in a hospital in which exercise myocardial perfusion imaging had recently been introduced and clinicians did not feel confident that a normal test result could exclude the presence of CAD. However, if in the same hospital, over a 5-year period, the exercise myocardial perfusion scan consistently detected 90 percent of patients with disease and was normal in 80 percent of patients with angiographically normal coronary arteries, clinicians might begin to apply the test in a different manner. Assume that 100 patients were now referred for exercise myocardial perfusion imaging and 70 of these patients had CAD. With a 90 percent sensitivity, exercise myocardial perfusion imaging would be abnormal in 63 of the 70 patients with disease. With a specificity of 80 percent, the test would also be falsely positive in 6 of the 30 patients without CAD. Because of the "known" high sensitivity of the test in that institution, if no clinician decided to send a patient with a negative exercise myocardial perfusion scan for coronary arteriography, there would be no angiographically proven true-negative results. Because the specificity is determined by the ratio of true-negative results to true-negative plus false-positive results, the apparent specificity will fall from 80 to 0 percent. This example illustrates the potential effect of posttest selection bias if a normal exercise scintigraphic test result is accepted as an end point for exclusion of clinically important CAD.

Two alternative approaches have been suggested to assess the ability of a noninvasive test to exclude the presence of CAD without the confounding effects of posttest selection bias. One approach is to calculate a normalcy rate for the test instead of the test specificity. This involves determination of the frequency with which

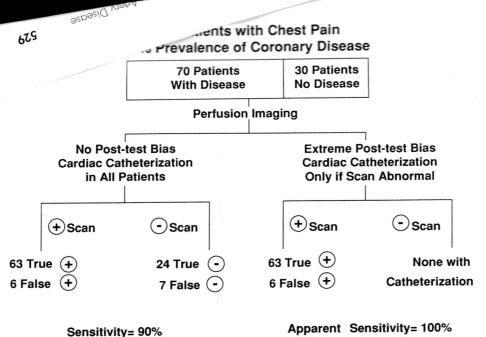

Figure 20-1 Effect of posttest selection bias on the apparent sensitivity and specificity of myocardial perfusion imaging.

the test is normal in a group of healthy individuals in whom the likelihood that CAD is present is very low, less than 5 percent. Because no verification (e.g., by coronary arteriography) of the noninvasive test result is indicated clinically, no posttest selection bias will occur. If populations with a very low likelihood of disease are selected by consistent criteria, the normalcy rate should permit comparison of results for different noninvasive tests. The problem with the use of the normalcy rate is that it measures test performance in a different population from that in which the test is indicated clinically. It cannot be assumed that the noninvasive test will perform in a similar manner in a population of patients with chest pain.

An alternative approach is to mathematically correct diagnostic test specificity for the confounding influence of posttest selection bias. This can be accomplished if the diagnostic results of the noninvasive test are known in all of the patients tested in the same laboratory who did not go on to verification of the diagnosis by coronary arteriography.[21] This approach has not entered into wide clinical use at this time.

Posttest selection bias can also inflate falsely the diagnostic sensitivity of a noninvasive test (see Fig. 20-1). If patients with a negative noninvasive test do not proceed to coronary arteriography, then falsely negative noninvasive test results will be underrepresented relative to the number of true positive results (in which a patient with an abnormal noninvasive test usually proceeds to coronary arteriography).

Sensitivity and specificity data reported in this chapter include data collected from early series in which pa-

tients had noninvasive testing before scheduled coronary arteriography, and posttest selection bias was probably less than might occur following longer experience with the noninvasive procedure. Because most patients in these early series were considered to have indications for coronary arteriography regardless of the noninvasive test outcome, early validation of noninvasive test accuracy was often carried out in populations with a relatively high prevalence of CAD.

It should also be noted that research studies that show superiority of a newer noninvasive test relative to an existing test are more likely to reach publication than is a "negative study." This has been referred to as "publication bias" and can falsely suggest improved accuracy of newer relative to established testing modalities.

Furthermore, diagnostic test sensitivity and specificity may vary substantially from one laboratory to another. Therefore, the sensitivity and specificity of each diagnostic test should be established for the laboratory in which testing is to be performed.

DETECTION OF CORONARY ARTERY DISEASE

Numerous studies document superior overall diagnostic accuracy for the postexercise ^{201}Tl myocardial scintigram, the exercise radionuclide ventriculogram, and the exercise echocardiogram compared to the exercise ECG.[22]

Sensitivity and Specificity for the Exercise ECG

In a tabulation of 30 reported series,[23-52] one or more millimeters of horizontal or downsloping ST-segment depression on the exercise ECG predicted the presence of angiographically important CAD in patients with chest pain with a sensitivity of 72 percent (positive exercise ECG in 2592 of 3583 patients with angiographic disease) and a specificity of 79 percent (negative exercise ECG in 1740 of 2213 patients without angiographic disease). In the present as well as previous[53] tabulations, patients with abnormal resting ECGs related to digitalis, or previous myocardial infarction, were excluded where possible. In many reports comparing the exercise ECG to the coronary arteriogram, comparison was made in male patients who were taking no cardiac medications, had no resting ST-segment or T-wave abnormalities, and were able to exercise to at least 85 percent of predicted maximal heart rate in the absence of diagnostic ECG changes. However, a majority of patients referred for evaluation of chest pain do not fulfill all of these criteria. The accuracy of the exercise ECG for detection of CAD must therefore be examined in a variety of test populations.

EFFECT OF DISEASE SEVERITY

The sensitivity of the exercise ECG for detection of CAD increases with the extent of disease. Tonkon et al[54] found 1.0 mm or greater of horizontal or downsloping ST-segment depression with exercise in 11 of 26 patients (42 percent) with single-vessel disease, 20 of 30 patients (66 percent) with double-vessel disease, and 28 of 35 patients (80 percent) with triple-vessel disease.

EXERCISE ECG ACCURACY IN WOMEN

It has been suggested that the exercise ECG is less accurate in women than in men. Numerous studies[24,30,41,49] have found poor predictive value of a positive exercise ECG for CAD detection in symptomatic women. In contrast, several series have noted that the predictive value of a negative exercise test (with an adequate level of exercise) is equivalent or higher in women than in men.[24,30,49] In the Coronary Artery Surgery Study (CASS)[51] the exercise ECG was compared in symptomatic men and women who were matched so that the prevalence of CAD was the same for both sexes. There was no difference between those symptomatic men and women in predictive value, sensitivity, or specificity of the exercise ECG for CAD detection.[51] It is concluded that reported differences in predictive value for the presence of CAD observed between symptomatic men and women are explained by differences in the prevalence of disease in the respective populations.[51] Robert et al[55] have shown that selection of multiple exercise variables by logistic discriminant analysis can improve diagnostic accuracy of exercise testing for CAD detection in women. A model including peak exercise work load, peak heart rate, and the number of millimeters of ST-segment depression measured at 60 msec after the J point provided improved diagnostic sensitivity without loss of specificity.

BASELINE ECG ABNORMALITIES

ST-segment depression in response to exercise has been found to be of little diagnostic value for detection of CAD in patients with left bundle branch block (LBBB),[56,57] Wolff-Parkinson-White syndrome,[58] or left ventricular hypertrophy.[59] In patients with right bundle branch block, ST-segment depression with exercise has been found to be a reliable predictor of CAD[60] when the depression is observed in a lateral precordial lead.

The presence of resting ST-segment and T-wave abnormalities resulted in a lower exercise ECG specificity as compared to patients with normal resting ST segments in the CASS study.[51] Symptomatic patients with abnormal resting ST segments and T waves have a higher prevalence of CAD than patients with a normal resting ECG. However, resting ST-segment and T-wave abnormalities are also commonly present in patients with a high prevalence of noncoronary heart disease (e.g., hypertensive heart disease), and these patients may develop ST-segment depression with exercise related to ischemia not caused by CAD, reducing test specificity. In symptomatic patients with abnormal resting ST segments and T waves, segmental myocardial hypoperfusion should be more specific than ECG changes for the presence of CAD.

In some asymptomatic populations metabolic and vasoregulatory disorders—as opposed to CAD—might be expected to account for more abnormal exercise ST-segment responses. The response of the resting ST segment to glucose loading, body position, and hyperventilation was a useful predictor of a false-positive exercise ST-segment response in one intermediate-prevalence, asymptomatic population,[44] but others have not confirmed this finding in asymptomatic men.[61]

LIMITED EXERCISE CAPACITY

Inability to exercise to at least 85 percent of predicted maximal heart rate may result in failure to produce ischemia in the distribution of a coronary artery containing a greater than 70 percent narrowing of the luminal diameter. The sensitivity of the exercise ECG for CAD detection is strongly dependent on the extent to which the heart is stressed. Patients with normal exercise ST segments but limited ability to exercise require an alternative method for excluding the presence of clinically important CAD.

CARDIAC DRUGS

Cardiac drugs can impair the diagnostic accuracy of exercise testing.[31] Antianginal drugs often enable patients to achieve a higher level of stress with less ischemia than is observed without medication.

Beta blockers Beta-adrenergic blockers can reduce myocardial oxygen requirements by reducing blood pressure and heart rate both at rest and with exercise and by decreasing ventricular contractility. Propranolol attenuates or delays the onset of ST-segment depression in response to exercise in patients with CAD.[62–64] In patients without CAD, propranolol also decreases the extent of ST-segment depression with exercise, reducing the number of false-positive test results and improving exercise test specificity.[65] Where there is a normal ST-segment response to exercise, beta-adrenergic blockade can prevent a patient from reaching the target heart rate and therefore produce an inconclusive test result. To avoid false-negative ST-segment responses and inadequate levels of exercise heart rate, propranolol may be tapered and withheld for 48 h prior to diagnostic exercise testing[62,66] in properly selected patients. Patients with angina pectoris may develop an acute ischemic complication (e.g., myocardial infarction) in response to sudden withdrawal of beta blockers.[67,68] This type of complication is uncommon[69] and is not likely to occur when the drug is withheld for 48 h or less, because adrenergic responsiveness is likely to remain decreased, because of persistent beta-blocker effect.[70] Nevertheless, patients should be carefully screened to exclude an unstable angina pattern before beta blockers are withheld prior to diagnostic exercise testing.

Long-acting nitrates, calcium channel blockers Treatment with long-acting nitrates may reduce, prevent, or delay the onset of ST-segment abnormalities in response to exercise testing.[71] Similar findings have been described for the calcium channel blockers nifedipine and diltiazem.[72,73]

Digitalis When normal subjects were placed on a maintenance dose of digoxin, greater than 1 mm of horizontal or downsloping ST-segment depression was observed in response to exercise.[74] The depth of ST-segment depression was roughly correlated with the serum digoxin level.[75] It has been suggested that a normal ST-segment response to exercise in a patient receiving digitalis provides good evidence against myocardial ischemia,[76] but this does not appear to be a common occurrence. Furthermore, Gianrossi et al[77] have reported a decrease in the sensitivity of the exercise ECG for detection of CAD in patients taking digitalis.

Other drugs False-negative ST-segment responses to exercise have been observed in patients receiving quinidine,[78,79] procainamide,[80] or phenothiazine tranquilizers.[78] Hypokalemia may produce horizontal or downsloping ST-segment depression in the absence of myocardial ischemia.[81]

ADDITIONAL EXERCISE TEST CRITERIA

For purposes of comparing the exercise ECG to other noninvasive tests, the presence of one or more millimeters of horizontal or downsloping ST-segment depression 0.08 s after the J point is defined as a positive test. This criterion alone has been extensively tested and proved to be clinically applicable in the detection of CAD. Numerous additional exercise test findings have been found to be predictive of CAD, including exercise-induced systolic hypotension,[82–85] rising postexercise systolic blood pressure,[86] systemic diastolic hypertension with exercise,[87] ST-segment elevation,[88–94] upsloping ST-segment depression,[95] time to onset of ST-segment depression, the response of the Q-T interval to exercise,[96,97] exercise-induced U-wave inversion,[98] exercise-related changes in R-wave amplitude,[96,99,100] abnormal ST-segment maps,[101] exercise duration,[102] and heart-rate-related extent of ST-segment depression.[103] Computer approaches to the measurement of ST-segment depression and slope have been reported to improve diagnostic accuracy.[104]

Sensitivity and Specificity of Exercise Myocardial Perfusion Scintigraphy

Radionuclide methods for assessment of myocardial perfusion have evolved dramatically over the last two decades. The resolution and sensitivity of gamma cameras have steadily improved. Tomographic methods have replaced planar methods in the majority of hospitals in the United States. Administered ^{201}Tl activity for myocardial imaging has been increased by 50 to 100 percent, improving counting statistics. Technetium 99m (^{99m}Tc) myocardial perfusion imaging agents are available with improved physical imaging properties compared to ^{201}Tl. Attenuation correction methods and gated myocardial perfusion imaging methods are becoming increasingly available, as are additional ^{99m}Tc myocardial imaging agents. The effects of these advances on the overall sensitivity and specificity of myocardial perfusion scintigraphy for determining the presence or absence of CAD are best documented in studies that directly compare newer to older imaging technologies in the same patients (Table 20-2). Despite evidence from these comparison studies,

Table 20-2   Reported Sensitivities and Specificities for Exercise Myocardial Perfusion Imaging Based on Studies Making Direct Comparisons in the Same Patients

	Method	Years	Sensitivity	Specificity	References
[201]Tl planar	Qualitative	1976–1981	1431/1711 (83.6%)	621/702 (88.4%)	39, 45, 47 105–131
	[a]Qualitative	1981–1985	255/333 (76.6%)	69/80 (87.4%)	131, 132, 134, 135
	[a]Quantitative		308/333 (92.5%)	74/80 (92.5%)	131, 132, 134, 135
[201]Tl SPECT	[a]Qual. Planar [a]Qual. SPECT[b]	1989	Receiver operating characteristic analysis (ROC)		145
	[a]Qualitative	1984–1990	442/482 (91.7%)	98/128 (76.6%)	137, 138, 140
	[a]Quantitative		442/482 (91.7%)	108/128 (84.4%)	137, 138, 140
[99m]Tc planar	[a]Sestamibi	1989–1992	154/171 (90.1%)	14/20 (70.0%)	150–154
	[a]Planar [201]Tl		157/171 (91.8%)	13/20 (65.0%)	150–154
	[a]Qual. sestamibi	1994–1995	74/82 (90.2%)	51/68 (75.0%)	157, 158
	[a]Quan. sestamibi		74/82 (90.2%)	55/68 (80.9%)	157, 158
[99m]Tc SPECT	[a]Sestamibi	1989–1992	225/250 (90.0%)	35/58 (60.3%)	149, 150, 166, 167, 169
	[a]SPECT [201]Tl		221/250 (88.4%)	29/58 (50.0%)	149, 150, 166, 167, 169
	[a]Qual. sestamibi	1995–1996	122/143 (85.3%)	11/14 (78.6%)	159, 173
	[a]Quan. sestamibi		121/143 (84.6%)	11/14 (78.6%)	159, 173
	[a]Not attenuation corrected	1996	50/60 (83.3%)	—	173
	[a]Attenuation corrected[b]		53/60 (88.3%)	—	173

[a] Direct comparison in the same patients
[b] Superior by receiver operating characteristic analysis
Qual, qualitative; Quan, quantitative; SPECT, single photon emission computed tomography

changes in patient selection criteria for myocardial perfusion tests over the last 20 years tend, at times, to obscure improvement in test accuracy.

QUALITATIVE PLANAR ^{201}Tl IMAGING WITH EXERCISE

Qualitatively interpreted planar ^{201}Tl myocardial perfusion imaging was validated in at least 30 studies between 1976 and 1981. For 2413 patients,[39,45,47,105–131] the mean sensitivity of qualitatively interpreted planar ^{201}Tl imaging was 83.6 percent with a mean specificity of 88.4 percent during that time frame (see Table 20-2). A normalcy rate for qualitative planar ^{201}Tl imaging with exercise is given in Table 20-3.

QUANTITATIVE PLANAR ^{201}Tl IMAGING WITH EXERCISE

Quantitation of planar ^{201}Tl images using an interpolative background subtraction followed by horizontal or

Table 20-3   Normalcy Rates Reported for Myocardial Perfusion Imaging

Method	Combined Normalcy Rate	References
[201]Tl—Qualitative planar	11/11 (100%)	132
[201]Tl—Quantitative planar	11/11 (100%)	132
[201]Tl—Qualitative SPECT	214/242 (88%)	139, 144, 150, 167
[201]Tl—Quantitative SPECT	94/115 (82%)	148
[99m]Tc sestamibi planar (qualitative)	21/22 (95%)	150, 155
[99m]Tc sestamibi SPECT (qualitative)	87/103 (84%)	150, 167
[99m]Tc sestamibi SPECT (quantitative)	30/37 (81%)	172
[99m]Tc sestamibi stress/^{201}Tl rest	119/124 (96%)	189, 190
[99m]Tc sestamibi SPECT (attenuation corrected)	58/59 (98%)	234

SPECT, single photon emission computed tomography

circumferential profile analysis has been clearly demonstrated to reduce interobserver variability in myocardial scintigram interpretation.[131-133] For 333 patients who were studied by both qualitative and quantitative exercise ^{201}Tl planar imaging, and in whom angiographic evidence of hemodynamically important coronary artery stenosis was present, the diagnostic sensitivity of ^{201}Tl imaging was 76.6 percent with qualitative assessment versus 92.5 percent for quantitative methods[131,132,134,135] (see Table 20-2). Specificity in 80 patients without angiographic evidence of CAD was 87.4 percent by qualitative analysis and 92.5 percent by quantitative analysis. It is not clear whether the somewhat lower apparent diagnostic sensitivity of qualitative ^{201}Tl imaging in the 1981–1985 interval compared to the 1976–1981 interval represents referral of patients with less extensive CAD for diagnostic testing (pretest selection bias), selective publication of studies showing improved accuracy of the newer, quantitative test relative to qualitative testing (publication bias), or other factors. Nevertheless, the available exercise ^{201}Tl testing literature strongly suggests that quantitative planar imaging is superior to qualitative planar imaging for establishing the presence or absence of CAD.[131-136]

QUALITATIVE TOMOGRAPHIC ^{201}Tl IMAGING WITH EXERCISE

The tomographic approach to myocardial perfusion imaging has produced a dramatic improvement in contrast resolution of myocardial images and has improved localization of perfusion defects. The sensitivity of exercise ^{201}Tl myocardial perfusion tomograms, interpreted subjectively, averaged 89.8 percent in a tabulation of 1394 patients reported between 1984 and 1994.[137-144] From those same studies, the diagnostic specificity in 307 patients was just 56.0 percent. This low mean specificity reflects the inclusion of a single study containing 110 patients with no angiographic stenosis greater than or equal to 50 percent of the luminal diameter in whom the diagnostic specificity was only 27 percent.[143] Patients presented in the latter study represented only 10 percent of the patients who underwent exercise ^{201}Tl scintigraphy in the same institution during that time interval. The authors[143] pointed out that the decision to proceed to coronary arteriography was influenced by the results of ^{201}Tl scintigraphy and that the specificity of ^{201}Tl scintigraphy may have been reduced significantly by posttest selection bias. Specificity in the other seven studies in the tabulation varied from 60 percent to 100 percent.

Direct support for the belief that qualitative interpretation of exercise ^{201}Tl myocardial tomograms provides improved diagnostic sensitivity without loss of specificity compared to qualitative planar ^{201}Tl images comes from a study by Fintel et al.[145] These authors used receiver operating analysis to compare qualitative planar to qualitative tomographic exercise ^{201}Tl imaging in 77 patients

with at least one 50 percent or greater coronary artery diameter stenosis, in 35 patients with no 50 percent or greater stenosis by coronary arteriography, and in 23 normal volunteers. Qualitative single photon emission computed tomography (SPECT) was more accurate than qualitative planar imaging over the entire range of decision thresholds for the overall detection and exclusion of CAD. On subgroup analysis, the authors showed that qualitative tomography was superior to qualitative planar imaging in male patients, in patients with no prior myocardial infarction, in patients with single-vessel disease, and in patients whose most severe stenosis was 50 percent to 69 percent of the luminal diameter.

Analysis of studies included in a tabulation by Detrano et al[146] suggests that tomographic myocardial perfusion imaging may be more specific than quantitative planar methods for CAD detection (91.1 percent versus 76.2 percent). Nevertheless, in the absence of adequate studies directly comparing tomographic to quantitative planar approaches to exercise ^{201}Tl scintigraphy, in the same patients, the relative capabilities of these approaches for determining the overall presence or absence of CAD remains speculative.

QUANTITATIVE TOMOGRAPHIC ^{201}Tl IMAGING WITH EXERCISE

Circumferential profile analysis and bull's-eye displays are used to add quantitation to myocardial perfusion tomograms (see Chap. 3 for description). These approaches reduce intra- and interobserver variability by making the process of image interpretation simpler and more objective.[138,140,147-149] However, interpretation of myocardial perfusion data from functional images (e.g., bull's-eye displays) should also include careful review of the raw data (i.e., planar projections) and of the reconstructed tomographic slices to detect artifacts related to body habitus, patient motion, and technical pitfalls of tomographic acquisition and reconstruction.

Using direct comparisons in the same patients, the sensitivities and specificities of quantitative compared to qualitative analysis of exercise ^{201}Tl tomograms have been analyzed in three large studies.[137,138,140] In these studies, the respective combined sensitivities in 482 patients and combined specificities in 128 patients were 91.7 percent and 76.6 percent for qualitative analysis and 91.7 percent and 84.4 percent for quantitative analysis (see Table 20-2).

IMAGING WITH ^{99m}Tc SESTAMIBI

Planar imaging with exercise As a result of the favorable physical properties of ^{99m}Tc for nuclear medicine imaging, ^{99m}Tc sestamibi images typically provide higher resolution, higher count rates, and less attenuation artifact compared to ^{201}Tl images acquired in the same patients. Regardless of these advantages in image quality, the diagnostic sensitivity and specificity of exercise myocardial perfusion scintigrams performed with ^{99m}Tc sestamibi has been similar to that obtained with ^{201}Tl for determining the presence or absence of angiographic CAD. For 316 patients studied by qualitative analysis of planar ^{99m}Tc sestamibi images, the sensitivity was 87 percent, whereas the specificity in 91 patients without angiographic evidence of significant CAD was 78 percent.[150-159] Taken together, two studies that directly compared qualitative to quantitative approaches to interpretation of planar exercise ^{99m}Tc sestamibi images demonstrated no clear advantage of the quantitative approaches.[157,158] Nevertheless, quantitative approaches to ^{99m}Tc sestamibi images may provide clinical advantages in the detection of viable myocardium.[160,161] Insufficient data are available to clarify the role of various quantitative approaches to planar ^{99m}Tc sestamibi imaging in determining the presence or absence of CAD.[162-165]

A few studies have directly compared exercise planar ^{201}Tl imaging to exercise planar ^{99m}Tc sestamibi imaging in the same patients.[150-154] For 171 patients with angiographic evidence of significant CAD and 20 patients without angiographic CAD, the respective diagnostic sensitivities and specificities were similar for [201]Tl (91.8 percent and 65.0 percent) and for ^{99m}Tc sestamibi (90.1 percent and 70.0 percent).

Tomographic imaging with exercise In a study of 43 patients without evidence of previous myocardial infarction, Jamar et al[159] found improved evaluation of CAD extent and improved disease localization with tomographic compared to planar ^{99m}Tc sestamibi imaging methods. Overall determination of the presence or absence of CAD was not improved significantly by tomography. In 9 studies[150,156,159,166-171] including 505 patients with angiographic evidence of CAD, the sensitivity of the qualitative approach to exercise ^{99m}Tc sestamibi imaging was 92.5 percent. In 145 patients without evidence of significant CAD by angiography, the specificity was 71.7 percent. Jamar et al[159] studied 97 patients with both qualitative and quantitative assessment of ^{99m}Tc sestamibi tomograms acquired following injection of tracer with exercise. Quantitative analysis, by comparing maximum count circumferential profiles to gender-matched normal data files, provided no advantage for overall detection of CAD compared to visual interpretation of the tomograms. Other quantitative studies of exercise ^{99m}Tc sestamibi tomograms[149,172] have also not provided any substantial improvement in overall determination of the presence or absence of CAD compared to the above noted mean values for qualitative methods.

Several studies have used treadmill exercise and either qualitative or quantitative methods to directly compare ^{201}Tl tomography to ^{99m}Tc sestamibi tomography in the overall detection of CAD.[149,150,166,167,169] Based on imaging

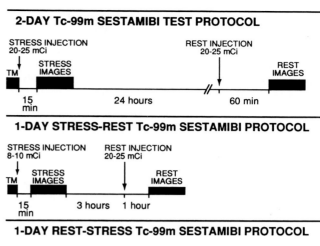

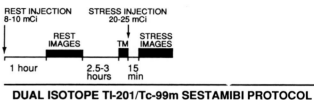

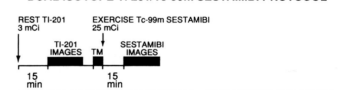

Figure 20-2 Four exercise and rest protocols that include ^{99m}Tc sestamibi in the detection of coronary artery disease.

in 250 patients with angiographic evidence of CAD and 58 patients without angiographic disease, the mean sensitivities and specificities were 88.4 percent and 50.0 percent for ^{201}Tl and 90.0 percent and 60.3 percent for ^{99m}Tc sestamibi. Thus, for tomographic as well as planar imaging methods, ^{201}Tl and ^{99m}Tc sestamibi appear to provide comparable detection of the overall presence or absence of CAD when testing is performed in conjunction with dynamic exercise.

Effect of various ^{99m}Tc sestamibi protocols in determining the overall presence of CAD Protocols for imaging ^{99m}Tc sestamibi are summarized in Fig. 20-2 and are discussed in Chap. 3.[173,174] One advantage of a 2-day protocol is that a full dose of ^{99m}Tc sestamibi can be administered prior to both exercise and rest images, resulting in high count rates for both studies. A second advantage of the 2-day protocol is that activity from the stress injection decays over three or four half-lives by the time of the second injection at rest, so that interference of residual activity from the stress injection is negligible. The principal limitation of the 2-day protocol is inconvenience for patients, although for patients with normal exercise ^{99m}Tc sestamibi images, rest imaging is usually unnecessary. Single-day ^{99m}Tc sestamibi imaging protocols consist of a stress–rest or rest–stress sequence. With a stress–rest ^{99m}Tc sestamibi protocol,[175] the stress images follow injection of a relatively small administered activity (8 to 10 mCi), and this may result in stress images that are of inferior quality compared to the rest images. In studies directly comparing stress–rest to rest–stress sequences in the same patients, Heo et al[176] and Taillefer et al[177] both showed that rest–stress studies result in identification of more myocardial segments with reversible ischemia than does a stress–rest imaging sequence. This is believed to be a consequence of persistence of the stress-induced perfusion defect on the subsequent rest images. For these reasons, a rest–stress sequence appears to be the preferred single-day, single-isotope ^{99m}Tc sestamibi imaging protocol.

The relative diagnostic accuracy of separate-day compared to single-day ^{99m}Tc sestamibi imaging protocols has been investigated. Taillefer et al[178] studied 15 patients with chest pain, at least one transient perfusion defect by ^{201}Tl perfusion imaging, and angiographic documentation of coronary artery stenosis. First, each patient was studied with an injection of 10 mCi ^{99m}Tc sestamibi at rest followed 1 h later by injection of 25 to 30 mCi sestamibi at peak treadmill exercise. Two to 3 days later a repeat exercise study was performed by injecting 10 mCi ^{99m}Tc sestamibi at peak exercise. Images from the two sestamibi protocols showed the same number of ischemic segments and also showed the same number of fixed defects. These findings suggest that a rest–stress 1-day protocol is an acceptable alternative to separate-day rest and stress sestamibi injections. It should be noted, however, that injection of 10 mCi ^{99m}Tc sestamibi for stress imaging on the separate-day protocol would not have yielded comparable counting statistics to the 25- to 30-mCi dose administered in the same-day protocol, resulting in a potential bias against the separate-day protocol. The findings of Taillefer et al[178] are supported by a study by Borges-Neto et al[179] in which similar myocardial-to-background organ ^{99m}Tc sestamibi activity was documented in 17 asymptomatic volunteers, studied with a 1-day rest–stress protocol and compared to target-to-nontarget activity ratios in 17 different volunteers studied with a 2-day protocol. Nevertheless, Whalley et al[180] observed a higher false-negative reporting rate for detection of CAD with a same-day rest–stress ^{99m}Tc sestamibi imaging sequence compared to a 2-day protocol. The latter study, however, compared the imaging protocols in matched patients rather than comparing both protocols in the same subjects. Therefore, documentation that a same-day ^{99m}Tc sestamibi imaging protocol provides comparable diagnostic information to a separate-day injection protocol must be considered suggestive rather than conclusive at this time.

A further variable that could alter the diagnostic ac-

curacy of ^{99m}Tc sestamibi imaging relates to the intervals between tracer injection and imaging. Although washout of ^{99m}Tc sestamibi is minimal, slight differential washout from ischemic versus normal myocardial segments does occur.[181,182] This resulted in a smaller ischemic-to-normal zone ratio at 1 h after tracer injection during exercise compared to the corresponding ratio in the same patient at 3 h.[182] Furthermore, it has been shown that ^{99m}Tc sestamibi can be imaged at 15 min following injection at peak exercise without loss of diagnostic accuracy or ischemic-to-normal wall contrast in comparison to images acquired 1 h following injection during peak exercise.[183] Although ^{99m}Tc sestamibi can be conveniently and accurately imaged at 15 min after injection during peak exercise, imaging following sestamibi injection at rest is ordinarily delayed for at least 60 min. This reflects the lower heart-to-background activity levels of ^{99m}Tc sestamibi that follow tracer injection at rest.

For same-day rest–stress ^{99m}Tc sestamibi imaging protocols, the optimal interval between tracer injections has not been determined. A longer interval between tracer injections allows more time for decay of the first dose and, therefore, less interference with imaging of the second dose. Delays of 1 to 4 h between tracer injections have been reported, but the effect of this variability on diagnostic accuracy, while presumed to be small, is not well documented.

DUAL-ISOTOPE REST ^{201}Tl/EXERCISE ^{99m}Tc SESTAMIBI IMAGING

Technetium-99m sestamibi provides excellent physical imaging properties for use with tomographic myocardial perfusion imaging, but ^{201}Tl injected at rest appears to provide superior detection of viable myocardium.[184-187] Consequently, dual-isotope imaging with ^{201}Tl injected at rest followed by ^{99m}Tc sestamibi injection at peak exercise provides an appealing method for accurate detection of CAD while facilitating identification of viable tissue. Although simultaneous imaging of ^{201}Tl and ^{99m}Tc sestamibi is possible using separate energy windows, Kiat et al[188] showed that 26.7 percent of activity in the ^{201}Tl energy window resulted from ^{99m}Tc cross talk, thereby degrading the ^{201}Tl images. A preferred dual-isotope method involves imaging resting ^{201}Tl activity prior to injection of ^{99m}Tc sestamibi at peak exercise (Fig. 20-2). Using this type of dual-isotope, separate imaging protocol, Berman et al[189] studied 63 patients without prior myocardial infarction who were also examined by coronary arteriography. In 55 patients with at least one coronary artery stenosis of 50 percent or greater, dual-isotope tomographic imaging was abnormal in 50 (sensitivity equals 91 percent). Corresponding specificity in 8 patients was 75 percent. Normalcy rate for dual-isotope tomographic imaging in 107 patients with a less than 5 percent likelihood of CAD was 95 percent. Rest ^{201}Tl/stress ^{99m}Tc sestamibi (as well as stress ^{201}Tl/rest

^{99m}Tc sestamibi) imaging was also evaluated by Heo et al[190] using either treadmill exercise or adenosine infusion. For 49 patients studied by the rest ^{201}Tl/stress ^{99m}Tc sestamibi protocol, a 50 percent or greater coronary stenosis was predicted from dual-isotope imaging with a sensitivity of 74 percent and specificity of 71 percent. The normalcy rate in 17 patients was 100 percent.

Additional advantages of dual-isotope rest ^{201}Tl/stress ^{99m}Tc sestamibi imaging include a brief total study time of less than 2 h. The principal disadvantages of this approach include the added complexity, cost, and radiation dose associated with administration of two tracers.

USE OF ^{99m}Tc SESTAMIBI TO MEASURE LEFT VENTRICULAR FUNCTION AND PERFUSION

First-pass radionuclide angiocardiography First-pass radionuclide angiocardiography can be performed in conjunction with ^{99m}Tc sestamibi injection. Technical aspects of first-pass radionuclide angiography are discussed in Chap. 10. Measurement of left ventricular ejection fraction (LVEF) at rest from first-pass imaging of a ^{99m}Tc sestamibi bolus compared well ($r = 0.93$, $p < 0.001$) to measurement of LVEF from first-pass imaging of a ^{99m}Tc diethylenetriamine pentaacetic acid bolus.[191] In one study, left ventricular regional wall motion from a ^{99m}Tc sestamibi first-pass study agreed with contrast ventriculography in 38 of 52 myocardial segments.[191] In addition, global and regional left ventricular function have been studied by first-pass angiography of a ^{99m}Tc sestamibi bolus during upright bicycle[192] or treadmill exercise.[192,193] The impact on diagnostic sensitivity and specificity of adding first-pass regional and global ventricular function assessment to exercise ^{99m}Tc sestamibi myocardial perfusion imaging remains to be documented.

Gated sestamibi imaging (See Chap. 3 for methods and Chap. 4 for examples.) Technetium-99m sestamibi provides a high count flux allowing ECG gating of planar or tomographic perfusion images. Typically, ^{99m}Tc sestamibi is injected during peak exercise and gated images are acquired at rest 15 to 60 min later. Therefore, ^{99m}Tc sestamibi images reflect myocardial perfusion during exercise, whereas regional wall thickening on the gated images reflects regional left ventricular function at rest. In myocardial segments with severe perfusion defects with exercise and normal wall thickening at rest, the presence of reversible myocardial ischemia can be inferred and a repeat injection of ^{99m}Tc sestamibi at rest may be obviated. The presence of a regional ^{99m}Tc sestamibi perfusion defect with stress with evidence of persistent impairment of regional wall thickening on gated images can result from either infarcted myocardium,

postexercise regional dysfunction related to stunned myocardium,[194] or an admixture of myocardial ischemia and scar. Therefore, if the gated sestamibi images show abnormal regional myocardial wall thickening at rest, a separate myocardial perfusion study at rest (probably with ^{201}Tl) is needed.[195] The presence of stunned myocardium can also produce impairment of regional myocardial thickening and an apparent myocardial perfusion defect in the presence of a patent coronary artery as a consequence of the partial volume effect.[196–198]

Left ventricular regional wall motion from gated ^{99m}Tc sestamibi images correlates highly with left ventricular regional wall motion from echocardiography.[199,200] In addition, left ventricular regional myocardial wall thickening can be assessed from gated ^{99m}Tc sestamibi images. As a result of the limited resolution of conventional gamma cameras, wall thickening is more accurately assessed from the increase in myocardial segmental count density instead of attempting to quantitate wall thickness from the apparent number of transmural pixels in a myocardial region.[199,201] In addition to assessment of regional left ventricular wall motion, global LVEF can be calculated from ^{99m}Tc sestamibi images using either planar[202] or tomographic[203] methods.

Preliminary data from a study of 115 women reported by Taillefer et al[204] strongly suggests that the combination of stress myocardial perfusion and stress left ventricular functional data from ^{99m}Tc sestamibi imaging provides improved diagnostic specificity and diagnostic sensitivity comparable to ^{201}Tl imaging for the detection of CAD in women. DePuey and Rozanski[205] and Smanio et al[206] also found evidence of improved diagnostic specificity of ^{99m}Tc sestamibi imaging when used in conjunction with ECG gating in the differentiation of soft-tissue attenuation artifacts from left ventricular myocardial scar in women with anterior wall fixed defects in ^{99m}Tc sestamibi activity. The presence of preserved left ventricular wall motion on gated images favors the presence of attenuation artifact, whereas the absence of left ventricular wall motion favors the presence of anterior myocardial scar. Similarly, inferoposterior wall fixed defects on ^{99m}Tc sestamibi images are likely to be a consequence of diaphragmatic attenuation when ECG gating demonstrates normal segmental wall motion.

IMAGING WITH ^{99m}Tc TEBOROXIME

The biological and kinetic properties of ^{99m}Tc teboroxime are presented in Chap. 1. Rapid myocardial clearance of teboroxime permits rapid exercise and rest imaging sequences with the potential for high patient throughput and substantial patient convenience in a busy nuclear cardiology laboratory. Rapid myocardial clearance of teboroxime also necessitates very brief imaging times to adequately visualize the myocardium prior to tracer clearance and prior to the presence of intense tracer activity adjacent to the heart in the liver.[207-211] Compared to ischemic myocardium, ^{99m}Tc teboroxime clears more rapidly from normal myocardium and this may provide additional information for detection of myocardial ischemia related to CAD. The rapid myocardial clearance of teboroxime, as well as the differential washout from normal and ischemic myocardial zones, has raised theoretical concerns with respect to the advisability of using ^{99m}Tc teboroxime for SPECT imaging with a single detector.[209]

Regardless of the logistic issues related to ^{99m}Tc teboroxime imaging, planar[154,207,208,210] and tomographic[211] teboroxime imaging sequences have been reported to provide comparable diagnostic accuracy for determining the presence or absence of CAD compared to ^{201}Tl in numerous small studies. In the Canadian exercise ^{99m}Tc-labeled teboroxime single-photon emission computed tomography study,[212] 108 patients were studied by both ^{99m}Tc teboroxime tomography and by ^{201}Tl tomography. Overall, agreement of ^{99m}Tc teboroxime versus ^{201}Tl segmental perfusion (i.e., normal versus abnormal) was present in 772 of 961 myocardial segments (80.3 percent, *kappa* = 0.51). Compared to coronary arteriography in 56 patients, the sensitivity and specificity of ^{99m}Tc teboroxime imaging were 80 percent and 67 percent compared to 84 percent and 67 percent for [201]Tl. Detection of stenoses in the distributions of individual coronary arteries was similar for ^{201}Tl and ^{99m}Tc teboroxime.[154,210-213,214] In particular, prominent hepatic ^{99m}Tc teboroxime activity did not appear to interfere with detection of disease in the inferior wall in this study. The principal advantage of ^{99m}Tc teboroxime in the multicenter Canadian study was the shorter imaging procedure time of 113.6 min compared to 240.5 min for [201]Tl.

NEWER ^{99m}Tc TRACERS

The biological and kinetic properties of ^{99m}Tc tetrofosmin, ^{99m}Tc furifosmin (Q12), and [99m]TcN-NOET are discussed in Chap. 1.

Imaging with ^{99m}Tc tetrofosmin Technetium-99m-tetrofosmin is a diphosphine imaging agent that shows little evidence of myocardial washout.[215,216] Rapid hepatic clearance of tetrofosmin results in favorable heart-to-liver activity ratios by 15 min after injection at rest or with exercise. This property facilitates acquisition of high-quality images in a single-day exercise and rest imaging protocol.[214,217,218] A potential disadvantage shared by ^{99m}Tc tetrofosmin[219] and ^{99m}Tc sestamibi[220-223] relative to ^{201}Tl relates to ischemic defect size. Exercise ^{99m}Tc tetrofosmin defect size determined either by visual or quantitative analysis of SPECT images is smaller than the corresponding defect on ^{201}Tl tomographic images. Planar imaging with ^{99m}Tc tetrofosmin was evaluated

in a phase III multicenter trial that included 252 patients with suspected CAD.[214] All patients underwent exercise and rest myocardial perfusion imaging with ^{99m}Tc tetrofosmin in a single-day protocol including two separate tracer injections 4 h apart. Exercise and rest ^{201}Tl images were obtained within 2 weeks of tetrofosmin imaging. Concordance of ^{99m}Tc tetrofosmin images with ^{201}Tl images for the presence of a normal versus abnormal scintigram was 80.4 percent (*kappa* = 0.55). Coronary arteriography was available in 181 study patients. The sensitivity and specificity for detection of at least one greater than 70 percent coronary stenosis were 77 percent and 58 percent for exercise ^{99m}Tc tetrofosmin imaging and were 83 percent and 48 percent for exercise ^{201}Tl imaging (differences not statistically significant). Sensitivities and specificities were also comparable for the two radiotracers in those study patients without a previous myocardial infarction. Technetium-99m-tetrofosmin and ^{201}Tl imaging provided comparable detection of perfusion defects in individual myocardial segments, although ^{99m}Tc tetrofosmin planar images tended nonsignificantly to provide higher sensitivity compared to ^{201}Tl images for detection of inferior wall defects, without loss of specificity. Comparable diagnostic accuracy of ^{99m}Tc tetrofosmin and ^{201}Tl exercise imaging has been reported by other investigators in conjunction with planar[223,224] or tomographic[225-228] imaging. The normalcy rate for ^{99m}Tc tetrofosmin images in 58 healthy subjects with a low likelihood of CAD was reported to be 97 percent.[214]

Although good correlation of defect reversibility by ^{99m}Tc tetrofosmin versus exercise and rest or reinjection ^{201}Tl imaging has been reported[214,225] data are needed to assess the ability of exercise and rest ^{99m}Tc tetrofosmin imaging to predict the recovery of segmental left ventricular function following revascularization. An alternative approach to the noninvasive assessment of myocardial viability, rest ^{201}Tl imaging followed by exercise ^{99m}Tc tetrofosmin imaging has been described. The latter study protocol may be completed in just 90 min.[229] In addition to assessment of myocardial perfusion, ^{99m}Tc tetrofosmin injection may be combined with first-pass radionuclide angiocardiography or ECG gating of the perfusion images to allow assessment of global and regional left ventricular function.[227]

Imaging with ^{99m}Tc furifosmin (Q12) Technetium-99m-furifosmin (Q12) is a mixed ligand complex that clears rapidly from the blood, is taken up into the myocardium in relation to myocardial blood flow,[230] and displays very rapid hepatic clearance. Rapid hepatic clearance of furifosmin has permitted clinical imaging within 15 min following tracer injection at exercise or at rest, without loss of diagnostic sensitivity and specificity compared to ^{201}Tl imaging in the same patients.[144]

In a phase III multicenter clinical study, tomographic furifosmin imaging following injection at peak exercise was directly compared to exercise ^{201}Tl imaging in 149 patients.[231] The agreement between ^{201}Tl and ^{99m}Tc furifosmin for the presence or absence of a perfusion abnormality was 86 percent ($p < 0.001$, *kappa* = 0.67). Concordance between ^{201}Tl and ^{99m}Tc furifosmin for detection of reversible perfusion defects was observed in 79 percent of patients ($p < 0.001$, *kappa* = 0.54). In comparison to coronary arteriography, the sensitivity of tomographic exercise ^{99m}Tc furifosmin images was found to be 85 percent (17 of 20 patients) in one study[144] and 98 percent (46 of 47 patients) in a larger study.[232] In the former study, the diagnostic sensitivity and normalcy rate was similar for ^{99m}Tc furifosmin and for ^{201}Tl in the same study patients.[144] In the phase III multicenter clinical study, the normalcy rate of furifosmin in 39 patients with a low likelihood of CAD was 100 percent.[231]

Imaging with [99m]TcN-NOET Technetium-99mN-NOET is a neutral, lipophilic technetium complex that has demonstrated good myocardial uptake in animals and in humans.[233] Prominent initial uptake of [99m]TcN-NOET in the lungs has been described. Because pulmonary clearance of tracer is more rapid than myocardial clearance, it has been recommended that clinical imaging begin 30 min following tracer injection. Technetium-99mN-NOET demonstrates evidence of differential washout from normal and ischemic myocardium over 4 h, suggesting its potential use as a tracer of myocardial viability.

In a multicenter European study, stress [99m]TcN-NOET and ^{201}Tl images were concordant for the presence of CAD in 22 of 25 patients (88 percent, *kappa* = 0.76). The overall sensitivity for detection of CAD was 79 percent (14 of 19 patients) with [99m]TcN-NOET versus 68 percent (13 of 19 patients) with [201]Tl ($p = $ NS). Specificity was 100 percent for both radiotracers. Segmental analysis of [99m]TcN-NOET and ^{201}Tl stress images showed concordance in 211 of 225 segments (94 percent, *kappa* = 0.82). Comparison of 4-h postinjection images showed a concordance of [99m]TcN-NOET and ^{201}Tl in 21 of 23 patients. Further investigation of [99m]TcN-NOET is needed to determine its full capability both in the detection of CAD and in the documentation of myocardial viability.

IMAGING WITH ATTENUATION CORRECTION

As has been emphasized in Chap. 4, attenuation artifacts on myocardial perfusion images are a common source of defects that may falsely suggest the presence of CAD. If the normal range of variability in regional myocardial tracer activity is broadened to avoid false-positive scans resulting from attenuation effects, then diagnostic sensitivity is likely to be reduced. The ideal approach to deal with attenuation artifacts is to eliminate these artifacts by correcting detected myocardial counts for activity lost to attenuation. Approaches to attenuation correction through the simultaneous acquisition of emission and

transmission nuclear images have been devised (see discussion in Chap. 3) and the method has entered into clinical use. An initial study comparing the use of attenuation-corrected versus nonattenuation-corrected myocardial perfusion imaging suggests that correction for attenuation can improve the diagnostic accuracy of myocardial perfusion imaging for detection of CAD.[234]

Ficaro et al[234] used a triple-detector SPECT system with an americium-241 transmission line source to perform simultaneous transmission and emission imaging in 60 patients with angiographic CAD and in 59 patients with a 5 percent or less likelihood of CAD. Iteratively reconstructed attenuation-corrected stress ^{99m}Tc sestamibi perfusion images were compared with uncorrected images. Gender-specific normal databases were calculated from the myocardial distributions of corrected and uncorrected myocardial counts. In the absence of correction for attenuation, significant regional differences in the distribution of myocardial activity were observed for both normal male and female patients. In most cases, regional inhomogeneity of detected tracer activity followed previously described[138] patterns of gender-specific soft-tissue attenuation. With attenuation correction, however, the distribution of detected myocardial activity around the circumference of the basal and mid-ventricular slices of the left ventricle was uniform, and did not vary by gender (Fig. 20-3, Plate 3). The apex of the left ventricle contained decreased counts per pixel, corresponding to the reduced myocardial mass of the left ventricular apex referred to as apical thinning. Visual interpretation of the attenuation-corrected and -uncorrected images was performed in random order by two observers who were unaware of whether the patient was from the group with low likelihood of disease or from the angiographically studied group. The observed normalcy rate improved from 88 ± 4 percent to 98 ± 2 percent with addition of attenuation correction ($p = 0.027$). By visual interpretation, the overall diagnostic sensitivity for detection of CAD was 78 percent without attenuation correction and 84 percent with attenuation correction ($p = $ NS). The diagnostic specificity was significantly better with attenuation correction (82 percent) compared to noncorrected images (46 percent, $p < 0.05$). Additionally, with attenuation correction, disease detection improved significantly for individual coronary artery distributions and for detection of individual coronary stenoses in patients with multivessel CAD. Similarly, with quantitative polar map analysis, overall assessment of the presence or absence of CAD, as well as detection of individual coronary artery stenoses was improved by attenuation correction.

SUMMARY

In direct comparison studies in the same patients, improved diagnostic accuracy for determining the presence

Non-Attenuation-Corrected (gender specific)

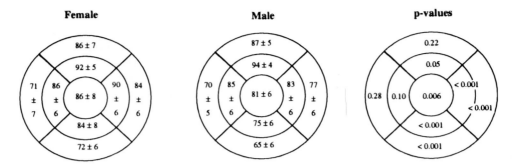

Attenuation-Corrected (gender specific)

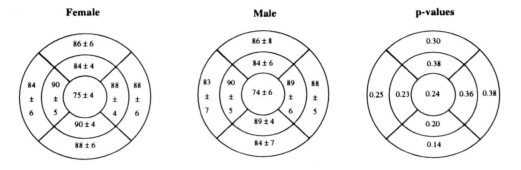

Attenuation-Corrected (gender composite)

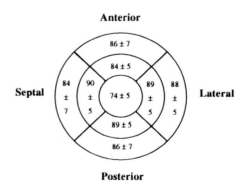

Figure 20-3 Stress ⁹⁹ᵐTc sestamibi tracer distribution in the myocardium of patients with a 5 percent or less pretest likelihood of CAD. Normal, gender-specific polar map distributions (20 subjects each) are presented for uncorrected (*top*) and attenuation-corrected (*bottom*) images. Significant differences (*p* values) between the gender maps are displayed on the right for the uncorrected and attenuation-corrected distributions. (From Ficaro et al,[234] by permission of the American Heart Association, Inc.)

or absence of CAD has been observed when comparing (1) quantitative planar to qualitative planar ²⁰¹Tl tests, (2) qualitative SPECT to qualitative planar ²⁰¹Tl tests, (3) quantitative SPECT to qualitative SPECT ²⁰¹Tl tests, (4) gated ⁹⁹ᵐTc sestamibi tomograms to ungated ⁹⁹ᵐTc sestamibi tomograms, and (5) attenuation-corrected to uncorrected ⁹⁹ᵐTc sestamibi SPECT tests. Direct comparisons in general chest pain populations of exercise myocardial perfusion imaging with ²⁰¹Tl to similar imaging with ⁹⁹ᵐTc sestamibi have not clearly demonstrated improved overall determination of the presence or absence of CAD with one tracer or the other.

If each of the five technical advances in myocardial perfusion imaging listed above has resulted in reports of improved sensitivity or specificity for determining the presence or absence of CAD, why are the reported levels of diagnostic sensitivity and specificity no greater in 1996 than in 1976–1981? The reason appears to be a combination of pretest selection bias, posttest selection bias, and, possibly, publication bias. In a meta-analysis of 56 publications (1977–1986) reporting on the sensitivity and specificity of exercise thallium scintigraphy, Detrano et al[146] found that the percentage of patients with a previous myocardial infarction (a pretest bias) had the highest correlation with diagnostic sensitivity of any of the 19 clinical and technical variables assessed. Both the presence of angiographic referral bias (a posttest bias) and publication year (a potential publication bias) adversely affected test specificity ($p < 0.05$). Despite efforts to eliminate selection biases,[235] different myocardial imaging modalities are best compared directly in the same patients. Direct comparison studies appear to indicate improving noninvasive diagnosis of CAD with advancing technology.

Severity of Disease

PREVIOUS MYOCARDIAL INFARCTION

The severity of disease in the study population will alter apparent test sensitivity. The postexercise myocardial perfusion scintigram is more likely to be abnormal in patients with a previous clinical myocardial infarction than in patients with ischemia only.[146,236] This results from the greater severity of perfusion defects in zones of Q-wave myocardial infarction compared to regions of reversible ischemia and is true for tomographic (see Table 21-4) as well as planar imaging.

NUMBER OF DISEASED VESSELS

Patients with multivessel CAD are more likely to have an exercise ^{201}Tl perfusion abnormality compared to patients with single-vessel CAD.[110,236] In a multicenter study[110] of planar myocardial imaging with ^{201}Tl, 37 of 59 patients (63 percent) with double-vessel disease and 33 of 43 patients (77 percent) with triple-vessel disease had exercise-induced perfusion defects, compared to 20 of 46 patients (43 percent) with single-vessel disease ($p < 0.05$). Although the diagnostic accuracy of myocardial perfusion imaging has been improved by tomographic imaging, multivessel CAD is still more readily detected than single-vessel disease. In nine studies[137,138,140–144,148,149] of exercise tomographic myocardial perfusion imaging (see Table 21-4), the sensitivity

for identifying patients with at least one coronary artery stenosis of greater than or equal to 50 percent of the luminal diameter was 84 percent in patients with one-vessel disease, 93 percent in patients with two-vessel disease, and 96 percent in patients with three-vessel disease.

An angiographic CAD score assesses the extent of myocardium in jeopardy by considering the amount of myocardium distal to each stenosis as well as the number of stenotic vessels. The angiographic score is correlated with an increasingly abnormal postexercise ^{201}Tl scintigram in terms of the number of abnormal left ventricular segments and the severity of hypoperfusion.[237]

SEVERITY OF INDIVIDUAL CORONARY ARTERY STENOSES

An exercise-induced ^{201}Tl perfusion defect will more likely be detected in the presence of a severe coronary artery stenosis consisting of a greater than 70 percent narrowing of the luminal diameter than in a moderate coronary artery stenosis consisting of a 50 to 70 percent narrowing.[238] In a tabulation of six reported studies using exercise tomographic myocardial perfusion imaging,[137,138,140–142,149] 473 of 543 (87 percent) severe coronary artery stenoses consisting of a 70 percent or greater luminal diameter reduction had a corresponding perfusion defect. Moderate coronary artery stenoses were detected significantly less frequently (196 of 309 arteries or 63 percent).

Addition of tomography and computer quantitation to qualitative planar ^{201}Tl imaging methods has been observed to improve detection of moderate coronary stenoses.[132,136] By receiver operating characteristic analysis, Fintel et al[145] documented improved detection of 50 to 69 percent coronary artery stenoses with qualitative tomographic compared to planar ^{201}Tl imaging methods. Kahn et al[149] compared postexercise quantitative tomographic imaging with ^{99m}Tc sestamibi to corresponding data acquired with ^{201}Tl. Tomography with ^{201}Tl identified 12 of 34 stenoses of 50 to 75 percent diameter reduction compared to 22 of 34 stenoses identified with ^{99m}Tc sestamibi ($p < 0.05$). Evidence also suggests that attenuation-corrected tomographic images provide superior detection of 50 to 69 percent luminal diameter stenoses compared to uncorrected images.[234]

Identification of "Surgical" Coronary Artery Disease

The presence of a 50 percent or greater stenosis in either the left main or all of the three major epicardial coronary arteries identifies a group of patients with improved survival with surgical compared to medical treatment.[239–242] Early in the history of exercise myocardial perfusion imaging, concern was expressed that a balanced pattern of myocardial ischemia in patients with severe three-vessel CAD could result in uniform myocardial tracer distribution on planar myocardial perfusion images. However, in a tabulation of 241 patients with angiographic three-vessel CAD, an abnormal qualitative planar ^{201}Tl scintigram was present in 223 patients (93 percent).[105,108,113,116,124,126,243–246] More recently, using tomographic methods in nine studies,[138–144,148,149] an abnormal exercise myocardial perfusion scan was present in 412 of 430 patients with three-vessel CAD (96 percent). Furthermore, it is likely that some of the remaining 4 percent of patients with three-vessel CAD would have been identified as abnormal if lung thallium activity and transient left ventricular cavity dilatation were considered in each of the studies. Thus, tomographic exercise myocardial perfusion imaging is rarely normal in the presence of three-vessel CAD. In most clinical settings, an abnormal exercise myocardial perfusion scintigram will lead to coronary angiography and identification of coronary anatomy that is best treated by surgical (or multivessel percutaneous transluminal angioplasty) therapy.

A noninvasive test that is highly accurate for discriminating between one-vessel and surgical three-vessel or left main CAD might, in theory, be used reliably to identify patients with minimal or no cardiac symptoms and one-vessel or two-vessel CAD who could be treated medically. Unfortunately, the ability of exercise perfusion scintigraphy alone to separate patients with one-vessel from those with severe three-vessel or left main CAD is often inadequate for exclusion of surgical coronary anatomy in individual patients.[143] Christian et al[143] examined the ability of exercise tomographic ^{201}Tl imaging to predict the presence of left main or three-vessel CAD in 688 patients who underwent both exercise ^{201}Tl testing and coronary arteriography. By logistic regression analysis of clinical, exercise, and scintigraphic variables, four factors were identified that were independently predictive for the presence of severe left main or three-vessel CAD: (1) presence or absence of diabetes mellitus, (2) magnitude of ST-segment depression with exercise, (3) change in systolic blood pressure with exercise, and (4) number of visually abnormal short-axis ^{201}Tl segments. Using these four variables, 205 of 492 patients (42 percent) were classified as having a high probability for severe CAD and 52 percent of these patients had severe CAD at angiography. A low probability of severe CAD was predicted in 170 patients (35 percent) and only 12 percent of these patients had three-vessel or left main disease. Only 29 percent of patients (n = 53) with three-vessel or left main CAD had perfusion abnormalities in the distributions of all three coronary arteries.[143] These data confirm the early observations of Patterson et al[247] who studied the ability of exercise planar ^{201}Tl scintigraphy to identify patients with left main or three-vessel CAD following a first transmural myocar-

dial infarction. An exercise ^{201}Tl perfusion defect outside the infarct zone was associated with high-risk angiographic anatomy with a sensitivity of 65 percent and specificity of 96 percent. Nevertheless, the sensitivity of myocardial perfusion imaging for detection of high-risk coronary anatomy was improved to 82 percent with a specificity of 83 percent by adding two exercise variables, peak heart rate less than 85 percent of that predicted in a patient not taking a beta blocker and blood pressure decrease during exercise. In summary, the ability of exercise myocardial perfusion imaging to identify specifically the presence of three-vessel or left main CAD is limited currently. The sensitivity can be improved significantly by considering selected clinical and exercise test variables.

Although exercise myocardial perfusion imaging alone may not currently be able to separate all patients with three-vessel or left main CAD from patients with less extensive CAD, several scintigraphic patterns have been described which, when present, indicate a high likelihood of multivessel (and, likely, surgical) CAD. These include: (1) the presence of perfusion defects in each of the three coronary artery distributions, (2) diffuse slow washout of ^{201}Tl, (3) prominent pulmonary thallium activity, (4) transient dilatation of the left ventricle, and (5) the "left main pattern" of perfusion defects in the anterior, septal, and posterolateral myocardial segments. Examples of these scintigraphic patterns are shown in Chap. 2.

DETECTION OF PERFUSION DEFECTS IN ALL THREE CORONARY TERRITORIES

Exercise myocardial perfusion imaging is highly efficient in inducing a defect in the distribution of the most severely stenotic coronary artery. Induction of further ischemia in the distribution of additional less severely stenosed coronary arteries is less consistently accomplished. Once ischemia is induced related to the most severe coronary narrowing, ischemic symptoms may prevent further exercise and the induction of additional perfusion defects. Scintigraphic demonstration of the full extent of jeopardized myocardium through exercise testing is unlikely to be accomplished unless the patient is unrestricted by noncardiac exercise limitations (e.g., musculoskeletal disease, claudication, pulmonary or psychiatric disease). In addition, to reveal the full extent of myocardial ischemic disease, the patient will usually need to be free of beta blockers, calcium antagonists, and other anti-ischemic drugs (see below). For these various reasons, induction and detection of ischemia in the distribution of all coronary artery stenoses greater than 50 percent of the luminal diameter has been less accurate in patients with three-vessel disease compared to patients with one-vessel disease. In a tabulation of six studies[137–142] that used tomographic exercise myocardial perfusion imaging, 300 of 363 (83 percent) stenotic coronary arteries were detected in patients with one-vessel disease, whereas 428 of 570 (75 percent) stenotic arteries were identified in patients with two-vessel disease and 307 of 444 (69 percent) stenotic arteries were detected in patients with three-vessel disease.

When myocardial perfusion defects are identified in each of the distributions of the three major coronary arteries, the likelihood that stenoses of 50 percent or greater will be found at angiography in all three coronary arteries is high. In one study, Iskandrian et al[139] detected exercise ^{201}Tl myocardial perfusion defects in the distributions of each of the three coronary arteries in 38 patients. A 50 percent or greater stenosis was found in each of the three major coronary arteries in 29 of the 38 patients (76 percent).

Additional scintigraphic signs have been described that suggest the presence of three-vessel CAD. The presence of prominent ^{201}Tl activity at the cardiac base relative to the apical two-thirds of the heart (see Fig. 2-14)[248] and perfusion defects with exercise involving 40 percent or more of the left ventricle[249] have been correlated with three-vessel CAD.

DIFFUSE SLOW WASHOUT OF [201]Tl

Following initial extraction during peak exercise, ^{201}Tl washes out of ischemic myocardium more slowly than from normal myocardium.[250] In 1265 consecutive patients having quantitatively analyzed stress-redistribution planar ^{201}Tl scintigrams, Bateman et al[251] identified 46 patients with diffuse slow washout of ^{201}Tl combined with no or at most one initial regional perfusion defect. Thirty-two patients with diffuse slow washout underwent clinically indicated coronary arteriography revealing three-vessel or left main CAD in 23 patients (72 percent). Of 30 similar patients without diffuse slow washout of ^{201}Tl and with no or at most one initial perfusion defect, only 5 (17 percent) had three-vessel or left main CAD. The authors demonstrated an independent relationship of diffuse slow washout to the presence of extensive CAD. The predictive value of diffuse slow washout of ^{201}Tl was maintained when the patient did not exercise to target heart rate.

A number of potential limitations of the diffuse slow washout pattern in the detection of three-vessel or left main CAD should be noted. Myocardial washout of ^{201}Tl following exercise is complex[252] and is altered by numerous factors including (1) exercise peak heart rate,[253-255] (2) blood ^{201}Tl level during washout, which in turn may be influenced by eating[256,257] (3) extra cardiac ^{201}Tl uptake in the lungs,[254] (4) patient gender,[258] (5) technical errors related to inconsistent stress and rest image registration,[259] (6) noncoronary heart disease,[260] (7) extravasation or "hangup" of the administered ^{201}Tl dose,[261] and (8) regional variability in myocardial ^{201}Tl clearance in normal individuals.[262] A practical limitation

of diffuse slow washout analysis in the detection of three-vessel and left main CAD is that washout analysis is seldom performed in conjunction with tomographic ^{201}Tl perfusion imaging because washout analysis has been found not to add significantly to the overall accuracy of initial ^{201}Tl distribution in determining the presence or absence of CAD with SPECT.[138] Nevertheless, several authors have confirmed the predictive value of diffuse slow washout analysis for identifying the presence of three-vessel or left main CAD from quantitative planar exercise ^{201}Tl scintigraphy.[263,264]

INCREASED PULMONARY ^{201}Tl ACTIVITY

The pathophysiologic correlation of increased pulmonary ^{201}Tl activity with prolonged pulmonary transit time and elevated left ventricular end-diastolic pressure is discussed in detail in Chap. 2, together with a description of methods used for detection of abnormal pulmonary ^{201}Tl activity. Compared to its absence, prominent pulmonary ^{201}Tl activity with exercise or pharmacologic stress has been correlated with an increased number of critical coronary artery stenoses,[265] a larger number of perfusion defects[266,267] evidence of left ventricular dysfunction,[265,268,269] prior myocardial infarction,[266] and multivessel compared to one-vessel disease.[267,270-274,275] For example, in a study of 306 patients with chest pain, Homma et al[271] assessed which of 23 clinical, exercise, planar thallium, and angiographic variables best discriminated between patients with increased lung-to-heart ratios of ^{201}Tl activity versus those with normal ratios. The number of diseased coronary arteries was the best discriminator between patients with increased heart-to-lung ratios compared to those with normal ratios.

In patients who undergo myocardial perfusion imaging by tomographic methods, most[269,270,275] but not all[276] studies have confirmed the relationship between increased pulmonary tracer activity and CAD severity. In one study, for example, patients with markedly increased lung-to-heart ratios of ^{201}Tl activity had three-vessel disease more frequently (67 percent) than those patients with slightly (14 percent) or moderately (35 percent) increased ratios.[277] Reported cut-off values for identifying an increased lung-to-heart ratio have differed for ratios calculated from anterior planar projections acquired for tomographic studies versus planar images acquired for a longer duration. By either method, the lung-to-heart ratio of ^{201}Tl counts provides valuable prediction for the presence of three-vessel CAD. In contrast, lung-to-heart ratios of ^{99m}Tc sestamibi following exercise have not been demonstrated convincingly to provide prediction of multivessel coronary disease.[278]

TRANSIENT LEFT VENTRICULAR CAVITY DILATION

In response to extensive myocardial ischemia during exercise or pharmacologic coronary artery vasodilation, the left ventricular cavity may dilate reflecting preload recruitment in diastole and declining LVEF, increasing systolic volumes. In addition, the left ventricular cavity may appear to increase in area as a result of reduced subendocardial tracer activity in the presence of subendocardial ischemia. From planar ^{201}Tl images, Weiss et al[279] calculated a ratio of left ventricular cavity area at stress to left ventricular cavity area at rest and designated it as the "transient dilation ratio." In 23 patients with a normal coronary arteriogram or less than 50 percent angiographic CAD, the transient dilation ratio was 1.02 ± 0.05 (mean $\pm$ 1 standard deviation). In patients with "mild" CAD (defined in that study as a 50 to 89 percent stenosis) or with a single coronary stenosis of 90 percent or greater, the transient dilation ratio was within 2 standard deviations of the mean for normals (i.e., 1.12 or less) in 35 of 36 patients (97 percent). However, in patients with a 90 percent or greater stenosis of all three coronary arteries, the transient ischemic dilation ratio exceeded 1.12 in 10 of 13 patients (77 percent). Similar findings have been reported with pharmacologic coronary vasodilation[280–282] as well as with exercise[248] and for tomographic as well as planar imaging.[282]

LEFT MAIN CORONARY ARTERY DISEASE PATTERN

Dash et al[116] described a scintigraphic pattern of reduced anterior, septal, and posterolateral myocardial activity on exercise ^{201}Tl planar images, corresponding to the proximal and distal distributions of the left coronary artery and referred to as a left main pattern. In that study, the authors observed that the majority of their 6 study patients with a 50 percent or greater stenosis of the left main coronary artery had additional severe disease in other coronary vessels so that a balanced pattern of hypoperfusion in the LAD and left circumflex coronary artery distributions was usually not present. Rehn et al[283] studied 24 patients with a 50 percent or greater stenosis of the left main coronary artery using exercise ^{201}Tl planar imaging and found an abnormal myocardial scintigram in 22 of 24 patients (92 percent). However, the left main pattern was only present in 3 of 24 patients (13 percent) with left main disease and was also present in 10 of 50 patients (20 percent) without left main disease.[283] The authors concluded that the pattern of perfusion defects in patients with left main CAD was determined by the location and severity of narrowings downstream from the left main lesion. In a study of 295 consecutive patients including 43 (14 percent) with a 50 percent or greater stenosis of the left main coronary artery, Nygaard et al[284] observed the left main pattern in just 14 percent of patients with significant left main CAD. On the other hand, a high-risk exercise planar ^{201}Tl scintigram consisting of either (1) a left main scintigraphic pattern, (2) abnormal ^{201}Tl uptake or washout in multiple coronary vascular territories, or (3) increased

pulmonary thallium uptake was present in 77 percent of 43 patients with left main disease and 58 percent of patients with three-vessel disease.

Using low-level exercise combined with dipyridamole infusion, Chikamori et al[285] studied 38 patients with 50 percent or greater left main coronary artery stenosis and 428 patients with at least one stenosis 75 percent or greater of the luminal diameter in a major coronary artery but without significant left main disease. The left main pattern was present in 6 of 9 patients (33 percent) with significant left main disease and a patent right coronary artery, but in only 3 of 29 patients (10 percent) with significant left main and right CAD ($p = 0.0005$). The left main pattern had a specificity of 91 percent in the 428 study patients without left main disease.

In summary, exercise myocardial perfusion imaging is seldom normal in patients with three-vessel or left main CAD. Exercise myocardial perfusion alone does not specifically identify the presence of high-risk coronary anatomy in a substantial proportion of patients with three-vessel or left main disease, but high-risk anatomy can often be suspected from the presence of high-risk clinical and exercise indicators taken together with the presence of high-risk scintigraphic findings. When present, ^{201}Tl defects in all three coronary artery distributions, diffuse slow washout of ^{201}Tl, increased pulmonary ^{201}Tl activity, transient left ventricular cavity dilation, and the left main pattern each provide strong evidence for the presence of three-vessel or left main CAD.

Identification of Stenoses in Individual Coronary Arteries

Detection of stenoses in individual coronary arteries from ^{201}Tl exercise myocardial perfusion images is summarized in Table 20-4. The studies listed differ in several important respects, making direct comparisons difficult. Few of the studies directly compare different approaches to exercise ^{201}Tl scintigraphy in the same patients. Importantly, detection of individual coronary artery stenoses by any of these methods will be more successful in patients with single-vessel CAD than for detecting a second or third stenotic coronary vessel, for the reasons discussed earlier. Scintigraphic detection of individual coronary artery stenoses will also be more readily accomplished in the presence of a severe (e.g., 70 percent or greater) stenosis compared to a moderate (e.g., 50 to 69 percent) stenosis. Nevertheless, several conclusions are suggested by available studies that directly compare in the same patients different methods for detection of individual coronary artery stenoses. A quantitative planar approach using circumferential profiles and ^{201}Tl washout kinetics produced a statistically significant improvement in detection of disease in indi-

Table 20-4 Detection of Stenoses in Individual Coronary Arteries by Various Thallium Imaging Methods

Method	Author	LAD	CIRC	RCA
			Sensitivity, %	
Planar (subjective)	Lenaers (105)	84	49	79
	Maddahi (132)	56	34	65
	Rigo (243)	83	35	62
	Massie (124)	78	45	73
	Starling (286)	61	32	64
	Fintel (145)	58	37	64
Planar (quantitative)	Maddahi (132)	80	63	94
Tomographic (subjective)	Tamaki (137)	83	63	88
	Mahmarian (140)	68	60	82
	Fintel (145)	70	55	66
	DePasquale (138)	70	50	88
Tomographic (quantitative)	Tamaki (137)	87	78	92
	Mahmarian (140)	81	77	75
	DePasquale (138)	78	65	89
	Kahn (149)	62	53	64
	Van Train (148)	78	71	83
			Specificity, %	
Planar (subjective)	Lenaers (105)	95	89	88
	Maddahi (132)	92	97	91
	Starling (286)	88	91	97
	Fintel (145)	~90	~90	~90
Planar (quantitative)	Maddahi (132)	85	94	82
Tomographic (subjective)	Tamaki (137)	95	96	89
	Mahmarian (140)	89	96	90
	Fintel (145)	~90	~90	~90
	DePasquale (138)	82	98	81
Tomographic (quantitative)	Tamaki (137)	98	96	93
	Mahmarian (140)	92	91	99
	DePasquale (138)	83	95	87
	Kahn (149)	83	63	71
	Van Train (148)	67	66	65

LAD, left anterior descending artery; CIRC, left circumflex artery; RCA, right coronary artery. Reference number given in parentheses.

vidual coronary arteries compared to subjective planar interpretation.[132] Compared to qualitative planar methods, qualitative interpretation of thallium tomograms has also been found to provide improved detection of individual coronary artery stenoses.[145] Quantitative approaches to thallium tomograms, using either circumferential profiles with thallium washout assessment or a bull's-eye method, have provided improved sensitivity for detection of individual coronary artery stenoses without associated loss of specificity when these methods were compared to both qualitative planar and qualitative tomographic interpretation.[137,140,286,287]

Technetium-99m-sestamibi and ^{201}Tl appear to provide similar detection of segmental myocardial hypoperfusion in the distribution of individual coronary artery stenoses.[149] Kahn et al[149] found superior detection of moderate stenoses (50 to 75 percent) in the distribution of the right coronary artery with ^{99m}Tc sestamibi compared to ^{201}Tl, but confirmation in a larger series is needed. Finally, using exercise ^{99m}Tc sestamibi myocardial perfusion imaging, Ficaro et al[234] found superior diagnostic sensitivity for detection of left anterior descending and left circumflex coronary artery stenoses of 50 percent or greater and superior diagnostic specificity

for right coronary lesions by using visually interpreted attenuation-corrected images compared to uncorrected images. Quantitative interpretation of attenuation-corrected images was also superior to quantitative interpretation of uncorrected images for detection of right coronary artery and left circumflex disease.

Accuracy of Exercise Myocardial Perfusion Scintigraphy in Women

Increased difficulty in interpreting scintigraphic studies in women often results from attenuation of myocardial activity by breast tissue. This problem can be alleviated, in part, by moving the breasts up to minimize attenuation of activity from the left ventricle[288] or by flattening the breasts against the chest wall with a breast binder so that soft-tissue attenuation is more evenly distributed over the heart. A further approach to the reduction of false-positive test results due to breast attenuation in women[289,290] is to consider as abnormal only exercise-induced anteroseptal or anterolateral perfusion abnormalities that show improved resting tracer activity. In women, "fixed" regions of diminished ^{201}Tl activity involving the base of the septum, the anterior wall, or the base of the posterolateral wall are likely to result from breast attenuation artifacts.[291] This approach improves test specificity. However, in one series[289] 5 of 6 women with reduced anteroseptal or anterolateral planar ^{201}Tl distribution plus subjective evidence of tracer redistribution in these areas had no angiographic evidence of CAD, suggesting that even "reversible" postexercise areas of decreased ^{201}Tl activity may occasionally result from soft-tissue attenuation. Fixed thallium defects involving the inferior or posterobasal walls are not likely to result from breast attenuation artifacts[291] but could result from diaphragm attenuation. In women and in men, fixed myocardial perfusion defects involving the anterior wall and the base of the septum are more likely to correspond to myocardial scar than to soft-tissue attenuation if the defect extends into the left ventricular apex. Lower diagnostic sensitivity of exercise ^{201}Tl scintigraphy has been reported in women as compared to men.[146,236] However, it should be pointed out that some authors have used "more stringent criteria for abnormality" in women to avoid false-positive results. The result of doing so is likely to be a decline in true-positive as well as false-positive test results and a fall in sensitivity.

It has been suggested that myocardial perfusion imaging with ^{99m}Tc sestamibi instead of ^{201}Tl should provide improved diagnostic accuracy for detection of CAD in women as a result of less soft-tissue attenuation with the ^{99m}Tc tracer.[292,293] Although breast attenuation artifacts remain a common problem in ^{99m}Tc sestamibi imaging in women,[294] a preliminary report[204] in 115 female patients noted a statistically significant improvement in diagnostic specificity from 59 percent for ^{201}Tl to 82 percent with ^{99m}Tc sestamibi ($p = 0.03$) for detection of coronary artery stenoses of 70 percent or greater without loss of diagnostic sensitivity.

Gated ^{99m}Tc sestamibi images provide a useful approach to the separation of stress and rest fixed anterior wall defects into those with associated preserved anterior wall contraction that are likely a result of breast attenuation, and those fixed defects with no associated contraction of the anterior wall that are likely to correspond to myocardial scar.[205] Gated ^{99m}Tc sestamibi studies are commonly acquired *following* injection of tracer at peak exercise or peak pharmacologic stress, but the gated images are acquired under resting conditions. Therefore, gated ^{99m}Tc sestamibi studies of regional wall motion can prove helpful in identifying myocardial scar versus breast attenuation as the basis for a fixed "perfusion" defect, but may not prove helpful in clarifying whether a reversible anterior wall defect is related to breast attenuation or to reversible myocardial ischemia. In theory, the optimal approach to elimination of breast attenuation artifacts should be accurate attenuation correc-

tion,[234,295] but further validation of current attenuation correction methods in women is needed.

In two studies using planar exercise ^{201}Tl scintigraphy for detection of CAD in a total of 149 women taken off antianginal medication for testing, the diagnostic sensitivities were 75 percent and 79 percent, with specificities of 91 percent and 88 percent, respectively.[289,290] Lower test sensitivity has been observed when ^{201}Tl testing is performed in women who are receiving antianginal drugs at the time of testing,[296] presumably related to prevention of ischemia by drugs. Seven of nine normal exercise thallium scintigrams in women with CAD were observed in those taking propranolol in the series reported by Ceretto et al.[296] Furthermore, reduced diagnostic specificity for CAD has also been reported by Osbakken et al[236] in patients who are receiving propranolol at the time of exercise ^{201}Tl testing. Propranolol use in 39 percent of study patients, as well as posttest selection bias, may have contributed to a relatively low specificity of 65 percent for tomographic exercise ^{201}Tl imaging in a study of 243 female patients by Chae et al.[297] The associated sensitivity of 71 percent is similar to that reported by others with planar ^{201}Tl imaging. However, in a study by Kong et al[298] of 43 women with dipyridamole ^{201}Tl testing, the diagnostic specificity was just 58 percent for CAD detection, suggesting that posttest selection bias and not inadequate stress may more often be responsible for reduced test specificity. Overall, a number of studies have suggested that similar exercise ^{201}Tl scintigraphic accuracy can be achieved in women as compared to men with a similar extent of disease provided that antianginal drugs, particularly beta-adrenergic blockers, are held prior to testing and provided that care is taken to avoid misinterpretation of findings related to attenuation by breast tissue.[236,289–291,296,299]

PATIENTS WITH NONDIAGNOSTIC EXERCISE ECGS

Several studies[124,130,300–302] have documented equivalent diagnostic accuracy of exercise ^{201}Tl scintigraphy in patients with conclusive, compared to nonconclusive, exercise ECG results. In particular, resting ST-segment abnormalities that interfered with the interpretation of exercise ECG changes did not impair the accuracy of exercise ^{201}Tl scintigraphy.[130]

Patients Receiving Cardiac Drugs During Testing

In some series,[124,130,146] equivalent sensitivity and specificity have been found for CAD detection with exercise ^{201}Tl scintigraphy in patients taking propranolol compared to patients not taking propranolol. The hazard of this type of analysis is that patients receiving propranolol may have more severe CAD than untreated patients. For example, patients who have had a previous myocardial infarction are likely to be treated with a beta-adrenergic blocker, but they are also more readily detected by ^{201}Tl scintigraphy than are patients without previous myocardial infarction. The findings of Pohost et al[115] are probably more clinically relevant. The sensitivity and specificity of exercise ^{201}Tl scintigraphy for CAD detection were no different in patients taking propranolol than in patients not taking propranolol provided that they exercised to diagnostic ischemic ST-segment depression. In patients not developing ischemic ST-segment depression with exercise[115] propranolol depressed diagnostic specificity ($p < 0.05$) and sensitivity (p not given). Decreased sensitivity[303] or specificity[236] of exercise ^{201}Tl scintigraphy in patients receiving propranolol has been confirmed by others. Steele et al,[304] Hockings et al,[305] and Narahara et al[306] have presented data from patients with angiographic CAD who were imaged with ^{201}Tl following maximal treadmill exercise while not receiving propranolol and again while receiving propranolol. Propranolol treatment reduced scintigraphic defect size and produced some false-negative tests both with planar and tomographic methods. Based on the results of the available reports, it is concluded that when exercise ^{201}Tl scintigraphy is performed in clinically stable patients for purposes of excluding the presence of CAD, it is desirable that propranolol be discontinued for 48 h prior to testing. In addition, Mahmarian et al[307] showed that transdermal nitroglycerin patch therapy produces a significant reduction in perfusion defect size on tomographic exercise ^{201}Tl images compared to placebo. Few data are available concerning the effect of calcium channel blockers on the diagnostic accuracy of exercise ^{201}Tl scintigraphy. Because the diagnosis of CAD requires the induction of ischemia, these drugs should be withheld for 24 h prior to diagnostic testing.

Level of Exercise During Testing

Exercise ^{201}Tl scintigraphy detects regional hypoperfusion in many patients with angiographic CAD who are unable to exercise to 85 percent of predicted maximal heart rate and who have no exertional ST-segment depression.[114] McLaughlin et al[308] reported results of ^{201}Tl scintigraphy in 8 patients with angiographic CAD who were exercised maximally and were also tested with exercise to 33 to 50 percent of the maximal work load achieved. The extent of coronary lesions was substantial, averaging at least two 50 percent luminal diameter nar-

rowings per patient. Each patient had a ^{201}Tl myocardial perfusion defect at both levels of exercise. However, in these patients the correlation of perfusion defects with diseased arteries increased from 13 of 19 for low-level exercise to 17 of 19 for maximal exercise. The importance of exercise to target heart rate (i.e., to greater than 85 percent of predicted maximal heart rate) for exercise thallium testing has been confirmed in a series of 272 patients studied by Iskandrian et al.[139] The sensitivity of thallium tomography was 88 percent in patients who reached target heart rate or had a positive exercise ECG compared to 73 percent in patients who failed to reach 85 percent of maximal predicted heart rate and did not have a positive exercise ECG ($p < 0.002$). Nevertheless, it appears that exercise ^{201}Tl scintigraphy is superior to exercise ECG in the diagnosis of chest pain in patients who are unable to exercise to 85 percent of predicted maximum heart rate.[309,310]

Effect of Coronary Collateral Vessels

High grade coronary collateral vessels[311] produce dense contrast opacification distal to a highly stenotic or occluded recipient coronary artery segment. Noncompromised coronary collateral vessels arise from a coronary artery with no significant (e.g., greater than 70 percent) narrowing of the luminal diameter. Noncompromised, high grade coronary collateral vessels permit a greater increase in resting regional myocardial blood flow during contrast-induced reactive hyperemia than do lesser grade collateral vessels.[312] Although data have been presented[313] demonstrating that coronary collateral vessels can in some cases prevent myocardial infarction during gradual coronary artery occlusion, the effectiveness of coronary collaterals in preventing exercise-induced ischemia is less clear. In patients undergoing exercise testing with ^{201}Tl, analysis of segments without ECG Q waves demonstrates perfusion defects more frequently in segments with collateral vessels compared to segments without collateral vessels,[314] apparently as a result of coronary collateral development in the regions of most severe myocardial ischemia.[315] Other investigators have found that noncompromised coronary collateral vessels may account for a normal-appearing ^{201}Tl scintigram in segments supplied by severely narrowed coronary arteries, suggesting a protective effect from exercise-induced ischemia.[316-320] Eng et al[320] studied patients with totally occluded coronary vessels subtending noninfarcted collateral-dependent myocardial segments. Nineteen of 41 of these segments manifested no evidence of ischemia with exercise. This "protective effect" of the collateral circulation was more likely to prevent the development of an exercise-induced ^{201}Tl scintigraphic defect in the distribution of the right or left circumflex coronary artery than that of the LAD coronary artery.[320] Iskandrian et al[321] found that noncompromised coronary collaterals reduced ^{201}Tl defect size in single-vessel CAD. In some cases, no exercise-induced perfusion defect occurred in the distribution of right or left circumflex coronary artery stenoses when noncompromised collaterals were present. For single-vessel LAD CAD, collateral circulation reduced the size of exercise-induced ^{201}Tl myocardial defects but did not generally eliminate them.

Causes of Abnormal Exercise [201]Tl Myocardial Perfusion in the Absence of Critical Atherosclerotic Coronary Artery Lesions

SUBCRITICAL CORONARY STENOSES

Brown et al[322] reported the results of exercise ^{201}Tl scintigraphy in 22 symptomatic patients with isolated subcritical coronary artery stenoses defined as a 21 to 40 percent luminal reduction in one or more coronary arteries measured in multiple projections. Thirteen of the 22 patients had an appropriately located ^{201}Tl defect in the distribution of a subcritical stenosis. In comparison, 21 of 28 patients with no coronary artery luminal narrowing greater than 20 percent had normal myocardial perfusion ($p < 0.01$ in contrast to patients with subcritical narrowings). Using a quantitative approach to planar ^{201}Tl imaging, Kaul et al[323] detected perfusion abnormalities in 7 of 8 patients with subcritical (0 to 49 percent) coronary stenoses only. It should be noted that subcritical coronary artery stenoses could, in theory, be flow restricting during exercise in patients with severe left ventricular hypertrophy. Further investigation of myocardial perfusion imaging is needed in patients with only subcritical coronary stenoses; however, the studies should include tomographic myocardial perfusion imaging and quantitative coronary arteriography.

CORONARY ARTERY SPASM

Exercise-induced ^{201}Tl defects have been observed in patients with coronary artery spasm in the absence of a fixed coronary artery stenosis.[324,325] Waters et al[324] described data on 5 patients with no fixed coronary artery stenosis who developed ST-segment elevation in the distribution of observed coronary artery spasm during coronary angiography. In each case, injection of ^{201}Tl during provocation of angina pectoris and ST-segment elevation by treadmill exercise resulted in a correspondingly located ^{201}Tl defect. Left ventricular ^{201}Tl myocardial defects during coronary artery spasm at rest in patients

with no fixed coronary artery stenosis were described by Maseri et al[326] and others.[15,327]

Recently, Nakajima et al[328] have reported the utility of a beta-methyl branched fatty acid, iodine 123 (^{123}I) BMIPP, in the diagnosis and follow-up of coronary artery spasm. Resting tomographic imaging following injection of ^{123}I BMIPP and stress and resting myocardial perfusion imaging with either ^{201}Tl or ^{99m}Tc sestamibi were performed within 1 week following coronary arteriography and a positive provocative test with ergonovine or acetylcholine in 32 patients. Reduced BMIPP activity was present in 25 of 32 patients (78 percent), whereas myocardial hypoperfusion was detected in 10 of 32 patients (31 percent). The authors postulated that unlike myocardial perfusion imaging with ^{201}Tl or ^{99m}Tc sestamibi, ^{123}I BMIPP imaging detected residual metabolic abnormalities from recent episodes of coronary artery spasm. They suggested that tomographic ^{123}I BMIPP imaging may prove helpful to monitor the response of coronary artery spasm to treatment.

LEFT BUNDLE BRANCH BLOCK

Ono et al[329] studied the physiologic correlates of LBBB in a canine model. Left bundle branch block was induced by pacing the heart from the right ventricle. Compared to the control state, during LBBB thickening of the interventricular septum was reduced, as measured by echocardiography. The intramyocardial pressure in the septum during LBBB, as measured by micromanometer catheters, was increased during diastole, likely raising coronary vascular resistance and impeding coronary blood flow. Although there was evidence for reduced coronary blood flow, evidence of septal ischemia was absent. Uptake of ^{18}F fluorodeoxyglucose was reduced and lactate production was absent.

Patients with LBBB and angiographically normal coronary arteries are commonly found to have an exercise-induced ^{201}Tl scintigraphic defect in the anteroseptal area, which returns to normal 4 h later.[330-334] Less frequently, a normal ^{201}Tl scan or a fixed anteroseptal defect may be present. Based on the findings of Ono et al,[329] it is likely that the reversible defects in the septum in patients with LBBB represent mechanical impairment of coronary blood flow resulting from the altered contractile sequence and not myocardial ischemia. Therefore, in patients with LBBB, rest or exercise-induced defects in the anteroseptal region do not accurately predict the presence of ischemia resulting from LAD CAD.[334,335] It appears that exercise-induced ^{201}Tl defects outside the anteroseptal and apical regions are specific for the presence of CAD in patients with LBBB.[331,334] Defects that extend from the anteroseptal segments into the left ventricular apex have been described as specific for the presence of CAD in patients with LBBB[336] but this could not be confirmed by others.[335] Normal rest and exercise ^{201}Tl myocardial scintigrams suggest the absence of angiographic CAD in patients with LBBB.[331,332]

Similar to dynamic exercise, dobutamine stress in combination with myocardial perfusion imaging results in elevated heart rates and anteroseptal perfusion defects in patients with LBBB and unobstructed coronary arteries.[337,338] Currently, the preferred method[339-343] for scintigraphic diagnosis of CAD in the presence of LBBB uses pharmacologic coronary artery vasodilation in place of dynamic exercise. Infusion of dipyridamole or adenosine allows scintigraphic detection of impaired coronary flow reserve without substantially elevating heart rate. This appears to minimize the direct effects of LBBB on septal blood flow. In reported series, pharmacologic stress has substantially improved the specificity of myocardial perfusion imaging compared to exercise testing for detection of CAD in patients with LBBB.[339-341]

In patients with angiographically normal coronary arteries and right bundle branch block, left anterior fascicular block, or Wolff-Parkinson-White syndrome, myocardial perfusion images are generally normal.[330,344] It has been reported in patients with angiographically normal coronary arteries and both right bundle branch block and left axis deviation, that perfusion defects may occur in the septum and inferior wall, but further confirmation is needed.[344]

MYOCARDIAL BRIDGES

The role of transient systolic coronary artery narrowing related to myocardial bridging in the production of exertional myocardial ischemia is unclear. In patients with no fixed coronary arterial stenoses, Ahmad et al[345] found normal exercise ^{201}Tl myocardial perfusion and a normal LVEF response to exercise in 3 patients with a 50 to 75 percent systolic narrowing of the coronary artery. Three of 4 patients with "no significant atherosclerotic disease" and a greater than 75 percent transient systolic narrowing of the coronary artery had a postexercise ^{201}Tl perfusion defect in the distribution of the narrowed coronary artery, and ^{201}Tl perfusion returned to normal 4 to 6 h later. The same 3 patients also had an abnormal response of the LVEF to exercise. Greenspan et al[346] found normal ^{201}Tl myocardial perfusion following exercise in 7 patients with transient systolic narrowing of 60 to 80 percent of the luminal diameter and no fixed coronary obstruction. A preliminary report by Raizner et al[347] described ^{201}Tl myocardial perfusion defects following exercise in the distribution of myocardial bridges in 7 patients. Following surgical interruption of the myocardial bridge in 3 of these patients, the ^{201}Tl scinti-

graphic findings returned to normal and cardiac symptoms were relieved.

ANOMALOUS LEFT CORONARY ARTERY ARISING FROM THE PULMONARY ARTERY

Verani et al[348] reported ^{201}Tl myocardial scintigraphic findings in a 28-year-old woman with anomalous origin of the left coronary artery from the pulmonary artery. Following exercise, hypoperfusion was apparent in the anterior wall of the left ventricle. Repeat postexercise ^{201}Tl scintigrams following surgical implantation of the left coronary artery into the aorta showed improvement but residual anterior wall exercise and resting hypoperfusion. Similar ^{201}Tl scintigraphic findings have been reported following exercise[349] and at rest[350,351] in children with anomalous origin of the left coronary artery from the pulmonary artery.

CHRONIC OBSTRUCTIVE PULMONARY DISEASE

Postexercise planar ^{201}Tl myocardial scintigraphic findings have been reported[352] in 6 selected patients with mild to moderate hypoxemia at rest and physiologic evidence of chronic obstructive pulmonary disease. The coronary arteries were angiographically normal in 5 patients and contained minimal luminal irregularity in a sixth patient. The defects on perfusion imaging corresponded to regions commonly associated with attenuation artifacts. Thus, conclusive evidence that chronic obstructive pulmonary disease is responsible for ^{201}Tl myocardial perfusion defects is not currently available. However, as illustrated in Fig. 2-19, it appears likely that severe right ventricular hypertrophy (e.g., as with cor pulmonale) may be associated with prominent myocardial perfusion tracer activity in the septum, suggesting falsely the presence of reduced perfusion in nonseptal left ventricular segments.

ANGINA PECTORIS WITH ANGIOGRAPHICALLY NORMAL CORONARY ARTERIES

The mechanism by which typical exertional angina pectoris occurs in the absence of (1) fixed coronary artery narrowing, (2) spasm of the epicardial coronary arteries, and (3) noncoronary heart disease is not clearly established. Recent studies suggest that this syndrome may result from reduced vasodilator reserve associated with endothelial dysfunction of the small coronary arteries.[353-360] Opherk et al[353] found no structural changes by myocardial biopsy in the coronary microvasculature. Yet, Wiedermann et al[361] have reported a relationship between the presence of atheromatous plaque or marked intimal thickening by coronary intravascular ultrasound and abnormal coronary vasoconstriction with exercise in patients with angina pectoris and a normal coronary arteriogram. Nonuniform ^{201}Tl myocardial distribution in response to exercise has been reported in numerous studies of patients with angina pectoris and normal coronary arteriograms.[362-365] In one study of 100 patients with typical angina, entirely normal coronary arteriograms, and no evidence of noncoronary heart disease, exercise-induced ST-segment depression was identified in 30 patients and 98 patients had defects on planar exercise ^{201}Tl images.[365] Patients with exercise-induced ST-segment depression had more extensive ^{201}Tl defects. It is difficult to document in these studies whether the perfusion defects were related to impaired endothelium-dependent coronary vasodilation. Epicardial coronary artery spasm was not excluded in most patients and ^{201}Tl defects could have resulted from attenuation or other artifacts. The presence of impaired endothelium-dependent coronary vasodilation was not investigated.

Geltman et al[359] evaluated 17 patients with chest pain and angiographically normal coronary arteries using positron emission tomography (PET) and ^{15}O-labeled water to quantitate coronary flow reserve. Eight of 17 patients had reduced coronary flow reserve (1.4 ± 0.5 versus 3.8 ± 1.1 in normals). Abnormalities of perfusion and perfusion reserve were spatially homogeneous without detectable regional disparities. Nevertheless, in a study by Galassi et al,[366] using PET and ^{15}O-labeled carbon dioxide to measure myocardial blood flow in 13 patients with angina pectoris and a normal coronary arteriogram, heterogeneous regional myocardial blood flow was detected, both at baseline and after dipyridamole. The authors analyzed smaller left ventricular regions of interest than in the Geltman study and postulated that the regional flow inhomogeneity in this syndrome was localized to small myocardial regions.

Legrand et al[367] compared coronary flow reserve, exercise ^{201}Tl scintigraphy, and exercise radionuclide ventriculography in 18 patients with chest pain and angiographically normal coronary arteries. In 9 of these patients, there was a history of chest pain at rest, but ergonovine administration produced coronary artery spasm in only 1 patient. Coronary flow reserve was measured by the flow response to administration of sodium meglumine diatrizoate as assessed by digital subtraction angiography. The coronary flow reserve of arterial distributions with abnormal perfusion or with regional dysfunction was lower ($p < 0.001$) than that of distributions associated with normal radionuclide results. This latter study strongly supports the concept that some patients with angina pectoris, angiographically normal coronary arteries, no evidence of coronary artery spasm, but scintigraphic evidence of impaired regional myocardial blood flow have abnormal regional coronary flow reserve.

LESIONS LIMITED TO THE SECONDARY BRANCHES OF THE CORONARY ARTERIES

Iskandrian et al[368] studied 19 patients with CAD (narrowing of 50 percent or more) confined to a diagonal branch of the LAD artery or to a marginal branch of the circumflex artery. Seven of the 19 patients (37 percent) had an exercise ^{201}Tl perfusion defect that normalized at rest. Iino et al[369] have described characteristic myocardial perfusion defects related to diagonal or marginal branch stenoses assessed by polar representations of ^{201}Tl tomograms.

OTHER CARDIAC DISEASES

Myocardial perfusion scintigraphic findings in valvular heart disease are discussed in Chap. 24, in cardiomyopathy are discussed in Chap. 25, in congenital heart disease are discussed in Chap. 27, and for hypertensive heart disease are discussed in Chap. 21.

SENSITIVITY AND SPECIFICITY OF EXERCISE RADIONUCLIDE VENTRICULOGRAPHY

Criteria for Detection of Coronary Artery Disease

The presence of normal global and regional left ventricular function at rest and with vigorous exercise is required to exclude the presence of CAD by radionuclide ventriculography. Most normal subjects will have a resting LVEF greater than 50 percent.[370] The exercise LVEF must rise by at least an additional 5 percent, with associated normal regional wall motion during peak exercise, to exclude the presence of CAD with a high level of certainty. This criterion, although most widely used, is not the only criterion proposed for separating normal from abnormal exercise LVEF responses. Jones et al[370] reported that for 60 patients with chest pain, angiographically normal coronary arteries, and no other evidence of cardiac disease, the most important predictors of the magnitude of increase in LVEF with exercise were (1) gender, (2) resting LVEF, and (3) rest-to-exercise changes in end-diastolic volume index. Regression equations based on these variables were derived to predict the absolute level of a normal exercise LVEF response for each patient.

In addition to normal global left ventricular function,

Table 20-5   Reported Results of Resting and Exercise Radionuclide Ventriculography for Detection of Coronary Artery Disease

Year	Investigator (Journal)	No. Patients	RWMA		EF		RWMA + EF	
			Sens.	Spec	Sens.	Spec.	Sens.	Spec.
1979	Borer (*Circulation*)	84	59/63	21/21	56/63	21/21	60/63	21/21
1979	Berger (*Am J Med*)	73	41/60	5/5	50/60	5/5	52/60	5/5
1979	Jengo (*Am J Cardiol*)	58	40/42	16/16	36/42	16/16	41/42	16/16
1979	Massie (*Am J Cardiol*)	16	10/10	6/6	9/10	6/6	10/10	6/6
1979	Brady (*Radiology*)	89	52/70	19/19	63/70	19/19	65/70	19/19
1980	Caldwell (*Circulation*)	52	—	—	39/41	6/11	—	—
1980	Slutsky (*Am J Cardiol*)	55	—	—	43/50	2/5	—	—
1981	Jones (*Circulation*)	387	—	—	—	—	256/284	60/103
1981	Uhl (*Circulation*)	32	—	—	11/13	16/19	—	—
1981	Dehmer (*Circulation*)	39	19/33	—	23/33	5/6	—	—
1981	Manyari (*J Appl Physiol*)	39	—	—	32/32	6/7	—	—
1981	Kirshenbaum (*Am Heart J*)	61	27/50	8/11	36/50	6/11	38/50	6/11
	Totals	985	248/328	75/78	398/464	108/126	522/579	133/181
			76%	96%	86%	86%	90%	73%

Note: RWMA, regional wall-motion abnormality at rest or exercise; EF, left ventricular ejection fraction less than 50 percent at rest or increased by less than 5 percent with exercise (except Jones et al[370], see text); SENS, sensitivity; SPEC, specificity (specificity data includes only patients with no angiographic evidence of significant coronary artery disease).

normal subjects have uniform left ventricular regional wall motion. Currently, there is no generally accepted and widely used radionuclide method for quantitating regional wall motion. Variation in cardiac position can produce major changes in apparent regional function based on criteria derived from normal subjects with normal cardiac position. Left ventricular dilation and hypertrophy are common in cardiac patients and also appear to alter left ventricular regional wall motion. For example, regional wall motion determined by contrast angiography is commonly different in patients with left heart failure related to valvular heart disease as compared to normal subjects.[371,372]

Patients with previous anterior wall myocardial infarction will generally have depressed resting LVEF as well as regional left ventricular dysfunction.[373,374] However, in patients with previous inferior or posterior myocardial infarction, resting left ventricular global function may be normal.[374] An isolated pattern of posterior wall left ventricular akinesis observed on a left lateral or left posterior oblique projection may be relatively specific for CAD because this finding is not typical for valvular heart disease or cardiomyopathy. Exercise-induced abnormalities of regional left ventricular function are also relatively specific for the presence of CAD and imply severe disease when they occur at a low heart rate.[375]

In 760 symptomatic patients[370,376–381] with indications for coronary arteriography, the resting and exercise radionuclide ventriculogram was 90 percent sensitive and 73 percent specific for the detection of CAD (Table 20-5). As noted by Rozanski et al,[20] more recent series document an apparent decline in test specificity for the

exercise radionuclide ventriculogram, apparently related to posttest selection bias. Okada et al[22] tabulated the results of seven reported series comparing directly the planar ^{201}Tl scintigram and exercise radionuclide ventriculography for detection of CAD in symptomatic patients. The two tests had similar diagnostic sensitivity but the exercise ^{201}Tl scintigram was more specific for the presence of CAD.

DETECTION OF SEVERE CORONARY ARTERY DISEASE

The exercise radionuclide ventriculogram is seldom normal in patients with either a 50 percent or greater stenosis of the left main coronary artery or significant stenoses of all three coronary arteries. Campos et al[382] detected a resting LVEF less than 50 percent, an increase in end-systolic volume of more than 20 ml during exercise, an exercise LVEF more than 5 percent below the predicted value or an exercise-induced regional wall-motion abnormality in 138 of 150 patients with significant left main or three-vessel disease (sensitivity, 92 percent). In a study of 681 patients who underwent both radionuclide ventriculography and coronary arteriography, Gibbons et al[383] used logistic regression analysis to identify variables that were independently predictive of three-vessel or left main disease. The four most important variables were the magnitude of ST-segment depression, peak exercise LVEF, male gender, and peak exercise rate–pressure product. Combination of these clinical and exercise variables with the exercise LVEF provided better predictive accuracy for the presence of significant left main or three-vessel disease compared to scintigraphic measurements alone.[383]

Wallis and Borer[384] used logistic regression analysis to evaluate the contribution of clinical, exercise, and radionuclide ventriculographic data in the identification of "surgical" coronary anatomy in 175 patients. In 128 of 175 patients (73 percent), a 50 percent or greater stenosis of the left main coronary artery, three vessels, or two vessels including the LAD artery was present. Severe CAD was predicted by the change in blood pressure with exercise, angina class, and exercise LVEF. A derived variable based on both change in blood pressure and change in LVEF proved most predictive. When the LVEF decreased by 10 percent or more with exercise, surgical anatomy was present in 83 percent of patients.[384]

Exercise Radionuclide Ventriculography: Accuracy in Women

Adams et al[385] measured the radionuclide LVEF at rest and during exercise to limiting fatigue in 54 normal volunteers (27 men and 27 women; mean age, 32 years). The mean rise in LVEF from rest to exercise was 14 percentage points in men compared to 7.3 percentage points in women ($p < 0.001$). A less than 5 percent rise in LVEF with exercise was frequently observed in normal female volunteers but not in male volunteers, suggesting lower specificity of the test in women.[385-387] Similarly, Jones et al[370] found poor diagnostic specificity for CAD detection of the first-pass exercise radionuclide angiogram in 56 women with chest pain and indications for coronary arteriography.

Intensity of Exercise

During exercise, radionuclide evidence of global or regional left ventricular dysfunction often precedes ECG ST-segment abnormalities in symptomatic patients with angiographic CAD.[388] Nevertheless, the sensitivity of the radionuclide ventriculogram for CAD detection is strongly dependent on achieving an adequate level of stress. Brady et al[380] studied 77 symptomatic patients with documented CAD. Among 35 of these patients who exercised to chest pain, to at least 1 mm of horizontal ECG ST-segment depression, or to a systolic blood pressure–heart rate product greater than 25,000, a global or regional radionuclide abnormality was found in 33 patients (sensitivity, 94 percent). Among 13 patients who failed to exercise adequately, the sensitivity was only 62 percent. Similarly, Mellendez et al[389] showed that symptomatic patients with CAD may have an initial rise in LVEF with an intermediate level of exercise. Maximal

exercise in the same patients produced a statistically significant fall in LVEF compared to the resting study.

Seaworth studied the effects of reducing the exercise work level at the time of measurement of left ventricular function.[390] In symptomatic men with documented CAD, the mean first-pass radionuclide LVEF fell from 53 percent at rest to 44 percent during peak exercise but then rose to 52 percent if the work load was reduced by a small increment averaging 33 watts. The study findings suggest that a reduction in work load during acquisition of a maximal exercise gated blood pool ventriculogram could result in clinically important overestimation of the exercise LVEF.

It has also been demonstrated that the exercise protocol should permit gradual adaptation to exercise. This is commonly done by beginning exercise at a low work level and gradually increasing the work load every 2 to 3 min. Sudden onset of exercise at high work loads can produce a fall in LVEF in normal subjects compared to resting levels.[391,392]

Effect of Body Position on Exercise Left Ventricular Performance

A number of investigators have performed gated blood pool studies in normal subjects[393] and in patients with CAD, both in the supine and upright positions.[394,395] In general, upright exercise produced higher heart rates and peak heart rate–systolic blood pressure products compared to supine exercise. Exercise duration was similar in both positions. Measurements of LVEF (rest, exercise, or change from rest to exercise) were similar—whether patients were in the upright or supine position—in patients with CAD. In normal subjects, upright LVEF measurements may be greater than, but were generally similar to, supine measurements. The resting left ventricular end-diastolic volume was smaller in the upright compared to the supine position in coronary patients and in normal subjects. During exercise, this continued to be the case for coronary patients. Coronary artery disease was detected by radionuclide ventriculography with equal sensitivity by upright compared to supine exercise.[394,395] Both global and regional wall-motion abnormalities have been detected with equivalent accuracy during supine versus upright exercise.[394,395]

Effect of Coronary Collateral Vessels

Angiographically demonstrated coronary collateral vessels can preserve myocardial function at rest in regions supplied by severely stenotic coronary arteries. Goldberg et al[396] demonstrated that the presence of good collaterals[315] can reduce (or prevent) exercise-induced global and regional left ventricular dysfunction as assessed by radionuclide ventriculography. When the collateral vessel was supplied by an artery containing a 75 percent or greater stenosis (i.e., a jeopardized collateral vessel), a protective effect related to that collateral vessel was less likely to be observed.[396]

Effect of Cardiac Drugs

Antianginal drugs may attenuate the global and regional ischemic response to exercise in patients with CAD, resulting in decreased detection of disease. Beta-adrenergic blockade can also reduce the normal rise in LVEF in response to exercise that is required to noninvasively determine that CAD is absent. The effects of cardiac drugs on radionuclide measures of left ventricular function are discussed in Chap. 17.

Causes of Abnormal Exercise Radionuclide Ventriculograms in the Absence of Atherosclerotic Coronary Artery Disease

ABNORMAL GLOBAL LEFT VENTRICULAR FUNCTION WITH EXERCISE

Port et al[397] observed a decline in the exertional change in LVEF with increasing age. In 24 of 29 healthy volunteers over age 60, the LVEF did not rise by 5 percent with exercise and actually declined with exercise in 21 of 29 subjects. A less than 5 percent rise in LVEF with exercise was also observed by Hitzhusen et al[398] in 34 healthy subjects age 70 or older. Twelve of 34 subjects had "minor" regional wall-motion abnormality with exercise. In the latter study, the presence of CAD was excluded by ^{201}Tl scintigraphy.

Patients with no evidence of CAD and with an elevated (75 percent or more) LVEF at rest not uncommonly have a less than 5 percent rise in LVEF with exercise.[399] A rise in LVEF with exercise of less than 5 percent is also common in patients with a resting LVEF greater than or equal to 75 percent and having CAD, limiting the diagnostic utility of the exercise radionuclide ventriculogram in patients with an elevated resting LVEF.

Conditions that may be associated with an abnormal LVEF response to exercise in the absence of CAD are listed in Table 20-6. A less than normal response of global left ventricular function to exercise is observed in a wide variety of patients with cardiac disease and is not specific for the presence of CAD.

ABNORMAL LEFT VENTRICULAR REGIONAL WALL MOTION WITH EXERCISE

Regional wall-motion abnormalities in response to exercise may be observed in apparently healthy elderly individuals. Port et al[397] observed such abnormalities in approximately 10 percent of asymptomatic volunteers in their sixth decade, increasing to 44 percent of volunteers in their eighth and ninth decades. Although no patient had historical or examination evidence of CAD, this condition was not excluded by arteriography. Similar findings were described by Hitzhusen et al[398] who excluded the presence of CAD by postexercise ^{201}Tl scintigraphy. Regional wall-motion abnormalities have also been described in patients with noncoronary heart disease, including valvular heart disease.[411]

Table 20-6   Conditions That May Be Associated with an Abnormal Left Ventricular Ejection Fraction Response to Exercise in the Absence of Coronary Artery Disease

Conditions	References
Age > 60 years	397, 398
Female gender	370, 385, 386
Beta blockers	See Chap. 17
Sudden exercise	391, 392
Elevated resting ejection fraction	399
Inadequate level of exercise	
Valvular heart disease (e.g., aortic regurgitation, aortic stenosis, mitral regurgitation, mitral valve prolapse)	See Chap. 24
Cardiomyopathy	See Chap. 25
Hypertrophic	
Restrictive	400, 401
Dilated	
Prior myocarditis	
	402
Hypertension	403–405
Congenital heart disease	See Chap. 27
Conduction system abnormality	
Chronic left bundle branch block	406, 407
Rate-dependent left bundle branch block	406
Complete heart block	408
Cystic fibrosis	409
?? chronic obstructive pulmonary disease	410

SUMMARY

The preceding data concerning the accuracy of noninvasive tests for detection of CAD lead to a number of conclusions:

1. Postexercise myocardial perfusion scintigraphy and exercise radionuclide ventriculography provide greater diagnostic sensitivity than does the exercise ECG.

2. For postexercise myocardial perfusion scintigraphy and, in some highly selected populations, exercise

radionuclide ventriculography, this increased sensitivity is not accompanied by loss of diagnostic specificity compared to the exercise ECG.

3. Quantitative planar and tomographic approaches to thallium scintigraphy improve diagnostic sensitivity and specificity compared to qualitative planar methods and reduce interobserver variability in test interpretation.

4. Since exercise tests identify CAD by inducing myocardial ischemia, poor exercise capacity and drugs that prevent myocardial ischemia interfere with test accuracy.

5. The prevalences of coronary and noncoronary heart disease in a study population influence the predictive value of a test result for the presence of CAD.

PREDICTION OF THE PRESENCE OR ABSENCE OF CORONARY DISEASE

The first portion of this chapter considered the accuracy of noninvasive tests for detecting CAD in populations of patients. The next consideration is the prediction of the presence or absence of disease in individual patients. Bayes' theorem can be used to illustrate the process by which such predictions can be made.[412]

Bayes' theorem describes the effect of a test result on the predicted likelihood that disease is present. If an estimate can be made of the likelihood that disease is present before the diagnostic test is performed (pretest likelihood of disease) and if the sensitivity and specificity of the test are known, then a new assessment of the likelihood of disease (posttest likelihood of disease) can be made that incorporates information gained from the test. The posttest likelihood of disease following a positive test result is given by

$$P_2 = \frac{P_1 Se}{P_1 Se + (1 - P_1)(1 - Sp)}$$

where P_1 = pretest likelihood of disease
P_2 = posttest likelihood of disease
Se = sensitivity
Sp = specificity

The posttest likelihood of disease following a negative test result is given by

$$P_2 = \frac{P_1(1 - Se)}{P_1(1 - Se) + (1 - P_1)Sp}$$

Assessment of Pretest Likelihood

In 1979, Diamond and Forrester[53] presented the use of probability analysis in the noninvasive diagnosis of CAD. In that study, the pretest likelihood of disease was assessed from three variables—age, gender, and type of chest pain. The authors summarized the prevalence of angiographically proven CAD in 4952 patients with typical angina, atypical angina, or nonanginal chest pain. In general *typical angina* is substernal in location, related to exertion, and has a usual duration of 2 to 10 min. *Atypical angina* has some but not all of these characteristics. *Nonanginal chest pain* or pain not suggestive of angina pectoris lacks the features of typical angina. Data describing the prevalence of CAD by symptoms were combined by the authors with autopsy data describing the prevalence of CAD by age and gender.

As Diamond and Forrester noted, assessment of the pretest likelihood of disease based on age, gender, and type of chest pain alone may neglect vital additional information. For example, the pretest likelihood of disease in a 32-year-old woman with typical angina is low—approximately 26 percent.[53] However, if that patient has insulin-requiring diabetes mellitus, hypertension, hyperlipidemia, and an abnormal resting ECG, the pretest likelihood of disease will be high. The clinical importance of assessing an adequate number of predictors is demonstrated by the work of Hlatky et al.[413] On a scale from 0 to 100, the likelihood of CAD was assessed in patients with chest pain by three methods, using the coronary arteriogram as the diagnostic standard. One method calculated the likelihood of CAD from a published table of data based on the patient's age, gender, symptoms, and extent of ST-segment change during exercise.[53] A second method calculated the mean likelihood of disease as estimated from clinical, laboratory, and exercise test data by 91 practicing cardiologists. The third method involved calculation of the likelihood of CAD from a computer program (CADENZA) that uses age, gender, coronary risk factors, resting ECG, and multiple exercise measurements.[414] Hlatky et al[413] found that the first method, using only three pretest variables and one exercise test variable, was less accurate than clinical assessment by cardiologists. Computer assessment of disease likelihood by the CADENZA program, using a large number of pretest and exercise test predictors, proved more accurate than the cardiologists' assessment for some subgroups of patients. The authors concluded that an adequate number of pretest predictors is necessary to achieve a diagnostic accuracy using Bayes' theorem that is comparable with that of cardiologists. Nevertheless, it is important that the predictive information provided by each variable be independent of that provided by other variables. Otherwise, the pretest likelihood of CAD will be overestimated, resulting in high sensitivity but reduced specificity for disease prediction.[415]

Continuous Versus Discrete Bayesian Analysis

Rifkin and Hood[416] suggested that *positive* and *negative* are inappropriate terms to describe most stress test results. Instead, results for the exercise ECG, for example, should be interpreted as a continuum of risk based on the number of millimeters and morphology of ST-segment depression. This observation was confirmed by Diamond et al,[417] who demonstrated a 41 percent increase in the information content of the exercise ECG when the specific magnitude of ST-segment depression is analyzed as opposed to a single, categorical 1-mm criterion. Similarly, Christopher et al[418] demonstrated that the diagnostic and prognostic information obtained from exercise radionuclide angiography was substantially greater when the likelihood of CAD was predicted from continuous variables (rest and exercise LVEF and end-systolic volume during exercise) compared to their previously determined discrete criteria for separating a positive or negative test result.

A second aspect of the continuous versus discrete test result is the level of certainty associated with the test findings. Consider a postexercise thallium scintigram from a patient with atypical angina. If two experienced readers interpret the scintigram as normal but two other experienced readers consider the test to be abnormal, then—regardless of the final reported result—the actual posttest likelihood of disease should change little from the pretest likelihood. In contrast, a scintigram that four observers agree demonstrates multiple distinct regions of decreased initial thallium distribution, accompanied by abnormal pulmonary thallium activity and evidence of thallium redistribution 4 h later, should substantially alter the posttest likelihood of disease. The most accurate effect of test results on the posttest likelihood of disease should occur when noninvasive test results are described as a continuous variable and the level of certainty of the test outcome is also considered.

Incremental Value

Before diagnostic testing is performed, extensive clinical information is already available. If a diagnostic test is to have clinical value, it must provide information that is not already available from assessment of clinical variables (e.g., age, gender, presence of diabetes, type of chest pain). Furthermore, exercise radionuclide imaging studies routinely incorporate exercise ECG assessment. Data from the exercise ECG test provide a statistically significant increase in diagnostic information regarding the presence and extent of CAD beyond that provided by standard clinical variables. Therefore, exercise ECG test variables (e.g., millimeters of ST-segment depression, exercise peak heart rate) provide incremental value in the assessment of CAD.[419–421] To provide clinically useful diagnostic information, exercise radionuclide imaging must provide incremental information beyond that already available from clinical data and beyond that which is obtained routinely and at lower cost from the concomitant exercise ECG test.

Morise et al[421] evaluated clinical, exercise ECG, and exercise ^{201}Tl tomographic data in 213 patients and developed incremental logistic algorithms designed to optimize noninvasive assessment of CAD presence and extent. The algorithms were then applied in a validation population of 865 patients at four centers. Predictive clinical variables included age, gender, cardiac symptoms, cholesterol level, diabetes, and smoking. Predictive exercise test variables included millimeters of ST-segment depression, downsloping ST-segment morphology, negative ST-segment response to exercise, peak heart rate, and change in systolic blood pressure from rest to peak exercise. Predictive exercise scintigraphic variables included scintigraphic evidence of hypoperfusion, absence of any perfusion defect, and evidence for defect reversibility. In the detection of disease presence (defined as at least one coronary stenosis greater than or equal to 50 percent of the luminal diameter), exercise ^{201}Tl imaging provided incremental value beyond clinical and exercise ECG data, both in men and in women. Incremental value of exercise ^{201}Tl imaging was also found in the detection of multivessel disease in patients of either gender. This confirms earlier findings of Oosterhuis et al[422] concerning the incremental value of exercise ^{201}Tl scintigraphy for establishing the presence and extent of coronary disease. Palmas et al[423] have demonstrated incremental value of data from ^{99m}Tc sestamibi imaging, beyond the information available from the exercise ECG, for diagnosis of multivessel CAD. Unfortunately, clinical variables were not considered in the predictive model for detection of multivessel disease. In addition to data from scintigraphic images of the myocardium, it has been shown that assessment of a ratio of lung-to-heart ^{201}Tl activity provides further incremental information concerning the presence of three-vessel or left main CAD.[424]

In addition to the incremental diagnostic value associated with exercise myocardial perfusion imaging, incremental prognostic value in patients with known or suspected CAD has also been demonstrated in multiple studies.[420,425–428] When the resting ECG is abnormal, the exercise myocardial perfusion scintigram is particularly likely to provide incremental prognostic data. However, in patients with a normal resting ECG, Christian et al[427] found little additional prognostic information from ^{201}Tl scintigraphy beyond that available from clinical and exercise ECG data. This is consistent with their previous observation that exercise radionuclide ventriculography provided little incremental diagnostic information in patients with a normal resting ECG beyond that derived from clinical and exercise ECG data.[429] Hachamovitch et al[425] observed incremental prognostic value of data from exercise dual-isotope myocardial perfusion images in a study of 2200 consecutive patients. Their study did consider whether the resting ECG was normal or abnormal[425]; however, patients with a normal resting ECG were not studied as a separate population.

A Reasonable Threshold for Deciding That Coronary Disease is Present or Absent

A potentially difficult aspect of the Bayesian approach to clinical decision making is the translation of a posttest likelihood of disease into a clinical course of action. If, for example, a 17-percent posttest likelihood of disease is found, several possible courses of action are available. First, the presence of CAD may be considered to be unlikely and no further diagnostic or therapeutic steps are taken. This course might be taken in the case of a patient thought to have only an intermediate likelihood of disease prior to testing, particularly if the patient had multiple severe medical problems, was a poor candidate for revascularization therapy, and had symptoms not so severe as to demand treatment. A second course in a different patient with a 17-percent posttest likelihood might be to do another noninvasive test to further exclude the presence of disease. Finally, if the 17-percent posttest likelihood of disease occurred in a young woman with typical angina and the noninvasive studies had been contradictory[430] or inconclusive, it might be elected to perform coronary arteriography.

For clinical decision making using Bayes' theorem, a threshold for decision making must be assumed. Perhaps the most widely used threshold is that proposed by Diamond et al.[431] In that study, 15 different combinations of four noninvasive tests provided a total of 645 estimates of posttest likelihood for 12 patients without subsequent angiographic evidence of CAD and 31 patients with CAD. Of the 645 posttest likelihood estimates, 441 consisted of a likelihood that was either less than 10 percent or greater than 90 percent. In 421 of these 441 likelihood estimates, the presence or absence of CAD was correctly identified (predictive accuracy, 95.5 percent). For the remainder of this discussion it will be assumed that a posttest likelihood less than 10 percent excludes the presence of CAD and a posttest likelihood greater than 90 percent demonstrates that disease is present. Although generally acceptable, there are instances in the course of clinical care when this level of certainty might not be acceptable to a clinician or a patient.

Infrequently, a patient with a very low posttest likelihood of disease (i.e., less than 10 percent) will have angiographically significant CAD but will not be treated as a result of Bayesian assessment. Diamond et al[414] have shown that when CAD is present in a patient with a very low posttest likelihood of disease, the disease is likely not to be multivessel and the patient has a favorable 1-year prognosis. Similarly, Christopher et al[418] prospectively assessed the posttest likelihood of CAD by exercise radionuclide ventriculography in 250 men. All 29 patients who died during a 35-month follow-up period had a posttest likelihood of CAD of 95 percent or greater. Even when Bayesian analysis led to an inaccurate assessment of the presence or absence of CAD, the outcome was accurately predicted.

Dans et al[432] retrospectively analyzed the pretest and posttest likelihood of CAD from the clinical history, exercise ECG, thallium scintigram, and coronary arteriogram in 96 patients with no documented myocardial infarction. Thirty-five of 36 patients with a preangiogram Bayesian likelihood less than or equal to 10 percent had no coronary luminal diameter narrowing of 50 percent or greater. Fifty-three of 60 patients (88 percent) with a preangiogram Bayesian likelihood greater than 10 percent had significant CAD by angiography. The authors concluded that a very low preangiogram Bayesian likelihood of CAD could have been successfully used to advise patients against coronary arteriography in their study. Patients having a less than 10 percent preangiogram likelihood of disease and a greater than or equal to 50 percent angiographic coronary artery narrowing have generally been found to have single-vessel CAD and a favorable 1-year prognosis.[431–433]

Test Selection for the Detection of Coronary Artery Disease

The calculation of disease likelihood using Bayes' theorem has led to a number of important observations concerning test selection. One important observation is that the posttest likelihood of disease can be altered most from the pretest likelihood in patients with an intermediate pretest likelihood of disease.[434,435] This concept is illustrated in Fig. 20-4. When the pretest likelihood of disease is high (e.g., 92 percent in a 55-year-old man with typical angina), a noninvasive test response indicative of disease will increase the likelihood of disease only slightly (e.g., 1 mm of horizontal ST-segment depression on the exercise ECG will raise the posttest likelihood to 98 percent). In a 65-year-old woman with atypical angina and a pretest likelihood of CAD of 54 percent, 1 mm of horizontal ST-segment depression with exercise will result in an 80 percent posttest likelihood of disease.[53] Noninvasive tests with a high level of sensitivity and specificity (e.g., postexercise myocardial scintigraphy) will have a greater influence on posttest likelihood than a less sensitive and specific test (e.g., exercise electrocardiography).

Figures 20-5 and 20-6 illustrate the effects of exercise

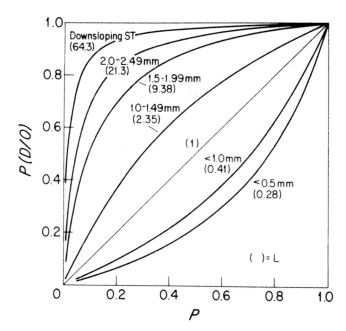

Figure 20-4 Posttest likelihood of coronary artery disease P (D/O) following exercise ECG testing as a function of the pretest likelihood (P). Curves are plotted for varying levels of ECG ST-segment depression. Greater degrees of ST-segment depression produce an increasing likelihood ratio (L) that coronary disease is present. For any given level of ST-segment change with exercise, the posttest likelihood will be altered most in comparison to the pretest likelihood for patients with an intermediate pretest likelihood of disease. (From Rifkin and Hood,[416] reproduced by permission.)

1. The pretest likelihood could be more accurately defined by considering a larger number of independent variables predictive of CAD.
2. Pretest or posttest selection biases may have altered the apparent test sensitivity and specificity.
3. No estimate of the level of certainty of noninvasive test results has been made or incorporated into the calculation of posttest likelihood.
4. For simplicity of presentation, only limited data from noninvasive tests are used (i.e., positive or negative results rather than the number of millimeters and morphology of ST-segment depression, percentage of the myocardial circumference with impaired perfusion, percentage change in radionuclide ventriculographic ejection fraction with exercise, etc.). Also, confounding factors such as baseline ST-segment abnormalities prior to exercise ECG are not addressed by the examples illustrated in Figs. 20-5 and 20-6.
5. The threshold for inclusion or exclusion of CAD may vary from patient to patient and may be different from the threshold for deciding on the use of a specific therapy such as coronary artery bypass surgery. With these limitations in mind, certain general observations may be made regarding test selection for patients with a high, low, or intermediate pretest likelihood of disease.

ECG and radionuclide test results on the likelihood of CAD. Pretest likelihood is computed from angiographic and autopsy data compiled by Diamond and Forrester.[53] The respective sensitivities and specificities used in preparing this table are 72 and 79 percent for the exercise ECG, 84 and 88 percent for the postexercise thallium scintigram, and 90 and 73 percent for the exercise radionuclide ventriculogram. It is assumed that when the posttest likelihood of disease is less than 10 percent or greater than 90 percent, a clinical decision can reasonably be made.[431] The posttest likelihood is computed from Bayes' theorem, first using the exercise ECG alone, provided that the resultant posttest likelihood of disease falls into one of the two extreme deciles. This initial approach reflects the low cost and general availability of the exercise ECG. Patients with an intermediate pretest likelihood of disease are tested with both the exercise ECG and the postexercise thallium scan (see Fig. 20-5)[436–438] or, alternatively, by exercise radionuclide ventriculography (see Fig. 20-6).

As the data from Figs. 20-5 and 20-6 are used to illustrate the test selection process, a number of limitations of this type of analysis must be kept in mind:

HIGH PRETEST LIKELIHOOD

In a patient with a high pretest likelihood (greater than 68 percent) of CAD, typical angina is usually present and further diagnostic efforts are often directed at determining the extent of disease with coronary arteriography. In patients with a high pretest likelihood of CAD and minimal or no symptoms on medical management, noninvasive testing can provide a valuable alternative to coronary arteriography for assessing cardiac prognosis. In this setting, a normal exercise ^{201}Tl scan predicts a favorable cardiac prognosis similar to that observed in patients presenting with chest pain and having a normal coronary arteriogram.[439] Conversely, a high-risk myocardial perfusion scan with reversible defects in multiple coronary artery distributions, increased pulmonary ^{201}Tl activity, or transient left ventricular cavity dilation suggests a substantial likelihood that three-vessel or left main CAD is present. Coronary arteriography and consideration for coronary revascularization should be given to the patient with a high-risk myocardial perfusion scintigram even if symptoms are controlled on medical therapy.[440]

Not all patients with typical angina have a high pretest likelihood of disease. A 35-year-old woman with typical angina will have a pretest likelihood of approximately 26 percent.

	NONANGINAL PAIN		ATYPICAL ANGINA		TYPICAL ANGINA	
	Men	Women	Men	Women	Men	Women
30–39	5.2 T-ECG(–) 1.9	0.8 T-ECG(–) 0.3	22.2 T-ECG(–) 9.2	4.2 T-ECG(–) 1.5	69.7 T-ECG(+) TH(+) 98.2	25.8 T-ECG(–) TH(–) 2.2
40–49	14.1 T-ECG(–) 5.5	2.8 T-ECG(–) 1.0	46.1 T-ECG(–) TH(–) 5.2	13.3 T-ECG(–) 5.2	87.3 T-ECG(+) 95.9	55.2 T-ECG(–) TH(–) 7.4
50–59	21.5 T-ECG(–) 8.8	8.4 T-ECG(–) 3.1	58.9 T-ECG(–) TH(–) 8.5	32.4 T-ECG(–) TH(–) 3.0	92.0 T-ECG(+) 97.5	79.4 T-ECG(+) 93.0
60–69	28.1 T-ECG(–) TH(–) 2.5	18.6 T-ECG(–) 7.5	67.1 T-ECG(+) TH(+) 98.0	54.4 T-ECG(–) TH(–) 7.1	94.3 T-ECG(+) 98.3	90.6 T-ECG(+) 97.1

Figure 20-5   Posttest likelihood of CAD following testing by treadmill exercise ECG with or without postexercise thallium scintigraphy. The effects of noninvasive testing are illustrated by decades of age (*horizontal lines*) and by chest pain description and gender (*vertical columns*). The top number in each square represents the pretest likelihood of CAD for the selected age, gender, and chest pain description.[53] A noninvasive test (or tests) is then selected which, if normal, will reduce the posttest likelihood of CAD to less than 10 percent. This test selection may consist of the treadmill ECG (T-ECG) alone (*white squares*) or in combination with postexercise thallium (TH) scintigraphy (*light gray squares*). The posttest likelihood of CAD is displayed at the bottom of each square. When the pretest likelihood of CAD is relatively high (in this table, greater than 67 percent), the posttest likelihood following negative test results will remain greater than 10 percent and it is assumed that CAD has not been adequately excluded. Therefore, the posttest likelihood is given following confirmation of the presence of CAD (greater than 90 percent posttest probability) by an abnormal treadmill ECG alone (*black squares*) or by a combination of abnormal exercise tests (*dark gray squares*). Calculation of posttest likelihood is based on a sensitivity for the treadmill ECG of 72 percent with a specificity of 79 percent and on a sensitivity for the postexercise thallium scintigram of 84 percent with a specificity of 88 percent. The assumptions and limitations of this type of tabulation are discussed in the text.

VERY LOW PRETEST LIKELIHOOD

In asymptomatic men and women without risk factors for CAD, the prevalence of CAD is very low. For an individual patient, the likelihood of disease may be so low (less than 10 percent) that no testing for CAD detection may be appropriate. If a population of asymptomatic patients with a 5 percent prevalence of CAD is tested using exercise ECG, the majority of abnormal test results will be falsely positive for the presence of CAD.[434] If the asymptomatic individuals under consideration have one or more risk factors for CAD, then the pretest likelihood of disease will rise and the predictive value of an abnormal noninvasive test result will also rise.[441]

LOW PRETEST LIKELIHOOD

In many patients with chest pain not suggestive of angina pectoris and in many asymptomatic patients with coronary risk factors, the pretest likelihood of CAD is low (10 to 25 percent). As shown by Figs. 20-5 and 20-6, a normal exercise ECG in this population will produce a posttest likelihood of CAD that is less than 10 percent and further testing for CAD is usually unnecessary.

In contrast, an abnormal noninvasive test result will usually prove less helpful in this group of patients with a low pretest likelihood. For example, in a 55-year-old man with chest pain not suggestive of angina and a 22 percent likelihood of CAD, the posttest likelihood following an abnormal exercise ECG will be 48 percent, leaving considerable diagnostic uncertainty.

INTERMEDIATE PRETEST LIKELIHOOD

Most patients with atypical angina have an intermediate (25 to 68 percent) likelihood of CAD. An intermediate pretest likelihood may also be observed in very young

	NONANGINAL PAIN		ATYPICAL ANGINA		TYPICAL ANGINA	
	Men	Women	Men	Women	Men	Women
30–39	5.2 T–ECG(–) 1.9	0.8 T–ECG(–) 0.3	22.2 T–ECG(–) 9.2	4.2 T–ECG(–) 1.5	69.7 RIV(+) T–ECG(+) 96.3	25.8 RIV(–) 4.5
40–49	14.1 T–ECG(–) 5.5	2.8 T–ECG(–) 1.0	46.1 RIV(–) T–ECG(–) 4.0	13.3 T–ECG(–) 5.2	87.3 T–ECG(+) 95.9	55.2 RIV(–) T–ECG(–) 5.6
50–59	21.5 T–ECG(–) 8.8	8.4 T–ECG(–) 3.1	58.9 RIV(–) T–ECG(–) 6.5	32.4 RIV(–) 6.2	92.0 T–ECG(+) 97.5	79.4 T–ECG(+) 93.0
60–69	28.1 RIV(–) 5.1	18.6 T–ECG(–) 7.5	67.1 RIV(–) T–ECG(–) 9.0	54.4 RIV(–) T–ECG(–) 5.5	94.3 T–ECG(+) 98.3	90.6 T–ECG(+) 97.1

Figure 20-6 Posttest likelihood of CAD following testing by treadmill exercise ECG and radionuclide ventriculography (RIV). The format is similar to that of Fig. 20-5. The radionuclide ventriculogram is assumed to have a diagnostic sensitivity of 90 percent and a specificity of 73 percent (see text).

patients with typical angina or in elderly men with chest pain not suggestive of angina. In patients with an intermediate pretest likelihood of CAD, an unacceptable level of diagnostic uncertainty will often remain whether or not 1 mm of horizontal ST-segment depression occurs on an exercise ECG.

In patients with an intermediate pretest likelihood, a noninvasive test that compares favorably to the exercise ECG in terms of sensitivity and specificity is needed (see Figs. 20-5 and 20-6). Alternatively, multiple noninvasive tests may be used. However, the use of multiple noninvasive tests can be disadvantageous. Multiple tests increase the cost of noninvasive testing and may delay diagnosis. Most importantly, conflicting noninvasive test results offer little useful diagnostic information.[442] For these reasons, it is not surprising that diagnostic strategies using thallium scintigraphy alone[443,444] or in combination with the exercise ECG[445] provided a more effective approach to the diagnosis of CAD compared to the treadmill ECG alone in patients with an intermediate pretest likelihood in reported series.

Gitler et al[446] studied the ordering patterns for exercise ECG and thallium testing in their hospital. Although combined testing produced the greatest shifts in disease likelihood in subjects with an intermediate pretest likelihood, the tests were most often applied in patients at the extremes of pretest likelihood. The authors concluded that clinicians "appear to value confirmatory test results in patients at the extremes of pretest disease likelihood."

A guide to exercise test selection based on Bayes' theorem is shown in Table 20-7.

Should Patient Care Decisions Be Made on the Basis of Bayesian Analysis?

Although progress has been made in the development of both Bayesian likelihood analysis and multivariate discriminant analysis[447] for the diagnosis of CAD, further data are needed before these approaches can be recommended for routine clinical use except, perhaps, as a supplemental aid to guide clinical judgment.[448,449] Despite the detailed approach taken by Hlatky et al,[413] computer-assisted likelihood calculations for CAD prediction achieved substantially less than 100 percent diagnostic accuracy and were only slightly more accurate as compared to the subjective judgment of cardiologists. In the subgroup of patients with atypical angina and a positive exercise ECG, computer-assisted Bayesian analysis offered no advantage over the cardiologists' judgment. Furthermore, the clinical value of likelihood analysis for CAD assessment in terms of patient outcome has not been clearly demonstrated. Hlatky and associates[413] pointed out that further studies were needed to determine whether these methods could improve patient care by reducing needless tests or by ensuring that findings suggestive of CAD are not overlooked.

Table 20-7 Test Selection for Determining the Presence or Absence of Coronary Artery Disease in Symptomatic, Clinically Stable Patients Aged 30 to 69 Years

Pretest Likelihood	Examples[a]	Recommended Test(s)
Very low (<10%)	Women <60 years or men <40 years and "nonanginal" chest pain	None (If confirmatory test needed, exercise ECG[b] recommended)
Low (10%–25%)	Men 40–59 years or women 60–69 years and "nonanginal" chest pain Men 30–39 years or women 40–49 years and atypical angina	Exercise ECG[b]
Moderate (25%–68%)	Men ≥40 years or women ≥ 50 years and atypical angina. Men ≥ 60 years and "nonanginal" chest pain. Women < 50 years and typical angina	Postexercise thallium scintigram or exercise radionuclide ventriculogram[c]
High (68%–100%)	Men ≥ 30 years or women ≥ 40 years and typical angina	Cardiac catheterization. (Alternatively,[d] combined exercise ECG and thallium scintigram)

Note: Test selection based in part on data presented in Figs. 20-5 and 20-6.
[a] Typical examples. This may not apply to similar patients with severe risk factors. Illustrations assume that the patient is able to exercise to target heart rate or double product. In patients who are unable to exercise adequately dipyridamole thallium testing will generally be more helpful than exercise testing.
[b] For patients without baseline ECG abnormality who are able to exercise vigorously.
[c] For patients with the conditions listed in Table 20-6, postexercise ^{201}Tl scintigraphy will usually be preferred to exercise radionuclide ventriculography. In obese patients exercise radionuclide ventriculography is often preferable. Exercise ECG data also evaluated.
[d] Assignment to high- and low-risk subsets of patients with typical angina and minimal or no symptoms on medical management.

What Should Be the Basis for Patient Care Decisions?

During the decades of the 1970s and 1980s, a major emphasis was placed on the use of noninvasive stress tests for estimating likelihood of the presence or absence of angiographic CAD. To the extent that patients with nonsurgical as well as surgical CAD may be benefitted by symptomatic relief of ischemic symptoms with coronary revascularization, this goal remains valid in the 1990s. However, there is now an increasing emphasis on cost containment in the delivery of health care. In the absence of convincing evidence that revascularization therapy with coronary artery bypass surgery or percutaneous transluminal coronary angioplasty improves survival in most patients with one-vessel or two-vessel coronary disease,[450] an increasing value will be placed on the abilities of noninvasive stress tests to predict the presence of surgical CAD and to assess cardiac prognosis. A combi-

nation of clinical, exercise, and radionuclide variables can provide useful stratification of patients to low-risk groups in which maximal medical therapy may be the most appropriate initial approach and to high-risk groups in which invasive studies and revascularization therapy may be most appropriate.

The available literature suggests that in most instances the best selection of noninvasive cardiac stress tests is the same whether the goal of testing is to assess the likelihood that CAD is present or absent (e.g., by Bayesian analysis), to identify patients with severe CAD who are best treated by revascularization therapy, or to assess cardiac prognosis as a basis for further diagnosis or treatment (Table 20-8). Depending on which of these diagnostic goals is pursued, different diagnostic information from the noninvasive tests may be applied. For example, if the goal of noninvasive testing is the identification of patients with surgical CAD for revascularization, then the presence of reversible perfusion defects in the distributions of multiple coronary arteries, pulmonary thallium uptake, and transient left ventricular cavity dilation would lead to coronary arteriography and consideration of revascularization. In this setting, a single small perfusion defect or a fixed, severe perfusion defect indicative of myocardial scar might indicate the appropriateness of medical therapy without initial coronary arteriography. Future studies are needed to document the cost effectiveness of the tests used to diagnose and guide treatment of CAD.[451,452]

MYOCARDIAL PERFUSION SCINTIGRAPHY VERSUS EXERCISE RADIONUCLIDE VENTRICULOGRAPHY IN THE DETECTION OF CORONARY DISEASE

Often, the choice between exercise radionuclide tests will be based on test availability and accuracy in the clinician's hospital. The choice between stress nuclear testing and stress echocardiography is discussed in detail in Chap. 21. Exercise radionuclide ventriculography is best avoided in patients who are likely to have an abnormal test result in the absence of CAD. Therefore, to diagnose CAD, patients over age 60, patients with an elevated resting LVEF at rest, patients with atrial fibrillation, and patients with hypertensive, valvular, or myocardial disease are usually better candidates for testing with postexercise myocardial perfusion scintigraphy. Patients with frequent premature beats require computer exclusion of premature beats and compensatory pauses. If this computer function is not available, then postexercise myocardial perfusion scintigraphy is the preferred method of testing. In patients with limited exercise capacity or in whom beta-adrenergic blockers cannot be safely withheld, myocardial perfusion imaging following

Table 20-8 Comparison of Noninvasive Test Selections

Pretest Likelihood	Presence or Absence of Coronary Disease (Bayes' Theorem)	Detection of Disease for Which Revascularization Improves Outcome	Prognostic Outcome
Very Low			
<10%	No test required	No test required	No test required
Low			
10–25% (normal rest ECG)	Exercise ECG[a]	Exercise ECG[a]	Exercise ECG[a]
10–25% (abnormal rest ECG)	Exercise imaging[a]	Exercise imaging[a]	Exercise imaging[a]
Moderate			
25–68% (normal rest ECG)	Exercise imaging[a]	Exercise ECG[a]	Exercise ECG or exercise imaging[a]
25–68% (abnormal rest ECG)	Exercise imaging[a]	Exercise imaging[a]	Exercise imaging[a]
High			
68–100% (symptomatic)	Coronary arteriogram	Coronary arteriogram	Coronary arteriogram
68–100% (asymptomatic)	Exercise imaging[a]	Exercise imaging[a]	Exercise imaging[a]

[a] Pharmacologic stress if patient unable to exercise to target heart rate

dipyridamole administration will generally be more productive than exercise radionuclide ventriculography. Because of difficulties related to soft-tissue attenuation of ^{201}Tl, exercise radionuclide ventriculography or ^{99m}Tc myocardial perfusion imaging may be preferable to ^{201}Tl scintigraphy in very obese patients.

EVALUATION OF PATIENTS WITH ABNORMAL EXERCISE ELECTROCARDIOGRAMS

The clinical implications of an abnormal exercise ECG strongly depend on the pretest likelihood of CAD.[434] In an asymptomatic 45-year-old man with a pretest likelihood of 5.5 percent, 1 mm of horizontal ST-segment depression with exercise will produce a posttest likelihood of 16.6 percent. A normal postexercise thallium scintigram will then yield a posttest likelihood of 3.5 percent. Therefore, in a patient with a very low pretest likelihood followed by an abnormal exercise ECG, a normal postexercise thallium scintigram will exclude the presence of CAD with a high level of certainty. This observation has been confirmed in a clinical study by Uhl et al.[453] If the same patient develops 2.5 mm of horizontal ST-segment depression with exercise, the posttest likelihood following exercise ECG will be 56

percent. A normal postexercise thallium scintigram will reduce the posttest likelihood of CAD to 19 percent, which, in some cases, may not produce a sufficient level of diagnostic certainty to enable the clinician to reassure the patient that no further evaluation is required.

In a 55-year-old man with atypical angina and an intermediate pretest likelihood (58.9 percent) of CAD, 1 mm of horizontal ST-segment depression will produce a posttest likelihood of 83.1 percent. If a postexercise thallium scintigram is performed and is normal, the posttest likelihood will fall to 47.2 percent. Therefore, in a patient with an intermediate pretest likelihood, a normal thallium scintigram will provide less insight as to whether the exercise ECG result was a true-positive or a false-positive result.

Finally, consider a 65-year-old man with typical angina pectoris and a pretest likelihood of CAD of 94.3 percent. If an abnormal exercise ECG is found with 1 mm of horizontal ST-segment depression, the posttest likelihood will be 98.3 percent. At this point, a normal postexercise thallium scintigram will reduce the posttest likelihood to 91.2 percent. Therefore, in a patient with a high pretest likelihood and an abnormal exercise ECG, exercise radionuclide testing will add little additional information concerning the presence or absence of CAD, although such testing may provide useful information concerning the extent of CAD and the location of individual lesions.

UNSTABLE ANGINA PECTORIS

Unstable angina pectoris is a heterogeneous group of chest pain syndromes that includes (1) crescendo angina, in which preexisting chest pain has become more frequent, more severe, more prolonged, or more easily provoked; (2) angina pectoris that occurs at rest as well as with activity; and (3) angina of recent onset (usually within 1 month) that is brought on with mild exertion. In the National Cooperative Study of Unstable Angina Pectoris,[454] it was found that patients with this syndrome could be managed acutely with intensive medical care, including the administration of nitrates and propranolol. This produced adequate early control of chest pain in most patients, with no increase in myocardial infarction or mortality compared to patients randomized to early surgical therapy. Elective cardiac surgery could be performed at a later time with low risk and good clinical results in patients with persistent angina despite intensive medical therapy. Although most patients with unstable angina pectoris can be stabilized in the coronary care unit, the subsequent natural history of this condition has been less favorable. Approximately 16 to 21 percent of patients with an episode of unstable angina have been reported to develop a myocardial infarction within 3 months,[455,456] and the mortality at 1 year has been reported to be 15 to 18 percent.[456,457] Although the clinical course with medical management of unstable angina appears to have improved over the years,[454] the continued high morbidity and mortality have led to the use of early coronary arteriography following initial stabilization by medical therapy. The coronary arteriographic findings have generally shown a similar percentage of patients having single-, double-, and triple-vessel severe (greater than 70 percent narrowing of the luminal diameter) CAD.[454,458] Approximately 10 percent of patients with a recent episode of unstable angina are found to have no significant coronary artery stenosis. Also, 10 to 15 percent of patients with unstable angina are found to have a greater than 50 percent stenosis of the left main coronary artery.

Resting ^{201}Tl myocardial perfusion imaging has been performed within hours following resting chest pain in patients with unstable angina. Resting scintigraphic defects have correlated well with the location of significant coronary artery stenosis and with the occurrence of in-hospital cardiac events.[459–462] Gregoire and Theroux[463] evaluated 43 patients with a presumptive diagnosis of unstable angina by injecting ^{99m}Tc sestamibi during chest pain. The presence or absence of a perfusion defect on ^{99m}Tc sestamibi images provided a sensitivity of 96 percent and specificity of 79 percent for detection of a 50 percent or greater coronary artery stenosis on angiography. In contrast, transient ECG ischemic changes during chest pain had a sensitivity of 35 percent and specificity

of 68 percent for CAD detection. Diagnostic exercise ECG, exercise myocardial perfusion imaging, and dipyridamole perfusion scintigraphy[255] have been safely performed after exclusion of acute myocardial infarction and after a pain-free period of at least 1 to 3 days following unstable angina in patients receiving medical treatment. Exercise-induced ST-segment depression, exercise-induced chest pain, and the extent of the stress-induced thallium myocardial perfusion defect have all been correlated with the extent of coronary artery stenosis.[464–467] However, in medically stabilized patients presenting with an unstable pattern of otherwise typical angina pectoris, no role has been satisfactorily demonstrated for the use of noninvasive diagnostic testing in place of coronary arteriography. On the other hand, following medical stabilization in patients presenting with an "unstable pattern" of chest pain that is subsequently thought not to be consistent with angina pectoris, exercise testing provides a potential alternative to coronary arteriography as a method of diagnosis.

SILENT ISCHEMIA

Increasingly, silent myocardial ischemia is being recognized as a major clinical factor in the diagnosis and prognosis of CAD.[468,469] Silent myocardial ischemia may be documented as transient left ventricular regional wall-motion abnormality or transient ischemic ST-segment changes in the absence of angina or usual angina equivalents.[468] It is a common phenomenon, occurring in approximately 2 to 15 percent of apparently healthy middle-aged men.[61,470–475] The pathophysiology of silent ischemic episodes is uncertain, but silent ischemia may result either from episodes of increased myocardial oxygen demand or diminished myocardial oxygen supply (e.g., coronary vasoconstriction).

The prognosis associated with silent ischemia appears to be similar to the prognosis of symptomatic myocardial ischemia.[476–478] In the Coronary Artery Surgery Study (CASS), 424 patients who demonstrated ischemic ST-segment depression but no angina during exercise testing were compared to 456 patients who had both ischemic ST-segment depression and angina.[476] At 7 years of follow-up, 20 percent of patients with silent ischemia and 18 percent of patients with symptomatic ischemia had developed an acute myocardial infarction (no significant difference). Similarly, at 7 years of follow-up, sudden cardiac death was absent in 91 percent of patients with silent ischemia and in 93 percent of patients with symptomatic ischemia. In the subgroup of patients with three-vessel CAD, myocardial infarction or sudden cardiac death over 7 years of follow-up occurred in 43 percent of patients with silent ischemia compared to 25 percent of patients with angina and ST-segment evidence of ischemia on the entry exercise test ($p = 0.007$). These observations are also supported by findings from Holter monitoring. Coronary patients who develop myocardial ischemia during routine daily activities are at greater risk for myocardial infarction and cardiac death than are patients who develop ischemia only during vigorous exercise on treadmill testing.[479-481] The prognostic importance of myocardial ischemia detected either during routine daily activities or during treadmill exercise testing is similar whether or not it is accompanied by angina pectoris.[479,482]

In myocardial ischemia, regional left ventricular hypoperfusion or hypokinesis often precedes the onset of ECG ST-segment depression, which then precedes angina pectoris.[388,483,484] In some instances, transient myocardial ischemia with regional alteration of left ventricular perfusion or function but without angina or ST-segment shifts may reflect myocardial ischemia that is relatively brief or relatively mild.[485,486] However, in other instances, severe myocardial ischemia may occur in the absence of angina pectoris or other cardiac symptoms.[487,488] For example, during balloon inflation with percutaneous transluminal coronary angioplasty, similar volumes of hypoperfused myocardium may result in symptomatic ischemia in some instances and silent ischemia in others. Several studies have suggested that diagnosis and treatment of silent myocardial ischemia can reduce risk for an adverse cardiac outcome in appropriately selected patients.[440,489-491]

SUMMARY

Approximately 30 percent of patients who undergo coronary arteriography are found to have normal coronary arteries.[492] In view of the high cost of coronary arteriography and the finite risk of associated morbidity and mortality, noninvasive exclusion of myocardial ischemia in patients with chest pain is an important goal. In addition, noninvasive tests can be used together with clinical data to separate patients with high-risk CAD who are best referred for coronary arteriography and possible revascularization, from patients with low-risk coronary lesions who can be appropriately treated medically.

REFERENCES

1. Zir LM, Miller SW, Dinsmore RE, et al: Interobserver variability in coronary angiography. *Circulation* 53:627, 1976.

2. Beauman GJ, Vogel RA: Accuracy of individual and panel visual interpretations. *Cardiology* 16:108, 1990.

3. Arnett EN, Isner JM, Redwood DR, et al: Coronary artery narrowing in coronary heart disease: Comparison of cineangiographic and necropsy findings. *Ann Intern Med* 91:350, 1979.

4. Sabbah HN, Stein PD: Hemodynamics of multiple versus single 50 percent coronary arterial stenoses. *Am J Cardiol* 50:276, 1982.

5. Feldman RL, Nichols WW, Pepine CJ, et al: Influence of aortic insufficiency on the hemodynamic significance of a coronary artery narrowing. *Circulation* 60:259, 1979.

6. Hoffman JIE: Determinants and prediction of transmural myocardial perfusion. *Circulation* 58:381, 1978.

7. Brown BG, Bolson E, Frimer M, et al: Quantitative coronary arteriography: Estimation of dimensions, hemodynamic resistance, and atheroma mass of coronary artery lesions using the arteriogram and digital computation. *Circulation* 55:329, 1977.

8. Gould KL, Kelley KO, Bolson EL: Experimental validation of quantitative coronary arteriography for determining pressure-flow characteristics of coronary stenosis. *Circulation* 66:930, 1982.

9. Spears JR, Sandor T, Als AV, et al: Computerized image analysis for quantitative measurement of vessel diameter from cineangiograms. *Circulation* 68:453, 1983.

10. Harrison DG, White CW, Hiratzka LF, et al: The value of lesion cross-sectional area determined by quantitative coronary angiography in assessing the physiologic significance of proximal left anterior descending arterial stenoses. *Circulation* 69:1111, 1984.

11. White CW, Wright CB, Doty DB, et al: Does visual interpretation of the coronary arteriogram predict the physiologic importance of a coronary stenosis? *N Engl J Med* 310:819, 1984.

12. Bateman T, Raymond M, Czer L, et al: Stenosis severity: Analysis using Tl-201 scintigraphy and intracoronary pressure gradients. *J Am Coll Cardiol* 3:606, 1984 (abstr).

13. Vincent GM, Anderson JL, Marshall HW: Coronary spasm producing coronary thrombosis and myocardial infarction. *N Engl J Med* 309:220, 1983.

14. Waters DD, Szlachcic J, Bourassa MG, et al: Exercise testing in patients with variant angina: Results, correlation with clinical and angiographic features and prognostic significance. *Circulation* 65:265, 1982.

15. Gerson MC, Noble RJ, Wann LS, et al: Noninvasive documentation of Prinzmetal's angina. *Am J Cardiol* 43:329, 1979.

16. Epstein SE: Limitations of electrocardiographic exercise testing. *N Engl J Med* 301:264, 1979.

17. Froehlicher VF Jr, Yanowitz FG, Thompson AJ, et al: The correlation of coronary angiography and the electrocardiographic response to maximal treadmill testing in 76 asymptomatic men. *Circulation* 48:597, 1973.

18. McHenry PL, Richmond HW, Weisenberger BL, et al: Evaluation of abnormal exercise electrocardiogram in apparently healthy subjects: Labile repolarization (ST-T) abnormalities as a cause of false positive responses. *Am J Cardiol* 47:1152, 1981.

19. Fleiss JL: *Statistical Methods for Rates and Proportions,* 2nd ed. New York, Wiley, 1981.

20. Rozanski A, Diamond GA, Berman D, et al: The declining specificity of exercise radionuclide ventriculography. *N Engl J Med* 309:518, 1983.

21. Begg CB, Greenes RA: Assessment of diagnostic tests when disease verification is subject to selection bias. *Biometrics* 39:207, 1983.

22. Okada RD, Boucher CA, Strauss HW, et al: Exercise radionuclide imaging approaches to coronary artery disease. *Am J Cardiol* 46:1188, 1980.

23. Ascoop CA, Simoons ML, Egmond WG, et al: Exercise test, history, and serum lipid levels in patients with chest pain and normal electrocardiogram at rest: Comparison to findings at coronary arteriography. *Am Heart J* 82:609, 1971.

24. Barolsky SM, Gilbert CA, Faruqui A, et al: Differences in electrocardiographic response to exercise of women and men: A non-Bayesian factor. *Circulation* 60:1021, 1979.

25. Bartel AG, Behar VS, Peter RH, et al: Graded exercise stress tests in angiographically documented coronary artery disease. *Circulation* 49:348, 1974.

26. Berman JL, Wynne J, Cohn PF: A multivariate approach for interpreting treadmill exercise tests in coronary artery disease. *Circulation* 58:505, 1978.

27. Borer JS, Brensike JF, Redwood DR, et al: Limitations of the electrocardiographic response to exercise in predicting coronary-artery disease. *N Engl J Med* 293:367, 1975.

28. Taradash M, Botvinick E, Shames D, et al: Tl-201 myocardial perfusion imaging for the clinical clarification of normal, abnormal, and equivocal stress tests. *Circulation* 54(suppl II):II-217, 1976 (abstr).

29. Chaitman BR, Bourassa MG, Wagniart P, et al: Improved efficiency of treadmill exercise testing using a multiple lead ECG system and basic hemodynamic exercise response. *Circulation* 57:71, 1978.

30. Detry JMR, Kapita BM, Cosyns J, et al: Diagnostic value of history and maximal exercise electrocardiography in men and women suspected of coronary heart disease. *Circulation* 56:756, 1977.

31. Goldschlager N, Selzer A, Cohn K: Treadmill stress tests as indicators of presence and severity of coronary artery disease. *Ann Intern Med* 85:277, 1976.

32. Val PG, Chaitman BR, Waters DD, et al: Diagnostic accuracy of exercise ECG lead systems in clinical subsets of women. *Circulation* 65:1465, 1982.

33. Harris FJ, Mason DT, Lee G, et al: Value and limitations of exercise testing in detecting coronary disease in the presence of ST-T abnormalities on standard 12-lead electrocardiogram. *Am J Cardiol* 37:141, 1976 (abstr).

34. Helfant RH, Banka VS, DeVilla MA, et al: Use of bicycle ergometry and sustained handgrip exercise in the diagnosis of presence and extent of coronary heart disease. *Br Heart J* 35:1321, 1973.

35. Hollenberg M, Budge WR, Wisneski JA, et al: Treadmill score quantifies electrocardiographic response to exercise and improves test accuracy and reproducibility. *Circulation* 61:276, 1980.

36. Kaplan MA, Harris CN, Aronow WS, et al: Inability of the submaximal treadmill stress test to predict the location of coronary disease. *Circulation* 47:250, 1973.

37. Kassebaum DG, Sutherland KI, Judkins MP: A comparison of hypoxemia and exercise electrocardiography in coronary artery disease: Diagnostic precision of the methods correlated with coronary angiography. *Am Heart J* 75:759, 1968.

38. Kelemen MH, Gillian RE, Bouchard RJ, et al: Diagnosis of obstructive coronary disease by maximal exercise and atrial pacing. *Circulation* 48:1227, 1973.

39. Klein GJ, Kostuk WJ: Diagnostic accuracy of noninvasive stress myocardial perfusion imaging. *Circulation* 54(suppl II):II-207, 1976 (abstr).

40. Linhart JW, Turnoff HB: Maximum treadmill exercise test in patients with abnormal control electrocardiograms. *Circulation* 49:667, 1974.

41. Linhart JW, Laws JG, Satinsky JD: Maximum treadmill exercise electrocardiography in female patients. *Circulation* 50:1173, 1974.

42. Martin CM, McConahay DR: Maximal treadmill exercise electrocardiography: Correlations with coronary arteriography and cardiac hemodynamics. *Circulation* 46:956, 1972.

43. Mason RE, Likar I, Biern RO, et al: Multiple-lead exercise electrocardiography: Experience in 107 normal subjects and 67 patients with angina pectoris, and comparison with coronary cinearteriography in 84 patients. *Circulation* 36:517, 1967.

44. McHenry PL, Phillips JF, Knoebel SB: Correlation of computer-quantitated treadmill exercise electrocardiogram with arteriographic location of coronary artery disease. *Am J Cardiol* 30:747, 1972.

45. Peterson K, Tsuji J, Schelbert H, et al: Improved diagnosis of coronary artery disease during exercise test using a computer processed thallium-201 image. *Circulation* 54(suppl II):II-207, 1976 (abstr).

46. Rios JC, Hurwitz LE: Electrocardiographic responses to atrial pacing and multistage treadmill exercise testing: Correlation with coronary arteriography. *Am J Cardiol* 34:661, 1974.

47. Ritchie JL, Trobaugh GB, Hamilton GW, et al: Myocardial imaging with thallium-201 at rest and during exercise: Comparison with coronary arteriography and resting and stress electrocardiography. *Circulation* 56: 66, 1977.

48. Roitman D, Jones WB, Sheffield LT: Comparison of submaximal exercise ECG test with coronary cineangiocardiogram. *Ann Intern Med* 72:641, 1970.

49. Sketch MH, Mohiuddin SM, Lynch JD, et al: Significant sex differences in the correlation of electrocardiographic exercise testing and coronary arteriograms. *Am J Cardiol* 36:169, 1975.

50. Vieweg WVR, Alpert JS, Johnson AD, et al: Electrocardiographic exercise stress testing and coronary arteriography: Correlation among 114 men with chest pain. *West J Med* 127:199, 1977.

51. Weiner DA, Ryan TJ, McCabe CH, et al: Exercise stress testing: Correlations among history of angina, ST-segment response and prevalence of coronary-artery disease in the Coronary Artery Surgery Study (CASS). *N Engl J Med* 301:230, 1979.

52. Zohman LP, Kattus AA: Exercise testing in the diagnosis of coronary heart disease: A perspective. *Am J Cardiol* 40:243, 1977.

53. Diamond GA, Forrester JS: Analysis of probability as an aid in the clinical diagnosis of coronary-artery disease. *N Engl J Med* 300:1350, 1979.

54. Tonkon MJ, Miller RR, DeMaria AN, et al: Multifactor evaluation of the determinants of ischemic electrocardiographic response to maximal treadmill testing in coronary disease. *Am J Med* 62:339, 1977.

55. Robert AR, Melin JA, Detry J-MR: Logistic discriminant analysis improves diagnostic accuracy of exercise testing for coronary artery disease in women. *Circulation* 83:1202, 1991.

56. Whinnery JE, Froelicher VF Jr, Stewart AJ, et al: The electrocardiographic response to maximal treadmill exercise of asymptomatic men with left bundle branch block. *Am Heart J* 94:316, 1977.

57. Orzan F, Garcia E, Mathur VS, et al: Is the treadmill exercise test useful for evaluating coronary artery disease in patients with complete left bundle branch block? *Am J Cardiol* 42:36, 1978.

58. Strasberg B, Ashley WW, Wyndham CRC, et al: Treadmill exercise testing in the Wolff-Parkinson-White syndrome. *Am J Cardiol* 45:742, 1980.

59. Harris CN, Aronow WS, Parker P, et al: Treadmill stress test in left ventricular hypertrophy. *Chest* 63: 353, 1973.

60. Tanaka T, Friedman MJ, Okada RD, et al: Diagnostic value of exercise-induced S-T segment depression in patients with right bundle branch block. *Am J Cardiol* 41:670, 1978.

61. Froehlicher VF, Thompson AJ, Longo MR, et al: Value of exercise testing for screening asymptomatic men for latent coronary artery disease. *Prog Cardiovasc Dis* 18:265, 1976.

62. Gianelly RE, Treister BL, Harrison DC: The effect of propranolol on exercise-induced ischemic S-T segment depression. *Am J Cardiol* 24:161, 1969.

63. Ho SWC, McComish J, Taylor RR: Effect of beta-adrenergic blockade on the results of exercise testing related to the extent of coronary artery disease. *Am J Cardiol* 55:258, 1985.

64. Thadani U, Parker JO: Propranolol in angina pectoris: Duration of improved exercise tolerance and circulatory effects after acute oral administration. *Am J Cardiol* 44:118, 1979.

65. Marcomichelakis J, Donaldson R, Green J, et al: Exercise testing after beta-blockade: Improved specificity and predictive value in detecting coronary heart disease. *Br Heart J* 43:252, 1980.

66. Braunwald E: *Heart Disease. A Textbook of Cardiovascular Medicine,* 2nd ed. Philadelphia, Saunders, 1984, p 270.

67. Alderman EL, Coltart J, Wettach GE, et al: Coronary artery syndromes after sudden propranolol withdrawal. *Ann Intern Med* 81:625, 1974.

68. Miller RR, Olson HG, Amsterdam EA, et al: Propranolol-withdrawal rebound phenomenon: Exacerbation of coronary events after abrupt cessation of antianginal therapy. *N Engl J Med* 293:416, 1975.

69. Myers MG, Wisenberg G: Sudden withdrawal of pro-

pranolol in patients with angina pectoris. *Chest* 71:24, 1977.

70. Lindenfeld J, Crawford MH, O'Rourke RA, et al: Adrenergic responsiveness after abrupt propranolol withdrawal in normal subjects and in patients with angina pectoris. *Circulation* 62:704, 1980.

71. Parker JO, Augustine RJ, Burton JR, et al: Effect of nitroglycerin ointment on the clinical and hemodynamic response to exercise. *Am J Cardiol* 38:162, 1976.

72. Mueller HS, Chahine RA: Interim report of multicenter double-blind, placebo-controlled studies of nifedipine in chronic stable angina. *Am J Med* 71:645, 1981.

73. Wagniart P, Ferguson RJ, Chaitman BR, et al: Increased exercise tolerance and reduced electrocardiographic ischemia with diltiazem in patients with stable angina pectoris. *Circulation* 66:23, 1982.

74. Kawai C, Hultgren HN: The effect of digitalis upon the exercise electrocardiogram. *Am Heart J* 68:409, 1964.

75. Tonkon MJ, Lee G, DeMaria AN, et al: Effects of digitalis on the exercise electrocardiogram in normal adult subjects. *Chest* 72:714, 1977.

76. Ellestad MH: *Stress Testing: Principles and Practice,* Philadelphia, Davis, 1975, p 253.

77. Gianrossi R, Detrano R, Mulvihill D, et al: Exercise-induced ST depression in the diagnosis of coronary artery disease. A meta-analysis. *Circulation* 80:87, 1989.

78. Surawicz B, Lasseter KC: Effect of drugs on the electrocardiogram. *Prog Cardiovasc Dis* 13:26, 1970.

79. Gey GO, Levy RH, Pettet G, et al: Quinidine plasma concentration and exertional arrhythmia. *Am Heart J* 90:19, 1975.

80. Gey GO, Levy RH, Fisher L, et al: Plasma concentration of procainamide and prevalence of exertional arrhythmias. *Ann Intern Med* 80:718, 1974.

81. Georgopoulos AJ, Proudfit WL, Page IH: Effect of exercise on electrocardiograms of patients with low serum potassium. *Circulation* 23:567, 1961.

82. Hammermeister KE, DeRouen TA, Dodge HT, et al: Prognostic and predictive value of exertional hypotension in suspected coronary heart disease. *Am J Cardiol* 51:1261, 1983.

83. Weiner DA, McCabe CH, Cutler SS, et al: Decrease in systolic blood pressure during exercise testing: Reproducibility, response to coronary bypass surgery and prognostic significance. *Am J Cardiol* 49:1627, 1982.

84. Morris SN, Phillips JF, Jordan JW, et al: Incidence and significance of decreases in systolic blood pressure during graded treadmill exercise testing. *Am J Cardiol* 41:221, 1978.

85. Dubach P, Froelicher VF, Klein J, et al: Exercise-induced hypotension in a male population: Criteria, causes, and prognosis. *Circulation* 78:1380, 1988.

86. Amon KW, Richards KL, Crawford MH: Usefulness of the postexercise response of systolic blood pressure in the diagnosis of coronary artery disease. *Circulation* 70:951, 1984.

87. Sheps DS, Ernst JC, Briese FW, et al: Exercise-induced increase in diastolic pressure: Indicator of severe coronary artery disease. *Am J Cardiol* 43:708, 1979.

88. Stiles GL, Rosati RA, Wallace AG: Clinical relevance of

exercise-induced S-T segment elevation. *Am J Cardiol* 46:931, 1980.

89. Waters DD, Chaitman BR, Bourassa MG, et al: Clinical and angiographic correlates of exercise-induced ST-segment elevation: Increased detection with multiple ECG leads. *Circulation* 61:286, 1980.

90. Sriwattanakomen S, Ticzon AR, Zubritsky SA, et al: S-T segment elevation during exercise: Electrocardiographic and arteriographic correlation in 38 patients. *Am J Cardiol* 45:762, 1980.

91. Longhurst JC, Kraus WL: Exercise-induced ST elevation in patients without myocardial infarction. *Circulation* 60:616, 1979.

92. Chahine RA, Raizner AE, Ishimori T: The clinical significance of exercise-induced ST-segment elevation. *Circulation* 54:209, 1976.

93. Fortuin NJ, Friesinger GC: Exercise-induced S-T segment elevation: Clinical, electrocardiographic and arteriographic studies in twelve patients. *Am J Med* 49:459, 1970.

94. Dunn RF, Freedman B, Kelly DT, et al: Exercise-induced ST-segment elevation in leads V1 or aV1: A predictor of anterior myocardial ischemia and left anterior descending coronary artery disease. *Circulation* 63:1357, 1981.

95. Rijneke RD, Ascoop CA, Talmon JL: Clinical significance of upsloping ST segments in exercise electrocardiography. *Circulation* 61:671, 1980.

96. O'Donnell J, Lovelace E, Knoebel SB, et al: Behavior of the terminal T wave during exercise in normal subjects, patients with symptomatic coronary artery disease and apparently healthy subjects with abnormal ST segment depression. *J Am Coll Cardiol* 5:78, 1985.

97. Greenberg PS, Friscia DA, Ellestad MH: Predictive accuracy of Q-X/Q-T ratio, Q-Tc interval, S-T depression and R wave amplitude during stress testing. *Am J Cardiol* 44:18, 1979.

98. Gerson MC, Phillips JF, Morris SN, et al: Exercise-induced U-wave inversion as a marker of stenosis of the left anterior descending coronary artery. *Circulation* 60:1014, 1979.

99. Bonoris PE, Greenberg PS, Christison GW, et al: Evaluation of R wave amplitude changes versus ST-segment depression in stress testing. *Circulation* 57:904, 1978.

100. Wagner S, Cohn K, Selzer A: Unreliability of exercise-induced R wave changes as indexes of coronary artery disease. *Am J Cardiol* 44:1241, 1979.

101. Fox K, Selwyn A, Shillingford J: Precordial electrocardiographic mapping after exercise in the diagnosis of coronary artery disease. *Am J Cardiol* 43:541, 1979.

102. Kansal S, Roitman D, Bradley EL Jr, et al: Enhanced evaluation of treadmill tests by means of scoring based on multivariate analysis and its clinical application: A study of 608 patients. *Am J Cardiol* 52:1155, 1983.

103. Elamin MS, Boyle R, Kardash MM, et al: Accurate detection of coronary heart disease by new exercise test. *Br Heart J* 48:311, 1982.

104. Bhargava V, Watanabe K, Froelicher VF: Progress in computer analysis of the exercise electrocardiogram. *Am J Cardiol* 47:1143, 1981.

105. Lenaers A, Block P, Van Thiel E, et al: Segmental analysis of Tl-201 stress myocardial scintigraphy. *J Nucl Med* 18:509, 1977.

106. Rosenblatt A, Lowenstein JM, Kerth W, et al: Post-exercise thallium-201 myocardial scanning: A clinical appraisal. *Am Heart J* 94:463, 1977.

107. Carrillo AP, Marks DS, Pickard D, et al: Correlation of exercise thallium-201 myocardial scan with coronary arteriograms and the maximal exercise test. *Chest* 73:321, 1978.

108. Verani MS, Marcus ML, Razzack MA, et al: Sensitivity and specificity of thallium-201 scintigrams under exercise in the diagnosis of coronary artery disease. *J Nucl Med* 19:773, 1978 (abstr).

109. Turner DA, Battle WE, Deshmukh H, et al: The predictive value of myocardial perfusion scintigraphy after stress in patients without previous myocardial infarction. *J Nucl Med* 19:249, 1978.

110. Ritchie JL, Zaret BL, Strauss HW, et al: Myocardial imaging with thallium-201: A multicenter study in patients with angina pectoris or acute myocardial infarction. *Am J Cardiol* 42:345, 1978.

111. Sternberg L, Wald RW, Feiglin DH, et al: Myocardial perfusion imaging with thallium-201: Correlation with coronary arteriography and electrocardiography. *Can Med Assoc J* 118:283, 1978.

112. Johnstone DE, Sands MJ, Reduto LA, et al: Comparison of exercise radionuclide ventricular performance and thallium-201 myocardial perfusion in coronary artery disease. *Circulation* 57,58(suppl II):II-132, 1978 (abstr).

113. Okada RD, Raessler KL, Woolfenden JM, et al: Clinical value of the thallium-201 stress test: Sensitivity and specificity in the detection of coronary artery disease. *Int J Nucl Med Biol* 5:211, 1978.

114. McCarthy DM, Blood DK, Sciacca RR, et al: Single dose myocardial perfusion imaging with thallium-201: Application in patients with nondiagnostic electrocardiographic stress tests. *Am J Cardiol* 43:899, 1979.

115. Pohost GM, Boucher CA, Zir LM, et al: The thallium stress test: The qualitative approach revisited. *Circulation* 59,60(suppl II):II-149, 1979 (abstr).

116. Dash H, Massie BM, Botvinick EH, et al: The noninvasive identification of left main and three-vessel coronary artery disease by myocardial stress perfusion scintigraphy and treadmill exercise electrocardiography. *Circulation* 60:276, 1979.

117. Vogel RA, Kirch DL, LeFree MT, et al: Thallium-201 myocardial perfusion scintigraphy: Results of standard and multipinhole tomographic technique. *Am J Cardiol* 43:787, 1979.

118. Meller J, Goldsmith SJ, Rudin A, et al: Spectrum of exercise thallium-201 myocardial perfusion imaging in patients with chest pain and normal coronary angiograms. *Am J Cardiol* 43:717, 1979.

119. Sonnemaker RE, Floyd JL, Nusynowitz ML, et al: Single injection thallium-201 stress and redistribution myocardial perfusion imaging: Comparison with stress electrocardiography and coronary arteriography. *Radiology* 131:199, 1979.

120. Stolzenberg J, London R: Reliability of stress thallium-

201 scanning in the clinical evaluation of coronary artery disease. *Clin Nucl Med* 4:225, 1979.

121. Hecht HS, Blumfield DE, Mirell SJ: Superiority of the single dose exercise and redistribution thallium-201 scan to the electrocardiogram in the diagnosis of myocardial ischemia and infarction. *Clin Res* 27:174, 1979.

122. Borer JS, Bacharach SL, Green MV: Sensitivity of stress radionuclide cineangiography and stress thallium perfusion scanning in detecting coronary artery disease. *Am J Cardiol* 43:431, 1979 (abstr).

123. Kirshenbaum HE, Okada RD, Kushner FG: The relation of global left ventricular function with exercise to thallium-201 exercise scintigrams. *Clin Res* 27:180, 1979.

124. Massie BM, Botvinick EH, Brundage BH: Correlation of thallium-201 scintigrams with coronary anatomy: Factors affecting region by region sensitivity. *Am J Cardiol* 44:616, 1979.

125. Caldwell JH, Hamilton GW, Sorensen SG, et al: The detection of coronary artery disease with radionuclide techniques: A comparison of rest-exercise thallium imaging and ejection fraction response. *Circulation* 61:610, 1980.

126. Ong YS, Quaife MA, Dzindzio BS, et al: Clinical decision-making with treadmill testing and thallium-201. *Am J Med* 69:31, 1980.

127. Johnstone DE, Sands MJ, Berger HJ, et al: Comparison of exercise radionuclide angiography and thallium-201 myocardial perfusion imaging in coronary artery disease. *Am J Cardiol* 45:1113, 1980.

128. Rigo P, Bailey IK, Griffith LSC, et al: Value and limitations of segmental analysis of stress thallium myocardial imaging for localization of coronary artery disease. *Circulation* 61:973, 1980.

129. Jengo JA, Freeman R, Brizedine M, et al: Detection of coronary artery disease: Comparisons of exercise stress radionuclide angiocardiography and thallium stress perfusion scanning. *Am J Cardiol* 45:535, 1980.

130. Iskandrian AS, Segal BL: Value of exercise thallium-201 imaging in patients with diagnostic and nondiagnostic exercise electrocardiograms. *Am J Cardiol* 48:233, 1981.

131. Berger BC, Watson DD, Taylor GJ, et al: Quantitative thallium-201 exercise scintigraphy for detection of coronary artery disease. *J Nucl Med* 22:585, 1981.

132. Maddahi J, Garcia EV, Berman DS, et al: Improved noninvasive assessment of coronary artery disease by quantitative analysis of regional stress myocardial distribution and washout of thallium-201. *Circulation* 64:924, 1981.

133. Pedersen F, Rabol A, Sorensen SS, et al: Planar 201Tl scintigraphy in ischaemic heart disease: A critical re-evaluation of qualitative and quantitative data analysis. *Clin Physiol* 13:397, 1993.

134. Faris JV, Burt RW, Graham MC, Knoebel SB: Thallium-201 myocardial scintigraphy: Improved sensitivity, specificity and predictive accuracy by application of a statistical image analysis algorithm. *Am J Cardiol* 49:733, 1982.

135. Wackers FJTh, Fetterman RC, Mattera JA, Clements JP: Quantitative planar thallium-201 stress scintigraphy: A critical evaluation of the method. *Semin Nucl Med* 15:46, 1985.

136. Kaul S, Chesler DA, Okada RD, Boucher CA: Computer versus visual analysis of exercise thallium-201 images: A critical appraisal in 325 patients with chest pain. *Am Heart J* 114:1129, 1987.

137. Tamaki N, Yonekura Y, Mukai T, et al: Stress thallium-201 transaxial emission computed tomography: Quantitative versus qualitative analysis for evaluation of coronary artery disease. *J Am Coll Cardiol* 4:1213, 1984.

138. DePasquale EE, Nody AC, DePuey EG, et al: Quantitative rotational thallium-201 tomography for identifying and localizing coronary artery disease. *Circulation* 77:316, 1988.

139. Iskandrian AS, Heo J, Kong B, Lyons E: Effect of exercise level on the ability of thallium-201 tomographic imaging in detecting coronary artery disease: Analysis of 461 patients. *J Am Coll Cardiol* 14:1477, 1989.

140. Mahmarian JJ, Boyce TM, Goldberg RK, et al: Quantitative exercise thallium-201 single photon emission computed tomography for the enhanced diagnosis of ischemic heart disease. *J Am Coll Cardiol* 15:318, 1990.

141. Fleming RM, Kirkeeide RL, Taegtmeyer H, et al: Comparison of technetium-99m teboroxime tomography with automated quantitative coronary arteriography and thallium-201 tomographic imaging. *J Am Coll Cardiol* 17:1297, 1991.

142. Tartagni F, Dondi M, Limonetti P, et al: Dipyridamole technetium-99m-2-methoxy isobutyl isonitrile tomoscintigraphic imaging for identifying diseased coronary vessels: Comparison with thallium-201 stress-rest study. *J Nucl Med* 32:369, 1991.

143. Christian TF, Miller TD, Bailey KR, Gibbons RJ: Noninvasive identification of severe coronary artery disease using exercise tomographic thallium-201 imaging. *Am J Cardiol* 70:14, 1992.

144. Gerson MC, Lukes J, Deutsch E, et al: Comparison of technetium 99m Q12 and thallium 201 for detection of angiographically documented coronary artery disease in humans. *J Nucl Cardiol* 1:499, 1994.

145. Fintel DJ, Links JM, Brinker JA, et al: Improved diagnostic performance of exercise thallium-201 single photon emission computed tomography over planar imaging in the diagnosis of coronary artery disease: A receiver operating characteristic analysis. *J Am Coll Cardiol* 13:600, 1989.

146. Detrano R, Janosi A, Lyons KP, et al: Factors affecting sensitivity and specificity of a diagnostic test: The exercise thallium scintigram. *Am J Med* 84:699, 1988.

147. Maddahi J, Van Train K, Prigent F, et al: Quantitative single photon emission computed thallium-201 tomography for detection and localization of coronary artery disease: Optimization and prospective validation of a new technique. *J Am Coll Cardiol* 14:1689, 1989.

148. Van Train KF, Maddahi J, Berman DS, et al: Quantitative analysis of tomographic stress thallium-201 myocardial scintigrams: A multicenter trial. *J Nucl Med* 31:1168, 1990.

149. Kahn JK, McGhie I, Akers MS, et al: Quantitative rotational tomography with 201Tl and 99mTc 2-methoxy-isobutyl-isonitrile. A direct comparison in normal individuals and patients with coronary artery disease. *Circulation* 79:1282, 1989.

150. Kiat H, Maddahi J, Roy LT, et al: Comparison of technetium 99m methoxy isobutyl isonitrile and thallium 201

for evaluation of coronary artery disease by planar and tomographic methods. *Am Heart J* 117:1, 1989.

151. Wackers FJTh, Berman DS, Maddahi J, et al: Technetium-99m hexakis 2-methoxyisobutyl isonitrile: Human biodistribution, dosimetry, safety, and preliminary comparison to thallium-201 for myocardial perfusion imaging. *J Nucl Med* 30:301, 1989.

152. Maisey MN, Lowry A, Bischof-Delaloye A, et al: European multi-centre comparison of thallium 201 and technetium 99m methoxyisobutylisonitrile in ischaemic heart disease. *Eur J Nucl Med* 16:869, 1990.

153. Verzijlbergen JF, Cramer MJ, Niemeyer MG, et al: ^{99}Tc^m-sestamibi for planar myocardial perfusion imaging; not as ideal as the physical properties. *Nucl Med Commun* 12:381, 1991.

154. Taillefer R, Lambert R, Essiambre R, et al: Comparison between thallium-201, technetium-99m-sestamibi and technetium-99m-teboroxime planar myocardial perfusion imaging in detection of coronary artery disease. *J Nucl Med* 33:1091, 1992.

155. Sporn V, Balino NP, Holman BL, et al: Simultaneous measurement of ventricular function and myocardial perfusion using the technetium-99m isonitriles. *Clin Nucl Med* 13:77, 1988.

156. Bisi G, Sciagra R, Santoro GM, et al: Evaluation of coronary artery disease extent using ^{99}Tc^m-sestamibi: Comparison of dipyridamole versus exercise and of planar versus tomographic imaging. *Nucl Med Commun* 14:946, 1993.

157. Verzijlbergen JF, van Oudheusden D, Cramer MJ, et al: Quantitative analysis of planar technetium-99m sestamibi myocardial perfusion images. Clinical application of a modified method for the subtraction of tissue crosstalk. *Eur Heart J* 15:1217, 1994.

158. Plachcinska A, Kusmierek J, Kosmider M, et al: Quantitative assessment of technetium-99m methoxyisobutylisonitrile planar perfusion heart studies: Application of multivariate analysis to patient classification. *Eur J Nucl Med* 22:193, 1995.

159. Jamar F, Topcuoglu R, Cauwe F, et al: Exercise gated planar myocardial perfusion imaging using technetium-99m sestamibi for the diagnosis of coronary artery disease: An alternative to exercise tomographic imaging. *Eur J Nucl Med* 22:40, 1995.

160. Altehoefer C, vom Dahl J, Biedermann M, et al: Significance of defect severity in technetium-99m-MIBI SPECT at rest to assess myocardial viability: Comparison with fluorine-18-FDG PET. *J Nucl Med* 35:569, 1994.

161. Marzullo P, Sambuceti G, Parodi O, et al: Regional concordance and discordance between rest thallium 201 and sestamibi imaging for assessing tissue viability: Comparison with postrevascularization functional recovery. *J Nucl Cardiol* 2:309, 1995.

162. Sinusas AJ, Beller GA, Smith WH, et al: Quantitative planar imaging with technetium-99m methoxyisobutyl isonitrile: Comparison of uptake patterns with thallium-201. *J Nucl Med* 30:1456, 1989.

163. Koster K, Wackers FJTh, Mattera JA, Fetterman RC: Quantitative analysis of planar technetium-99m-sestamibi myocardial perfusion images using modified background subtraction. *J Nucl Med* 31:1400, 1990.

164. Najm YC, Maisey MN, Clarke SM, et al: Exercise myocardial perfusion scintigraphy with technetium-99m methoxy isobutylisonitrile: A comparative study with thallium-201. *Int J Cardiol* 26:93, 1990.

165. Maisey MN, Mistry R, Sowton E: Planar imaging techniques used with technetium-99m sestamibi to evaluate chronic myocardial ischemia. *Am J Cardiol* 66:47E, 1990.

166. Iskandrian AS, Heo J, Kong B, et al: Use of technetium-99m isonitrile (RP-30A) in assessing left ventricular perfusion and function at rest and during exercise in coronary artery disease, and comparison with coronary arteriography and exercise thallium-201 SPECT imaging. *Am J Cardiol* 64:270, 1989.

167. Maddahi J, Kiat H, Van Train KF, et al: Myocardial perfusion imaging with technetium-99m sestamibi SPECT in the evaluation of coronary artery disease. *Am J Cardiol* 66:55E, 1990.

168. Liu X-J, Wang X-B, Gao R-L, et al: Clinical evaluation of ^{99}Tc^m-MIBI SPECT in the assessment of coronary artery disease. *Nucl Med Commun* 13:776, 1992.

169. Camargo EE, Hironaka FH, Giorgi MCP, et al: Amplitude analysis of stress technetium-99m methoxy isobutylisonitrile images in coronary artery disease. *Eur J Nucl Med* 19:484, 1992.

170. Solot G, Hermans J, Merlo P, et al: Correlation of ^{99}Tc^m-sestamibi SPECT with coronary angiography in general hospital practice. *Nucl Med Commun* 14:23, 1993.

171. Herman SD, LaBresh KA, Santos-Ocampo CD, et al: Comparison of dobutamine and exercise using technetium-99m sestamibi imaging for the evaluation of coronary artery disease. *Am J Cardiol* 73:164, 1994.

172. Van Train KF, Garcia EV, Maddahi J, et al: Multicenter trial validation for quantitative analysis of same-day rest-stress technetium-99m-sestamibi myocardial tomograms. *J Nucl Med* 35:609, 1994.

173. Berman DS, Kiat HS, Van Train KF, et al: Myocardial perfusion imaging with technetium-99m-sestamibi: Comparative analysis of available imaging protocols. *J Nucl Med* 35:681, 1994.

174. Udelson JE: Choosing a thallium-201 or technetium 99m sestamibi imaging protocol. *J Nucl Cardiol* 1:S99, 1994.

175. Buell U, Dupont F, Uebis R, et al: ^{99}Tc^m-methoxy-isobutyl-isonitrile SPECT to evaluate a perfusion index from regional myocardial uptake after exercise and at rest. Results of a four hour protocol in patients with coronary heart disease and in controls. *Nucl Med Commun* 11:77, 1990.

176. Heo J, Kegel J, Iskandrian AS, et al: Comparison of same-day protocols using technetium-99m-sestamibi myocardial imaging. *J Nucl Med* 33:186, 1992.

177. Taillefer R, Gagnon A, Laflamme L, et al: Same day injections of Tc-99m methoxy isobutyl isonitrile (hexamibi) for myocardial tomographic imaging: Comparison between rest-stress and stress-rest injection sequences. *Eur J Nucl Med* 15:113, 1989.

178. Taillefer R, Laflamme L, Dupras G, et al: Myocardial perfusion imaging with ^{99m}Tc-methoxy-isobutyl-isonitrile (MIBI): Comparison of short and long time intervals between rest and stress injections. Preliminary results. *Eur J Nucl Med* 13:515, 1988.

179. Borges-Neto S, Coleman RE, Jones RH: Perfusion and function at rest and treadmill exercise using technetium-99m-sestamibi: Comparison of one- and two-day protocols in normal volunteers. *J Nucl Med* 31:1128, 1990.

180. Whalley DR, Murphy JJ, Frier M, et al: A comparison of same day and separate day injection protocols for myocardial perfusion SPECT using $^{99}Tc^m$-MIBI. *Nucl Med Commun* 12:99, 1991.

181. Franceschi M, Guimond J, Zimmerman RE, et al: Myocardial clearance of Tc-99m-hexakis-2-methoxy-2-methylpropylisonitrile (MIBI) in patients with coronary artery disease. *Clin Nucl Med* 15:307, 1990.

182. Taillefer R, Primeau M, Costi P, et al: Technetium-99m-sestamibi myocardial perfusion imaging in detection of coronary artery disease: Comparison between initial (1-hour) and delayed (3-hour) postexercise images. *J Nucl Med* 32:1961, 1991.

183. Taillefer R, Lambert R, Bisson G, et al: Myocardial technetium 99m-labeled sestamibi single-photon emission computed tomographic imaging in the detection of coronary artery disease: Comparison between early (15 minutes) and delayed (60 minutes) imaging. *J Nucl Cardiol* 1:441, 1994.

184. Cuocolo A, Pace L, Ricciardelli B, et al: Identification of viable myocardium in patients with chronic coronary artery disease: Comparison of thallium-201 scintigraphy with reinjection and technetium-99m-methoxyisobutyl isonitrile. *J Nucl Med* 33:505, 1992.

185. Marzullo P, Sambuceti G, Parodi O: The role of sestamibi scintigraphy in the radioisotopic assessment of myocardial viability. *J Nucl Med* 33:1925, 1992.

186. Dilsizian V, Arrighi JA, Diodati JG, et al: Myocardial viability in patients with chronic coronary artery disease. Comparison of ^{99m}Tc-sestamibi with thallium reinjection and [^{18}F]fluorodeoxyglucose. *Circulation* 89:578, 1994.

187. Udelson JE, Coleman PS, Metherall J, et al: Predicting recovery of severe regional ventricular dysfunction. Comparison of resting scintigraphy with ^{201}Tl and ^{99m}Tc-sestamibi. *Circulation* 89:2552, 1994.

188. Kiat H, Germano G, Friedman J, et al: Comparative feasibility of separate or simultaneous rest thallium-201/stress technetium-99m-sestamibi dual-isotope myocardial perfusion SPECT. *J Nucl Med* 35:542, 1994.

189. Berman DS, Kiat H, Friedman JD, et al: Separate acquisition rest thallium-201/stress technetium-99m sestamibi dual-isotope myocardial perfusion single-photon emission computed tomography: A clinical validation study. *J Am Coll Cardiol* 22:1455, 1993.

190. Heo J, Wolmer I, Kegel J, Iskandrian AS: Sequential dual-isotope SPECT imaging with thallium-201 and technetium-99m-sestamibi. *J Nucl Med* 35:549, 1994.

191. Baillet GY, Mena IG, Kuperus JH, et al: Simultaneous technetium-99m MIBI angiography and myocardial perfusion imaging. *J Nucl Med* 30:38, 1989.

192. Villanueva-Meyer J, Mena I, Narahara KA: Simultaneous assessment of left ventricular wall motion and myocardial perfusion with technetium-99m-methoxy isobutyl isonitrile at stress and rest in patients with angina: Comparison with thallium-201 SPECT. *J Nucl Med* 31:457, 1990.

193. Benari B, Kiat H, Erel J, et al: Repeatability of treadmill exercise ejection fraction and wall motion using techne-tium 99m-labeled sestamibi first-pass radionuclide ventriculography. *J Nucl Cardiol* 2:478, 1995.

194. Kloner RA, Allen J, Cox TA, et al: Stunned left ventricular myocardium after exercise treadmill testing in coronary artery disease. *Am J Cardiol* 68:329, 1991.

195. Chua T, Kiat H, Palmas W, et al: Can assessment of stress perfusion/rest function by single injection gated SPECT Tc-99m sestamibi substitute for separate injection stress/rest perfusion studies? *Circulation* 86:I-507, 1992 (abstr).

196. Sinusas AJ, Shi QX, Vitols PJ, et al: Impact of regional ventricular function, geometry, and dobutamine stress on quantitative ^{99m}Tc-sestamibi defect size. *Circulation* 88:2224, 1993.

197. Eisner RL, Schmarkey LS, Martin SE, et al: Defects on SPECT "perfusion" images can occur due to abnormal segmental contraction. *J Nucl Med* 35:638, 1994.

198. Mannting F, Morgan-Mannting MG: Gated SPECT with technetium-99m-sestamibi for assessment of myocardial perfusion abnormalities. *J Nucl Med* 34:601, 1993.

199. Chua T, Kiat H, Germano G, et al: Gated technetium-99m sestamibi for simultaneous assessment of stress myocardial perfusion, postexercise regional ventricular function and myocardial viability. Correlation with echocardiography and rest thallium-201 scintigraphy. *J Am Coll Cardiol* 23:1107, 1994.

200. Tischler MD, Niggel JB, Battle RW, et al: Validation of global and segmental left ventricular contractile function using gated planar technetium-99m sestamibi myocardial perfusion imaging. *J Am Coll Cardiol* 23:141, 1994.

201. Marzullo P, Marcassa C, Parodi O, et al: Noninvasive quantitative assessment of segmental myocardial wall motion using technetium-99m 2-methoxy-isobutyl-iso-nitrile scintigraphy. *Am J Noninvas Cardiol* 4:22, 1990.

202. Williams KA, Taillon LA: Gated planar technetium 99m-labeled sestamibi myocardial perfusion image inversion for quantitative scintigraphic assessment of left ventricular function. *J Nucl Cardiol* 2:285, 1995.

203. DePuey EG, Nichols K, Dobrinsky C: Left ventricular ejection fraction assessed from gated technetium-99m-sestamibi SPECT. *J Nucl Med* 34:1871, 1993.

204. Taillefer R, DePuey EG, Udelson J, et al: Comparative diagnostic accuracy of thallium-201 and Tc-99m ses-tamibi (perfusion and gated SPECT) in detecting coronary artery disease in women. *J Nucl Med* 37:69P, 1996 (abstr).

205. DePuey EG, Rozanski A: Using gated technetium-99m-sestamibi SPECT to characterize fixed myocardial defects as infarct or artifact. *J Nucl Med* 36:952, 1995.

206. Smanio PE, Watson DD, Segalla D, et al: Is it worthwhile to add gating to SPECT sestamibi perfusion imaging? *Circulation* 92(suppl I):I-11, 1995 (abstr).

207. Seldin DW, Johnson LL, Blood DK, et al: Myocardial perfusion imaging with technetium-99m SQ30217: Comparison with thallium-201 and coronary anatomy. *J Nucl Med* 30:312, 1989.

208. Hendel RC, McSherry B, Karimeddini M, Leppo JA: Diagnostic value of a new myocardial perfusion agent, teboroxime (SQ 30,217), utilizing a rapid planar imaging protocol: Preliminary results. *J Am Coll Cardiol* 16:855, 1990.

209. Weinstein H, Dahlberg ST, McSherry BA, et al: Rapid redistribution of teboroxime. *Am J Cardiol* 71:848, 1993.

210. Dahlberg ST, Weinstein H, Hendel RC, et al: Planar myocardial perfusion imaging with technetium-99m-teboroxime: Comparison by vascular territory with thallium-201 and coronary angiography. *J Nucl Med* 33:1783, 1992.

211. Fleming RM, Kirkeeide RL, Taegtmeyer H, et al: Comparison of technetium-99m teboroxime tomography with automated quantitative coronary arteriography and thallium-201 tomographic imaging. *J Am Coll Cardiol* 17:1297, 1991.

212. Burns RJ, Iles S, Fung AY, et al: The Canadian exercise technetium 99m-labeled teboroxime single-photon emission computed tomographic study. *J Nucl Cardiol* 2:117, 1995.

213. Oshima M, Ishihara M, Ohno M, et al: Myocardial SPECT and left ventricular performance study using a single Tc-99m teboroxime injection. Comparison with thallium-201 myocardial SPECT. *Clin Nucl Med* 18:844, 1993.

214. Zaret BL, Rigo P, Wackers FJTh, et al: Myocardial perfusion imaging with ^{99m}Tc tetrofosmin. Comparison to ^{201}Tl imaging and coronary angiography in a phase III multicenter trial. *Circulation* 91:313, 1995.

215. Jain D, Wackers FJTh, Mattera J, et al: Biokinetics of technetium-99m-tetrofosmin: Myocardial perfusion imaging agent: Implications for a one-day imaging protocol. *J Nucl Med* 34:1254, 1993.

216. Sridhara BS, Braat S, Rigo P, et al: Comparison of myocardial perfusion imaging with technetium-99m tetrofosmin versus thallium-201 in coronary artery disease. Am *J Cardiol* 72:1015, 1993.

217. Braat SH, Leclercq B, Itti R, et al: Myocardial imaging with technetium-99m-tetrofosmin: Comparison of one-day and two-day protocols. *J Nucl Med* 35:1581, 1994.

218. Sridhara B, Sochor H, Rigo P, et al: Myocardial single-photon emission computed tomographic imaging with technetium 99m tetrofosmin: Stress-rest imaging with same-day and separate-day rest imaging. *J Nucl Cardiol* 1:138, 1994.

219. Matsunari I, Fujino S, Taki J, et al: Comparison of defect size between thallium-201 and technetium-99m tetrofosmin myocardial single-photon emission computed tomography in patients with single-vessel coronary artery disease. *Am J Cardiol* 77:350, 1996.

220. Leon AR, Eisner RL, Martin SE, et al: Comparison of single-photon emission computed tomographic (SPECT) myocardial perfusion imaging with thallium-201 and technetium-99m sestamibi in dogs. *J Am Coll Cardiol* 20:1612, 1992.

221. Glover DK, Ruiz M, Edwards NC, et al: Comparison between ^{201}Tl and ^{99m}Tc sestamibi uptake during adenosine-induced vasodilation as a function of coronary stenosis severity. *Circulation* 91:813, 1995.

222. Narahara KA, Villanueva-Meyer J, Thompson CJ, et al: Comparison of thallium-201 and technetium-99m hexakis 2-methoxyisobutyl isonitrile single-photon emission computed tomography for estimating the extent of myo-cardial ischemia and infarction in coronary artery disease. *Am J Cardiol* 66:1438, 1990.

223. Maublant JC, Marcaggi X, Lusson J-R, et al: Comparison between thallium-201 and technetium-99m methoxyisobutyl isonitrile defect size in single-photon emission computed tomography at rest, exercise and redistribution in coronary artery disease. *Am J Cardiol* 69:183, 1992.

224. Rigo P, Leclercq B, Itti R, et al: Technetium-99m-tetrofosmin myocardial imaging: A comparison with thallium-201 and angiography. *J Nucl Med* 35:587, 1994.

225. Heo J, Cave V, Wasserleben V, Iskandrian AS: Planar and tomographic imaging with technetium 99m-labeled tetrofosmin: Correlation with thallium 201 and coronary angiography. *J Nucl Cardiol* 1:317, 1994.

226. Nakajima K, Taki J, Shuke N, et al: Myocardial perfusion imaging and dynamic analysis with technetium-99m tetrofosmin. *J Nucl Med* 34:1478, 1993.

227. Takahashi N, Tamaki N, Tadamura E, et al: Combined assessment of regional perfusion and wall motion in patients with coronary artery disease with technetium 99m tetrofosmin. *J Nucl Cardiol* 1:29, 1994.

228. Tamaki N, Takahashi N, Kawamoto M, et al: Myocardial tomography using technetium-99m-tetrofosmin to evaluate coronary artery disease. *J Nucl Med* 35:594, 1994.

229. Mahmood S, Gunning M, Bomanji JB, et al: Combined rest thallium-201/stress technetium-99m-tetrofosmin SPECT: Feasibility and diagnostic accuracy of a 90-minute protocol. *J Nucl Med* 36:932, 1995.

230. Gerson MC, Millard RW, Roszell NJ, et al: Kinetic properties of ^{99m}Tc-Q12 in canine myocardium. *Circulation* 89:1291, 1994.

231. Hendel RC, Verani MS, Miller DD, et al: Diagnostic utility of tomographic myocardial perfusion imaging with technetium-99m furifosmin (Q12) compared with thallium-201: Results of a phase III multicenter trial. *J Nucl Cardiol* 3:291, 1996.

232. Rossetti C, Vanoli G, Paganelli G, et al: Human biodistribution, dosimetry and clinical use of technetium(III)-99m-Q12. *J Nucl Med* 35:1571, 1994.

233. Fagret D, Marie P-Y, Brunotte F, et al: Myocardial perfusion imaging with technetium-99m-Tc NOET: Comparison with thallium-201 and coronary angiography. *J Nucl Med* 36:936, 1995.

234. Ficaro EP, Fessler JA, Shreve PD, et al: Simultaneous transmission/emission myocardial perfusion tomography. Diagnostic accuracy of attenuation-corrected ^{99m}Tc-sestamibi single-photon emission computed tomography. *Circulation* 93:463, 1996.

235. Diamond GA: Affirmative actions: Can the discriminate accuracy of a test be determined in the face of selection bias? *Med Decis Making* 11:48, 1991.

236. Osbakken MD, Okada RD, Boucher CA, et al: Comparison of exercise perfusion and ventricular function imaging: An analysis of factors affecting the diagnostic accuracy of each technique. *J Am Coll Cardiol* 3:272, 1984.

237. DePace NL, Iskandrian AS, Hakki AH: Relation between the extent of coronary artery disease and exercise-induced thallium-201 perfusion abnormalities. *J Cardiac Rehabil* 3:611, 1983.

238. Turner JD, Schwartz KM, Logic JR, et al: Detection of residual jeopardized myocardium 3 weeks after myocardial infarction by exercise testing with thallium-201 myocardial scintigraphy. *Circulation* 61: 729, 1980.

239. Takaro T, Hultgren HN, Lipton MJ, et al: The VA cooperative randomized study of surgery for coronary arterial occlusive disease: II. Subgroup with significant left main lesions. *Circulation* 54(suppl III):III-107, 1976.

240. Detre K, Peduzzi P, Murphy M, et al: Effect of bypass surgery on survival in patients in low- and high-risk subgroups delineated by the use of simple clinical variables. *Circulation* 63:1329, 1981.

241. European Coronary Surgery Study Group: Long-term results of prospective, randomized study of coronary-artery bypass surgery in stable angina pectoris. *Lancet* 2:1173, 1982.

242. Passamani E, Davis KB, Gillespie MJ, et al: A randomized trial of coronary artery bypass surgery. Survival of patients with a low ejection fraction. *N Engl J Med* 312:1665, 1985.

243. Rigo P, Bailey IK, Griffith LSC, et al: Stress thallium-201 myocardial scintigraphy for the detection of individual coronary arterial lesions in patients with and without previous myocardial infarction. *Am J Cardiol* 48:209, 1981.

244. McKillop JH, Murray RG, Turner JG, et al: Can the extent of coronary artery disease by predicted from thallium-201 myocardial images? *J Nucl Med* 20:715, 1979.

245. Iskandrian AS, Segal BL, Haaz W, Kane S: Effects of coronary artery narrowing, collaterals, and left ventricular function on the pattern of myocardial perfusion. *Cathet Cardiovasc Diagn* 6:159, 1980.

246. Corne RA, Gotsman MS, Weiss A, et al: Thallium-201 scintigraphy in diagnosis of coronary stenosis. Comparison with electrocardiography and coronary arteriography. *Br Heart J* 41:575, 1979.

247. Patterson RE, Horowitz SF, Eng C, et al: Can noninvasive exercise test criteria identify patients with left main or 3-vessel coronary disease after a first myocardial infarction? *Am J Cardiol* 51:361, 1983.

248. Canhasi B, Dae M, Botvinick E, et al: Interaction of "supplementary" scintigraphic indicators of ischemia and stress electrocardiography in the diagnosis of multivessel coronary disease. *J Am Coll Cardiol* 6:581, 1985.

249. Iskandrian AS, Hakki A-H, Segal BL, et al: Assessment of the myocardial perfusion pattern in patients with multivessel coronary artery disease. *Am Heart J* 106:1089, 1983.

250. Sklar J, Kirch D, Johnson T, et al: Slow late myocardial clearance of thallium: A characteristic phenomenon in coronary artery disease. *Circulation* 65:1504, 1982.

251. Bateman TM, Maddahi J, Gray RJ, et al: Diffuse slow washout of myocardial thallium-201: A new scintigraphic indicator of extensive coronary artery disease. *J Am Coll Cardiol* 4:55, 1984.

252. Bergmann SR, Hack SN, Sobel BE: "Redistribution" of myocardial thallium-201 without reperfusion: Implications regarding absolute quantification of perfusion. *Am J Cardiol* 49:1691, 1982.

253. Kaul S, Chesler DA, Pohost GM, et al: Influence of peak exercise heart rate on normal thallium-201 myocardial clearance. *J Nucl Med* 27:26, 1986.

254. Nishimura T, Uehara T, Hayashida K, et al: Quantitative assessment of thallium myocardial washout rate: Importance of peak heart rate and lung thallium uptake in defining normal values. *Eur J Nucl Med* 13:67, 1987.

255. Nordrehaug JE, Danielsen R, Vik-Mo H: Effects of heart rate on myocardial thallium-201 uptake and clearance. *J Nucl Med* 30:1972, 1989.

256. Wilson RA, Sullivan PJ, Okada RD, et al: The effect of eating on thallium myocardial imaging. *Chest* 89:195, 1986.

257. Angello DA, Wilson RA, Palac RT: Effect of eating on thallium-201 myocardial redistribution after myocardial ischemia. *Am J Cardiol* 60:528, 1987.

258. Rabinovitch M, Suissa S, Elstein J, et al: Sex-specific criteria for interpretation of thallium-201 myocardial uptake and washout studies. *J Nucl Med* 27:1837, 1986.

259. Lancaster JL, Starling MR, Kopp DT, et al: Effect of errors in reangulation on planar and tomographic thallium-201 washout profile curves. *J Nucl Med* 26:1445, 1985.

260. Kimball BP, Shurvell BL, Mildenberger RR, et al: Abnormal thallium kinetics in postoperative coarctation of the aorta: Evidence for diffuse hypertension-induced vascular pathology. *J Am Coll Cardiol* 7:538, 1986.

261. Gal R, Niazi I, Port SC: Importance of the site and technique of intravenous thallium injection during exercise. *J Am Coll Cardiol* 7:23A, 1986 (abstr).

262. Kaul S, Chesler DA, Newell JB, et al: Regional variability in the myocardial clearance of thallium-201 and its importance in determining the presence or absence of coronary artery disease. *J Am Coll Cardiol* 8:95, 1986.

263. Gewirtz H, Paladino W, Sullivan M, Most AS: Value and limitations of myocardial thallium washout rate in the noninvasive diagnosis of patients with triple-vessel coronary artery disease. *Am Heart J* 106:681, 1983.

264. Abdulla A, Maddahi J, Garcia E, et al: Slow regional clearance of myocardial thallium-201 in the absence of perfusion defect: Contribution to detection of individual coronary artery stenoses and mechanism for occurrence. *Circulation* 71:72, 1985.

265. Hurwitz GA, O'Donoghue JP, Powe JE, et al: Pulmonary thallium-201 uptake following dipyridamole-exercise combination compared with single modality stress testing. *Am J Cardiol* 69:320, 1992.

266. Villanueva FS, Kaul S, Smith WH, et al: Prevalence and correlates of increased lung/heart ratio of thallium-201 during dipyridamole stress imaging for suspected coronary artery disease. *Am J Cardiol* 66:1324, 1990.

267. Nishimura S, Mahmarian JJ, Verani MS: Significance of increased lung thallium uptake during adenosine thallium-201 scintigraphy. *J Nucl Med* 33:1600, 1992.

268. Baccelli G, Terrani S, Pacenti P, et al: A new method for evaluating lung uptake of thallium-201 during stress myocardial scintigraphy. *Am J Cardiol* 70:940, 1992.

269. Takeishi Y, Chiba J, Abe S, Tomoike H: Ratio of lung to heart thallium-201 uptake on exercise and dipyridamole stress imaging in coronary artery disease. Implication of SPECT. *Jpn Circ J* 57:379, 1993.

270. Levy R, Rozanski A, Berman DS, et al: Analysis of the degree of pulmonary thallium washout after exercise in patients with coronary artery disease. *J Am Coll Cardiol* 2:719, 1983.

271. Homma S, Kaul S, Boucher CA: Correlates of lung/heart ratio of thallium-201 in coronary artery disease. *J Nucl Med* 28:1531, 1987.

272. Gibson RS, Watson DD, Carabello BA, et al: Clinical implications of increased lung uptake of thallium-201 during exercise scintigraphy 2 weeks after myocardial infarction. *Am J Cardiol* 49:1586, 1982.

273. Brown KA, Boucher CA, Okada RD, et al: Quantification of pulmonary thallium-201 activity after upright exercise in normal persons: Importance of peak heart rate and propranolol usage in defining normal values. *Am J Cardiol* 53:1678, 1984.

274. Wahl RL, Kumar B, Biello DR, Miller TR: The (F)utility of the thallium-201 quantitative lung/myocardial ratio in the detection of coronary artery disease. *Eur J Nucl Med* 12:5, 1986.

275. Aksut SV, Mallavarapu C, Russell J, et al: Implications of increased lung thallium uptake during exercise single photon emission computed tomography imaging. *Am Heart J* 130:367, 1995.

276. Kahn JK, Carry MM, McGhie I, et al: Quantitation of postexercise lung thallium-201 uptake during single photon emission computed tomography. *J Nucl Med* 30:288, 1989.

277. Kurata C, Tawarahara K, Taguchi T, et al: Lung thallium-201 uptake during exercise emission computed tomography. *J Nucl Med* 32:417, 1991.

278. Hurwitz GA, Fox SP, Driedger AA, et al: Pulmonary uptake of sestamibi on early post-stress images: Angiographic relationships, incidence and kinetics. *Nucl Med Commun* 14:15, 1993.

279. Weiss AT, Berman DS, Lew AS, et al: Transient ischemic dilation of the left ventricle on stress thallium-201 scintigraphy: A marker of severe and extensive coronary artery disease. *J Am Coll Cardiol* 9:752, 1987.

280. Chouraqui P, Rodrigues EA, Berman DS, Maddahi J: Significance of dipyridamole-induced transient dilation of the left ventricle during thallium-201 scintigraphy in suspected coronary artery disease. *Am J Cardiol* 66:689, 1990.

281. Lette J, Lapointe J, Waters D, et al: Transient left ventricular cavitary dilation during dipyridamole-thallium imaging as an indicator of severe coronary artery disease. *Am J Cardiol* 66:1163, 1990.

282. Iskandrian AS, Heo J, Nguyen T, et al: Left ventricular dilatation and pulmonary thallium uptake after single-photon emission computer tomography using thallium-201 during adenosine-induced coronary hyperemia. *Am J Cardiol* 66:807, 1990.

283. Rehn T, Griffith LSC, Achuff SC, et al: Exercise thallium-201 myocardial imaging in left main coronary artery disease: Sensitive but not specific. *Am J Cardiol* 48:217, 1981.

284. Nygaard TW, Gibson RS, Ryan JM, et al: Prevalence of high- risk thallium-201 scintigraphic findings in left main coronary artery stenosis: Comparison with patients with multiple- and single-vessel coronary artery disease. *Am J Cardiol* 53:462, 1984.

285. Chikamori T, Doi YL, Yonezawa Y, et al: Noninvasive identification of significant narrowing of the left main coronary artery by dipyridamole thallium scintigraphy. *Am J Cardiol* 68:472, 1991.

286. Starling MR, Dehmer GJ, Lancaster JL, et al: Comparison of quantitative SPECT vs planar thallium-201 myocardial scintigraphy for detecting and localizing segmental coronary artery disease. *J Am Coll Cardiol* 5:531, 1985 (abstr).

287. Kasabali B, Woodard ML, Bekerman C, et al: Enhanced sensitivity and specificity of thallium-201 imaging for the detection of regional ischemic coronary disease by combining SPECT with "bull's eye" analysis. *Clin Nucl Med* 14:484, 1989.

288. Dunn RF, Wolff L, Wagner S, et al: The inconsistent pattern of thallium defects: A clue to the false positive perfusion scintigram. *Am J Cardiol* 48:224, 1981.

289. Hung J, Chaitman BR, Lam J, et al: Noninvasive diagnostic test choices for the evaluation of coronary artery disease in women: A multivariate comparison of cardiac fluoroscopy, exercise electrocardiography and exercise thallium myocardial perfusion scintigraphy. *J Am Coll Cardiol* 4:8, 1984.

290. Friedman TD, Greene AC, Iskandrian AS, et al: Exercise thallium-201 myocardial scintigraphy in women: Correlation with coronary arteriography. *Am J Cardiol* 49:1632, 1982.

291. Goodgold HM, Rehder JG, Samuels LD, Chaitman BR: Improved interpretation of exercise Tl-201 myocardial perfusion scintigraphy in women: Characterization of breast attenuation artifacts. *Radiology* 165: 361, 1987.

292. Cerqueira MD: Diagnostic testing strategies for coronary artery disease: Special issues related to gender. *Am J Cardiol* 75:52D, 1995.

293. Johnson LL: Sex specific issues relating to nuclear cardiology. *J Nucl Cardiol* 2:339, 1995.

294. Lette J, Caron M, Cerino M, et al: Normal qualitative and quantitative Tc-99m sestamibi myocardial SPECT: Spectrum of intramyocardial distribution during exercise and at rest. *Clin Nucl Med* 19:336, 1994.

295. Manglos SH, Thomas FD, Gagne GM, Hellwig BJ: Phantom study of breast tissue attenuation in myocardial imaging. *J Nucl Med* 34:992, 1993.

296. Ceretto W, Vieweg V, Slutsky R, et al: Thallium-201 myocardial perfusion imaging in women: Correlation with coronary arteriography. *Am J Cardiol* 47:422, 1981 (abstr).

297. Chae HC, Heo J, Iskandrian AS, et al: Identification of extensive coronary artery disease in women by exercise single-photon emission computed tomographic (SPECT) thallium imaging. *J Am Coll Cardiol* 21:1305, 1993.

298. Kong BA, Shaw L, Miller DD, Chaitman BR: Comparison of accuracy for detecting coronary artery disease and side-effect profile of dipyridamole thallium-201 myocardial perfusion imaging in women versus men. *Am J Cardiol* 70:168, 1992.

299. Pacold I, Maier PT, Moran JF, et al: Exercise testing of women with chest pain with and without thallium tomography. *Am J Cardiol* 47:422, 1981 (abstr).

300. Bailey IK, Griffith LSC, Rouleau J, et al: Thallium-201 myocardial perfusion imaging at rest and during exercise: Comparative sensitivity to electrocardiography in coronary artery disease. *Circulation* 55:79, 1977.

301. Botvinick EH, Taradash MR, Shames DM, et al: Thallium-201 myocardial perfusion scintigraphy for the clinical clarification of normal, abnormal and equivocal electrocardiographic stress tests. *Am J Cardiol* 41:43, 1978.

302. Iskandrian AS, Wasserman LA, Anderson GS, et al: Merits of stress thallium-201 myocardial perfusion imaging in patients with inconclusive exercise electrocardiograms: Correlation with coronary arteriograms. *Am J Cardiol* 46:553, 1980.

303. Martin GJ, Henkin RE, Scanlon PJ: Beta blockers and the sensitivity of the thallium treadmill test. *Chest* 92:486, 1987.

304. Steele P, Sklar J, Kirch D, et al: Thallium-201 myocardial imaging during maximal and submaximal exercise: Comparison of submaximal exercise with propranolol. *Am Heart J* 106:1353, 1983.

305. Hockings B, Saltissi S, Croft DN, et al: Effect of beta adrenergic blockade on thallium-201 myocardial perfusion imaging. *Br Heart J* 49:83, 1983.

306. Narahara KA, Thompson CJ, Hazen JF, et al: The effect of beta blockade on single photon emission computed tomographic (SPECT) thallium-201 images in patients with coronary disease. *Am Heart J* 117:1030, 1989.

307. Mahmarian JJ, Fenimore NL, Marks GF, et al: Transdermal nitroglycerin patch therapy reduces the extent of exercise-induced myocardial ischemia: Results of a double-blind, placebo-controlled trial using quantitative thallium-201 tomography. *J Am Coll Cardiol* 24:25, 1994.

308. McLaughlin PR, Martin RP, Doherty P, et al: Reproducibility of thallium-201 myocardial imaging. *Circulation* 55:497, 1977.

309. Esquivel L, Pollock SG, Beller GA, et al: Effect of the degree of effort on the sensitivity of the exercise thallium-201 stress test in symptomatic coronary artery disease. *Am J Cardiol* 63:160, 1989.

310. Heller GV, Ahmed I, Tilkemeier PL, et al: Influence of exercise intensity on the presence, distribution, and size of thallium-201 defects. *Am Heart J* 123:909, 1992.

311. Goldstein RE, Stinson EB, Scherer JL, et al: Intraoperative coronary collateral function in patients with coronary occlusive disease. *Circulation* 49:298, 1974.

312. Cohn PF, Maddox DE, Holman BL, et al: Effect of coronary collateral vessels on regional myocardial blood flow in patients with coronary artery disease. *Am J Cardiol* 46:359, 1980.

313. Gregg DE: The natural history of coronary collateral development. *Circ Res* 35:335, 1974.

314. Berger BC, Watson DD, Taylor GJ, et al: Effect of coronary collateral circulation on regional myocardial perfusion assessed with quantitative thallium-201 scintigraphy. *Am J Cardiol* 46:365, 1980.

315. Goldberg HL, Goldstein J, Borer JS, et al: Determination of the angiographic appearance of coronary collateral vessels: The importance of supplying and recipient arteries. *Am J Cardiol* 51:434, 1983.

316. Rigo P, Becker LC, Griffith LSC, et al: Influence of coronary collateral vessels on the results of thallium-201 myocardial stress imaging. *Am J Cardiol* 44:452, 1979.

317. Tubau JF, Chaitman BR, Bourassa MG, et al: Importance of coronary collateral circulation in interpreting exercise test results. *Am J Cardiol* 47:27, 1981.

318. Kolibash AJ, Bush CA, Wepsic RA, et al: Coronary collateral vessels: Spectrum of physiologic capabilities with respect to providing rest and stress myocardial perfusion, maintenance of left ventricular function and protection against infarction. *Am J Cardiol* 50:230, 1982.

319. Wainwright RJ, Maisey MN, Edwards AC, et al: Functional significance of coronary collateral circulation during dynamic exercise evaluated by thallium-201 myocardial scintigraphy. *Br Heart J* 43:47, 1980.

320. Eng C, Patterson RE, Horowitz SF, et al: Coronary collateral function during exercise. *Circulation* 66:309, 1982.

321. Iskandrian AS, Lichtenberg R, Segal BL, et al: Assessment of jeopardized myocardium in patients with one-vessel disease. *Circulation* 65:242, 1982.

322. Brown KA, Osbakken M, Boucher CA, et al: Positive exercise thallium-201 test response in patients with less than 50% maximal coronary stenosis: Angiographic and clinical predictors. *Am J Cardiol* 55:54, 1985.

323. Kaul S, Newell JB, Chesler DA, et al: Quantitative thallium imaging findings in patients with normal coronary angiographic findings and in clinically normal subjects. *Am J Cardiol* 57:509, 1986.

324. Waters DD, Chaitman BR, Dupras G, et al: Coronary artery spasm during exercise in patients with variant angina. *Circulation* 59:580, 1979.

325. Fuller CM, Raizner AE, Chahine RA, et al: Exercise-induced coronary arterial spasm: Angiographic demonstration, documentation of ischemia by myocardial scintigraphy and results of pharmacologic intervention. *Am J Cardiol* 46:500, 1980.

326. Maseri A, Parodi O, Severi S, et al: Transient transmural reduction of myocardial blood flow, demonstrated by thallium-201 scintigraphy, as a cause of variant angina. *Circulation* 54:280, 1976.

327. Ricci DR, Orlick AE, Doherty PW, et al: Reduction of coronary blood flow during coronary artery spasm occurring spontaneously and after provocation by ergonovine maleate. *Circulation* 57:392, 1978.

328. Nakajima K, Shimizu K, Taki J, et al: Utility of iodine-123-BMIPP in the diagnosis and follow-up of vasospastic angina. *J Nucl Med* 36:1934, 1995.

329. Ono S, Nohara R, Kambara H, et al: Regional myocardial perfusion and glucose metabolism in experimental left bundle branch block. *Circulation* 85:1125, 1992.

330. McGowan RL, Welch TG, Zaret BL, et al: Noninvasive myocardial imaging with potassium-43 and rubidium-81 in patients with left bundle branch block. *Am J Cardiol* 38:422, 1976.

331. Braat SH, Brugada P, Bar FW, et al: Thallium-201 exercise scintigraphy and left bundle branch block. *Am J Cardiol* 240:224, 1985.

332. Johnson RE, Williams BR, Liberman HA, et al: Stress thallium scintigraphy in patients with left bundle branch block. *Circulation* 64(suppl IV):IV-105, 1981 (abstr).

333. Hirzel HO, Senn M, Nuesch K, et al: Thallium-201 scin-

tigraphy in complete left bundle branch block. *Am J Cardiol* 53:764, 1984.

334. DePuey EG, Guertler-Krawczynska E, Robbins WL: Thallium-201 SPECT in coronary artery disease patients with left bundle branch block. *J Nucl Med* 29:1479, 1988.

335. Larcos G, Gibbons RJ, Brown ML: Diagnostic accuracy of exercise thallium-201 single-photon emission computed tomography in patients with left bundle branch block. *Am J Cardiol* 68:756, 1991.

336. Matzer L, Kiat H, Friedman JD, et al: A new approach to the assessment of tomographic thallium-201 scintigraphy in patients with left bundle branch block. *J Am Coll Cardiol* 17:1309, 1991.

337. Mairesse GH, Marwick TH, Arnese M, et al: Improved identification of coronary artery disease in patients with left bundle branch block by use of dobutamine stress echocardiography and comparison with myocardial perfusion tomography. *Am J Cardiol* 76:321, 1995.

338. Tighe DA, Hutchinson HG, Park CH, et al: False-positive reversible perfusion defect during dobutamine-thallium imaging in left bundle branch block. *J Nucl Med* 35:1989, 1994.

339. Burns RJ, Galligan L, Wright LM, et al: Improved specificity of myocardial thallium-201 single-photon emission computed tomography in patients with left bundle branch block by dipyridamole. *Am J Cardiol* 68:504, 1991.

340. O'Keefe JH Jr, Bateman TM, Barnhart CS: Adenosine thallium- 201 is superior to exercise thallium-201 for detecting coronary artery disease in patients with left bundle branch block. *J Am Coll Cardiol* 21:1332, 1993.

341. Ebersole DG, Heironimus J, Toney MO, Billingsley J: Comparison of exercise and adenosine technetium-99m sestamibi myocardial scintigraphy for diagnosis of coronary artery disease in patients with left bundle branch block. *Am J Cardiol* 71:450, 1993.

342. Krishnan R, Lu J, Zhu YY, et al: Myocardial perfusion scintigraphy in left bundle branch block: A perspective on the issue from image analysis in a clinical context. *Am Heart J* 126:578, 1993.

343. Larcos G, Brown ML, Gibbons RJ: Role of dipyridamole thallium-201 imaging in left bundle branch block. *Am J Cardiol* 68:1097, 1991.

344. Tawarahara K, Kurata C, Taguchi T, et al: Exercise testing and thallium-201 emission computed tomography in patients with intraventricular conduction disturbances. *Am J Cardiol* 69:97, 1992.

345. Ahmad M, Merry SL, Haibach H: Evidence of impaired myocardial perfusion and abnormal left ventricular function during exercise in patients with isolated systolic narrowing of the left anterior descending coronary artery. *Am J Cardiol* 48:832, 1981.

346. Greenspan M, Iskandrian AS, Catherwood E, et al. Myocardial bridging of the left anterior descending artery: Evaluation using exercise thallium-201 myocardial scintigraphy. *Cathet Cardiovasc Diagn* 6:173, 1980.

347. Raizner AE, Ishimori T, Verani MS, et al: Surgical relief of myocardial ischemia due to myocardial bridges. *Am J Cardiol* 45:417, 1980 (abstr).

348. Verani MS, Marcus ML, Ehrhardt JC, et al: Demonstra-tion of improved myocardial perfusion following aortic implantation of anomalous left coronary artery. *J Nucl Med* 19:1032, 1978.

349. Raifer SI, Oetgen WJ, Weeks KD Jr, et al: Thallium-201 scintigraphy after surgical repair of hemodynamically significant primary coronary artery anomalies. *Chest* 81:687, 1982.

350. Gutgesell HP, Pinsky WW, DePuey EG: Thallium-201 myocardial perfusion imaging in infants and children: Value in distinguishing anomalous left coronary artery from congestive cardiomyopathy. *Circulation* 61:596, 1980.

351. Finley JP, Howman-Giles R, Gilday DL, et al: Thallium-201 myocardial imaging in anomalous left coronary artery arising from the pulmonary artery: Applications before and after medical and surgical treatment. *Am J Cardiol* 42:675, 1978.

352. Mehrotra PP, Weaver YJ, Higginbotham EA: Myocardial perfusion defect on thallium-201 imaging in patients with chronic obstructive pulmonary disease. *J Am Coll Cardiol* 2:233, 1983.

353. Opherk D, Zebe H, Weihe E, et al: Reduced coronary dilatory capacity and ultrastructural changes of the myocardium in patients with angina pectoris but normal coronary arteriograms. *Circulation* 63:817, 1981.

354. Cannon RO, Watson RM, Rosing DR, et al: Angina caused by reduced vasodilator reserve of the small coronary arteries. *J Am Coll Cardiol* 1:1359, 1983.

355. Ouyyumi AA, Cannon RO III, Panza JA, et al: Endothelial dysfunction in patients with chest pain and normal coronary arteries. *Circulation* 86:1864, 1992.

356. Egashira K, Inou T, Hirooka Y, et al: Evidence of impaired endothelium-dependent coronary vasodilatation in patients with angina pectoris and normal coronary angiograms. *N Engl J Med* 328:1659, 1993.

357. Vrints CJM, Bult H, Hitter E, et al: Impaired endothelium-dependent cholinergic coronary vasodilation in patients with angina and normal coronary arteriograms. *J Am Coll Cardiol* 19:21, 1992.

358. Chauhan A, Mullins PA, Petch MC, Schofield PM: Is coronary flow reserve in response to papaverine really normal in syndrome X? *Circulation* 89:1998, 1994.

359. Geltman EM, Henes CG, Senneff MJ, et al: Increased myocardial perfusion at rest and diminished perfusion reserve in patients with angina and angiographically normal coronary arteries. *J Am Coll Cardiol* 16:586, 1990.

360. Rosen SD, Uren NG, Kaski J-C, et al: Coronary vasodilator reserve, pain perception, and sex in patients with syndrome X. *Circulation* 90:50, 1994.

361. Wiedermann JG, Schwartz A, Apfelbaum M: Anatomic and physiologic heterogeneity in patients with syndrome X: An intravascular ultrasound study. *J Am Coll Cardiol* 25:1310, 1995.

362. Korhola O, Valle M, Frick MH, et al: Regional myocardial perfusion abnormalities on xenon-133 imaging in patients with angina pectoris and normal coronary arteries. *Am J Cardiol* 39:355, 1977.

363. Meller J, Goldsmith SJ, Rudin A, et al: Spectrum of exercise thallium-201 myocardial perfusion imaging in patients with chest pain and normal coronary angiograms. *Am J Cardiol* 43:717, 1979.

364. Berger BC, Abramowitz R, Park CH, et al: Abnormal thallium-201 scans in patients with chest pain and angiographically normal coronary arteries. *Am J Cardiol* 52:365, 1983.

365. Tweddel AC, Martin W, Hutton I: Thallium scans in syndrome X. *Br Heart J* 68:48, 1992.

366. Galassi AR, Crea F, Araujo LI, et al: Comparison of regional myocardial blood flow in syndrome X and one-vessel coronary artery disease. *Am J Cardiol* 72:134, 1993.

367. Legrand V, Hodgson J McB, Bates ER, et al: Abnormal coronary flow reserve and abnormal radionuclide exercise test results in patients with normal coronary angiograms. *J Am Coll Cardiol* 6:1245, 1985.

368. Iskandrian AS, Scherer H, Croll MN, et al: Exercise thallium-201 myocardial scans in patients with disease limited to the secondary branches of the left coronary system. *Clin Cardiol* 2:121, 1979.

369. Iino T, Toyosaki N, Katsuki TA, et al: Evaluation of diseased coronary arterial branches by polar representations of thallium-201 rotational myocardial imaging. *Clin Nucl Med* 12:688, 1987.

370. Jones RH, McEwan P, Newman GE, et al: Accuracy of diagnosis of coronary artery disease by radionuclide measurement of left ventricular function during rest and exercise. *Circulation* 64:586, 1981.

371. Osbakken MD, Bove AA, Spann JF: Left ventricular regional wall motion and velocity of shortening in chronic mitral and aortic regurgitation. *Am J Cardiol* 47:1005, 1981.

372. Hecht HS, Hopkins JM: Exercise induced regional wall motion abnormalities on radionuclide angiography are not specific for coronary artery disease. *Circulation* 62(suppl III):III-147, 1980 (abstr).

373. Borer JS, Rosing DR, Miller RH, et al: Natural history of left ventricular function during 1 year after acute myocardial infarction: Comparison with clinical, electrocardiographic and biochemical determinations. *Am J Cardiol* 46:1, 1980.

374. Hirsowitz GS, Lakier JB, Marks DS, et al: Comparison of radionuclide and enzymatic estimate of infarct size in patients with acute myocardial infarction. *J Am Coll Cardiol* 1:1405, 1983.

375. Kimchi A, Rozanski A, Fletcher C, et al: The clinical significance of exercise-induced left ventricular wall motion abnormality occurring at a low heart rate. *Am Heart J* 114:724, 1987.

376. Borer JS, Kent KM, Bacharach SL, et al: Sensitivity, specificity and predictive accuracy of radionuclide cineangiography during exercise in patients with coronary artery disease: Comparison with exercise electrocardiography. *Circulation* 60:572, 1979.

377. Berger HJ, Reduto LA, Johnstone DE, et al: Global and regional left ventricular response to bicycle exercise in coronary artery disease: Assessment of quantitative radionuclide angiocardiography. *Am J Med* 66:13, 1979.

378. Jengo JA, Freeman R, Brizendine M, et al: Detection of coronary artery disease: Comparison of exercise stress radionuclide angiocardiography and thallium stress perfusion scanning. *Am J Cardiol* 45:535, 1980.

379. Massie B, Botvinick E, Shames D, et al: Correlation of myocardial perfusion with global and segmental ventricular function during exercise: Increased sensitivity of exercise blood pool scintigraphy for coronary disease. *Am J Cardiol* 43:343, 1979 (abstr).

380. Brady TJ, Thrall JH, Lo K, et al: The importance of adequate exercise in the detection of coronary heart disease by radionuclide ventriculography. *J Nucl Med* 21:1125, 1980.

381. Kirshenbaum HD, Okada RD, Boucher CA, et al: Relationship of thallium-201 myocardial perfusion pattern to regional and global left ventricular function with exercise. *Am Heart J* 101:734, 1981.

382. Campos CT, Chu HW, D'Agostino HJ Jr, Jones RH: Comparison of rest and exercise radionuclide angiocardiography and exercise treadmill testing for diagnosis of anatomically extensive coronary artery disease. *Circulation* 67:1204, 1983.

383. Gibbons RJ, Fyke FE III, Clements IP, et al: Noninvasive identification of severe coronary artery disease using exercise radionuclide angiography. *J Am Coll Cardiol* 11:28, 1988.

384. Wallis JB, Borer JS: Identification of "surgical" coronary anatomy by exercise radionuclide cineangiography. *Am J Cardiol* 68:1150, 1991.

385. Adams KF, Vincent LM, Kimrey S, et al: Sex influences ventricular response to exercise in normals free of chest pain. *Circulation* 72(suppl III):III-425, 1985 (abstr).

386. Greenberg PS, Berge RD, Johnson KD, et al: The value and limitations of radionuclide angiocardiography with stress in women. *Clin Cardiol* 6:312, 1983.

387. Hanley PC, Zinsmeister AR, Clements IP, et al: Gender-related differences in cardiac response to supine exercise assessed by radionuclide angiography. *J Am Coll Cardiol* 13:624, 1989.

388. Upton MT, Rerych SK, Newman GE, et al: Detecting abnormalities in left ventricular function during exercise before angina and ST-segment depression. *Circulation* 62:341, 1980.

389. Mellendez LJ, Manyari DE, Driedger AA, et al: Left ventricular function during graded exercise in patients with coronary artery disease and in control subjects. *Can Med Assoc J* 124:569, 1981.

390. Seaworth JF, Higginbotham MB, Coleman RE, et al: Effect of partial decreases in exercise work load on radionuclide indexes of ischemia. *J Am Coll Cardiol* 2:522, 1983.

391. Foster C, Anholm JD, Hellman CK, et al: Left ventricular function during sudden strenuous exercise. *Circulation* 63:592, 1981.

392. Foster C, Dymond DS, Anholm JD, et al: Effect of exercise protocol on the left ventricular response to exercise. *Am J Cardiol* 51:859, 1983.

393. Poliner LR, Dehmer GJ, Lewis SE, et al: Left ventricular performance in normal subjects: A comparison of the responses to exercise in the upright and supine positions. *Circulation* 62:528, 1980.

394. Manyari DE, Kostuk WJ, Purves PP: Left and right ventricular function at rest and during bicycle exercise in the supine and sitting positions in normal subjects and patients with coronary artery disease: Assessment by

radionuclide ventriculography. *Am J Cardiol* 51:36, 1983.

395. Freeman MR, Berman DS, Staniloff H, et al: Comparison of upright and supine bicycle exercise in the detection and evaluation of extent of coronary artery disease by equilibrium radionuclide ventriculography. *Am Heart J* 102:182, 1981.

396. Goldberg HL, Goldstein J, Borer JS, et al: Functional importance of coronary collateral vessels. *Am J Cardiol* 53:694, 1984.

397. Port S, Cobb FR, Coleman RE, et al: Effect of age on the response of the left ventricular ejection fraction to exercise. *N Engl J Med* 303:1133, 1980.

398. Hitzhusen JC, Hickler RB, Alpert JS, et al: Exercise testing and hemodynamic performance in healthy elderly persons. *Am J Cardiol* 54:1082, 1984.

399. Chen DCP, Rapp JS, Lindsay JL Jr, et al: Cardiac response to exercise in the hyperkinetic heart. *Radiology* 149:181, 1983 (abstr).

400. Leon MB, Borer, JS, Bacharach SL, et al: Detection of early cardiac dysfunction in patients with severe beta-thalassemia and chronic iron overload. *N Engl J Med* 301:1143, 1979.

401. Covitz W, Eubig C, Balfour IC, et al: Exercise-induced cardiac dysfunction in sickle cell anemia: A radionuclide study. *Am J Cardiol* 51:570, 1981.

402. Das SK, Brady TJ, Thrall JH, et al: Cardiac function in patients with prior myocarditis. *J Nucl Med* 21:689, 1980.

403. Wasserman AG, Katz RJ, Varghese PJ, et al: Exercise radionuclide ventriculographic responses in hypertensive patients with chest pain. *N Engl J Med* 311:1276, 1984.

404. Miller DD, Ruddy TD, Zusman RM, et al: Left ventricular ejection fraction response during exercise in asymptomatic systemic hypertension. *Am J Cardiol* 59:409, 1987.

405. Christian TF, Zinsmeister AR, Miller TD, et al: Left ventricular systolic response to exercise in patients with systemic hypertension without left ventricular hypertrophy. *Am J Cardiol* 65:1204, 1990.

406. Bramlet DA, Morris KG, Coleman RE, et al: Effects of rate-dependent left bundle branch block on global and regional left ventricular function. *Circulation* 67:1059, 1983.

407. Rowe DW, DePuey EG, Sonnemaker RE, et al: Left ventricular performance during exercise in patients with LBBB. *Circulation* 62(suppl III):III-147, 1980 (abstr).

408. Manno BV, Hakki A-H, Eshaghpour E, et al: Left ventricular function at rest and during exercise in congenital complete heart block: A radionuclide angiographic evaluation. *Am J Cardiol* 52:92, 1983.

409. Chipps BE, Alderson PO, Roland JMA, et al: Noninvasive evaluation of ventricular function in cystic fibrosis. *J Pediatr* 95:379, 1979.

410. Slutsky R, Ackerman W, Hooper W, et al: The response of left ventricular ejection fraction and volume to supine exercise in patients with severe COPD. *Circulation* 59,60(suppl II):II-234, 1979 (abstr).

411. Hecht HS, Hopkins JM: Exercise-induced regional wall motion abnormalities on radionuclide angiography: Lack of reliability for detection of coronary artery disease in the presence of valvular heart disease. *Am J Cardiol* 47:861, 1981.

412. Detrano R, Yiannikas J, Salcedo EE, et al: Bayesian probability analysis: A prospective demonstration of its clinical utility in diagnosing coronary disease. *Circulation* 69:541, 1984.

413. Hlatky M, Botvinick E, Brundage B: Diagnostic accuracy of cardiologists compared with probability calculations using Bayes' rule. *Am J Cardiol* 49:1927, 1982.

414. Diamond GA, Staniloff HM, Forrester JS, et al: Computer-assisted diagnosis in the noninvasive evaluation of patients with suspected coronary artery disease. *J Am Coll Cardiol* 1:444, 1983.

415. Morise AP, Duval RD: Comparison of three Bayesian methods to estimate posttest probability in patients undergoing exercise stress testing. *Am J Cardiol* 64:1117, 1989.

416. Rifkin RD, Hood WB Jr: Bayesian analysis of electrocardiographic exercise stress testing. *N Engl J Med* 297:681, 1977.

417. Diamond GA, Hirsch M, Forrester JS, et al: Application of information theory to clinical diagnostic testing. The electrocardiographic stress test. *Circulation* 63:915, 1981.

418. Christopher TD, Konstantinow G, Jones RH: Bayesian analysis of data from radionuclide angiocardiograms for diagnosis of coronary artery disease. *Circulation* 69:65, 1984.

419. Ladenheim ML, Kotler TS, Pollock BH, et al: Incremental prognostic power of clinical history, exercise electrocardiography and myocardial perfusion scintigraphy in suspected coronary artery disease. *Am J Cardiol* 59:270, 1987.

420. Pollock SG, Abbott RD, Boucher CA, et al: Independent and incremental prognostic value of tests performed in hierarchical order to evaluate patients with suspected coronary artery disease. Validation of models based on these tests. *Circulation* 85:237, 1992.

421. Morise AP, Diamond GA, Detrano R, et al: Incremental value of exercise electrocardiography and thallium-201 testing in men and women for the presence and extent of coronary artery disease. *Am Heart J* 130:267, 1995.

422. Oosterhuis WP, Niemeyer MG, Kuijper AFM, et al: Evaluation of the incremental diagnostic value and impact on patient treatment of thallium scintigraphy. *J Nucl Med* 33:1727, 1992.

423. Palmas W, Friedman JD, Diamond GA, et al: Incremental value of simultaneous assessment of myocardial function and perfusion with technetium-99m sestamibi for prediction of extent of coronary artery disease. *J Am Coll Cardiol* 25:1024, 1995.

424. Morise AP: An incremental evaluation of the diagnostic value of thallium single-photon emission computed tomographic imaging and lung/heart ratio concerning both the presence and extent of coronary artery disease. *J Nucl Cardiol* 2:238, 1995.

425. Hachamovitch R, Berman DS, Kiat H, et al: Exercise myocardial perfusion SPECT in patients without known coronary artery disease. Incremental prognostic value and use in risk stratification. *Circulation* 93:905, 1996.

426. Iskandrian AS, Chae SC, Heo J, et al: Independent and

incremental prognostic value of exercise single-photon emission computed tomographic (SPECT) thallium imaging in coronary artery disease. *J Am Coll Cardiol* 22:665, 1993.

427. Christian TF, Miller TD, Bailey KR, Gibbons RJ: Exercise tomographic thallium-201 imaging in patients with severe coronary artery disease and normal electrocardiograms. *Ann Intern Med* 121:825, 1994.

428. Berman DS, Hachamovitch R, Kiat H, et al: Incremental value of prognostic testing in patients with known or suspected ischemic heart disease: A basis for optimal utilization of exercise technetium-99m sestamibi myocardial perfusion single-photon emission computed tomography. *J Am Coll Cardiol* 26:639, 1995.

429. Simari RD, Miller TD, Zinsmeister AR, Gibbons RJ: Capabilities of supine exercise electrocardiography versus exercise radionuclide angiography in predicting coronary events. *Am J Cardiol* 67:573, 1991.

430. Melin JA, Piret LJ, Vanbutsele RJM, et al: Diagnostic value of exercise electrocardiography and thallium myocardial scintigraphy in patients without previous myocardial infarction: A Bayesian approach. *Circulation* 63: 1019, 1981.

431. Diamond GA, Forrester JS, Hirsch M, et al: Application of conditional probability analysis to the clinical diagnosis of coronary artery disease. *J Clin Invest* 65:1210, 1980.

432. Dans PE, Weiner JP, Melin JA, et al: Conditional probability in the diagnosis of coronary artery disease: A future tool for eliminating unnecessary testing? *South Med J* 76:1118, 1983.

433. Patterson RE, Horowitz SF, Eng C, et al: Can exercise electrocardiography and thallium-201 myocardial imaging exclude the diagnosis of coronary artery disease? Bayesian analysis of the clinical limits of exclusion and indications for coronary angiography. *Am J Cardiol* 49:1127, 1982.

434. Epstein SE: Implications of probability analysis on the strategy used for noninvasive detection of coronary artery disease: Role of single or combined use of exercise electrocardiographic testing, radionuclide cineangiography and myocardial perfusion imaging. *Am J Cardiol* 46:491, 1980.

435. Weintraub WS, Madeira SW Jr, Bodenheimer MM, et al: Critical analysis of the application of Bayes' theorem to sequential testing in the noninvasive diagnosis of coronary artery disease. *Am J Cardiol* 54:43, 1984.

436. Detrano R, Leatherman J, Salcedo EE, et al: Bayesian analysis versus discriminant function analysis: Their relative utility in the diagnosis of coronary disease. *Circulation* 73:970, 1986.

437. Charuzi Y, Diamond GA, Pichler M, et al: Analysis of multiple noninvasive test procedures for the diagnosis of coronary artery disease. *Clin Cardiol* 4:67, 1981.

438. Pollock SG, Watson DD, Gibson RS, et al: A simplified approach for evaluating multiple test outcomes and multiple disease states in relation to the exercise thallium-201 stress test in suspected coronary artery disease. *Am J Cardiol* 64:466, 1989.

439. Brown KA: Prognostic value of thallium-201 myocardial

perfusion imaging. A diagnostic tool comes of age. *Circulation* 83:363, 1991.

440. Weiner DA, Ryan TJ, McCabe CH, et al: Comparison of coronary artery bypass surgery and medical therapy in patients with exercised-induced silent myocardial ischemia: A report from the coronary artery surgery study (CASS) registry. *J Am Coll Cardiol* 12:595, 1988.

441. Hopkirk JAC, Uhl GS, Hickman JR Jr, et al: Discriminant value of clinical and exercise variables in detecting significant coronary artery disease in asymptomatic men. *J Am Coll Cardiol* 3:887, 1984.

442. Trobaugh GB, Wackers FJTh, Sokole EB, et al: Thallium-201 myocardial imaging: An interinstitutional study of observer variability. *J Nucl Med* 19:359, 1978.

443. Patterson RE, Eng C, Horowitz SF, et al: Bayesian comparison of cost-effectiveness of different clinical approaches to diagnose coronary artery disease. *J Am Coll Cardiol* 4:278, 1984.

444. Hung J, Chaitman BR, Lam J, et al: Noninvasive diagnostic test choices for the evaluation of coronary artery disease in women: A multivariate comparison of cardiac fluoroscopy, exercise electrocardiography and exercise thallium myocardial perfusion scintigraphy. *J Am Coll Cardiol* 4:8, 1984.

445. Melin JA, Wijns W, Vanbutsele RJ, et al: Alternative diagnostic strategies for coronary artery disease in women: Demonstration of the usefulness and efficiency of probability analysis. *Circulation* 71:535, 1985.

446. Gitler B, Fishbach M, Steingart RM: Use of electrocardiographic-thallium exercise testing in clinical practice. *J Am Coll Cardiol* 3:262, 1984.

447. Detrano R, Janosi A, Steinbrunn W, et al: International application of a new probability algorithm for the diagnosis of coronary artery disease. *Am J Cardiol* 64:304, 1989.

448. Feinstein AR: XXXIX. The haze of Bayes, the aerial palaces of decision analysis, and the computerized Ouija board. *Clin Pharmacol Ther* 21:482, 1979.

449. Marcus FI: A critical appraisal of the Bayesian approach to diagnose coronary artery disease. *J Am Coll Cardiol* 4:292, 1984.

450. Mark DB, Nelson CL, Califf RM, et al: Continuing evolution of therapy for coronary artery disease. Initial results from the era of coronary angioplasty. *Circulation* 89:2015, 1994.

451. Gibbons RJ: Role of nuclear cardiology for determining management of patients with stable coronary artery disease. *J Nucl Cardiol* 1:S118, 1994.

452. Stein JH, Uretz EF, Parrillo JE, Barron JT: Cost and appropriateness of radionuclide exercise stress testing by cardiologists and non-cardiologists. *Am J Cardiol* 77:139, 1996.

453. Uhl GS, Kay TN, Hickman JR Jr: Computer-enhanced thallium scintigrams in asymptomatic men with abnormal exercise tests. *Am J Cardiol* 48:1037, 1981.

454. Russell RO Jr, Moraski RE, Kouchoukos N, et al: Unstable angina pectoris: National cooperative study group to compare surgical and medical therapy: II. In-hospital experience and initial follow-up results in patients with one, two and three vessel disease. *Am J Cardiol* 42: 839, 1978.

455. Fulton M, Lutz W, Donald KW, et al: Natural history of unstable angina. *Lancet* 1:860, 1972.

456. Gazes PC, Mobley EM Jr, Faris HM Jr, et al: Preinfarctional (stable) angina—a prospective study: Ten-year follow-up. Prognostic significance of electrocardiographic changes. *Circulation* 48:331, 1973.

457. Krauss KR, Hutter AM, DeSanctis RW: Acute coronary insufficiency: Course and follow-up. *Circulation* 45(suppl I):66, 1972.

458. Alison HW, Russell RO Jr, Mantle JA, et al: Coronary anatomy and arteriography in patients with unstable angina pectoris. *Am J Cardiol* 41:204, 1978.

459. Freeman MR, Williams AE, Chisholm RJ, et al: Role of resting thallium-201 perfusion in predicting coronary anatomy, left ventricular wall motion, and hospital outcome in unstable angina pectoris. *Am Heart J* 117:306, 1989.

460. Brown KA, Okada RD, Boucher CA, et al: Serial thallium-201 imaging at rest in patients with unstable and stable angina pectoris: Relationship of myocardial perfusion at rest to presenting clinical syndrome. *Am Heart J* 106:70, 1983.

461. Berger BC, Watson DD, Burwell LR, et al: Redistribution of thallium at rest in patients with stable and unstable angina and the effect of coronary artery bypass surgery. *Circulation* 60:1114, 1979.

462. Wackers FJTh, Lie KI, Liem KL, et al: Thallium-201 scintigraphy in unstable angina pectoris. *Circulation* 57:738, 1978.

463. Gregoire J, Theroux P: Detection and assessment of unstable angina using myocardial perfusion imaging: Comparison between technetium-99m sestamibi SPECT and 12-lead electrocardiogram. *Am J Cardiol* 66:42E, 1990.

464. Zhu YY, Chung WS, Botvinick EH, et al: Dipyridamole perfusion scintigraphy: The experience with its application in one hundred seventy patients with known or suspected unstable angina. *Am Heart J* 121:33, 1991.

465. Freeman MR, Chisholm RJ, Armstrong PW: Usefulness of exercise electrocardiography and thallium scintigraphy in unstable angina pectoris in predicting the extent and severity of coronary artery disease. *Am J Cardiol* 62:1164, 1988.

466. Swahn E, Areskog M, Berglund U, et al: Predictive importance of clinical findings and a predischarge exercise test in patients with suspected unstable coronary artery disease. *Am J Cardiol* 59:208, 1987.

467. Butman SM, Olson HG, Gardin JM, et al: Submaximal exercise testing after stabilization of unstable angina pectoris. *J Am Coll Cardiol* 4:667, 1984.

468. Cohn PF: Silent myocardial ischemia: Present status. *Mod Concepts Cardiovasc Dis* 56:1, 1987.

469. Epstein SE, Quyyumi AA, Bonow RO: Myocardial ischemia—silent or symptomatic. *N Engl J Med* 318:1038, 1988.

470. McHenry PL, O'Donnell J, Morris SN, Jordan JJ: The abnormal exercise electrocardiogram in apparently healthy men: A predictor of angina pectoris as an initial coronary event during long-term follow-up. *Circulation* 70:547, 1984.

471. Bruce RA, DeRouen TA, Hossack KF, et al: Value of maximal exercise tests in risk assessment of primary coronary heart disease events in healthy men: Five years' experience of the Seattle Heart Watch Study. *Am J Cardiol* 46:371, 1980.

472. Erikssen J, Enge I, Forfang K, Storstein O: False positive diagnostic tests and coronary angiographic findings in 105 presumably healthy males. *Circulation* 54:371, 1976.

473. Langou RA, Huang EK, Kelley MJ, Cohen LS: Predictive accuracy of coronary artery calcification and abnormal exercise test for coronary artery disease in asymptomatic men. *Circulation* 62:1196, 1980.

474. Fleg JL, Gerstenblith G, Zonderman AB, et al: Prevalence and prognostic significance of exercise-induced silent myocardial ischemia detected by thallium scintigraphy and electrocardiography in asymptomatic volunteers. *Circulation* 81:428, 1990.

475. Cohn PF: Total ischemic burden: Pathophysiology and prognosis. *Am J Cardiol* 59:3C, 1987.

476. Weiner DA, Ryan TJ, McCabe CH, et al: Risk of developing an acute myocardial infarction or sudden coronary death in patients with exercise-induced silent myocardial ischemia: A report from the Coronary Artery Surgery Study (CASS) Registry. *Am J Cardiol* 62:1155, 1988.

477. Callaham PR, Froelicher VF, Klein J, et al: Exercise-induced silent ischemia: Age, diabetes mellitus, previous myocardial infarction and prognosis. *J Am Coll Cardiol* 14:1175, 1989.

478. Assey ME, Walters GL, Hendrix GH, et al: Incidence of acute myocardial infarction in patients with exercise-induced silent myocardial ischemia. *Am J Cardiol* 59:497, 1987.

479. Tzivoni D, Weisz G, Gavish A, et al: Comparison of mortality and myocardial infarction rates in stable angina pectoris with and without ischemic episodes during daily activities. *Am J Cardiol* 63:273, 1989.

480. Rocco MB, Nabel EG, Campbell S, et al: Prognostic importance of myocardial ischemia detected by ambulatory monitoring in patients with stable coronary artery disease. *Circulation* 78:877, 1988.

481. Deedwania PC, Carbajal EV: Silent ischemia during daily life is an independent predictor of mortality in stable angina. *Circulation* 81:748, 1990.

482. Travin MI, Flores AR, Boucher CA, et al: Silent versus symptomatic ischemia during a thallium-201 exercise test. *Am J Cardiol* 68:1600, 1991.

483. Chierchia S, Lazzari M, Freedman B, et al: Impairment of myocardial perfusion and function during painless myocardial ischemia. *J Am Coll Cardiol* 1:924, 1983.

484. Rozanski A, Bairey CN, Krantz DS, et al: Mental stress and the induction of silent myocardial ischemia in patients with coronary artery disease. *N Engl J Med* 318:1005, 1988.

485. Cecchi AC, Dovellini EV, Marchi F, et al: Silent myocardial ischemia during ambulatory electrocardiographic monitoring in patients with effort angina. *J Am Coll Cardiol* 1:934, 1983.

486. Quyyumi AA, Mockus L, Wright C, et al: Morphology of ambulatory ST changes in patients with varying severity of coronary artery disease: Investigation of the fre-

quency of nocturnal ischaemia and coronary spasm. *Br Heart J* 53:186, 1985.

487. Droste C, Roskamm H: Experimental pain measurement in patients with asymptomatic myocardial ischemia. *J Am Coll Cardiol* 1:940, 1983.

488. Ambepityia G, Kopelman PG, Ingram D, et al: Exertional myocardial ischemia in diabetes: A quantitative analysis of anginal perceptual threshold and the influence of autonomic function. *J Am Coll Cardiol* 15:72, 1990.

489. Rogers WJ, Bourassa MG, Andrews TC, et al: Asymptomatic cardiac ischemia pilot (ACIP) study: Outcome at 1 year for patients with asymptomatic cardiac ischemia randomized to medical therapy or revascularization. *J Am Coll Cardiol* 26:594, 1995.

490. Pepine CJ, Cohn PF, Deedwania PC, et al: Effects of treatment on outcome in mildly symptomatic patients with ischemia during daily life. The atenolol silent ischemia study (ASIST). *Circulation* 90:762, 1994.

491. Mouratidis B, Vaughan-Neil EF, Gilday DL, et al: Detection of silent coronary artery disease in adolescents and young adults with familial hypercholesterolemia by single-photon emission computed tomography thallium-201 scanning. *Am J Cardiol* 70:1109, 1992.

492. Davis K, Kennedy JW, Kemp HG Jr, et al: Complications of coronary arteriography from the collaborative study of coronary artery surgery (CASS). *Circulation* 59: 1105, 1979.

Comparison of Stress Myocardial Perfusion Imaging and Stress Echocardiography in Assessment of Coronary Artery Disease

Myron C. Gerson
Brian D. Hoit

If detection of anatomic coronary artery stenoses was the only objective in the evaluation of the patient with suspected coronary artery disease (CAD), then all of these patients would be examined by coronary arteriography alone. There is, however, a continuing need for noninvasive tests that clarify the physiologic significance of coronary artery stenosis,[1] provide powerful prognostic data,[2] and permit accurate detection of coronary artery stenosis with lower cost and greater patient convenience compared with coronary arteriography.

Myocardial perfusion imaging and echocardiography each provide numerous favorable and some unfavorable properties for noninvasive diagnosis of CAD. These are discussed in the next section. The diagnostic accuracy of stress myocardial perfusion imaging and stress echocardiography as reported in the literature is then reviewed, leading to a number of conclusions.

THEORETICAL ADVANTAGES AND DISADVANTAGES OF MYOCARDIAL PERFUSION IMAGING AND ECHOCARDIOGRAPHY

Pathophysiology (Table 21-1)

FLOW VERSUS CONTRACTION

Myocardial nuclear perfusion imaging is based on assessment of myocardial blood flow, whereas stress echocardiography is primarily based on evaluation of left ven-tricular regional wall motion. When acute myocardial ischemia occurs in a patient with coronary artery stenosis, the initial abnormality is an imbalance in myocardial blood flow between the hypoperfused and normally perfused myocardial segments. In response to increasingly severe regional myocardial hypoperfusion, regional myocardial relaxation becomes impaired, providing an early functional indication of myocardial ischemia. Impairment of left ventricular relaxation may be followed by abnormalities of regional left ventricular contraction during systole,[3–8] and, subsequently, by ischemic electrocardiographic (ECG) ST-segment depression and ischemic chest pain.[9] Because abnormal regional myocardial blood flow precedes regional contractile abnormalities in patients with CAD, myocardial perfusion imaging may become abnormal earlier in the course of myocardial ischemia compared with stress echocardiography, which is dependent on induction of abnormal regional contraction. It has also been theorized that coronary artery stenosis may, under some conditions, impair myocardial blood flow during exercise or pharmacologic stress without producing sufficient myocardial ischemia to produce a regional contractile abnormality. The latter hypothesis is supported by clinical studies documenting abnormal regional left ventricular myocardial relaxation in the absence of contractile dysfunction in the distribution of a coronary artery stenosis.[3–6] If some patients with coronary artery stenosis develop substantial imbalances of regional myocardial blood flow in the absence of, or prior to, regional wall motion abnormality, then it is reasonable to anticipate that imaging of myocardial

Table 21-1 Characteristics of Stress Myocardial Perfusion Imaging and Stress Echocardiography

	Perfusion Imaging	Stress Echocardiography
Mechanism	Altered blood flow	Altered myocardial wall motion
Normal variability	Decreased inferior and septal activity	Inferobasilar hypokinesia
Abnormalities in noncoronary heart disease	Yes	Yes
Unique problems	Relative flow not absolute	Effects of whole heart motion
Advantages	Quantitative, automated, mature technology, superior prognostic and myocardial viability information	Cost, versatility ("one stop shopping"), availability
Disadvantages	Technically demanding, expensive, radiation	Subjective, technically difficult

perfusion may provide more sensitive detection of coronary artery stenoses compared with imaging of stress-induced abnormalities of regional left ventricular contraction. This property might be particularly valuable in the noninvasive detection of moderate coronary artery stenoses (e.g, 50 to 70 percent luminal diameter reduction), in the detection of coronary disease despite inadequate stress to produce regional contractile abnormalities (e.g., submaximal dynamic exercise), or with exercise tests in which an ischemic response is blunted by antianginal drugs.

If a relatively severe imbalance in regional myocardial blood flow is required to induce abnormal regional myocardial contraction or wall thickening, then it is likely that diagnostic imaging modalities that assess left ventricular regional wall motion will be more specific for the presence of ischemia, as judged by an independent reference standard, compared with assessment of regional myocardial perfusion. Thus, from these theoretical considerations alone, one could speculate that stress myocardial perfusion imaging might be more sensitive than stress echocardiography for detection of coronary artery stenoses, whereas stress echocardiography may provide higher diagnostic specificity.

NORMAL VARIABILITY IN REGIONAL MYOCARDIAL PERFUSION AND CONTRACTION

Detection of CAD by myocardial perfusion imaging requires differentiation of uniform from nonuniform myocardial blood flow.[10–12] DePasquale et al[12] studied the postexercise regional left ventricular distribution of thallium 201 (^{201}Tl) using tomographic data displayed in a bull's-eye format. For 20 men with a less than 5 percent likelihood that clinically significant CAD was present, ^{201}Tl activity in the inferior wall was 78 ± 5 percent and septal activity 80 ± 6 percent of activity in the lateral left ventricular wall. For 16 women with a less than 5 percent likelihood of CAD, inferior wall activity was 87 ± 5 percent and septal activity 84 ± 4 percent of lateral wall activity. Therefore, in this study and in others,[10,11] the regional variability of myocardial tracer activity in normal subjects is significant, and this variability is a factor in attempting to separate normal from abnormal myocardial segments. However, the regional pattern of tomographic ^{201}Tl distribution in the left ventricle shows substantial predictability among members of a normal population. Therefore, when tomographic myocardial perfusion scans are interpreted either by subjective or quantitative criteria, the anticipated reduction in inferior and septal activity observed in normal populations can be incorporated into the criteria for detecting stress-induced myocardial perfusion defects.

Detection of CAD by stress echocardiography requires differentiation of normal from abnormal regional myocardial contraction or wall thickening. In normal subjects, the coefficient of variation for echocardiographic resting regional wall motion of 24 percent and of regional wall thickening of 48 percent[13] is not different from reported coefficients of variation for resting radionuclide regional myocardial perfusion of 16 to 35 percent.[10,11] Gintzon et al[14] assessed the percent area reduction between diastolic and systolic left ventricular endocardial contours in 25 healthy adults studied at rest and during upright bicycle exercise. The left ventricular contour was divided into 32 segments. At rest, the percent area reduction was 54 ± 4 percent for the septum, 67 ± 3 percent for the left ventricular apex, and 67 ± 8 percent for the lateral wall. At peak exercise, the percent area reduction was 84 ± 5 percent for the septum, 88 ± 2 percent for the apex, and 83 ± 6 percent for the lateral wall. However, because the range of standard deviation of normal endocardial motion and the degree of variability between radial segments in the same healthy individuals were substantial, the authors concluded that hypokinetic wall motion "may be a normal event." In a preliminary report, Hausnerova et al[15] measured end-diastolic and end-systolic regional wall thickness by echocardiography in 16 normal subjects during infusion of 30 μg/kg/min of the positive inotropic beta-adrenergic agonist, dobutamine. Average percent wall thickening during drug infusion was greater in the septum (59 ± 22 percent) compared with the free wall segments (51 ± 19 percent, $p = 0.05$). The authors concluded that echocardiographic quantitation of percent myocardial wall thickening should be used with caution to detect regional myocardial ischemia. Recently, Carstensen et al[16] examined the response of echocardiographic left ventricular wall motion to infusion of dobutamine combined with atropine injection in 42 asymptomatic volunteers. In these healthy subjects, quantitative measures of wall motion and wall thickening increased from baseline to low-dose infusion, but decreased from low-dose to peak infusion. The authors called for a revision of the assumptions on which analysis of dobutamine–atropine stress echocardiography are based. Furthermore, external factors may alter the apparent extent of left ventricular regional contraction. Hypokinesia of the inferobasilar segment may result from tethering to the mitral annulus.[17] In addition, abnormal interventricular septal motion may be seen in patients with interventricular conduction abnormalities and after cardiac surgery. Thus, significant heterogeneity of regional left ventricular contraction and wall thickening have been observed in normal subjects who undergo stress echocardiography and this may have implications for identification of left ventricular hypokinesis resulting from CAD, for minimizing interobserver variability in test interpretation, and for applying current quantitative methods to stress echocardiography.

REGIONAL ABNORMALITIES IN NONCORONARY HEART DISEASE

Stress imaging tests must also be capable of separating regional perfusion or contractile abnormalities resulting from CAD from those resulting from noncoronary forms of heart disease. Characteristic myocardial perfusion defects have been described in the absence of coronary artery stenosis, in the left ventricular apex in some patients with volume overload related to aortic regurgitation,[18] in the interventricular septum in some patients with left ventricular pressure overload related to aortic stenosis[19] or in hypertrophic cardiomyopathy,[20–22] and in the septum and anterior walls in patients with asynchronous left ventricular contraction resulting from left bundle branch block.[23–25]

Reports of left ventricular regional wall motion by stress echocardiography in patients with noncoronary heart disease have been limited to date. Sharp et al[26] used dobutamine echocardiography and coronary arteriography to study 54 subjects with left ventricular dilatation and systolic dysfunction. Dobutamine stress echocardiography had a sensitivity of 83 percent and a specificity of 71 percent for detection of CAD—a lower specificity than that previously reported in patients with normal resting regional wall motion. Bach et al[27] have confirmed that left ventricular regional wall motion, as assessed by echocardiography, in patients with dilated cardiomyopathy, is heterogeneous relative to controls, and that this

heterogeneity is correlated with measures of regional oxidative metabolism. Left ventricular regional wall motion abnormalities may also occur in patients with valvular heart disease in the absence of coronary artery stenosis.[28] Thus, myocardial perfusion and regional contraction may be abnormal in noncoronary heart disease and this will likely pose some diagnostic difficulties for either modality. However, the versatility and efficiency of stress echocardiography (i.e., the ability to discriminate wall motion from wall thickening and to identify noncoronary cardiac disease) offers a clear advantage in this regard.

ASSESSMENT OF RELATIVE VERSUS ABSOLUTE MYOCARDIAL BLOOD FLOW

At present, a potential limitation of myocardial perfusion imaging with single-photon tracers is that absolute myocardial blood flow in mL/min/kg is not measured. Instead, relative myocardial blood flow to different left ventricular segments is represented. Early in the history of myocardial perfusion imaging, concern was expressed that balanced myocardial hypoperfusion could lead to images with uniform tracer distribution in a setting of proximal three-vessel CAD. However, with current single-photon tomographic imaging technology, abnormal myocardial perfusion is detected in approximately 96 percent of patients with three-vessel CAD.[12,29–35] If, in fact, delineation of relative rather than absolute regional myocardial blood flow is disadvantageous diagnostically, the problem is most likely to occur in attempting to identify ischemia in the distribution of the least severely diseased coronary artery in patients with hemodynamically significant three-vessel CAD. In theory, stress echocardiography may avert this problem because the change in regional myocardial wall motion is compared between rest and stress for each of the three coronary artery distributions. Nevertheless, when exercise-induced ischemia is produced, patients with three-vessel CAD often must discontinue exercise before ischemia is induced in the distribution of all three coronary arteries. Thus, it is possible that limited exercise owing to ischemic symptoms may prevent detection of the full extent of myocardial ischemia.

Effects of Cardiac Motion on Assessment of Segmental Contraction

Normal cardiac physiology as well as pathophysiologic states may compromise assessment of left ventricular regional wall motion by echocardiography. Cardiac motion is complex, including cardiac rotational and translational motion resulting from respiration. At any given time, two-dimensional echocardiography visualizes a single slice through the left ventricular endocardium. As a result of rotational and translational motion, as well as the echocardiographic beam not being oriented parallel to the direction of contractile motion of the ventricular walls, the endocardial surface visualized at the end of systole may not be the same endocardial surface visualized in that plane at end diastole. In theory, visualization of different areas of endocardium in diastole and systole may result in underestimation of left ventricular regional contraction or wall thickening. In patients with a prior myocardial infarction, impaired left ventricular regional wall motion may result in a "tethering" of adjacent normal myocardial segments.[36] This has been observed to result in overestimation of the extent of left ventricular involvement from CAD.

Type of Intervention

EXERCISE STRESS

An advantage of myocardial perfusion testing is that the resultant images display what is fundamentally the distribution of myocardial blood flow at the time of peak exercise. In some patients with ischemic heart disease, myocardial ischemia resolves rapidly with cessation of exercise. Using first-pass radionuclide angiography, Seaworth et al[37] showed that exercise-induced abnormalities of global left ventricular ejection fraction (LVEF) and of left ventricular regional wall motion had resolved in the majority of their 43 study patients within 1 min of cessation of maximal exercise. Similarly, with exercise echocardiography performed during peak exercise, Presti et al[38] observed exercise-induced regional wall-motion abnormalities in 29 patients with CAD, but there was no detectable wall-motion abnormality in 7 of the 29 patients (24 percent) during imaging performed within 3 min postexercise. Ciniglio et al[39] examined regional myocardial wall thickening by echocardiography at 0 to 2, 2 to 4, and 5 to 7 min following treadmill exercise. Wall thickening was increased at 0 to 2 min following treadmill exercise in comparison to the pre-exercise baseline recording. By 2 to 4 min following completion of treadmill exercise, regional myocardial wall thickening, as detected by two-dimensional echocardiography, had returned to pre-exercise levels. Therefore, imaging during peak dynamic exercise appears to be required to provide the highest level of diagnostic sensitivity and exercise echocardiographic data collected in the postexercise period only provides very limited information for detection of CAD after the first 2 min of the recovery period.

In the United States, patients are more often accustomed to performing walking rather than bicycle exercise. Unfortunately, technically adequate echocardiograms cannot be acquired during treadmill exercise with current instrumentation. Supine bicycle exercise provides the most convenient exercise position for recording high quality echocardiograms, but the heart rate response is generally lower in comparison to maximal upright exercise in the same patient.[40] Supine exercise to a slightly lower heart rate may provide a comparable stress to upright bicycle exercise in some coronary patients as a result of augmented left ventricular preload in the supine position. Nevertheless, the necessary level of peak (target) heart rate required to achieve optimal diagnostic accuracy for supine exercise echocardiography has not been clearly established and may not be achievable in many patients.

PHARMACOLOGIC STRESS

Pharmacologic stress testing, with coronary artery vasodilators (e.g., dipyridamole or adenosine) or with positive inotropic drugs (e.g., dobutamine), provides a valuable alternative approach for noninvasive detection of CAD in the patient who is unable to perform vigorous physical exercise. In an open-chest, anesthetized canine model, Fung et al[41] observed the effects of dobutamine and dipyridamole infusions on regional myocardial blood flow measured by radiolabeled microspheres and regional left ventricular wall thickening by two-dimensional echocardiography in the distributions of a highly stenotic left circumflex artery and an unobstructed left anterior descending (LAD) artery. The ratio of LAD to left circumflex subendocardial blood flow was threefold greater with dipyridamole compared with dobutamine infusion. Dobutamine induced wall thickening abnormalities in all dogs but dipyridamole induced dysfunction in only 55 percent of the animals studied ($p < 0.01$). Therefore, the authors concluded that pharmacologic coronary artery vasodilation is the pharmacologic intervention of choice in conjunction with myocardial perfusion imaging, whereas inotropic stress with dobutamine may be the intervention of choice for noninvasive detection of CAD with echocardiographic imaging of regional wall motion. However, clinical implications of the study are severely limited because the dipyridamole (0.56 mg/kg) and dobutamine (15 μg/kg/min) doses used were substantially lower than the doses of these drugs used currently (i.e., up to 0.84 mg/kg for dipyridamole echocardiography and up to 40 to 50 μg/kg/min of dobutamine with addition of up to 1 mg atropine for either dobutamine echocardiography or dobutamine perfusion imaging). Similarly, Kumar et al[42] reported a randomized crossover study of dipyridamole and dobutamine thallium stress imaging in humans. However, their conclusion that dipyridamole is more effective than dobutamine in producing perfusion defects detectable by ^{201}Tl perfusion imaging cannot be extrapolated to current dobutamine–thallium imaging protocols that use dobutamine infusion doses higher than

20 μg/kg/min and include atropine injection when required to raise the heart rate.

The diagnostic sensitivity of dipyridamole echocardiography for detection of CAD is improved significantly by increasing the dipyridamole dose from 0.56 mg/kg to 0.84 mg/kg.[43] However, Martin et al[44] compared dobutamine (40 μg/kg/min) echocardiography with high-dose dipyridamole (0.84 mg/kg) echocardiography and found the former to be more sensitive ($p < 0.05$) for detection of coronary artery stenosis. Because the diagnostic specificity was slightly higher for dipyridamole compared with dobutamine echocardiography, the overall accuracy of dobutamine compared to dipyridamole echocardiography did not differ to a statistically significant extent.

In summary, current data suggest that pharmacologic coronary artery vasodilation produces greater maldistribution of coronary blood flow beyond a coronary artery stenosis compared with inotropic stimulation with dobutamine, but that dobutamine produces more consistent appearance of regional wall motion abnormalities. Dobutamine is also favored by some echocardiography investigators because it provides a graded response simulating exercise.

Image Acquisition

Acquisition of high quality echocardiographic or nuclear cardiac images is highly dependent on the availability of experienced, skilled technical personnel to acquire and process the imaging data. In a well equipped nuclear cardiology laboratory staffed by experienced personnel, myocardial perfusion images that are technically satisfactory for interpretation can be obtained in nearly all patients and high quality images can be obtained in the majority of patients.

SOFT-TISSUE ATTENUATION

Quality of the myocardial perfusion imaging data is primarily compromised by soft-tissue attenuation resulting from tissues interposed between the heart and the nuclear medicine camera. When soft-tissue attenuation interferes with tracer activity detection in some myocardial segments to a greater extent than with tracer activity from other myocardial segments, spurious defects may result. A variety of imaging maneuvers have been developed to diminish attenuation artifacts. This includes the use of breast binders to more evenly distribute soft-tissue attenuation in women and decubitus or prone imaging positions to minimize diaphragmatic attenuation of myocardial activity.[45-47] Also, the lower limits of "normal" tracer activity are usually extended in myocardial segments that are commonly affected by attenuation artifact. There-

fore, bull's-eye displays of myocardial perfusion commonly include lower limits for normal tracer activity in the anterior (relative to the lateral) left ventricular wall in women and in the inferior wall, particularly in men.[12] This reflects the observed effects of soft-tissue attenuation in individuals who comprise a normal reference population.[12] However, broad normal ranges in myocardial regions involved by soft-tissue attenuation may result in underdetection of CAD in those segments. In a study by Quinones et al,[48] in which exercise echocardiography and exercise tomographic myocardial perfusion imaging were compared in the same patients, it was observed that resting echocardiographic abnormalities that were unchanged with exercise, and were undetected by perfusion scintigraphy, were localized to the inferior wall in 76 percent of cases. Tomographic perfusion imaging of the inferior left ventricular wall is often compromised by soft-tissue attenuation related to the diaphragm.[46,47]

Attenuation correction is a more appealing approach to the problem of soft-tissue attenuation. It involves measurement of attenuation through the use of a transmission scan and then restoring to the emission scan data scintillation counts lost to attenuation. Methods for simultaneous emission–transmission data collection and attenuation correction are described in Chap. 3. Attenuation correction holds substantial promise for elimination of spurious perfusion defects resulting from soft-tissue attenuation. With quantitative tomographic methods that use a normal reference file, attenuation correction offers the prospect of narrowing the range of cardiac scintigraphic findings in normal subjects, permitting an increase in diagnostic accuracy for detection of CAD. Further validation of simultaneous emission–transmission methods for attenuation correction is currently needed.

RADIOACTIVE MATERIALS

In comparison to echocardiography, nuclear imaging methods have the intrinsic disadvantage of requiring the use of radioactive materials. No clinically significant adverse medical effects have been documented resulting from the use of radioactive materials in standard diagnostic nuclear medicine procedures. However, assurance of safe use of radioactive materials requires a detailed radiation safety program, which adds to the costs of nuclear medicine procedures.

TEST DURATION

In comparison to echocardiography, stress and rest myocardial perfusion imaging requires more patient time. A typical stress and rest nuclear cardiology imaging sequence is completed over approximately 4 h of the patient's time compared with approximately 1 h for interventional echocardiographic studies. In patients with a normal stress myocardial perfusion scintigram, total duration of the diagnostic test can be reduced to approximately 1 h if the corresponding rest imaging sequence is omitted. Imaging time for stress and rest myocardial perfusion imaging can be reduced through the use of dual-radioisotope imaging (e.g., rest ^{201}Tl followed by stress technetium 99m (^{99m}Tc) sestamibi imaging[49]) or by imaging with a radioisotope with a brief myocardial half-time (e.g., teboroxime[50]). At present, these approaches have not been applied widely and myocardial perfusion imaging with single-photon tracers usually requires more patient time compared with stress echocardiography.

TECHNICALLY INADEQUATE ECHOCARDIOGRAMS

Before the advent of computer processing methods, exercise echocardiography was accompanied by an unacceptably high incidence of technically inadequate studies. Selection of technically optimal cardiac cycles during intervention for side-by-side continuous loop display with the corresponding resting and recovery images has substantially improved the yield in terms of technically adequate echocardiograms.[51] Selection of cardiac cycles with minimal respiratory artifact has helped to reduce the frequency of poor quality echocardiograms in patients with chronic obstructive pulmonary disease. Regardless of these technical advances, the left ventricular endocardium is incompletely visualized in a high proportion of echocardiographic studies. Lindower et al[52] studied 46 patients with computer-assisted two-dimensional echocardiography to evaluate LVEF at rest. Visualization of 75 percent or more of the left ventricular endocardium could only be accomplished in 27 of 46 patients (59 percent).

With current stress echocardiographic methods, including cine-loop quad-screen computer display, echocardiographic images that are technically unsatisfactory for diagnostic purposes have been reported in approximately 1 to 9 percent of studies.[48,53–61] However, Ryan et al[59] have noted that the proportion of patients with technically inadequate resting echocardiograms who, consequently, are not referred for stress echocardiography is currently undefined.

Data Display, Quantitation, and Interpretation

Tomographic myocardial perfusion imaging is a technologically complex procedure. However, with modern nuclear medicine computers, image reconstruction, quantitation, and display can be achieved rapidly. A major strength of myocardial perfusion imaging is that the data are collected in a nuclear medicine computer in a digital format. This facilitates display of myocardial perfusion tomograms in three orthogonal and highly standardized series of projection slices. Because the tomographic projections are readily standardized from patient to patient, quantitation of myocardial tomograms and comparison of the tomograms to normal limits established in populations of healthy subjects can be readily accomplished.[12,29,30] Most current nuclear medicine computers permit an individual nuclear cardiology laboratory to develop a database of regional myocardial tracer activity observed in healthy subjects. This type of normal database allows quantitative comparison of tomographic myocardial perfusion images with a normal reference range of values developed in the same laboratory. Quantification of myocardial perfusion images has made it possible to document objectively specific patterns of abnormal perfusion or soft-tissue attenuation that could only be suspected from subjective image interpretation.

A further advantage of a quantitative approach to myocardial perfusion imaging is the resultant standardization of image interpretation and resultant reduction of interobserver variability.[62] In a study involving 11 academic centers and community hospitals, in which the same bull's-eye quantitation program was used to evaluate ^{201}Tl myocardial tomograms, Van Train et al[30] found that this diverse group of hospital nuclear cardiology laboratories accomplished the same high level of diagnostic sensitivity and specificity compared with the institution that developed the quantitative method.

In addition to myocardial perfusion data, the high photon flux associated with myocardial imaging of ^{99m}Tc sestamibi and other nonredistributing ^{99m}Tc tracers allows ECG gating of perfusion images, thereby allowing estimation of regional myocardial wall thickening. This is currently best assessed from the change in regional myocardial count density.[63–65] Supplementation of myocardial perfusion data with scintigraphic regional wall thickening data has already proven valuable in separating fixed inferior wall defects related to myocardial scar from those related to diaphragm attenuation of inferior wall activity. Inferior wall defects on stress and rest tomograms, when related to diaphragm attenuation, have preserved inferior myocardial wall thickening.[64] At the time of writing, limited data document improved detection of the presence or absence of CAD through the addition of gated myocardial perfusion wall motion or wall thickening studies to data from myocardial perfusion imaging alone.[66] Furthermore, Palmas et al[67] have shown that addition of first-pass radionuclide angiographic imaging of the ^{99m}Tc sestamibi injection bolus can provide regional wall-motion data that significantly improve the prediction of extent of CAD compared with ^{99m}Tc sestamibi perfusion images alone.

As alluded to earlier, echocardiographic images provide cardiac visualization with excellent spatial resolution. All cardiac chambers and valves, as well as the ascending aorta and pericardium, are well visualized in most patients. In addition, Doppler echocardiography can provide clinically useful estimates of stenotic valve orifice area, severity of valvular regurgitation, pulmonary artery pressures, and pressure gradients within cardiac chambers (e.g., in hypertrophic cardiomyopathy). Thus, in the patient with cardiac chest pain unrelated to CAD, the combined two-dimensional echocardiographic and Doppler echocardiographic examinations can often rapidly detect other cardiac disorders.

Lack of an easily quantifiable normal response of echocardiographic regional wall motion to exercise[68] or to dobutamine infusion has resulted in a continuing lack of consensus regarding the criteria for a normal stress echocardiographic examination.[69] In some series, the presence of a baseline regional wall-motion abnormality at rest has been defined as a criterion for an abnormal stress echocardiogram.[57,59] There is a general consensus that normal resting regional wall motion that becomes hypokinetic, akinetic, or dyskinetic in response to exercise or pharmacologic stress is indicative of an abnormal response consistent with myocardial ischemia.[48,53–61,70–72] Some investigators have suggested that normal resting regional wall motion that is not augmented by exercise or pharmacologic stress is indicative of myocardial ischemia.[55,57] Moreover, others have indicated that left ventricular contraction that is augmented with stress but is segmentally delayed in onset (i.e., tardokinesis) is a useful predictor for the presence of underlying CAD.[55] However, no consensus has developed regarding the applicability of these latter two criteria in the interpretation of stress echocardiograms.

When left ventricular myocardial segments contract abnormally at rest by echocardiographic criteria, detection of myocardial ischemia with stress may be compromised.[73] Worsening of a segmental wall-motion abnormality with stress has been difficult to quantitate and the interobserver variability of this determination has not been defined. The influence of adjacent hyperkinetic motion of a normally perfused myocardial segment or the tethering effect of adjacent myocardial scar may alter the motion of a myocardial segment. Furthermore, myocardial segments that are akinetic at rest may become dyskinetic with pharmacologic stress in the absence of demonstrable segmental ischemia, apparently as a mechanical effect of bulging of a myocardial scar.[74] Thus, in its present form, nuclear stress is more quantitative and automated and, as a result, offers important advantages over stress echocardiography in identifying inducible ischemia in areas of previous infarction.

Utility of Results

Although determination of the presence or absence of CAD is the principal role for noninvasive stress tests, these procedures should also be capable of detecting stenoses in individual coronary arteries, determining the physiologic significance of an angiographic lesion, identifying high-risk three-vessel and left main disease, distinguishing viable myocardium from myocardial scar, and, perhaps most importantly, assessing prognosis. By virtue of the relatively longer availability of highly accurate myocardial perfusion imaging procedures, more extensive prognostic data are available currently in the stress nuclear compared with the stress echocardiographic literature. Based on the literature available at present, it appears that stress myocardial perfusion imaging provides a number of advantages compared with stress echocardiography in the prediction of coronary events. In a tabulation of 3266 patients with a normal exercise thallium scan, the incidence of cardiac death or nonfatal myocardial infarction was 0.9 percent per year[75–86] with progression to late coronary artery bypass surgery in 0.2 percent of 1274 patients per year.[76,80–82] Among 443 patients with a normal exercise echocardiogram, the annualized event-rates were 2.2 percent for cardiac death or nonfatal myocardial infarction and 2.1 percent for late coronary artery bypass surgery.[87,88] In a direct comparison of exercise echocardiography and exercise ^{201}Tl myocardial perfusion imaging for prediction of cardiac death, myocardial infarction or refractory ischemic symptoms requiring revascularization, Amanullah et al[89] found ^{201}Tl imaging to be the only independent predictor. The prognostic implications of stress myocardial perfusion defects and of stress echocardiographic regional wall-motion abnormalities are discussed in detail in Chap. 23.

Few studies of exercise echocardiography have been published examining its ability to predict recovery of segmental regional wall motion following revascularization or comparing its findings to viability determined from assessment of myocardial metabolism with positron emission tomography. In comparison, exercise myocardial perfusion imaging and dobutamine echocardiography have undergone extensive investigation in the detection of myocardial viability. Assessment of myocardial viability by stress echocardiography and by single-photon myocardial perfusion imaging is reviewed in Chap. 5.

Although there is institutional variability, the cost (both per patient and startup costs) of stress echocardiography should be less than exercise myocardial perfusion imaging. Stress echocardiography requires no radiopharmaceutical, no radiation safety program, and currently requires less postprocedural processing time. The cost of stress echocardiography instrumentation is not substantially different from the cost of a single-detector nuclear medicine camera and computer configuration, but it is less costly compared with multiple-detector nuclear imaging systems.

Table 21-2   Considerations in Comparing Noninvasive Tests

Patient Population
1. Tests should be compared in the same patients.
2. Tests should be performed under comparable experimental conditions (e.g., no change in medications).
3. Eligible patients should be consecutively entered into the comparative study without pretest selection bias (e.g., not excluded on a basis of a prior technically unsatisfactory resting echocardiogram, not preferentially included based on presence of prior myocardial infarction).
4. Posttest selection bias should be absent (e.g., the noninvasive test result should not be the determinant of which potential study patients undergo coronary arteriography).

Test Performance—Technical Aspects
5. Testing should be carried out using comparable high quality, state-of-the-art instrumentation and equivalent high levels of technical expertise for both tests.

Test Interpretation
6. Tests should be interpreted by objective, reproducible criteria.
7. Tests should be interpreted in blinded fashion.

CONSIDERATIONS IN COMPARING NONINVASIVE TESTS

To ensure accurate comparison of noninvasive tests, numerous conditions must be satisfied. These are summarized in Table 21-2. Unfortunately, such conditions are rarely met in published studies. The concepts of pretest and posttest[90] selection bias are presented in detail with examples in Chap. 20.

DETECTION OF CORONARY ARTERY DISEASE BY EXERCISE ECHOCARDIOGRAPHY AND EXERCISE MYOCARDIAL PERFUSION IMAGING—REVIEW OF AVAILABLE REPORTS

Numerous studies have compared exercise echocardiography with coronary arteriography. The present analysis emphasizes recent studies in which rest and exercise echocardiograms were viewed side by side in a computerized continuous-loop format. Similarly, extensive literature has compared exercise myocardial perfusion scintigraphy with coronary arteriography, but the present analysis focuses on studies using single photon emission computed tomography (SPECT). Indirect comparisons of exercise echocardiography and exercise myocardial perfusion imaging for detection of CAD can incorporate relatively large numbers of patients, but only limited conclusions can be drawn because echocardiography and perfusion imaging are not compared with coronary arteriography in the same patients. Conversely, studies in which both exercise echocardiography and exercise myocardial perfusion imaging are compared with coronary arteriographic findings in the same patients permit more

valid comparisons of these noninvasive tests, but the number of patients studied in this manner is small.

Presence or Absence of Coronary Artery Disease

Overall diagnostic sensitivities and specificities for detection of a 50 percent or greater luminal diameter coronary artery stenosis are summarized for exercise echocardiography in Table 21-3 and for tomographic exercise myocardial perfusion imaging in Table 21-4. Data are presented in a format previously reported by Mahmarian and Verani.[91] The reported sensitivities and specificities are similar for exercise echocardiography and for tomographic exercise myocardial perfusion imaging. These two diagnostic tests provided comparable sensitivities and specificities to one another in the presence or absence of prior myocardial infarction and in the presence of one-, two-, or three-vessel CAD. Available data defining the normalcy rate for exercise echocardiography are limited but appear to be highly favorable.

Direct comparison of exercise echocardiography and exercise myocardial perfusion imaging to coronary arteriography in the same patients has been reported in the series listed in Table 21-5. In each of these five studies, diagnostic sensitivity for overall detection of CAD tended to be higher with exercise myocardial perfusion imaging, and in four of five studies the specificity tended to be higher with exercise echocardiography. The differences in disease detection were not statistically significant for any individual published study.[48,70,71,92,93] Two additional studies with comparable overall results are not included in Table 21-3 because continuous loop echocardiographic display was not included[94] or full echocardiographic and myocardial imaging data were not available[95] for study patients with technically inadequate echocardiograms. In the largest available study that directly compares the diagnostic performance of exercise echocardiography and exercise myocardial perfusion imaging,[48] both tests yielded diagnostic sensitivities substantially below the average levels of sensitivity in reported series for either test. Therefore, additional large direct comparison studies of exercise echocardiography and exercise myocardial imaging to coronary arteriography are needed. However, the available studies suggest that these noninvasive tests provide comparable overall diagnostic accuracy for detection of CAD, although exercise myocardial perfusion imaging may be slightly more sensitive, whereas exercise echocardiography may be slightly more specific.

Individual Coronary Artery Stenoses

Detection of a 50 percent or greater coronary artery stenosis in the distribution of an individual coronary

Table 21-3 Sensitivity and Specificity of Exercise Echocardiography

Study	% with MI	Sensitivity						Specificity	Normalcy Rate
		Overall	MI	No MI	1-Vessel Disease	2-Vessel Disease	3-Vessel Disease		
Crouse[53] (n = 225)	0	168/172 (97%)	—	168/172 (97%)	61/66 (92%)	65/65 (100%)	41/41 (100%)	34/53 (64%)	—
Hecht[54] (n = 222)[a]	17	127/137 (93%)	36/37 (97%)	91/100 (91%)	46/55 (84%)	42/42 (100%)	40/40 (100%)	37/43 (86%)	42/42 (100%)
Quinones[48] (n = 112)[a]	—	64/86 (74%)	—	—	24/41 (58%)	25/29 (86%)	15/16 (94%)	23/26 (88%)	—
Marwick[55] (n = 179)	31	96/114 (84%)	49/55 (89%)	47/59 (80%)	46/60 (77%)	—	—	31/36 (86%)	27/29 (93%)
Beleslin[56] (n = 136)	57	105/119 (88%)	66/72 (92%)	39/47 (83%)	95/108 (88%)	—	—	14/17 (82%)	—
Armstrong[57] (n = 123)	41	89/101 (88%)	49/50 (98%)	40/51 (78%)	34/42 (81%)	—	—	19/22 (86%)	—
Galanti[71] (n = 53)[a]	0	25/27 (93%)	—	25/27 (93%)	13/14 (93%)	—	—	25/26 (96%)	—
Pozzoli[70] (n = 75)	0	35/49 (71%)	—	35/44 (71%)	20/33 (61%)	—	—	25/26 (96%)	—
Blomstrand[58] (n = 65)[a]	—	51/61 (84%)	—	—	21/23 (91%)	12/18 (67%)	18/20 (90%)	1/4 (25%)	—
Ryan[59] (n = 309)[a]	43	193/211 (91%)	—	—	73/85 (86%)	—	—	76/98 (78%)	—
Sheikh[60] (n = 34)	0	17/23 (74%)	—	17/23 (74%)	17/23 (74%)	—	—	10/11 (91%)	—
Marangelli[61] (n = 60)[a]	—	31/35 (89%)	—	—	13/16 (81%)	13/14 (93%)	5/5 (100%)	22/25 (88%)	—
Total (n = 1593)		1001/1135 (88%)	200/214 (93%)	461/523 (88%)	463/566 (82%)	157/168 (93%)	119/122 (98%)	317/411 (77%)	69/71 (97%)

[a] Technically inadequate tests deleted: 1–9% of tests
MI, myocardial infarction

Table 21-4 Sensitivity and Specificity of Exercise Tomographic Perfusion Imaging

Study	% with MI	Sensitivity						Specificity	Normalcy Rate
		Overall	MI	No MI	1-Vessel Disease	2-Vessel Disease	3-Vessel Disease		
Tamaki[105] (n = 104)	31	80/82 (98%)	32/32 (100%)	48/50 (96%)	39/40 (98%)	—	—	20/22 (91%)	—
DePasquale[12] (n = 210)	22	170/179 (95%)	47/47 (100%)	123/132 (93%)	85/93 (91%)	72/73 (99%)	13/13 (100%)	23/31 (74%)	—
Mahmarian[29] (n = 296)	43	192/221 (87%)	73/74 (99%)	68/86 (79%)	119/142 (84%)	60/66 (91%)	13/13 (100%)	65/75 (87%)	—
Van Train[30] (n = 486)	26	290/307 (94%)	127/128 (99%)	163/179 (91%)	76/88 (86%)	109/113 (96%)	105/106 (99%)	32/64 (50%)	94/115 (82%)
Iskandrian[31] (n = 461)	12	224/272 (82%)	50/50 (100%)	174/222 (78%)	45/70 (64%)	93/107 (87%)	86/95 (91%)	36/58 (62%)	123/131 (93%)
Kahn[32] (n = 50)	53	32/38 (84%)	20/20 (100%)	12/18 (67%)	10/13 (75%)	11/13 (85%)	11/12 (92%)	—	9/12 (75%)
Tartagni[33] (n = 30)	57	26/26 (100%)	17/17 (100%)	9/9 (100%)	8/8 (100%)	12/12 (100%)	6/6 (100%)	3/4 (75%)	—
Fleming[34] (n = 21)	55	14/16 (88%)	8/8 (100%)	6/8 (75%)	8/10 (80%)	5/5 (100%)	1/1 (100%)	3/5 (60%)	—
Gerson[35] (n = 30)	37	18/20 (90%)	11/11 (100%)	7/9 (78%)	12/13 (92%)	3/4 (75%)	3/3 (100%)	2/2 (100%)	7/8 (88%)
Total (n = 1688)		1046/1161 (90%)	385/387 (99%)	610/713 (86%)	402/477 (84%)	365/393 (93%)	238/249 (96%)	184/261 (70%)	233/266 (88%)

MI, myocardial infarction

Table 21-5   Direct Comparison in the Same Patients of Exercise Echocardiography and Exercise Nuclear Myocardial Perfusion Imaging for Coronary Disease Detection

Study	Sensitivity		Specificity	
	Echo	Nuclear	Echo	Nuclear
Pozzoli[70]	35/49 (71%)	41/49 (84%)	25/26 (96%)	23/26 (88%)
Quinones[48]	64/86 (74%)	65/86 (76%)	23/26 (88%)	21/26 (81%)
Amanullah[92]	18/22 (82%)	21/22 (95%)	4/15 (80%)	5/5 (100%)
Galanti[71]	25/27 (93%)	27/27 (100%)	25/26 (96%)	24/26 (92%)
Hecht[93]	46/51 (90%)	47/51 (92%)	16/20 (80%)	13/20 (65%)
Total	188/235 (80%)	201/235 (86%)	93/103 (90%)	86/103 (83%)

artery is summarized in Tables 21-6 and 21-7. Disease detection in the LAD and right coronary arterial distributions appears to be similar for exercise echocardiography and exercise myocardial perfusion imaging, but left circumflex CAD was underdetected by exercise echocardiography.[57,59,70,96] This parallels the early experience reported for subjectively interpreted planar myocardial perfusion imaging in which left circumflex CAD was underdetected.[97–102] With the use of quantitative planar and tomographic myocardial perfusion imaging methods, similar high diagnostic sensitivities and specificities have been accomplished for each of the three major coronary arteries.[101–104]

Detection of coronary artery stenosis in individual major epicardial coronary arteries has been directly compared in the same patients for exercise echocardiography and exercise myocardial perfusion imaging with coronary arteriography as the reference standard (Table 21-8). In the study of Galanti et al,[71] the sensitivity of ^{201}Tl myocardial imaging for the classification of individual diseased coronary arteries was 85 percent and that of exercise echocardiography was 63 percent ($p < 0.01$). The corresponding specificities were 98 percent for both methods. The differences were in large part attributable

to higher sensitivity of myocardial perfusion imaging (88 percent) compared with exercise echocardiography (58 percent, $p < 0.05$) for detection of right coronary artery stenoses. Others[54,70] have reported higher sensitivity of one method or the other for detection of coronary artery stenosis in the distribution of a single coronary artery, but the gain has been offset by a relatively lower diagnostic specificity in the same coronary artery resulting in no improvement in diagnostic accuracy for that artery.

Moderate Coronary Stenosis

Indirect comparison of exercise echocardiography and exercise myocardial perfusion imaging for detection of moderate (i.e., 50 to approximately 70 percent) coronary artery stenoses has been severely compromised by the use of subjective criteria for determining percent luminal diameter stenosis. Thus, the "gold standard" for assessment of stenosis severity against which these noninvasive tests have been compared is itself characterized by a high level of measurement uncertainty and interobserver variability. Despite this limitation, exercise echocardiog-

Table 21-6   Individual Vessel Disease Detection with Exercise Echocardiography

Study	Left Anterior Descending		Right Coronary		Left Circumflex		Overall	
	Sensitivity	Specificity	Sensitivity	Specificity	Sensitivity	Specificity	Sensitivity	Specificity
Hecht[54]	102/107 (95%)	61/73 (84%)	64/79 (81%)	91/101 (90%)	56/72 (78%)	100/108 (93%)	222/258 (86%)	252/282 (89%)
Armstrong[57]	48/74 (65%)	21/21 (100%)	52/66 (79%)	22/29 (69%)	11/49 (22%)	34/34 (100%)	111/189 (59%)	77/84 (92%)
Salustri[96]	11/15 (73%)	26/29 (89%)	2/8 (75%)	35/36 (97%)	3/7 (42%)	34/37 (97%)	16/30 (53%)	95/102 (93%)
Pozzoli[70]	20/29 (69%)	45/46 (98%)	11/17 (65%)	52/58 (89%)	11/24 (45%)	49/51 (96%)	42/70 (60%)	146/155 (94%)
Ryan[59]	119/150 (79%)	—	105/133 (79%)	—	39/109 (36%)	—	263/392 (67%)	—
Total	300/375 (80%)	153/169 (90%)	234/303 (77%)	200/224 (89%)	120/361 (33%)	172/230 (75%)	654/939 (70%)	570/623 (91%)

Table 21-7   Individual Vessel Disease Detection with Tomographic Perfusion Imaging

Study	Left Anterior Descending		Right Coronary		Left Circumflex		Overall	
	Sensitivity	Specificity	Sensitivity	Specificity	Sensitivity	Specificity	Sensitivity	Specificity
Tamaki[105]	55/63 (87%)	40/41 (98%)	45/49 (92%)	51/55 (93%)	25/32 (78%)	69/72 (96%)	125/144 (87%)	160/168 (95%)
DePasquale[12]	75/96 (78%)	95/114 (83%)	93/104 (89%)	92/106 (87%)	51/78 (65%)	125/132 (95%)	219/278 (79%)	312/352 (89%)
Mahmarian[29]	79/98 (81%)	130/142 (92%)	103/137 (75%)	145/147 (99%)	60/78 (77%)	178/196 (91%)	242/313 (77%)	453/485 (93%)
Van Train[30]	186/240 (78%)	88/131 (67%)	185/223 (83%)	96/148 (65%)	119/167 (71%)	134/204 (66%)	490/630 (78%)	318/483 (66%)
Kahn[32]	21/34 (62%)	5/6 (83%)	14/22 (64%)	12/17 (71%)	10/19 (53%)	10/16 (63%)	45/75 (60%)	27/39 (69%)
Fleming[34]	9/12 (75%)	8/9 (89%)	7/8 (88%)	7/13 (54%)	2/3 (67%)	16/18 (89%)	18/23 (78%)	31/40 (78%)
Gerson[35]	8/10 (80%)	17/20 (85%)	7/10 (70%)	17/20 (85%)	9/10 (90%)	15/20 (75%)	24/30 (80%)	49/60 (82%)
Total	433/553 (78%)	383/463 (83%)	454/553 (82%)	420/506 (83%)	276/387 (71%)	547/658 (83%)	1163/1493 (78%)	1350/1627 (83%)

raphy and exercise myocardial perfusion imaging have been reported to provide similar accuracy in the detection of moderate coronary artery stenosis. In six reported series,[12,29,32–34,105] exercise myocardial perfusion imaging provided 63 percent mean sensitivity (196 of 309 patients) and 87 percent mean specificity (473 of 543 patients) for detection of moderate coronary artery stenoses. In four series,[48,54,60,96] exercise echocardiography provided 67 percent mean sensitivity (82 of 123 patients) and 89 percent mean specificity (204 of 228 patients). Additional data directly comparing exercise echocardiography and exercise myocardial perfusion imaging for detection of moderate coronary artery stenoses in the same patients are needed, but should be performed with quantitative coronary arteriography as the reference standard.

Effect of Coronary Collaterals

Few data are available concerning the influence of angiographically demonstrated coronary collateral vessels on the results of exercise echocardiography. Stone et al[106] studied 21 consecutive patients referred for coronary arteriography who also underwent either exercise or dobutamine echocardiography. Echocardiographic images were interpreted in blinded fashion with a closed cineloop, quad-screen format. Echocardiography revealed stress-induced regional wall-motion abnormalities in the distribution of seven of nine obstructed coronary arteries without angiographic collaterals, but in only one of seven vessels with collaterals ($p = 0.02$). The authors concluded that angiographically demonstrated coronary collaterals can prevent the development of stress-induced

regional wall-motion abnormalities as evaluated by echocardiography. The reported influence of coronary collateral vessels on the detection of coronary artery stenoses by myocardial perfusion imaging has been more variable. Rigo et al[107] detected a greater than 50 percent coronary artery stenosis in 19 of 29 myocardial regions (66 percent) in the presence of angiographic coronary collaterals. Wainwright et al[108] observed a 50 percent or greater reduction in ^{201}Tl distribution with exercise in the distribution of 41 of 41 (100 percent) severely stenotic coronary arteries when coronary collaterals were of poor quality or absent and in the distribution of 41 of 54 (76 percent) severe coronary stenoses when coronary collaterals to the jeopardized territory were graded as moderate, good, or excellent. However, in a small series including 10 patients with a 90 percent or greater reduction in coronary artery luminal diameter and large intercoronary collateral vessels, Tubau et al[109] found a postexercise myocardial perfusion defect in only 4 patients. Overall, these limited data suggest that the presence of substantial coronary collateral vessels may interfere with the noninvasive detection of severe coronary artery stenosis and that induction of wall-motion abnormalities with stress may be compromised to a greater extent than induction of regional hypoperfusion. However, direct comparison studies of the diagnostic accuracy of stress echocardiography and stress myocardial perfusion imaging in patients with coronary collateral vessels are needed.

Extent of Disease

Attempts based on noninvasive tests to identify all coronary arteries containing a 50 percent or greater luminal

Table 21-8 Direct Comparison of Exercise Echocardiography and Exercise Myocardial Perfusion Imaging in Detection of Stenosis in Individual Coronary Arteries

Study	Method	Total		LAD		LCX		RCA	
		Sensitivity	Specificity	Sensitivity	Specificity	Sensitivity	Specificity	Sensitivity	Specificity
Hecht[93]	Echocardiography	84/95 (88%)	103/118 (87%)	38/39 (97%)[a]	26/32 (81%)	21/26 (81%)	41/45 (91%)	25/30 (83%)	36/41 (88%)[a]
	²⁰¹Tl	76/95 (80%)	99/118 (84%)	32/39 (82%)[a]	30/32 (94%)	17/26 (65%)	42/45 (93%)	27/30 (90%)	28/41 (68%)[a]
Pozzoli[70]	Echocardiography	42/70 (60%)	146/155 (95%)	20/29 (69%)	45/46 (98%)	11/24 (45%)	49/51 (96%)	11/17 (65%)	52/58 (81%)
	Sestamibi	47/70 (64%)	145/155 (94%)	19/29 (66%)	44/46 (96%)	16/24 (67%)	49/51 (96%)	12/17 (70%)	52/58 (81%)
Galanti[71]	Echocardiography	29/46 (63%)[b]	111/113 (98%)	15/20 (75%)	—	6/10 (60%)	—	9/16 (58%)[b]	—
	²⁰¹Tl	39/46 (85%)[b]	111/113 (98%)	19/20 (95%)	—	6/10 (60%)	—	14/16 (88%)[b]	—

[a] p < 0.05, but accuracy not different for that vessel
[b] p < 0.05
LAD, left anterior descending artery; LCX, left circumflex artery; RCA, right coronary artery

diameter stenosis have resulted in widely discrepant results.[59,110] Correct prediction of disease in each stenotic vessel by use of exercise echocardiography has ranged from 78 to 92 percent in single-vessel disease, 59 to 90 percent in double-vessel disease, and 25 to 93 percent in triple-vessel disease.[53,54,59] With exercise myocardial perfusion imaging, accurate detection of all individual coronary artery stenoses of greater than 50 percent of the luminal diameter have ranged from 64 to 100 percent for single-vessel disease, 71 to 93 percent for double-vessel disease, and 65 to 85 percent in triple-vessel disease.[12,29,31,33,34,105] These variable results are likely to reflect the importance of the level of exercise achieved and the influence of antianginal drugs in determining how many diseased coronary arteries will produce myocardial ischemia during exercise testing. In two studies in which exercise echocardiography and exercise myocardial perfusion imaging were directly compared in the same patients for identification of the exact number of diseased coronary arteries, Hecht et al[93] concluded that exercise echocardiography was superior, but Galanti et al[71] came to the opposite conclusion.

Detection of Myocardial Viability

The capability of exercise myocardial perfusion imaging to identify viable myocardium has been extensively documented and is reviewed in detail in Chap. 5. The presence of a reversible myocardial perfusion defect[111-115] or of a mild to moderate myocardial perfusion defect at rest (i.e., a resting perfusion defect with less than 50 percent reduction in activity compared with the normal segment with maximum myocardial activity[116]) is evidence for myocardial viability. These scintigraphic findings have identified hypocontractile myocardial segments that improve measurably with coronary artery revascularization.[112,113] In addition, these scintigraphic signs of viable myocardium also correspond to myocardial segments with retained glucose metabolism measured by positron emission tomography.[111,114-116]

By echocardiography, myocardial segments that contract normally at rest but become hypokinetic, akinetic, or dyskinetic with exercise are classified as containing viable myocardium. Myocardial segments that contract abnormally at rest and develop worsening regional myocardial contraction with exercise are also considered to show reversible myocardial ischemia, but data confirming improvement of these myocardial segments after coronary artery revascularization are needed. Separation of myocardial ischemia from myocardial scar by exercise echocardiography has proven to be problematic in myocardial segments with a resting regional wall-motion abnormality that is unchanged with dynamic exercise. Some authors have chosen to identify these left ventricular segments as containing myocardial scar and have excluded the segments from evaluation for the presence of residual myocardial ischemia.[117]

Difficulty in the assessment of myocardial viability by exercise echocardiography in the presence of a resting regional wall-motion abnormality is illustrated by the study of Quinones et al.[48] In that study, exercise echocardiography and exercise myocardial perfusion imaging were directly compared in the same patients. A fixed echocardiographic regional wall-motion abnormality was defined as a segmental contraction abnormality that was unchanged with exercise compared with rest. Of 81 patients with a fixed echocardiographic wall-motion abnormality, 30 patients had evidence of ^{201}Tl redistribution in the same myocardial segment, suggesting the presence of reversible myocardial ischemia. Because ^{201}Tl reinjection methods were not used in that study, it is likely that additional ischemic myocardial segments went undetected by myocardial perfusion imaging[111,113] and, hence, by exercise echocardiography. These studies suggest that exercise echocardiography is of limited utility for detection of inducible myocardial ischemia in myocardial segments that contract abnormally at rest. Consequently, exercise echocardiography is currently of limited utility for detection of viable myocardium in segments with resting regional wall-motion abnormalities. By contrast, clinical studies suggest that low-dose dobutamine echocardiography may identify viable myocardium.[118]

Accuracy in Women

The diagnostic accuracy of exercise echocardiography has been evaluated in women with typical angina pectoris, atypical angina pectoris, and a medium pretest probability that CAD is present.[119-121] Among 19 women with typical angina pectoris examined by exercise echocardiography, Sawada et al[119] correctly identified the presence of angiographic disease in 15 of 16 women (94 percent) and the absence of angiographic disease in 2 of 3 women (67 percent). Among 38 women with atypical chest pain, the presence of angiographic CAD was identified in 9 of 12 women (75 percent) and the absence of angiographic disease in 23 of 26 women (88 percent).[119] In an exercise echocardiographic study of 70 women having a pretest probability of CAD of 53 ± 30 percent, Williams et al[120] found a sensitivity of 88 percent and specificity of 84 percent for detection of CAD. A similar level of diagnostic accuracy of myocardial perfusion imaging for detection of CAD in women is detailed in Chap. 20, together with comments on the importance of the level of exercise achieved in female patients. Direct comparison studies of exercise echocardiography and exercise myocardial perfusion imaging in the same female patients are needed.

Level of Exercise and Effect of Beta Blockers

Both exercise echocardiography and exercise myocardial perfusion imaging provide a superior level of diagnostic sensitivity for CAD compared with exercise ECG in patients who fail to exercise to 85 percent of predicted maximal heart rate.[31,122,123] The effect of exercise to less than 85 percent of predicted maximum heart rate on the accuracy of exercise echocardiography has been controversial. Neither Ryan et al[59] nor Hecht et al[54] observed any difference in diagnostic accuracy when comparing the results of exercise echocardiography in patients who did versus those who did not reach target heart rate. However, Marwick et al[55] detected angiographic CAD in 90 percent of patients (96 of 107) who achieved 85 percent or more of predicted maximum heart rate with exercise echocardiography, whereas the sensitivity was 0 percent in the 7 patients who exercised inadequately. These analyses are of limited value because patients who stop exercise early as a result of ischemic symptoms may have more extensive disease that may be more readily detected by noninvasive imaging.[122] More informative is the type of analysis of exercise level reported by Iskandrian et al.[31] In that study, the sensitivity of tomographic ^{201}Tl myocardial perfusion imaging in patients who reached 85 percent of predicted maximum heart rate or who had ischemic ST-segment depression was 88 percent (145 of 164 patients), whereas the sensitivity of thallium imaging was significantly lower (73 percent, 79 of 108 patients, $p < 0.002$) in patients who had an inadequate exercise peak heart rate and no ischemic ST-segment changes. The same considerations apply in the analysis of the effect of beta-adrenergic blockers on the accuracy of exercise imaging.[124,125] Thus, the effects of submaximal exercise and beta-adrenergic blockade on the diagnostic accuracy of exercise echocardiography and exercise myocardial perfusion imaging might better be assessed in patients who do not stop exercise as a result of ischemic symptoms or ECG changes. Until studies are available that isolate the effects of exercise level or beta blockade on the diagnostic accuracy of exercise imaging studies, it would appear preferable to use pharmacologic stress as an alternative to dynamic exercise in patients who are unable to exercise to target heart rate or discontinue the use of beta-adrenergic blockers.

PHARMACOLOGIC STRESS TESTING WITH DOBUTAMINE

In patients either unable to reach target heart rate, or to reproduce predictably ischemic symptoms during exercise, pharmacologic stress testing provides a valuable alternative to dynamic exercise. The mode of pharmacologic stress may consist of positive inotropic and chronotropic stimulation or pharmacologic coronary artery vasodilation. Dobutamine hydrochloride infusion, with stepwise infusions up to 40 or 50 μg/kg/min, has been the most widely used positive inotropic drug in this setting. In instances in which high-dose dobutamine infusion has not produced heart rates of 85 percent of predicted maximum for age, atropine sulfate in doses of 0.25 to 1.0 mg intravenously has been added to further augment heart rate.[126–128] Studies in open-chest dogs have led to the suggestion that 5-min dobutamine dose stages produce a larger heart rate response for a 10 μg/kg/min infusion compared with 3-min dose stages, but the optimal dobutamine dose stage duration for dobutamine imaging in man remains uncertain.[129]

Mertes et al[130] have reported the safety profile of dobutamine infusions to 30 to 50 μg/kg/min in 118 consecutive patients. There were no deaths, myocardial infarctions, or episodes of sustained ventricular tachycardia related to dobutamine testing in their study. Pingitore et al[131] have reported a series of 2554 echocardiographic tests using dobutamine (up to 40 μg/kg/min) plus atropine (up to 1 mg). No deaths or episodes of cardiac asystole occurred, but there were two episodes of ventricular fibrillation, three periprocedural myocardial infarctions, one episode of sustained (90 s) ventricular tachycardia, and one episode of unstable angina pectoris. Paradoxical hypotension may also occur in approximately 20 percent of dobutamine stress echocardiograms and is unrelated to the presence of underlying CAD.[132,133] Dobutamine stress testing is contraindicated in the presence of hypertrophic cardiomyopathy, critical aortic stenosis, or uncontrolled cardiac arrhythmias.

Interruption of dobutamine infusion has been recommended for 2 mm or more of ECG ST-segment depression, for severe or extensive regional wall-motion abnormalities, and for significant hypotension or arrhythmia.[127,130,134,135] In three reported series, the drug infusion was stopped prior to reaching the maximum dose as a result of noncardiac side effects in 2 to 11 percent of patients.[127,130,131] Target heart rate was achieved in 91 percent of patients if an inadequate heart response to dobutamine infusion was followed by atropine administration.[127] Dobutamine infusion has also been used in combination with transesophageal echocardiography in an attempt to provide superior images to transthoracic echocardiography for detection of regional wall-motion abnormalities.[136,137] In one series,[137] the transesophageal echocardiogram could not be performed in 4 percent of patients because of patient discomfort and the echocardiograms were technically inadequate for interpretation in an additional 8 percent of study patients. It has not been demonstrated that the transesophageal approach to dobutamine echocardiography provides any significant improvement in diagnostic accuracy for CAD detection compared with the transthoracic approach, but it may provide a useful alternative approach in patients with technically inadequate transthoracic echocardiograms. Dobutamine infusion has also been used in numerous studies in conjunction with myocardial perfusion imaging. It may be particularly applicable in patients who are unable to exercise vigorously and in whom the pharmacologic coronary artery vasodilators, dipyridamole and adenosine, may be contraindicated as a result of reactive airway obstruction.[138,139]

Presence or Absence of Coronary Disease

In a tabulation of 12 reported series,[95,126,140–149] dobutamine echocardiography detected the presence of angiographic CAD in 512 of 643 patients yielding a diagnostic sensitivity of 80 percent. Dobutamine echocardiography was normal in 232 of 284 patients in whom angiographic CAD was absent, producing a specificity of 82 percent. The criteria for significant coronary stenosis varied from 50 to 70 percent in these reports. Other reports,[150–152] in which there is or appears to be a substantial overlap of study patients with these tabulated series, have been excluded. The tabulated series are heterogeneous in that atropine was added if necessary to the dobutamine infusion in some[95,126] but not most of these studies. McNeill et al[126] have reported improved diagnostic sensitivity for CAD detection with the administration of atropine in patients not reaching 85 percent of predicted maximal heart rate with dobutamine infusion alone. However, in the present tabulation, the overall diagnostic accuracy was no better with atropine (122 of 156 tests, 78 percent) than without atropine (622 of 771 tests, 81 percent).

Although one would expect motion of the thorax during echocardiographic acquisition to be a greater technical problem with exercise rather than dobutamine echocardiography, the use of a quad-screen, continuous-loop computer display was associated with a higher diagnostic sensitivity in these 12 studies. Thus, the sensitivity of dobutamine echocardiography with continuous-loop display for CAD detection was 84 percent (338 of 404 tests) versus 73 percent (74 of 239 tests) without continuous-loop display. The respective specificities were 83 percent and 81 percent. As noted for exercise echocardiography, the criteria used to define an abnormality of segmental left ventricular contraction with dobutamine echocardiography have been variable. Worsening echocardiographic segmental wall motion or wall thickening with dobutamine infusion was considered to be abnormal in these studies, but myocardial segments in which contraction was unchanged from rest to dobutamine infusion were variously classified as normal[95,126,141,142,144,145,148] or abnormal.[140,142,147,149] The preva-

lence of a nonischemic dobutamine echocardiographic response, defined as absence of resting wall-motion abnormality and absence of a new or worsened wall-motion abnormality with dobutamine infusion, in a low-risk population of patients with a less than 5 percent likelihood of CAD (i.e., normalcy rate) was 92.1 percent in a study by Bach et al.[153]

Myocardial perfusion tracers can be injected during peak dobutamine infusion and high quality scintigraphic images produced. For nine reported studies,[139,146–149,152,154–156] the mean diagnostic sensitivity of dobutamine myocardial perfusion imaging for detection of angiographic CAD was 87 percent (322 of 371 patients) with a mean specificity of 73 percent (99 of 135 patients). Thus, the diagnostic sensitivity reported with dobutamine myocardial perfusion imaging is similar to that reported for dobutamine echocardiography. Although the specificity of dobutamine echocardiography tends to be higher than for dobutamine myocardial perfusion imaging, the influence of posttest selection bias on test specificity in these studies is undefined.

In patients with normal regional wall motion by echocardiography at rest, CAD was detected by the presence of a new regional wall-motion abnormality during dobutamine infusion in 210 of 280 patients from six studies[140–143,147,148] yielding a sensitivity of 75 percent. The corresponding specificity in 158 patients without angiographic CAD was 90 percent. Corresponding data for dobutamine myocardial perfusion imaging are limited because baseline regional wall motion is not reported in most perfusion imaging studies. However, the sensitivity of dobutamine myocardial perfusion imaging for CAD detection in 46 patients[139,152] with no evidence of prior myocardial infarction was 78 percent with a specificity of 89 percent. Therefore, from indirect evidence, it appears that the diagnostic accuracies of dobutamine echocardiography in patients with normal baseline regional wall motion and from dobutamine myocardial perfusion imaging in patients without evidence of prior myocardial infarction were similar.

A few studies have directly compared both dobutamine echocardiography and dobutamine myocardial perfusion imaging with coronary arteriography in the same patients (Table 21-9). The combined diagnostic sensitivity for detection of a 50 percent or greater angiographic coronary artery stenosis, from five available direct comparison studies, was 76 percent for dobutamine echocardiography and 83 percent for dobutamine myocardial perfusion imaging. In these studies, the diagnostic accuracy was the same (79 percent) for dobutamine echocardiograms displayed with a continuous-loop, quad-screen display[147,149] and for images displayed without computer techniques.[146,148,152] The diagnostic sensitivity for detection of angiographic CAD in patients with no prior ECG[147,148,152] or historical[147,152] evidence of myocardial infarction was 73 percent (126 of 172 patients)

Table 21-9   Direct Comparison in the Same Patients of Dobutamine Echocardiography and Dobutamine Myocardial Perfusion Imaging for Coronary Disease Detection

Study	Sensitivity		Specificity	
	Echo	Nuclear	Echo	Nuclear
Marwick[147]	102/142 (72%)	108/142 (76%)	62/75 (83%)[a]	50/75 (67%)
Gunalp[148]	15/18 (83%)	17/18 (94%)	8/9 (89%)	8/9 (89%)
Warner[146]	8/13 (62%)	14/15 (93%)	1/1 (100%)	1/1 (100%)
Forster[152]	9/12 (75%)	10/12 (83%)	8/9 (89%)	8/9 (89%)
Senior[149]	41/44 (93%)	42/44 (95%)	16/17 (94%)	12/17 (71%)
Total	175/229 (76%)	191/231 (83%)	95/111 (86%)	79/111 (71%)

[a] $p < 0.05$ versus nuclear imaging

for dobutamine echocardiography and 78 percent (135 of 172 patients) for dobutamine myocardial perfusion imaging. Correct identification of the presence or absence of angiographic CAD in patients with single-vessel disease was accomplished in 55 of 81 patients (68 percent) by dobutamine echocardiography and in 61 of 81 patients (75 percent) by dobutamine myocardial perfusion imaging, whereas the presence of CAD was detected in 71 of 91 patients with multivessel disease (78 percent) by echocardiography and 74 of these 91 patients (81 percent) by perfusion imaging.[147,148,152]

Individual Coronary Artery Stenoses

Using dobutamine echocardiography, Mazeika et al[142] were able to identify a 70 percent or greater angiographic coronary artery stenosis in only 41 percent of 29 diseased LAD coronary arteries. Correct localization of a coronary stenosis by dobutamine echocardiography to either the right or left circumflex arterial territory was accomplished in only 45 percent of arteries. Specificity for disease detection was 95 percent in both LAD and non-LAD coronary artery distributions. Others have reported sensitivities for dobutamine echocardiography in the LAD territory of 62 percent[147] to 82 percent[126] with sensitivities in the posterior circulation of 57 percent[126] to 77 percent,[152] but corresponding specificities were not provided. It has been suggested that dobutamine-enhanced myocardial contractility impairs blood flow through the septal perforators. Because the (generally) nondominant left circumflex does not supply septal perforators, ischemia may be difficult to identify in this vascular territory using dobutamine.[140]

In a tabulation of three reported series,[139,146,154] dobutamine myocardial perfusion imaging yielded a diagnostic sensitivity of 77 percent for detecting 60 LAD artery stenoses, of 53 percent for detecting 66 left circumflex stenoses, and of 87 percent in detecting 75 right coronary artery stenoses. The corresponding specificities were 92 percent in 74 arteries, 88 percent in 52 arteries, and 73 percent in 44 arteries, respectively. The available dobu-

tamine echocardiography and dobutamine myocardial perfusion imaging series vary widely in methodology and are limited in terms of reported data. To date, direct comparison studies of dobutamine echocardiography and dobutamine myocardial perfusion imaging for assessment of sensitivity and specificity of disease detection in individual coronary arteries have not been reported, making any meaningful comparison difficult based on the available data.

Extent of Disease

Coronary artery revascularization provides a survival advantage compared with medical therapy in subgroups of patients with multivessel CAD. Several investigators have provided data describing the ability of dobutamine imaging studies to detect specifically the presence of multivessel CAD[140–142,148] or of left main coronary disease.[157] In four studies of patients with resting regional wall-motion abnormalities by echocardiography, including 58 patients with and 26 patients without multivessel CAD, the sensitivity of dobutamine echocardiography was 74 percent with a specificity of 77 percent for detection of multivessel disease.[140–142,148] In two studies including 56 patients with and 31 patients without multivessel CAD, the sensitivity of dobutamine myocardial perfusion imaging was 71 percent with a specificity of 94 percent for identification of multivessel CAD.[139,149] Two studies have directly compared the ability of dobutamine echocardiography and dobutamine myocardial perfusion imaging to identify the presence of multivessel CAD in the same 203 study patients.[147,149] In these studies, dobutamine infusion with echocardiography and with ^{99m}Tc sestamibi myocardial perfusion imaging provided sensitivities for detection of multivessel CAD of 33 percent and 46 percent, respectively, with specificity for multivessel disease identification of 91 percent and 86 percent. Thus, the reported diagnostic sensitivities and specificities for dobutamine echocardiographic and perfusion imaging studies have been variable, with a trend to slightly better overall accuracy for detection of CAD extent with nuclear imaging.

Detection of Myocardial Viability

(see Chap. 5)

Accuracy in Women

In a study by Marwick et al,[147] which directly compared the diagnostic performances of dobutamine echocardiography and dobutamine myocardial perfusion imaging in the same patients, it was observed that both tests provided a lower diagnostic sensitivity (55 percent for both tests) in women compared with men (76 percent and 81 percent, respectively). The lower diagnostic sensitivity observed in women compared with men was attributed to a higher prevalence of single-vessel disease in women.

Left Ventricular Hypertrophy

Marwick et al[147] and others[149] have suggested that myocardial perfusion imaging with ^{99m}Tc sestamibi tomography and dobutamine infusion may result in perfusion defects in the absence of angiographic coronary artery stenosis in patients with echocardiographic documentation of left ventricular hypertrophy. In 17 patients with these clinical characteristics studied by Marwick, the specificity of dobutamine echocardiography was 94 percent and that of dobutamine scintigraphy was 59 percent ($p = 0.02$). The sensitivity of dobutamine myocardial perfusion imaging was 78 percent in their 37 study patients with both left ventricular hypertrophy and angiographic CAD compared with 73 percent by dobutamine echocardiography. In patients with left ventricular hypertrophy, the overall accuracies of dobutamine echocardiography and dobutamine myocardial perfusion imaging did not differ significantly. One possible explanation for these findings comes from the study of DePuey et al[158] in which 100 patients with chronic systemic hypertension underwent tomographic ^{201}Tl myocardial perfusion imaging in conjunction with either treadmill exercise or pharmacologic coronary artery vasodilation by dipyridamole infusion. A fixed decrease in the normal lateral-to-septal count density was observed in the hypertensive patients both on immediate poststress images and on 3-h delayed images. This resulted in apparent lateral wall fixed defects in 35 of the 100 hypertensive patients. The basis for this variation in distribution of ^{201}Tl counts in hypertensive patients has not been established. Patients with renovascular hypertension have been reported to have disproportionate septal-to-lateral wall thickness,[159] which could result in relatively greater ra-

diotracer activity in the septum compared with the lateral wall; however, echocardiographic evidence of asymmetric septal hypertrophy was not found in the patients studied by DePuey et al. An alternative explanation might relate to the effect of left ventricular hypertrophy on regional wall motion. If excursion of the hypertrophied ventricular septum was decreased relative to the lateral wall, the septum might have a higher count density on ungated tomographic images because lateral wall count density would be spread across more pixels in response to greater lateral wall excursion.[158] However, other authors have examined myocardial perfusion imaging in patients with hypertension[160–162] or left ventricular hypertrophy[161,163] and found excellent diagnostic sensitivity and good to excellent specificity with no fixed lateral wall defects. Using primarily planar methods, Chin et al[161] studied 30 asymptomatic hypertensive men with exercise ^{201}Tl myocardial perfusion imaging and reported a diagnostic sensitivity of 89 percent and specificity of 90 percent for detection of angiographic CAD. In the subgroup of 10 patients with left ventricular hypertrophy by echocardiographic criteria, the diagnostic accuracy of exercise ^{201}Tl myocardial imaging was 100 percent.

Whether performed in combination with myocardial perfusion imaging or with echocardiography, pharmacologic stress testing with dobutamine infusion offers a theoretical advantage compared with stress imaging with a pharmacologic coronary artery vasodilator. In response to left ventricular hypertrophy, resting coronary blood flow increases so that blood flow per gram of myocardium remains relatively constant.[164] Maximum coronary blood flow in response to a potent coronary artery vasodilator (e.g., papaverine, adenosine, or dipyridamole) does not change. Therefore, the coronary flow reserve, which is the difference between maximal coronary blood flow and resting coronary blood flow, decreases in the presence of left ventricular hypertrophy.[164–170] In some instances, coronary flow reserve may decrease greatly, so that myocardial blood flow through patent coronary arteries cannot be augmented substantially by pharmacologic agents. Consequently, in theory, pharmacologic coronary artery vasodilators may not induce sufficiently large differences in myocardial blood flow in the distributions of stenotic compared with nonstenotic coronary arteries to produce a defect by myocardial perfusion imaging in patients with severe left ventricular hypertrophy.[169,170] The frequency with which false-negative myocardial perfusion images may occur by this mechanism is not clear, but must be infrequent in general populations investigated for diagnosis of chest pain because myocardial perfusion imaging following pharmacologic coronary artery vasodilation has produced comparable diagnostic accuracy to myocardial perfusion imaging with exercise in several studies.[171,172] Dobutamine infusion, by inducing myocardial ischemia through increased myocardial oxygen demand, would be expected to induce perfusion defects related to coronary artery stenoses despite the presence of diminished coronary flow reserve in patients with ventricular hypertrophy. However, Carlson et al[173] showed that dobutamine-induced (demand) ischemia produced smaller wall-motion abnormalities compared with similar sized ischemic zones produced by a decrease in myocardial oxygen supply. This may be an explanation for false-negative dobutamine stress studies.

Beta-Adrenergic Blockade and Failure to Complete the Pharmacologic Stress Protocol

The effect of beta-adrenergic blocking drugs on the diagnostic accuracy of dobutamine echocardiography has been controversial. Among the 12 series cited earlier comparing the results of dobutamine echocardiography with coronary arteriography, in 7 studies beta-adrenergic blockers were discontinued prior to dobutamine infusion[95,141,142,145,146,148,149] and in 1 study the number of patients on beta-adrenergic blockers was not specified.[143] Thus, only 124 patients from those studies were documented to have been receiving a beta-adrenergic blocker at the time of dobutamine echocardiography.[95,140,144,147] Sawada et al[140] reported a diagnostic sensitivity of 88 percent for CAD in the 28 patients they studied with dobutamine echocardiography during beta-blocker therapy. They concluded that the sensitivity of dobutamine echocardiography was not affected by beta-adrenergic blocker therapy. A larger series of patients receiving a beta-adrenergic blocker ($n = 64$) was studied with dobutamine echocardiography in a report by McNeill et al.[126] Among 31 patients whose heart rate reached 85 percent of predicted maximum for age in response to dobutamine infusion alone, 58 percent were receiving a beta-adrenergic blocker at the time of testing. Of 49 patients who required addition of atropine to the dobutamine infusion to reach target heart rate, 94 percent were receiving a beta-adrenergic blocker at the time of testing. In this latter group of patients, use of atropine in addition to the dobutamine infusion was accompanied by an increase in diagnostic sensitivity from 7 percent to 65 percent with minimal effect on specificity.[126]

Marwick et al[147] have reported that a "submaximal" test, in which the stress was limited by side effects, was the most important correlate of a false-negative dobutamine echocardiogram. In 43 percent of 40 patients with angiographic CAD in whom dobutamine echocardiography demonstrated no abnormality, dobutamine infusion had to be stopped before the full infusion protocol could be completed. A submaximal dobutamine infusion was significantly less frequent (24 percent) in 102 patients in whom echocardiographic evidence of angio-

graphic CAD was correctly identified. In the same study patients, failure to complete the full dobutamine infusion protocol was not associated with a loss of diagnostic sensitivity by dobutamine myocardial perfusion imaging.

In summary, the available study data suggest that use of beta-adrenergic blockers may impair the diagnostic sensitivity of dobutamine echocardiography but that addition of atropine may, at least in part, overcome this limitation of dobutamine stress testing. Dobutamine myocardial perfusion imaging appears to be less compromised compared with dobutamine echocardiography in patients who are unable to complete the full dobutamine infusion protocol,[147] or who reach a lower peak rate-pressure product.[174]

PHARMACOLOGIC STRESS TESTING WITH DIPYRIDAMOLE OR ADENOSINE

Myocardial perfusion imaging detects angiographic coronary artery stenoses with similar accuracy whether it is performed in combination with pharmacologic coronary artery vasodilation or with dynamic exercise.[171,172,175–179] The literature related to myocardial perfusion imaging with pharmacologic coronary artery vasodilation is reviewed in detail in Chap. 6. With pharmacologic coronary artery vasodilation using dipyridamole or adenosine infusion, coronary blood flow is increased through patent coronary arteries,[180–182] but cannot be augmented fully beyond a hemodynamically significant coronary artery stenosis.[183] An intravenous infusion over 4 min of 0.56 mg/kg of dipyridamole or of adenosine 0.14 mg/kg/minute for 6 min is adequate for induction of myocardial perfusion defects in most patients with an angiographically significant coronary artery stenosis but does not induce a corresponding regional wall-motion contractile abnormality in a high proportion of patients.[184–187] Consequently, in studies directly comparing myocardial perfusion imaging with echocardiography for detection of angiographic coronary artery stenosis following adenosine[184–186] or standard-dose (0.56 mg/kg) dipyridamole[187] infusion, perfusion imaging has provided superior diagnostic sensitivity and, in the adenosine studies, superior diagnostic accuracy. As noted earlier, in an attempt to induce regional wall-motion abnormalities in a higher proportion of patients with coronary artery stenosis, high-dose (0.84 mg/kg over 10 min) dipyridamole infusion was introduced and improved the diagnostic sensitivity of stress echocardiography compared with standard-dose infusion.[43] A study by Picano et al[188] suggested that echocardiography following high-dose (0.84 mg/kg) dipyridamole infusion could provide comparable accuracy for detection of CAD to myocardial perfusion imaging with bicycle exercise. In that study, 98 percent of patients stopped exercise without reaching target heart rate and the symptoms or ECG changes for which they stopped bore little relationship to the presence or absence of angiographic CAD. Using high-dose dipyridamole echocardiography, Mazeika et al[189] found inducible left ventricular asynergy in only 16 of 40 patients (40 percent) with angiographic CAD and observed no inducible wall-motion abnormality in 10 study patients with single-vessel CAD. Beleslin and colleagues[56] directly compared echocardiography with dobutamine infusion (up to 40 μg/kg/min), echocardiography with high-dose dipyridamole infusion (up to 0.84 mg/kg over 10 min) and echocardiography following treadmill exercise in 136 consecutive patients with documented angiographic coronary anatomy. For overall detection of angiographic CAD, exercise echocardiography was significantly more sensitive (88 percent) and accurate (87 percent) compared with high-dose dipyridamole echocardiography (74 percent and 77 percent, respectively, $p < 0.01$), whereas dobutamine echocardiography and exercise echocardiography did not differ significantly. In 108 patients with single-vessel CAD, exercise echocardiography detected evidence of coronary stenosis in 95 patients (88 percent), whereas high-dose dipyridamole echocardiography detected disease in 78 patients (72 percent, $p = 0.002$). In 59 patients receiving beta-adrenergic blocking drugs, accuracy for detection of angiographic CAD was significantly worse by stress echocardiography following high-dose dipyridamole infusion compared with echocardiography with dobutamine infusion or following treadmill exercise. Recently, the Echo Persantine International Cooperative (EPIC) study group reported that addition of atropine to high-dose (0.84 mg/kg) dipyridamole infusion can provide echocardiographic assessment for CAD detection that is comparable to echocardiographic testing with atropine injection and dobutamine infusion.[190] Confirmatory studies are needed.

In a recent review, O'Keefe et al[191] tabulated the results of 8 studies of myocardial perfusion imaging with adenosine infusion and 14 studies of dobutamine echocardiography. They found a higher composite sensitivity for detection of angiographic CAD of 89 percent for adenosine perfusion imaging compared with 81 percent for dobutamine echocardiography. The respective specificities of 81 percent and 83 percent were not significantly different. The authors also concluded that adenosine myocardial perfusion imaging was significantly more sensitive for detection of right CAD (85 percent versus 57 percent, $p < 0.001$), tended to be more sensitive for left circumflex disease (69 percent versus 54 percent, $p < 0.06$), and had comparable sensitivity for LAD disease (78 percent versus 69 percent, $p = NS$) relative to dobutamine echocardiography. Recently, Ho et al[192] directly compared dobutamine echocardiography and dipyridamole ^{201}Tl SPECT in the detection of CAD in 54 pa-

tients who also underwent coronary arteriography. Overall, CAD was detected with a sensitivity of 93 percent and specificity of 73 percent for dobutamine echocardiography and of 98 percent and 73 percent for dipyridamole thallium imaging (all values $p = NS$). The sensitivity for detecting individual coronary artery stenosis with dobutamine echocardiography was 81 percent (30 of 37) for the LAD artery, 75 percent (24 of 32) for the right coronary artery, and 61 percent (17 of 28) for the left circumflex artery. For SPECT perfusion imaging, it was 89 percent, 97 percent ($p < 0.05$ versus dobutamine echocardiography) and 75 percent, respectively. Both methods provided comparable detection of coronary stenoses greater than or equal to 70 percent of the luminal diameter. However, SPECT perfusion imaging detected 82 percent (14 of 17) of moderate coronary stenoses (i.e., 50 to 69 percent), whereas dobutamine echocardiography detected 53 percent ($p < 0.05$). Before firm conclusions can be drawn concerning the relative diagnostic accuracies of myocardial perfusion imaging with pharmacologic coronary artery vasodilation versus dobutamine echocardiography, larger direct comparison studies are needed.

In summary, echocardiography with pharmacologic coronary artery vasodilation has generally produced lower diagnostic sensitivity and similar specificity compared with echocardiographic testing with dynamic exercise or dobutamine infusion. With myocardial perfusion imaging, overall diagnostic sensitivity, specificity, and accuracy appear to be comparable with pharmacologic coronary vasodilation, dobutamine infusion, and dynamic exercise.[171,172,175–179,193]

CONCLUSIONS

Stress echocardiographic and stress myocardial perfusion imaging methods for determining the presence, extent, and prognosis of CAD have evolved rapidly over the last 5 years. Although divergent results have at times been reported, certain trends have been identified. In laboratories with investigative experience in the performance of these noninvasive tests, similar diagnostic accuracy for detection of angiographic coronary artery stenosis has been achieved with exercise echocardiography and exercise myocardial perfusion imaging. Overall diagnostic sensitivity for detection of angiographic CAD tends to be greater with exercise myocardial perfusion imaging and diagnostic specificity tends to be greater with exercise echocardiography. These observations have been most apparent in studies directly comparing the two noninvasive methods in the same patients. Improved sensitivity of exercise myocardial perfusion imaging relative to exercise echocardiography without loss of specificity has resulted largely from superior detection of disease in the posterior coronary circulation (left circumflex or right coronary artery or both). Myocardial perfusion imaging with exercise may be superior to exercise echocardiography in patients with coronary artery collaterals but few data are available. When resting regional wall-motion abnormalities are present, assessment of myocardial viability appears to be limited with exercise echocardiography. In comparison, exercise and resting myocardial perfusion imaging have proven to be reliable in assessment of viable myocardium. Perhaps most importantly, the available studies suggest that the more mature technique, exercise myocardial perfusion imaging, provides superior prognostic information relative to exercise echocardiography. Most notably, a normal exercise myocardial perfusion scintigram has been followed by fewer coronary events per year compared with a normal exercise echocardiogram.

Similar overall results have been described when pharmacologic inotropic stress with dobutamine infusion has been substituted for dynamic exercise. With dobutamine stress, myocardial perfusion imaging tends to yield higher diagnostic sensitivity but lower specificity relative to echocardiography, resulting in comparable overall accuracy. Dobutamine myocardial perfusion imaging appears to hold some advantage over dobutamine echocardiography in determining the extent of CAD. It also appears to be advantageous diagnostically in patients who are unable to complete the full dobutamine infusion protocol. Compared with dobutamine myocardial perfusion imaging, dobutamine echocardiography may provide better diagnostic specificity in patients with left ventricular hypertrophy; however, reported results have been variable.

When pharmacologic coronary artery vasodilation is used, myocardial perfusion imaging provides superior diagnostic sensitivity to echocardiography for detection of angiographic CAD. Based on tabulations of reported series, myocardial perfusion imaging with pharmacologic coronary artery vasodilation has been reported to be superior to dobutamine echocardiography for detection of angiographic coronary stenoses; however, direct comparison of these methods in the same patients is needed.

How does the clinician decide between two noninvasive modalities, nuclear and echocardiographic, with similar indications and overall accuracies? Although the importance of local expertise cannot be overstated, several factors, such as cost, versatility, and efficiency also merit serious consideration. Thus, in patients in whom noncoronary heart disease is suspected, when left ventricular hypertrophy or left bundle branch block is present, or when the goal of the exercise test is to determine the time to ischemia, stress echocardiography may be advantageous. A major advantage of nuclear methods is that they are readily quantifiable and quantitative criteria

for normal and abnormal studies are widely available. Therefore, stress nuclear imaging may be preferable in patients after myocardial infarction. Although dobutamine stress echocardiography can detect viable myocardium, nuclear imaging is more established in this regard, and at present, is the preferable test.

The competitive roles of stress myocardial perfusion imaging and stress echocardiography for noninvasive detection of CAD will likely stimulate rapid technical advances for both approaches. Correction for attenuation and Compton scatter on myocardial perfusion images provides promise for substantial improvement in diagnostic specificity. Combination of attenuation correction methods with ECG gating should result in radionuclide methods that provide increasingly accurate assessment of left ventricular perfusion and wall thickening. Quantitative approaches to stress echocardiography will likely include on-line edge detection algorithms and automated quantitation of wall-motion abnormalities. Echocardiographic contrast agents[194] will be available to enhance endocardial definition. Color-coded images may be used to assess regional wall motion based on ultrasound backscatter. These advances should further improve the accuracy of stress echocardiography. In the era of cost containment, these advances and others will ensure an expanding role for noninvasive detection of CAD and for noninvasive cardiac risk stratification.

REFERENCES

1. Miller DD, Donohue TJ, Younis LT, et al: Correlation of pharmacological ^{99m}Tc-sestamibi myocardial perfusion imaging with poststenotic coronary flow reserve in patients with angiographically intermediate coronary artery stenoses. *Circulation* 89:2150, 1994.
2. Brown KA: Prognostic value of thallium-201 myocardial perfusion imaging: A diagnostic tool comes of age. *Circulation* 83:363, 1991.
3. Gibson DG, Prewitt TA, Brown DJ: Analysis of left ventricular wall movement during isovolumic relaxation and its relation to coronary artery disease. *Br Heart J* 38:1010, 1976.
4. Gibson DG, Traill TA, Brown DJ: Changes in left ventricular free wall thickness in patients with ischaemic heart disease. *Br Heart J* 39:1312, 1977.
5. Bonow RO, Bacharach SL, Green MV, et al: Impaired left ventricular diastolic filling in patients with coronary artery disease: Assessment with radionuclide angiography. *Circulation* 64:315, 1981.
6. Bonow RO, Kent KM, Rosing DR, et al: Improved left ventricular diastolic filling in patients with coronary artery disease after percutaneous transluminal coronary angioplasty. *Circulation* 66:1159, 1982.
7. Lawson WE, Seifert F, Anagnostopoulos C, et al: Effect

of coronary artery bypass grafting on left ventricular diastolic function. *Am J Cardiol* 61:283, 1988.

8. Poliner LR, Farber SH, Glaeser DH, et al: Alteration of diastolic filling rate during exercise radionuclide angiography: A highly sensitive technique for detection of coronary artery disease. *Circulation* 70:942, 1984.

9. Upton MT, Rerych SK, Newman GE, et al: Detecting abnormalities in left ventricular function during exercise before angina and ST-segment depression. *Circulation* 62:341, 1980.

10. Cannon PJ, Dell RB, Dwyer EM Jr: Regional myocardial perfusion rates in patients with coronary artery disease. *J Clin Invest* 51:978, 1972.

11. Bergmann SR, Herrero P, Markham J, et al: Noninvasive quantitation of myocardial blood flow in human subjects with oxygen-15-labeled water and positron emission tomography. *J Am Coll Cardiol* 14:639, 1989.

12. DePasquale EE, Nody AC, DePuey EG, et al: Quantitative rotational thallium-201 tomography for identifying and localizing coronary artery disease. *Circulation* 77:316, 1988.

13. Pandian NG, Skorton DJ, Collins SM, et al: Heterogeneity of left ventricular segmental wall thickening and excursion in 2-dimensional echocardiograms of normal human subjects. *Am J Cardiol* 51:1667, 1983.

14. Ginzton LE, Conant R, Brizendine M, et al: Quantitative analysis of segmental wall motion during maximal upright dynamic exercise: variability in normal adults. *Circulation* 73:268, 1986.

15. Hausnerova E, Gottdiener JS, Hecht GM, Hausner PF: Heterogeneity of regional left ventricular wall thickening during dobutamine stress echocardiography in normal subjects. *Circulation* 90:I-391, 1994 (abstr).

16. Carstensen S, Ali SM, Stensgaard-Hansen FV, et al: Dobutamine-atropine stress echocardiography in asymptomatic healthy individuals. The relativity of stress-induced hyperkinesis. *Circulation* 92:3453, 1995.

17. Bach DS, Muller DWM, Gros BJ, Armstrong WF: False positive dobutamine stress echocardiograms: Characterization of clinical, echocardiographic and angiographic findings. *J Am Coll Cardiol* 24:928, 1994.

18. Pfisterer M, Muller-Brand J, Brundler H, et al: Prevalence and significance of reversible radionuclide ischemic perfusion defects in symptomatic aortic valve disease patients with or without concomitant coronary disease. *Am Heart J* 103:92, 1982.

19. Bailey IK, Come PC, Kelly DT, et al: Thallium-201 myocardial perfusion imaging in aortic valve stenosis. *Am J Cardiol* 40:889, 1977.

20. Rubin KA, Morrison J, Padnick MB, et al: Idiopathic hypertrophic subaortic stenosis: Evaluation of anginal symptoms with thallium-201 myocardial imaging. *Am J Cardiol* 44:1040, 1979.

21. O'Gara PT, Bonow RO, Maron BJ, et al: Myocardial perfusion abnormalities in patients with hypertrophic cardiomyopathy: Assessment with thallium-201 emission computed tomography. *Circulation* 76:1214, 1987.

22. von Dohlen TW, Prisant LM, Frank MJ: Significance of positive or negative thallium 201 scintigraphy in hypertrophic cardiomyopathy. *Am J Cardiol* 64:498, 1989.

23. Braat SH, Brugada P, Bar FW, et al: Thallium-201 exercise scintigraphy and left bundle branch block. *Am J Cardiol* 55:224, 1985.

24. Hirzel HO, Senn M, Nuesch K, et al: Thallium-201 scintigraphy in complete left bundle branch block. *Am J Cardiol* 53:764, 1984.

25. DePuey EG, Guertler-Krawczysnka E, Robbins WL: Thallium-201 SPECT in coronary artery disease patients with left bundle branch block. *J Nucl Med* 29:1479, 1988.

26. Sharp SM, Sawada SG, Segar DS, et al: Dobutamine stress echocardiography: Detection of coronary artery disease in patients with dilated cardiomyopathy. *J Am Coll Cardiol* 24:934, 1994.

27. Bach DS, Beanlands RSB, Schwaiger M, Armstrong WF: Heterogeneity of ventricular function and myocardial oxidative metabolism in nonischemic dilated cardiomyopathy. *J Am Coll Cardiol* 25:1258, 1995.

28. Hecht HS, Hopkins JM: Exercise-induced regional wall motion abnormalities on radionuclide angiography: Lack of reliability for detection of coronary artery disease in the presence of valvular heart disease. *Am J Cardiol* 47:861, 1981.

29. Mahmarian JJ, Boyce TM, Goldberg RK, et al: Quantitative exercise thallium-201 single photon emission computed tomography for the enhanced diagnosis of ischemic heart disease. *J Am Coll Cardiol* 15:318, 1990.

30. Van Train KF, Maddahi J, Berman DS, et al: Quantitative analysis of tomographic stress thallium-201 myocardial scintigrams: A multicenter trial. *J Nucl Med* 31:1168, 1990.

31. Iskandrian AS, Heo J, Kong B, Lyons E: Effect of exercise level on the ability of thallium-201 tomographic imaging in detecting coronary artery disease: Analysis of 461 patients. *J Am Coll Cardiol* 14:1477, 1989.

32. Kahn JK, McGhie I, Akers MS, et al: Quantitative rotational tomography with ^{201}Tl and ^{99m}Tc 2-methoxy- isobutyl-isonitrile. A direct comparison in normal individuals and patients with coronary artery disease. *Circulation* 79:1282, 1989.

33. Tartagni F, Dondi M, Limonetti P, et al: Dipyridamole technetium-99m-2-methoxy isobutyl isonitrile tomoscintigraphic imaging for identifying diseased coronary vessels: Comparison with thallium-201 stress-rest study. *J Nucl Med* 32:369, 1991.

34. Fleming RM, Kirkeeide RL, Taegtmeyer H, et al: Comparison of technetium-99m teboroxime tomography with automated quantitative coronary arteriography and thallium-201 tomographic imaging. *J Am Coll Cardiol* 17:1297, 1991.

35. Gerson MC, Lukes J, Deutsch E, et al: Comparison of technetium 99m Q12 and thallium 201 for detection of angiographically documented coronary artery disease in humans. *J Nucl Cardiol* 1:499, 1994.

36. Force T, Kemper A, Perkins L, et al: Overestimation of infarct size by quantitative two-dimensional echocardiography: The role of tethering and of analytic procedures. *Circulation* 73:1360, 1986.

37. Seaworth JF, Higginbotham MB, Coleman RE, et al: Effect of partial decreases in exercise work load on radionuclide indexes of ischemia. *J Am Coll Cardiol* 2:522, 1983.

38. Presti CF, Armstrong WF, Feigenbaum H: Comparison of echocardiography at peak exercise and after bicycle exercise in evaluation of patients with known or suspected coronary artery disease. *J Am Soc Echocardiogr* 1:119, 1988.

39. Ciniglio R, Kime M, Burns TL, Vandenberg BF: Rapid resolution of hyperkinesis after exercise. Two-dimensional echocardiographic studies in normal subjects. *Chest* 104:712, 1993.

40. Freeman MR, Berman DS, Staniloff H, et al: Comparison of upright and supine bicycle exercise in the detection and evaluation of extent of coronary artery disease by equilibrium radionuclide ventriculography. *Am Heart J* 102:182, 1981.

41. Fung AY, Gallagher KP, Buda AJ: The physiologic basis of dobutamine as compared with dipyridamole stress interventions in the assessment of critical coronary stenosis. *Circulation* 76:943, 1987.

42. Kumar EB, Steel SA, Howey S, et al: Dipyridamole is superior to dobutamine for thallium stress imaging: A randomised crossover study. *Br Heart J* 71:129, 1994.

43. Picano E, Lattanzi F, Masini M, et al: High dose dipyridamole echocardiography test in effort angina pectoris. *J Am Coll Cardiol* 8:848, 1986.

44. Martin TW, Seaworth JF, Johns JP, et al: Comparison of adenosine, dipyridamole, and dobutamine in stress echocardiography. *Ann Intern Med* 116:190, 1992.

45. Stolzenberg J, Kaminsky J: Overlying breast as cause of false-positive thallium scans. *Clin Nucl Med* 3:229, 1978.

46. Gordon DG, Pfisterer M, Williams R, et al: The effect of diaphragmatic attenuation on ^{201}Tl images. *Clin Nucl Med* 4:150, 1979.

47. Johnstone DE, Wackers FJTh, Berger HJ, et al: Effect of patient positioning on left lateral thallium-201 myocardial images. *J Nucl Med* 20:183, 1979.

48. Quinones MA, Verani MS, Haichin RM, et al: Exercise echocardiography versus ^{201}Tl single-photon emission computed tomography in evaluation of coronary artery disease. Analysis of 292 patients. *Circulation* 85:1026, 1992.

49. Kiat H, Germano G, Friedman J, et al: Comparative feasibility of separate or simultaneous rest thallium-201/stress technetium-99m-sestamibi dual-isotope myocardial perfusion SPECT. *J Nucl Med* 35:542, 1994.

50. Hendel RC, McSherry B, Karimeddini M, Leppo JA: Diagnostic value of a new myocardial perfusion agent, teboroxime (SQ 30,217), utilizing a rapid planar imaging protocol: Preliminary results. *J Am Coll Cardiol* 16:855, 1990.

51. Feigenbaum H: Exercise echocardiography. *J Am Soc Echocardiogr* 1:161, 1988.

52. Lindower PD, Rath L, Preslar J, et al: Quantification of left ventricular function with an automated border detection system and comparison with radionuclide ventriculography. *Am J Cardiol* 73:195, 1994.

53. Crouse LJ, Harbrecht JJ, Vacek JL, et al: Exercise echocardiography as a screening test for coronary artery disease and correlation with coronary arteriography. *Am J Cardiol* 67:1213, 1991.

54. Hecht HS, DeBord L, Shaw R, et al: Digital supine bicycle stress echocardiography: A new technique for evaluating coronary artery disease. *J Am Coll Cardiol* 21:950, 1993.

55. Marwick TH, Nemec JJ, Pashkow FJ, et al: Accuracy and limitations of exercise echocardiography in a routine clinical setting. *J Am Coll Cardiol* 19:74, 1992.

56. Beleslin BD, Ostojic M, Stepanovic J, et al: Stress echocardiography in the detection of myocardial ischemia. Head-to-head comparison of exercise, dobutamine, and dipyridamole tests. *Circulation* 90:1168, 1994.

57. Armstrong WF, O'Donnell J, Ryan T, Feigenbaum H: Effect of prior myocardial infarction and extent and location of coronary disease on accuracy of exercise echocardiography. *J Am Coll Cardiol* 10:531, 1987.

58. Blomstrand P, Engvall J, Karlsson JE, et al: Exercise echocardiography: A methodological study comparing peak-exercise and post-exercise image information. *Clin Physiol* 12:553, 1992.

59. Ryan T, Segar DS, Sawada SG, et al: Detection of coronary artery disease with upright bicycle exercise echocardiography. *J Am Soc Echocardiogr* 6:186, 1993.

60. Sheikh KH, Bengtson JR, Helmy S, et al: Relation of quantitative coronary lesion measurements to the development of exercise-induced ischemia assessed by exercise echocardiography. *J Am Coll Cardiol* 15:1043, 1990.

61. Marangelli K, Iliceto S, Piccinni G, et al: Detection of coronary artery disease by digital stress echocardiography: Comparison of exercise, transesophageal atrial pacing and dipyridamole echocardiography. *J Am Coll Cardiol* 24:117, 1994.

62. Prigent FM, Berman DS, Elashoff J, et al: Reproducibility of stress redistribution thallium-201 SPECT quantitative indexes of hypoperfused myocardium secondary to coronary artery disease. *Am J Cardiol* 70:1255, 1992.

63. Marcassa C, Marzullo P, Parodi O, et al: A new method for noninvasive quantitation of segmental myocardial wall thickening using technetium-99m 2-methoxy-isobutyl-isonitrile scintigraphy — Results in normal subjects. *J Nucl Med* 31:173, 1990.

64. Mochizuki T, Murase K, Fujiwara Y, et al: Assessment of systolic thickening with thallium-201 ECG-gated single-photon emission computed tomography: A parameter for local left ventricular function. *J Nucl Med* 32:1496, 1991.

65. Cooke CD, Garcia EV, Cullom SJ, et al: Determining the accuracy of calculating systolic wall thickening using a fast Fourier transform approximation: A simulation study based on canine and patient data. *J Nucl Med* 35:1185, 1994.

66. Sciagra R, Bisi G, Santoro GM, et al: Evaluation of coronary artery disease using technetium-99m-sestamibi first-pass and perfusion imaging with dipyridamole infusion. *J Nucl Med* 35:1254, 1994.

67. Palmas W, Friedman JD, Diamond GA, et al: Incremental value of simultaneous assessment of myocardial function and perfusion with technetium-99m sestamibi for prediction of extent of coronary artery disease. *J Am Coll Cardiol* 25:1024, 1995.

68. Agati L, Arata L, Luongo R, et al: Assessment of severity of coronary narrowings by quantitative exercise echocar-

diography and comparison with quantitative arteriography. *Am J Cardiol* 67:1201, 1991.

69. Hoffmann R, Lethen H, Marwick T, et al: Analysis of interinstitutional observer agreement in interpretation of dobutamine stress echocardiograms. *J Am Coll Cardiol* 27:330, 1996.

70. Pozzoli MMA, Fioretti PM, Salustri A, et al: Exercise echocardiography and technetium-99m MIBI single-photon emission computed tomography in the detection of coronary artery disease. *Am J Cardiol* 67:350, 1991.

71. Galanti G, Sciagra R, Comeglio M, et al: Diagnostic accuracy of peak exercise echocardiography in coronary artery disease: Comparison with thallium-201 myocardial scintigraphy. *Am Heart J* 122:1609, 1991.

72. Amanullah AM, Lindvall K, Bevegard S: Exercise echocardiography after stabilization of unstable angina: Correlation with exercise thallium-201 single photon emission computed tomography. *Clin Cardiol* 15:585, 1992.

73. Feigenbaum H: Evolution of stress testing. *Circulation* 85:1217, 1992.

74. Arnese M, Fioretti PM, Cornel JH, et al: Akinesis becoming dyskinesis during high-dose dobutamine stress echocardiography: A marker of myocardial ischemia or a mechanical phenomenon? *Am J Cardiol* 73:896, 1994.

75. Brown KA, Boucher CA, Okada RD, et al: Prognostic value of exercise thallium-201 imaging in patients presenting for evaluation of chest pain. *J Am Coll Cardiol* 1:994, 1983.

76. Staniloff HM, Forrester JS, Berman DS, Swan HJC: Prediction of death, myocardial infarction, and worsening chest pain using thallium scintigraphy and exercise electrocardiography. *J Nucl Med* 27:1842, 1986.

77. Iskandrian AS, Hakki AH, Kane-Marsch S: Exercise thallium-201 scintigraphy in men with nondiagnostic exercise electrocardiograms: Prognostic implications. *Arch Intern Med* 146:2189, 1986.

78. Gill JB, Ruddy TD, Newell JB, et al: Prognostic importance of thallium uptake by the lungs during exercise in coronary artery disease. *N Engl J Med* 317:1485, 1987.

79. Kaul S, Finkelstein DM, Homma S, et al: Superiority of quantitative exercise thallium-201 variables in determining long-term prognosis in ambulatory patients with chest pain: A comparison with cardiac catheterization. *J Am Coll Cardiol* 12:25, 1988.

80. Wahl JM, Hakki A-H, Iskandrian AS: Prognostic implications of normal exercise thallium-201 images. *Arch Intern Med* 145:263, 1985.

81. Pamelia FX, Gibson RS, Watson DD, et al: Prognosis with chest pain and normal thallium-201 exercise scintigrams. *Am J Cardiol* 55:920, 1985.

82. Wackers FJTh, Russo DJ, Russo D, Clements JP: Prognostic significance of normal quantitative planar thallium-201 stress scintigraphy in patients with chest pain. *J Am Coll Cardiol* 6:27, 1985.

83. Heo J, Thompson WO, Iskandrian AS: Prognostic implications of normal exercise thallium images. *Am J Noninvas Cardiol* 1:209, 1987.

84. Bairey CN, Rozanski A, Maddahi J, et al: Exercise thallium-201 scintigraphy and prognosis in typical angina pectoris and negative exercise electrocardiography. *Am J Cardiol* 64:282, 1989.

85. Fleg JL, Gerstenblith G, Zonderman AB, et al: Prevalence and prognostic significance of exercise-induced silent myocardial ischemia detected by thallium scintigraphy and electrocardiography in asymptomatic volunteers. *Circulation* 81:428, 1990.

86. Koss JH, Kobren SM, Grunwald AM, Bodenheimer MM: Role of exercise thallium-201 myocardial perfusion scintigraphy in predicting prognosis in suspected coronary artery disease. *Am J Cardiol* 59:531, 1987.

87. Krivokapich J, Child JS, Gerber RS, et al: Prognostic usefulness of positive or negative exercise stress echocardiography for predicting coronary events in ensuing twelve months. *Am J Cardiol* 71:646, 1993.

88. Sawada SG, Ryan T, Conley MJ, et al: Prognostic value of a normal exercise echocardiogram. *Am Heart J* 120:49, 1990.

89. Amanullah AM, Lindvall K, Bevegard S: Prognostic significance of exercise thallium-201 myocardial perfusion imaging compared to stress echocardiography and clinical variables in patients with unstable angina who respond to medical treatment. *Int J Cardiol* 39:71, 1993.

90. Rozanski A, Diamond GA, Berman D, et al: The declining specificity of exercise radionuclide ventriculography. *N Engl J Med* 309:518, 1983.

91. Mahmarian JJ, Verani MS: Exercise thallium-201 perfusion scintigraphy in the assessment of coronary artery disease. *Am J Cardiol* 67:2D, 1991.

92. Amanullah AM, Lindvall K, Bevegard S: Exercise echocardiography after stabilization of unstable angina: Correlation with exercise thallium-201 single photon emission computed tomography. *Clin Cardiol* 15:585, 1992.

93. Hecht HS, DeBord L, Shaw R, et al: Supine bicycle stress echocardiography versus tomographic thallium-201 exercise imaging for the detection of coronary artery disease. *J Am Soc Echocardiogr* 6:177, 1993.

94. Maurer G, Nanda NC: Two dimensional echocardiographic evaluation of exercise-induced left and right ventricular asynergy: Correlation with thallium scanning. *Am J Cardiol* 48:720, 1981.

95. Hoffmann R, Lethen H, Kleinhans E, et al: Comparative evaluation of bicycle and dobutamine stress echocardiography with perfusion scintigraphy and bicycle electrocardiogram for identification of coronary disease. *Am J Cardiol* 72:555, 1993.

96. Salustri A, Pozzoli MMA, Hermans W, et al: Relationship between exercise echocardiography and perfusion single-photon emission computed tomography in patients with single-vessel coronary artery disease. *Am Heart J* 124:75, 1992.

97. Starling MR, Dehmer GJ, Lancaster JL, et al: Comparison of quantitative SPECT vs planar thallium-201 myocardial scintigraphy for detecting and localizing segmental coronary artery disease. *J Am Coll Cardiol* 5:531, 1985 (abstr).

98. Rigo P, Bailey IK, Griffith LSC, et al: Stress thallium-201 myocardial scintigraphy for the detection of individual coronary arterial lesions in patients with and without previous myocardial infarction. *Am J Cardiol* 48:209, 1981.

99. Massie BM, Botvinick EH, Brundage BH: Correlation of thallium-201 scintigrams with coronary anatomy: Fac-

tors affecting region by region sensitivity. *Am J Cardiol* 44:616, 1979.

100. Lenaers A, Block P, van Thiel E, et al: Segmental analysis of Tl-201 stress myocardial scintigraphy. *J Nucl Med* 18:509, 1977.

101. Maddahi J, Garcia EV, Berman DS, et al: Improved noninvasive assessment of coronary artery disease by quantitative analysis of regional stress myocardial distribution and washout of thallium-201. *Circulation* 64:924, 1981.

102. Tamaki N, Yonekura Y, Mukai T, et al: Segmental analysis of stress thallium myocardial emission tomography for localization of coronary artery disease. *Eur J Nucl Med* 9:99, 1984.

103. Kasabali B, Woodard ML, Bekerman C, et al: Enhanced sensitivity and specificity of thallium-201 imaging for the detection of regional ischemic coronary disease by combining SPECT with "bull's eye" analysis. *Clin Nucl Med* 14:484, 1989.

104. Fintel DJ, Links JM, Brinker JA, et al: Improved diagnostic performance of exercise thallium-201 single photon emission computed tomography over planar imaging in the diagnosis of coronary artery disease: A receiver operating characteristic analysis. *J Am Coll Cardiol* 13:600, 1989.

105. Tamaki N, Yonekura Y, Mukai T, et al: Stress thallium-201 transaxial emission computed tomography: Quantitative versus qualitative analysis for evaluation of coronary artery disease. *J Am Coll Cardiol* 4:1213, 1984.

106. Stone DA, Corretti MC, Hawke MW, et al: The influence of angiographically demonstrated coronary collaterals on the results of stress echocardiography. *Clin Cardiol* 18:205, 1995.

107. Rigo P, Becker LC, Griffith LSC, et al: Influence of coronary collateral vessels on the results of thallium-201 myocardial stress imaging. *Am J Cardiol* 44:452, 1979.

108. Wainwright RJ, Maisey MN, Edwards AC, Sowton E: Functional significance of coronary collateral circulation during dynamic exercise evaluated by thallium-201 myocardial scintigraphy. *Br Heart J* 43:47, 1980.

109. Tubau JF, Chaitman BR, Bourassa MG, et al: Importance of coronary collateral circulation in interpreting exercise test results. *Am J Cardiol* 47:27, 1981.

110. Roger VL, Pellikka PA, Oh JK, et al: Identification of multivessel coronary artery disease by exercise echocardiography. *J Am Coll Cardiol* 24:109, 1994.

111. Bonow RO, Dilsizian V, Cuocolo A, Bacharach SL: Identification of viable myocardium in patients with chronic coronary artery disease and left ventricular dysfunction. Comparison of thallium scintigraphy with reinjection and PET imaging with ^{18}F-fluorodeoxyglucose. *Circulation* 83:26, 1991.

112. Tamaki N, Ohtani H, Yonekura Y, et al: Significance of fill-in after thallium-201 reinjection following delayed imaging: Comparison with regional wall motion and angiographic findings. *J Nucl Med* 31:1617, 1990.

113. Ohtani H, Tamaki N, Yonekura Y, et al: Value of thallium-201 reinjection after delayed SPECT imaging for predicting reversible ischemia after coronary artery bypass grafting. *Am J Cardiol* 66:394, 1990.

114. Perrone-Filardi P, Bacharach SL, Dilsizian V, et al: Regional left ventricular wall thickening. Relation to re-

gional uptake of ^{18}Fluorodeoxyglucose and ^{201}Tl in patients with chronic coronary artery disease and left ventricular dysfunction. *Circulation* 86:1125, 1992.

115. Dilsizian V, Perrone-Filardi P, Arrighi JA, et al: Concordance and discordance between stress-redistribution-reinjection and rest-redistribution thallium imaging for assessing viable myocardium. Comparison with metabolic activity by positron emission tomography. *Circulation* 88:941, 1993.

116. Dilsizian V, Freedman NMT, Bacharach SL, et al: Regional thallium uptake in irreversible defects. Magnitude of change in thallium activity after reinjection distinguishes viable from nonviable myocardium. *Circulation* 85:627, 1992.

117. Crouse LJ, Vacek JL, Beauchamp GD, et al: Exercise echocardiography after coronary artery bypass grafting. *Am J Cardiol* 70:572, 1992.

118. Baer FM, Voth E, Deutsch HJ, et al: Assessment of viable myocardium by dobutamine transesophageal echocardiography and comparison with fluorine-18 fluorodeoxyglucose positron emission tomography. *J Am Coll Cardiol* 24:343, 1994.

119. Sawada SG, Ryan T, Fineberg NS, et al: Exercise echocardiographic detection of coronary artery disease in women. *J Am Coll Cardiol* 14:1440, 1989.

120. Williams MJ, Marwick TH, O'Gorman D, Foale RA: Comparison of exercise echocardiography with an exercise score to diagnose coronary artery disease in women. *Am J Cardiol* 74:435, 1994.

121. Marwick TH, Anderson T, Williams MJ, et al: Exercise echocardiography is an accurate and cost-efficient technique for detection of coronary artery disease in women. *J Am Coll Cardiol* 26:335, 1995.

122. Esquivel L, Pollock SG, Beller GA, et al: Effect of the degree of effort on the sensitivity of the exercise thallium-201 stress test in symptomatic coronary artery disease. *Am J Cardiol* 63:160, 1989.

123. Travin MI, Emaus SP, Korr KS, et al: Detection of coronary artery disease as assessed by electrocardiogram or thallium-201 imaging: Impact of achieved heart rate during exercise testing. *Am J Noninvas Cardiol* 5:40, 1991.

124. Martin GJ, Henkin RE, Scanlon PJ: Beta blockers and the sensitivity of the thallium treadmill test. *Chest* 92:486, 1987.

125. Rainwater J, Steele P, Kirch D, et al: Effect of propranolol on myocardial perfusion images and exercise ejection fraction in men with coronary artery disease. *Circulation* 65:77, 1982.

126. McNeill AJ, Fioretti PM, El-Said E-SM, et al: Enhanced sensitivity for detection of coronary artery disease by addition of atropine to dobutamine stress echocardiography. *Am J Cardiol* 70:41, 1992.

127. Poldermans D, Fioretti PM, Boersma E, et al: Safety of dobutamine-atropine stress echocardiography in patients with suspected or proven coronary artery disease. *Am J Cardiol* 73:456, 1994.

128. McNeill AJ, Fioretti PM, El-Said E-SM, et al: Dobutamine stress echocardiography before and after coronary angioplasty. *Am J Cardiol* 69:740, 1992.

129. Weissman NJ, Nidorf SM, Guerrero JL, et al: Optimal

stage duration in dobutamine stress echocardiography. *J Am Coll Cardiol* 25:605, 1995.

130. Mertes H, Sawada SG, Ryan T, et al: Symptoms, adverse effects, and complications associated with dobutamine stress echocardiography. Experience in 1118 patients. *Circulation* 88:15, 1993.

131. Pingitore A, Bigi R, Mathias W, et al: The safety and tolerability of dobutamine-atropine stress echocardiography. *Circulation* 90:I-659, 1994.

132. Marcovitz PA, Bach DS, Mathias W, et al: Paradoxic hypotension during dobutamine stress echocardiography: Clinical and diagnostic implications. *J Am Coll Cardiol* 21:1080, 1993.

133. Mazeika PK, Nadazdin A, Oakley CM: Clinical significance of abrupt vasodepression during dobutamine stress echocardiography. *Am J Cardiol* 69:1484, 1992.

134. Lombardo A, Loperfido F, Pennestri F, et al: Significance of transient ST-T segment changes during dobutamine testing in Q wave myocardial infarction. *J Am Coll Cardiol* 27:599, 1996.

135. Sorrentino MJ, Marcus RH, Lang RM: Left ventricular outflow tract obstruction as a cause for hypotension and symptoms during dobutamine stress echocardiography. *Clin Cardiol* 19:225, 1996.

136. Panza JA, Laurienzo JM, Curiel RV, et al: Transesophageal dobutamine stress echocardiography for evaluation of patients with coronary artery disease. *J Am Coll Cardiol* 24:1260, 1994.

137. Frohwein S, Klein JL, Lane A, Taylor WR: Transesophageal dobutamine stress echocardiography in the evaluation of coronary artery disease. *J Am Coll Cardiol* 25:823, 1995.

138. Pennell DJ, Underwood SR, Ell PJ: Safety of dobutamine stress for thallium-201 myocardial perfusion tomography in patients with asthma. *Am J Cardiol* 71:1346, 1993.

139. Hays JT, Mahmarian JJ, Cochran AJ, Verani MS: Dobutamine thallium-201 tomography for evaluating patients with suspected coronary artery disease unable to undergo exercise or vasodilator pharmacologic stress testing. *J Am Coll Cardiol* 21:1583, 1993.

140. Sawada SG, Segar DS, Ryan T, et al: Echocardiographic detection of coronary artery disease during dobutamine infusion. *Circulation* 83:1605, 1991.

141. Previtali M, Lanzarini L, Fetiveau R, et al: Comparison of dobutamine stress echocardiography, dipyridamole stress echocardiography and exercise stress testing for diagnosis of coronary artery disease. *Am J Cardiol* 72:865, 1993.

142. Mazeika PK, Nadazdin A, Oakley CM: Dobutamine stress echocardiography for detection and assessment of coronary artery disease. *J Am Coll Cardiol* 19:1203, 1992.

143. Marcovitz PA, Armstrong WF: Accuracy of dobutamine stress echocardiography in detecting coronary artery disease. *Am J Cardiol* 69:1269, 1992.

144. Martin TW, Seaworth JF, Johns JP, et al: Comparison of adenosine, dipyridamole, and dobutamine in stress echocardiography. *Ann Intern Med* 116:190, 1992.

145. Cohen JL, Ottenweller JE, George AK, Duvvuri S: Comparison of dobutamine and exercise echocardiography for detecting coronary artery disease. *Am J Cardiol* 72:1226, 1993.

146. Warner MF, Pippin JJ, DiSciascio G, et al: Assessment of thallium scintigraphy and echocardiography during dobutamine infusion for the detection of coronary artery disease. *Cathet Cardiovasc Diagn* 29:122, 1993.

147. Marwick T, D'Hondt A-M, Baudhuin T, et al: Optimal use of dobutamine stress for the detection and evaluation of coronary artery disease: Combination with echocardiography or scintigraphy, or both? *J Am Coll Cardiol* 22:159, 1993.

148. Gunalp B, Dokumaci B, Uyan C, et al: Value of dobutamine technetium-99m-sestamibi SPECT and echocardiography in the detection of coronary artery disease compared with coronary angiography. *J Nucl Med* 34:889, 1993.

149. Senior R, Sridhara BS, Anagnostou E, et al: Synergistic value of simultaneous stress dobutamine sestamibi single-photon-emission computerized tomography and echocardiography in the detection of coronary artery disease. *Am Heart J* 128:713, 1994.

150. Mairesse GH, Marwick TH, Vanoverschelde J-LJ, et al: How accurate is dobutamine stress electrocardiography for detection of coronary artery disease? Comparison with two-dimensional echocardiography and technetium-99m methoxyl isobutyl isonitrile (Mibi) perfusion scintigraphy. *J Am Coll Cardiol* 24:920, 1994.

151. Segar DS, Brown SE, Sawada SG, et al: Dobutamine stress echocardiography: Correlation with coronary lesion severity as determined by quantitative angiography. *J Am Coll Cardiol* 19:1197, 1992.

152. Forster T, McNeill AJ, Salustri A, et al: Simultaneous dobutamine stress echocardiography and technetium-99m isonitrile single-photon emission computed tomography in patients with suspected coronary artery disease. *J Am Coll Cardiol* 21:1591, 1993.

153. Bach DS, Hepner A, Marcovitz PA, Armstrong WF: Dobutamine stress echocardiography: Prevalence of a non-ischemic response in a low-risk population. *Am Heart J* 125:1257, 1993.

154. Pennell DJ, Underwood SR, Swanton RH, et al: Dobutamine thallium myocardial perfusion tomography. *J Am Coll Cardiol* 18:1471, 1991.

155. Herman SD, LaBresh KA, Santos-Ocampo CD, et al: Comparison of dobutamine and exercise using technetium-99m sestamibi imaging for the evaluation of coronary artery disease. *Am J Cardiol* 73:164, 1994.

156. Elliott BM, Robison JG, Zellner JL, Hendrix GH: Dobutamine-201Tl imaging. Assessing cardiac risks associated with vascular surgery. *Circulation* 84(suppl III):III-54, 1991.

157. Attenhofer CH, Pellikka PA, Oh JK, et al: Comparison of ischemic response during exercise and dobutamine echocardiography in patients with left main coronary artery disease. *J Am Coll Cardiol* 27:1171, 1996.

158. DePuey EG, Guertler-Krawczynska E, Perkins JV, et al: Alterations in myocardial thallium-201 distribution in patients with chronic systemic hypertension undergoing single-photon emission computed tomography. *Am J Cardiol* 62:234, 1988.

159. Vensel LA, Devereux RB, Pickering TG, et al: Cardiac

structure and function in renovascular hypertension produced by unilateral and bilateral renal artery stenosis. *Am J Cardiol* 58:575, 1986.

160. Grogan M, Christian TF, Miller TD, et al: The effect of systemic hypertension on exercise tomographic thallium-201 imaging in the absence of electrocardiographic left ventricular hypertrophy. *Am Heart J* 126:327, 1993.

161. Chin WL, O'Kelly B, Tubau JF, et al: Diagnostic accuracy of exercise thallium-201 scintigraphy in men with asymptomatic essential hypertension. *Am J Hypertens* 5:465, 1992.

162. Prisant LM, von Dohlen TW, Houghton JL, et al: A negative thallium (± dipyridamole) stress test excludes significant obstructive epicardial coronary artery disease in hypertensive patients. *Am J Hypertens* 5:71, 1992.

163. Ambrosi P, Habib G, Kreitman B, et al: Thallium perfusion and myocardial hypertrophy in transplanted heart recipients with normal or near-normal coronary arteriograms. *Eur Heart J* 15:1119, 1994.

164. Marcus ML, Mueller TM, Gascho JA, Kerbr RE: Effects of cardiac hypertrophy secondary to hypertension on the coronary circulation. *Am J Cardiol* 44:1023, 1979.

165. Wicker P, Tarazi RC: Coronary blood flow in left ventricular hypertrophy: a review of experimental data. *Eur Heart J* 3(suppl A):111, 1982.

166. Goldstein RA, Haynie M: Limited myocardial perfusion reserve in patients with left ventricular hypertrophy. *J Nucl Med* 31:255, 1990.

167. Opherk D, Mall G, Zebe H, et al: Reduction of coronary reserve: A mechanism for angina pectoris in patients with arterial hypertension and normal coronary arteries. *Circulation* 69:1, 1984.

168. Antony I, Nitenberg A, Foult J-M, Aptecar E: Coronary vasodilator reserve in untreated and treated hypertensive patients with and without left ventricular hypertrophy. *J Am Coll Cardiol* 22:514, 1993.

169. Houghton JL, Frank MJ, Carr AA, et al: Relations among impaired coronary flow reserve, left ventricular hypertrophy and thallium perfusion defects in hypertensive patients without obstructive coronary artery disease. *J Am Coll Cardiol* 15:43, 1990.

170. Marwick TH, Cook SA, Lafont A, et al: Influence of left ventricular mass on the diagnostic accuracy of myocardial perfusion imaging using positron emission tomography with dipyridamole stress. *J Nucl Med* 32:2221, 1991.

171. Timmis AD, Lutkin JE, Fenney LJ, et al: Comparison of dipyridamole and treadmill exercise for enhancing thallium-201 perfusion defects in patients with coronary artery disease. *Eur Heart J* 1:275, 1980.

172. Varma SK, Watson DD, Beller GA: Quantitative comparison of thallium-201 scintigraphy after exercise and dipyridamole in coronary artery disease. *Am J Cardiol* 64:871, 1989.

173. Carlson RE, Kavanaugh KM, Buda AJ: The effect of different mechanisms of myocardial ischemia on left ventricular function. *Am Heart J* 116:536, 1988.

174. Elhendy A, Geleijnse ML, Roelandt JRTC, et al: Dobutamine-induced hypoperfusion without transient wall motion abnormalities: Less severe ischemia or less severe stress? *J Am Coll Cardiol* 27:323, 1996.

175. Verani MS, Mahmarian JJ, Hixson JB, et al: Diagnosis of coronary artery disease by controlled coronary vasodilation with adenosine and thallium-201 scintigraphy in patients unable to exercise. *Circulation* 82:80, 1990.

176. Nishimura S, Mahmarian JJ, Boyce TM, Verani MS: Equivalence between adenosine and exercise thallium-201 myocardial tomography: A multicenter, prospective, crossover trial. *J Am Coll Cardiol* 20:265, 1992.

177. Coyne EP, Belvedere DA, Vande Streek PR, et al: Thallium-201 scintigraphy after intravenous infusion of adenosine compared with exercise thallium testing in the diagnosis of coronary artery disease. *J Am Coll Cardiol* 17:1289, 1991.

178. Gupta NC, Esterbrooks DJ, Hilleman DE, et al: Comparison of adenosine and exercise thallium-201 single-photon emission computed tomography (SPECT) myocardial perfusion imaging. *J Am Coll Cardiol* 19:248, 1992.

179. Cuocolo A, Soricelli A, Pace L, et al: Adenosine technetium-99m-methoxy isobutyl isonitrile myocardial tomography in patients with coronary artery disease: Comparison with exercise. *J Nucl Med* 35:1110, 1994.

180. Wilson RF, Wyche K, Christensen BV, et al: Effects of adenosine on human coronary arterial circulation. *Circulation* 82:1595, 1990.

181. Rossen JD, Quillen JE, Lopez AG, et al: Comparison of coronary vasodilation with intravenous dipyridamole and adenosine. *J Am Coll Cardiol* 18:485, 1991.

182. Chan SY, Brunken RC, Czernin J, et al: Comparison of maximal myocardial blood flow during adenosine infusion with that of intravenous dipyridamole in normal men. *J Am Coll Cardiol* 20:979, 1992.

183. Kern MJ, Deligonul U, Tatineni S, et al: Intravenous adenosine: Continuous infusion and low dose bolus administration for determination of coronary vasodilator reserve in patients with and without coronary artery disease. *J Am Coll Cardiol* 18:718, 1991.

184. Nguyen T, Heo J, Ogilby JD, Iskandrian AS: Single photon emission computed tomography with thallium-201 during adenosine-induced coronary hyperemia: Correlation with coronary arteriography, exercise thallium imaging and two-dimensional echocardiography. *J Am Coll Cardiol* 16:1375, 1990.

185. Marwick T, Willemart B, D'Hondt A-M, et al: Selection of the optimal nonexercise stress for the evaluation of ischemic regional myocardial dysfunction and malperfusion. Comparison of dobutamine and adenosine using echocardiography and ^{99m}Tc-MIBI single photon emission computed tomography. *Circulation* 87:345, 1993.

186. Amanullah AM, Bevegard S, Lindvall K, Aasa M: Assessment of left ventricular wall motion in angina pectoris by two-dimensional echocardiography and myocardial perfusion by technetium-99m sestamibi tomography during adenosine-induced coronary vasodilation and comparison with coronary angiography. *Am J Cardiol* 72:983, 1993.

187. Di Bello V, Gori E, Bellina CR, et al: Incremental diagnostic value of dipyridamole echocardiography and exercise thallium 201 scintigraphy in the assessment of presence and extent of coronary artery disease. *J Nucl Cardiol* 1:372, 1994.

188. Picano E, Parodi O, Lattanzi F, et al: Comparison of dipyridamole-echocardiography test and exercise thal-

lium-201 scanning for diagnosis of coronary artery disease. *Am J Noninvas Cardiol* 3:85, 1989.

189. Mazeika P, Nihoyannopoulos P, Joshi J, Oakley CM: Uses and limitations of high dose dipyridamole stress echocardiography for evaluation of coronary artery disease. *Br Heart J* 67:144, 1992.

190. Pingitore A, Picano E, Quarta Colosso M, et al: The atropine factor in pharmacologic stress echocardiography. *J Am Coll Cardiol* 27:1164, 1996.

191. O'Keefe JH Jr, Barnhart CS, Bateman TM: Comparison of stress echocardiography and stress myocardial perfusion scintigraphy for diagnosing coronary artery disease and assessing its severity. *Am J Cardiol* 75:25D, 1995.

192. Ho FM, Huang PJ, Liau CS, et al: Dobutamine stress echocardiography compared with dipyridamole thallium-201 single-photon emission computed tomography in detecting coronary artery disease. *Eur Heart J* 16:570, 1995.

193. Wallbridge DR, Tweddel AC, Martin W, Hutton I: A comparison of dobutamine and maximal exercise as stress for thallium scintigraphy. *Eur J Nucl Med* 20:319, 1993.

194. Ismail S, Jayaweera AR, Goodman NC, et al: Detection of coronary stenoses and quantification of the degree and spatial extent of blood flow mismatch during coronary hyperemia with myocardial contrast echocardiography. *Circulation* 91:821, 1995.

Radionuclide Assessment of Coronary Artery Disease Following Revascularization

D. Douglas Miller

As is the case in other subsets of coronary artery disease, the use of radionuclide cardiac imaging is a valuable tool for the assessment of patients who have undergone recent or remote coronary revascularization procedures. In this setting, the diagnosis of coronary artery disease is self-evident and, as such, the principal value of nuclear cardiac imaging procedures in the postrevascularization patient is twofold:

1. Assessment of the initial adequacy and sustained benefit of coronary revascularization, as reflected by myocardial perfusion and ventricular function.
2. Determination of the risk of future cardiac events (short-term prognosis and long-term prognosis) in patients with varying degrees of revascularization.

Whether nuclear cardiac imaging is performed following percutaneous transluminal coronary angioplasty (PTCA) or coronary artery bypass graft (CABG) surgery, the importance of acquiring serial studies cannot be over-emphasized. The comparison of an initial prerevascularization cardiac nuclear scan with a postrevascularization study can provide important information as to the initial success and completeness of the revascularization procedure. The timing and indications for postrevascularization imaging are variable and remain controversial in the setting of PTCA. However, it is generally accepted that patients with recurrent ischemic symptoms following a revascularization procedure (PTCA or CABG) are good candidates for nuclear myocardial perfusion imaging, and that these studies are most valuable when

compared with previous studies performed either before or early after the index revascularization procedure. Routine postrevascularization cardiac imaging studies are usually not recommended outside the setting of clinical investigation, but some investigators have used myocardial perfusion studies to evaluate CABG patency at 5 to 7 years following surgery, even in the absence of recurrent symptoms suggestive of myocardial ischemia.[1]

The current accepted indications for the use of radionuclide cardiac imaging studies following angioplasty and bypass graft surgery are listed in Tables 22-1 and 22-2. When used in this fashion, myocardial perfusion imaging (with or without assessment of regional left ventricular function) can provide useful information that will assist in the clinical management of patients who have undergone either PTCA or CABG procedures.

To date, no study has demonstrated the cost effectiveness of routine pre- and/or postrevascularization cardiac imaging. Most investigators appropriately reserve these studies for patients with recurrent symptoms of myocardial ischemia of mild-to-moderate severity, or for the evaluation of patients with absent or difficult-to-evaluate symptoms of myocardial ischemia in whom the indications for proceeding directly to coronary angiography are not clear. Patients whose symptoms indicate a high likelihood of recurrent myocardial ischemia are generally referred directly to cardiac catheterization, as are those patients whose noninvasive cardiac imaging studies suggest moderate-to-extensive myocardial jeopardy in zones

Table 22-1 Stress Myocardial Imaging After Percutaneous Transluminal Coronary Angioplasty (PTCA)

Indications
  Assessment for post-PTCA improvement in coronary blood flow
    Direct: reduced perfusion defect size and severity
    Indirect: improved regional left ventricular function (gated SPECT and radionuclide ventriculography)
  Confirmation of angiographic success
    Questionable initial angiographic result
    Adequacy of subsequent vascular remodeling
  Detection of residual ischemia (with or without angina recurrence)
    Unmasking of less severe secondary (nonculprit) stenoses
    Prediction/early detection of restenosis
      Predictive value higher with typical angina
      Predictive value lower with atypical or no angina

Limitations
  Optimal timing uncertain
    Immediate (1 to 3 days): limited exercise tolerance
    Early (2 to 4 weeks): more false-positive results
    Later (3 months): restenosis potential increased
  Expense compared with stress ECG
    ECG favored: single-vessel left anterior descending PTCA with normal rest ECG
    Stress imaging favored: multivessel disease and/or abnormal rest ECG
  Prognostic value from small populations
    Negative predictive value of normal scan: excellent
    Positive predictive value: varies widely
  Post-PTCA vasodilator reserve
    Attenuated response to coronary vasodilators
    Few intravenous stress imaging studies

ECG, electrocardiograph; SPECT, single photon emission computed tomography.

that have been previously revascularized, or in vascular territories that suggest the progression of coronary disease in nonrevascularized myocardial territories.

PERCUTANEOUS TRANSLUMINAL CORONARY ANGIOPLASTY

Andreas Gruentzig was among the first actively to advocate and perform functional assessments of poststenotic myocardial perfusion before and after angioplasty. The performance of interventional cardiology has since grown dramatically as the result of several factors, including (1) expansion of indications from single-vessel to multivessel disease and from stable to acute chest pain syndromes, (2) improved angioplasty devices for coronary interventions, (3) increased referral and acceptance of PTCA as a nonsurgical alternative to CABG, and (4) the need for repeat procedures to treat restenosis. The applications of myocardial perfusion imaging have kept pace with the evolution of PTCA. These techniques have had a significant impact on each other in the last two decades.

The recognized limitations of coronary angiographic assessments of functional stenosis severity, and the occurrence of significant rheologic vascular changes immediately following angioplasty (i.e., elastic recoil, remodeling, dynamic vasomotion, and so on), render the initial post-PTCA angiogram a procedurally important but prognostically and functionally limited study.

In the PTCA setting, stress myocardial perfusion imaging is of value for primary "culprit" lesion identification and documentation of myocardial viability before PTCA. As in other coronary artery disease subsets, perfusion imaging following PTCA has been useful for the prognostication of early restenosis and future ischemic cardiac events.

Current Indications (Table 22-1)

ASSESSMENT OF POSTSTENOTIC PERFUSIONAL IMPROVEMENT

After PTCA for medically unresponsive angina pectoris, stress imaging studies are performed to confirm that

Table 22-2 Stress Imaging After Coronary Bypass Grafting (CABG)

Indications
  Assessment of conduit patency and completeness of revascularization
    Direct: myocardial perfusion
      Target vascular beds
      Perioperative infarction
    Indirect: ventricular function improvement
      Regional wall motion
      Global ejection fraction
  Evaluation of recurrent angina (with or without abnormal rest ECG)
    Conduit failure (early and late)
    Incomplete revascularization (early)
    Comparison with early post-CABG baseline study (if available)
  Planning for repeat revascularization
    Limited jeopardy: PTCA or medical therapy
    Extensive jeopardy: repeat CABG
  Prediction of function improvement after revascularization
    Preoperative extent of ischemia
    Preoperative left ventricular function impairment
    Viability indices

Limitations
  Factors affecting left ventricular function improvement
    Post-CABG septal wall-motion abnormality
    Concomitant valvular disease on left ventricular function (i.e., mitral regurgitation)
    Negatively inotropic medications
  Factors reducing myocardial perfusion defect specificity
    Higher frequency of left bundle branch block
    Left ventricular dilation
    Postpericardiotomy syndromes (effusion/constriction)
  Postoperative debility limiting exercise performance (reduced sensitivity)
  Complexity of native and post-CABG anatomy (anatomic: perfusion correlates)
    Need for serial studies
    Vascular territory overlap
    Collateralization and backflow of occluded vessels
    Interval myocardial infarction (perioperatively or later)

ECG, electrocardiograph; PTCA, percutaneous transluminal coronary angioplasty.

procedural (i.e., angiographic) success has produced a concomitant improvement in poststenotic myocardial perfusion. This improvement in perfusion is frequently associated with improved exercise cardiac functional capacity.

DOCUMENTATION OF POSTINFARCTION MYOCARDIAL SALVAGE

Following infarct-related coronary artery angioplasty (either primary PTCA or as an adjunct to thrombolysis), perfusion imaging studies reflect myocardial *salvage* in the infarction zone. Improved thrombolysis in myocardial infarction grade flow and infarct zone reperfusion are covariables of subsequent regional wall-motion recovery and prognosis in this setting.

DETECTION AND PREDICTION OF CORONARY RESTENOSIS

Despite an angiographically optimal PTCA result, up to 45 percent of patients develop restenosis following their initial dilatation.[2] Myocardial perfusion imaging has been shown to predict whether beneficial early vascular "remodeling" or undesirable restenosis due to mechanical "recoil" or biologic intimal growth will occur.

EVALUATION OF RECURRENT CHEST PAIN SYNDROMES

Myocardial perfusion studies can confirm that recurrent chest pain is due to residual myocardial ischemia in the perfusion bed subtended by a restenotic vessel. In addition to detecting recurrent ischemia due to restenosis, myocardial perfusion data may also be useful in the evaluation of patients with defective anginal warning mechanisms or recurrent atypical chest pain.

Optimum Timing of Myocardial Perfusion Imaging After Percutaneous Transluminal Coronary Angioplasty

The optimal timing for postangioplasty stress testing and myocardial perfusion imaging has been controversial. Practical considerations (i.e., arteriotomy site discomfort and hemorrhagic potential following removal of sheaths) usually preclude maximal exercise stress imaging until more than 48 h after the index PTCA procedure. The application of postangioplasty stress perfusion imaging to predict restenosis varies from exercise or rapid-pacing studies 24 h or sooner after the intervention to more numerous studies performed 2 to 4 weeks later.

As such, the rate of "false-positive" perfusion defects that subsequently improve is highest in imaging studies done early (12 to 48 h) following PTCA.[3,4] While only 25 to 75 percent of myocardial perfusion zones with an early post-PTCA defect subsequently develop restenosis,[3,4] the negative predictive value of a normal study in this early time frame is much higher. The negative

predictive value of a normal early post-PTCA stress perfusion study is approximately 85 to 95 percent, while the positive predictive value of an abnormal scan is much lower (approximately 50 percent).

Abnormalities of coronary vessel tone and inadequate early vascular remodeling[5] can contribute to incomplete 3- to 4-h postexercise thallium redistribution, creating apparent fixed defects at 1 to 4 days after successful PTCA that subsequently improve with delayed imaging[6] or repeat studies in the ensuing weeks and months.[7,8] The differentiation of myocardial scarring from myocardial ischemia may be difficult early after the reestablishment of nutritive blood flow by PTCA. In general, most published studies indicate that a minimum of 2- to 4-week delay following angioplasty is required to determine the extent of recovery of nutritive myocardial perfusion and to distinguish reversible hypoperfusion from infarction in the PTCA zone.[9-13] This timing algorithm assumes that the post-PTCA perfusion study is being performed in an asymptomatic population as a mechanism to predict future restenosis, an indication that is not widely accepted in the current clinical management of PTCA patients.

The recurrence of angina after 1 month following PTCA is a strong correlate of restenosis, and patients with recurrent typical angina are frequently triaged directly to coronary angiography in lieu of myocardial perfusion imaging. In the patient population with recurrent atypical symptoms, stress perfusion imaging should be performed soon after the onset of symptoms in order to determine whether persistent myocardial ischemia is the cause of the chest pain. In patients with typical recurrent angina, in whom coronary angiography demonstrates intermediate stenosis severity, a functional study such as a stress myocardial perfusion scan can be valuable to determine the physiologic significance of the recurrent coronary stenosis early following cardiac catheterization. Because these recurrent symptoms generally appear sooner than 1 month following the PTCA procedure, the confounding effects of vessel remodeling and persistent myocardial hibernation on thallium uptake and clearance are generally less significant.[14,15]

In summary, a continuum of mildly to severely ischemic (but viable) to infarcted myocardial tissues exists distal to angioplasty sites. This produces marked differences in thallium-201 (^{201}Tl) clearance and can create the appearance of 3- to 4-h poststress "fixed" defects that can slowly improve weeks after reestablishment of blood flow by PTCA.

Radionuclide Imaging Comparisons with Routine Exercise Electrocardiographic Stress Testing

Exercise treadmill testing is a widely available and inexpensive noninvasive approach with proven diagnostic and prognostic value in populations with known or suspected coronary artery disease. Exercise treadmill testing was used to follow the original Gruentzig PTCA population of 169 patients, of whom 97 percent had abnormal results on exercise treadmill testing prior to their angioplasty procedure.[16] At 5 to 8 years of follow-up, only 10 percent of patients with successfully dilated arteries in this original series had abnormal results on exercise treadmill testing.[17] Ischemia during electrocardiographic (ECG) testing occurs at a significantly higher cardiac workload after successful PTCA compared with those patients with restenosis after 1 month following PTCA.[18] Patients with post-PTCA restenosis have significantly reduced exercise work capacities, angina, and ST-segment depression.[12,19] A strong association exists between clinical, scintigraphic, and exercise ECG data in the post-PTCA population.

Despite the widespread availability and relative technical ease of exercise treadmill testing, its sensitivity is suboptimal and its predictive value for ischemic events is low (13.6 percent) in asymptomatic patients compared with ^{201}Tl perfusion imaging.[20] Exercise treadmill testing may be cost-effective in patients with single-vessel left anterior descending PTCA and a normal resting ECG, whereas other asymptomatic patients are optimally studied with exercise myocardial perfusion imaging.

Functional and Perfusional Correlates of Postangioplasty Outcome

Several studies have demonstrated variable improvement in exercise ECG and rest–stress scintigraphic abnormalities after successful coronary angioplasty.[21,22] Pre-PTCA agreement between exercise ECG and ^{201}Tl data is improved after PTCA (Kappa = 0.45).

In patients undergoing rest–exercise radionuclide ventriculography, 52 percent still had abnormal results after PTCA, raising the possibility of subclinical residual ischemia or false-positive radionuclide ventriculographic findings in these patients.[22]

Peak exercise workload, heart rate, and systolic blood pressure increase significantly in patients at 1 week after successful single-vessel left anterior descending PTCA,[21] in association with significant improvements in ^{201}Tl uptake and redistribution kinetics, exercise ECG ST-segment abnormalities, decreased ^{201}Tl lung uptake, and exercise radionuclide ventriculographic regional and global ventricular function improvements.[22]

The prognostic advantages of perfusion imaging over exercise treadmill testing have been noted in several studies,[12,23] in which the sensitivity of exercise treadmill testing for restenosis detection averages 40 to 59 percent as compared with 67 to 96 percent with perfusion imaging. The positive predictive values of abnormal results on

4-week symptom-limited exercise treadmill testing for recurrent angina and restenosis (greater than 50 percent luminal diameter reduction) at 6 months after PTCA were 60 and 50 percent, respectively,[11] as compared with 82 and 74 percent for exercise ^{201}Tl defect redistribution in the same patients.

The relatively low sensitivity and predictive value of recurrent chest pain alone[23] or of exercise treadmill testing data for recurrent ischemia following angioplasty suggest that 4-week post-PTCA stress perfusion imaging detects restenosis in more patients destined for this adverse outcome. Routine exercise ECG testing may suffice to screen patients with single-vessel left anterior descending disease and a normal resting ECG, but functional perfusion studies are required to define future risk and offer several proven advantages in multivessel coronary artery disease patients with resting ECG abnormalities.

Prognostication by Postangioplasty Perfusion Imaging

Despite numerous studies detailing the clinical and angiographic natural history of postangioplasty restenosis, the prediction of this phenomenon based on clinical and procedural parameters remains limited. Noninvasive imaging has proven to be a useful adjunct for the prediction of restenosis following PTCA. The high restenosis rate indicates that the PTCA population is an intermediate-risk population in which nuclear studies have been demonstrated to perform optimally. Abnormal findings on post-PTCA cardiac imaging, particularly in association with recurrent symptoms suggestive of myocardial ischemia, can indicate hemodynamically significant restenosis at the index angioplasty site. Conversely, normal maximal stress imaging findings have an excellent negative predictive value for excluding restenosis, regardless of patient symptomatology. Unfortunately, most studies evaluating the prognostic value of post-PTCA perfusion imaging have been performed in relatively small numbers of patients. However, the cumulative weight of these data is significant and clearly demonstrates the incremental value of post-PTCA stress perfusion imaging for predicting restenosis over clinical and postprocedural angiographic parameters alone.

For example, exercise-induced abnormalities of regional myocardial thallium clearance and the presence of post-PTCA redistribution thallium defects are highly predictive of restenosis within 6 months following PTCA.[10] These findings are correlated with postangioplasty evidence of abnormal stenosis rheology (elevated translesional pressure gradient) that identifies patients at significantly greater risk for future ischemic cardiac events and angiographic restenosis. A similar relationship between thallium imaging, coronary rheology, and exercise left ventricular function has also been demonstrated.[24] As such, the analysis of thallium-washout kinetics on planar imaging studies may identify patients at a greater future risk for restenosis.[21,25] This may represent a relative advantage of the planar technique over tomographic myocardial imaging, which itself is better for the localization of multivessel disease and culprit-vessel identification.[26]

Several studies have demonstrated a high positive predictive value for restenosis in association with exercise-induced or drug-induced stress perfusion defects.[9,27–30] The positive predictive value of a 4-week postangioplasty perfusion defect for 6-month restenosis ranges from 77 to 86 percent. Chest pain alone carries a positive predictive value of 70 percent, which is incremented to 86 percent in association with ischemic ST changes and 93 percent in association with thallium defect reversibility.[9] By contrast, the negative predictive value of a normal thallium scan for restenosis is high (93 percent). In asymptomatic patients studied at 2 weeks following PTCA, the positive predictive value and negative predictive value of an exercise thallium stress study are generally lower (69 percent and 75 percent, respectively[28]).

Pharmacologic stress is a valuable alternative to exercise stress in patients with physical or psychologic limitations to exercise. The administration of dipyridamole may demonstrate abnormalities of coronary flow reserve early following successful PTCA[29,30] As is the case with exercise stress following PTCA, coronary vasodilator stress imaging studies should be delayed for approximately 2 to 4 weeks following PTCA, at which time their predictive value for restenosis approaches that of maximal exercise stress imaging studies.

Summary: Percutaneous Transluminal Coronary Angioplasty

In patients with a good angioplasty result, as judged by postprocedural angiography, there is no need for routine post-PTCA stress cardiac imaging studies. These studies are indicated if recurrent symptoms consistent with angina occur, and are particularly useful if the symptomatology is not typical of angina pectoris. Patients with typical angina should be referred for coronary angiography. Patients with less typical symptoms and intermediate probability of restenosis can be accurately assessed for this PTCA complication by myocardial perfusion imaging studies. Maximal stress imaging studies have a high positive predictive value for restenosis and excellent negative predictive value, particularly when they are delayed for a minimum of 2 to 4 weeks following the index PTCA procedure. Myocardial imaging studies offer several advantages over stress ECG, particularly in patients with abnormalities of the resting ECG, multivessel coronary disease, or a limitation to exercise stress testing. The exercise stress test may be of some value for screening of patients with good exercise tolerance, left anterior descending PTCA, and a normal resting ECG. Routine use of post-PTCA myocardial perfusion imaging following angiographically successful procedures is not feasible, nor cost-efficient, outside of the setting of clinical investigation. Patients with suboptimal angioplasty results should undergo early post-PTCA stress perfusion imaging studies to determine whether desirable remodeling or restenosis has occurred following the index revascularization procedure.

CORONARY ARTERY BYPASS GRAFT SURGERY

Indications (Table 22-2)

The most common causes of recurrent angina following CABG surgery are incomplete revascularization and conduit closure. The natural history of conduit survival has been defined for saphaneous vein grafts and internal mammary arteries. It is well recognized that perioperative myocardial infarction and subsequent conduit closure may be clinically silent events, and that stress perfusion imaging studies provide important information about the functional impact of bypass graft stenoses that may not be available based on a clinical or angiographic assessment alone.

Nuclear cardiac imaging studies are not generally recommended in the absence of recurrent symptoms, particularly since imaging abnormalities would not likely result in a change in therapy or repeat revascularization (unless the zone of myocardial jeopardy was large). During prolonged follow-up (more than 5 years), a noninvasive assessment of conduit patency may be more useful in view of the high rate of attrition at this time point (greater than 50 percent for saphenous vein grafts). In this setting, exercise thallium SPECT (single photon emission computed tomography) imaging has been demonstrated to predict the 1-year cardiac event-free survival following CABG surgery.[31]

Prior to this time point, the lower rate of graft stenosis does not argue for the performance of routine noninvasive testing in asymptomatic patients.[32–35] The high incidence of chronic myocardial hibernation in the CABG population also argues against the routine use of early (less than 3-month) postoperative myocardial perfusion or ventricular function assessment. These parameters might take several months to normalize after revascularization, and abnormalities of noninvasive imaging studies may not truly reflect the status of the conduit in this time frame.

Several studies have demonstrated significant improvements in myocardial perfusion following revascularization by coronary bypass surgery. Early postoperative studies may demonstrate improvements when compared with preoperative studies, although the impact of myocardial hibernation on perfusion and functional recovery should not be underestimated in the first 3 months following CABG surgery. Early (less than 3-month) post-CABG myocardial imaging may be useful for the detection of perioperative infarction or if early graft closure with recurrence of angina symptoms is suspected.

Beyond 3 months, and following the recovery of hibernation effects, noninvasive cardiac imaging is useful to detect asymptomatic graft attrition and the recurrence of myocardial ischemia. However, this approach cannot be routinely recommended in all post-CABG patients because it would not be cost-effective to screen this large population in the 1 to 2 years following CABG surgery. If an early postoperative study is performed following the recovery from myocardial hibernation effects, this can be used as a baseline for future assessments of functional capacity and myocardial ischemia and may be particularly useful if angina recurs. Any significant perfusion abnormality on an early postoperative study would be an indication for more frequent follow-up studies and would lower the threshold for coronary angiography, particularly if ischemic symptoms recurred. Serial studies in such patients would also enable the future identification of newly ischemic myocardial zones suggestive of progressive coronary disease in the ungrafted native circulation.

Comparison of Radionuclide Imaging with Exercise Stress Testing

A comparison of precoronary and postcoronary bypass surgery ECG exercise treadmill testing usually demonstrates a concomitant improvement in functional capacity and reduced exercise-induced ischemia. Preoperative impairment in the exercise heart rate response is improved following bypass surgery, leading to improved cardiac output and myocardial oxygen extraction, while reducing ischemic symptoms and ST-segment depression.[36]

Exercise ECG and radionuclide imaging variables indicative of high-risk coronary artery disease have been derived from patients *without* previous coronary artery bypass surgery (Table 22-3). The recurrence of these high-risk markers following bypass surgery indicates continued or recurrent evidence of significant ischemia. As with perfusion studies, comparison of a late postoperative stress ECG study with an immediate postoperative stress ECG study will be valuable to determine whether a serial change has occurred. These serial changes are

Table 22-3 Exercise Electrocardiographic (ECG) Stress Test and Radionuclide Variables Indicative of High-Risk Coronary Artery Disease

Exercise ECG stress test
    Failure to achieve 4 or more metabolic equivalents
    Low exercise heart rate off beta blockers
    Abnormal or inadequate blood pressure response
    ST depression of 2.0 mm or more
    ST depression of 1.0 mm or more at low exercise workloads
    ST depression persisting for 5 min or longer after recovery

Myocardial perfusion imaging
    Left main thallium scan pattern (see Chap. 2)
    Multiple thallium defects in more than one coronary supply region
    Thallium-201 redistribution at low heart rate or workload
    Abnormal lung thallium uptake
    Exercise left ventricular cavity dilation
    Thallium redistribution in zone of recent infarction

Exercise radionuclide angiography
    Exercise left ventricular ejection fraction less than 50 percent
    Decreased in left ventricular ejection fraction by 10 percent or more
    Exercise-induced multiple wall-motion abnormalities

generally associated with recurrent exertional angina pectoris. Thallium-201 imaging is generally more useful than the exercise ECG in patients who demonstrate significant ST-T-wave changes caused by drugs (e.g., digitalis) or conduction abnormalities (e.g., left bundle branch block) following bypass surgery. In addition, stress imaging findings objectify identification of myocardial ischemia and reflect the extent of jeopardized and dysfunctional myocardium following bypass surgery in a manner that stress ECG studies cannot.

Myocardial Perfusion Imaging

Although numerous studies have been performed, the practical clinical role for exercise radionuclide perfusion imaging following CABG surgery remains poorly defined. Institutional data suggest that there may be utility for serial assessment of myocardial perfusion, even in asymptomatic patients, when graft attrition rates rise at more than 5 years following the index procedure.

Serial stress myocardial imaging studies (before and after CABG) have clearly demonstrated improved myocardial perfusion in a high percentage of preoperative perfusion defects.[37-41] More than 90 percent of totally redistributing (i.e., ischemic) myocardial segments become normal postoperatively, while the percentage of segments with partial redistribution or a relatively fixed appearance preoperatively that demonstrate improvement following CABG is lower (50 to 75 percent). The degree of regional wall-motion improvement in corresponding segments is correlated with the pre- to postoperative improvement in myocardial perfusion in the same segments.

Table 22-4   Factors Affecting Improvement in Left Ventricular Function After Coronary Revascularization

Presence and degree of preoperative myocardial hibernation or stunning

Coronary anatomy

Complete revascularization

Presence and degree of perioperative necrosis

Graft patency

Reliable method to detect improvement

Left ventricle size

Presence of concomitant primary cardiomyopathy

Studies evaluating pre- to postoperative improvements in regional myocardial perfusion have been generally performed at 4 to 8 weeks postoperatively, in part to improve exercise performance and to reduce the likelihood of residual chronic myocardial hibernation effects on the postoperative recovery. The factors potentially influencing the degree of recovery are summarized in Table 22-4. One or more of these factors may be operative in any patient. However, the reversibility of postoperative perfusion defects is generally correlated with the degree of improvement in nutritive myocardial blood flow and the restoration of normal myocyte metabolism. Both of these factors are strongly correlated with subsequent improvements in regional wall motion.[40] While planar imaging is of limited value for the localization of graft stenoses, tomographic imaging can be very useful in this regard.[41]

As is the case following PTCA, the recurrence of typical angina is generally an indication for coronary angiography, while the recurrence of atypical chest pain or a change in chest pain pattern may be an indication for noninvasive stress cardiac imaging. The presence of a normal stress myocardial perfusion study in a patient with atypical chest pain is correlated with a low likelihood of significant graft stenosis and a good short-term cardiac event-free survival. The likelihood of a significant graft occlusion in a patient without a new perfusion defect and no chest pain is less than 5 percent. Even in the presence of atypical chest pain, the likelihood of significant graft occlusion without a new perfusion defect is less than 10 percent. As such, the negative predictive value of a normal post-CABG study for significant graft occlusion is high (greater than 90 percent).

Ventricular Functional Improvement

During the interval between the initial bypass and reoperation, approximately one-third of patients suffer a decrease in resting left ventricular function (i.e., ejection fraction) in association with progressive age

or coronary artery disease or with the onset of microvascular disease. The presence of a new exercise-induced transient regional wall-motion abnormality in a zone perfused by a bypass graft frequently reflects graft stenosis or occlusion. Resting wall motion alone is not generally predictive of graft patency status. The presence of new exercise-induced global or regional ventricular dysfunction in a patient with recurrent angina following bypass surgery is strongly suggestive of myocardial ischemia.

Previous studies have demonstrated a variable effect of revascularization on resting left ventricular function, with the greatest improvement observed in patients with preoperative unstable angina. There may be no significant postoperative improvement in global left ventricular ejection fraction following limited revascularization (single- or double-vessel bypass). However, more complete revascularization usually improves both rest and exercise ejection fractions, in addition to improving regional wall motion. Following successful coronary bypass surgery, an abnormal exercise ejection-fraction response (any decrease or failure to rise of more than 5 percent) is also often reversed[42] in association with the disappearance of exercise-related ischemia and exercise-induced regional wall-motion abnormalities.[43] This global ejection-fraction improvement is greater in patients with normal perfusion scans or with a reversible defect and is less common in patients with a fixed defect.

The degree of improvement in ventricular function after bypass surgery depends on the extent of prerevascularization ischemia and myocardial fibrosis and the completeness of surgical revascularization. The resting left ventricular ejection fraction is unlikely to improve in a patient with normal resting left ventricular function preoperatively or with inadequate revascularization. Conversely, patients who have decreased resting left ventricular function, scintigraphic evidence of viable myocardium, and a technically satisfactory revascularization frequently have an improvement in resting left ventricular ejection fraction postoperatively.[38] However, in patients with depressed left ventricular ejection fraction due to scarring (without evidence of viability), functional improvement should not be anticipated following surgery. Functional abnormalities (global or regional) usually persist, even after complete revascularization, in akinetic segments without evidence of viability on reinjection or late thallium redistribution studies.[40]

While coronary bypass surgery patients with chronic stable angina frequently demonstrate no improvement in rest ejection fraction, exercise ejection fraction often improves in association with a higher maximum workload and rate–pressure product.[44] This increase in exercise ejection fraction following bypass surgery is principally the result of decreased exercise end-systolic volumes. Patients with severe preoperative exercise-induced ischemia (greater than 2-mm ST-segment depression) have the greatest postoperative improvement in ventricular function.

In summary, only the improvement in nutritive blood flow associated with coronary revascularization can reproducibly improve left ventricular function in chronically ischemic (hibernating) myocardium. Perfusion defects noted in the immediate postoperative period may be associated with dysfunctional areas of myocardial stunning or hibernation that can require up to 6 months to reverse.[45] Patients with a reduced exercise left ventricular ejection fraction preoperatively demonstrated improved survival with successful revascularization. Conversely, patients with a normal exercise left ventricular ejection fraction regardless of coronary anatomy were not found to have improved survival.[46]

Summary: Coronary Artery Bypass Graft Surgery

Numerous studies have demonstrated that postoperative myocardial perfusion imaging is useful to assess the functional status of bypass grafts.[47-50] The majority of preoperative ischemic perfusion defects are associated with preserved resting wall motion, and subsequent improvement in both myocardial perfusion and recruitable ventricular function can be expected postoperatively. However, without a baseline study, either preoperatively or in the immediate postoperative state, subsequent observations lose their predictive accuracy for the detection and localization of graft stenoses.

Radionuclide imaging abnormalities may precede the development of angina by several months and may be the only clues to conduit occlusion in patients with silent ischemia. Stress imaging may distinguish patients with noncoronary chest pain from those with significant myocardial ischemia. Regardless of symptoms, normal results on a post-CABG stress perfusion scan essentially exclude significant graft stenosis. Patients with patent bypass grafts who have not suffered an intraoperative myocardial infarction should eventually normalize their regional perfusion and function following surgery.

While most data on the perfusion correlates of bypass grafting have been accrued from exercise stress studies, the choice of stress modality in this population (exercise versus pharmacologic) must be individually assessed in view of the patient's ability to exercise adequately. A maximal pharmacologic stress test can be useful to assess perfusional improvement following bypass graft surgery but lacks information on the cardiac functional capacity that is provided by exercise stress.

ROLE OF POSITRON EMISSION TOMOGRAPHY

Metabolic imaging using positron emission tomography (PET) can distinguish hypoperfused but viable myocar-

dium from infarcted tissue. The discordance between increased fluorodeoxyglucose (FDG) and decreased nitrogen-13–ammonia uptake, which reflects a change to increased anaerobic glycolysis in the ischemic zone, can be used preoperatively to predict recovery of function following myocardial revascularization procedures.[51] Return of segmental myocardial perfusion and FDG activity to normal following bypass surgery is a reliable sign of successful revascularization of hibernating myocardium.[52]

Preoperative and postoperative PET imaging may be useful for noninvasively serially following the myocardial metabolic response to coronary revascularization. The relationship of metabolic activity to prognosis and functional recovery has been assessed.[53] The expense and technical complexity of PET imaging has limited the widespread applicability of this technique. Less expensive and more widely applicable single-photon perfusion imaging, with ^{201}Tl reinjection or late (24-h) studies to determine viability, may provide a more practical, albeit less sensitive, alternative to PET imaging in this setting. Newer metabolic imaging techniques such as PET and single-photon myocardial tomography with iodine-123-labeled fatty-acid analysis remain promising but are less well validated for the evaluation of unselected patient populations who have recurrent angina following revascularization surgery.[39,54]

REFERENCES

1. Berman DS, Kiat H, Friedman JD, Diamond G: Clinical applications of exercise nuclear cardiology studies in the era of healthcare reform. *Am J Cardiol* 75:3D, 1995.
2. Nobuyoshi N, Kimura T, Ohishi H, et al: Restenosis after PTCA: Pathologic observation in 20 patients. *J Am Coll Cardiol* 17:433, 1991.
3. Powelson SW, DePuey EG, Roubin GS, et al: Discordance of coronary angiography and 201-thallium tomography early after transluminal coronary angioplasty. *J Nucl Med* 27:900, 1986.
4. Hardoff R, Shefer A, Gips S, et al: Predicting late restenosis after coronary angioplasty by very early (12 to 24 h) thallium-201 scintigraphy: Implications with regard to mechanisms of late coronary restenosis. *J Am Coll Cardiol* 15:1486, 1990.
5. Bates ER, McGillem MJ, Beals TF, et al: Effect of angioplasty-induced endothelial denudation compared with medial injury on regional coronary blood flow. *Circulation* 76:710, 1987.
6. Cloninger KG, DePuey EG, Garcia EV, et al: Incomplete redistribution in delayed thallium-201 single photon emission computed tomographic (SPECT) images: An overestimation of myocardial scarring. *J Am Coll Cardiol* 12:955, 1988.
7. Liu P, Kiess MC, Okada RD, et al: The persistent detection on exercise thallium imaging and its fate after myocardial

revascularization: Does it represent scar or ischemia? *Am Heart J* 110:996, 1985.

8. Manyari DE, Knudtson M, Kloiber R, Roth D: Sequential thallium-201 myocardial perfusion studies after successful percutaneous transluminal coronary artery angioplasty: Delayed resolution of exercise-induced scintigraphic abnormalities. *Circulation* 77:86, 1988.

9. Breisblatt WM, Weiland FL, Spaccavento LJ: Stress thallium-201 imaging after coronary angioplasty predicts restenosis and recurrent symptoms. *J Am Coll Cardiol* 12:1199, 1988.

10. Miller DD, Liu P, Strauss HW, et al: Prognostic value of computer-quantitated exercise thallium imaging early after percutaneous transluminal coronary angioplasty. *J Am Coll Cardiol* 10:275, 1987.

11. Wijns W, Serruys PW, Reiber JHC, et al: Early detection of restenosis after successful percutaneous transluminal coronary angioplasty by exercise-redistribution thallium scintigraphy. *Am J Cardiol* 55:357, 1985.

12. Scholl JM, Chaitman BR, David PR, et al: Exercise electrocardiography and myocardial scintigraphy in the serial evaluation of the results of percutaneous transluminal coronary angioplasty. *Circulation* 66:380, 1982.

13. Hirzel HO, Gruentzig A, Neusch K, et al: Thallium-201 imaging for the evaluation of myocardial perfusion after percutaneous transluminal angioplasty of coronary artery stenosis. *Circulation* 57 and 58(suppl II):II-180, 1978.

14. Nienaber CA, Brunken RC, Sherman CT, et al: Metabolic and functional recovery of ischemic human myocardium after coronary angioplasty. *J Am Coll Cardiol* 18:966, 1991.

15. Cohen M, Charney R, Hershman R, et al: Reversal of chronic ischemic myocardial dysfunction after transluminal coronary angioplasty. *J Am Coll Cardiol* 12:1193, 1988.

16. Meier B, Gruentzig AR, Siegenthaler WE, Schlumpf M: Long-term exercise performance after percutaneous transluminal coronary angioplasty and coronary artery bypass grafting. *Circulation* 68:796, 1983.

17. Gruentzig AR, King SB, Schlumpf M, Siegenthaler W: Long-term follow-up after percutaneous transluminal coronary angioplasty. *N Engl J Med* 316:1127, 1987.

18. El-Tamimi H, Davies GJ, Hackett D, et al: Very early prediction of restenosis after successful coronary angioplasty: Anatomic and functional assessment. *J Am Coll Cardiol* 15:259, 1990.

19. DePuey G, Leatherman LL, Leachman RD, et al: Restenosis after transluminal coronary angioplasty detected with exercise-gated radionuclide ventriculography. *J Am Coll Cardiol* 4:1103, 1984.

20. Ellestad MH, Cooke BM Jr, Greenberg PS: Stress testing: Clinical application and predictive capacity. *Prog Cardiovasc Dis* 21:431, 1979.

21. Okada RD, Lim YL, Boucher CA, et al: Clinical, angiographic, hemodynamic, perfusional and function changes after one-vessel left anterior descending coronary angioplasty. *Am J Cardiol* 55:347, 1985.

22. Rosing DR, Van Raden MJ, Mincemoyer RM, et al: Exercise, electrocardiographic and function responses after percutaneous transluminal coronary angioplasty. *Am J Cardiol* 53:36C, 1984.

23. Hecht HS, Shaw RS, Chin HL, et al: Silent ischemia after coronary angioplasty: Evaluation of restenosis and extent of ischemia in asymptomatic patients by tomographic thallium-201 exercise imaging and comparison with symptomatic patients. *J Am Coll Cardiol* 17:670, 1991.

24. Legrand V, Aueron FM, Bates ER, et al: Value of exercise radionuclide ventriculography and thallium-201 scintigraphy in evaluated successful coronary angioplasty: Comparison with coronary flow reserve, translesional gradient and percent diameter stenosis. *Eur Heart J* 8:329, 1987.

25. Verani MS, Tadros S, Raizner AE, et al: Quantitative analysis of thallium-201 uptake and washout before and after transluminal coronary angioplasty. *Int J Cardiol* 13:109, 1986.

26. Breisblatt WM, Barnes JV, Weiland F, Spaccavento LJ: Incomplete revascularization in multivessel percutaneous transluminal coronary angioplasty: The role of stress thallium-201 imaging. *J Am Coll Cardiol* 11:1183, 1988.

27. Wijns W, Serruys PW, Simoons ML, et al: Predictive value of early maximal exercise test in thallium scintigraphy after successful percutaneous transluminal coronary angioplasty. *Br Heart J* 53:194, 1985.

28. Stuckey TD, Burwell LR, Nygaard TW, et al: Quantitative exercise thallium-201 scintigraphy for predicting angina recurrence after percutaneous transluminal coronary angioplasty. *Am J Cardiol* 63:517, 1989.

29. Jain A, Mahmarian JJ, Borges-Neto S, et al: Clinical significance of perfusion defects by thallium-201 single photon emission tomography following oral dipyridamole early after coronary angioplasty. *J Am Coll Cardiol* 11:970, 1988.

30. LeGrand V, Aueron FM, Bates ER, et al: Significance of radionuclide stress tests in patients undergoing a successful coronary angioplasty. *Circulation* 70(suppl II):II-298, 1984.

31. Palmas W, Bingham S, Diamond GA, et al: Incremental prognostic value of exercise thallium-201 myocardial single-photon emission computed tomography late after coronary artery bypass surgery. *J Am Coll Cardiol* 25:403, 1995.

32. Weisz D, Hamby RI, Aintablian A, et al: Late coronary bypass graft flow: Quantitative assessment by roentgendensitometry. *Ann Thorac Surg* 28:429, 1979.

33. Stinson EB, Olinger GN, Glancy DL: Anatomical and physiological determinants of blood flow through aortocoronary vein bypass grafts. *Surgery* 74:390, 1979.

34. Bittar N, Kroncke GM, Dacumos GC: Vein graft flow and reactive hyperemia in the human heart. *J Thorac Cardiovasc Surg* 64:855, 1972.

35. Greenfield JC, Rembert JC, Young WG: Studies of blood flow in aorta-to-coronary venous bypass grafts in man. *J Clin Invest* 51:2724, 1972.

36. Hossack KF, Bruce RA, Ivey TD: Changes in cardiac functional capacity after coronary bypass surgery in relation to adequacy of revascularization. *J Am Coll Cardiol* 3:47, 1984.

37. Kiat H, Berman DS, Maddahi J, et al: Late reversibility of tomographic myocardial thallium-201 defects: An accurate marker of myocardial viability. *J Am. Coll Cardiol* 12:1456, 1988.

38. Gibson RS, Watson DD, Taylor GJ, et al: Prospective

assessment of regional myocardial perfusion before and after coronary revascularization surgery by quantitative thallium-201 scintigraphy. *J Am Coll Cardiol* 1:804, 1983.

39. Iskandrian AS, Heo J, Stanberry C: When is myocardial viability an important clinical issue? *J Nucl Med* 35(suppl I):45, 1994.

40. Brundage BH, Bassie BM, Botvinick EH: Improved regional ventricular function after successful surgical revascularization. *J Am Coll Cardiol* 3:902, 1984.

41. Pfisterer M, Emmenegger H, Schmitt HE, et al: Accuracy of serial myocardial perfusion scintigraphy with thallium-201 for prediction of graft patency early and late after coronary artery bypass surgery. *Circulation* 66:1017, 1982.

42. Kent KM, Borer JS, Green MV: Effects of coronary artery bypass on global and regional left ventricular function during exercise. *N Engl J Med* 298:1434, 1978.

43. Iskandrian AS, Hakki AH, Kane SA, et al: Rest and redistribution thallium-201 myocardial scintigraphy to predict improvement in LV function after coronary arterial bypass grafting. *Am J Cardiol* 51:1312, 1983.

44. Lim LY, Kalff V, Kelly MJ: Radionuclide angiographic assessment of global and sequential left ventricular function at rest and during exercise after coronary artery bypass surgery. *Circulation* 66:972, 1982.

45. Cohen M, Charney R, Hershman R: Reversal of chronic ischemic myocardial dysfunction after transluminal coronary angioplasty. *J Am Coll Cardiol* 12:1193, 1988.

46. Jones RH, Floyd RD, Austin EH, Sabiston DC: The role of radionuclide angiocardiography in the preoperative prediction of pain relief and prolonged survival following coronary artery bypass grafting. *Ann Surg* 197:743, 1983.

47. Ritchie JL, Narahara KA, Trobaugh JB, et al: Thallium-201 myocardial imaging before and after coronary revascularization: Assessment of regional myocardial blood flow and graft patency. *Circulation* 56:830, 1977.

48. Verani MS, Marcus ML, Spoto G, et al: Thallium-201 myocardial perfusion scintigrams in the evaluation of aorto-coronary saphenous bypass surgery. *J Nucl Med* 19:765, 1978.

49. Sbarbaro JA, Karunarantne H, Cantez S, et al: Thallium-201 imaging and assessment of aorto-coronary artery bypass graft patency. *Br Heart J* 42:553, 1979.

50. Hirzel HO, Nuesch K, Siale RG, et al: Thallium-201 exercise myocardial imaging to evaluate myocardial perfusion after coronary bypass surgery. *Br Heart J* 43:426, 1980.

51. Brunken R, Schwaiger M, Grover-McKay M, et al: Positron emission tomography detects tissue metabolic activity in myocardial segments with persistent thallium perfusion defects. *J Am Coll Cardiol* 10:557, 1987.

52. Tamaki N, Yonekura Y, Yamashita K, et al: Positron emission tomography using fluorine-18 deoxyglucose in evaluation of coronary artery bypass grafting. *Am J Cardiol* 64:860, 1989.

53. DiCarli M, Davidson M, Little R, et al: Value of metabolic imaging with PET for evaluating prognosis in patients with coronary artery disease and left ventricular dysfunction. *Am J Cardiol* 73:527, 1994.

54. Hansen CL: Preliminary report of an ongoing phase I/II dose range, safety and efficacy study of iodine-123–phenylpentadecanoic acid for the identification of viable myocardium. *J Nucl Med* 35(suppl 4):38S, 1994.

Prognostic Value of Nuclear Cardiology Techniques

Kenneth A. Brown

As the expense of interventional technologic advances in cardiology continues to grow in an environment of contracting resources available for health care, the need to identify which patients can best benefit from such expensive procedures has never been greater. In this setting, the now well established prognostic power of nuclear cardiology techniques has become a valuable adjunct to clinical decision making by allowing the clinician to distinguish patients at high risk for future cardiac events who may benefit from further interventions from those at low risk who are unlikely to benefit.

MYOCARDIAL PERFUSION IMAGING

The powerful prognostic value of myocardial perfusion imaging appears to be related to its unique ability to identify the presence and extent of jeopardized viable myocardium and has been shown to be applicable to a wide spectrum of patients with coronary artery disease.[2]

PATIENTS PRESENTING WITH KNOWN OR SUSPECTED CORONARY ARTERY DISEASE

The relationship between the presence and extent of jeopardized viable myocardium determined from myo-

cardial perfusion imaging and the risk of future cardiac events was first reported by Brown and colleagues in 1983.[1] In a series of 100 patients without known prior myocardial infarction who presented for evaluation of chest pain, the predictive value of exercise thallium-201 imaging results was compared with clinical, exercise electrocardiographic, and angiographic data using a multivariate approach. The best predictor of subsequent cardiac death or myocardial infarction was the extent of jeopardized viable myocardium reflected in the number of myocardial segments with transient ^{201}Tl defects (Fig. 23-1). Although the number of coronary vessels with angiographic disease was a significant univariate predictor of cardiac events, angiographic data added no significant prognostic value to the myocardial perfusion imaging data. Thus it appeared that noninvasive functional data had at least as good prognostic value for identifying patients at risk for future cardiac events as invasive, anatomic data.

These initial observations have subsequently been confirmed and extended by many other investigators. Ladenheim and colleagues found that among clinical and scintigraphic variables the number of reversible ^{201}Tl defects was the best predictor of future cardiac events in a large series of patients presenting with suspected but not documented coronary disease (Fig. 23-2).[3] Similarly, Staniloff et al showed that patients having any or multiple transient defects had a 6- to 12-fold increased risk of cardiac death by myocardial infarction compared to patients with normal ^{201}Tl studies.[4] A series of studies by Iskandrian and colleagues demonstrated that the pres-

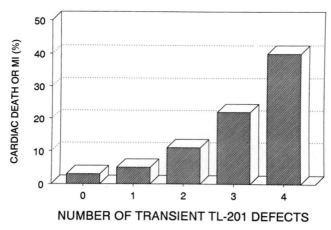

Figure 23-1 Risk of cardiac death or nonfatal myocardial infarction (MI) as a function of the number of myocardial segments with transient ^{201}Tl defects. Risk of cardiac events increases as the extent of jeopardized viable myocardium (reflected in the number of transient ^{201}Tl defects) increases. (Adapted from Brown et al,[1] reproduced with permission from the American College of Cardiology, Journal of the American College of Cardiology, 1:994, 1983.)

ence and extent of perfusion defects (transient or fixed) were the only significant predictors of cardiac events when compared to clinical and exercise electrocardiographic data, although the prognostic value of transient defects alone was not described.[5-7] However, more recently these investigators reported that the presence of reversible ^{201}Tl defects, multivessel territory perfusion abnormalities, and extensive perfusion abnormalities each has significant univariate predictive value for cardiac death or nonfatal myocardial infarction.[8]

Two large long-term follow-up studies have compared exercise ^{201}Tl imaging data to electrocardiographic, cardiac catheterization, and clinical data.[9,10]

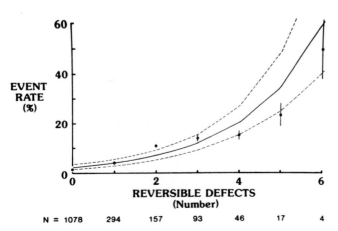

Figure 23-2 Risk of future cardiac events plotted as a function of the number of reversible ^{201}Tl defects. The relationship is exponential (R = 0.99, p < 0.001). (Reprinted from Ladenheim et al[3] with permission of the American College of Cardiology.)

Kaul and colleagues found that among all variables examined, increased ^{201}Tl lung uptake was the best predictor of cardiac events, although the number of angiographically diseased vessels and the presence of transient defects had significant multivariate predictive value when lung uptake was not considered.[9] Importantly, consistent with prior studies, the overall predictive value of ^{201}Tl data was significantly superior to angiographic and exercise electrocardiographic data. In a separate investigation at a different institution, Kaul et al found that although the number of diseased anigiographic vessels was the best predictor of cardiac events, the extent of jeopardized viable myocardium reflected in the number of transient perfusion defects added significant prognostic value.[10] The authors concluded that both overall exercise ^{201}Tl test data (including the number of transient defects, ST-segment depression, change in heart rate during exercise, and exercise-induced ventricular ectopy) and catheterization data were highly significant predictors of cardiac events ($p < 0.0001$) and were equal in predictive value. Importantly, each was significantly superior to exercise electrocardiographic data alone.

Scintigraphic Indices of Left Ventricular Dysfunction

Increased lung uptake on exercise ^{201}Tl imaging has been shown to reflect exercise-induced left ventricular dysfunction, resting left ventricular dysfunction, and extensive angiographic coronary disease.[11-16] It is therefore not surprising that increased ^{201}Tl lung uptake has been associated with an adverse prognosis. As described previously, Kaul et al found that increased ^{201}Tl lung uptake was the overall best predictor of cardiac events.[9] In addition, Gill and colleagues found that increased lung uptake of ^{201}Tl on exercise studies was the best predictor of cardiac events in a series of patients with suspected coronary artery disease.[17] Although the presence and extent of transient defects was also a powerful univariate predictor of cardiac events, these variables did not add any prognostic value to increased lung uptake of ^{201}Tl in this study.[17]

Left ventricular dilatation can also be determined from myocardial perfusion imaging studies and has been shown to be a marker of extensive coronary artery disease and left ventricular dysfunction.[18,19] Recently, Krawczynska and colleagues reported the outcome of a series of 291 patients with large perfusion defects in the left anterior descending coronary territory as a function of the presence or absence of left ventricular dilatation.[20] They found that patients with significant left ventricular dilatation on stress images had a reduced 3-y survival compared to patients with nondilated left ventricles.[20] Similarly, Lette and colleagues found transient left ventricular dilation during dipyridamole infusion to be associated with a high risk of perioperative or long-term

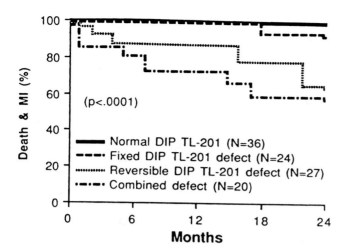

Figure 23-3 Actuarial survival free of myocardial infarction in 107 asymptomatic patients with coronary artery disease stratified by intravenous dipyridamole (DIP) ^{201}Tl imaging results. Reversible defect or combined reversible plus fixed defect significantly increased the risk of death or infarction (p < 0.0001). (Reprinted from Younis et al[23] with permission of the American College of Cardiology.)

cardiac events.[21] An association between extensive coronary artery disease and transient, exercise-induced left ventricular dilatation seen on stress myocardial perfusion imaging compared to rest images has also been described.[22] However, although it is reasonable to infer that such a marker of extensive underlying coronary disease would have significant adverse prognostic implications, no confirmatory data currently exist.

Pharmacological Stress Imaging

(For additional discussion, see Chap. 6)
Thallium-201 imaging performed in conjunction with dipyridamole-induced coronary hyperemia also has important prognostic value.[23–25] In a series of asymptomatic patients with documented angiographic coronary disease,[23] reversible defects on dipyridamole ^{201}Tl imaging studies were found to be the only significant predictors of cardiac events when compared with angiographic and clinical variables (Fig. 23-3). Patients with only fixed defects or normal studies had low cardiac event rates.[23] A larger, more recent study also found that an abnormal dipyridamole ^{201}Tl study was a significant independent predictor of subsequent myocardial infarction or cardiac death.[24] The presence of ^{201}Tl redistribution significantly increased the likelihood of developing a cardiac event.[24] However, there were no angiographic data available for comparison in this study. Significant prognostic value of reversible defects has also been reported in patients undergoing ^{201}Tl atrial pacing stress studies.[26,27]

Normal Myocardial Perfusion Imaging Studies

The clinical value of myocardial perfusion imaging derives not only from its ability to identify high-risk patients who might benefit from further interventions, but also from its ability to identify *low-risk patients* for whom any intervention, particularly invasive, is unlikely to produce benefit. Many clinical series of patients with known or suspected coronary artery disease have consistently shown that patients with normal myocardial perfusion imaging have a very low cardiac event rate. A recent review[2] summarized the outcome of 3573 patients with normal myocardial perfusion imaging. Future death or myocardial infarction averaged less than 1 percent per year, an event rate similar to the general population.[28] The benign prognostic implications of a normal ^{201}Tl study appear to be maintained even over a very long follow-up. Steinberg and colleagues reported the outcome on 309 patients with normal stress ^{201}Tl imaging over an average follow-up of 10 y.[29] In this group, the annualized cardiac event rate was 0.1 percent for cardiac death and 0.6 percent for nonfatal myocardial infarction.

Furthermore, even in populations of patients with exercise electrocardiographic (ST-segment depression) or angiographic (multivessel disease) markers of adverse outcome, when myocardial perfusion imaging is normal, the prognosis continues to be benign.[30–32] Fagan and colleagues reported that in 70 patients with an abnormal exercise electrocardiogram but normal exercise ^{201}Tl study, the annual cardiac event rate was 0.7 percent.[30] Even when marked ST-segment depression is present on exercise electrocardiography, prognosis remains benign when myocardial perfusion imaging is normal. Schalet and colleagues reported that among 154 patients with ≥2 mm of ST-segment depression on exercise electrocardiography but normal ^{201}Tl imaging, there were no cardiac events (death or myocardial infarction) over a mean follow-up of 34 ± 17 mo.[31] Similarly, in a smaller group of 32 patients with markedly positive stress electrocardiography (≥2 mm ST depression) but no reversible ^{201}Tl defects on exercise myocardial perfusion imaging, there were no cardiac events observed over a mean follow-up of 38 mo.[32]

When myocardial perfusion imaging is normal in patients with documented angiographic coronary disease, the clinician is faced with a dilemma. Is the myocardial perfusion imaging a false-negative study underestimating the cardiac risk? Or is myocardial perfusion imaging a true "physiologic negative" indicating that the angiographic disease is not hemodynamically significant and that the patient remains at low risk? Brown and colleagues reported their findings in a series of 75 patients with angiographic coronary disease (including 36 with multivessel disease) who had normal exercise ^{201}Tl imaging.[32] Over a mean follow-up of two years, there was only one cardiac death or myocardial infarction,

Table 23-1 Outcome of Patients with Angiographic CAD and Normal Myocardial Perfusion Imaging

Study	n	Cardiac Events	Annual Event Rate (%/y)
Wahl[34a]	8	0	0
Pamelia[34b]	22	2	3.2
Younis[22]	36	0	0
Brown[32]	75	1	0.75
Abdel Fattah[37]	97	3	1.1
Doat[34]	52	2	0.7
Summary	290	8	0.9%/y

CAD = coronary artery disease
y = year

yielding an annual cardiac event rate of 0.7 percent. The outcome was not significantly different from that observed in a contemporaneous series of 101 patients with normal exercise ^{201}Tl studies and no coronary disease based on angiographic data or a less than 1 percent probability of coronary artery disease based on age, symptoms, and stress electrocardiogram results: 2 of 101 patients developed cardiac events for an annual rate of 1.0 percent. Abdel Fattah et al subsequently confirmed these observations in a series of 97 patients with angiographic coronary disease (45 with multivessel disease) who had normal exercise SPECT ^{201}Tl imaging.[34] Over a mean follow-up of 32 mo, there were three cardiac deaths or myocardial infarctions yielding an annual cardiac event rate of 1 percent per year.[34] Similarly, in a preliminary report, Doat and colleagues reported a 5-y mean follow-up of patients undergoing exercise ^{201}Tl and coronary angiography.[35] When significant angiographic disease (greater than 70 percent stenosis) was present but ^{201}Tl imaging was normal, the combined annual cardiac death or myocardial infarction rate was 0.7 percent, which was not different from that noted in patients who had normal ^{201}Tl studies and no significant angiographic disease (annual event rate 0.6 percent).[35] However, among patients with angiographic disease who had ischemic ^{201}Tl studies, the annual cardiac death or myocardial infarction rate was 6.5 percent. Table 23-1 summarizes the annual cardiac event rate of patients with a normal ^{201}Tl study and significant angiographic disease based on these studies and smaller series of patients culled from earlier reports.

IMPACT OF ANTIANGINAL MEDICATIONS AND LEVEL OF STRESS

Although the previously cited studies firmly establish that the risk of cardiac events is low in patients with a normal exercise myocardial perfusion imaging study, it is not clear whether the same low risk would be predicted by a normal study when a patient is taking antianginal

medications or when the level of exercise achieved is low. It is possible that in such patients antianginal therapy or a poor level of stress could result in a normal ^{201}Tl study that could underestimate the extent of angiographic coronary artery disease and therefore the risk of subsequent cardiac events. Brown and Rowen recently reported their findings in a series of 261 patients with normal exercise ^{201}Tl studies followed for approximately two years.[38] They found an overall cardiac death or nonfatal myocardial infarction rate of 1.2 percent per year comparable to previous studies. Importantly, they found that antianginal therapy, including β-blocker use, and level of stress (reflected by peak heart rate or final Bruce stage) did not affect the benign prognosis in patients with normal ^{201}Tl imaging (Table 23-2). This study confirmed that the risk of cardiac death or nonfatal myocardial infarction is very low in patients with a normal exercise ^{201}Tl study and that the risk is not affected by concurrent antianginal medications or by the level of stress achieved.

In summary, normal myocardial perfusion imaging identifies patients with a very low risk of future cardiac death or nonfatal myocardial infarction, even when stress electrocardiography is markedly positive or when significanct angiographic disease is present. This suggests that the hemodynamic significance of a coronary lesion is more important than anatomic considerations alone (depicted on angiography) and that the results of myocardial perfusion imaging are more specific for cardiac events than stress electrocardiography. Furthermore, concurrent use of antianginal medications and low peak level of stress do not appear to result in an underestimation of cardiac risk when myocardial perfusion imaging is normal. The important clinical implication of these data is that a group of patients can be identified who are at such a low risk for cardiac events, even when angiographic disease is present, that the expense and risk of further intervention such as revascularization are not justified because such intervention is very unlikely to improve prognosis.

Incremental Value of Myocardial Perfusion Imaging

Although the previously cited studies have clearly established important prognostic value of myocardial perfusion imaging, the recent evolution of the health care environment has changed the way we judge such value. It is no longer adequate simply to demonstrate that a procedure such as myocardial perfusion imaging has prognostic value. It is now necessary to demonstrate what such testing adds to the predictive value of data that is less expensive to obtain, such as clinical data and results of stress electrocardiography. In an analogous way, we are now asking what more invasive and expensive procedures such as coronary angiography add to

Table 23-2 Annual Cardiac Death or Nonfatal Myocardial Infarction Rate as a Function of Antianginal Therapy or Stress Indices in Patients with a Normal Myocardial Perfusion Scan

	Cardiac Death or Nonfatal MI	(%/y)	p Value
Antianginal therapy	3/133	1.2	ns (≥0.6)
No antianginal therapy	3/128	1.2	
Beta-blocker use	2/77	1.4	ns (≥0.6)
No beta-blocker use	4/184	1.1	
Peak HR ≥85% MPHR	4/178	1.2	ns (≥0.6)
<85% MPHR	2/82	1.2	
≥60% MPHR	6/249	1.3	
<60% MPHR	0/12	0	
Final Bruce stage ≥3	3/152	1.0	ns (≥0.6)
≤2	3/109	1.4	
≤1	0/39	0	

HR = heart rate; MI = myocardial infarction; MPHR = maximal predicted heart rate

the value of less expensive noninvasive testing with myocardial perfusion imaging. An important first step to address these issues was taken by Pollock and colleagues,[39] who evaluated the additive incremental prognostic information obtained in hierarchial order from clinical, exercise electrocardiography, ^{201}Tl imaging, and coronary angiography in a series of patients suspected to have coronary disease originally described by Kaul et al.[10] Using the global chi-square obtained from the Cox proportional hazards regression model as an index of the relative predictive value, the results from stress electrocardiography added significantly to the prognostic value of clinical data alone (Fig. 23-4). However, the addition of ^{201}Tl data (reversible defects) to stress electrocardiography almost doubled the ability to predict cardiac events (Fig. 23-4). Importantly, the addition of coro-

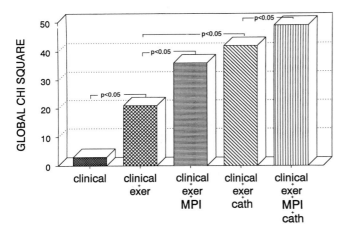

Figure 23-4 Incremental prognostic value (depicted by global chi-squared on Y axis) of tests performed in hierarchial order at the University of Virginia. exer = exercise electrocardiography; MPI = myocardial perfusion imaging; cath = cardiac catheterization. (Adapted from Pollock et al[39] with permission of the American Heart Association, Inc.)

nary angiographic data did not add any significant prognostic value to the combination of clinical, stress electrocardiographic, and ^{201}Tl imaging data. Thus, this study was the first to show that although it is more expensive, ^{201}Tl imaging data greatly increase the ability to predict cardiac events compared with stress electrocardiographic and clinical data alone. Furthermore, it showed that the addition of angiographic data did not add any significant prognostic value, consistent with previous studies. Subsequently, Iskandrian and colleagues looked at the incremental prognostic value of exercise SPECT ^{201}Tl imaging in patients with known coronary disease.[40] They found that when all patient variables (including clinical, exercise electrocardiographic, myocardial perfusion imaging, and cardiac catheterization data) were analyzed, myocardial perfusion imaging had the greatest predictive value. More importantly, when variables were evaluated in an incremental, hierarchial manner, they found that exercise testing did not add any significant predictive value to clinical variables, but that the addition of myocardial perfusion imaging data improved prognostic value by a factor of greater than four (Fig. 23-5). In addition, the increment in prognostic value was greater with myocardial perfusion imaging data than with cardiac catheterization data. Furthermore, the cardiac catheterization data did not add any significant prognostic value to the ^{201}Tl data. Thus, myocardial perfusion imaging data greatly improved the prognostic value of the less expensive stress electrocardiography. However, compared with myocardial perfusion imaging data, the more expensive cardiac catheterization data did not.

More recently, Palmas and colleagues reported the incremental prognostic value of exercise SPECT ^{201}Tl imaging in patients who had undergone previous coronary bypass surgery.[41] They found that the extent of jeopardized viable myocardium reflected in a summed ^{201}Tl reversibility score added significant prognostic in-

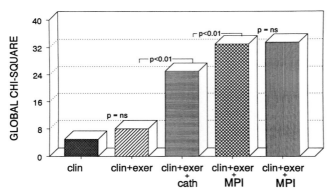

Figure 23-5 Hierarchial incremental prognostic value of clinical (clin), exercise electrocardiography (exer), cardiac catheterization (cath), and myocardial perfusion imaging (MPI) variables. The addition of myocardial perfusion imaging data to clinical and exercise testing data significantly increased the prognostic power of the predictive model and added significantly more prognostic value than cardiac catheterization data. However, addition of catheterization data to myocardial perfusion imaging data did not provide any additional prognostic value. (Adapted from Iskandrian et al[40] with permission of the American College of Cardiology.)

formation to the clinical and exercise data, doubling the chi-square value. Thus, there are now compelling data that myocardial perfusion imaging does not simply have statistically significant prognostic value in patients with known or suspected coronary disease. More importantly, it *adds* statistically significant and substantial predictive value to more easily obtained and less expensive clinical and exercise testing data. Equally important, compared with myocardial perfusion imaging, more expensive cardiac catheterization and angiographic data do not appear to add any significant incremental prognostic value.

Technetium-99m-Sestamibi Myocardial Perfusion Imaging

Technetium-99m sestamibi is a new myocardial perfusion imaging agent that has been shown to have important imaging advantages over ^{201}Tl for myocardial perfusion scintigraphy.[42] Previous data have established that the sensitivity and specificity of ^{99m}Tc sestamibi for detecting coronary artery disease is comparable to ^{201}Tl imaging.[43-48] However, because of the growing use of myocardial perfusion imaging for risk stratification as an adjunct for clinical decision making, it will be important to establish comparable prognostic value for this new agent. Recent data suggests that the prognostic value of ^{99m}Tc sestamibi myocardial perfusion imaging will indeed be comparable to that for ^{201}Tl imaging.[49-52] Given the comparable sensitivity for the detection of coronary disease, it would not be surprising to find that normal ^{99m}Tc sestamibi imaging carries a benign prognosis comparable to normal ^{201}Tl imaging. Brown and colleagues

recently reported the outcome of 234 patients who had undergone exercise or dipyridamole ^{99m}Tc sestamibi myocardial perfusion imaging.[49] Cardiac death or nonfatal myocardial infarction occurred in only one patient for an annualized event rate of 0.5 percent per year. Similar to ^{201}Tl studies described earlier, the prognosis remained benign even among patients who had exercise- or dipyridamole-induced ST-segment depression.

More recently, Raiker and colleagues confirmed these observations, demonstrating in 208 patients undergoing stress ^{99m}Tc sestamibi myocardial perfusion imaging that only one patient developed cardiac death or nonfatal myocardial infarction for an annualized event rate of 0.5 percent per year.[50] Strattman and colleagues evaluated the prognostic value of ^{99m}Tc sestamibi myocardial perfusion imaging in a series of 548 patients with stable angina.[51] Using multivariate analysis, they found that myocardial perfusion abnormalities and reversible myocardial perfusion defects had independent predictive value for cardiac events. This group of investigators has also reported similar findings with dipyridamole ^{99m}Tc sestamibi myocardial imaging.[52] In a series of 534 patients with stable chest pain, they found that an abnormal scan or a reversible defect had the greatest prognostic value compared with clinical electrocardiographic or angiographic data. Although more data are needed to confirm these initial observations, these studies suggest that risk stratification using ^{99m}Tc sestamibi myocardial perfusion imaging will have comparable value to ^{201}Tl imaging.

SPECT Imaging

Almost all the previously cited studies demonstrating the prognostic value of myocardial perfusion imaging have used planar imaging. Nevertheless, SPECT imaging would be expected to have at least as good predictive value as planar imaging because of its greater sensitivity and ability to distinguish coronary artery territories. A growing body of data now appears to be confirming this expectation. In a large series of 1926 patients undergoing stress SPECT ^{201}Tl imaging reported by Machecourt and colleagues, the extent of initial perfusion defect provided the best imaging variable for prediction of long-term prognosis and added significant prognostic value to clinical variables and exercise electrocardiography.[53] Furthermore, the cardiac event rate in patients with normal SPECT ^{201}Tl studies was 0.4 percent per year, comparable to previous planar studies described earlier. In addition, several other studies already cited have used SPECT imaging and have shown significant prognostic value.[31,32,40,50-52]

Fixed [201]Tl Defects

Standard dogma for many years after the introduction of ^{201}Tl imaging has been that reversible defects reflect jeopardized viable myocardium whereas fixed defects reflect infarction or scar.[54] In support of this construct has been the very consistent observation that the presence and extent of reversible defects predict future cardiac events whereas defects that are fixed at 2–4 h delayed imaging do not.[1,7,10,23,24,26,55–72] Recently, however, several studies have challenged the concept that all fixed defects represent myocardial scar or infarction.[73–76] An earlier study suggested that some fixed defects will show improved perfusion after coronary revascularization but that the more severe the defect, the less likely that improvement is to occur.[77] Furthermore, regional or global improvement in left ventricular contractile function was far more likely to occur after revascularization when transient defects were present compared with fixed defects.[78,79] More recently, Liu and colleagues reported that 75 percent of fixed defects showed improved perfusion after coronary angioplasty.[79] However, this was a highly selected group of patients, since only 8 percent had electrocardiographic evidence of myocardial infarction despite having fixed defects.[73] In a larger prospective study, 22 percent of all fixed defects at 4 h showed redistribution at 18–72 late imaging.[71] Interestingly, approximately 10 percent of defects that were transient at 4 h appeared fixed on late imaging.[74] Importantly, this study did not differentiate partial redistribution from fixed defects. This is an important issue because most of the previously cited prognostic studies have found significant prognostic value for the presence of *any* significant reversibility, lumping partial and complete reversibility together. In addition, Dilsizian and colleagues have reported that approximately 50 percent of defects that appear fixed on standard stress-delayed ^{201}Tl imaging will show reversibility with reinjection of a second dose of [201]Tl.[80]

Although technical considerations may explain some of these observations, it is evident that some defects that do not show redistribution at 2–4 h probably do not represent infarction or scar, particularly in the absence of Q waves or with known normal regional wall motion. However, regardless of these observations, as already pointed out, prior studies have shown a remarkably consistent lack of prognostic value for defects that are fixed at standard 2- to 4-h delayed imaging. In a recent large study comprising 896 patients with known coronary disease, 217 patients with defects that were fixed at standard delayed imaging had an outcome identical to 310 patients with normal ^{201}Tl images (death rate <1 percent) whereas in 369 patients with reversible defects, death was substantially more frequent (5 percent, $p >$ 0.001)(Fig. 23-6).[81] In addition, Brown and colleagues evaluated the prognosis of 100 patients with isolated fixed ^{201}Tl defects on standard stress 2- to 4-h delayed imaging and no prior myocardial infarction.[82] These patients represent a cohort very likely to show defect reversibility with reinjection or late imaging since the fixed defects in these cases do not represent scarring.

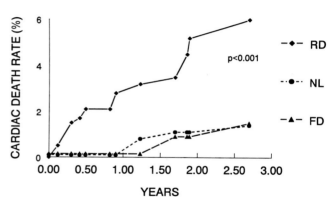

Figure 23-6 Actuarial cardiac death rate in 896 patients with known coronary disease as a function of myocardial perfusion imaging results. Patients with reversible defects (RD) had a significantly greater cardiac death rate than patients with normal studies or with fixed defects (FD) (p < 0.001).

Over a mean follow-up period of 2 y, only 1 patient developed a nonfatal myocardial infarction and no patient developed cardiac death. The annual cardiac event rate was 0.5 percent per year. Thus, even in a cohort of patients in whom the fixed defect probably does not represent scar or infarction, the prognosis remained benign, comparable to patients with a normal ^{201}Tl study. Furthermore, a preliminary report suggests that the presence of fixed defects that become reversible after reinjection does not identify patients at higher risk for cardiac events.[83] Therefore, although reinjection or late imaging may result in new reversibility and thus identify fixed defects with viable myocardium, these defects appear unlikely to have the same clinical significance as do those showing reversibility on standard 2- to 4-h delayed imaging. Some laboratories now advocate substituting a reinjection image for the standard 2- to 4-h delayed redistribution image. However, caution should be used in changing standard imaging protocols until the prognostic significance of this phenomenon is demonstrated. Since prior reinjection studies have shown that some defects that would otherwise be reversible on 2- to 4-h delayed imaging will become fixed with reinjection,[80] it is possible that changes in protocol to the use of only stress and reinjection imaging (omitting standard delayed imaging) could result in an underestimation of cardiac risk in patient populations evaluated.

POST MYOCARDIAL INFARCTION RISK STRATIFICATION

The primary goal of noninvasive risk stratification following an acute myocardial infarction is to identify the presence and extent of residual, jeopardized viable myo-

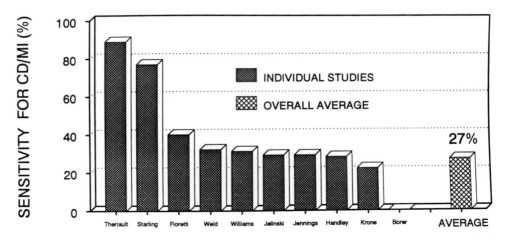

Figure 23-7 Sensitivity of submaximal exercise electrocardiography following acute myocardial infarction for detection of patients who develop subsequent cardiac death or myocardial infarction. The results of individual studies and the overall weighted average are displayed. Although there are exceptions, sensitivity of stress electrocardiography for identification of patients at risk for cardiac death or infarction was low, averaging 27 percent.

cardium and thereby identify patients at risk for future cardiac events.

Submaximal (heart rate– or work load–limited) exercise electrocardiography has been used widely for risk stratification before hospital discharge following acute myocardial infarction. However, although some studies have found predischarge submaximal stress testing to have prognostic value, many other studies have not.[84] Several factors play a role in limiting the utility of such an approach. Under the best conditions, exercise electrocardiography has a modest sensitivity for detecting coronary disease: 60 to 70 percent.[85] Furthermore, the sensitivity is very dependent on the peak heart rate achieved. When the peak heart rate achieved is less than 85 percent of maximal predicted heart rate, the sensitivity becomes so low that a negative test is categorized as "indeterminate."

Submaximal stress testing will therefore have intrinsic limitations for detecting noninfarct zone coronary artery disease and thus for identifying residual myocardium at risk. In addition, the interpretation of the significance of ST-segment changes is frequently limited because ST-segment elevation may occur in electrocardiogram leads with Q waves, reflecting regional asynergy rather than ischemia, and may be associated with reciprocal ST-segment depression that may also not reflect ischemia.[86] A review by Froelicher and colleagues[87] of prior studies evaluating submaximal exercise testing post-infarction[88–97] found that the overall sensitivity of ST-segment depression for detecting patients at risk for future cardiac events was very low, averaging only 27 percent (Fig. 23-7).

Myocardial perfusion imaging offers several poten-

tial advantages over submaximal exercise electrocardiography:

1. Increased sensitivity for detecting provokable ischemia and multivessel coronary disease. The sensitivity for myocardial perfusion imaging is much less affected by peak level of heart rate achieved than exercise electrocardiography.[98,99,100]
2. The ability to localize ischemia to individual coronary territories is frequently helpful in making management decisions regarding revascularization.
3. The ability to distinguish infarct from non–infarct zone myocardium, and, importantly, the ability to quantitate extent of jeopardized viable myocardium can help quantify risk of cardiac events and may play an important role in making management decisions for an individual patient.
4. The ability to identify resting and exercise-induced left ventricular dysfunction using myocardial perfusion imaging may be of particular added value since left ventricular function has important independent prognostic implications.[101,102]
5. The ability to perform myocardial perfusion imaging with pharmacological stress can allow application of risk stratification much earlier post-myocardial infarction than exercise testing. This may have important implications regarding cost savings. It also can allow risk stratification of patients who are unable to exercise.

The predictive value of myocardial perfusion imaging following acute myocardial infarction was first reported by Gibson and colleagues who compared predischarge

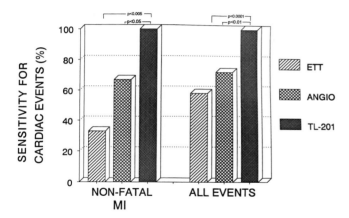

Figure 23-8 Sensitivity of exercise testing (ETT), coronary angiography (ANGIO), and ^{201}Tl imaging for detection of patients who develop subsequent cardiac events is displayed for nonfatal myocardial infarction (MI) and for all cardiac events. The sensitivity of ^{201}Tl imaging was significantly greater than stress testing and angiography for both end points. (Adapted from Gibson et al[103] with permission of the American Heart Association, Inc.)

submaximal exercise ^{201}Tl imaging with clinical, exercise electrocardiographic, and coronary angiographic data.[103] Among ^{201}Tl imaging variables, the presence of reversible defects involving multiple vascular territories and increased lung uptake had the most important prognostic value. The combination of these ^{201}Tl variables had a significantly greater sensitivity for predicting future cardiac events (defined as cardiac death, recurrent myocardial infarction, or development of rapidly progressive angina pectoris) than submaximal exercise testing or coronary angiography (Fig. 23-8). Furthermore, the ability to distinguish high-risk from low-risk groups was greatest for the ^{201}Tl criteria (Fig. 23-9). The superior sensitivity for detecting patients at risk for further cardiac events was reflected in the substantially lower probability of cardiac events in the "low-risk" subgroups for thallium scintigraphy compared with stress testing or coronary angiography (Fig. 23-9). Two subsequent studies evaluating postinfarction risk stratification reported that exercise ^{201}Tl imaging had significant prognostic value but that the ^{201}Tl predictors were not additive to exercise radionuclide ventriculographic data[104] or were significant only when used in combination with stress electrocardiography.[105] However, exercise testing for each of these studies was done at 3 wk post–myocardial infarction and were subject to selection bias. More recently, a study of patients with acute myocardial infarction and single-vessel coronary artery disease found that late cardiac events (cardiac death, recurrent myocardial infarction, or severe angina requiring hospitalization) were significantly related to the presence and number of transient defects on a submaximal predischarge ^{201}Tl imaging study and that no exercise electrocardiographic or clinical variables had any significant prognostic value.[55]

Myocardial perfusion imaging performed in conjunc-

tion with pharmacological stress may have particular advantage for risk stratification following acute myocardial infarction. It has been shown that ^{201}Tl imaging performed with maximal coronary hyperemia induced by dipyridamole has improved sensitivity for detecting coronary artery disease compared with submaximal stress ^{201}Tl imaging where the hyperemic stimulus is presumably less than maximal.[106] Leppo and colleagues compared the prognostic value of dipyridamole thallium imaging at 10–16 d following acute myocardial infarction with clinical, electrocardiographic and radionuclide ventriculographic data and found that the presence

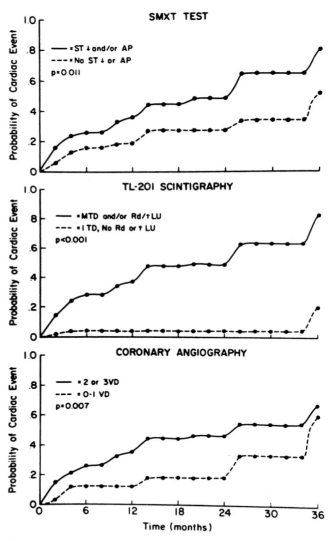

Figure 23-9 Actuarial probability of cardiac event in patients after myocardial infarction based on submaximal exercise testing (SMXT)(top panel), ^{201}Tl scintigraphy criteria (middle panel), and coronary angiography (bottom panel). Solid and dashed lines represent the high- and low-risk group cumulative probabilities, respectively. AP = angina pectoris; LU = lung uptake; MTD = multiple vascular territory ^{201}Tl defects; Rd = ^{201}Tl redistribution; ST ↓ = ST segment depression; VD = coronary vessels diseased. (Reprinted from Gibson et al[103] with permission of the American Heart Association, Inc.)

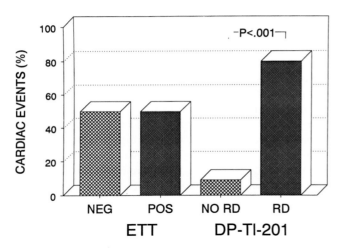

Figure 23-10 Frequency of cardiac events as a function of results of exercise electrocardiography (ETT) and dipyridamole ^{201}Tl imaging (DP-Tl-201). The presence of ^{201}Tl redistribution was associated with a significantly increased risk of cardiac events whereas stress electrocardiogram results had no significant prognostic value. NEG = negative stress electrocardiogram; POS = positive stress electrocardiogram; RD = ^{201}Tl redistribution.

of ^{201}Tl reversible defects was the only significant predictor of postdischarge cardiac death or recurrent infarction.[56] Furthermore, in the subgroup of patients undergoing submaximal stress testing, ST-segment depression had no predictive value (Fig. 23-10). Similarly, patients with transient defects on dipyridamole ^{201}Tl imaging 5–13 d after myocardial infarction had a much higher incidence of late cardiac events (64 percent) compared with those without transient defects (8 percent; $p < 0.005$).[57] In a study by Younis et al of patients who presented with acute myocardial infarction or unstable angina, the presence of a transient ^{201}Tl defect was again the best predictor of overall cardiac events, although catheterization data were better predictors of death or myocardial infarction.[58] Gimple and colleagues found that in patients with an uncomplicated myocardial infarction the presence of ^{201}Tl redistribution outside the infarct was the only significant predictor of cardiac events among scintigraphic, clinical, and electrocardiographic data.[59]

Early Post–Myocardial Infarction Risk Stratification

In addition to its greater sensitivity for detecting coronary disease than submaximal exercise, vasodilator-myocardial perfusion imaging has advantages that may allow this technique to play an important part in early, in-hospital management of acute myocardial infarction. Unlike exercise, pharmacologic stress with vasodilators induces only modest changes in determinants of myocardial oxygen demand[60,107–109] but provides superior quality

images compared with resting studies, maintaining a sensitivity for coronary disease detection equal to that of maximal exercise ^{201}Tl imaging.[107,108,110–112] Furthermore, the hemodynamic effects of dipyridamole are brief when used intravenously, and its actions can be rapidly reversed with theophylline.[109] Adenosine has an ultra-short half-life of only several seconds, and its effects rapidly diminish within 1–2 min after cessation of infusion.[113] Thus vasodilator-myocardial perfusion imaging may be particularly well suited for evaluating patients within the first few days after acute myocardial infarction when exercise testing is not appropriate. Brown and colleagues first reported a series of 50 patients undergoing dipyridamole-^{201}Tl imaging 1–4 d (mean 2.6) post–myocardial infarction.[60] Half the patients had received thrombolytic therapy. There were no serious adverse effects observed during the dipyridamole protocol. The prognostic value of ^{201}Tl imaging data was compared with clinical, electrocardiographic, and cardiac catheterization data. Using multivariate analysis, the only significant predictor of in-hospital ischemic cardiac events was the presence of infarct zone ^{201}Tl redistribution ($p = 0.00001$): 9 of 20 patients (45 percent) with infarct zone redistribution had in-hospital cardiac events compared with 0 of 30 patients without infarct zone redistribution (Fig. 23-11). During a mean 12-mo follow-up, 3 additional patients with infarct zone ^{201}Tl redistribution had ischemic cardiac events compared with 0 patients without infarct zone redistribution (Fig. 11). On a more extended follow-up to a mean of 33 mo, only 1 patient without infarct zone redistribution developed a cardiac event, yielding an annualized cardiac event rate of approximately 1 percent a year.[114] Angiographic variables were not significant predictors of cardiac events. Thus, it appears that the presence of jeopardized viable myocardium, regardless of underlying coronary angiographic anatomy, may be the best predictor of early and late cardiac events after an acute myocardial infarction.

These observations were recently confirmed by Mahmarian and colleagues, who examined the value of quantitative ^{201}Tl SPECT imaging using adenosine-induced coronary hyperemia at 5 ± 3 d after acute myocardial infarction.[115] They found that adenosine SPECT ^{201}Tl imaging had a high sensitivity for detecting stenosed noninfarct arteries (>80 percent) and that ^{201}Tl redistribution, reflecting jeopardized viable myocardium, was observed in 59 percent of infarct zones and 92 percent of noninfarct zones supplied by stenotic arteries. Importantly, the angiographic patency status of the arteries did not predict the presence or extent of jeopardized viable myocardium. The authors confirmed that thallium redistribution is an important predictor of in-hospital cardiac events. The presence of significant ^{201}Tl redistribution identified a subgroup of patients with a 43 percent probability of developing ischemic in-hospital cardiac events compared to only 9 percent in patients without

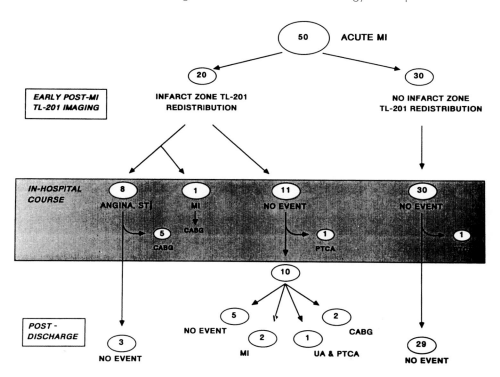

Figure 23-11 Flow chart of in-hospital and postdischarge outcome for patients as a function of the presence or absence of infarct zone ²⁰¹Tl redistribution seen on early post–myocardial infarction dipyridamole ²⁰¹Tl imaging. CABG = coronary artery bypass graft surgery; MI = myocardial infarction; PTCA = percutaneous transluminal coronary angioplasty; ST↓ = ST-segment depression, UA = unstable angina. (Reprinted by permission of the publisher from ability of dipyridamolethallium-201 imaging one to four days after acute myocardial infarction to predict in-hospital and late recurrent myocardial ischemic events, Brown et al, *American Journal of Cardiology*, Vol. 65, pp. 160–167. Copyright 1990 by Excerpta Medica Inc.)

significant redistribution.[115] These investigators recently reported their observations regarding long-term follow-up in an expanded population of 146 patients who had undergone adenosine SPECT ²⁰¹Tl imaging 5 ± 3 d after myocardial infarction.[116] They found that over a mean of 16 mo of follow-up that the best predictors of overall cardiac events as well as the hard end points of death or recurrent myocardial infarction were the extent of reversible ²⁰¹Tl redistribution and the left ventricular ejection fraction.

Importantly, myocardial perfusion imaging data (including perfusion defect size and extent of reversible defects) had significant incremental prognostic value when added to clinical and angiographic variables, improving the global chi-square of the predictive model by a factor of two to three (Fig. 23-12). Thus, the presence and extent of residual jeopardized viable myocardium detected by vasodilator-myocardial perfusion imaging performed early after acute myocardial infarction can identify a subgroup of patients at high risk for early and late cardiac events who may most benefit from an aggressive intervention. In contrast, patients without significant jeopardized viable myocardium appear to be at very low risk for both early and late cardiac events and may be candidates for early hospital discharge.

Non-Q Wave Myocardial Infarction

Historically, clinicians have generally preferred a more aggressive interventional approach in patients with non-

Q wave myocardial infarctions because such infarctions are often considered to be "incomplete," placing the patient at increased risk for recurrent cardiac events. However, patients with non-Q wave infarctions in fact represent a heterogeneous group, many of whom have a transmural or completed infarction.[117] Residual jeopardized viable myocardium has been shown to be absent in 30 to 40 percent of patients with non-Q wave infarction.[115,59] The ability of myocardial perfusion imaging to identify the presence and extent of jeopardized viable

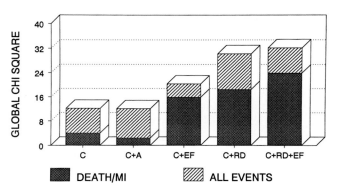

Figure 23-12 Hierarchal incremental prognostic value of clinical (C), angiographic (A), ejection fraction (EF), and ²⁰¹Tl redistribution (RD) with postinfarction adenosine dipyridamole ²⁰¹Tl imaging. Stipple bar graph shows the prognostic value (indicated by global chi-square) for death or reinfarction. Total bar graph including the cross-hatched bar indicates relative global chi-square for all cardiac events. Thallium-201 redistribution significantly improved the predictive value of clinical data and the combination of clinical plus ejection fraction data for both end points.

myocardium may be useful in evaluating patients with non-Q wave myocardial infarction by distinguishing patients at high risk, who would most likely benefit from further interventions, from patients at low risk, who would do as well with conservative management. The recent Thrombolysis in Myocardial Infarction (TIMI) IIIB trial showed that the outcome of patients treated with a conservative approach, in whom catheterization and revascularization were reserved only for patients who showed evidence of provocable ischemia on stress ^{201}Tl imaging, was the same as the outcome of patients undergoing early cardiac catheterization.[118] Furthermore, a study by Gibson and colleagues of patients with non-Q wave myocardial infarction undergoing predischarge submaximal exercise ^{201}Tl imaging showed that infarct zone ^{201}Tl redistribution was present in 15 of 16 patients who later developed recurrent infarction and in 18 of 21 patients who suffered a late cardiac death.[62] Thus, myocardial perfusion imaging may provide important information regarding risk of future cardiac events and hence guide a rational approach to the treatment of patients with non-Q wave infarction.

Unstable Angina

Patients with unstable angina are another subgroup for whom traditional management has generally involved an invasive and aggressive approach because of the concern that it is a precurser to myocardial infarction. However, it is important to distinguish between "unstable" and "stable" subgroups of this population. Patients who continue to have recurrent angina despite medical treatment obviously require coronary revascularization. However, many patients who present with unstable angina become stabilized with institution or intensification of medical treatment. In this group of patients, it is reasonable to question whether proceeding to cardiac catheterization and revascularization is necessary or whether continued medical treatment with noninvasive risk stratification is a reasonable alternative. Several studies have shown that heparin, aspirin, β-blockers, and nifedipine can all reduce the rate of death or myocardial infarction in patients who present with unstable angina.[119,120] Furthermore, intensification of medical treatment can reduce the "medically refractory rate."[121] Several randomized trials have failed to demonstrate an overall improvement in survival or infarction rate with coronary bypass surgery compared with medical treatment of unstable angina.[122-124] The recent TIMI-IIIB trial described earlier also showed no advantage of an early invasive approach compared with a conservative approach reserving catheterization for refractory angina or evidence of provocable ischemia on submaximal exercise ^{201}Tl imaging.[118]

Several studies have examined the prognostic value of myocardial perfusion imaging in patients presenting with unstable angina.[125-127] Hilliard and colleagues performed submaximal exercise ^{201}Tl imaging in patients who stabilized after admission for unstable angina and found that 15 of 19 patients with ^{201}Tl redistribution developed myocardial infarction or had Class III/IV angina pectoris at 12 wk after discharge compared to only 2 of 18 patients without ^{201}Tl redistribution ($p <$ 0.001).[125] In a series of 158 patients admitted with chest pain but who were ruled out for myocardial infarction and underwent symptom limited exercise ^{201}Tl imaging, transient defects were associated with a 21 percent frequency of nonfatal myocardial infarction or cardiac death compared to only 3 percent in patients without transient defects.[126] Marmur et al described 54 patients with unstable angina who became responsive to medical treatment and compared ^{201}Tl imaging, Holter data, stress electrocardiogram data, and cardiac catheterization for predicting cardiac events over a short follow-up of only 6 mo.[127] The only significant multivariable predictors in this study were a history of prior myocardial infarction and the extent of transient ^{201}Tl defects.[127] More recently, Brown reported a series of 52 patients presenting with unstable angina who became responsive to medical treatment and underwent symptom limited exercise ^{201}Tl imaging before hospital discharge.[128] Over a mean follow-up of 39 mo, 7 patients developed cardiac death or nonfatal myocardial infarction, and 17 additional patients required revascularization for recurrent unstable angina.

Using multivariate logistic regression analysis, the only significant predictor of cardiac death or nonfatal myocardial infarction was the presence of ^{201}Tl redistribution (Fig. 23-13). When thallium redistribution was present, 26 percent of patients developed cardiac death or nonfatal myocardial infarction. However, when no ^{201}Tl redistribution was present, the cardiac event rate was only 3 percent, yielding an annualized cardiac event rate of <1 percent per year. Importantly, stress electrocardiography had no significant prognostic value. Thus, consistent with prior studies, the presence of jeopardized viable myocardium identified patients at high risk for cardiac events whereas the absence identified low-risk patients. Therefore, myocardial perfusion imaging can be very helpful in distinguishing patients who deserve additional intervention from patients who can be managed medically and for whom further intervention is unlikely to be of benefit.

Postthrombolysis Patients

With introduction of thrombolytic therapy to the treatment of acute myocardial infarction, attention has been focused on identifying patients who have residual "sal-

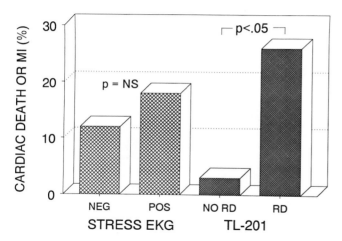

Figure 23-13 Prognostic value of exercise electrocardiography and ^{201}Tl imaging in patients presenting with unstable angina. The presence of ^{201}Tl redistribution (RD) was associated with a significantly increased risk of subsequent cardiac death or myocardial infarction (MI). However, stress electrocardiography had no significant predictive value. NEG = negative for ST-segment depression; POS = positive for ST-segment depression.

vaged" viable myocardium that remains potentially threatened by a significant residual coronary stenosis. As with non-Q wave myocardial infarction and unstable angina described earlier, the initial conventional approach was to use coronary angiography to define high-risk groups. However, accumulating data including those of the TIMI-IIB, Should We Intervene Following Thrombolysis (SWIFT), and Treatment Of Postthrombolytic Stenoses (TOPS) trials[129-131] showed that such an invasive strategy did not have any advantage over a more conservative approach where cardiac catheterization and intervention was reserved for patients who manifest spontaneous ischemia or who have provocable ischemia on stress testing (generally with myocardial perfusion imaging).

Myocardial perfusion imaging may be particularly well suited for risk stratification of patients following thrombolytic therapy for acute myocardial infarction because of its ability to identify (a) the presence of residual viable myocardium in the infarct zone, (b) the presence of a hemodynamically significant coronary lesion threatening such viable myocardium, and (c) identification of jeopardized viable myocardium outside of the infarct zone. Ellis and colleagues reported their observations in patients receiving thrombolytic therapy who had a residual coronary stenosis in the infarct vessel and who were randomized to either coronary angioplasty or to risk stratification with stress testing (primarily ^{201}Tl imaging).[125] In the subgroup undergoing risk stratification, when provocable ischemia was not present, subsequent infarct-free survival was 98 percent at 12 mo compared with 91 percent in patients who were randomized to coronary angioplasty at the time of discharge ($p = 0.07$).

Thus, noninvasive risk stratification was able to identify the low-risk patient for whom further intervention is unnecessary.

However, several recent studies have suggested that risk stratification with myocardial perfusion imaging may have less value in the "thrombolytic era" compared to studies performed before the advent of thrombolysis.[132,134] Tilkemeier and colleagues described the prognostic value of submaximal exercise thallium imaging in 64 patients receiving thrombolysis.[132] The sensitivity and specificity of ^{201}Tl for cardiac events in this group was 55 percent and 63 percent, respectively. The authors concluded that ^{201}Tl was a weak predictor of cardiac events in patients receiving thrombolysis. However, 14 patients had undergone revascularization based on ^{201}Tl results and 10 of the 64 patients in the "thrombolysis" group had actually undergone coronary angioplasty. Other studies have shown that early following coronary angioplasty transient defects occur that resolve with normal vascular remodeling and would therefore not be expected to have predictive value for cardiac events.[133] In a report by Miller and colleagues, ^{201}Tl did not have any significant prognostic value in 210 patients undergoing coronary angioplasty or thrombolytic therapy for acute myocardial infarction.[134] However, the results of ^{201}Tl imaging were used by clinicians in 36 patients who underwent early revascularization based on the ^{201}Tl imaging. These studies point out the current difficulty in performing prognostic studies with myocardial perfusion imaging. Since earlier studies have firmly established the prognostic value of myocardial perfusion imaging and this approach has become widely accepted by clinicians, the technique now forms a basis for making management decision regarding coronary revascularization. As a result, the large majority of patients with high-risk myocardial perfusion imaging results undergo coronary revascularization, and thus the natural outcome in such patients cannot be known. In these recent reports of patients undergoing thrombolytic therapy, the highest-risk patients based on the myocardial perfusion imaging data underwent coronary revascularization. This type of posttest bias greatly limits any conclusions based on the remaining patient cohort regarding the prognostic value of myocardial perfusion imaging.

Furthermore, as Gimple and Beller have pointed out,[135] the type of patients receiving thrombolytic therapy that have been reported in the literature tend to be generally a low-risk cohort with a low mortality in both treated and placebo groups. In addition, thrombolytic cohorts have a much lower incidence of three vessel coronary artery disease (10 percent) and prior myocardial infarction (7 percent) than prethrombolytic cohorts (30 to 50 percent and 17 percent, respectively).[135] These trends of lower risk and less severe coronary disease probably represent patient selection rather than any major change in coronary demographics in the current "thrombolytic era" compared to the prethrombolytic era. It is important to remember that in the United States, still only a minority of patients who present with acute myocardial infarction are candidates to receive thrombolytic therapy.[136] There is no reason to think that the prognostic value of myocardial perfusion imaging, which is based primarily on its intrinsic ability to detect the presence and extent of jeopardized viable myocardium, has changed in recent years. Any lessened observed predictive value is much more readily explained by a very strong posttest bias reflecting revascularization in the highest-risk patients based on myocardial perfusion imaging results, an overall low extent of coronary disease, and a low mortality in patients who actually receive thrombolysis.

Late Post–Myocardial Infarction

The presence of transient thallium defects on exercise studies in patients who present with recurrent angina late (post-discharge) after prior myocardial infarction also predicts future cardiac events.[63] Thallium-201 redistribution in the infarct zone was found to be the only significant predictor of cardiac death, nonfatal myocardial infarction, or overall cardiac events (including recurrent unstable angina) during a 37-mo mean follow-up.[63] Whereas most patients (10 of 15) with evidence of jeopardized viable myocardium outside the infarct zone by ^{201}Tl were sent to coronary revascularization without antecedent ischemic events, only 6 of 29 patients with infarct zone–only ischemia were referred for coronary revascularization by their treating physicians. This suggests that infarct zone ischemia was considered to be less threatening than noninfarct zone ischemia. However, patients with jeopardized viable myocardium limited to the infarct zone cannot be considered to be low risk: 28 percent (8 of 29) developed recurrent cardiac events compared to 0 of 15 patients without thallium redistribution ($p < 0.05$).[63]

Technetium-99m Sestamibi Imaging

Since the primary determinants of prognosis following acute myocardial infarction are the presence and extent of residual jeopardized viable myocardium and global left ventricular contractile function, myocardial perfusion imaging using ^{99m}Tc sestamibi may be particularly advantageous. In addition to being able to identify jeopardized viable myocardium, technetium-based agents offer the opportunity to evaluate regional and global left ventricular contractile function through first-pass studies or gated image acquisitions. However, at this time few data are available regarding risk stratification with this

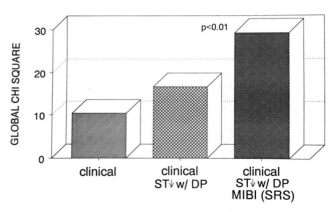

Figure 23-14 Incremental predictive value of dipyridamole myocardial perfusion imaging (MPI) with ^{99m}Tc sestamibi imaging performed 2–4 d post–myocardial infarction. A summed reversibility score (SRS) based on the myocardial perfusion imaging study significantly increased the prognostic power for predicting in-hospital cardiac events compared with clinical and dipyridamole (DP) data.

perfusion agent in the post–myocardial infarction setting. A preliminary report by Brown and colleagues described the prognostic value of intravenous dipyridamole ^{99m}Tc sestamibi SPECT imaging performed early post–myocardial infarction for prediction of in-hospital cardiac events.[137] Imaging was performed 2–4 d post–myocardial infarction in 265 patients enrolled in a multicenter study. A summed reversibility sestamibi score reflecting extent and degree of jeopardized viable myocardium provided significant incremental prognostic value to clinical and dipyridamole variables for predicting ischemic in-hospital cardiac events, improving global chi-square of the predictive model by a factor of three (Fig. 23-14).

The prognostic value of predischarge submaximal exercise SPECT sestamibi imaging was recently reported by Travin and colleagues involving 134 patients post–myocardial infarction.[138] Over a mean 15-mo follow-up, 13 patients developed a cardiac event. Reversible defects on sestamibi imaging identified 11 of these patients (85 percent) compared to only 4 (31 percent) for ST-segment depression on stress electrocardiography ($p < 0.02$)(Fig. 23-15). Using multivariate analysis of clinical, stress electrocardiographic, and myocardial perfusion imaging data, the number of reversible defects on SPECT imaging was the only significant predictor of future cardiac events. Furthermore, the extent of jeopardized viable myocardium on myocardial perfusion imaging remained a strong predictor of cardiac events in the subgroup of 54 patients who had received thrombolytic therapy. It is important to note that myocardial perfusion imaging retained important prognostic value despite the potential influence of significant posttest bias: 25 percent of patients were referred for coronary revascularization, often

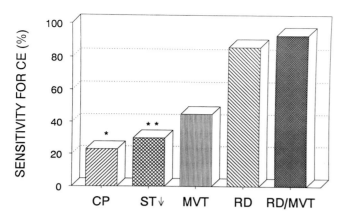

* p<0.01 compared with RD & RD/MVT
** p<0.05 compared with RD & RD/MVT

Figure 23-15 Relative sensitivity for detecting patients who developed cardiac events following acute myocardial infarction. Reversible defects (RD) and reversible defects with multiple vascular territories (MVT) had significantly greater sensitivity than chest pain or ST-segment depression during stress. (Adapted from Travin et al[138] with permission of the *American Journal of Cardiology*, Copyright 1995, Excerpta Medica, Inc.)

those with the most extensive ischemia by myocardial perfusion imaging.

Summary

The potential advantages of myocardial perfusion imaging for risk stratification of patients following acute myocardial infarction are listed in Table 23-3. Multiple studies now establish that the presence and extent of transient defects, reflecting residual jeopardized viable myocardium, have important prognostic value in predischarge risk stratification following acute myocardial infarction and unstable angina. Both infarct zone and noninfarct zone myocardium at risk appear to have important adverse prognostic implications.[105,59,60,62,63] Several studies have compared myocardial perfusion imaging with cardiac catheterization and clinical data

Table 23-3 Advantages of Myocardial Perfusion Imaging for Post-MI Risk Stratification

1. Increased sensitivity for MVD
2. Ability to localize ischemia to coronary territories
3. Ability to distinguish infarct from noninfarct zone myocardium at risk
4. Ability to quantify amount of jeopardized viable myocardium
5. Ability to define global and regional LV function (^{99m}Tc-based agents)
6. Vasodilator-stress as adjunct, allowing risk stratification earlier and in patients unable to exercise

LV = left ventricular.
MVD = multivessel coronary artery disease

showing that presence and extent of jeopardized viable myocardium detected on myocardial perfusion imaging is consistently the best predictor of cardiac events.[103,55,58,60,63] When examined in a hierarchial incremental model, myocardial perfusion imaging results, again, in particular, presence and extent of transient defects add substantially to both clinical and cardiac catheterization data for predicting future cardiac events.[116] Fewer studies have directly compared predischarge submaximal exercise testing with myocardial perfusion imaging. However, each of these has shown myocardial perfusion imaging data to be superior predictors of cardiac events consistent with their greater sensitivity for coronary artery disease.[103,55,59]

The prognostic value of postdischarge maximal exercise myocardial perfusion imaging has been less consistent,[98,99] which may reflect a selection bias toward a very low risk group. In contrast, among patients who present late after myocardial infarction with recurrent angina, which defines a higher-risk group, maximal exercise ^{201}Tl imaging has significant and superior prognostic value when compared with clinical, electrocardiographic, and cardiac catheterization data.[63] As a general rule, the earlier risk stratification can be applied, the greater the value since more cardiac events, including in-hospital events, can be prevented. The ability of vasodilator-myocardial perfusion imaging to identify apparently stable patients who are at high risk for in-hospital and late ischemic cardiac events as early as 24 h after myocardial infarction[57] offers potential marked advantages over routine predischarge risk stratification since management strategies and the need for cardiac catheterization can be determined as much as 1 wk earlier. If standard predischarge submaximal exercise testing is elected, the cost of using myocardial perfusion imaging instead of stress electrocardiography alone can be justified by (1) the improved sensitivity for identifying patients at risk for cardiac events evident in prior studies; (2) the ability to distinguish infarct zone from noninfarct zone ischemia and to quantify extent of jeopardized viable myocardium, thereby better defining risk and the likely benefit of further intervention; and (3) the difficulty in interpreting exercise-induced ST-segment change in the setting of Q wave infarctions and baseline ST-segment abnormalities.

PREOPERATIVE RISK STRATIFICATION

It has long been recognized that underlying coronary artery disease plays a major role in determining perioperative morbidity or mortality, particularly in patients with a high prevalence of coronary disease such as those undergoing vascular surgery. Prior studies have shown that 40 to 80 percent of patients undergoing vascular surgery have significant angiographic or clinical evidence of coronary artery disease.[139-141] Despite improvements in patient treatment, the primary cause of perioperative death remains cardiac in a large majority of previously reported studies.[142-147] Given the impact of ischemic heart disease on the welfare of patients undergoing vascular surgery, a great deal of attention has been focused on identifying the high-risk cardiac patient before undergoing surgery to better prevent perioperative cardiac events.

Although standard cardiac risk indices based on clinical factors such as the Goldman Index have been shown to be valuable for risk stratification of general patient populations undergoing noncardiac surgery,[148,149] such clinical indices have been very disappointing in their ability to identify high-risk patients undergoing vascular surgery. MacEnroe and colleagues found no correlation between the Goldman Index classification and perioperative cardiac events, need for preoperative revascularization, or myocardial ischemia demonstrated by myocardial perfusion imaging in patients undergoing elective abdominal aortic aneurysm repair.[150] In addition, Jeffery et al[151] found that the Goldman Index markedly underestimated the perioperative risk of important cardiac events in patients undergoing elective abdominal aortic surgery: the perioperative cardiac morbidity and mortality was approximately 8 percent in Goldman Class I patients predicted to have a <1 percent risk of a cardiac event. A number of other studies have also found low Goldman indices in the subgroup of patients who develop perioperative cardiac events.[66-69]

A major limitation of such clinical indices is that the patient population from which they were developed generally has had a very low prevalence of coronary artery disease and a low incidence of ischemic perioperative cardiac events.[149,150] The validity of applying such derived clinical criteria to populations of patients that have a much higher frequency of underlying coronary artery disease and ischemic perioperative events, such as those undergoing peripheral vascular disease surgery, is problematic and has never been confirmed. It is well known that many patients with underlying coronary artery disease may be asymptomatic.[152] Therefore, clinical criteria based on presence or absence of angina, myocardial infarction, or abnormal resting electrocardiograms may have insufficient sensitivity or specificity to be of value in analyzing patient populations where there is a high prevalence of coronary disease. The high frequency of occult coronary artery disease in vascular surgery patients has led to the development of myocardial perfusion imaging for risk stratification in the preoperative setting given its high sensitivity for coronary artery disease detection and established prognostic value in other settings. Furthermore, because myocardial perfusion imaging can be performed with vasodilator stress, it may be particularly valuable in this subgroup of patients who are often unable to exercise.

Boucher and colleagues first reported their experience

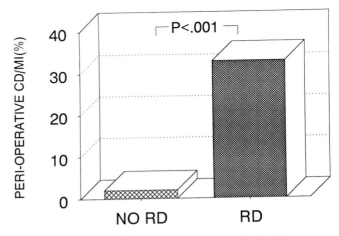

Figure 23-16 Risk of perioperative cardiac death (CD) or myocardial infarction (MI) as a function of the results of preoperative intravenous dipyridamole ^{201}Tl imaging. The presence of reversible defects (RD) was associated with significantly increased risk of perioperative cardiac death or myocardial infarction compared with patients without reversible defects.

with preoperative dipyridamole ^{201}Tl imaging in a series of 48 patients undergoing nonemergent peripheral vascular disease surgery who had clinical evidence of coronary disease.[64] Perioperative ischemic cardiac events, which occurred in 8 patients, could not be predicted by clinical data. However, 8 of 16 patients (50 percent) with ^{201}Tl defects that showed redistribution had cardiac events compared with 0 of 32 patients with fixed defects only ($n = 12$) or with normal studies ($n = 20$)($p < 0.0001$).[64] Thus, consistent with prior studies in other clinical settings, the presence of jeopardized viable myocardium had important prognostic value. This landmark study has now been confirmed by many subsequent studies.[64,65,66,68-72,154,158-163,168-170] Leppo and colleagues took the next logical step by comparing the relative predictive value of dipyridamole ^{201}Tl imaging with clinical and stress electrocardiogram variables using a multivariate analysis in patients undergoing peripheral vascular disease surgery.[65] In this cohort, patients were not selected on the basis of suspected coronary disease; only 51 percent had clinical evidence of coronary disease. Among the many patient variables examined, multivariate analysis showed that the presence of ^{201}Tl redistribution was the best predictor of perioperative cardiac events: 14 of 42 patients (33 percent) with thallium redistribution developed perioperative death or nonfatal myocardial infarction compared with only 1 of 47 patients (2 percent) with only fixed defects or normal studies ($p < 0.001$)(Fig. 23-16). In the subgroup of patients who also had exercise testing, the presence of thallium redistribution remained the best predictor of cardiac events. Watters and colleagues showed a significant relationship between reversible defects on preoperative dipyridamole myocardial perfusion imaging and intraoperative development of new wall motion abnormalities seen on transesophageal echocardiography.[153] These data confirm the relationship between myocardium at risk determined with myocardial perfusion imaging and segmental ischemia induced during noncardiac surgery.

Although it is clear that clinical criteria alone are inadequate for risk stratification of patients undergoing noncardiac vascular surgery, it remains a goal to use clinical and electrocardiographic data to define a subgroup of patients at such low risk of cardiac events that preoperative myocardial perfusion imaging may not be necessary, thereby allowing a more selective approach. Eagle and colleagues examined a cohort of 61 patients scheduled for major abdominal aortic vascular surgery who underwent preoperative dipyridamole ^{201}Tl imaging.[63] Among patients with clinical risk factors of coronary disease (angina, prior myocardial infarction, congestive heart failure, diabetes mellitus, or Q waves on their electrocardiogram), approximately half (15 of 32) had reversible ^{201}Tl defects. Of these patients, nearly half (7 of 15) had perioperative cardiac events compared with 0 of 17 patients without reversible defects ($p = 0.002$). In contrast, only 10 percent of patients (3 of 29) without such clinical coronary risk factors had reversible ^{201}Tl defects. Although 1 of the 3 patients had a perioperative cardiac event compared with 0 of 26 patients without reversible defects, the incidence of reversible defects and perioperative events was substantially lower in this group. The authors observed similar findings when these criteria were applied prospectively to an additional 50 patients. This study suggested that certain clinical criteria may be helpful in selecting those patients who would most benefit from the time and expense of preoperative myocardial perfusion imaging.

Subsequently, Eagle and colleagues reported their observations using a multivariate logistic regression approach to compare the prognostic value of dipyridamole ^{201}Tl imaging to clinical variables.[68] The cohort consisted of 200 patients undergoing dipyridamole ^{201}Tl imaging before planned peripheral vascular surgery, including carotid or femoral-popliteal bypass surgery, which constituted 34 percent of the total. Cardiac events were defined as cardiac death, myocardial infarction, congestive heart failure, and unstable angina. Among all patient variables, ^{201}Tl redistribution was the best predictor of perioperative cardiac events. Additional multivariate predictors included dipyridamole-induced ST-segment depression and five clinical variables (history of angina, Q waves, ventricular ectopy requiring treatment, diabetes, and age greater than 70 y). Using the clinical factors for screening, ^{201}Tl imaging appeared to be of most benefit in patients with one or two clinical risk factors or an intermediate risk of coronary disease (Fig. 23-17). In this subgroup, patients with ^{201}Tl redistribution had a 10-fold increased risk of perioperative cardiac events compared to those without redistribution. Patients with three or more clinical risk factors (high risk of underlying coronary artery disease) had a high perioperative risk regardless of ^{201}Tl results. The authors argued that this group, which constituted only 10 percent of the overall cohort, did not require additional risk stratification because its members were already identified to be at high risk. Patients with no clinical risk factors, representing nearly one-third of the overall cohort, had a relatively low risk of perioperative cardiac events (3 percent), and the authors suggested that this group also did not require additional risk stratification with ^{201}Tl imaging. This type of approach allows a rational application of myocardial perfusion imaging (which although minimally invasive has significant cost) to preoperative risk stratification.

An approach that allows selective application of a superior but more expensive test to risk stratification has a great potential value, but some caution should be taken in accepting the specific algorithms of these studies as a new "gold standard." Additional corroboration with larger studies, preferably applied prospectively, is needed. However, it may be difficult to obtain such data in the current environment since the prognostic value of myocardial perfusion imaging is so well established that it influences patient management. Thus, as discussed earlier for postinfarction risk stratification, it is now difficult to determine the natural history of patients with "high-risk" imaging results since these patients generally un-

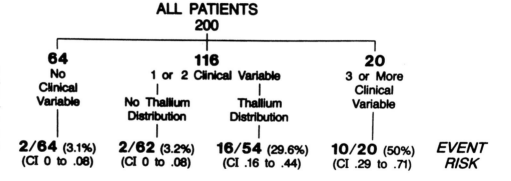

Figure 23-17 Flow chart depicting risk of perioperative cardiac events as a function of the number of clinical risk factors and the presence or absence of ^{201}Tl redistribution. CI = confidence interval. (Reprinted from Eagle et al[68] with permission of the American College of Physicians.)

ALL PATIENTS
200

64 No Clinical Variable

116 1 or 2 Clinical Variable

20 3 or More Clinical Variable

No Thallium Distribution

Thallium Distribution

2/64 (3.1%) (CI 0 to .08)

2/62 (3.2%) (CI 0 to .08)

16/54 (29.6%) (CI .16 to .44)

10/20 (50%) (CI .29 to .71)

EVENT RISK

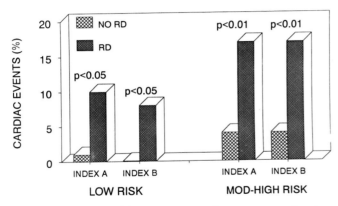

Figure 23-18 Risk of perioperative cardiac events as a function of results of preoperative dipyridamole ^{201}Tl imaging and clinical risk based on two Eagle indices: (Q waves on EKG, history of congestive heart failure, diabetes mellitus, prior myocardial infarction, history of angina pectoris);[63] (Q waves on EKG, history of angina, history of ventricular ectopic activity requiring treatment, diabetes requiring treatment, advanced age).[65] The presence of ^{201}Tl redistribution (RD) was associated with a significantly increased risk of perioperative cardiac events for both the moderate-to-high-risk patients and the low-risk patients using either index. (Adapted from Hendel et al[154] with permission of the *Journal of Nuclear Cardiology*.)

dergo invasive evaluation and intervention before noncardiac surgery.

Furthermore, the subgroup of patients with no clinical risk factors may be problematic. As previously discussed, in many patients with peripheral vascular disease, underlying coronary artery disease may be occult. Thus, clinical risk stratification may lack sufficient sensitivity to identify patients at risk for cardiac events, and myocardial perfusion imaging may still have important prognostic value. In the Eagle study,[68] although the overall risk of cardiac events in patients without clinical variables was low (3 percent), 2 of 17 patients (12 percent) with thallium redistribution had perioperative cardiac events compared with 0 of 47 without redistribution. Similarly, Hendel and Leppo[154] found that in patients undergoing vascular surgery who were predicted to have a low cardiac risk by the clinical criteria proposed by Eagle et al, the presence of reversible thallium defects increased the risk of cardiac events by a factor of four to eight (Fig. 23-18). Another problem with the Eagle study[68] may be patient selection. Approximately one-third of the patient cohort underwent nonaortic surgery including carotid artery surgery, which has a substantially lower perioperative cardiac risk than aortic surgery. However, the prevalence of such carotid surgery among each clinical risk subgroup, particularly the low-risk subgroup, was not reported. It is therefore not known whether the same overall low risk found in patients without clinical risk factors in the Eagle study[68] would apply to patients undergoing major aortic reconstructive surgery. Importantly, in a series of patients undergoing major vascular and general surgery,[69] no clinical risk factor stratification scheme, including Eagle's crite-

ria,[68] Goldman,[148,149] Detsky modified,[155,156] or Dripps ASA score,[157] was of value in predicting perioperative cardiac death or myocardial infarction. However, 9 of 21 patients (42 percent) with transient ^{201}Tl defects had perioperative cardiac death or infarction compared with 0 of 30 patients without reversible defects ($p < 0.0001$).[69]

Extent of Jeopardized Viable Myocardium

Prior studies in other patient populations, as discussed earlier, have established the concept that the risk of cardiac events is not simply related to the presence or absence of jeopardized viable myocardium, but rather is directly proportional to the *extent* of myocardium at risk. Recent data now suggest that this same principle applies to risk stratification before noncardiac surgery as well. Lane and colleagues found that perioperative cardiac risk was directly related to the number of reversible thallium defects in diabetic patients undergoing vascular surgery.[70] Patients with five or more (of a possible 10) transient defects had a 44 percent probability of a perioperative event compared with a 14 percent probability in patients with one or more reversible defects, and only a 3 percent probability in patients without reversible defects ($p < 0.01$). Other investigators identified a subgroup of patients based on the extent and severity of reversible ^{201}Tl defects comprising 17 percent of all patients undergoing major vascular and general surgery, which had an 80 percent probability of perioperative death or myocardial infarction.[71] Furthermore, on reanalysis of previous studies,[68] Eagle and colleagues found that perioperative cardiac risk was related to the extent of myocardium with transient defects.[158] Similarly, in a study by Lette and associates, high-, medium-, and low-risk patient subgroups were defined in a series of 355 patients undergoing major vascular or nonvascular surgery based on the number of myocardial segments with transient defects.[159]

More recently, Brown and Rowen[160] demonstrated that in patients undergoing dipyridamole ^{201}Tl imaging before noncardiac surgery the risk of perioperative cardiac death or nonfatal myocardial infarction is directly proportional to the extent of jeopardized viable myocardium reflected in the number of myocardial segments with transient ^{201}Tl defects (Fig. 23-19). In addition, for a given amount of myocardium at risk, the perioperative risk of cardiac events was increased by a history of diabetes mellitus. Thus, assessment of perioperative risk must take into consideration not simply the presence or absence of transient defects but rather the extent. Patients who have only a small amount of jeopardized viable myocardium appear to be at low risk for perioperative cardiac events, and probably do not require additional intervention such as cardiac catheterization or revascularization.

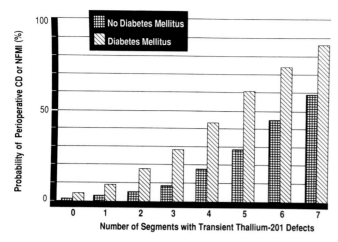

Figure 23-19 Probability of perioperative cardiac death (CD) or nonfatal myocardial infarction (NFMI) as a function of the number of myocardial segments with transient ^{201}Tl defects and the presence or absence of diabetes mellitus. Risk increases incrementally as the extent of jeopardized viable myocardium reflected in the number of transient ^{201}Tl defects increases. In addition, for any degree of jeopardized viable myocardium the presence of diabetes mellitus significantly increases the risk of cardiac events. (Reprinted from Brown and Rowen[160] with permission of the American College of Cardiology.)

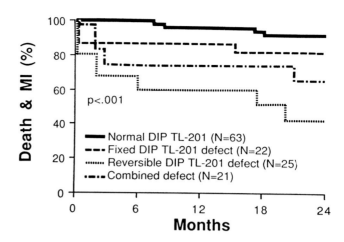

Figure 23-20 Long-term actuarial survival free of myocardial infarction (MI) in patients following peripheral vascular disease surgery stratified by results of preoperative dipyridamole ^{201}Tl imaging (DIP). Patients with reversible defects had significantly greater incidence of death or myocardial infarction than patients with other tests results. (Reprinted from Younis et al[162] by permission of the *American Heart Journal*.)

Late Cardiac Events

Since patients with peripheral vascular disease define a cohort with a high prevalence of coronary artery disease, they will remain at increased risk for cardiac events over subsequent years even if they remain event-free during the immediate postoperative period. Several studies have now shown that myocardial perfusion imaging also has significant predictive value for late cardiac events. Hendel and colleagues reported their experience with 360 patients undergoing dipyridamole ^{201}Tl imaging before elective vascular surgery.[161] Consistent with prior studies, the best predictor of early perioperative cardiac events was transient ^{201}Tl defects: cardiac death or nonfatal myocardial infarction occurred in 14 percent of patients with transient ^{201}Tl defects compared with only 1 percent with a normal scan ($p < 0.001$). For late cardiac events over a mean follow-up period of 31 mo, transient defects also had a significant univariate predictive value.

However, the best predictor of outcome was the presence of persistent defects. Younis and colleagues also examined the late outcome of patients undergoing dipyridamole ^{201}Tl imaging before peripheral vascular disease surgery.[162] Using multivariate analysis for the overall cohort, they found that the best predictor of cardiac death or myocardial infarction was the presence of reversible ^{201}Tl defects (Fig. 23-20). Importantly, the actuarial event-free survival rate for patients with transient ^{201}Tl defects was approximately 50 percent. The ability to identify such a high-risk group can potentially influence

decisions about whether to proceed with planned peripheral vascular disease surgery given such a poor long-term outcome. More recently, Urbinati and colleagues reported their findings regarding the early and late outcome of patients undergoing exercise ^{201}Tl myocardial perfusion imaging before carotid endarterectomy.[163] This patient cohort had a very low perioperative risk with no cardiac death or myocardial infarction reported within 30 d of surgery. However, after a 7-y follow-up the probability of developing a fatal or nonfatal cardiac event was 49 percent in patients with concordant reversible ^{201}Tl defects and a positive stress electrocardiogram compared with only 2 percent of patients without such findings (Fig. 23-21).

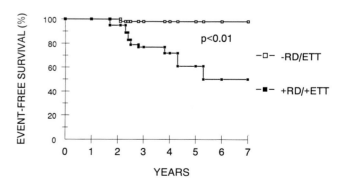

Figure 23-21 Long-term follow-up in patients undergoing exercise ^{201}Tl imaging before carotid endarterectomy. Event-free survival was significantly lower in patients with reversible ^{201}Tl defects and a positive stress electrocardiogram compared with patients without such results. (Adapted from Urbinati et al[163] with permission of the *American Journal of Cardiology*. Copyright 1992 by Excerpta Medica, Inc.)

Other Noncardiac Surgery

Although the literature is slowly growing, there is as yet little data regarding the value of myocardial perfusion imaging for risk stratification of patients undergoing *nonvascular*, noncardiac surgery. Several studies have included subgroups of nonvascular, noncardiac surgery in their overall predominantly vascular surgery cohorts.[69,71,160] However, although some have found the type of surgery to be unrelated to patient outcome,[154] these studies have not separately evaluated the prognostic value of myocardial perfusion imaging in the nonvascular subgroup. Brown and colleagues compared the perioperative and long-term prognostic value of dipyridamole ^{201}Tl, radionuclide ventriculography, and clinical variables in a series of patients with renal failure who were candidates for renal allograft surgery.[72]

Similar to vascular surgery cohorts, such a population of patients is known to be at increased risk for clinical or occult coronary artery disease and ischemic complications.[164-166] Multivariate regression analysis showed that the presence of a transient ^{201}Tl defect and left ventricular ejection fraction were the only significant predictors of future cardiac death or myocardial infarction. Only patients without transient ^{201}Tl defects underwent allograft surgery. There were no perioperative cardiac events among these 35 patients, although 13 (37 percent) had depressed left ventricular ejection fractions. Some investigators have found dipyridamole ^{201}Tl imaging to be insensitive for angiographic coronary disease or long-term cardiac events in patients with end-stage renal failure.[167] However, another study found that pretransplant and postoperative cardiac death and myocardial infarction were related to results of myocardial perfusion imaging, occurring only in patients with transient defects and not in patients with only fixed defects or normal images.[168]

More recently, Coley and colleagues described 100 patients undergoing nonvascular noncardiac surgery who had preoperative dipyridamole ^{201}Tl imaging.[169] Multivariate analysis showed that thallium redistribution, along with age greater than 70 y and a history of heart failure, remained the best predictor of cardiac events. Similar to previous observations of vascular surgery, they also found that clinical assessment may be helpful in identifying patients most appropriate for preoperative myocardial perfusion imaging. Among 45 patients with neither significant clinical variable (age or heart failure), no patient developed cardiac events. However, among the 55 patients with at least one clinical marker, outcome was directly related to the presence or absence of thallium redistribution: 8 of 24 (33 percent) patients with redistribution had a cardiac event compared with only 1 of 31 (3 percent) without thallium redistribution (*p* < 0.01)(Fig. 23-22).

In the absence of more specific data, two general

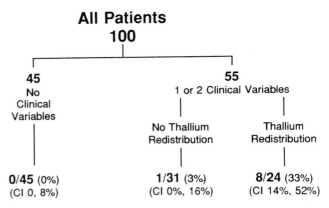

Figure 23-22   Flow chart relating risk of perioperative cardiac events in patients undergoing noncardiac surgery as a function of results of dipyridamole ^{201}Tl imaging and number of clinical variables. Patients without clinical variables had no cardiac events. Among patients with one or two clinical variables, the presence of ^{201}Tl redistribution was associated with a 10-fold increased risk of perioperative cardiac events (p < 0.01). (Reprinted by permission of the publisher from usefulness of dipyridamole-thallium scanning for preoperative evaluation of cardiac risk for nonvascular surgery, Coley et al,[169] *American Journal of Cardiology*, Vol. 69, pp. 1280–1285, copyright 1992 by Excerpta Medica, Inc.)

principles may guide patient selection for using myocardial perfusion imaging in preoperative risk stratification of patients undergoing nonvascular, noncardiac surgery. First, myocardial perfusion imaging, like any other risk stratifier, will be most useful in patients preparing for noncardiac surgical procedures that are associated with a substantial likelihood of perioperative cardiac complications. Therefore, myocardial perfusion imaging will be more useful in risk stratification of patients undergoing major orthopedic procedures, bowel resections, or major thoracic surgery compared with patients undergoing such low-stress procedures as herniorrhaphy or transurethral resection of prostate.[148,149,170] Secondly, myocardial perfusion imaging will be most likely to be helpful in patients with a high prevalence of underlying coronary disease. For example, patients with known prior myocardial infarction or with a history of angina will more likely benefit from risk stratification than patients without clinical evidence of cardiac disease. Although asymptomatic coronary disease could be problematic, unlike peripheral vascular disease, in which the patient population itself defines a cohort of patients with a high prevalence of coronary disease independent of symptomatology, in nonvascular surgery the prevalence of coronary disease is much lower, comparable to a normal population. Therefore, in nonvascular noncardiac surgery it may be more appropriate to use clinical evidence of coronary disease to determine whether to proceed with myocardial perfusion imaging for risk stratification.

Impact of Therapy on the High-risk Patient

Although it is now clear that myocardial perfusion imaging can identify patients at high risk for perioperative cardiac events, it is not fully established whether such risk stratification can be translated into better outcome for patients following surgery. However, initial data suggest that intervention based on the results of myocardial perfusion imaging can have beneficial results.[171,172] Golden and colleagues reported their findings in a consecutive series of 500 patients undergoing abdominal aortic aneurysm repair.[171] A subgroup of 212 patients had either symptoms or electrocardiographic evidence of coronary disease and underwent further cardiac evaluation, including myocardial perfusion imaging, but were felt to be "stable" and did not undergo coronary revascularization before vascular surgery. In this subgroup, 12 patients developed perioperative death or myocardial infarction. An additional 28 patients based on coronary angiography and noninvasive testing were felt to have "unstable" coronary artery disease and to be at high risk for perioperative cardiac events. Consequently, they underwent coronary revascularization before abdominal aortic aneurysm repair. There were no perioperative cardiac events in this group. Although the numbers are obviously small, this study provides evidence that coronary revascularization of the highest-risk group may prevent perioperative cardiac events. More recently, Younis and colleagues described the impact of preoperative risk modification in patients undergoing major noncardiovascular surgery.[172] Preoperative revascularization or medical interventions were implemented in 36 of 72 patients, based on the results of dipyridamole ^{201}Tl imaging, primarily reversible defects. They found that preoperative interventions were associated with a significant reduction in all perioperative cardiac events and in death or myocardial infarction (Fig. 23-23). Furthermore, in patients undergoing cardiac catheterization based on an abnormal dipyridamole ^{201}Tl study, cardiac events occurred in 0 of 6 patients undergoing coronary angioplasty compared with 7 of 19 (37 percent) patients not undergoing revascularization.

Contrary Studies

Although the weight of evidence based now on dozens of articles has clearly established the prognostic value of myocardial perfusion imaging for risk stratification of patients undergoing noncardiac surgery, two recent studies found contrary findings of no predictive value and require examination.[173,174] Mangano and colleagues prospectively studied 60 patients undergoing elective vascular surgery.[173] Thallium-201 results were blinded to

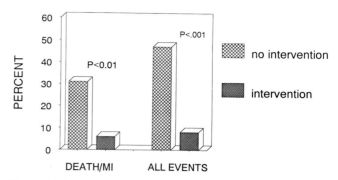

Figure 23-23 Incidence of perioperative cardiac events including death or myocardial infarction (MI) and all cardiac events as a function of preoperative intervention. Patients who receive preoperative intervention including revascularization or escalation of medical treatment had a significantly lower risk of perioperative death or myocardial infarction and all cardiac events.

treating physicians and compared to historical, clinical, laboratory, and physiologic data. They found no association between reversible ^{201}Tl perfusion defects and adverse cardiac outcomes. However, this study suffers from a small overall cohort ($n = 60$) and an extremely small percentage of important adverse outcomes: only 3 patients developed myocardial infarction or cardiac death. This extremely low incidence greatly limits any meaningful statistical analysis of any predictors. Baron and colleagues reported a larger group of 457 patients undergoing elective abdominal aortic aneurysm surgery who had preoperative dipyridamole ^{201}Tl studies and radionuclide angiography.[174] They found that cardiac imaging data did not predict adverse cardiac outcomes. However, this study also suffers from important methodological flaws. For example, 10 of the 20 deaths used as clinical outcomes were clearly described as noncardiac. To include as end points noncardiac deaths greatly diminishes the value of their analysis because myocardial perfusion imaging could not be expected to predict noncardiac events. In addition, only 16 percent of the cohort had a prior myocardial infarction. However, reversible defects were described in only 39 percent of patients with definite coronary artery disease, only 22 percent of patients with a history of angina, and only 18 percent of patients with ischemic ST- and T-wave abnormalities. This very low proportion of reversible defects in a subset of patients that one would expect to have a much higher frequency of reversible defects raises important questions regarding whether reversibility of perfusion defects was greatly underestimated by those interpreting the studies. This may explain the lack of predictive value of reversible defects in this study. In addition, the authors did not evaluate the extent of reversible defects as potential predictors of cardiac events.

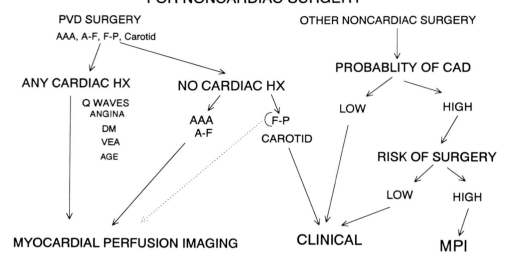

Figure 23-24 Algorithm for using clinical criteria versus ^{201}Tl imaging for risk stratification of patients before noncardiac surgery. AAA = abdominal aortic aneurysm repair; A-F = aortobifemoral bypass surgery; CAD = coronary artery disease; DM = diabetes mellitus requiring treatment; F-P = femoral-popliteal bypass surgery; PVD = peripheral vascular disease; VEA = ventricular ectopic activity requiring treatment.

Summary and Proposed Algorithm for Preoperative Risk Stratification

Previous studies have now firmly established that myocardial perfusion imaging has important prognostic value in the preoperative risk stratification of patients undergoing noncardiac, particularly vascular, surgery. A remarkably consistent observation has been that the presence and extent of jeopardized viable myocardium reflected in transient myocardial perfusion imaging defects can distinguish high- from low-risk patients. In addition, clinical variables may be helpful in identifying subgroups of patients in whom myocardial perfusion imaging may be most helpful.

It is reasonable to recommend risk stratification with vasodilator myocardial perfusion imaging in all patients undergoing aortic reconstructive surgery who have clinical evidence of coronary disease (Fig. 23-24). Patients without clinical risk factors who are scheduled to have aortic reconstructive surgery are also likely to benefit from such risk stratification because of the major cardiovascular stress of this surgery, its overall relatively high ischemic perioperative cardiac event rate, and the known high prevalence of asymptomatic coronary disease. Patients undergoing infrainguinal (e.g., femoral-popliteal bypass) peripheral vascular procedures could be expected to have lower perioperative cardiac stress and therefore be at lower cardiac risk. It might, therefore, be appropriate to rely initially on clinical assessment of cardiac risk in this group. However, there is evidence

that infrainguinal operations have a surprisingly similar cardiac morbidity and mortality compared with aortic surgery.[175] Therefore, these patients may also benefit from additional noninvasive risk stratification. Patients undergoing carotid endarterectomy appear to have a substantially lower cardiac risk,[163] and it probably would be reasonable to rely on clinical assessment for screening.

For patients undergoing nonvascular, noncardiac surgery, risk stratification with myocardial perfusion imaging is probably best reserved for patients who have both a high probability of underlying coronary artery disease based on clinical assessment and who are undergoing a major surgical procedure with a high level of associated cardiac stress (Fig. 23-24).

STRESS ECHOCARDIOGRAPHY

The temporal sequence of coronary ischemia is such that hypoperfusion precedes diastolic and systolic ventricular dysfunction. In some cases hypoperfusion may occur that is insufficient to cause ventricular dysfunction. Therefore, independent from other considerations, myocardial perfusion imaging, which detects the primary insult (hypoperfusion), would be expected to be potentially more sensitive for the detection of coronary artery disease than echocardiography, which is dependent on the development of a secondary phenomenon (abnormal

Table 23-4   Distinguishing Jeopardized Viable Myocardium from Scar: Myocardial Perfusion Imaging Versus Stress Echocardiography

| | Frequency of Jeopardized Viable Myocardium | | | |
| | Patients | | Myocardial Segments | |
Study	MPI	Echocardiography	MPI	Echocardiography
Quinones et al[172]	87/289	54/289	120/867	14/867
Forster et al[175]	45/102	38/102	58/306	50/306
Simeck et al[177]	18/51	7/52	—	—
Pozolli et al[171]	44/75	36/75	—	—
Summary	194/517 (38%*)	135/518 (26%*)	178/1,173 (15%+)	124/1,173 (11%+)

*p < 0.0001
+p < 0.002
See Table 4 for abbreviation

wall motion). Review of the current literature[176-182] suggests that this hypothesis is true. The reported sensitivities and specificities for stress myocardial perfusion imaging are presented in detail in Chap. 21, and confirm that stress myocardial perfusion imaging tends to be more sensitive for detection of coronary artery disease compared with stress echocardiography. However, stress echocardiography tends to be more specific.

Detection of Reversible Ischemia

Perhaps more importantly, stress echocardiography appears to be less sensitive than myocardial perfusion imaging for distinguishing jeopardized viable myocardium from myocardial scar (Table 23-4). In four studies comprising over 500 patients, each consistently detected approximately 30 percent less "ischemia," or jeopardized viable myocardium, by stress echocardiography compared with myocardial perfusion imaging either by patient or myocardial segment analysis.[177,178,181,183] Furthermore, 20 to 46 percent of individual segments showing jeopardized viable myocardium by myocardial perfusion imaging show normal contraction or scar by stress echocardiography.[178,181]

Prognostic Implications

Previous myocardial perfusion imaging studies have rather consistently shown that the most powerful predictor of future cardiac events is the presence and extent of jeopardized viable myocardium. If stress echocardiography is less sensitive for detecting such ischemia, it would be anticipated that the technique might consequently be less sensitive for identifying patients at risk for future cardiac events. In particular, the ability of a negative study to predict a low risk of cardiac events may be compromised. Early studies provide some foundation for this concern.[184-187] Brown recently summarized

available data regarding the outcome for patients based on stress echocardiography compared with a representative sample of myocardial perfusion imaging studies.[188] The cardiac event rate appears to be substantially higher among patients with negative stress echocardiography (at least 12 percent per year) compared with myocardial perfusion imaging (4 percent per year). The difference between the two techniques is probably greatest when the prevalence of coronary artery disease is highest. Among patients with a pretest probability of coronary disease of only 39 percent, Sawada and colleagues[189] found a low cardiac event rate in patients with normal stress echocardiography: 4.1 percent over 2 y. Similarly, among patients without known coronary artery disease, Bateman et al[190] found a low cardiac event rate in patients with normal stress echocardiography or myocardial perfusion imaging (Fig. 23-25). However, among patients

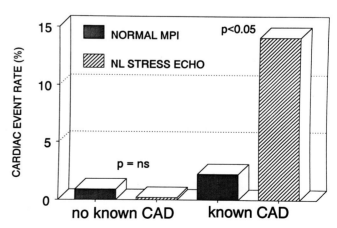

Figure 23-25 Cardiac event rate in patients with normal myocardial perfusion imaging (MPI) or stress echocardiography (ECHO) as a function of whether patients had known or no known coronary artery disease (CAD). In patients without known CAD the event rate was very low in both groups; however, among patients with known CAD, the cardiac event rate was significantly higher in patients with normal stress echocardiography compared with myocardial perfusion imaging.

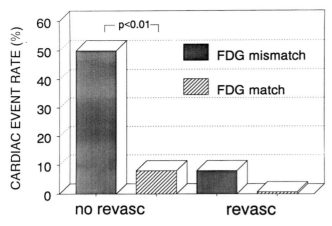

Figure 23-26 Cardiac event rate in patients undergoing positron emission tomography imaging. The cardiac event rate was significantly higher in patients with a fluorodeoxyglucose (FDG)-perfusion mismatch who did not undergo coronary revascularization (revasc) compared with other groups (p < 0.01).

with documented coronary artery disease, whereas a low event rate was seen with normal myocardial perfusion imaging, patients with normal stress echocardiography had a greater than six fold increase in cardiac events (*p* < 0.05) (Fig. 23-25). Therefore, in contrast to myocardial perfusion imaging, normal stress echocardiography may not reliably identify a low-risk group, especially in patients with known coronary artery disease. Although stress echocardiography appears to have a higher positive predictive value for cardiac events,[188] myocardial perfusion imaging has a sufficiently high predictive value (nearly 20 percent per year) that aggressive management strategies are mandated. Thus, patients are not likely to be managed differently based on a positive stress echocardiogram as compared with positive stress perfusion imaging data, whereas they might be managed differently based on negative studies.

POSITRON EMISSION TOMOGRAPHY (PET)

Even fewer studies have evaluated the prognostic value of PET imaging, but the findings appear to be consistent with anticipated results. The potential strengths of PET imaging lie in its high sensitivity for detection of coronary disease and its ability to distinguish viable from nonviable myocardium, for which it is often considered a gold standard. Eitzman and colleagues[191] found that patients with evidence of jeopardized viable myocardium, manifested by perfusion-metabolism mismatches, had a significantly higher cardiac event rate compared with patients without such findings, particularly when coronary revascularization was not performed (Fig. 23-26). Cardiac events were defined as death, myocardial infarction,

cardiac arrest, or late revascularization precipated by development of new symptoms during 12 mo of follow-up. This study also provides some evidence that patients identified as high risk by PET imaging can have the risk ameliorated by revascularization. Among patients with fluorodeoxyglucose (FDG) mismatching, the cardiac event rate was significantly lower in patients who subsequently underwent revascularization compared with those who did not (Fig. 23-26). A subsequent study by Lee and colleagues reported similar results.[192] In a series of 137 patients undergoing PET imaging following myocardial infarction, the outcome was related to presence or absence of resting FDG-perfusion mismatches and to revascularization versus medical treatment. Like Eitzman et al,[191] the authors found that among patients treated medically, those with FDG mismatching had a much greater incidence of future ischemic events (cardiac death, myocardial infarction, or unstable angina) than patients without mismatching. Furthermore, patients with FDG mismatching fared significantly better if they subsequently underwent revascularization compared with medical treatment.

These findings are also very similar to those of Di Carli and colleagues,[186] who evaluated the prognostic value of PET imaging in patients with coronary artery disease and severe left ventricular dysfunction (mean ejection fraction 25 percent). Among patients with resting FDG mismatching, those who underwent revascularization had an 88 percent survival rate compared with only 50 percent for patients treated medically (*p* = 0.03). In addition, the annual survival rate of patients treated medically was lower among those with FDG mismatching (50 percent) compared with those without FDG mismatching (92 percent, *p* = 0.07). In contrast, using only death as an end point, Yoshida and Gould found that cardiac events during 3 y of follow-up were more common in patients without viable myocardium in the infarct zone compared with those with FDG mismatching.[194] However, 80 percent of the patients in this study who had evidence of viable myocardium by PET imaging subsequently underwent coronary revascularization. The authors suggested that the improved survival in the group with viable myocardium was a result of successful coronary revascularization. In the group of patients with evidence of only myocardial scar, there did not appear to be any difference in outcome with revascularization (2 of 20 deaths) versus without (0 of 5 deaths). Such observations are limited by the small size of the cohort.

Tamaki and colleagues compared the prognostic value of PET and ^{201}Tl imaging in patients with prior myocardial infarction.[195] The authors found that perfusion-metabolism mismatching on PET imaging was the best predictor of future cardiac events, which they defined as cardiac death, myocardial infarction, unstable angina, or late myocardial revascularization at 23 mo

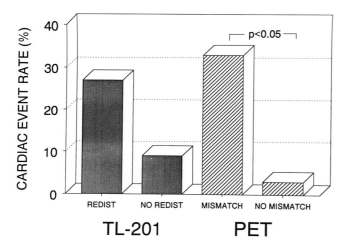

Figure 23-27 Cardiac event rate in patients undergoing ^{201}Tl and positron emission tomography (PET) imaging. Cardiac event rate was significantly higher in patients with metabolic-perfusion mismatches by PET imaging compared with the absence of these abnormalities ($p < 0.05$).

of follow-up (Fig. 23-27). The number of myocardial segments with transient ^{201}Tl defects was also a highly significant predictor by univariate statistical testing, but it did not add incrementally to the prognostic value of PET imaging.

Taken as a whole, these studies suggest that ischemic cardiac events are more common in patients with resting hypoperfused viable myocardium manifested by FDG mismatching than in patients without such findings, particularly in the setting of prior myocardial infarction. Furthermore, revascularization appears to improve the prognosis of the high-risk group with jeopardized viable myocardium. However, these studies are not randomized trials, and firm conclusions will require further investigation. Nevertheless, although additional data are needed, these early studies suggest that PET imaging will have important prognostic value, probably related to its ability (as with single photon myocardial perfusion imaging) to detect the presence and extent of jeopardized viable myocardium.

EXERCISE RADIONUCLIDE CINEANGIOGRAPHY

Exercise radionuclide cineangiography has been demonstrated to have important value for the detection of coronary artery disease. Ejection fraction and regional wall motion response to exercise have been shown to reflect the presence, site, and extent of underlying coronary artery disease.[196-200] Resting left ventricular ejection fraction determined by either first-pass or equilibrium radionuclide cineangiography has been shown to have important prognostic implications, particularly regarding cardiac death.[201-226] The Multicenter Postinfarction Re-

search Group[207] study showed a strong inverse relationship between ejection fraction and mortality rate (Fig. 23-28). Changes in global and regional left ventricular function with exercise as a result of inducible ischemia would be expected to show significant prognostic value, since it potentially reflects the extent of additional myocardium at risk.

Chronic Stable Coronary Artery Disease

Jones and colleagues were the first to describe a relationship between radionuclide cineangiography results and outcome in patients with coronary artery disease.[227] They demonstrated that an exercise-induced fall in left ventricular ejection fraction was the best predictor of outcome following coronary bypass surgery. In patients with an abnormal left ventricular ejection fraction response to exercise, outcome was better with coronary artery bypass surgery than with medical treatment. In contrast, among patients with a normal left ventricular ejection fraction response to exercise, bypass surgery showed no advantage over medical treatment for survival or chest pain relief. Bonow and colleagues also demonstrated that an abnormal ejection fraction response was an important determinant of outcome in patients with three-vessel disease.[228] Survival at 4 y was only 71 percent in patients who had an abnormal left ventricular ejection fraction response to exercise, ST-segment depression, and low exercise tolerance. In contrast, no deaths occurred in patients with three-vessel disease who had a normal left ventricular ejection fraction response to exercise (Fig. 23-29).

Peak Exercise Ejection Fraction

A number of studies have suggested that the exercise radionuclide cineangiographic variable with greatest

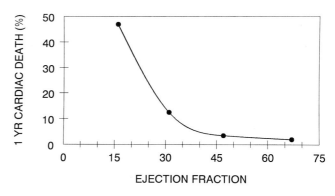

Figure 23-28 One-year cardiac death rate following acute myocardial infarction as a function of resting left ventricular ejection fraction. Risk of cardiac death increases substantially when ejection fraction falls below 35 percent. (Adapted from the *New England Journal of Medicine*, the Multicenter Postinfarction Research Group, 309:331, 1983. Copyright 1983. Massachusetts Medical Society. All rights reserved.)

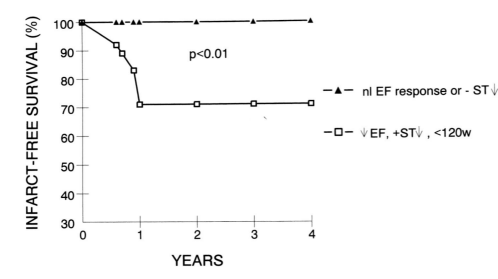

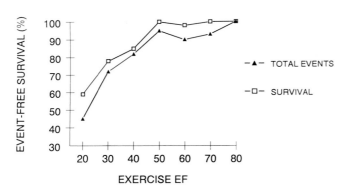

Figure 23-29 Actuarial infarct-free survival as a function of exercise radionuclide ventriculography results. Patients with a fall in ejection fraction (EF), ST-segment depression, and low exercise tolerance had a significantly increased risk of death or myocardial infarction compared with patients without these findings. (Adapted from Bonow et al[228] with permission of the *New England Journal of Medicine*.)

prognostic value is the ejection fraction at peak exercise.[229–237] Pryor and colleagues[229] found that the exercise ejection fraction was the best predictor of cardiac events over a 2-y follow-up (Fig. 23-30). The major cut-off for an increase in cardiac events was seen with exercise ejection fractions less than 50 percent. They found that no other patient variable including resting ejection fraction, regional wall motion abnormalities, or angiographic data added any significant prognostic value. These observations were confirmed by Iskandrian et al, who found that an exercise ejection fraction less than 50 percent was the best predictor of cardiac events.[230,231] In an important study by Lee and colleagues from Duke, the prognostic utility of first-pass radionuclide cineangiography was compared with clinical and angiographic data in 571 patients with stable coronary disease over a median follow-up of 5 y.[232] Among radionuclide predictors, the exercise ejection fraction

was again the best predictor of cardiac death. Neither resting ejection fraction nor change in ejection fraction with exercise added any significant prognostic value. Importantly, the prognostic value of radionuclide data was compared in a hierarchal, additive manner to clinical and cardiac catheterization data. Radionuclide cineangiographic data added substantially to clinical data for predicting clinical events (Fig. 23-31). Furthermore, the incremental value was equal to cardiac catheterization data. In an expanded Duke study of 1663 patients, reported by Jones et al, exercise ejection fraction remained the best predictor of cardiac death.[233] Exercise ejection fractions greater than 50 percent were associated with a very benign outcome, whereas when the exercise ejection fraction fell below 35 percent, mortality increased substantially. Several other investigators have also found exercise ejection fraction to be a significant predictor of cardiac events.[234–237]

The apparent superior prognostic value of absolute ejection fraction (particularly exercise ejection fraction) compared with exercise-induced changes in ejection fraction has fostered much discussion in the literature. Borer and colleagues argue that the most likely explanation for this observation is the failure of many studies to account for patients with a low resting ejection fraction.[238] They observe that ejection fraction during exercise is related to resting ejection fraction, with the relationship strongest and change in ejection fraction from rest to exercise the least among patients with markedly abnormal resting ejection fractions.[238,239] In addition, prior studies have shown that coronary artery disease mortality is strongly related to resting ejection fraction with a hyperbolic relationship, such that mortality increases markedly when resting ejection fraction falls below 30 percent.[207] Borer et al have reported that among patients with resting ejection fraction greater than 30 percent the change in ejection fraction with exercise was

Figure 23-30 Event-free survival as a function of left ventricular ejection fraction at peak exercise. Death and all cardiac events increase substantially when peak exercise ejection fraction falls below 50 percent. (Adapted from Pryor et al[229] with permission of the *American Journal of Cardiology*. Copyright 1984 by Excerpta Medica, Inc.)

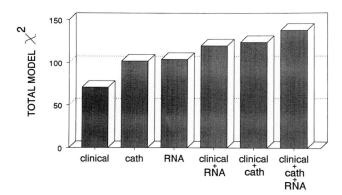

Figure 23-31 Incremental hierarchial prognostic value of exercise radionuclide angiography (RNA). The prognostic value associated with radionuclide angiography was superior to clinical data and comparable to cardiac catheterization (cath) data.

highly predictive of cardiac events.[240,241] A fall in ejection fraction with exercise of 10 percent or more identified a group of patients with an annual mortality rate of approximately 6 percent in the absence of bypass surgery. There was a relative risk of approximately 12:1 compared with patients with a less than 5 percent decrease in ejection fraction with exercise.

Post–Myocardial Infarction Risk Stratification

As previously noted, resting ejection fraction is an important predictor of cardiac events following an acute myocardial infarction.[207,222] In addition, a number of studies have established that exercise radionuclide cineangiography before hospital discharge has important prognostic value in patients following acute myocardial infarction.[214,238,242–246] Corbett and colleagues showed that failure of ejection fraction to rise by at least 5 percent with exercise had a 95 percent sensitivity and 96 percent specificity for identifying patients who develop cardiac events over a 10-mo follow-up.[206] Several other investigators have also found that the left ventricular ejection fraction response to exercise, particularly a failure to improve by at least 5 percent, is an important predictor of future cardiac events following myocardial infarction.[238,242,243] Some investigators have found peak exercise ejection fraction to be the best predictor of cardiac events, with a cut-off of less than 40 percent associated with a substantially increased risk of cardiac events.[244–246]

Summary

The ability to define resting and peak functions and changes in left ventricular ejection fraction with exercise using radionuclide cineangiography has now been estab-

lished to have important prognostic implications. A major determinate of cardiac outcome across all subsets of patients with coronary artery disease is resting left ventricular function. Ischemia-induced changes in left ventricular function during exercise allows the potential definition of jeopardized myocardium. These responses would be expected to carry prognostic implications similar to the presence and extent of jeopardized viable myocardium defined by myocardial perfusion imaging. Among patients with stable coronary artery disease, peak exercise ejection fraction appears to be the best determinate of outcome (particularly when resting function is depressed); among patients with recent myocardial infarction, changes in ejection fraction in response to exercise appear to be the best predictor of cardiac events. On one hand, exercise radionuclide cineangiography has significant incremental prognostic value compared with clinical and exercise data. On the other hand, cardiac catheterization data does not appear to add significantly to the predictive value of radionuclide data. As with myocardial perfusion imaging, the ability to define high-risk and low-risk patient groups can greatly facilitate patient management decisions.

CONCLUSIONS

The prognostic value of myocardial perfusion imaging and radionuclide cineangiography has now been firmly established across a wide spectrum of patients with coronary disease and with different stress modalities. These radionuclide techniques have evolved into powerful risk stratifiers that have significant and substantial incremental value compared with standard clinical and stress electrocardiogram data for predicting future cardiac events. These techniques now have a major impact on patient management decisions by allowing a rational application of further, more invasive and costly diagnostic and therapeutic interventions.

REFERENCES

1. Brown KA, Boucher CA, Okada RD, et al: Prognostic value of exercise thallium 201 imaging in patients presenting for evaluation of chest pain. *J Am Coll Cardiol* 1:994, 1983.
2. Brown KA: Prognostic value of thallium 201 myocardial perfusion imaging: A diagnostic tool comes of age. *Circulation* 83:363, 1991.
3. Ladenheim ML, Pollack BH, Rozanski A, et al: Extent and severity of myocardial reperfusion as predictors of

prognosis in patients with suspected coronary artery disease. *J Am Coll Cardiol* 7:464, 1986.

4. Staniloff HM, Forrester JS, Berman DS, Swan HJC: Prediction of death, myocardial infarction, and worsening chest pain using thallium scintigraphy and exercise electrocardiography. *J Nucl Med* 27:1842, 1986.

5. Iskandrian AS, Hakki AH, Kane-Marsch S: Prognostic implications of exercise thallium 201 scintigraphy in patients with suspected or known coronary artery disease. *Am Heart J* 110:135, 1985.

6. Iskandrian AS, Hakki AH, Kane-Marsch S: Exercise thallium 201 scintigraphy in men with nondiagnostic exercise electrocardiograms: Prognostic implications. *Arch Intern Med* 146:2189, 1986.

7. Felsher J, Meissner MD, Hakki AH, et al: Exercise thallium imaging in patients with diabetes mellitus: Prognostic implications. *Arch Intern Med* 147:313, 1987.

8. Iskandrian AS, Heo J, Decoskey D, et al: Use of exercise thallium 201 imaging for risk stratification of elderly patients with coronary artery disease. *Am J Cardiol* 61:269, 1988.

9. Kaul S, Finkelstein DM, Homma S, et al: Superiority of quantitative exercise thallium 201 variables in determining long-term prognosis in ambulatory patients with chest pain: A comparison with cardiac catheterization. *J Am Coll Cardiol* 12:25, 1988.

10. Kaul S, Lilly DR, Gasho JA, et al: Prognostic utility of the exercise thallium 201 test in ambulatory patients with chest pain. *Circulation* 77:745, 1988.

11. Boucher CA, Zir LM, Beller GA, et al: Increased lung uptake of thallium 201 during exercise myocardial imaging: Clinical, hemodynamic and angiographic implications in patiens with coronary artery disease. *Am J Cardiol* 46:189, 1980.

12. Bingham JB, McKusick KA, Strauss HW, et al: Influence of coronary artery disease on pulmonary uptake of thallium 201. *Am J Cardiol* 46:821, 1980.

13. Kushner FG, Okada RD, Kirshenbaum HD, et al: Lung thallium 201 uptake after stress testing in patients with coronary artery disease. *Circulation* 63:341, 1981.

14. Gibson RS, Watson DD, Carabello BA, et al: Clinical implications of increased lung uptake of thallium 201 during exercise scintigraphy 2 weeks after myocardial infarction. *Am J Cardiol* 49:1586, 1982.

15. Brown KA, Boucher CA, Okada RD, et al: Quantification of pulmonary thallium 201 activity after upright exercise in normal persons: Importance of peak heart rate and propranolol usage in defining normal values. *Am J Cardiol* 53:1678, 1984.

16. Liu P, Kiess M, Okada RD, et al: Increased thallium lung uptake after exercise in isolated left anterior descending coronary artery disease. *Am J Cardiol* 55:1469, 1985.

17. Gill JB, Ruddy TD, Newell JB, et al: Prognostic importance of thallium uptake by the lungs during exercise coronary artery disease. *N Engl J Med* 317:1485, 1987.

18. Stolzenberg J: Dilatation of left ventricular cavity on stress thallium scan as an indicator of ischemic disease. *Clin Nucl Med* 5:289, 1980.

19. Lette J, Lapointe J, Waters D, et al: Transient left ventricular cavity dilatation during dipyridamole-thallium imaging as an indicator of severe coronary artery disease. *Am J Cardiol* 66:1163, 1990.

20. Krawczynska EG, Weintraub WS, Garcia EV, et al: Left ventricular dilatation and multivessel coronary artery disease on thallium 201 SPECT are important prognostic indicators in patients with large defects in the left anterior descending distribution. *Am J Cardiol* 74:1233, 1994.

21. Lette J, Lapointe J, Waters D, et al: Transient left ventricular cavitary dilation during dipyridamole-thallium imaging as an indicator of severe coronary artery disease. *Am J Cardiol* 66:1163, 1990.

22. Weiss AT, Berman DS, Lew AS, et al: Transient ischemic dilation of the left ventricle on stress thallium 201 scintigraphy: A marker of severe and extensive coronary artery disease. *J Am Coll Cardiol* 9:752, 1987.

23. Younis LT, Byers S, Shaw L, et al: Prognostic importance of silent myocardial ischemia detected by intravenous dipyridamole-thallium myocardial imaging in asymptomatic patients with coronary artery disease. *J Am Coll Cardiol* 14:1635, 1989.

24. Hendel RC, Layden JJ, Leppo JA: Prognostic value of dipyridamole-thallium scintigraphy for evaluation of ischemic heart disease. *J Am Coll Cardiol* 15:109, 1990.

25. Shaw L, Chaitman BR, Hilton TC, et al: Prognostic value of dipyridamole thallium 201 imaging in elderly patients. *J Am Coll Cardiol* 19:1390, 1992.

26. Stratman HG, Mark AL, Walter KE, Williams GA: Prognostic value of atrial pacing and thallium 201 scintigraphy in patients with stable chest pain. *Am J Cardiol* 64:985, 1989.

27. LeFeuvre C, Vacheron A, Metzger JP, et al: Prognostic value of thallium 201 myocardial scintigraphy after atrial transesophageal pacing in patients wtih suspected coronary artery disease. *Eur Heart J* 14:1195, 1993.

28. National Center for Health Statistics: *Vital Statistics of the United States, 1979: Vol II, Mortality, Part A.* Washington, DC, US Government Printing Office, DHHS publication No. (PHS) 84-1101, 1984.

29. Steinberg EH, Koss JH, Lee M, et al: Prognostic significance from 10-year follow-up of a qualitatively normal planar exercise thallium test in suspected coronary artery disease. *Am J Cardiol* 71:1270, 1993.

30. Fagan LF Jr, Shaw L, Kong BA, et al: Prognostic value of exercise thallium scintigraphy in patients with good exercise tolerance and a normal or abnormal exercise electrocardiogram and suspected or confirmed coronary artery disease. *Am J Cardiol* 69:607, 1992.

31. Schalet BD, Kegel JG, Heo J, et al: Prognostic implications of normal exercise SPECT thallium images in patients with strongly positive exercise electrocardiograms. *Am J Cardiol* 72:1201, 1993.

32. Krishnan R, Lu J, Dae MW, Botvinick EH: Does myocardial perfusion scintigraphy demonstrate clinical usefulness in patients with markedly positive exercise tests? An assessment of the method in a high-risk subset. *Am Heart J* 127:804, 1994.

33. Brown KA, Rowen M: Prognostic value of a normal exercise myocardial perfusion imaging study in patients

with angiographically significant coronary artery disease. *Am J Cardiol* 71:865, 1993.

34. Abdel Fattah A, Kamal AM, Pancholy S, et al: Prognostic implications of normal exercise tomographic thallium images in patients with angiographic evidence of significant coronary artery disease. *Am J Cardiol* 74:769, 1994.

35. Doat M, Podio V, Pavin D, et al: Long term prognostic significance of normal or abnormal exercise ^{201}Tl myocardial scintigraphy in patients with or without significant coronary stenosis (abstr). *J Am Coll Cardiol* 158A, February 1994.

36. Wahl JM, Hakki A-H, Iskandrian AS: Prognostic implications of normal exercise thallium 201 images. *Arch Intern Med* 145:263, 1985.

37. Pamelia FX, Gibson RS, Watson DD, et al: Prognosis with chest pain and normal thallium 201 exercise scintigrams. *Am J Cardiol* 55:920, 1985.

38. Brown K, Rowen M: Impact of antianginal medications, peak heart rate and stress level on the prognostic value of a normal exercise myocardial perfusion imaging study. *J Nucl Med* 34:1467, 1993.

39. Pollock SG, Abbott RD, Boucher CA, et al: Independent and incremental prognostic value of tests performed in hierarchical order to evaluate patients with suspected coronary artery disease. *Circulation* 85:237, 1992.

40. Iskandrian AS, Chae SC, Heo J, et al: Independent and incremental prognostic value of exercise single photon emission computed tomographic (SPECT) thallium imaging in coronary artery disease. *J Am Coll Cardiol* 22:665, 1993.

41. Palmas W, Bingham S, Diamond GA, et al: Incremental prognostic value of exercise thallium 201 myocardial single photon emission computed tomography late after coronary artery bypass surgery. *J Am Coll Cardiol* 25:403, 1995.

42. Leppo JA, DePuey EG, Johnson LL: A review of cardiac imaging with sestamibi and teboroxime. *J Nucl Med* 32:2012, 1991.

43. Wackers FJTh, Berman DS, Maddahi J, et al: Technetium 99m hexakis 2-methoxyisobutyle isonitrile: Human biodistribution, dosimetry, safety, and preliminary comparison to thallium 201 for myocardial perfusion imaging. *J Nucl Med* 30:301, 1989.

44. Kahn JK, McGhie I, Akers MS, et al: Quantitative rotational tomography with ^{201}Tl and [99m]Tc 2-methoxy-isobutyl-isonitrile: A direct comparison in normal individuals and patients with coronary artery disease. *Circulation* 79:1282, 1989.

45. Najm YC, Maisey MN, Clarke SM, et al: Exercise myocardial perfusion scintigraphy with technetium-99m-methoxy isobutyl-isonitrile: A comparative study with thallium 201. *Int J Cardiol* 26:93, 1990.

46. Kiat H, Maddahi J, Toy LT, et al: Comparison of technetium-99m-methoxy isobutyl isonitrile and thallium 201 for evaluation of coronary artery disease by planar and tomographic methods. *Am Heart J* 117:1, 1989.

47. Iskandrian AS, Heo J, Kong B, et al: Use of technetium-99m-isonitrile (RP-30A) in assessing left ventricular perfusion and function at rest and during exercise in coronary artery disease and comparison with coronary arteriography and exercise thallium 201 SPECT imaging. *Am J Cardiol* 64:270, 1989.

48. Inglese E, Galli M, Parodi O, et al: Sensitivity of ^{99m}Tc hexakis 2-methoxyisobutyl isonitrile (^{99m}Tc-sestamibi) at rest and during exercise for detection of coronary artery disease and comparison with [201]Tl: A multicenter study. *Am J Noninvas Cardiol* 6:285, 1992.

49. Brown KA, Altland E, Rowen M: Prognostic value of normal technetium 99m sestamibi cardiac imaging. *J Nucl Med* 35:554, 1994.

50. Raiker K, Sinusas AJ, Wackers FJTh, Zaret BL: One-year prognosis of patients with normal planar or single photon emission computed tomographic technetium-99m-labeled sestamibi exercise imaging. *J Nucl Med* 1:449, 1994.

51. Stratmann HG, Williams GA, Wittry MD, et al: Exercise technetium 99m sestamibi tomography for cardiac risk stratification of patients with stable chest pain. *Circulation* 89:615, 1994.

52. Stratmann HG, Tamesis BR, Younis LT, et al: Prognostic value of dipyridamole technetium 99m sestamibi myocardial tomography in patients with stable chest pain who are unable to exercise. *Am J Cardiol* 73:647, 1994.

53. Machecourt J, Longere P, Fagret D, et al: Prognostic value of thallium 201 single photon emission computed tomograpic myocardial perfusion imaging according to extent of myocardial defect: Study in 1,926 patients with follow-up at 33 months. *J Am Coll Cardiol* 23:1096, 1994.

54. Pohost GM, Alpert NS, Ingwall JS, Strauss HW: Thallium redistribution: Mechanisms and clinical utility. *Semin Nucl Med* 20:70, 1980.

55. Wilson WW, Gibson RS, Nygaard TW, et al: Acute myocardial infarction associated with single vessel coronary artery disease: An analysis of clinical outcome and the prognostic importance of vessel patency and residual ischemic myocardium. *J Am Coll Cardiol* 11:223, 1988.

56. Leppo JA, O'Brien J, Rothendler JA, et al: Dipyridamole-thallium-201 scintigraphy in the prediction of future cardiac events after acute myocardial infarction. *N Engl J Med* 310:1014, 1984.

57. Pirelli S, Inglese E, Suppa M, et al: Dipyridamole-thallium-201 scintigraphy in the early post-infarction period. *Eur Heart J* 9:1324, 1988.

58. Younis LT, Byers S, Shaw L, et al: Prognostic value of intravenous dipyridamole-thallium scintigraphy after acute myocardial ischemic events. *Am J Cardiol* 64:161, 1989.

59. Gimple LW, Hutter AM, Guiney TE, Boucher CA: Prognostic utility of predischarge dipyridamole-thallium imaging after uncomplicated acute myocardial infarction. *Am J Cardiol* 64:1243, 1989.

60. Brown KA, O'Meara J, Chambers CE, Plante DA: Ability of dipyridamole-thallium-201 imaging 1 to 4 hours after acute myocardial infarction to predict in-hospital and later recurrent myocardial ischemic events. *Am J Cardiol* 65:160, 1990.

61. Bosch X, March R, Magrina J, et al: Prediction of in-hospital cardiac events using dipyridamole perfusion

scintigraphy after myocardial infarction (abstr). *Circulation* 80(suppl II):II, 1989.

62. Gibson RS, Beller GA, Gheorghiade M, et al: The prevalence and clinical significance of residual myocardial ischemia 2 weeks after uncomplicated non-Q-wave myocardial infarction: A prospective natural history study. *Circulation* 73:1186, 1986.

63. Brown KA, Weiss RM, Clements JP, Wackers FJTh: Usefulness of residual ischemic myocardium within prior infarct zone for identifying patients at high risk late after acute myocardial infarction. *Am J Cardiol* 60:15, 1987.

64. Boucher CA, Brewster DC, Darling RC, et al: Determination of cardiac risk by dipyridamole-thallium imaging before peripheral vascular surgery. *N Engl J Med* 312:389, 1985.

65. Leppo J, Plaja J, Gionet M, et al: Noninvasive evaluation of cardiac risk before elective vascular surgery. *J Am Coll Cardiol* 9:269, 1987.

66. Eagle KA, Singer DE, Brewster DC, et al: Dipyridamole-thallium scanning in patients undergoing vascular surgery: Optimizing pre-operative evaluation of cardiac risks. *JAMA* 257:2185, 1987.

67. Sachs RN, Tellier P, Larmignat P, et al: Assessment by dipyridamole-thallium-201 myocardial scintigraphy of coronary risk before peripheral vascular surgery. *Surgery* 103:584, 1988.

68. Eagle KA, Coley CM, Newell JB, et al: Combining clinical and thallium data optimizes preoperative assessment of cardiac risk before major vascular surgery. *Ann Intern Med* 110:859, 1989.

69. Lette J, Waters D, Lassonde J, et al: Postoperative myocardial infarction and cardiac death. *Ann Surg* 211:84, 1990.

70. Lane SE, Lewis SM, Pippin JJ, et al: Predictive value of quantitative dipyridamole-thallium scintigraphy in assessing cardiovascular risk after vascular surgery in diabetes mellitus. *Am J Cardiol* 64:1275, 1989.

71. Lette J, Waters D, Lapointe J, et al: Usefulness of the severity and extent of reversible perfusion defects during thallium-dipyridamole imaging for cardiac risk assessment before noncardiac surgery. *Am J Cardiol* 64:276, 1989.

72. Brown KA, Rimmer J, Haisch C: Noninvasive cardiac risk stratifications of diabetic and nondiabetic uremic renal allograft candidates using dipyridamole-thallium-201 imaging and radionuclide ventriculography. *Am J Cardiol* 64:1017, 1989.

73. Liu P, Kiess MC, Okada RD, et al: The persistent defect on exercise thallium imaging and its fate after myocardial revascularization: Does it represent scar or ischemia? *Am Heart J* 110:996, 1985.

74. Yang LD, Berman DS, Kiat H, et al: The frequency of late reversibility in SPECT thallium 201 stress-redistribution studies. *J Am Coll Cardiol* 15:334, 1990.

75. Botvinick EH: Late reversibility: A viability issue. *J Am Coll Cardiol* 15:341, 1990.

76. Brunken R, Schwaiger M, Grover McKay M, et al: Positron emission tomography detects tissue metabolic activity in myocardial segments with persistent thallium perfusion defects. *J Am Coll Cardiol* 10:557, 1987.

77. Gibson RS, Watson DD, Taylor GJ, et al: Prospective assessment of regional myocardial perfusion before and after coronary revascularization surgery by quantitative thallium 201 scintigraphy. *J Am Coll Cardiol* 1:804, 1983.

78. Rozanski A, Berman DS, Gray R, et al: Use of thallium 201 redistribution scintigraphy in the pre-operative differentiation of reversible and nonreversible myocardial asynergy. *Circulation* 64:936, 1981.

79. Iskandrian AS, Hakki A-H, Kane SA, et al: Rest and redistribution thallium 201 myocardial scintigraphy to predict improvement in left ventricular function after coronary arterial bypass grafting. *Am J Cardiol* 51:312, 1983.

80. Dilsizian V, Rocco TP, Freedman NMT, et al: Enhanced detection of ischemic but viable myocardium by the reinjection of thallium after stress-redistribution imaging. *N Engl J Med* 323:141, 1990.

81. Bodenheimer MM, Wackers FJTh, Schwartz RG, et al: Prognostic significance of a fixed thallium defect one to six months after onset of acute myocardial infarction or unstable angina. *Am J Cardiol* 74:1196, 1994.

82. Brown KA, Rowen M, Altland E: Prognosis of patients with an isolated fixed thallium 201 defect and no prior myocardial infarction. *Am J Cardiol* 72:1199, 1993.

83. Pieri PL, Tisselli A, Moscatelli G, et al: Prognostic value of ^{201}Tl reinjection (RI) in patients with chronic myocardial infarction (abstr). *J Nuc Cardiol* 2:S89, 1995.

84. Froelicher VF, Perdue S, Pewen W, Risch M: Application of meta-analysis using an electronic spread sheet to exercise testing in patients after myocardial infarction. *Am J Cardiol* 83:1045, 1987.

85. Froelicher VF: *Exerise Testing and Training*. New York, LeJacq Publishing. 1983, pp. 74–111.

86. Dunn RF, Bailey IK, Uren R, Kelly DT: Exercise-induced ST segment elevation: Correlation of thallium 201 myocardial perfusion scanning and coronary arteriography. *Circulation* 61:989, 1980.

87. Froelicher VF, Perdue S, Pewen W, Rich M: Meta-analysis using electronic spread sheet: Application to exercise testing in post-MI patients. *Am J Med* 83:1045, 1987.

88. Froelicher ES: Usefulness of exercise testing shortly after acute myocardial infarction for predicting 10-year mortality. *Am J Cardiol* 74:318, 1994.

89. Williams WL, Nair RC, Higginson LAJ, et al: Comparison of clinical and treadmill variables for the prediction of outcome after myocardial infarction. *J Am Coll Cardiol* 4:477, 1984.

90. Weld FM, Chu KL, Bigger JT, Rolnitzky LM: Risk stratification with low-level exercise testing 2 weeks after acute myocardial infarction. *Circulation* 64:306, 1991.

91. Krone RJ, Gillespie JA, Weld FM, et al: Low-level exercise testing after myocardial infarction: Usefulness in enhancing clinical risk stratification. *Circulation* 71:80, 1985.

92. Jennings K, Reid DS, Hawkins T, Julian DJ: Role of exercise testing early after myocardial infarction in identifying candidates for coronary surgery. *Br Med J* 288:185, 1984.

93. Jelinek VM, McDonald IG, Ryan WF, et al: Assessment

of cardiac risk 10 days after uncomplicated myocardial infarction. *Br Med J* 284:227, 1982.

94. Starling MR, Crawford MH, Kennedy GT, O'Rourke RA: Exercise testing early after myocardial infarction: Predictive value for subsequent unstable angina and death. *Am J Cardiol* 46:909, 1980.

95. Handler CE: Submaximal predischarge exercise testing after myocardial infarction: Prognostic value and limitations. *Eur Heart J* 6:510, 1985.

96. Fioretti P, Brower RW, Simoons ML, et al: Prediction of mortality during the first year after acute myocardial infarction from clinical variables and stress test at hospital discharge. *Am J Cardiol* 55:1313, 1985.

97. Borer JS, Rosing DR, Miller RH, et al: Natural history of left ventricular function during 1 year after acute myocardial infarction: Comparison with clinical, electrocardiographic and biochemical determinations. *Am J Cardiol* 46:1, 1980.

98. Pohost GM, Alpert NS, Ingwall JS, Strauss HW: Thallium redistribution: Mechanisms and clinical utility. *Semin Nucl Med* 20:70, 1980.

99. Esquivel L, Pollock SG, Beller GA, et al: Effect of the degree of effort on the sensitivity of the exercise thallium 201 stress test in symptomatic coronary artery disease. *Am J Cardiol* 63:160, 1989.

100. Iskandrian AS, Heo J, Kong B, Lyons E: Effect of exercise level on the ability of thallium 201 tomograpic imaging in detecting coronary artery disease: Analysis of 461 patients. *J Am Coll Cardiol* 14:1477, 1989.

101. Hammermeister KE, DeRouen TA, Dodge HT: Variables predictive of survival in patients with coronary disease: Selection by univariate and multivariate analyses from the clinical, electrocardiographic, exercise, arteriographic, and quantitative angiographic evaluations. *Circulation* 59:421, 1979.

102. Harris PJ, Harrell FE Jr, Lee KL, et al: Survival in medically treated coronary artery disease. *Circulation* 60:1259, 1979.

103. Gibson RS, Watson DD, Craddock GB, et al: Predication of cardiac events after uncomplicated myocardial infarction: A prospective study comparing predischarge exercise thallium 201 scintigraphy and coronary angiography. *Circulation* 68:321, 1983.

104. Hung J, Goris ML, Nash E, et al: Comparative value of maximal treadmill testing, exercise thallium myocardial perfusion scintigraphy and exercise radionuclide ventriculography for distinguishing high- and low-risk patients soon after acute myocardial infarction. *Am J Cardiol* 53:1221, 1984.

105. Abraham RD, Freedman SB, Dunn RF, et al: Prediction of multivessel coronary artery disease and prognosis early after acute myocardial infarction by exercise electrocardiography and thallium 201 myocardial perfusion scanning. *Am J Cardiol* 58:423, 1986.

106. Young DZ, Guiney TE, McKusick KA, et al: Unmasking potential myocardial ischemia with dipyridamole-thallium imaging in patients with normal submaximal exercise thallium tests. *Am J Noninvas Cardiol* 1:11, 1987.

107. Leppo JA, Boucher CA, Okada RD, et al: Serial ^{201}Tl myocardial imaging after dipyridamole infusion: Diag-

nostic utility in detecting coronary stenoses and relationship to regional wall motion. *Circulation* 66:649, 1982.

108. Iskandrian AS, Heo J, Askenase A, et al: Dipyridamole cardiac imaging. *Am Heart J* 115:432, 1988.

109. Homma S, Gilliland Y, Guiney TE, et al: Safety of intravenous dipyridamole for stress testing with thallium imaging. *Am J Cardiol* 59:152, 1987.

110. Gould KL: Noninvasive assessment of coronary stenoses by myocardial perfusion imaging during pharmacologic coronary vasodilation: I. Physiologic basis and experimental validation. *Am J Cardiol* 41:267, 1978.

111. Gould KL, Wescott RJ, Albro PC, Hamilton GW: Noninvasive assessment of coronary stenosis by myocardial imaging during pharmacologic coronary vasodilatation. II. Clinical methodology and feasibility. *Am J Cardiol* 41:279, 1978.

112. Albro PC, Gould KL, Wescott RJ, et al: Noninvasive assessment of coronary stenoses by myocardial imaging during pharmacologic coronary vasodilation. III. Clinical trial. *Am J Cardiol* 42:751, 1978.

113. Bellardinelli L, Linden J, Berne R: Cardiac effects of adenosine. *Progr Cardiovasc Dis* 32:73, 1989.

114. Brown KA: Unpublished data.

115. Mahmarian JJ, Pratt CM, Nishimura S, et al: Quantitative adenosine ^{201}Tl single photon emission computed tomography for the early assessment of patients surviving acute myocardial infarction. *Circulation* 87:1197, 1993.

116. Mahmarian JJ, Mahmarian AC, Marks GF, et al: Role of adenosine thallium 201 tomography for defining long-term risk in patients after acute myocardial infarction. *J Am Coll Cardiol* 25:1333, 1995.

117. Phipps B: "Transmural" versus "subendocardial" myocardial infarction: An electrocardiographic myth. *J Am Coll Cardiol* 1:561, 1983.

118. The TIMI IIIB Investigators: Effects of tissue plasminogen activator and a comparison of early invasive and conservative strategies in unstable angina and non-Q-wave myocardial infarction: Results of the TIMI IIIB trial. *Circulation* 89:1545, 1994.

119. Theroux P, Ouimet H, McCans J, et al: Aspirin, heparin, or both in unstable angina. *N Engl J Med* 313:1369, 1985.

120. HINT Research Group: Early treatment of unstable angina in the coronary care unit: A randomized, double blind, placebo controlled comparison of recurrent ischemia in patients treated with nifedipine or metoprolol or both. *Br Heart J* 56:400, 1986.

121. Grambow DW, Topol EJ: Effect of maximal medical therapy on refractoriness of unstable angina pectoris. *Am J Cardiol* 70:577, 1992.

122. National Cooperative Study Group: Unstable angina: National cooperative study group to compare surgical and medical therapy. II. In-hospital experience and initial follow-up results in patients with one, two and three vessel disease. *Am J Cardiol* 42:839, 1978.

123. Luchi RJ, Scott SM, Deupree RH: Comparison of medical and surgical treatment for unstable angina pectoris. *N Engl J Med* 316:977, 1987.

124. Parisi AF, Khuri S, Deupree RH, et al: Medical compared

with surgical management of unstable angina: 5-year mortality and morbidity in the Veterans Administration study. *Circulation* 80:1176, 1989.

125. Hillert MC, Narahara KA, Smitherman TC, et al: Thallium 201 perfusion imaging after the treatment of unstable angina pectoris: Relationship to clinical outcome. *West J Med* 145:355, 1986.

126. Madsen JK, Stubgaard M, Utne HE, et al: Prognosis and thallium 201 scintigraphy in patients admitted with chest pain without confirmed acute myocardial infarction. *Br Heart J* 59:184, 1988.

127. Marmur JD, Freeman MR, Langer A, et al: Prognosis in medically stabilized unstable angina: Early Holter ST segment monitoring compared with predischarge exercise thallium tomography. *Ann Int Med* 113:575, 1990.

128. Brown KA: Prognostic value of thallium 201 myocardial perfusion imaging in patients with unstable angina who respond to medical treatment. *J Am Coll Cardiol* 17:1053, 1991.

129. The TIMI Study Group: Comparison of invasive and conservative strategies after treatment with intravenous tissue plasminogen activator in acute myocardial infarction: Results of the thrombolysis in myocardial infarction (TIMI) Phase II trial. *N Engl J Med* 320:618, 1989.

130. SWIFT (Should we intervene following thrombolysis) Trial Study Group: Trial of delayed elective intervention vs conservative treatment after thrombolysis with anti-streplase in acute myocardial infarction. *Br Med J* 302:555, 1991.

131. Ellis SG, Moonly MR, George BS, et al: Randomized trial of late elective angioplasty versus conservative management for patients with residual stenoses after thrombolytic treatment of myocardial infarction: Treatment of post-thrombolytic stenoses (TOPS) Study Group. *Circulation* 86:1400, 1992.

132. Tilkemeier PL, Guiney TE, LaRaia PJ, Boucher CA: Prognostic value of predischarge low-level exercise thallium testing after thrombolytic treatment of acute myocardial infarction. *Am J Cardiol* 1990; 66:1203, 1990.

133. Manyari DE, Kundtson M, Kloiber R, Roth D: Sequential thallium 201 myocardial perfusion studies after successful percutaneous transluminal coronary angioplasty: Delayed resolution of exercise-induced scintigraphic abnormalities. *Circulation* 77:86, 1988.

134. Miller TD, Gersh BJ, Christian TF, et al: Limited prognostic value of thallium 201 exercise treadmill testing early after myocardial infarction in patients treated with thrombolysis. *Am Heart J* 130:259, 1995.

135. Gimple LW, Beller GA: Assessing prognosis after myocardial infarction in the thrombolytic era. *J Nuc Cardiol* 1:198, 1994.

136. Anderson HW, Willerson JT: Thrombolysis in acute myocardial infarction. *N Engl J Med* 329:703, 1993.

137. Brown KA, Heller GV, Landin RJ, et al: Prognostic value of IV dipyridamole ^{99m}Tc sestamibi SPECT imaging early post myocardial infarction for prediction of in-hospital cardiac events. *Circulation* 92(I):I-522, 1995.

138. Travin MI, Dessouki A, Cameron T, Heller GV: Use of exercise technetium 99m sestamibi SPECT imaging to detect residual ischemia and for risk stratification after acute myocardial infarction. *Am J Cardiol* 75:665, 1995.

139. Hertzer NR, Beven EG, Young JR, et al: Coronary artery disease in peripheral vascular patients: A classification of 1000 coronary angiograms and results of surgical management. *Ann Surg* 199:223, 1984.

140. Brown OW, Hollier LH, Pairolero RC, et al: Abdominal aortic aneurysm and coronary artery disease: A reassessment. *Arch Surg* 116:1484, 1981.

141. Blombery PA, Ferguson IA, Rosengarten DS, et al: The role of coronary artery disease in complications of abdominal aortic aneurysm surgery. *Surgery* 101:150, 1987.

142. Young AE, Sanberg GW, Couch NP: The reduction of mortality of abdominal aortic aneurysm resection. *Am J Surg* 134:585, 1977.

143. Hertzer NR: Fatal myocardial infarction following abdominal aortic aneurysm resection: Three hundred forty-three patients followed 6–11 years post-operatively. *Ann Surg* 192:667, 1980.

144. Crawford ES, Saleh SA, Babb JW III, et al: Infrarenal abdominal aortic aneurysms: Factors influencing survival after operation performed over a 25-year period. *Ann Surg* 193:699, 1981.

145. Jamieson WRE, Janusz MT, Miyagishima RT, Gerein AN: Influence of ischemic heart disease on early and late mortality after surgery for peripheral vascular disease. *Circulation* 66(suppl I):I, 1982.

146. Yeager RA, Weigel RM, Murphy ES, et al: Application of clinically valid cardiac risk factors to aortic aneurysm surgery. *Arch Surg* 121:278, 1986.

147. Lundqvist BW, Bergstrom R, Enghoff E, et al: Cardiac risk in abdominal aortic surgery. *Acta Chir Scand* 155:321, 1989.

148. Goldman L, Caldera DL, Nussbaum SR, et al: Multifactorial index of cardiac risk in noncardiac surgical procedures. *N Engl J Med* 297:845, 1977.

149. Goldman L, Caldera DL, Southwick FS, et al: Cardiac risk factors and complications in non-cardiac surgery. *Medicine* 57:357, 1978.

150. McEnroe CS, O'Donnell TF Jr, Yeager A, et al: Comparison of ejection fraction and Goldman risk factor analysis to dipyridamole-thallium-201 studies in the evaluation of cardiac morbidity after aortic aneurysm surgery. *J Vasc Surg* 11:497, 1990.

151. Jeffrey CC, Kunsman J, Cullen DJ, Brewster DC: A prospective evaluation of cardiac risk index. *Anesthesiology* 58:462, 1983.

152. Cohn PF: Asymptomatic coronary artery disease: Pathophysiology, diagnosis, management. *Mod Concepts Cardiovasc Dis* 50:55, 1981.

153. Watters TA, Botvinick EH, Dae MW, et al: Comparison of the findings on preoperative dipyridamole perfusion scintigraphy and intraoperative transesophageal echocardiography: Implications regarding the identification of myocardium at ischemic risk. *J Am Coll Cardiol* 18:93, 1991.

154. Hendel RC, Leppo JA: The value of perioperative clinical indexes and dipyridamole thallium scintigraphy for the prediction of myocardial infarction and cardiac death

in patients undergoing vascular surgery. *J Nucl Cardiol* 2:18, 1995.

155. Detsky AS, Abrama HB, Forbath N, et al: Cardiac assessment for patients undergoing noncardiac surgery: A multifactorial clinical risk index. *Arch Intern Med* 146:2131, 1986.

156. Detsky AS, Abrams HB, McLaughlin JR: Prediction of cardiac complications in patients undergoing noncardiac surgery. *J Gen Intern Med* 1:211, 1986.

157. Dripps RD, Lamont A, Eckenhoff JE: The role of anesthesia in surgical mortality. *JAMA* 178:261, 1961.

158. Levinson JR, Boucher CA, Coley CM, et al: Usefulness of semiquantitative analysis of dipyridamole-thallium-201 redistribution for improving risk stratification before vascular surgery. *Am J Cardiol* 66:406, 1990.

159. Lette J, Waters D, Cerino M, et al: Preoperative coronary artery disease risk stratification based on dipyridamole imaging and a simple three-step, three-segment model for patients undergoing noncardiac vascular surgery or major general surgery. *Am J Cardiol* 69:1553, 1992.

160. Brown, KA, Rowen M: Extent of jeopardized viable myocardium determined by myocardial perfusion imaging best predicts perioperative cardiac events in patients undergoing noncardiac surgery. *J Am Coll Cardiol* 21:325, 1993.

161. Hendel RC, Whitfield SS, Billegas BJ, et al: Prediction of late cardiac events by dipyridamole thallium imaging in patients undergoing elective vascular surgery. *Am J Cardiol* 70:1243, 1992.

162. Younis LT, Aguirre F, Byers S, et al: Perioperative and long-term prognostic value of intravenous dipyridamole thallium scintigraphy in patients with peripheral vascular disease. *Am Heart J* 119:1287, 1990.

163. Urbinati S, DiPasquale G, Andreoli A, et al: Frequency and prognostic significance of silent coronary artery disease in patients with cerebral ischemia undergoing carotid endarterectomy. *Am J Cardiol* 69:1166, 1992.

164. Weinrauch LA, D'Elia JA, Healy RW, et al: Asymptomatic coronary disease: Angiography in diabetic patients before renal transplantation: Relation of findings to postoperative survival. *Ann Intern Med* 88:346, 1978.

165. Weinrauch L, D'Elia J, Healy RW, et al: Asymptomatic coronary artery disease: Angiographic assessment of diabetics evaluated for renal transplantation. *Circulation* 58:1184, 1973.

166. Bruan WE, Phillips DF, Vidt DG, et al: Coronary artery disease in 100 diabetics with end-stage renal failure. *Transplant Proc* 16:603, 1984.

167. Marwick TH, Steinmuller DR, Underwood DA, et al: Ineffectiveness of dipyridamole SPECT thallium imaging as a screening technique for coronary artery disease in patients with end-stage renal failure. *Transplantation* 49:100, 1990.

168. Camp AD, Garvin PJ, Hoff J, et al: Prognostic value of intravenous dipyridamole thallium imaging in patients with diabetes mellitus considered for renal transplantation. *Am J Cardiol* 65:1459, 1990.

169. Coley CM, Field TS, Abraham SA, et al: Usefulness of dipyridamole-thallium scanning for preoperative evalua-

tion of cardiac risk for nonvascular surgery. *Am J Cardiol* 69:1280, 1992.

170. Skinner JF, Pierce ML: Surgical risk in the cardiac patient. *J Chron Dis* 17:57, 1964.

171. Golden MA, Whittemore AD, Donaldson MC, Mannick JA: Selective evaluation and management of coronary artery disease in patients undergoing repair of abdominal aortic aneurysms. *Ann Surg* 212:415, 1990.

172. Younis L, Stratmann H, Takase B, et al: Preoperative clinical assessment and dipyridamole thallium 201 scintigraphy for prediction and prevention of cardiac events in patients having major noncardiovascular surgery and known or suspected coronary artery disease. *Am J Cardiol* 74:311, 1994.

173. Mangano DT, London MJ, Tubau JF, et al: Dipyridamole thallium 201 scintigraphy as a preoperative screening test: A reexamination of its predictive potential. *Circulation* 84:493, 1991.

174. Baron JF, Mulder O, Bertrand M, et al: Dipyridamole-thallium scintigraphy and gated radionuclide angiography to assess cardiac risk before abdominal aortic surgery. *N Engl J Med* 330:663, 1994.

175. Krupski WC, Layug EL, Reilly LM, et al: Comparison of cardiac morbidity between aortic and infrainguinal operations. *J Vasc Surg* 15:354, 1992.

176. Galanti G, Sciagra R, Comeglio M, et al: Diagnostic accuracy of peak exercise echocardiography in coronary artery disease: Comparison with thallium 201 myocardial scintigraphy. *Am Heart J* 122:1609, 1991.

177. Pozzoli MMA, Fioretti PM, Salustri A, et al: Exercise echocardiography and technetium 99m MIBI single photon emission computed tomography in the detection of coronary artery disease. *Am J Cardiol* 67:350, 1991.

178. Quinones MA, Verani MS, Haichin RM, et al: Exercise echocardiography versus ^{201}Tl single photon emission computed tomography in evaluation of coronary artery disease: Analysis of 292 patients. *Circulation* 85:1026, 1992.

179. Salustri A, Pozzoli MMA, Hermans W, et al: Relationship between exercise echocardiography and perfusion single photon emission computed tomography in patients with single-vessel coronary artery disease. *Am Heart J* 124:74, 1992.

180. Hoffman R, Lethen H, Kleinhans E, et al: Comparative evaluation of bicycle and dobutamine stress echocardiography with perfusion scintigraphy and bicycle electrocardiogram for identification of coronary artery disease. *Am J Cardiol* 72:555, 1993.

181. Forester T, McNeill AJ, Salustri A, et al: Simultaneous dobutamine stress echocardiography and technetium 99m isonitrile single photon emission computed tomography in patients with suspected coronary artery disease. *J Am Coll Cardiol* 21:1591, 1993.

182. Marwick T, D'Hondt A, Baudhuin T, et al: Optimal use of dobutamine stress for the detection and evaluation of coronary artery disease: Combination with echocardiography or scintigraphy, or both? *J Am Coll Cardiol* 22:159, 1993.

183. Simeck CL, Watson D, Smith WH, et al: Dipyridamole thallium 201 imaging versus dobutamine echocardiogra-

phy for the evaluation of coronary artery disease in patients unable to exercise. *Am J Cardiol* 72:1257, 1993.

184. Jaarsma W, Visser CA, Kupper AJF, et al: Usefulness of two-dimensional exercise echocardiography shortly after myocardial infarction. *Am J Cardiol* 57:86, 1986.

185. Ryan T, Armstrong WF, O'Donnell JA, Feigenbaum H: Risk stratification after acute myocardial infarction by means of exercise two-dimensional echocardiography. *Am Heart J* 114:1305, 1987.

186. Applegate RJ, Dell'Italia IJ, Crawford MH: Usefulness of two-dimensional echocardiography during low-level exercise testing early after uncomplicated acute myocardial infarction. *Am J Cardiol* 60:10, 1987.

187. Krivokapich J, Child JS, Gerber RS, et al: Prognostic usefulness of positive or negative exercise stress echocardiography for predicting coronary events in ensuing twelve months. *Am J Cardiol* 71:646, 1993.

188. Brown KA: Prognostic value of cardiac imaging in patients with known or suspected coronary artery disease: Comparison of myocardial perfusion imaging, stress echocardiography, and positron emission tomography. *Am J Cardiol* 75:35D, 1995.

189. Sawada SG, Ryan T, Conley MJ, et al: Prognostic value of normal exercise echocardiogram. *Am Heart J* 120:49, 1990.

190. Bateman TM, O'Keff J, Barnhart C, et al: Clinical comparison of cardiac events during follow up after a nonischemic exercise test suggests superiority of SPECT ^{201}Tl over echocardiography (abstr). *J Am Coll Cardiol* 21:67A, 1993.

191. Eitzman D, Al-Aour Z, Kanter HL, et al: Clinical outcome of patients with advanced coronary artery disease after viability studies with positron emission tomography. *J Am Coll Cardiol* 20:559, 1992.

192. Lee KS, Marwick TH, Cook SA, et al: Prognosis of patients with left ventricular dysfunction, with and without viable myocardium after myocardial infarction. *Circulation* 90:2687, 1994.

193. DiCarli MF, Davidson M, Little R, et al: Value of metabolic imaging with positron emission tomography for evaluating prognosis in patients with coronary artery disease and left ventricular dysfunction. *Am J Cardiol* 73:527, 1994.

194. Yoshida K, Gould LK: Quantitative relation of myocardial infarction size and myocardial viability by positron emission tomography to left ventricular ejection fraction and 3-year mortality with and without revascularization. *J Am Coll Cardiol* 22:984, 1993.

195. Tamaki N, Kawamoto M, Takahashi N, et al: Prognostic value of an increase in fluorine 18 deoxyglucose uptake in patients with myocardial infarction: Comparison with stress thallium imaging. *J Am Coll Cardiol* 22:1621, 1993.

196. Gibbons RJ: Rest and exercise radionuclide angiography for diagnosis in chronic ischemic heart disease. *Circulation* 84:193, 1991.

197. Beller GA, Gibson RS: Sensitivity, specificity and prognostic significance of noninvasive testing for occult or known coronary disease. *Prog Cardiovasc Dis* 29:241, 1987.

198. Borer JS, Bacharach SL, Green MV: Radionuclide cineangiography in the evaluation of patients with heart disease: The perspective of the decade. *Cardiovasc Rev Rep* 12:14,31,70, 1991.

199. Dymond DS: Radionuclide assessment of ventricular function in patients with coronary artery disease: Clinical perspective. *Br Med Bull* 45:881, 1989.

200. Iskandrian AS, Hakki AH: Radionuclide evaluation of exercise left ventricular performance in patients with coronary artery disease. *Am Heart J* 110:851, 1985.

201. Rigo P, Murray M, Strauss HW, et al: Left ventricular function in acute myocardial infarction by gated scintiphotography. *Circulation* 50:678, 1974.

202. Schelbert HR, Henning H, Ashburn W, et al: Serial measurements of left ventricular ejection fraction by radionuclide angiography early and late after myocardial infarction. *Am J Cardiol* 38:407, 1976.

203. Schulze RA, Strauss HW, Pitt B: Sudden death in the year following myocardial infarction: Relation to ventricular premature contractions in the late hospital phase and left ventricular ejection fraction. *Am J Med* 62:192, 1977.

204. Reduto LA, Berger HJ, Cohen LS, et al: Sequential radionuclide assessment of left and right ventricular performance after acute transmural myocardial infarction. *Ann Intern Med* 89:441, 1978.

205. Borer JS, Rosing DR, Miller RH, et al: Natural history of left ventricular function during 1 year after acute myocardial infarction: Comparison with clinical, electrocardiographic and biochemical determinations. *Am J Cardiol* 46:1, 1980.

206. Corbett JR, Dehmer GJ, Lewis SE, et al: The prognostic value of submaximal exercise testing with radionuclide ventriculography before hospital discharge in patients with recent myocardial infarction. *Circulation* 64:535, 1981.

207. Multicenter Postinfarction Research Group: Risk stratification and survival after myocardial infarction. *N Engl J Med* 309:331, 1983.

208. Nicod P, Corbett JR, Firth BG, et al: Prognostic value of resting and submaximal exercise radionuclide ventriculogram after acute myocardial infarction in high-risk patients wtih single and multivessel disease. *Am J Cardiol* 52:30, 1983.

209. Dewhurst NG, Muir AL: Comparative prognostic value of radionuclide ventriculography at rest and during exercise in 100 patients after first myocardial infarction. *Br Heart J* 49:111, 1983.

210. Morris KG, Palmeri ST, Califf RM, et al: Value of radionuclide angiography for predicting specific cardiac events after acute myocardial infarction. *Am J Cardiol* 55:318, 1985.

211. Ong L, Green S, Reiser P, Morrison J: Early prediction of mortality in patients with acute myocardial infarction: A prospective study of clinical and radionuclide risk factors. *Am J Cardiol* 57:33, 1986.

212. Starling MR, Crawford MH, Henry RL, et al: Prognostic value of electrocardiographic exercise testing and noninvasive assessment of left ventricular ejection fraction soon after acute myocardial infarction. *Am J Cardiol* 57:532, 1986.

213. Stadius ML, Davis K, Maynard C, et al: Risk stratifica-

tion for 1 year survival based on characteristics identified in the early hours of acute myocardial infarction: The western Washington intracoronary streptokinase trial. *Circulation* 74:703, 1986.

214. Ahnve S, Gilpin E, Henning H, et al: Limitations and advantages of the ejection fraction for defining high risk after acute myocardial infarction. *Am J Cardiol* 58:872, 1986.

215. White HD, Norris RM, Brown MA, et al: Left ventricular end-systolic volume as the major determinant of survival after recovery from myocardial infarction. *Circulation* 76:44, 1987.

216. Kuchar DL, Thorburn CW, Sammel NL: Prediction of serious arrhythmic events after myocardial infarction: Signal averaged electrocardiogram, Holter monitoring and radionuclide ventriculography. *J Am Coll Cardiol* 9:531, 1987.

217. Hakki AH, Nestico PF, Heo J, et al: Relative prognostic value of rest thallium 201 imaging radionuclide ventriculography and 24-hour ambulatory electrocardiogaphic monitoring after acute myocardial infarction. *J Am Coll Cardiol* 10:25, 1987.

218. Gomes JA, Winters SL, Steward D, et al: A new noninvasive index to predict sustained ventricular tachycardia and sudden death in the first year after myocardial infarction: Based on signal-averaged electrocardiogram, radionuclide ejection fraction and Holter monitoring. *J Am Coll Cardiol* 10:3498, 1987.

219. Abraham RD, Harris PJ, Roubin GS, et al: Usefulness of ejection fraction response to exercise one month after acute myocardial infarction in predicting coronary anatomy and prognosis. *Am J Cardiol* 60:225, 1987.

220. Kuchar DL, Freund J, Yeates M, Sammel N: Enhanced prediction of major cardiac events after myocardial infarction using exercise radionuclide ventriculography. *Aust NZ J Med* 17:228, 1987.

221. Gabsboll N, Hoilund-Carlsen PF, Madsen EB, et al: Right and left ventricular ejection fractions: Relation to one-year prognosis in acute myocardial infarction. *Eur Heart J* 8:1201, 1987.

222. Zaret BL, Wackers FJ, Terrin M, et al: Does left ventricular ejection fraction following thrombolytic therapy have the same prognostic impact described in the prethrombolytic era? Results of the TIMI II Trial (abstr). *J Am Coll Cardiol* 17:214A, 1991.

223. Mazzotta G, Camerini A, Scopinaro G, et al: Predicting cardiac mortality after uncomplicated myocardial infarction by exercise radionuclide ventriculography and exercise-induced ST-segment elevation. *Eur Heart J* 13:330, 1992.

224. Harris PJ, Harrell FE, Lee KI, et al: Survival in medically treated coronary artery disease. *Circulation* 60:1259, 1979.

225. Mock MB, Ringqvist I, Fisher LD, et al: Survival of medically treated patients in the coronary artery surgery study (CASS) registry. *Circulation* 66:562, 1982.

226. Bonow RO, Epstein SE: Indications for coronary artery bypass surgery: Implications of the multicenter randomized trials. *Circulation* 72(suppl):V, 1985.

227. Jones RH, Floyd RD, Austin EH, Sabiston DC: The role of radionuclide angiocardiography in the preoperative prediction of pain relief and prolonged survival following coronary artery bypass grafting. *Ann Surg* 197:743, 1983.

228. Bonow RO, Kent KM, Rosing DR, et al: Exercise-induced ischemia in mildly symptomatic patients with coronary artery disease and preserved left ventricular function: Identification of subgroups at risk of death during medical therapy. *N Engl J Med* 311:1339, 1984.

229. Pryor DB, Harrell FE Jr, Lee KL, et al: Prognostic indicators from radionuclide angiography in medically treated patients with coronary artery disease. *Am J Cardiol* 53:18, 1984.

230. Iskandrian AS, Hakki AH, Goel IP, et al: The use of rest and exercise radionuclide ventriculography in risk stratification in patients with suspected coronary artery disease. *Am Heart J* 110:864, 1985.

231. Iskandrian AS, Hakki AH, Schwartz JS, et al: Prognostic implications of rest and exercise radionuclide ventriculography in patiens with suspected or proven coronary heart disease. *Int J Cardiol* 6:707, 1984.

232. Lee KL, Pryor DB, Pieper KS, et al: Prognostic value of radionuclide angiography in medically treated patients with coronary artery disease: A comparison with clinical and catheterization variables. *Circulation* 82:1705, 1990.

233. Jones RH, Johnson SH, Bigelow C, et al: Exercise radionuclide angiocardiography predicts cardiac death in patients with coronary artery disease. *Circulation* 84:I52, 1991.

234. Clements IP, Brown ML, Zinsmeister AR, et al: Influence of left ventricular diastolic filling on symptoms and survival in patients with decreased left ventricular systolic function. *Am J Cardiol* 67:1245, 1991.

235. Johnson SH, Bigelow C, Lee KL, et al: Prediction of death and myocardial infarction by radionuclide angiocardiography in patients with suspected coronary artery disease. *Am J Cardiol* 67:919, 1991.

236. Mazzotta G, Bonow RO, Pace L, et al: Relation between exertional ischemia and prognosis in mildly symptomatic patients with single or double vessel coronary artery disease and left ventricular dysfunction at rest. *J Am Coll Cardiol* 13:567, 1989.

237. Wallis JB, Holmes JR, Borer JS: Prognosis in patients with coronary artery disease and low ejection fraction at rest: Impact of exercise ejection fraction. *Am J Cardiol Imaging* 4:1, 1990.

238. Borer JS, Supino P, Wencker D, et al: Assessment of coronary artery disease by radionuclide cineangiography: History, current applications, and new directions, in Crawford MH (ed): *Cardiology Clinics, Nuclear Cardiology: State of the Art.* Philadelphia, WB Saunders Company, 1994, pp 333–357.

239. Braegelmann F, Herrold EM, Wallis J, et al: Ejection fraction change with exercise: Variation dependent on ejection fraction at rest (abstr). *Clin Res* 40:272A, 1992.

240. Borer JS, Wallis J, Hochreiter C, et al: Prognostic value of left ventricular dysfunction at rest and during exercise in patients with coronary artery disease. *Adv Cardiol* 34:179, 1986.

241. Borer JS, Wallis J, Holmes J, et al: Prognostication in

patients with coronary artery disease: Preliminary results of radionuclide cineangiographic studies. *Bull NY Acad Med* 59:847, 1983.

242. Dewhurst NG, Muir AL: Comparative prognostic value of radionuclide ventriculography at rest during exercise in 100 patients after first myocardial infarction. *Br Heart J* 49:111, 1983.

243. Roig E, Magrina J, Armengol X, et al: Prognostic value of exercise radionuclide angiography in low-risk acute myocardial infarction survivors. *Eur Heart J* 14:213, 1993.

244. Abraham RD, Harris PJ, Roubin GS, et al: Usefulness of ejection fraction response to exercise one month after acute myocardial infarction in predicting coronary anatomy and prognosis. *Am J Cardiol* 60:225, 1987.

245. Candell-Riera J, Permanyer-Miralda G, Castell J, et al: Uncomplicated first myocardial infarction: Strategy for comprehensive prognostic studies. *J Am Coll Cardiol* 18:1207, 1991.

246. Morris KG, Palmeri ST, Califf RM, et al: Value of radionuclide angiography for predicting specific cardiac events after acute myocardial infarction. *Am J Cardiol* 55:318, 1985.

Valvular Heart Disease

Claire S. Duvernoy
Mark R. Starling

The role of cardiac nuclear studies in the assessment of valvular heart disease is generally felt to be secondary to Doppler and two-dimensional echocardiography. Nuclear techniques can offer useful additional information, however, as well as data not available by other means to aid in assessing the functional consequences of each valve lesion. This chapter focuses primarily on left-sided regurgitant lesions because radionuclide angiography has proven most useful in defining the effect of these valve lesions on both right and left ventricular performance. Both right and left ventricular size and performance can be assessed serially, and the degree of regurgitation can be quantitated. Biventricular function can further be evaluated during exercise and after surgical or medical interventions. Moreover, the scintigraphic evaluation of myocardial perfusion in both regurgitant and stenotic valve lesions is examined.

ASSESSMENT OF THE SEVERITY OF VALVULAR REGURGITATION

The development of methods to quantitate the degree of valvular regurgitation has relied on the assumption that, in the absence of any right-sided regurgitation or intracardiac shunts, the left ventricular (LV) and right ventricular (RV) stroke volumes should be equal. In radionuclide angiography, stroke counts can be subsituted for stroke volumes because the two are proportional. Thus, the change in counts between systole and diastole over the right and left ventricles can be used to determine whether significant regurgitation is present. If left-sided valvular regurgitation is present, the LV stroke volume (or stroke counts) should exceed the RV stroke volume, or stroke counts, and the ratio of the two should be proportional to the degree of regurgitation. This assumption will be valid only if there is no right-sided regurgitant lesion or left-to-right intracardiac shunt. If there is concomitant mitral and aortic regurgitation, the ratio will reflect the sum of the regurgitant lesions; it is, therefore, valid chiefly for patients with isolated valvular lesions.

The technique was first described by Rigo et al in 1979. This group analyzed stroke count ratios in the left anterior oblique (LAO) 40° to 45° projection and compared their findings with an angiographic assessment of the extent of valvular regurgitation in 19 patients and 11 control subjects. They found good agreement between the two methods, when using semiquantitative groupings of stroke index ratio and a qualitative assessment of angiographic regurgitation.[1] This technique was subsequently described by several investigators[2,3] with generally good agreement between the noninvasive technique and invasive measurements. Urquhart et al further described the use of stroke count ratios to assess the success or failure of valve surgery. In 3 patients with clinical evidence of residual postoperative regurgitation, the

End Diastole	Mid Systole	End Systole

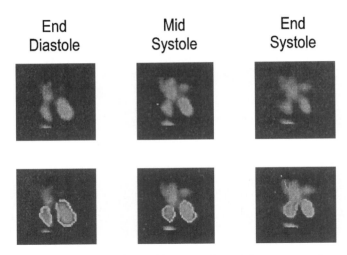

Figure 24-1 Gated equilibrium radionuclide angiography. Counts are obtained from end-diastole and end-systole for each ventricle by the varying region-of-interest method that minimizes overlap of ventricular and atrial activity. (From Sorensen et al,[6] by permission of the American Heart Association, Inc.)

stroke index ratio was greater than 2 standard deviations above the mean value in the control subjects.[2] In animal experiments performed by Baxter et al, the LV/RV stroke count ratio correlated closely with the direct measurement of regurgitant flow using electromagnetic flow-meters in a model of acutely induced aortic regurgitation.[4]

However, despite the initial enthusiasm, technique limitations quickly became apparent. Lam et al described discordant regurgitant indices in 12 of 100 patients whose radionuclide indices were compared with angiographic assessments. Factors that led to an inaccurate measurement were mitral valve prolapse with frequent premature ventricular contractions in 3 patients, and an LV ejection fraction (LVEF) of less than 0.30. In fact, discordance occurred in 8 of 10 patients with LV dysfunction.[5]

Refinements in the technique were subsequently described by a number of investigators. Sorensen et al described a "variable region-of-interest" approach, which required separate regions-of-interest constructed manually for each ventricle at end-diastole and end-systole.[6] (Fig. 24-1) Nicod et al modified the index further by measuring ventricular stroke counts from the stroke volume image, or the reverse stroke image, if the boundary of the stroke image could not be clearly defined. They then calculated regurgitant index directly from the ratio of the ventricular stroke counts.[7] Their assessment of all three methods revealed equivalent, very high specificities (> 97 percent), and greater sensitivity with their method than with the earlier methods, especially for less severe regurgitation. All three methods were less sensitive with greater LV dysfunction, as had been demonstrated earlier by Lam et al.[5]

First-pass radionuclide angiography was subsequently used to derive both right and left ventricular stroke counts, which then could be used to calculate the regurgitant fraction according to the formula:

$$\text{Regurgitant fraction (RF)} = (C_L - C_R)/C_L$$

where C_L and C_R refer to LV and RV ejected counts, respectively. Janowitz and Fester found good correlation ($r = 0.86$) between this method and invasive angiographic data.[8] Henze et al attempted to correct for the inevitable contamination of RV counts by right atrial activity by subtracting one-half of the right atrial counts obtained from the RV counts in the standard LAO projection.[9] They found good separation between normals and patients with known aortic or mitral regurgitation, and they were further able to document a significant decrease in regurgitant fraction with exercise.

A combination of first-pass and equilibrium radionuclide ventriculography was used by Klepzig et al to permit the quantitation of effective left ventricular stroke volume (SV_{eff}). This value was then used to calculate a radionuclide regurgitant fraction, defined as the difference between total and effective stroke volume as a fraction of total LV stroke volume:

$$(EF \times EDV - SV_{eff})/EF \times EDV$$

Comparison of the radionuclide regurgitant fraction and LV/RV stroke count ratio with angiographic regurgitant fraction revealed superior sensitivity and equal specificity for the former method (100 percent versus 87 percent sensitivity, 100 percent specificity for both). The correlation coefficient for angiographic and radionuclide regurgitant fraction was 0.79 ($p < 0.001$), while that for angiography and LV/RV stroke count ratio was much lower ($r = 0.47$, $p < 0.05$).[10] Further refinements in the radionuclide evaluation of valvular regurgitation were carried out by Makler et al using first-harmonic Fourier analysis of gated blood pool scans.[11,12] This method generates two functional images of the heart. The phase image provides pixel-by-pixel information on timing of contraction, and the amplitude image, which was used for the calculation of regurgitant fraction by these investigators, gives the magnitude of the count–density change during the cardiac cycle. It clearly separates the four chambers of the heart, a noted drawback in the stroke count ratio method. Good agreement ($r = 0.84$) was found between the radionuclide and hemodynamic determination of the degree of regurgitation using this method (Fig. 24-2).

There is not a great deal of information available regarding the quantitation of right-sided regurgitant lesions, but a determination of stroke count ratio should intuitively offer analogous information to that gained in the assessment of left-sided regurgitant lesions. Thus,

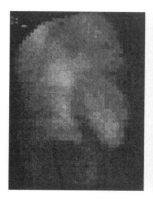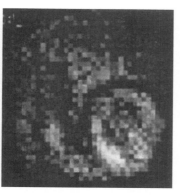

Figure 24-2 First-harmonic Fourier analysis of gated cardiac blood pool. Left panel shows a 40° left anterior oblique view of the heart. Separation of the chambers is difficult, as is precise determination of the location of ventricular boundaries. Right panel shows the amplitude image generated from this study. Clear separation between atria and ventricles is evident. (From Makler et al,[11] Fourier amplitude ratio: a new way to assess valvular regurgitation, reprinted with permission from the *Journal of Nuclear Medicine,* 24:204, 1983.)

Handler et al described the detection of tricuspid insufficiency using the ratio of RV − LV stroke counts to RV stroke counts.[13] Left-to-right shunts can also be accurately quantified using gated radionuclide angiography. Sorensen et al evaluated 9 patients undergoing cardiac catheterization for the evaluation of left-to-right shunts, and found good correlation between pulmonary/systemic flow ratios (Qp/Qs) calculated by radionuclide angiography, and Qp/Qs defined by oximetry ($r = 0.87$). In 5 patients who subsequently underwent successful surgical repair, the radionuclide angiography Qp/Qs declined from a mean of 2.9 ± 1.0 to 1.1 ± 0.2. The authors concluded that shunt ratios, as well as RV performance and relative ventricular enlargement, can be noninvasively defined and followed serially before and after therapeutic intervention using gated radionuclide angiography.[14]

Comparison between Radionuclide and Echocardiographic Assessment of the Severity of Valvular Regurgitation

Color-flow imaging is commonly used in echocardiography to semiquantitatively assess the degree of valvular regurgitation. The severity of regurgitation is determined by the width and area of the regurgitant jet.[15] Caution must be used, however, when estimating regurgitant volume by means of color-flow Doppler imaging. Losordo et al experimented with known volumes of echogenic material ejected from one chamber into another and found that the volume of material ejected appeared greater at faster velocities. They concluded that color-flow analysis may be more a reflection of the velocity,

rather than the volume, of a regurgitant jet.[16] Other methods require the use of continuous- and pulsed-wave Doppler echocardiography. In aortic regurgitation (AR), continuous-wave Doppler determination of the pressure half-time of the AR signal, and pulsed-wave analysis of the mitral inflow velocity deceleration time allow for accurate assessment of the severity of the regurgitant lesion.[17,18] Actual calculation of the regurgitant fraction can also be performed. The echocardiographic regurgitant volume is the difference between systemic flow volume (determined from another valve with little or no regurgitation) and forward flow through the regurgitant valve. The regurgitant fraction then becomes the percentage of regurgitant volume compared to total forward flow across the valve.[19] A direct comparison of Doppler-derived regurgitant fraction (DOPRF) and radionuclide regurgitant fraction (RIRF) was carried out by Kurokawa et al. These investigators analyzed patients with both AR and mitral regurgitation (MR) and compared Doppler, radionuclide, and cineangiographic assessments of regurgitant severity. They found a good correlation between DOPRF and RIRF ($r = 0.79$, $p < 0.01$), and generally good agreement between cineangiographic severity of regurgitation (graded mild, moderate, and severe) and increasing DOPRF.[20]

A newer technique described by Recusani et al looks at the region of flow convergence proximal to the regurgitant lesion and is known as proximal isovelocity surface area (PISA). Blood flow accelerates progressively as it converges toward the regurgitant orifice, at which point it attains its maximal velocity (Fig. 24-3). The severity of regurgitation can be related quantitatively to the region of proximal flow convergence.[21] This method can give an accurate estimate of regurgitant flow rates and can be used in conjunction with continuous-wave Doppler measurements of the maximal velocity of flow through the orifice to calculate the orifice area. This calculation, which is analogous to the orifice area calculated in stenotic lesions, may be less dependent on loading conditions than both regurgitant flow rate and regurgitant volume or fraction and may, therefore, be a more accurate parameter for grading regurgitant lesion severity.[22,23] A further modification of the flow convergence method, called the centerline velocity profile method, was tested by Shiota et al, to overcome the potential limitations caused by the variable shape of the regurgitant orifice. They were able to show a clear separation of flow profiles for three different flow rates analyzed in their orifice models, when using this method.[24]

Evaluation of right-sided regurgitant lesions is commonly carried out using color-flow and Doppler echocardiography. As with left-sided lesions, semiquantitative assessment using color-flow imaging is by far the most prevalent technique, and it is very sensitive for even trivial amounts of regurgitation, which may be considered normal.[25] Severe tricuspid regurgitation is also deter-

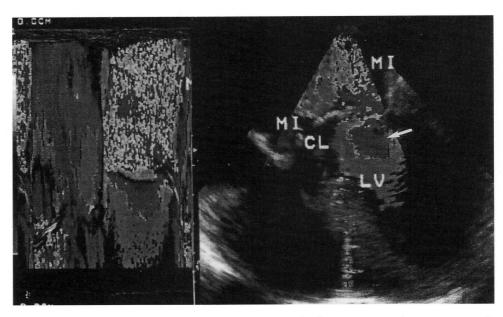

Figure 24-3 Transesophageal intraoperative color Doppler flow map image from a patient with mitral regurgitation demonstrating the region of proximal flow convergence (*arrow*) seen within the left ventricular cavity. MI, mitral valve; LV, left ventricle; CL, cleft. (From Simpson and Sahn,[239] by permission of the American Heart Association, Inc.)

mined by increased tricuspid inflow velocity, and by systolic flow reversal in the hepatic vein, as assessed by Doppler echocardiography.

Because the velocity at a regurgitant valve is a direct representation of pressure drop across that valve, Doppler analysis can be used to arrive at intracardiac pressures as well. Thus, the tricuspid regurgitation (TR) velocity reflects the pressure difference between the right ventricle and atrium, and can be used to calculate right ventricular systolic pressure (RVSP) using the formula:

$$(\text{TR velocity}^2 \times 4) + \text{estimated right atrial pressure}$$

Currie et al compared RVSP derived in this fashion with right-sided cardiac pressure measurements performed during cardiac catheterization; they found an excellent correlation between the two methods ($r = 0.96$) in those patients in whom TR was adequately analyzable by continuous-wave Doppler echocardiography. This was the case in approximately 80 percent of patients with increased, and 57 percent of patients with normal RV pressures.[26]

In summary, both radionuclide angiography and Doppler echocardiography offer accurate noninvasive methods whereby the severity of valvular regurgitation can be quantitated. Radionuclide angiography offers excellent reproducibility for serial measurements of ventricular size and performance, as will be discussed below; it is also advantageous in patients with poor echocardiographic windows due to body habitus or pulmonary disease. In clinical practice, it is much less commonly

used to quantify valvular regurgitation for several reasons. Echocardiography is a more portable, generally less expensive technique, which allows the clinician the ability to evaluate valve morphology by two-dimensional analysis in addition to measuring chamber sizes, estimating LV mass, and analyzing the severity of valvular regurgitation by Doppler technique. Color Doppler analysis is most commonly used semiquantitatively to stratify the severity of the regurgitant lesion as mild, moderate, or severe. Regurgitant fraction is not generally calculated in clinical practice. In patients with lesions of questionable severity, it is certainly reasonable to obtain regurgitant fraction by either method to provide a more complete assessment of disease status.

AORTIC REGURGITATION

Pathophysiology

The classical features of chronic AR include the presence of LV (stroke) volume overload, which initially results in LV dilation with a normal ejection fraction. In contrast to MR, aortic insufficiency also leads to increased afterload as measured by systolic wall stress. The left ventricle dilates to provide increased LV systolic tension and maintain an adequate level of systolic pressure. Increases in wall stress lead to the replication of sarcomeres in series and elongation of fibers, and to the replication

Relationship of EF and Stress in Aortic Regurgitation

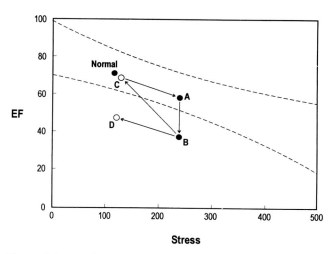

Figure 24-4   Relationship of ejection fraction (EF) and stress in aortic regurgitation. Point A indicates asymptomatic, untreated patients with aortic regurgitation; there is a mild decline in EF, and a marked increase in wall stress. Point B shows the development of LV contractile dysfunction in these patients. Point C shows the result of aortic valve replacement in patients with a brief (≤ 14 months) period of contractile dysfunction, indicating the removal of the heightened wall stress, and the capacity of the left ventricle to recover contractile performance. Point D shows the result of aortic valve replacement in patients with prolonged (> 18 months) contractile dysfunction; wall stress diminishes, but the ejection fraction remains abnormal.

of sarcomeres in parallel, both to decrease systolic and diastolic wall stress in this valve lesion manifest by persistent afterload excess. The ratio of ventricular wall thickness to cavity radius remains normal.[27] With time, myocardial hypertrophy and fibrosis develop, and progressive, eventually irreversible LV dysfunction will result if the lesion is not corrected. Symptoms of congestive heart failure (CHF) will develop when the compensatory mechanisms noted above—dilation of the ventricle, increased LV muscle mass, and wall thickness—can no longer maintain forward cardiac output. Unfortunately, symptom onset is variable from patient to patient, and an irreversible decline in LV performance can occur before the manifestation of significant symptoms[28] (Fig. 24-4).

Optimal management of patients with AR requires precise knowledge of the patient's LV size and performance under a variety of loading conditions in addition to knowledge regarding the severity of the regurgitant lesion. Patients may not manifest cardiac symptoms despite increasing LV dysfunction because of progressive lifestyle changes; it is, therefore, crucial to serially assess LV performance to define disease progression to make the best decision regarding the need for and timing of valve replacement. With the onset of CHF, the course

is progressive and the prognosis is poor without valve replacement.[29] Unfortunately, valve replacement in patients with symptoms is associated with higher operative risk and a greater chance for persistence of symptoms or death after surgery compared to patients without preoperative symptoms. The presence of both LV dysfunction and cardiac symptoms in patients with severe AR predicts an increased risk of cardiac death following AR replacement.[30–32]

Resting Left Ventricular Performance in Aortic Regurgitation—Radionuclide Assessment

Numerous investigators have attempted to use radionuclide ventriculography in the assessment of patients with AR, both to serially evaluate LVEF and to determine optimal timing for valve replacement. From angiographic studies in symptomatic and asymptomatic patients with severe AR and abnormal resting LV performance, it appears that valve replacement is usually indicated if the LVEF is less than 45 percent.[30,33–36]

Radionuclide ventriculography can provide serial noninvasive measurements of LVEF and can, therefore, play a useful role in the selection of patients for aortic valve replacement. Serial radionuclide measurements of resting LVEF show virtually no mean change over 3 months in groups of clinically stable patients with chronic AR. In contrast, in individual patients with AR and stable hemodynamics, the resting LVEF can fluctuate substantially with serial measurements 3 months apart. In a study of 22 clinically stable patients with chronic AR studied on two occasions 3 months apart, Cornyn et al found that an 8 percent change in resting LVEF was required to be 95 percent certain that the change was not due to the variability inherent in the radionuclide technique.[37] Therefore, the decision for surgical intervention should not be based on minor differences in repeated measurements of LVEF.

Radionuclide assessment of left ventricular end-diastolic volume (LVEDV) in relation to regurgitant volume has also been proposed as a useful marker for determining timing of aortic valve replacement. Kress et al studied a group of 54 patients with chronic AR, 24 of whom underwent surgical repair during the study, and 30 of whom remained clinically stable. They found that an LVEDV greater than 300 ml was a marker for appearance of symptoms and fall in LVEF. They also noted that if the ratio of LVEDV to regurgitant volume remained normal, even if both increased, patients generally remained asymptomatic.[38] Analysis of LV geometry by radionuclide angiography can also be performed; Starling et al have suggested that LV contractile dysfunction is in part related to a configurational change in the ventricle from ellipsoid to spherical, reflecting inadequate eccentric hypertrophy.[39]

In contrast, others have found that radionuclide angiography at rest has not proven useful for predicting which asymptomatic patients with a normal resting LVEF will develop progressive hemodynamic deterioration or symptoms requiring valve replacement. Bonow et al followed 77 asymptomatic patients with severe AR, a normal resting radionuclide LVEF, and a normal echocardiographic LV percent fractional shortening. During a mean follow-up of 49 months (range 6 to 114), no patient died; 11 patients underwent aortic valve replacement following the onset of symptoms and 1 patient, who remained asymptomatic, underwent valve replacement for LV dysfunction.[40] All 12 patients survived surgery and all showed improvement in resting and exercise LVEF postoperatively. One can conclude from this study that aortic valve replacement is not indictated in the asymptomatic patient with a normal resting LVEF. Surgery can be postponed until symptoms appear or until resting LV performance deteriorates. Patients in whom the duration of LV dysfunction is relatively brief (approximately 14 months or less) will generally show a greater increase in both short- and long-term postoperative LVEF, a greater postoperative decrease in LV dilation, and increased overall postoperative survival, when compared with patients in whom LV dysfunction has been present for a prolonged period[41–43] (Fig. 24-5). In patients with normal resting LV performance and recent onset of symptoms, surgery will carry minimal risk and will produce excellent results. Thus, an abnormal resting LVEF is useful for determining the timing of aortic valve replacement, but a normal resting LVEF measurement is not. Serial assessment of asymptomatic patients with an initially normal LVEF should be carried out at yearly intervals; when the resting LVEF falls below normal, reassessment in 1 to 3 months should be done to confirm the abnormal finding, followed by aortic valve replacement if indicated by a persistently abnormal value.[44]

Left ventricular contractility can be evaluated separately from changes in LV preload by analyzing LV end-systolic pressure–volume relations, which are used to evaluate LV contractility separately from changes in LV preload.

Left Ventricular End-Systolic Pressure–Volume Relations

The LVEF is altered by changes in preload and afterload, as well as myocardial contractility. In AR, LV dilatation (increased preload) is an important mechanism for maintaining cardiac output. The LV end-systolic pressure–volume relation offers an alternative method for evaluating LV contractility that is independent of loading conditions. The slope of the line connecting the upper left corners of LV pressure–volume loops changes with inotropic intervention, is minimally dependent on loading conditions, and, thus, is a useful index for the evaluation of LV contractility.[45–47] The ratio of the end-systolic pressure to end-systolic volume has been used as an estimate of contractility. Further, in previous studies, the peak systolic pressure has been used as a substitute for end-systolic pressure in the evaluation of the pressure–volume relationship. Such an approximation permits the noninvasive evaluation of the pressure–volume relationship by using the cuff method to measure the peak systolic pressure and radionuclide angiography to calculate end-systolic volume. However, on theoretical grounds, one would expect a peak systolic pressure to end-systolic volume ratio, which is derived from a single point on the pressure–volume loop, to be a less reliable index of contractility than the slope of the end-systolic pressure–volume relationship, which is derived over a range of loading conditions.

Schuler et al performed gated equilibrium radionuclide angiography in 9 normal subjects and 14 asymptomatic patients with isolated AR who had normal resting LV performance. The LVEDV was measured by a method based on counts. The peak systolic pressure, measured by the cuff method, was used instead of the end-systolic pressure. The slope of the pressure–volume relation was determined in each patient at various levels of systolic blood pressure by infusing a diluted methoxamine solution. The slope of the peak systolic pressure to end-systolic volume relationship was significantly lower in patients with AR than in normal subjects (3.1 ± 1.1 versus 4.1 ± 0.5) (mean ± SD)[48] (Fig. 24-6). Patients with AR could be classified into two subgroups with respect to the slope. In one group, the slope was within the normal range as defined by control subjects, and all patients in this group had a normal LVEF response to exercise. In the second group, the slope was significantly lower than the normal slope, indicating depressed contractility. The latter patients had an abnormal LVEF response to exercise. Therefore, an abnormal baseline contractile state in asymptomatic patients with AR may be revealed by noninvasive determination of the end-systolic pressure–volume relation, and may be uncovered in an abnormal LVEF response to exercise. These observations have been confirmed by others.[49,50] An abnormality in the end-systolic pressure–volume relationship may be evoked by increasing afterload in some patients with mild or no symptoms even if echocardiographic parameters of LV size and performance are normal.[51] Thus, abnormalities in the end-systolic pressure–volume relationship may represent one of the earliest markers of depressed LV performance in patients with AR. It is a parameter that can be useful to explain the pathophysiologic mechanisms behind depressed LV performance, that is, depressed myocardial contractility, increased LV wall stress, and depressed LVEF.[52] An abnormal end-systolic pressure–volume slope has, however, been found in a majority of patients with AR in

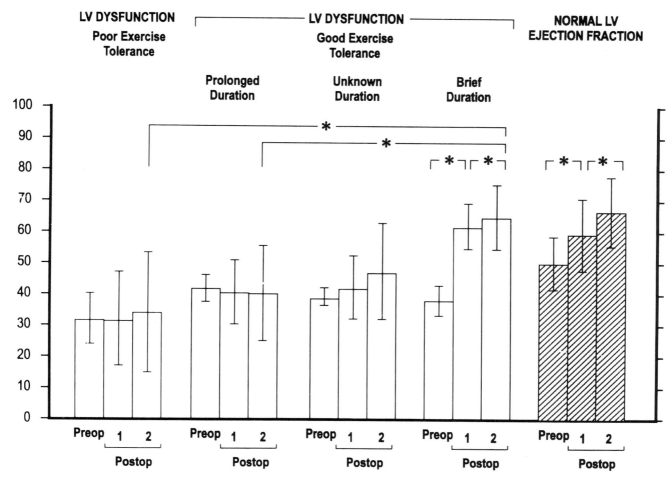

Figure 24-5   Resting left ventricular (LV) ejection fraction before (preop) and after (postop) operation in patients with normal and abnormal LV performance. Postoperative data are shown at 6 to 8 months (1) and 3 to 7 years (2). Patients who had a brief duration of preoperative LV dysfunction were significantly more likely to show a postoperative increase in LV ejection fraction than those who had either a prolonged or an unknown period of LV dysfunction preoperatively. Patients with poor exercise tolerance and preoperative LV dysfunction did not show a postoperative improvement in LV performance. Asterisks indicate significant differences. (From Bonow et al,[43] by permission of the American Heart Association, Inc.)

some studies,[50] making it too sensitive to be used clinically in guiding the timing of aortic valve replacement.

Left Ventricular Performance During Atrial Pacing

In patients with severe AR, rapid atrial pacing or dynamic exercise can be used to detect LV dysfunction that may precede symptoms. Radionuclide ventriculography has been used in numerous studies designed to elucidate the effects of these interventions on ejection phase indices and forward cardiac output. Atrial pacing alters not only the heart rate but also the LVEDV (preload). The effects of heart rate in AR were described by Corrigan in 1832:

The nature of the disease (aortic regurgitation) is in proportion to the quantity of blood that regurgitates, and the quantity that regurgitates will be large in proportion to the degree of inadequacy of the valves and to the length of the pause between the contractions of the ventricle, during which the blood can be pouring back. If the action of the heart be rendered very slow, the pause after each contraction will be long and consequently the regurgitation of blood must be considerable. Frequent action of the heart on the contrary makes the pause after each contraction short and in proportion as the pauses are shortened, the regurgitation must be lessened.[53]

Thus, more than 150 years ago, the changes in end-diastolic volume during tachycardia in patients with AR were thought to be directionally opposite to those ob-

A

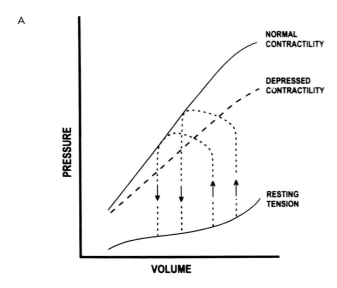

END-SYSTOLIC PRESSURE-VOLUME RELATION -- SCHULER ET AL

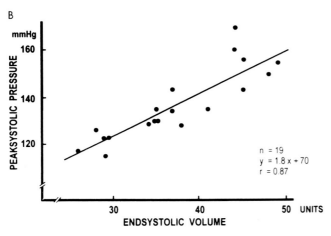

$n = 19$
$y = 1.8 x + 70$
$r = 0.87$

Figure 24-6 Depiction of the end-systolic pressure–volume relation. **Panel A:** The physiologic basis is the Frank-Starling diagram. End points of all LV contractions arising from any point on the resting tension curve are described by a straight line whose slope (LV chamber elastance) is an index of myocardial contractility. **Panel B:** Depiction of the end-systolic pressure–volume relation determined by radionuclide angiography and cuff pressure measurements in a patient with severe aortic regurgitation. (From Schuler et al,[48] by permission from the American Heart Association, Inc.)

served in normal subjects or in patients with coronary artery disease (CAD). This is an important observation because changes in LVEDV (preload) and changes in blood pressure may substantially alter ejection phase indices such as the LVEF irrespective of any change in LV contractility. Judge et al used atrial pacing in 8 patients with AR and measured LVEDV by contrast angiography. His group confirmed that rapid atrial pacing caused a decrease in the end-diastolic volume.[54] Forward cardiac output increases with increasing heart rate dur-

ing atrial pacing in patients with AR, and LVEDV and total and forward stroke volume typically decrease during pacing-induced tachycardia. There is a decrease in the time available per cardiac cycle for regurgitant flow. Although the regurgitant volume per stroke decreases, the regurgitant volume per minute does not. Thus, the decrease in end-diastolic volume produced by rapid atrial pacing is accompanied by a decrease in regurgitant flow per stroke but not in regurgitant fraction.[55]

Left Ventricular Performance During Exercise

Numerous investigators have used exercise testing with or without echocardiography or radionuclide angiography in an attempt to define the optimum timing of valve replacement in asymptomatic patients with AR and to identify predictors of outcome after surgery. The exercise test can be used to measure functional capacity and to provide an objective assessment of the presence or absence of symptoms. Unfortunately, no level of exercise capacity has been identified which can, by itself, be used to determine the timing of aortic valve replacement. Kligfield et al observed that horizontal or downsloping ST-segment depression on treadmill testing correlated with the presence of severely impaired LV performance and geometry in patients with AR, even if they were clinically asymptomatic.[56] Whether exercise-induced ST-segment depression can provide clinically useful information for the timing of aortic valve replacement in patients with AR is currently unknown. Presently, exercise testing in patients with AR is commonly performed in addition to a test for measurement of LV performance, such as echocardiography or radionuclide angiography.

Results of surgery in symptomatic patients with AR depend on the preoperative functional class and can be predicted by the level of exercise tolerance. In symptomatic patients with AR and a subnormal preoperative shortening fraction by echocardiography, Bonow et al showed that limited treadmill exercise capacity was associated with a poor long-term survival after aortic valve replacement and with limited reversibility of LV dysfunction.[57] In symptomatic patients with severe AR but no evidence of resting LV dysfunction, patients with equivocal or inconsistent symptoms, or patients in whom there is reason to suspect that symptoms might be underestimated or overestimated, exercise testing may be helpful.

Exercise testing is useful for detecting early evidence of LV dysfunction as well as for uncovering early symptoms in patients with AR. Multiple hemodynamic mechanisms are involved because dynamic exercise produces important changes in myocardial contractility and in loading conditions in addition to changes in heart rate. Several groups have found that the observed reduction in regurgitant fraction with exercise is most likely due

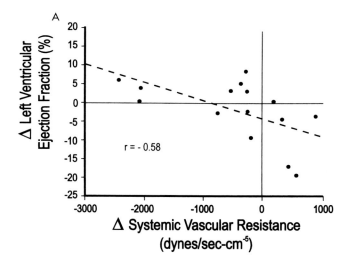

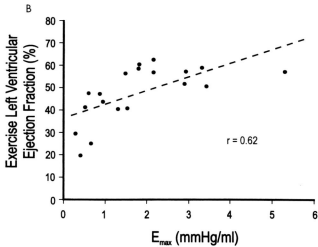

Figure 24-7 **Panel A:** Relationship between the change in LV ejection fraction from rest to exercise and the change in systemic vascular resistance (SVR). The greater the decline in SVR, the larger the increase in LV ejection fraction with exercise. **Panel B:** Relationship between the exercise LV ejection fraction and LV chamber elastance (E_{max}). Individual data points, regression lines, and correlation coefficients are noted. (From Stewart et al,[52] reproduced with permission.)

to the reduction in systemic vascular resistance with exercise[52,58] (Fig. 24-7). Dehmer et al found that while LV diastolic and systolic volume indices increased significantly with supine bicycle exercise in patients with AR and cardiac symptoms, patients with minimal or no symptoms showed no change in LV volume in response to exercise.[59] A decrease in LV diastolic volume is more likely to be observed with upright exercise, in younger patients, in patients with normal exercise tolerance, and in patients with large LVEDV at rest.[60–62] It is possible that a decrease in LVEDV with exercise may limit the increase in LV end-diastolic pressure (LVEDP) in these patients and, therefore, preserve exercise capacity.

In contrast to findings during atrial pacing, forward stroke volume (defined as total LV stroke volume minus

regurgitant volume) may increase during exercise in patients with AR and normal LV performance. This may relate to the inotropic effects associated with exercise. Also, in contrast to the measurements made during atrial pacing, numerous studies have demonstrated that the regurgitant fraction decreases with dynamic exercise.[63–65] Although total stroke volume is unchanged (or may even fall related to decreasing LVEDV), forward stroke volume may increase in the face of a decreasing regurgitant volume. These findings may further explain the preservation of exercise capacity in many patients with AR.

Borer et al in 1978 reported the first study using rest and exercise radionuclide angiography in patients with AR. In their study, the resting LVEF was abnormal in 7 of 21 symptomatic patients and in 1 of 22 asymptomatic patients. During exercise, however, all but 1 patient in the symptomatic group had an abnormal LVEF response (exercise LVEF ≤ 55 percent), whereas only 9 asymptomatic patients had an abnormal LVEF during exercise.[66] This study demonstrated that an abnormal exercise LVEF may be seen in asymptomatic patients with normal resting LV performance, and suggested that abnormalities in exercise LV performance often precede the development of resting LV dysfunction. Hecht et al pointed out that, in patients with volume overload related to AR, LV regional wall-motion abnormalities can be seen in the absence of concomitant CAD.[67]

Some authors have suggested that the exercise LVEF is a more sensitive indicator of LV dysfunction than resting echocardiographic parameters such as LV end-systolic volume and percent fractional shortening. In a study performed by Lewis et al, angiographic and echocardiographic data were compared with the LVEF response to exercise in 15 patients with AR who had no or minimal symptoms. During exercise, 5 patients had a normal LVEF response to exercise and 10 had an abnormal response. However, only 4 of 10 patients with an abnormal LVEF response to exercise had an angiographic LV end-systolic volume index (LVESVI) of 60 ml/m² or more, and only one had an echocardiographic end-systolic dimension of 55 mm or more.[68] Siemienczuk et al identified several LV parameters that were important prognostically in patients progressing to surgery. They included LV end-diastolic volume index (LVEDVI), LVESVI, LV end-systolic wall stress, and LVEF at maximal exercise[69] (Fig. 24-8). Therefore, it may be that exercise radionuclide ventriculography identifies LV dysfunction in patients with AR earlier than traditional methods using contrast angiography or echocardiography. In contrast, when Bonow et al performed a multivariate Cox analysis of factors associated with adverse outcome in a cohort of asymptomatic patients with AR, only age and LV end-systolic dimension were significant predictors.[44]

In interpreting the results of these various reports, it should be kept in mind that patient selection may have an important influence on exercise radionuclide LVEF.

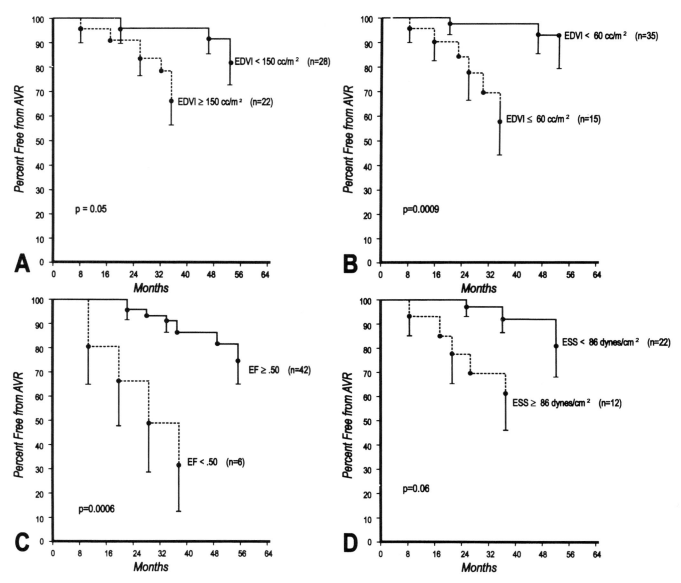

Figure 24-8 Univariate life-table analysis showing the progression to aortic valve replacement (AVR) in groups segregated by variables measured at baseline. Standard error bars are shown. **Panel A:** Left ventricular end-diastolic volume index (EDVI) of 150 cc/m² or more compared with less than 150 cc/m². **Panel B:** Left ventricular end-systolic volume index (ESVI) of 60 cc/m² or more compared with less than 60 cc/m². **Panel C:** Left ventricular ejection fraction (EF) at maximal exercise of 0.50 or more compared with less than 0.50. **Panel D:** End-systolic wall stress (ESS) of 86 dynes/cm² or more compared with less than 86 dynes/cm². Progression to surgery was earlier in patients with larger ventricles, higher ESS, or lower exercise LVEF. (From Siemienczuk et al,[69] reproduced with permission.)

Thus, the age of the patient, the severity of AR, the presence of associated diseases [such as aortic stenosis, (AS), MR, or CAD], medications, the functional class of the patient, the type of exercise (upright versus supine), the adequacy of LV hypertrophy for reducing wall stress, and the intensity of exercise might all be important factors that modify the response of LVEF to exercise.[44,61,70-72] For example, Shen et al demonstrated that a sublingual dose of 20 mg nifedipine resulted in im-

provement in the exercise LVEF, with a decrease in regurgitant index at rest and during exercise. It is also important to keep in mind that the response of the LVEF to exercise fluctuates somewhat over time in the absence of a change in clinical status. In 22 clinically stable patients with chronic AR studied on two occasions 3 months apart, Cornyn et al noted only a 2 percent difference in mean exercise LVEF measurements. However, the standard deviation for the group differences in exercise LVEF was 5 percent, and a difference of 10 percent in the LVEF from one study to the next was required to establish with 95 percent confidence that a significant serial change was present in an individual patient.[37]

In the analysis of asymptomatic AR patients with normal resting LV performance performed by Bonow et al, the exercise LVEF did identify a subgroup of patients who were likely to develop cardiac symptoms and require valve replacement. Of 24 patients, who had a greater than 5-unit decrease in LVEF from rest to exercise in the initial study, 33 percent required aortic valve replacement within 4 years. Although certain echocardiographic measurements—such as the LV end-systolic dimension, end-diastolic dimension, and percent fractional shortening—were also found to be predictors of subsequent requirement for surgery, it was evident that no single measurement at one point in time (other than an abnormal resting LVEF, measured on two occasions) could be used as the sole criterion for aortic valve replacement.[40]

The precise clinical role of the exercise radionuclide ventriculogram in asymptomatic patients with AR remains to be clarified. It may be that a totally normal rest and exercise LVEF response excludes clinically important impairment of LV contractility and predicts a relatively slow progression of disease, permitting follow-up at longer intervals than in patients with an abnormal response. Alternatively, an abnormal exercise LVEF response may signal a phase of relatively rapid progression to resting LV dysfunction, and herald the need for frequent follow-up and testing.[73] Although Bonow et al followed some asymptomatic patients with normal resting but abnormal exercise radionuclide LV performance for up to 4 years and found no deterioration of resting or exercise LV performance,[74] others have observed more rapid deterioration in this group. Peter and Jones observed a 6-unit mean decline in exercise LVEF by radionuclide determination over a 1-year period in 10 patients with severe AR. Most, but not all, of the patients were asymptomatic or minimally symptomatic.[62]

An improved understanding of the hemodynamic mechanisms underlying changes in LVEF with exercise could clarify the usefulness of this parameter in predicting the need for aortic valve replacement. Massie et al reported the hemodynamic correlates of radionuclide ventriculography during exercise in asymptomatic or mildly symptomatic patients with severe AR. Patients having a greater than 5-unit decrease in LVEF with exercise had a smaller rise in cardiac output and a greater rise in pulmonary capillary wedge pressure (PCWP) with exercise than did patients in whom the LVEF increased or did not decrease by more than 5 units ($p < 0.01$).[75] Boucher et al noted that a peak exercise PCWP of 15 mmHg or greater identified patients with AR who had significantly lower LVEFs and higher LVESV at peak exercise, compared to patients with AR who had more

normal PCWPs at peak exercise.[76] Stewart et al further defined the mechanisms responsible for an abnormal LVEF response to exercise as increased exercise LVESV, and abnormal LV chamber elastance.[52]

Symptomatic patients with AR and resting LV dysfunction have been observed to have higher levels of LV end-systolic wall stress compared to asymptomatic patients with normal resting LV performance or to normal subjects. Reichek et al concluded that afterload excess contributed to the reduced LVEF response to exercise in patients with AR.[77] Others have extended this observation by demonstrating that estimates of peak systolic stress at rest were higher in patients with AR who had an abnormal exercise LVEF response compared to patients with normal exercise reserve.[61,68,78] There was, however, significant overlap in echocardiographic measurements of systolic stress between patients with normal and abnormal exercise LV reserve, suggesting that M-mode echocardiographic parameters cannot be used in place of exercise radionuclide angiography to assess LV reserve.

In an attempt to measure LV contractility during exercise, while minimizing the effects of loading conditions, Iskandrian et al have extended observations concerning the end-systolic pressure–volume relation to the exercise state.[50] Fifteen normal subjects were compared to 21 AR patients with a resting radionuclide LVEF of 50 percent or more (group one) and to 18 AR patients with a resting LVEF less than 50 percent (group two). Both the resting and exercise systolic blood pressure/end-systolic volume index ratios (SBP/ESVI) were higher in normal subjects than in patients in group one and, similarly, higher in group one patients than in group two patients. Twelve patients (57 percent) in group one and 16 patients (89 percent) in group two had a resting SBP/ESVI that was below the lower limit of normal. During exercise, 17 patients in group one (81 percent) and all patients in group two (100 percent) had a SBP/ESVI that was below the lower limit of normal. Abnormality in the SBP/ESVI was significantly more frequent than abnormality in the LVEF response to exercise, because 43 percent of the patients with a normal resting LVEF and 39 percent of those patients with an abnormal resting LVEF had a normal response to exercise ($\geq$ 5-unit increase). The 4 patients in group one who had exercise pressure–volume ratios that were within the normal range also had normal LVEF responses to exercise. A significant correlation was found between the change in SBP/ESVI and the change in LVEF with exercise ($r = -0.79$, $p < 0.001$). Although the LV systolic pressure–volume relation during exercise may detect impaired LV functional reserve at an earlier stage than the exercise LVEF in some patients, the prognostic significance of this index and its role in the timing of aortic valve replacement in patients with severe AR is currently unknown.[79]

Changes in coronary blood flow may also be important in determining transient dysfunction during exercise or pharmacologic intervention.[80,81] Thus, though the baseline coronary blood flow (measured by coronary sinus thermodilution technique) has been found to be higher in AR than normal (presumably because of higher muscle mass), the dipyridamole-induced hyperemic-to-basal flow ratio is reduced in AR. Others have found resting perfusion defects in a majority of patients with AR, and have correlated abnormal resting thallium 201 (^{201}Tl) single photon emission computed tomography (SPECT) results with increased LVEDVI and LVESVI, in those patients.[82] Repeated episodes of ischemia in the presence of normal coronary arteries may lead to fibrosis and dysfunction. In a study by Pfisterer et al, 29 patients with aortic valve disease underwent rest and exercise ^{201}Tl myocardial scintigraphy. Among 16 patients with pure or predominant AR, reversible apical perfusion abnormalities were commonly observed in the absence of associated CAD. These apical abnormalities were most likely related to extreme volume overload and LV dilatation with exaggerated apical thinning. Similar apical abnormalities were not observed in patients with pure or predominant aortic stenosis.[83]

Value and Limitations of Echocardiography

Numerous studies have looked at the value of echocardiographic measurements as prognostic indicators in both symptomatic and asymptomatic patients with AR. Henry et al found that LV end-systolic dimension, fractional shortening, and ejection fraction were significantly associated ($p < 0.05$) with overall postoperative mortality in symptomatic patients.[84] Nine of 14 patients with LV fractional shortening less than 25 percent either died at surgery or developed symptoms of CHF and died during the 44-month follow-up period. In contrast, only 2 of 35 symptomatic patients with a preoperative fractional shortening of at least 25 percent died at operation or developed symptoms of CHF and died during follow-up. Similarly, perioperative or postoperative cardiac death occurred during the follow-up period in 9 of 17 patients with a perioperative LV end-systolic dimension greater than 55 mm. In contrast, perioperative or late cardiac death occurred in only 2 of 32 patients with an LV end-systolic dimension of 55 mm or less.

The LV end-diastolic dimension, end-systolic dimension, and fractional shortening as measured by echocardiography have also been proposed as prognostic indicators in asymptomatic patients with AR. After a mean of 43 months of follow-up, 4 of 5 initially asymptomatic patients with a LV end-systolic dimension greater than 55 mm, studied by Henry et al, became symptomatic and came to valve replacement, whereas only 4 of 20

asymptomatic patients with an LV end-systolic dimension of 55 mm or less developed symptoms leading to valve replacement.[85] This observation led to the recommendation that asymptomatic patients with AR and an echocardiographic LV end-systolic dimension greater than 55 mm undergo aortic valve replacement. More recent work in symptomatic patients has not, however, confirmed the predictive usefulness of the echocardiographic LV end-systolic dimension greater than 55 mm or of the fractional shortening less than 25 percent.[86,87] In 47 symptomatic patients with AR, who underwent aortic valve replacement, Fioretti et al observed no perioperative or postoperative deaths during a mean follow-up period of 41 months. The study population included 20 patients with a preoperative LV end-systolic dimension greater than 55 mm and 11 patients with a fractional shortening less than 25 percent. The latter group of patients had similar symptomatic improvement compared to patients with more normal preoperative echocardiographic measurements. Postoperative normalization of LV performance was also not precluded by a preoperative LV end-systolic dimension greater than 55 mm or a fractional shortening less than 25 percent.[86] Similarly, in a study of 84 patients with AR, Daniel et al found that a preoperative LV end-systolic dimension greater than 55 mm or a fractional shortening less than 25 percent did not provide statistically significant prediction of early or late postoperative death, did not correlate with postoperative symptoms, and did not preclude postoperative regression of LV dilatation or hypertrophy. Nevertheless, Bonow and Epstein have pointed out that the 2.5-year survival following aortic valve replacement in Daniel's series fell progressively from 90.5 percent in patients with a preoperative LV end-systolic dimension less than or equal to 55 mm and a fractional shortening greater than 25 percent to 78.5 percent in patients with *either* a preoperative LV end-systolic dimension greater than 55 mm *or* a fractional shortening less than or equal to 25 percent, and to 70 percent in patients with *both* a preoperative LV end-systolic dimension greater than 55 mm and a fractional shortening less than or equal to 25 percent.[88] Thus, the prognostic usefulness of the echocardiographic LV end-systolic dimension and fractional shortening for assessing the timing of aortic valve replacement for AR continues to be a source of controversy.[89,90]

In addition to LV systolic and diastolic dimensions and percent fractional shortening, other echocardiographic indices have been obtained in an attempt to predict postoperative clinical outcome and postoperative LV size and performance. The ratio of LV volume to mass can be estimated from M-mode echocardiographic determination of the LV end-diastolic radius-to-wall thickness ratio. The product of the systolic arterial blood pressure and the end-diastolic radius-to-wall thickness ratio is referred to as the "corrected" end-diastolic radius-to-wall thickness ratio and is an index of peak systolic wall stress. Gaasch et al have suggested that these indices increase if LV volume increases out of proportion to LV hypertrophy.[91] These investigators found an LV end-diastolic radius-to-wall thickness ratio greater than 3.8 or a corrected LV end-diastolic radius-to-wall thickness ratio greater than 600 to be predictive of persistent LV enlargement following aortic valve replacement. In contrast to the findings of Gaasch et al, Fioretti et al found the preoperative LV radius-to-wall thickness ratio to be a poor predictor of persistent LV enlargement 3 years after surgery.[92] The LV end-diastolic dimension was a more useful predictor in their study.

Elevated LV end-systolic stress as measured by M-mode or two-dimensional echocardiography has been associated with progression to aortic valve replacement and with persistent LV dilatation following surgery.[69,93] It is not clear, however, that echocardiographic measurement of LV end-systolic stress provides predictive information in patients with AR beyond that provided by the LV end-systolic dimension. Similar to radionuclide angiography, echocardiography can also provide insight into changes in LV shape that occur with volume overload related to severe AR. Vandenbossche et al calculated end-systolic and end-diastolic ratios of LV long axis to minor axis in patients with chronic AR. These authors suggested that when myocardial hypertrophy becomes inadequate to normalize increased wall stress, and LV volume increases disproportionately to myocardial mass, LV shape is transformed from ellipsoidal to spherical.[94] Whether assessment of LV shape provides information useful for timing of aortic valve replacement in patients with AR remains to be demonstrated.

Thus, although controversy regarding the prognostic utility of echocardiographic measurements for selecting the correct time for aortic valve replacement remains, the echocardiogram is an important tool for monitoring LV size and performance. Echocardiography is noninvasive, relatively inexpensive, and involves no exposure to ionizing radiation. The echocardiogram may be successfully used to follow the progress of patients with AR and to demonstrate when these patients are entering a stage of increased risk for irreversible LV dysfunction.

Selection of Patients with Aortic Regurgitation for Valve Replacement: An Integrated Approach

SYMPTOMATIC PATIENTS WITH ABNORMAL LEFT VENTRICULAR PERFORMANCE

Symptomatic patients with a resting LVEF less than 45 percent are candidates for cardiac catheterization and aortic valve replacement.[33,36] Even when severe LV dysfunction is present, improvement in symptoms and decrease in LV size and mass are common following sur-

gery.[95] The preoperative radionuclide LVEF at rest, the echocardiographic LV end-diastolic and end-systolic dimensions, the echocardiographic LV percent fractional shortening, the ability to complete stage one of the National Institutes of Health treadmill exercise protocol, and the length of time during which symptoms have been present all provide predictive information regarding outcome following aortic valve replacement. Patients who have demonstrated LV dysfunction for a relatively brief period (approximately 14 months or less) will generally show a greater increase in both short- and long-term postoperative LVEF, a greater postoperative decrease in LV dilation, and increased overall postoperative survival, when compared with patients in whom LV dysfunction has been present for a prolonged period.[41-43]

SYMPTOMATIC PATIENTS WITH NORMAL LEFT VENTRICULAR PERFORMANCE

A graded exercise test can verify that limiting symptoms (New York Heart Association class III or IV) are present. Patients with one or more episodes of CHF or with limiting symptoms are candidates for cardiac catheterization and aortic valve replacement. Patients with mild symptoms (New York Heart Association class II) and normal exercise capacity on a graded exercise test provide a more difficult management problem. Athletic or other physically active individuals may be considered for early valve replacement for relatively mild symptoms, whereas more sedentary patients will in some cases await progression of symptoms or development of early evidence of resting LV dysfunction before proceeding to invasive studies. Although the indications for valve replacement in this latter group are not clearly defined, frequent noninvasive monitoring of symptoms and LV size and performance is advisable.

ASYMPTOMATIC PATIENTS WITH ABNORMAL LEFT VENTRICULAR PERFORMANCE

Although fewer data are available in asymptomatic patients compared to symptomatic patients, existing data suggest that asymptomatic patients with abnormal resting LV performance are at increased risk of developing postoperative CHF and having decreased survival after aortic valve replacement compared to those without resting LV dysfunction. Some authors have suggested that evidence for both a decreased resting LVEF and echocardiographically severe LV systolic or diastolic enlargement, or inadequate LV hypertrophy, be required before proceeding to aortic valve replacement.[96] Data are needed to evaluate the latter recommendation. In view of the unfavorable prognostic implications of progressive resting LV dysfunction in symptomatic patients with AR, it does not appear advisable to delay surgery until further deterioration in LV performance develops in asymptomatic patients with an LVEF less than 45 percent.[33,36]

ASYMPTOMATIC PATIENTS WITH NORMAL LEFT
VENTRICULAR PERFORMANCE

The majority of asymptomatic patients with AR and
normal LV systolic performance will remain clinically
stable for many years. This favorable clinical course has
led a number of authors to recommend that "prophylactic" aortic valve replacement not be carried out in asymptomatic patients with normal resting LV performance.[40,95,96] These patients can be followed with exercise
testing to objectively document the appearance of symptoms or evidence of decreasing exercise capacity. Noninvasive testing can provide evidence of new LV dysfunction.

The selection of a noninvasive test or tests for serial
assessment of LV size or performance will, in some cases,
depend on test availability and local experience with the
test procedure. Echocardiography provides an inexpensive, widely available tool for measuring LV size and
performance and does not require ionizing radiation.
Patients with an echocardiographic preoperative LV
fractional shortening greater than 26 percent, an LV end-
systolic dimension less than 55 mm, and an LV end-
diastolic dimension less than 80 mm will generally have
normal LV performance following aortic valve replacement for AR.[95] This suggests that asymptomatic patients
with these findings can be successfully followed with
serial echocardiograms until one of these measurements
is approached. When echocardiographic indices cannot
reliably be measured, radionuclide LVEF can be used to
determine whether resting LV performance has become
abnormal. Although the frequency of follow-up with
noninvasive testing must be individualized, the response
of the radionuclide LVEF to exercise may have a role in
identifying high-risk patients who require closer observation. Patients having a greater than 5-unit increase in
LVEF with exercise have a relatively low rate of progression to resting LV dysfunction. On the other hand, in
the study by Bonow et al, one third of patients with a
greater than 5-unit decrease in LVEF during exercise
required aortic valve replacement within 4 years.[40]
Therefore, exercise radionuclide ventriculography may
provide a practical method for determining the frequency
of clinical follow-up in asymptomatic patients with AR.

Response to Medical Therapy in Asymptomatic Patients With Aortic Regurgitation

Treatment of chronic AR with cardiac glycosides has in
the past been a mainstay of medical therapy for this
disease. Beneficial effects of digitalis included improvement in resting LVEF as well as exercise LV performance.[97] A number of recent studies have assessed the
effects of vasodilator therapy on the natural history of
patients with chronic, moderate to severe AR. It has now

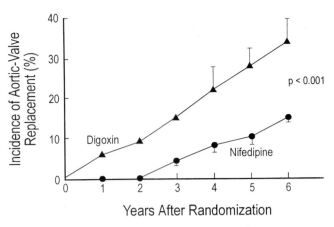

Figure 24-9 Cumulative actuarial incidence of progression to
aortic valve replacement in the nifedipine and digoxin treatment
groups. (From Scognamiglio et al,[99] reproduced with permission.)

become apparent that long-term therapy with vasodilators can prolong the asymptomatic period, retard the
onset of LV dysfunction, and thus delay the need for
aortic valve replacement.[98,99] All vasodilators act to decrease systemic vascular resistance and thereby increase
forward flow and reduce regurgitant volume. Dumesnil
et al were able to show a decrease in LV end-diastolic
and end-systolic dimensions in a small group of asymptomatic patients with significant AR.[100] Stopping hydralazine therapy in a group of 17 patients with stable aortic
insufficiency did not, however, lead to clinical deterioration in a study performed by Nauman et al. These authors concluded that discontinuation of vasodilators
would not lead to an altered progression to valve replacement.[101] Since then, however, the preponderance of
evidence has favored the beneficial effects of long-term
vasodilator therapy in patients with AR. Angiotensin-
converting enzyme inhibitors, alpha-1 blockers, and calcium channel antagonists have all produced favorable
effects on the left ventricle, whether assessment was carried out with serial echocardiographic studies or with
serial radionuclide ventriculograms.[98,102-104] When different vasodilator classes were compared, calcium channel
antagonists were somewhat more beneficial in one study
because of their incremental improvement in forward
LV stroke volume and cardiac output over angiotensin-
converting enzyme inhibitors.[105] Scognamiglio et al ce-
mented the role of nifedipine as the vasodilator of choice
in the long-term treatment of severe AR in their recently
published study. Their study compared nifedipine, 20
mg twice daily, with digoxin, 0.25 mg daily, in 143
asymptomatic patients followed for a mean of 6 years.
They showed that significantly fewer patients progressed
to aortic valve replacement in the nifedipine group versus
the digoxin group (15 ± 3 percent versus 34 ± 6 percent,
$p < 0.001$) (Fig. 24-9). Echocardiographic parameters
such as LVEDVI and LVESVI, LVEF, and LV mass were
all significantly improved in the nifedipine group by the

end of the study.[99] Thus, it appears that long-term therapy with a vasodilating agent, most probably nifedipine, should be instituted in most asymptomatic patients with significant AR who present with normal LV performance. These patients should continue to be monitored for the appearance of symptoms or of LV dysfunction and should be considered for aortic valve replacement when either symptoms or LV dysfunction supervenes.

Left Ventricular Performance After Aortic Valve Replacement

Numerous studies have documented improvements in LV performance in patients who have undergone aortic valve replacement for AR. Borer et al observed that the resting LVEF and exercise LVEF improved in 16 patients after surgery for AR. In their study, the postoperative LVEF during exercise, although improved, was still lower than that seen in normal subjects.[106] Therefore, preoperative LV dysfunction is at least partially reversible after aortic valve replacement for AR. Boucher et al examined 20 patients with AR 2 to 4 weeks after aortic valve replacement and found that the resting LVEF decreased in the early postoperative period from a mean of 55 percent preoperatively to 40 percent postoperatively. However, when the LVEF was measured 1 to 2 years after valve replacement, it was found that it had increased to a level comparable to that seen preoperatively.[107] This late improvement in LV performance may correspond temporally to the gradual regression over many years of LV hypertrophy following aortic valve replacement for severe chronic AR.[108] It seems that a sudden decrease in LVEDV immediately after valve replacement may be responsible for the early decline in LVEF. Further, because many of these patients also have sinus tachycardia soon after surgery, the decrease in preload may be more pronounced because, in addition to the elimination of the leak across the valve, the decrease in diastolic filling period may contribute to a further decrease in volume. Although the LVEDV decreased early postoperatively in many of the patients studied by Boucher et al, it did remain higher than normal, suggesting that LV dilatation was only partly reversible.[107] The reversible part may be ascribed to regurgitation, while the irreversible part may result from LV contractile dysfunction. Bonow et al have shown that in severe AR, patients with an improved LVEF at 6 to 8 months after aortic valve replacement are likely to have a further improvement in LVEF, with further decrease in LV end-diastolic dimension, at 3 to 7 years after valve replacement. Patients with no improvement in resting LVEF during the first 6 months after operation are not likely to have a late improvement in postoperative LV performance.[43] Regional wall-motion abnormalities may be

seen quite commonly following aortic valve replacement and should not be mistaken for myocardial ischemia, according to van der Wall et al.[109]

The recurrence of symptoms of CHF after aortic valve replacement may be due to LV dysfunction or to prosthetic valve dysfunction. Goldman et al found that radionuclide ventriculography is useful for differentiating between the two causes of CHF.[110] If the LVEF is normal, then CHF is most likely due to mechanical dysfunction of the valve, which should be evident on clinical evaluation of the patient. On the other hand, if LV performance is abnormal, then CHF is most likely due to LV contractile dysfunction.

Survival following aortic valve replacement for chronic AR has improved substantially over the past two decades. Nevertheless, preoperative resting LV dysfunction continues to accurately identify patients with AR at risk for death following aortic valve replacement. In a series from 1976 to 1983 reported from the National Institutes of Health, 5-year survival following aortic valve replacement in 30 patients with chronic severe AR and a preoperative radionuclide LVEF greater than 45 percent was 95 ± 3 percent. In contrast, among 50 patients with chronic severe AR and a preoperative LVEF less than or equal to 45 percent, 5-year survival following aortic valve replacement was only 63 ± 12 percent.[42]

AORTIC STENOSIS

In adult patients with severe valvular AS, the onset of symptoms of angina pectoris, syncope, or CHF predicts an average survival of 2 to 5 years in medically treated patients.[111-113] Symptomatic patients with severe AS who undergo valve replacement will have considerably improved survival.[31] For this reason, patients with an aortic valve area less than 0.75 cm² or less than or equal to 0.4 cm²/m² body surface area and symptoms of syncope, angina pectoris, or left heart failure are best treated with aortic valve replacement.[96] M-mode and two-dimensional echocardiography have demonstrated limited accuracy in estimating the severity of AS.[114,115] Doppler techniques, on the other hand, are now accepted as reliable methods for assessment of the instantaneous gradient across the aortic valve and for measurement of aortic valve area.[116]

Several authors have suggested that traditional invasive calculations of aortic valve area may not accurately quantify hemodynamic impairment under varying conditions of flow and have proposed hemodynamic resistance across the valve as a more accurate functional parameter.[117,118] Aortic valve resistance is defined by Ford et al as the mean pressure gradient across the valve divided by the mean flow rate during systolic ejection. Calculation of resistance as a stenotic index has the advantage of not requiring any assumptions, as does calculation of the valve area.[117] Cannon et al found the aortic valve resistance to be less susceptible to hemodynamic manipulation than the calculated valve area. Using valve resistance measurements, they were able to distinguish more precisely between a group of patients with AS who had truly critical disease (confirmed at surgery) and those patients with milder disease and a lower gradient, in whom calculated aortic valve area at rest failed to make this separation.[118]

If the degree of AS is determined to be severe, however, surgery should not be denied to that patient, regardless of the level of resting LV performance. Although not all patients with AS and LV dysfunction have an improvement in LV performance following aortic valve replacement, nearly all patients are clinically improved.[119] Improvement in LV performance (often marked) is more common after aortic valve replacement for AS than for AR.

Patients with AS may be markedly symptomatic despite the presence of a normal or elevated resting LVEF. The symptoms in these patients are due to mechanical obstruction, a disparity between myocardial oxygen supply and demand, and an increase in LV stiffness. When present, LV dysfunction at rest can be due to impaired LV contractility or to inappropriate afterload.[30,120] Hypertrophy in these patients is a compensatory mechanism to maintain normal wall stress. Thus, an abnormal resting LVEF in a patient with LV hypertrophy is more likely to be due to a decrease in contractility than in a patient with no hypertrophy.

Pressure overload hypertrophy of the LV is associated with abnormal LV diastolic filling.[121-123] Murakami et al analyzed LV performance indices in a group of patients with AS and grouped patients according to degree of hypertrophy.[123] Patients with severe hypertrophy, defined as a muscle mass index greater than or equal to 180 g/m², had increased LVEDV and LVESV and a decreased LVEF. Peak diastolic filling rate and percent LV volume increase in the first half of diastole were greater in patients with severe compared to those with moderate LV hypertrophy. The time constant of LV pressure decline—an index of the rate of relaxation—was prolonged in patients with severe hypertrophy. In patients with moderate LV hypertrophy, early diastolic LV filling was decreased or normal, and the peak filling rate in the second half of diastole was increased. Thus, in severe LV hypertrophy, increased early diastolic driving pressure allows early filling to remain normal despite prolonged LV relaxation and decreased elastic recoil. In patients with AS and moderate LV hypertrophy, diastolic filling is maintained by a forceful atrial contraction. Lavine et al observed that the peak filling rate (PFR) assessed by radionuclide ventriculography was significantly lower

than control in a group of patients with AS. They found augmentation of the rapid filling period in a subgroup of patients with depressed LVEF, however.[122] Hess et al further analyzed abnormalities in diastolic function in patients with aortic valve disease by performing myocardial biopsies in patients with AS, mixed aortic valve disease (stenosis/insufficiency), and those with AR. They found a significant increase in interstitial fibrosis in those patients with isolated AS and a slight increase in patients with stenosis/insufficiency and those with isolated AR.[124]

Abnormalities in diastolic LV performance may be responsible for episodes of angina in patients with AS in the absence of associated CAD. In a simultaneous echocardiographic-hemodynamic evaluation, angina was produced by rapid atrial pacing in 8 patients with AS and no CAD.[121] During isovolumic relaxation, the time constant of LV pressure decline increased without changes in LV end-diastolic and end-systolic dimensions or fractional shortening. Impaired diastolic distensibility appeared to account for the observed increase in end-diastolic pressure.

Assessment of coronary anatomy is essential in patients with aortic valve disease prior to proceeding with valve replacement. Angina pectoris commonly occurs in adult patients with AS and associated CAD, but it is also frequently a manifestation in patients with AS alone.[115,125-129] The mechanism of angina in patients with AS without significant CAD is generally thought to be related to diffuse subendocardial ischemia caused by a reduced diastolic pressure–time index relative to myocardial oxygen demand. In patients with AS and angina pectoris, the exercise electrocardiogram is generally not useful because of the presence of LV hypertrophy and diffuse ST-segment abnormalities. Careful exercise testing may, however, have a role in defining symptoms and objectively assessing limitations in effort tolerance.

Relatively little information is available about LV performance during exercise in patients with severe AS, possibly because of the fear of exercising such patients. This fear, however, is not entirely justified, because these patients, especially if asymptomatic, are likely to participate in physical activities that may be strenuous and unsupervised in their daily lives. A number of studies have reported exercise testing without complications in patients with severe AS.[130] Several groups have attempted to quantify exercise LV performance using radionuclide ventriculography at rest and with exercise.[131,132] In patients referred for angiographic evaluation of AS, Milanes et al reported that a 5-unit or greater increase in LVEF with supine bicycle exercise was only observed in those with an aortic valve area greater than 0.8 cm² and in the absence of any 50 percent or greater reduction in the luminal diameter of the major coronary arteries.[132] Archer et al used rest and exercise radionuclide angiography to assess patients with symptomatic and asymptomatic AS. They found several distinguishing factors between the two groups. Both sets of patients demonstrated exercise-evoked functional limitations, but symptomatic patients exercised to significantly lower work levels than asymptomatic subjects. Symptomatic patients also demonstrated higher mean aortic gradients and enhanced early diastolic filling versus asymptomatic patients.[133] Clyne et al found that asymptomatic patients with AS demonstrated reduced exercise tolerance, as well as decreased maximal oxygen consumption, and decreased systolic blood pressure response to exercise, when compared with age- and gender-matched controls. Although their study did not address long-term follow-up in these patients, the authors theorized that exercise testing might identify a subgroup of asymptomatic patients at relatively high risk of adverse outcomes because of abnormal exercise hemodynamics, in whom early valve replacement should be recommended.[134] At the present time, however, radionuclide ventriculography with exercise probably should not be recommended for routine clinical use in patients with AS.

Several groups have attempted to noninvasively exclude significant coronary artery stenoses in patients with moderate to severe AS, with conflicting results. Bailey et al evaluated 22 patients with AS, 11 with and 11 without associated significant CAD. The ^{201}Tl myocardial perfusion abnormalities at rest and at exercise were characterized by the following findings: (1) presence of fixed focal defects; (2) presence of fixed defects plus exercise-induced reversible defects; and (3) exercise-induced LV myocardial thinning.[135] The fixed focal defects could represent scar due to previous infarction or fibrosis related to chronic pressure overload. Myocardial perfusion abnormalities were present in patients both with and without associated CAD and, therefore, the results of exercise ^{201}Tl imaging did not allow adequate separation of patients with AS and CAD from those with AS alone. Possible reasons are that (1) angiographically significant CAD may not always produce focal ischemia before diffuse subendocardial ischemia develops and (2) angiographically insignificant CAD may become functionally important in the presence of AS and, thus, produce focal ischemia. Seven of the patients studied by Bailey et al underwent repeat exercise ^{201}Tl myocardial scintigraphy after aortic valve replacement. In 2 patients, new focal defects were seen consistent with perioperative infarction; and in the remaining patients the preoperative abnormalities (either focal or diffuse) were no longer visible postoperatively. Thus, the results of ^{201}Tl myocardial imaging may be of value in assessing the results of surgery in patients with AS.[83,135] Other groups have demonstrated more accurate exercise ^{201}Tl myocardial scintigraphy results in patients with AS. Using bicycle ergometry, Kupari et al evaluated 44 patients with moderate to severe AS and normal LV systolic performance.

They reported sensitivity and specificity of an abnormal scintigram as 100 percent and 57 percent, respectively. If only segmental defects typical of CAD were considered abnormal, specificity rose to 70 percent.[136]

Often patients with severe valvular heart disease are unable to exercise sufficiently to permit accurate exclusion of CAD. Aubry et al evaluated the predictive accuracy of ^{201}Tl myocardial scintigraphy with dipyridamole infusion for detecting concomitant CAD in patients with aortic and mitral stenosis. Ten of 13 patients in the group of 34 patients studied had positive ^{201}Tl myocardial scintigrams. The sensitivity and specificity of perfusion imaging for detecting CAD were 69 percent and 95 percent, respectively. Positive predictive value of the study was 90 percent. The authors concluded, however, that because of the relatively low sensitivity, basing indications for coronary angiography before valve surgery on the results of ^{201}Tl myocardial perfusion scinitigraphy with pharmacologic stress could not be advised.[137] Huikuri et al have combined intravenous dipyridamole infusion and isometric hand grip with ^{201}Tl myocardial scintigraphy and detected concomitant coronary stenoses in 11 of 13 patients with mild to severe AS (associated specificity 86 percent) and 10 of 11 patients with mild to severe mitral stenosis (associated specificity 82 percent).[138,139] Recently, Rask et al used computer-assisted evaluation of dipyridamole ^{201}Tl SPECT to establish normal distribution patterns for patients with AS without CAD and to validate these patterns in a group of patients with AS and angiographically verified CAD. They achieved a sensitivity of 88 percent for detecting CAD in 16 patients with known coronary artery stenoses.[140] These promising results require confirmation in larger series. Currently, cardiac catheterization and coronary angiography are still considered necessary before aortic valve replacement to define coronary anatomy in elderly patients or in patients with angina pectoris.[141]

Assessment of Surgical and Percutaneous Therapy for Aortic Stenosis

Balloon valvuloplasty has provided short-term improvement in cardiac symptoms and hemodynamics—mediated through a decrease in aortic valve gradient—and an increase in cardiac output and aortic valve area.[142-144] A high restenosis rate has largely limited the procedure to elderly patients with an unacceptably high risk for aortic valve replacement. Individual responses to aortic valvuloplasty vary in terms of improvement in aortic valve area and in systolic LV performance.[143] The immediate response to percutaneous aortic balloon valvuloplasty has been assessed via first-pass radionuclide ventriculography.[145] As expected, immediate decreases were seen in the peak and mean aortic valve gradients, with concomitant increases in the aortic valve area. The LVEF increased significantly, and LVEDV and LVESV both decreased significantly. Left ventricular systolic wall stress, end-diastolic pressure, and stroke work all decreased significantly. Thus, the LV outflow obstruction is decreased and cardiac output is maintained at a lower level of LV filling. These trends continue when LV performance is assessed serially in the days after the procedure.[145,146]

The appropriate management of asymptomatic patients with hemodynamically severe AS is not clear. Ross and Braunwald noted that 3 to 5 percent of patients with acquired AS die suddenly without preceding symptoms.[111] Kelly et al studied 51 initially asymptomatic patients with severe AS and found that syncope or sudden cardiac death was not observed as a first symptom during follow-up.[147] In view of the postoperative improvement in LV performance observed in most patients with severe AS and preoperative LV dysfunction, it is not justified to replace the aortic valve in an asymptomatic patient to preserve LV performance.[96,148] When the presence or absence of cardiac symptoms is in doubt, cautious use of exercise testing, as described above, may be helpful. The decision to replace the aortic valve in asymptomatic patients with an aortic valve area less than 0.75 cm^2 depends on clinical judgment, weighing the small risk of sudden death against the morbidity and mortality of valve replacement and life with a prosthetic valve.

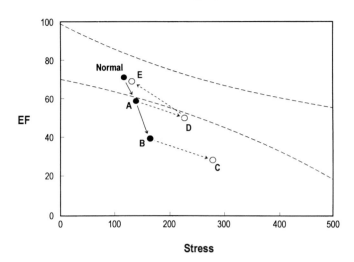

Figure 24-10 Relationship of ejection fraction (EF) and stress in mitral regurgitation. Point A shows untreated, asymptomatic patients with severe mitral regurgitation; there is little or no change in EF and in wall stress. Point B shows that continued severe mitral regurgitation will lead to contractile dysfunction and a decline in EF, again with little increase in wall stress. Point C shows the result of mitral valve surgery after irreversible contractile dysfunction has supervened; wall stress increases with the removal of the low impedance leak into the left atrium, and EF declines. Point D shows the immediate postoperative result of mitral valve surgery before irreversible contractile dysfunction has supervened; there is a temporary decline in EF associated with the postoperative increase in wall stress. Point E shows the eventual recovery of ventricular contractility and return towards normal of EF and wall stress.

MITRAL REGURGITATION

Pathophysiology

Mitral regurgitation is a condition characterized by primary LV volume overload. Preload is elevated due to excess volume, and eccentric hypertrophy develops. Left ventricular ejection performance is initially normal or even elevated, because the decrease in afterload caused by unloading into a low-pressure left atrium leads to increased velocity and extent of fiber shortening. In a canine model, acute MR results in an increase in LVEF.[149] In the chronic, compensated state, there is progressive LV enlargement and continued eccentric hypertrophy, and LVEDV and mass increase. Gradually, LV radius increases without a significant change in LV wall thickness, and the initially reduced wall stress normalizes. Subsequently, there is an increase in the LVESV, and, therefore, a reduction in LV emptying and a decline in LVEF toward normal levels. When the LV decompensates late in the course of the disease, there is an irreversible decline in contractile function, leading to a down-

ward spiral characterized by progressive increases in LVESV and a decline in LVEF[150,151] (Fig. 24-10). Measurements of LV contractility that are relatively independent of ventricular loading conditions (e.g., end-systolic elastance, or E_{max}, and the end-systolic stress–volume relationship) document a decrease in LV contractility in response to chronic MR. Thus, LV emptying into the low-pressure left atrium may maintain a normal or mildly elevated LVEF despite abnormal LV contractility. Several animal studies have analyzed myocardial changes in response to surgically created MR in an attempt to pinpoint the level of abnormality responsible for abnormal contractile function. Urabe et al analyzed LV contractile performance in dogs after 3 months of severe MR. They concluded that, first, chronic LV volume overload from MR led to contractile defects at both the ventricular and cellular levels. Second, no quantitative interstitial change resulted from MR. Together, these two findings suggested that the contractile defect must be intrinsic to the cardiocyte. Third, while the contractile abnormality in MR was as yet undefined, the most basic defects appeared to be a combination of myofibrillar loss with the failure of compensatory hypertrophy to occur

Group II

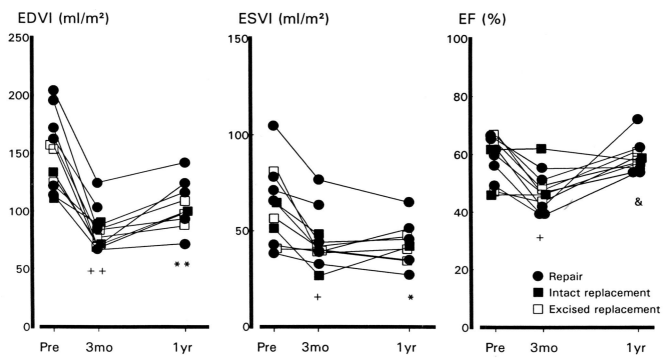

Figure 24-11 Preoperative (Pre) to postoperative (at 3 months, 3mo, and 1 year) responses in left ventricular (LV) indices in group II patients (those with impaired LV contractile performance but normal ejection fraction). EDVI, end-diastolic volume index; ESVI, end-systolic volume index; EF, ejection fraction. Solid circles represent those who had mitral valve repair; solid squares, those with mitral valve replacement with preservation of the submitral apparatus; open squares, those with mitral valve replacement without chordal preservation.
+ $p \leq 0.001$ versus Pre
++ $p < 0.0001$ versus Pre
* $p < 0.01$ versus Pre
** $p < 0.001$ versus Pre and 3mo and $p < 0.01$ versus 3mo
(From Starling et al,[153] reprinted with permission from the American College of Cardiology, *Journal of the American College of Cardiology*, 22:239, 1993.)

in response to progressive decrements in cellular and ventricular function.[152] Starling et al verified this hypothesis in a group of 28 patients with chronic MR. Using micromanometer-measured LV pressures, biplane contrast ventriculography, and radionuclide ventriculography, they were able to construct pressure–volume loops under a variety of loading conditions for each patient. Patients could be divided into three groups: group one consisted of patients with no impairment of LV contractile function, as evidenced by a normal heart size-corrected E_{max}; group two was composed by patients with impaired contractile function (reduced E_{max}) but normal LVEF; and group three consisted of patients with reduced E_{max}, reduced systolic myocardial stiffness, and low LVEF. Mitral valve surgery caused no appreciable changes in short- or long-term measurement of LVEF in group one, whereas patients in group two showed a decline in LVEF at 3 months, with a return toward normal values at 1 year (Fig. 24-11). Patients in group three

manifested an immediate postoperative decline in LVEF which was sustained at 1 year.[153] These results, as well as animal studies performed by Nakano et al, suggest that contractile dysfunction is potentially reversible after mitral valve surgery in a subset of patients.[154] More recent work by Starling has shown conclusively that LV contractility can improve after mitral valve surgery, even in long-term MR[155] (Fig. 24-12). The challenge, therefore, remains to identify patients before irreversible contractile dysfunction supervenes.

Assessment of Left Ventricular Performance in Mitral Regurgitation

Numerous studies have attempted to identify echocardiographic or angiographic parameters predictive of clinical outcome following mitral valve surgery for MR.

Ees (mmHg/ml)

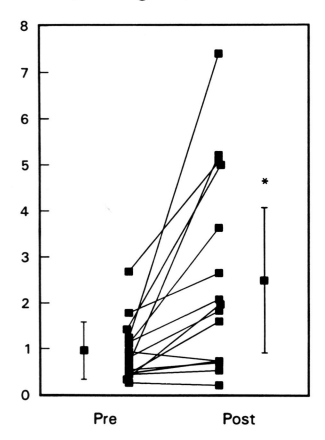

* p < 0.05

Figure 24-12 Plot of individual and mean left ventricular chamber elastance (E_{es}) values pre- and postoperatively. Significant improvement is shown. (From Starling MR,[155] by permission of the American Heart Association, Inc.)

Preoperative angiographic parameters predictive of postoperative clinical status have included measurement of the LVESVI and the ratio of LV end-systolic wall stress to end-systolic volume index.[32,156-158] Preoperative echocardiographic variables predictive of postoperative clinical outcome have included the LV end-systolic dimension, fractional shortening, and end-systolic wall stress index. Zile et al found that when LV dimension at end-systole exceeded 2.6 cm/m², fractional shortening was less than 31 percent, or end-systolic wall stress index exceeded 195 mmHg, patients showed no functional improvement after mitral valve surgery.[157] Donovan and Starling have, after a careful scrutiny of the world literature, proposed an end-systolic dimension greater than 45 mm as an echocardiographic index for proceeding with mitral valve surgery.[151]

Radionuclide ventriculography can also be used for serial assessment of LV performance in asymptomatic patients with chronic MR. Two technical points should be remembered when studying these patients. First, patients with mitral valve disease are often in atrial fibrillation, which results in uncertainty in radionuclide ventriculographic measurements. Second, the enlarged left atrium may interfere with the determinations of LV counts. Therefore, every effort should be made to optimize the separation of the left atrium and the left ventricle, including the use of caudal detector angulation. Fourier analysis may be useful in defining the boundary between the two chambers, but cannot prevent overlap. Because of the limited reliability of measurement of LVEF as an index of LV contractility in patients with MR, several investigators have used other indices, such as the LVESV, the end-systolic pressure–volume relation, and the end-systolic stress–volume relation, to evaluate contractile performance in a load-independent fashion. Carabello et al found that the ratio of LV end-systolic wall stress to end-systolic volume index (ESWS/ESVI) was the only independent predictor of outcome in a group of patients with chronic, symptomatic MR.[156] In the previously described study by Starling et al, the LVESVI rose progressively as LV contractile dysfunction became more marked. Patients who had irreversible contractile dysfunction after surgery all had an LVESVI greater than 60 ml/m².[153]

Despite the theoretical limitations of the LVEF in patients with MR, Ramanathan et al found the LVEF at rest to be a more accurate predictor of cardiac morbidity and mortality than the ratio of peak systolic blood pressure to LV end-systolic volume in medically treated patients with MR.[159]

Right Ventricular Performance in the Assessment of Mitral Regurgitation

Right ventricular ejection fraction (RVEF) also appears to predict cardiac morbidity and mortality in chronic MR. In 53 patients with chronic MR, treadmill exercise time correlated with RVEF during exercise ($r = 0.48$, $p < 0.005$). In 23 of these patients in whom hemodynamic data were also available, an inverse correlation between RVEF and pulmonary artery wedge and pulmonary artery systolic pressures was also found. Asymptomatic patients with chronic MR had a higher RVEF both at rest and during exercise than did symptomatic patients. Patients with an RVEF of 30 percent or less at entry made up a subgroup of patients at high mortality risk ($p < 0.0001$ versus patients with RVEF > 30 percent).[160] Rosen et al found that the RVEF response to exercise was the best predictor of disease progression in a group of patients with severe MR and normal resting right and left ventricular performance. The annual risk of progression to a surgical end point was 4.9 percent in the subgroup in which this parameter increased with exercise and 14.7 percent in the subgroup without an increase ($p = 0.04$).[161]

Medical versus Surgical Therapy for Mitral Regurgitation

Animal data showing that depressed LV contractility is reversible have led to intriguing mechanistic approaches to correct this abnormality on a cellular level. Evidence that beta-receptor downregulation may play a significant role in the progressive decline in LV contractile function is provided by experiments in which contractile impairment was improved with beta-adrenergic blocker therapy.[162] In the clinical setting, however, no study to date has been able to document improved survival in patients with chronic MR treated with medical therapy, despite documented decreases in regurgitant volume in patients treated with vasodilators.[163–166] Surgical therapy for MR appears to offer a clear survival benefit, when compared with medical therapy.[29,167–169] Hammermeister et al found significantly improved 5- and 9- to-10-year survival rates for surgically treated versus medically treated patients (72 percent and 63 percent versus 55 percent and 22 percent). Delahaye et al reported 8-year survival rates of 74 percent for the surgically treated group versus 33 percent for the group treated with medical therapy. Thus, although survival is reduced in patients with impaired LV pump function, overall mortality is significantly improved with surgery compared with medical therapy, and surgery should therefore not be withheld in any patient with MR, even if LVEF is reduced at baseline.[151]

Mechanisms responsible for clinical improvement after surgery have been analyzed by several groups. Zile et al recently looked at LV diastolic parameters before and after mitral valve surgery and found that although there was incomplete regression of LV hypertrophy 3 months after valve replacement, the enhanced diastolic function seen preoperatively returned to normal after correction of the chronic volume overload.[170] Objective improvement in LV contractile performance was documented in 15 patients with chronic MR 1 year after successful valve surgery by Starling. While LVEF fell slightly in these patients, both the LV contractile index (E_{es}) and LV pump efficiency (expressed as the ratio of forward LV stroke work to the corresponding pressure–volume area) increased significantly[155] (see Fig. 24-12).

Evaluation of Mitral Valve Surgery

Mitral valve replacement will result in elimination of the low-pressure outflow pathway from the left ventricle,

thereby increasing afterload and, thus, resulting in a lower LVEF.[107,171] Boucher et al found a mean decrease in LVEF of 18 percent early after mitral valve replacement in 20 patients with MR. This decrease persisted when the patients were reevaluated late after mitral valve replacement. The decrease was more evident in patients whose resting LVEF preoperatively was 50 to 60 percent than in those whose LVEF was greater than 60 percent, implying that a low normal LVEF preoperatively indicates LV dysfunction, whereas a high normal resting LVEF implies better preserved LV performance.[107,172] In contrast to mitral valve replacement, surgical repair of the regurgitant mitral valve may not result in a decrease in LVEF postoperatively.[173] Furthermore, it has now been shown that postoperative survival and exercise capacity are improved in patients who undergo mitral valve replacement with chordal preservation, compared with traditional mitral valve replacement with excision of the submitral apparatus.[174,175] Rozich et al have identified several mechanisms responsible for preservation of LV pump performance following mitral valve replacement with chordal preservation. Conventional mitral valve replacement disrupts the submitral apparatus, and thereby disturbs the continuity between the mitral annulus and LV wall through the leaflets, chordae tendinae, and papillary muscles, resulting in significant increases in LVESV and end-systolic stress.[176] Furthermore, the ratio of the LV major axis to minor axis dimension decreases significantly, resulting in a loss of ellipsoidal LV geometry, and creation of a more spherical left ventricle.[177,178]

In conclusion, the following points should be remembered when evaluating patients with MR for surgery.[151]

1. A progressive decline in LV pump performance will be the consequence of chronic severe MR.
2. There is a prolonged asymptomatic period with a normal LVEF in these patients.
3. Contractile dysfunction may be occult in patients who remain asymptomatic and continue to show normal LVEFs, and it may or may not be reversible.
4. Patients who undergo mitral valve replacement or reconstruction while LV performance is normal, or while contractile dysfunction is reversible, will have a favorable long-term prognosis.
5. Those patients in whom irreversible contractile dysfunction has supervened are at risk of postoperative LV dysfunction and death due to CHF.

Despite the last point, patients treated with surgery enjoy improved long-term survival compared with patients treated medically. Furthermore, newer surgical techniques such as mitral valve reconstruction can preserve LV pump performance and reduce mortality and should be attempted preferentially whenever possible, especially in patients with reduced preoperative LV performance. Thus, the following generalizations can be made regarding patient groups with mitral regurgitation.

SYMPTOMATIC PATIENTS WITH REDUCED LEFT VENTRICULAR PERFORMANCE

Patients presenting with CHF, decreased exercise tolerance, or atrial arrhythmias should be referred for surgery, regardless of the status of the left ventricle. This is particularly true when mitral valve reconstruction can be performed.

ASYMPTOMATIC PATIENTS WITH BORDERLINE LEFT VENTRICULAR PERFORMANCE

Patients who manifest an LVEF in the low normal range (50 to 55 percent) or show LV dilatation (end-systolic dimension > 40 mm) are likely to have occult contractile dysfunction, and should be referred for surgery before irreversible contractile dysfunction supervenes.

ASYMPTOMATIC PATIENTS WITH NORMAL LEFT VENTRICULAR PERFORMANCE

Those patients who have a high normal LVEF (> 60%) and small left ventricles (end-systolic dimension < 40 mm) can be followed at 6- to 12-month intervals with echocardiography or radionuclide ventriculography. Should these patients deteriorate clinically or develop abnormal LV performance indices, they may then be considered for mitral valve surgery due to the assumed development of occult contractile dysfunction. In general, because MR has come to be recognized as a problem of contractile performance, it is appropriate, especially in the era of mitral valve repair, to consider mitral valve surgery earlier than previously thought (adapted from Donovan and Starling, with permission).[151]

MITRAL VALVE PROLAPSE

Mitral valve prolapse (MVP) is characterized morphologically by systolic billowing into the left atrium of either the posterior or anterior mitral valve leaflet or both. The disease occurs in about 6 percent of apparently normal subjects, is more common in women than in men, and has been reported in all age groups. Most patients are asymptomatic, and a systolic ejection click or a late systolic murmur or both are often observed on routine clinical evaluation.[179-188] Patients may manifest cardiac symptoms such as angina pectoris, palpitations, fatigue, dyspnea, and syncope. The angina is often atypical but may occasionally be confused with that due to concomitant CAD. The palpitations are often due to arrhythmias, both supraventricular and ventricular. Sud-

den death has been reported in these patients, but it is a rare complication. Symptoms of heart failure may occur in the subset of patients with MVP who have significant MR, now the most common cause for mitral valve surgery in this country.[189] Infrequently, embolic episodes, especially those involving the central nervous system, have been reported. The contrast left ventriculogram in these patients has variously been noted to demonstrate normal wall motion, regional asynergy, or diffuse asynergy.[190-192] Left ventricular performance is not directly related to the severity of MVP or to the presence and severity of MR.[184]

Chest pain in patients with MVP has been studied by the radionuclide LVEF response to exercise and by ^{201}Tl myocardial perfusion scintigraphy. Although many patients with MVP have normal LV performance, there is a subgroup without MR in whom diminished LV functional reserve is suggestive of a cardiomyopathic process in the absence of CAD.[193] Both RVEF and LVEF responses to exercise have been found to be abnormal in symptomatic patients with MVP. Assessment of radionuclide regurgitant fraction during rest and exercise also has revealed the development of MR with exercise in a significant proportion of symptomatic patients.[194] Some groups have found that men with MVP are more likely to have a normal LVEF response to exercise than are women, and a normal exercise LVEF response is more commonly observed in patients under 40 years of age than in older patients.[195,196] Additionally, during upright exercise, symptomatic women with MVP, but without associated CAD or MR, have been observed to have a significantly reduced LVEDV, stroke volume, and cardiac output compared to normal subjects.[196] These hemodynamic findings may explain the reduced exercise capacity observed in some women with MVP. Overall, a normal resting LVEF with a normal LVEF response to exercise in a patient with MVP indicates that the patient is unlikely to have associated CAD. An abnormal response, however, is not diagnostic of associated CAD and may instead indicate abnormal LV filling, hemodynamically significant MR, or an associated myocardial abnormality.[190,193,197]

Myocardial Perfusion Scintigraphy in Mitral Valve Prolapse

Several reports have examined the use of exercise ^{201}Tl scintigraphy to determine the coexistence of CAD and MVP.[198-204] In general, patients with MVP and no associated CAD have normal exercise ^{201}Tl images. Occasionally, fixed defects are noted. In some cases, these defects may be due to attenuation artifacts such as those due to breast attenuation in women. Others have found fixed defects that are localized to the inferior and posterior walls and may relate to diaphragm attenuation resulting from the use of a supine left lateral image or uniform background subtraction techniques.[200] Rarely, patients with MVP in the absence of associated CAD have exercise-induced reversible ^{201}Tl perfusion defects. This may be seen in about 5 percent of patients with MVP. Myocardial ischemia in patients with MVP has been inferred from the presence of chest pain and abnormal myocardial lactate metabolism.[205] LeWinter et al have shown that intravenous phenylephrine may induce chest pain in patients with MVP. They suggest that phenylephrine increases myocardial wall tension, which may result in a discrepancy between myocardial oxygen supply and demand.[206] A number of investigators have suggested that the increased tension of the taut chordae tendineae is transmitted to the papillary muscles and produces ischemia either by impairing blood supply or by causing an imbalance between supply and demand. The mechanism for exercise-induced myocardial ischemia in patients with MVP is not known. However, during exercise, the increase in sympathetic activity and tachycardia may augment the prolapse, increase the stretch of the chordae tendineae on the papillary muscles, and produce ischemia of the papillary muscles and surrounding myocardium. These factors may, in turn, lead to the appearance of MR, as documented by Lumia et al.[194] Coronary artery spasm has also been implicated as an important factor in the pathogenesis of pain in patients with MVP.[207] Chesler et al postulated that coronary artery spasm might be responsible for acute myocardial infarctions noted in 4 patients with MVP in whom postinfarction coronary angiography failed to show significant CAD.[208] Therefore, myocardial perfusion defects in patients with MVP may represent cellular loss, cellular dysfunction, or regional malperfusion. In general, the presence of an exercise-induced perfusion defect in patients with MVP suggests the presence of associated CAD, although infrequently this finding may be seen in the absence of significant CAD.

MITRAL STENOSIS

Cardiac nuclear imaging has not played a major role in the evaluation of mitral stenosis. Doppler and two-dimensional echocardiography can be used to assess the mitral valve orifice area noninvasively in most patients with this disease. Two-dimensional echocardiographic imaging allows the operator to define leaflet anatomy and dynamics, presence or absence of subvalvular disease and biventricular performance, functional orifice area (by valve planimetry), associated valvular regurgitation, and pulmonary artery pressures.[209] Doppler color-flow imaging allows accurate estimation of mitral valve area

and has been shown to correlate better with measurements obtained invasively than valve planimetry or the Doppler pressure half-time method.[210] Others have also evaluated the accuracy of the proximal isovelocity surface area (PISA) method for estimating mitral valve area and have found that it compares favorably with both pressure half-time estimates and valve planimetry.[211] Nishimura et al compared Doppler-derived mitral valve gradients with invasively measured gradients using both the directly measured left atrial (LA) pressure (obtained by transseptal catheterization) versus LV pressure, and the more commonly used PCWP approximation of LA pressure. They found that the Doppler-derived mean gradient correlated better with the directly measured LA–LV gradient than did the PCWP–LV gradient. They concluded that the Doppler-derived gradient is more accurate than that obtained by conventional cardiac catheterization techniques, and should be considered the reference standard.[212]

The stenotic mitral valve area has, however, been estimated from radionuclide ventriculography using a ratio of peak to mean LV filling rate, cardiac cycle length, and ejection fraction.[213] The appearance on radionuclide ventriculography of a normal-sized left ventricle, a dilated left atrium, a dilated hypocontractile right ventricle, and a normal stroke-count ratio represents a constellation of findings suggestive of mitral stenosis. The presence or absence of left atrial thrombi may also be demonstrated by radionuclide angiography.[214]

Radionuclide Assessment of Right Ventricular Performance in Mitral Valve Disease

Radionuclide techniques for the measurement of RV performance can assist in the assessment of disease severity in mitral stenosis. Several noninvasive techniques have been used to evaluate for the presence or absence of RV pressure or volume overload in patients with valvular heart disease. These include electrocardiography, vectorcardiography, chest roentgenography, ^{201}Tl myocardial scintigraphy, echocardiography, contrast ventriculography, and radionuclide ventriculography. Contrast cineventriculography may still be the "gold standard" for evaluating RV function, but there are several limitations that include the geometric shape of the right ventricle, the depressant effect of contrast material on ventricular function, and the risk and inconvenience of invasive testing. These are all factors that make RV cineventriculography unsuitable for serial evaluations. Echocardiography shares some of the disadvantages of cineventriculography because the RVEF and RV volumes are measured on the basis of geometric assumptions.

In contrast, the ejection fraction of the right ventricle with radionuclide ventriculography is determined from count changes that are independent of geometric assumptions. The first-pass method is probably the method of choice for measuring the RVEF and offers an advantage compared to multigated blood pool imaging because it allows temporal separation of the right ventricle from the left ventricle. In addition, the multicrystal camera may offer additional advantages over the single-crystal camera because of its high count rate efficiency. However, the first-pass method permits analysis of only a limited number of cardiac cycles. It requires careful quality control and a significant amount of computer processing time. The analysis of wall motion is not ideal with this method and multiple projections or studies require multiple injections with an increase in radiation dose to the patient. Single-beat RVEF measurement changes with variation in the concentration of the tracer in the right ventricle; underestimation occurs when tracer rapidly enters and overestimation when it rapidly leaves the right ventricle.[215] This effect may be attenuated by using a relative time–activity curve derived by dividing the original time–activity curve by a gamma variate function representing the time–concentration curve. Using this modified method, good agreement with a phantom ejection fraction was found. In addition to global RV performance, regional function may be determined using a chordal method. The combination of the first-pass method in the right anterior oblique projection and the gated method in the LAO projection permits biplane regional function analysis.[216] Most of the difficulty with the gated equilibrium technique is due to the overlap of the right ventricle and the right atrium. However, the method is easier, the processing time is shorter, and it permits evaluation of the right ventricle in multiple projections. Thus, the gated equilibrium method provides important information about RV size and wall motion as well.[217] It is also well suited for making serial measurements after interventions. Both the gated first-pass and gated equilibrium blood pool measurements of RVEF appear to correlate well with measurements from contrast ventriculography.[218]

There are several possible factors that influence RV performance in patients with mitral valve disease. These include an increase in afterload, an increase in preload (because of concomitant tricuspid regurgitation or pulmonic valve regurgitation), an interaction between the left and right ventricles through the common septum, and a decrease in contractility. In some patients, rheumatic myocarditis may be a cause of depressed RV performance.

Iskandrian et al measured intracardiac pressures and forward cardiac output during cardiac catheterization in 43 patients with mitral valve disease and measured the RVEF in these patients by first-pass radionuclide ventriculography with a multicrystal camera.[219] As has been described by others, a linear correlation between the pulmonary artery pressure and the right atrial pres-

sure was found.[220] The RVEF was abnormal in 88 percent of the patients with mitral valve disease. The RVEF correlated inversely with RVEDV, potentially an important compensatory mechanism to maintain cardiac output. In 22 of the 43 patients, the RV circumferential wall stress was measured using the equation:

$$Stress = (pressure \times radius)/thickness$$

where the pressure is the RV systolic pressure and the radius and thickness were measured by M-mode echocardiography. The circumferential wall stress of the right ventricle was abnormal in 15 patients with mitral valve disease compared to that obtained in normal subjects, and in 14 of these 15 patients the RVEF was also abnormal (<40 percent). Thus, an increase in afterload may be an important determinant of abnormal RV performance in patients with mitral valve disease, confirming that mitral valve disease adversely affects both RV and LV performance.

Several studies have examined the relationship between intra-cardiac pressures and the RVEF in patients with valvular heart disease. Winzelberg et al found no significant correlation between RVEF and RV systolic pressure or between the RVEF and right atrial pressure.[221] Others, however, have observed a significant inverse relationship between mean pulmonary arterial pressure and the RVEF.[222-224] Nonetheless, Morrison et al concluded that changes in resting RVEF could be explained only to a minor extent by changes in the mean pulmonary artery pressure. The presence of a normal RVEF (>45 percent) did not exclude the presence of pulmonary hypertension in patients with valvular heart disease.[222] Furthermore, the hemodynamic RV abnormalities in valvular heart disease are also influenced by diastolic as well as systolic LV performance, interactions between the left and right ventricles, and pericardial compressing effects.

Abnormal RV functional reserve in patients with mitral valve disease has been observed. Henze et al found a significant decrease in RVEF from a mean of 49 percent at rest to 37 percent during exercise in patients with MR. The RVEF response to exercise, however, was normal in patients with aortic valve disease, increasing from 49 percent at rest to 64 percent during exercise.[9] These results again imply that abnormal RV performance may play an important role in the progression of mitral valve but not aortic valve disease. Morise and Goodwin used radionuclide ventriculography to study 26 patients with mitral stenosis. An RVEF less than 40 percent at rest was noted in 9 patients, and an additional 13 patients had an abnormal RVEF response to exercise. The observed abnormal RVEF with exercise was related to an increase in RV end-systolic volume (counts). Most study patients also had a less than 5-unit increase in LVEF with exercise, reflecting a decrease in LVEDV (counts) rather than an increase in end-systolic volume.[225]

Radionuclide Assessment of Percutaneous or Surgical Correction of Mitral Stenosis

At present, the timing of mitral valvuloplasty or surgery for mitral stenosis is based on the presence or absence of limiting symptoms and on the mitral valve orifice area measured by cardiac catheterization. Balloon valvuloplasty has produced improvement in cardiac output and mitral valve area associated with a decrease in transvalvular gradient, pulmonary artery wedge pressure, and pulmonary artery pressure. The technique compares favorably with both closed and open mitral commissurotomy, for those patients with optimal mitral valve morphologic features (mobile, thin, noncalcified leaflets, little or no MR.)[226,227] The radionuclide-derived LV peak filling rate improves after mitral valvuloplasty.[228] The effects of mitral valve surgery on RV performance in patients with mitral valve disease have also been studied. In 14 patients who had radionuclide RVEF studies before and after mitral valve replacement, the RVEF improved significantly following surgery. Such improvement substantiates the effect of alleviation of abnormal wall stress on RV performance. However, complete normalization of RVEF was uncommon after mitral valve surgery, perhaps related to irreversible depression of RV inotropy, substantiating biventricular contractile dysfunction as the root problem in mitral valve disease. Perhaps the persistence of symptoms in some patients after successful mitral valve surgery for mitral stenosis or MR may be primarily an RV consequence, which limits an increase in cardiac output and conceivably affects the exercise tolerance in these patients.

Radionuclide Assessment of Right-Sided Valvular Lesions

Although tricuspid regurgitation is generally best evaluated by echocardiographic methods, several authors have described the use of radionuclide techniques for the diagnosis and serial assessment of this valvular lesion.[229-233] When systemic venous reflux is noted on radionuclide ventriculography, the diagnosis of tricuspid regurgitation is strongly suggested. [221,234,235] Radionuclide assessment of RV performance permits confirmation of the etiology of tricuspid insufficiency; if the lesion is a primary disorder, RV systolic function should be preserved, because the RV is unloaded into the right atrium. If severe pulmonary hypertension is present, ventriculography will show an enlarged, hypocontrac-

tile RV with an enlarged outflow tract and pulmonary artery.

Radionuclide ventriculography has also been used in the diagnosis of congenital right-sided disorders such as tricuspid atresia.[236-238] Huckell et al concluded from their analysis of a patient with tricuspid atresia and a malfunctioning shunt that first-pass radionuclide angiography could be used to demonstrate anatomic configurations not obvious at cardiac catheterization, and thus could be useful in the evaluation of adults with complex congenital lesions.[237]

SUMMARY

Radionuclide techniques can be used in the management of patients with valvular heart disease in a variety of ways. Although not as commonly applied as echocardiographic techniques, quantitative radionuclide evaluation of the severity of regurgitant lesions provides an accurate noninvasive method for assessing the severity and consequences of both right- and left-sided regurgitant lesions. Radionuclide ventriculography has been most widely applied in the serial assessment of right and left ventricular performance to determine the most appropriate timing for valve surgery in patients with aortic and mitral regurgitation, as well as those with stenotic lesions. Exercise radionuclide ventriculography may further clarify this subject in a subset of patients. Finally, ^{201}Tl myocardial perfusion scintigraphy, either with exercise or pharmacologic stress, allows for the accurate determination of coexisting CAD in patients with valvular lesions.

ACKNOWLEDGEMENT

The authors wish to acknowledge Dr. A.S. Iskandrian and Dr. M.C. Gerson, authors of this chapter in the second edition of *Cardiac Nuclear Medicine*, some of whose text they have retained in this edition.

REFERENCES

1. Rigo P, Alderson PO, Robertson RM, et al: Measurement of aortic and mitral regurgitation by gated cardiac blood pool scans. *Circulation* 60:306, 1979.
2. Urquhart J, Patterson RE, Packer M, et al: Quantification of valve regurgitation by radionuclide angiography be-

fore and after valve replacement surgery. *Am J Cardiol* 47:287, 1981.

3. Bough EW, Gandsman EJ, North DL, Shulman RS: Gated radionuclide angiographic evaluation of valve regurgitation. *Am J Cardiol* 46:423, 1980.

4. Baxter RH, Becker LC, Alderson PO, et al: Quantification of aortic valvular regurgitation in dogs by nuclear imaging. *Circulation* 61:404, 1980.

5. Lam W, Pavel D, Byrom E, et al: Radionuclide regurgitant index: Value and limitations. *Am J Cardiol* 47:292, 1981.

6. Sorensen SG, O'Rourke RA, Chaudhuri TK: Noninvasive quantitation of valvular regurgitation by gated equilibrium radionuclide angiography. *Circulation* 62:1089, 1980.

7. Nicod P, Corbett JR, Firth BG, et al: Radionuclide techniques for valvular regurgitant index: Comparison in patients with normal and depressed ventricular function. *J Nucl Med* 23:763, 1982.

8. Janowitz WR, Fester A: Quantitation of left ventricular regurgitant fraction by first pass radionuclide angiocardiography. *Am J Cardiol* 49:85, 1982.

9. Henze E, Schelbert HR, Wisenberg G, et al: Assessment of regurgitant fraction and right and left ventricular function at rest and during exercise: A new technique for determination of right ventricular stroke counts from gated equilibrium blood pool studies. *Am Heart J* 104:953, 1982.

10. Klepzig H Jr, Standke R, Nickelsen T, et al: Combined first-pass and equilibrium radionuclide ventriculography and comparison with left ventricular/right ventricular stroke count ratio in mitral and aortic regurgitation. *Am J Cardiol* 55:1048, 1985.

11. Makler P Jr, McCarthy DM, Velchik MG, et al: Fourier amplitude ratio: A new way to assess valvular regurgitation. *J Nucl Med* 24:204, 1983.

12. Makler P Jr, McCarthy DM, Kleaveland JP, et al: Validation of Fourier amplitude ratio to quantitate valvular regurgitation. *J Am Coll Cardiol* 3:1482, 1984.

13. Handler B, Pavel DG, Lam W, et al: Tricuspid insufficiency detected by equilibrium gated radionuclide study. *Clin Nucl Med* 6:485, 1981.

14. Sorensen SG, Starling MR, Chaudhuri TK, O'Rourke RA: Noninvasive quantitation of right-ventricular volume overload in adults by gated equilibrium radionuclide angiography. *J Nucl Med* 23:957, 1982.

15. Oh J, Seward J, Tajik A: Valvular heart disease, in Oh J, Seward J, Tajik A (eds): *The Echo Manual*. Rochester, MN, Little, Brown, 1994, p. 101.

16. Losordo DW, Pastore JO, Coletta D, et al: Limitations of color flow Doppler imaging in the quantification of valvular regurgitation: Velocity of regurgitant jet, rather than volume, determines size of color Doppler image. *Am Heart J* 126:168, 1993.

17. Samstad SO, Hegrenaes L, Skjaerpe T, Hatle L: Half time of the diastolic aortoventricular pressure difference by continuous wave Doppler ultrasound: A measure of the severity of aortic regurgitation? *Br Heart J* 61:336, 1989.

18. Oh JK, Hatle LK, Sinak LJ, et al: Characteristic Doppler echocardiographic pattern of mitral inflow velocity in severe aortic regurgitation [see comments]. *J Am Coll Cardiol* 14:1712, 1989.

19. Rokey R, Sterling LL, Zoghbi WA, et al: Determination of regurgitant fraction in isolated mitral or aortic regurgitation by pulsed Doppler two-dimensional echocardiography. *J Am Coll Cardiol* 7:1273, 1986.

20. Kurokawa S, Takahashi M, Sugiyama T, et al: Noninvasive evaluation of the magnitude of aortic and mitral regurgitation by means of Doppler two-dimensional echocardiography. *Am Heart J* 120:638, 1990.

21. Recusani F, Bargiggia GS, Yoganathan AP, et al: A new method for quantification of regurgitant flow rate using color Doppler flow imaging of the flow convergence region proximal to a discrete orifice. An in vitro study. *Circulation* 83:594, 1991.

22. Enriquez-Sarano M, Seward JB, Bailey KR, Tajik AJ: Effective regurgitant orifice area: A noninvasive Doppler development of an old hemodynamic concept. *J Am Coll Cardiol* 23:443, 1994.

23. Vandervoort PM, Rivera JM, Mele D, et al: Application of color Doppler flow mapping to calculate effective regurgitant orifice area. An in vitro study and initial clinical observations. *Circulation* 88:1150, 1993.

24. Shiota T, Teien D, Deng YB, et al: Estimation of regurgitant flow volume based on centerline velocity/distance profiles using digital color M-Q Doppler: Application to orifices of different shapes. *J Am Coll Cardiol* 24:440, 1994.

25. Klein AL, Burstow DJ, Tajik AJ, et al: Age-related prevalence of valvular regurgitation in normal subjects: A comprehensive color flow examination of 118 volunteers. *J Am Soc Echocardiogr* 3:54, 1990.

26. Currie PJ, Seward JB, Chan KL, et al: Continuous wave Doppler determination of right ventricular pressure: A simultaneous Doppler-catheterization study in 127 patients. *J Am Coll Cardiol* 6:750, 1985.

27. Grossman W, Jones D, McLaurin LP: Wall stress and patterns of hypertrophy in the human left ventricle. *J Clin Invest* 56:56, 1975.

28. Wisenbaugh T, Spann JF, Carabello BA: Differences in myocardial performance and load between patients with similar amounts of chronic aortic versus chronic mitral regurgitation. *J Am Coll Cardiol* 3:916, 1984.

29. Rapaport E: Natural history of aortic and mitral valve disease. *Am J Cardiol* 35:221, 1975.

30. Gaasch WH, Andrias CW, Levine HJ: Chronic aortic regurgitation: The effect of aortic valve replacement on left ventricular volume, mass and function. *Circulation* 58:825, 1978.

31. Copeland JG, Griepp RB, Stinson EB, Shumway NE: Long-term follow-up after isolated aortic valve replacement. *J Thorac Cardiovasc Surg* 74:875, 1977.

32. Borow KM, Green LH, Mann T, et al: End-systolic volume as a predictor of postoperative left ventricular performance in volume overload from valvular regurgitation. *Am J Med* 68:655, 1980.

33. Turina J, Turina M, Rothlin M, Krayenbuehl HP: Improved late survival in patients with chronic aortic regurgitation by earlier operation. *Circulation* 70:I147, 1984.

34. Toussaint C, Cribier A, Cazor JL, et al: Hemodynamic

and angiographic evaluation of aortic regurgitation 8 and 27 months after aortic valve replacement. *Circulation* 64:456, 1981.

35. Hwang MH, Hammermeister KE, Oprian C, et al: Preoperative identification of patients likely to have left ventricular dysfunction after aortic valve replacement. Participants in the Veterans Administration Cooperative Study on Valvular Heart Disease. *Circulation* 80:I65, 1989.

36. Greves J, Rahimtoola SH, McAnulty JH, et al: Preoperative criteria predictive of late survival following valve replacement for severe aortic regurgitation. *Am Heart J* 101:300, 1981.

37. Cornyn JW, Massie BM, Greenberg B, et al: Reproducibility of rest and exercise left ventricular ejection fraction and volumes in chronic aortic regurgitation. *Am J Cardiol* 59:1361, 1987.

38. Kress P, Adam WE, Hombach V: Timing of valve replacement in chronic aortic regurgitation. A pathophysiological approach. *Clin Physiol Biochem* 8:38, 1990.

39. Starling MR, Kirsh MM, Montgomery DG, Gross MD: Mechanisms for left ventricular systolic dysfunction in aortic regurgitation: Importance for predicting the functional response to aortic valve replacement [see comments]. *J Am Coll Cardiol* 17:887, 1991.

40. Bonow RO, Rosing DR, McIntosh CL, et al: The natural history of asymptomatic patients with aortic regurgitation and normal left ventricular function. *Circulation* 68:509, 1983.

41. Bonow RO, Rosing DR, Maron BJ, et al: Reversal of left ventricular dysfunction after aortic valve replacement for chronic aortic regurgitation: Influence of duration of preoperative left ventricular dysfunction. *Circulation* 70:570, 1984.

42. Bonow RO, Picone AL, McIntosh CL, et al: Survival and functional results after valve replacement for aortic regurgitation from 1976 to 1983: Impact of preoperative left ventricular function. *Circulation* 72:1244, 1985.

43. Bonow RO, Dodd JT, Maron BJ, et al: Long-term serial changes in left ventricular function and reversal of ventricular dilatation after valve replacement for chronic aortic regurgitation. *Circulation* 78:1108, 1988.

44. Bonow RO, Lakatos E, Maron BJ, Epstein SE: Serial long-term assessment of the natural history of asymptomatic patients with chronic aortic regurgitation and normal left ventricular systolic function. *Circulation* 84:1625, 1991.

45. Mehmel HC, Stockins B, Ruffmann K, et al: The linearity of the end-systolic pressure-volume relationship in man and its sensitivity for assessment of left ventricular function. *Circulation* 63:1216, 1981.

46. Sagawa K, Suga H, Shoukas AA, Bakalar KM: End-systolic pressure/volume ratio: A new index of ventricular contractility. *Am J Cardiol* 40:748, 1977.

47. Suga H, Sagawa K, Shoukas AA: Load independence of the instantaneous pressure-volume ratio of the canine left ventricle and effects of epinephrine and heart rate on the ratio. *Circ Res* 32:314, 1973.

48. Schuler G, von Olshausen K, Schwarz F, et al: Noninvasive assessment of myocardial contractility in asymptomatic patients with severe aortic regurgitation and normal

left ventricular ejection fraction at rest. *Am J Cardiol* 50:45, 1982.

49. Shen WF, Roubin GS, Choong CY, et al: Evaluation of relationship between myocardial contractile state and left ventricular function in patients with aortic regurgitation. *Circulation* 71:31, 1985.

50. Iskandrian AS, Hakki AH, Kane-Marsch S: Left ventricular pressure/volume relationship in aortic regurgitation. *Am Heart J* 110:1026, 1985.

51. Branzi A, Lolli C, Piovaccari G, et al: Echocardiographic evaluation of the response to afterload stress test in young asymptomatic patients with chronic severe aortic regurgitation: Sensitivity of the left ventricular end-systolic pressure-volume relationship. *Circulation* 70:561, 1984.

52. Stewart RE, Gross MD, Starling MR: Mechanisms for an abnormal radionuclide left ventricular ejection fraction response to exercise in patients with chronic, severe aortic regurgitation. *Am Heart J* 123:453, 1992.

53. Corrigan D: On permanent patency of the mouth of the aorta or inadequacy of the aortic valves. *Edinburgh Med Surg J* 37:225, 1832.

54. Judge TP, Kennedy JW, Bennett LJ, et al: Quantitative hemodynamic effects of heart rate in aortic regurgitation. *Circulation* 44:355, 1971.

55. Firth BG, Dehmer GJ, Nicod P, et al: Effect of increasing heart rate in patients with aortic regurgitation. Effect of incremental atrial pacing on scintigraphic, hemodynamic and thermodilution measurements. *Am J Cardiol* 49:1860, 1982.

56. Kligfield P, Ameisen O, Okin PM, et al: Relationship of the electrocardiographic response to exercise to geometric and functional findings in aortic regurgitation. *Am Heart J* 113:1097, 1987.

57. Bonow RO, Borer JS, Rosing DR, et al: Preoperative exercise capacity in symptomatic patients with aortic regurgitation as a predictor of postoperative left ventricular function and long-term prognosis. *Circulation* 62:1280, 1980.

58. Kawanishi DT, McKay CR, Chandraratna PA, et al: Cardiovascular response to dynamic exercise in patients with chronic symptomatic mild-to-moderate and severe aortic regurgitation. *Circulation* 73:62, 1986.

59. Dehmer GJ, Firth BG, Hillis LD, et al: Alterations in left ventricular volumes and ejection fraction at rest and during exercise in patients with aortic regulation. *Am J Cardiol* 48:17, 1981.

60. Johnson LL, Powers ER, Tzall WR, et al: Left ventricular volume and ejection fraction response to exercise in aortic regurgitation. *Am J Cardiol* 51:1379, 1983.

61. Iskandrian AS, Hakki AH, Manno B, et al: Left ventricular function in chronic aortic regurgitation. *J Am Coll Cardiol* 1:1374, 1983.

62. Peter CA, Jones RH: Cardiac response to exercise in patients with chronic aortic regurgitation. *Am Heart J* 104:85, 1982.

63. Iskandrian AS, Hakki AH, Amenta A, et al: Regulation of cardiac output during upright exercise in patients with aortic regurgitation. *Cathet Cardiovasc Diagn* 10:573, 1984.

64. Gerson MC, Engel PJ, Mantil JC, et al: Effects of dynamic

and isometric exercise on the radionuclide-determined regurgitant fraction in aortic insufficiency. *J Am Coll Cardiol* 3:98, 1984.

65. Steingart RM, Yee C, Weinstein L, Scheuer J: Radionuclide ventriculographic study of adaptations to exercise in aortic regurgitation. *Am J Cardiol* 51:483, 1983.

66. Borer JS, Bacharach SL, Green MV, et al: Exercise-induced left ventricular dysfunction in symptomatic and asymptomatic patients with aortic regurgitation: Assessment with radionuclide cineangiography. *Am J Cardiol* 42:351, 1978.

67. Hecht HS, Hopkins JM: Exercise-induced regional wall motion abnormalities on radionuclide angiography. Lack of reliability for detection of coronary artery disease in the presence of valvular heart disease. *Am J Cardiol* 47:861, 1981.

68. Lewis SM, Riba AL, Berger HJ, et al: Radionuclide angiographic exercise left ventricular performance in chronic aortic regurgitation: Relationship to resting echographic ventricular dimensions and systolic wall stress index. *Am Heart J* 103:498, 1982.

69. Siemienczuk D, Greenberg B, Morris C, et al: Chronic aortic insufficiency: Factors associated with progression to aortic valve replacement. *Ann Intern Med* 110:587, 1989.

70. Goldman ME, Packer M, Horowitz SF, et al: Relation between exercise-induced changes in ejection fraction and systolic loading conditions at rest in aortic regurgitation. *J Am Coll Cardiol* 3:924, 1984.

71. Port S, Cobb FR, Coleman RE, Jones RH: Effect of age on the response of the left ventricular ejection fraction to exercise. *N Engl J Med* 303:1133, 1980.

72. Shen WF, Roubin GS, Hirasawa K, et al: Noninvasive assessment of acute effects of nifedipine on rest and exercise hemodynamics and cardiac function in patients with aortic regurgitation. *J Am Coll Cardiol* 4:902, 1984.

73. Greenberg B, Massie B, Thomas D, et al: Association between the exercise ejection fraction response and systolic wall stress in patients with chronic aortic insufficiency. *Circulation* 71:458, 1985.

74. Bonow RO, Rosing DR, Kent KM, Epstein SE: Timing of operation for chronic aortic regurgitation. *Am J Cardiol* 50:325, 1982.

75. Massie BM, Kramer BL, Loge D, et al: Ejection fraction response to supine exercise in asymptomatic aortic regurgitation: Relation to simultaneous hemodynamic measurements. *J Am Coll Cardiol* 5:847, 1985.

76. Boucher CA, Wilson RA, Kanarek DJ, et al: Exercise testing in asymptomatic or minimally symptomatic aortic regurgitation: Relationship of left ventricular ejection fraction to left ventricular filling pressure during exercise. *Circulation* 67:1091, 1983.

77. Reichek N, Wilson J, St John Sutton M, et al: Noninvasive determination of left ventricular end-systolic stress: validation of the method and initial application. *Circulation* 65:99, 1982.

78. Shen W, Fletcher PJ, Roubin GS, et al: Relation between left ventricular functional reserve during exercise and resting systolic loading conditions in chronic aortic regurgitation. *Am J Cardiol* 58:757, 1985.

79. Wilson RA, Greenberg BH, Massie BM, et al: Left ventricular response to submaximal and maximal exercise in asymptomatic aortic regurgitation. *Am J Cardiol* 62:606, 1988.

80. Nitenberg A, Foult JM, Antony I, et al: Coronary flow and resistance reserve in patients with chronic aortic regurgitation, angina pectoris and normal coronary arteries. *J Am Coll Cardiol* 11:478, 1988.

81. Kawachi K, Kitamura S, Oyama C, et al: Relations of preoperative hemodynamics and coronary blood flow to improved left ventricular function after valve replacement for aortic regurgitation. *J Am Coll Cardiol* 11:925, 1988.

82. Nies R, Hanke H, Helber U, et al: [Perfusion of the left ventricular myocardium in patients with aortic valve diseases using single photon emission computerized tomography (published erratum appears in *Z Kardiol* 84:77, 1995)]. *Z Kardiol* 83:864, 1994.

83. Pfisterer M, Muller-Brand J, Brundler H, Cueni T: Prevalence and significance of reversible radionuclide ischemic perfusion defects in symptomatic aortic valve disease patients with or without concomitant coronary disease. *Am Heart J* 103:92, 1982.

84. Henry WL, Bonow RO, Borer JS, et al: Observations on the optimum time for operative intervention for aortic regurgitation. I. Evaluation of the results of aortic valve replacement in symptomatic patients. *Circulation* 61:471, 1980.

85. Henry WL, Bonow RO, Rosing DR, Epstein SE: Observations on the optimum time for operative intervention for aortic regurgitation. II. Serial echocardiographic evaluation of asymptomatic patients. *Circulation* 61:484, 1980.

86. Fioretti P, Roelandt J, Bos RJ, et al: Echocardiography in chronic aortic insufficiency. Is valve replacement too late when left ventricular end-systolic dimension reaches 55 mm? *Circulation* 67:216, 1983.

87. Daniel WG, Hood W Jr, Siart A, et al: Chronic aortic regurgitation: Reassessment of the prognostic value of preoperative left ventricular end-systolic dimension and fractional shortening. *Circulation* 71:669, 1985.

88. Bonow RO, Epstein SE: Is preoperative left ventricular function predictive of survival and functional results after aortic valve replacement for chronic aortic regurgitation? *J Am Coll Cardiol* 10:713, 1987.

89. Carabello BA, Usher BW, Hendrix GH, et al: Predictors of outcome for aortic valve replacement in patients with aortic regurgitation and left ventricular dysfunction: A change in the measuring stick. *J Am Coll Cardiol* 10:991, 1987.

90. Borow KM: Surgical outcome in chronic aortic regurgitation: a physiologic framework for assessing preoperative predictors. *J Am Coll Cardiol* 10:1165, 1987.

91. Gaasch WH, Carroll JD, Levine HJ, Criscitiello MG: Chronic aortic regurgitation: Prognostic value of left ventricular end-systolic dimension and end-diastolic radius/thickness ratio. *J Am Coll Cardiol* 1:775, 1983.

92. Fioretti P, Roelandt J, Sclavo M, et al: Postoperative regression of left ventricular dimensions in aortic insufficiency: A long-term echocardiographic study. *J Am Coll Cardiol* 5:856, 1985.

93. Kumpuris AG, Quinones MA, Waggoner AD, et al: Im-

portance of preoperative hypertrophy, wall stress and end-systolic dimension as echocardiographic predictors of normalization of left ventricular dilatation after valve replacement in chronic aortic insufficiency. *Am J Cardiol* 49:1091, 1982.

94. Vandenbossche JL, Massie BM, Schiller NB, Karliner JS: Relation of left ventricular shape to volume and mass in patients with minimally symptomatic chronic aortic regurgitation. *Am Heart J* 116:1022, 1988.

95. Stone PH, Clark RD, Goldschlager N, et al: Determinants of prognosis of patients with aortic regurgitation who undergo aortic valve replacement. *J Am Coll Cardiol* 3:1118, 1984.

96. Ross J Jr: Afterload mismatch in aortic and mitral valve disease: Implications for surgical therapy. *J Am Coll Cardiol* 5:811, 1985.

97. Crawford MH, Wilson RS, O'Rourke RA, Vittitoe JA: Effect of digoxin and vasodilators on left ventricular function in aortic regurgitation. *Int J Cardiol* 23:385, 1989.

98. Lin M, Chiang HT, Lin SL, et al: Vasodilator therapy in chronic asymptomatic aortic regurgitation: Enalapril versus hydralazine therapy. *J Am Coll Cardiol* 24:1046, 1994.

99. Scognamiglio R, Rahimtoola SH, Fasoli G, et al: Nifedipine in asymptomatic patients with severe aortic regurgitation and normal left ventricular function [see comments]. *N Engl J Med* 331:689, 1994.

100. Dumesnil JG, Tran K, Dagenais GR: Beneficial long-term effects of hydralazine in aortic regurgitation. *Arch Intern Med* 150:757, 1990.

101. Nauman D, Greenberg B, Massie B, et al: Effects of stopping long-term vasodilator therapy in patients with chronic aortic insufficiency. *Chest* 102:720, 1992.

102. Leenen FH, Strauss MH, Chan YK, Burns RJ: Cardiac effects of prazosin in chronic aortic insufficiency. *Can J Cardiol* 7:265, 1991.

103. Scognamiglio R, Fasoli G, Ponchia A, Dalla-Volta S: Long-term nifedipine unloading therapy in asymptomatic patients with chronic severe aortic regurgitation [see comments]. *J Am Coll Cardiol* 16:424, 1990.

104. Schon HR, Schomig A. [Long-term treatment with quinapril in chronic aortic and mitral insufficiency]. *Dtsch Med Wochenschr* 120:429, 1995.

105. Rothlisberger C, Sareli P, Wisenbaugh T: Comparison of single-dose nifedipine and captopril for chronic severe aortic regurgitation. *Am J Cardiol* 72:799, 1993.

106. Borer JS, Rosing DR, Kent KM, et al: Left ventricular function at rest and during exercise after aortic valve replacement in patients with aortic regurgitation. *Am J Cardiol* 44:1297, 1979.

107. Boucher CA, Bingham JB, Osbakken MD, et al: Early changes in left ventricular size and function after correction of left ventricular volume overload. *Am J Cardiol* 47:991, 1981.

108. Monrad ES, Hess OM, Murakami T, et al: Time course of regression of left ventricular hypertrophy after aortic valve replacement. *Circulation* 77:1345, 1988.

109. van der Wall EE, Kasim M, Camps JA, et al: Abnormal septal motion after aortic valve replacement for chronic aortic regurgitation: No evidence for myocardial isch-

aemia by exercise radionuclide angiography. *Eur J Nucl Med* 17:252, 1990.

110. Goldman MR, Boucher CA, Block PC, et al: Spectrum of congestive heart failure late after aortic valve or mitral replacement: Differentiation of valvular versus myocardial cause by radionuclide ventriculogram-ejection fraction. *Am Heart J* 102:751, 1981.

111. Ross J Jr, Braunwald E: Aortic stenosis. *Circulation* 38:Suppl 5:V61+, 1968.

112. Frank S, Johnson A, Ross J Jr: Natural history of valvular aortic stenosis. *Br Heart J* 35:41, 1973.

113. Chizner MA, Pearle DL, deLeon A Jr: The natural history of aortic stenosis in adults. *Am Heart J* 99:419, 1980.

114. DePace NL, Ren JF, Iskandrian AS, et al: Correlation of echocardiographic wall stress and left ventricular pressure and function in aortic stenosis. *Circulation* 67:854, 1983.

115. Nadell R, DePace NL, Ren JF, et al: Myocardial oxygen supply/demand ratio in aortic stenosis: Hemodynamic and echocardiographic evaluation of patients with and without angina pectoris. *J Am Coll Cardiol* 2:258, 1983.

116. Richards KL, Cannon SR, Miller JF, Crawford MH: Calculation of aortic valve area by Doppler echocardiography: A direct application of the continuity equation. *Circulation* 73:964, 1986.

117. Ford LE, Feldman T, Chiu YC, Carroll JD: Hemodynamic resistance as a measure of functional impairment in aortic valvular stenosis. *Circ Res* 66:1, 1990.

118. Cannon J Jr, Zile MR, Crawford F Jr, Carabello BA: Aortic valve resistance as an adjunct to the Gorlin formula in assessing the severity of aortic stenosis in symptomatic patients. *J Am Coll Cardiol* 20:1517, 1992.

119. Rediker DE, Boucher CA, Block PC, et al: Degree of reversibility of left ventricular systolic dysfunction after aortic valve replacement for isolated aortic valve stenosis. *Am J Cardiol* 60:112, 1987.

120. Fischl SJ, Gorlin R, Herman MV: Cardiac shape and function in aortic valve disease: physiologic and clinical implications. *Am J Cardiol* 39:170, 1977.

121. Fifer MA, Bourdillon PD, Lorell BH: Altered left ventricular diastolic properties during pacing-induced angina in patients with aortic stenosis. *Circulation* 74:675, 1986.

122. Lavine SJ, Follansbee WP, Shreiner DP, Amidi M: Left ventricular diastolic filling in valvular aortic stenosis. *Am J Cardiol* 57:1349, 1986.

123. Murakami T, Hess OM, Gage JE, et al: Diastolic filling dynamics in patients with aortic stenosis. *Circulation* 73:1162, 1986.

124. Hess OM, Ritter M, Schneider J, et al: Diastolic stiffness and myocardial structure in aortic valve disease before and after valve replacement. *Circulation* 69:855, 1984.

125. Mandal AB, Gray IR: Significance of angina pectoris in aortic valve stenosis. *Br Heart J* 38:811, 1976.

126. Marcus ML, Doty DB, Hiratzka LF, et al: Decreased coronary reserve: A mechanism for angina pectoris in patients with aortic stenosis and normal coronary arteries. *N Engl J Med* 307:1362, 1982.

127. Hakki AH, Kimbiris D, Iskandrian AS, et al: Angina pectoris and coronary artery disease in patients with severe aortic valvular disease. *Am Heart J* 100:441, 1980.

128. Graboys TB, Cohn PF: The prevalence of angina pectoris

and abnormal coronary arteriograms in severe aortic valvular disease. *Am Heart J* 93:683, 1977.

129. Basta LL, Raines D, Najjar S, Kioschos JM: Clinical, haemodynamic, and coronary angiographic correlates of angina pectoris in patients with severe aortic valve disease. *Br Heart J* 37:150, 1975.

130. Anderson FL, Tsagaris TJ, Tikoff G, et al: Hemodynamic effects of exercise in patients with aortic stenosis. *Am J Med* 46:872, 1969.

131. Borer J, Bacharach SL, Green MV, et al: Left ventricular function in aortic stenosis: Response to exercise and effects of operation. *Am J Cardiol* 41:382, 1978 (abstr).

132. Milanes JC, Paldi J, Romero M, et al: Detection of coronary artery disease in aortic stenosis by exercise gated nuclear angiography. *Am J Cardiol* 54:787, 1984.

133. Archer SL, Mike DK, Hetland MB, et al: Usefulness of mean aortic valve gradient and left ventricular diastolic filling pattern for distinguishing symptomatic from asymptomatic patients. *Am J Cardiol* 73:275, 1994.

134. Clyne CA, Arrighi JA, Maron BJ, et al: Systemic and left ventricular responses to exercise stress in asymptomatic patients with valvular aortic stenosis. *Am J Cardiol* 68:1469, 1991.

135. Bailey IK, Come PC, Kelly DT, et al: Thallium-201 myocardial perfusion imaging in aortic valve stenosis. *Am J Cardiol* 40:889, 1977.

136. Kupari M, Virtanen KS, Turto H, et al: Exclusion of coronary artery disease by exercise thallium-201 tomography in patients with aortic valve stenosis. *Am J Cardiol* 70:635, 1992.

137. Aubry P, Assayag P, Faraggi M, et al: [Detection of coronary disease before valve surgery. Contribution of myocardial scintigraphy with dipyridamole]. *Ann Cardiol Angeiol* 40:9, 1991.

138. Huikuri HV, Korhonen UR, Ikaheimo MJ, et al: Detection of coronary artery disease by thallium imaging using a combined intravenous dipyridamole and isometric handgrip test in patients with aortic valve stenosis. *Am J Cardiol* 59:336, 1987.

139. Huikuri HV, Airaksinen KE, Ikaheimo MJ, et al: Detection of coronary artery disease by dipyridamole thallium tomography in mitral valve stenosis. *Am J Cardiol* 63:124, 1989.

140. Rask P, Karp K, Edlund B, et al: Computer-assisted evaluation of dipyridamole thallium-201 SPECT in patients with aortic stenosis. *J Nucl Med* 35:983, 1994.

141. Vandeplas A, Willems JL, Piessens J, De Geest H: Frequency of angina pectoris and coronary artery disease in severe isolated valvular aortic stenosis. *Am J Cardiol* 62:117, 1988.

142. Cribier A, Savin T, Berland J, et al: Percutaneous transluminal balloon valvuloplasty of adult aortic stenosis: Report of 92 cases. *J Am Coll Cardiol* 9:381, 1987.

143. Isner JM, Salem DN, Desnoyers MR, et al: Treatment of calcific aortic stenosis by balloon valvuloplasty. *Am J Cardiol* 59:313, 1987.

144. McKay RG, Safian RD, Lock JE, et al: Assessment of left ventricular and aortic valve function after aortic balloon valvuloplasty in adult patients with critical aortic stenosis. *Circulation* 75:192, 1987.

145. Harpole DH, Davidson CJ, Skelton TN, et al: Changes in left ventricular systolic performance immediately after percutaneous aortic balloon valvuloplasty. *Am J Cardiol* 65:1213, 1990.

146. Harpole DH, Davidson C, Skelton T, et al: Serial evaluation of ventricular function after percutaneous aortic balloon valvuloplasty. *Am Heart J* 119:130, 1990.

147. Kelly TA, Rothbart RM, Cooper CM, et al: Comparison of outcome of asymptomatic to symptomatic patients older than 20 years of age with valvular aortic stenosis. *Am J Cardiol* 61:123, 1988.

148. Harpole DH, Jones RH: Serial assessment of ventricular performance after valve replacement for aortic stenosis. *J Thorac Cardiovasc Surg* 99:645, 1990.

149. Berko B, Gaasch WH, Tanigawa N, et al: Disparity between ejection and end-systolic indexes of left ventricular contractility in mitral regurgitation. *Circulation* 75:1310, 1987.

150. Carabello BA: Mitral valve disease. *Curr Probl Cardiol* 18:423, 1993.

151. Donovan CL, Starling MR: The role of echocardiography in the timing of surgical intervention for chronic mitral and aortic regurgitation, in Otto CM (ed.), *Textbook of Clinical Echocardiography*, Philadelphia, WB Saunders, In press.

152. Urabe Y, Mann DL, Kent RL, et al: Cellular and ventricular contractile dysfunction in experimental canine mitral regurgitation. *Circ Res* 70:131, 1992.

153. Starling MR, Kirsh MM, Montgomery DG, Gross MD: Impaired left ventricular contractile function in patients with long-term mitral regurgitation and normal ejection fraction. *J Am Coll Cardiol* 22:239, 1993.

154. Nakano K, Swindle MM, Spinale F, et al: Depressed contractile function due to canine mitral regurgitation improves after correction of the volume overload [published erratum appears in *J Clin Invest* 88:723, 1991]. *J Clin Invest* 87:2077, 1991.

155. Starling MR: Effects of valve surgery on left ventricular contractile function in patients with long-term mitral regurgitation. *Circulation* 92:811, 1995.

156. Carabello BA, Nolan SP, McGuire LB: Assessment of preoperative left ventricular function in patients with mitral regurgitation: Value of the end-systolic wall stress-end-systolic volume ratio. *Circulation* 64:1212, 1981.

157. Zile MR, Gaasch WH, Carroll JD, Levine HJ: Chronic mitral regurgitation: Predictive value of preoperative echocardiographic indexes of left ventricular function and wall stress. *J Am Coll Cardiol* 3:235, 1984.

158. Carabello BA, Williams H, Gash AK, et al: Hemodynamic predictors of outcome in patients undergoing valve replacement [published erratum appears in *Circulation* 75:650, 1989]. *Circulation* 74:1309, 1986.

159. Ramanathan KB, Knowles J, Connor MJ, et al: Natural history of chronic mitral insufficiency: Relation of peak systolic pressure/end-systolic volume ratio to morbidity and mortality. *J Am Coll Cardiol* 3:1412, 1984.

160. Hochreiter C, Niles N, Devereux RB, et al: Mitral regurgitation: Relationship of noninvasive descriptors of right and left ventricular performance to clinical and hemodynamic findings and to prognosis in medically and surgically treated patients. *Circulation* 73:900, 1986.

161. Rosen SE, Borer JS, Hochreiter C, et al: Natural history of

the asymptomatic/minimally symptomatic patient with severe mitral regurgitation secondary to mitral valve prolapse and normal right and left ventricular performance. *Am J Cardiol* 74:374, 1994.

162. Tsutsiu H NM, Ishihara K, DeFreyte G, et al: Ameliorative effects of β-adrenoceptor blockade on contractile dysfunction in chronic mitral regurgitation. *Circulation* 86(Suppl II):II-16, 1992.

163. Greenberg BH, Massie BM, Brundage BH, et al: Beneficial effects of hydralazine in severe mitral regurgitation. *Circulation* 58:273, 1978.

164. Greenberg BH, DeMots H, Murphy E, Rahimtoola SH: Arterial dilators in mitral regurgitation: Effects on rest and exercise hemodynamics and long-term clinical follow-up. *Circulation* 65:181, 1982.

165. Yoran C, Yellin EL, Becker RM, et al: Mechanism of reduction of mitral regurgitation with vasodilator therapy. *Am J Cardiol* 43:773, 1979.

166. Wisenbaugh T, Essop R, Sareli P: Short-term vasodilator effect of captopril in patients with severe mitral regurgitation is parasympathetically mediated. *Circulation* 84:2049, 1991.

167. Munoz S, Gallardo J, Diaz-Gorrin JR, Medina O: Influence of surgery on the natural history of rheumatic mitral and aortic valve disease. *Am J Cardiol* 35:234, 1975.

168. Hammermeister KE, Fisher L, Kennedy W, et al: Prediction of late survival in patients with mitral valve disease from clinical, hemodynamic, and quantitative angiographic variables. *Circulation* 57:341, 1978.

169. Delahaye JP, Gare JP, Viguier E, et al: Natural history of severe mitral regurgitation. *Eur Heart J* 12:5, 1991.

170. Zile MR, Tomita M, Ishihara K, et al: Changes in diastolic function during development and correction of chronic LV volume overload produced by mitral regurgitation. *Circulation* 87:1378, 1993.

171. Huikuri HV, Ikaheimo MJ, Linnaluoto MM, Takkunen JT: Left ventricular response to isometric exercise and its value in predicting the change in ventricular function after mitral valve replacement for mitral regurgitation. *Am J Cardiol* 51:1110, 1983.

172. Wisenbaugh T: Does normal pump function belie muscle dysfunction in patients with chronic severe mitral regurgitation? *Circulation* 77:515, 1988.

173. Goldman ME, Mora F, Guarino T, et al: Mitral valvuloplasty is superior to valve replacement for preservation of left ventricular function: An intraoperative two-dimensional echocardiographic study. *J Am Coll Cardiol* 10:568, 1987.

174. Komeda M, David TE, Rao V, et al: Late hemodynamic effects of the preserved papillary muscles during mitral valve replacement. *Circulation* 90:suppl II-190, 1994.

175. Hennein HA, Swain JA, McIntosh CL, et al: Comparative assessment of chordal preservation versus chordal resection during mitral valve replacement. *J Thoracic Cardiovasc Surg* 99:828, discussion 836, 1990.

176. Rozich JD, Carabello BA, Usher BW, et al: Mitral valve replacement with and without chordal preservation in patients with chronic mitral regurgitation. Mechanisms for differences in postoperative ejection performance. *Circulation* 86:1718, 1992.

177. David TE, Uden DE, Strauss HD: The importance of the mitral apparatus in left ventricular function after correction of mitral regurgitation. *Circulation* 68:suppl II-76, 1983.

178. Gaasch WH, Zile MR: Left ventricular function after surgical correction of chronic mitral regurgitation. *Eur Heart J* 12:48, 1991.

179. Barlow JB, Bosman CK: Aneurysmal protrusion of the posterior leaflet of the mitral valve. An auscultatory-electrocardiographic syndrome. *Am Heart J* 71:166, 1966.

180. Jeresaty RM: Mitral valve prolapse—Click syndrome. *Prog Cardiovasc Dis* 15:623, 1973.

181. Devereux RB, Perloff JK, Reichek N, Josephson ME: Mitral valve prolapse. *Circulation* 54:3, 1976.

182. Lobstein HP, Horwitz LD, Curry GC, Mullins CB: Electrocardiographic abnormalities and coronary arteriograms in the mitral click-murmur syndrome. *N Engl J Med* 289:127, 1973.

183. Gilbert BW, Schatz RA, VonRamm OT, et al: Mitral valve prolapse. Two-dimensional echocardiographic and angiographic correlation. *Circulation* 54:716, 1976.

184. Iskandrian AS, Kotler MN, Kimbiris D, et al: Prolapse of the mitral valve: Clinical, hemodynamic, angiographic and echocardiographic correlations. *Cardiology* 63:321, 1978.

185. Pocock WA, Barlow JB: Etiology and electrocardiographic features of the billowing posterior mitral leaflet syndrome. Analysis of a further 130 patients with a late systolic murmur or nonejection systolic click. *Am J Med* 51:731, 1971.

186. Procacci PM, Savran SV, Schreiter SL, Bryson AL: Prevalence of clinical mitral-valve prolapse in 1169 young women. *N Engl J Med* 294:1086, 1976.

187. Raizada V, Benchimol A, Desser KB, et al: Mitral valve prolapse in patients with coronary artery disease. Echocardiographic-angiographic correlation. *Br Heart J* 39:53, 1977.

188. Ruwitch J Jr, Weiss AN, Fleg JL, et al: Insensitivity of echocardiography in detecting mitral valve prolapse in older patients with chest pain. *Am J Cardiol* 40:686, 1977.

189. Cosgrove D: Surgery for degenerative valve disease. *Semin Thorac Cardiovasc Surg* 1:183, 1989.

190. Gulotta SJ, Gulco L, Padmanabhan V, Miller S: The syndrome of systolic click, murmur, and mitral valve prolapse—A cardiomyopathy? *Circulation* 49:717, 1974.

191. Scampardonis G, Yang SS, Maranhao V, et al: Left ventricular abnormalities in prolapsed mitral leaflet syndrome. Review of eighty-seven cases. *Circulation* 48:287, 1973.

192. Liedtke AJ, Gault JH, Leaman DM, Blumenthal MS: Geometry of left ventricular contraction in the systolic click syndrome. Characterization of a segmental myocardial abnormality. *Circulation* 47:27, 1973.

193. Gottdiener JS, Borer JS, Bacharach SL, et al: Left ventricular function in mitral valve prolapse: Assessment with radionuclide cineangiography. *Am J Cardiol* 47:7, 1981.

194. Lumia FJ, LaManna MM, Atfeh M, Maranhao V: Exercise first-pass radionuclide assessment of left and right

ventricular function and valvular regurgitation in symptomatic mitral valve prolapse [see comments]. *Angiology* 40:443, 1989.

195. Iskandrian AS, Hakki AH: Scintigraphic evaluation of patients with valvular heart disease. *Cardiovasc Clin* 16:211, 1986.

196. Bashore TM, Grines CL, Utlak D, et al: Postural exercise abnormalities in symptomatic patients with mitral valve prolapse. *J Am Coll Cardiol* 11:499, 1988.

197. Mason JW, Koch FH, Billingham ME, Winkle RA: Cardiac biopsy evidence for a cardiomyopathy associated with symptomatic mitral valve prolapse. *Am J Cardiol* 42:557, 1978.

198. Gaffney FA, Wohl AJ, Blomqvist CG, et al: Thallium-201 myocardial perfusion studies in patients with the mitral valve prolapse syndrome. *Am J Med* 64:21, 1978.

199. Greenspan M, Iskandrian AS, Mintz GS, et al: Exercise myocardial scintigraphy with 201-thallium. Use in patients with mitral valve prolapse without associated coronary artery disease. *Chest* 77:47, 1980.

200. Butman S, Chandraratna PA, Milne N, et al: Stress myocardial imaging in patients with mitral valve prolapse: Evidence of a perfusion abnormality. *Cathet Cardiovasc Diagn* 8:243, 1982.

201. Massie B, Botvinick EH, Shames D, et al: Myocardial perfusion scintigraphy in patients with mitral valve prolapse: Its advantage over stress electrocardiography in diagnosing associated coronary artery disease and its implications for the etiology of chest pain. *Circulation* 57:19, 1978.

202. Klein GJ, Kostuk WJ, Boughner DR, Chamberlain MJ: Stress myocardial imaging in mitral leaflet prolapse syndrome. *Am J Cardiol* 42:746, 1978.

203. Tresch D, Soin JS, Siegel R, et al: Mitral valve prolapse: Evidence for a myocardial perfusion abnormality. *Am J Cardiol* 41:441, 1978 (abstr).

204. Padmanabhan V, Margouleff D, Binder A, et al: Thallium-201 imaging during exercise in mitral valve prolapse. *Circulation* 55:iii, 1977 (abstr).

205. Duca P, Gottlieb R, Kasparian H, et al: Abnormal myocardial lactate metabolism as an additional feature of the syndrome of mitral valve prolapse. *Am J Cardiol* 35:133, 1975 (abstr).

206. LeWinter MM, Hoffman JR, Shell WE, et al: Phenylephrine-induced atypical chest pain in patients with prolapsing mitral valve leaflets. *Am J Cardiol* 34:12, 1974.

207. Buda AJ, Levene DL, Myers MG, et al: Coronary artery spasm and mitral valve prolapse. *Am Heart J* 95:457, 1978.

208. Chesler E, Matisonn RE, Lakier JB, et al: Acute myocardial infarction with normal coronary arteries: A possible manifestation of the billowing mitral leaflet syndrome. *Circulation* 54:203, 1976.

209. Pearlman AS: Role of echocardiography in the diagnosis and evaluation of severity of mitral and tricuspid stenosis. *Circulation* 84:I193, 1991.

210. Kawahara T, Yamagishi M, Seo H, et al: Application of Doppler color flow imaging to determine valve area in mitral stenosis [see comments]. *J Am Coll Cardiol* 18:85, 1991.

211. Rifkin RD, Harper K, Tighe D: Comparison of proximal isovelocity surface area method with pressure half-time and planimetry in evaluation of mitral stenosis. *J Am Coll Cardiol* 26:458, 1995.

212. Nishimura RA, Rihal CS, Tajik AJ, Holmes D Jr: Accurate measurement of the transmitral gradient in patients with mitral stenosis: A simultaneous catheterization and Doppler echocardiographic study. *J Am Coll Cardiol* 24:152, 1994.

213. Burns RJ, Armitage DL, Fountas PN, et al: Usefulness of radionuclide angiocardiography in predicting stenotic mitral orifice area. *Am J Cardiol* 58:1218, 1986.

214. Uehara T, Nishimura T, Hayashida K, Kozuka T: Diagnostic value of technetium-99m radionuclide angiography for detecting thrombosis in left atrial appendage. *J Nucl Med* 33:365, 1992.

215. Iwata K: Alternative method for calculating right ventricular ejection fraction from first-pass time-activity curves [see comments]. *J Nucl Med* 29:1990, 1988.

216. Ratner SJ, Huang PJ, Friedman MI, Pierson R Jr: Assessment of right ventricular anatomy and function by quantitative radionuclide ventriculography. *J Am Coll Cardiol* 13:354, 1989.

217. Manno BV, Iskandrian AS, Hakki AH: Right ventricular function: Methodologic and clinical considerations in noninvasive scintigraphic assessment. *J Am Coll Cardiol* 3:1072, 1984.

218. Morrison DA, Turgeon J, Ovitt T: Right ventricular ejection fraction measurement: Contrast ventriculography versus gated blood pool and gated first-pass radionuclide methods. *Am J Cardiol* 54:651, 1984.

219. Iskandrian AS, Hakki AH, Ren JF, et al: Correlation among right ventricular preload, afterload and ejection fraction in mitral valve disease: Radionuclide, echocardiographic and hemodynamic evaluation. *J Am Coll Cardiol* 3:1403, 1984.

220. Weiner BH, Alpert JS, Dalen JE, Ockene IS: Response of the right ventricle to exercise in patients with chronic heart disease. *Am Heart J* 105:386, 1983.

221. Winzelberg GG, Boucher CA, Pohost GM, et al: Right ventricular function in aortic and mitral valve disease. *Chest* 79:520, 1981.

222. Morrison DA, Lancaster L, Henry R, Goldman S: Right ventricular function at rest and during exercise in aortic and mitral valve disease. *J Am Coll Cardiol* 5:21, 1985.

223. Korr KS, Gandsman EJ, Winkler ML, et al: Hemodynamic correlates of right ventricular ejection fraction measured with gated radionuclide angiography. *Am J Cardiol* 49:71, 1982.

224. Grose R, Strain J, Yipintosoi T: Right ventricular function in valvular heart disease: relation to pulmonary artery pressure. *J Am Coll Cardiol* 2:225, 1983.

225. Morise AP, Goodwin C: Exercise radionuclide angiography in patients with mitral stenosis: Value of right ventricular response. *Am Heart J* 112:509, 1986.

226. Reyes VP, Raju BS, Wynne J, et al: Percutaneous balloon valvuloplasty compared with open surgical commissurotomy for mitral stenosis [see comments]. *N Engl J Med* 331:961, 1994.

227. Turi ZG, Reyes VP, Raju BS, et al: Percutaneous balloon

versus surgical closed commissurotomy for mitral stenosis. A prospective, randomized trial [see comments]. *Circulation* 83:1179, 1991.

228. McKay RG, Lock JE, Safian RD, et al: Balloon dilation of mitral stenosis in adult patients: Postmortem and percutaneous mitral valvuloplasty studies. *J Am Coll Cardiol* 9:723, 1987.

229. Mishkin FS, Mishkin ME: Documentation of tricuspid regurgitation by radionuclide angiocardiography. *Br Heart J* 36:1019, 1974.

230. Lumia FJ, Patil A, Germon PA, Maranhao V: Tricuspid regurgitation by radionuclide angiography and contrast right ventriculography: A preliminary observation. *J Nucl Med* 22:804, 1981.

231. Mishkin FS, Prosin MA: Radionuclide angiocardiographic confirmation of tricuspid insufficiency. *J Nucl Med* 15:205, 1974.

232. Kress P, Waitzinger J, Seibold H, et al: [Radionuclide ventriculography—A noninvasive method of diagnosis and quantification of tricuspid valve insufficiency]. *Nuklearmedizin* 26:177, 1987.

233. Grossmann G, Otto L, Felder C, et al: [Quantification of tricuspid insufficiency—Comparison of Doppler echocardiography and radionuclide ventriculography]. *Z Kardiol* 81:9, 1992.

234. Jacobson AF, Whitley MA, Harrison SD, Cerqueira MD: Massive tricuspid regurgitation identified on renal flow scintigraphy. *Clin Nucl Med* 16:767, 1991.

235. Spiegler EJ, Ratliff C Jr, Gillilan R: Detection of tricuspid regurgitation by Tc-99m DTPA renal scintigraphy. *Clin Nucl Med* 16:92, 1991.

236. Baker EJ, Jones OD, Joseph MC, et al: Radionuclide measurement of left ventricular ejection fraction in tricuspid atresia. *Br Heart J* 52:572, 1984.

237. Huckell VF, Sprangers MA, Horne BD, et al: Leaking Glenn anastomosis demonstrated by first pass radionuclide angiography. *Clin Nucl Med* 7:58, 1982.

238. Lopez-Majano V, Dulay CC, Sansi P: Radionuclide angiocardiography in tricuspid atresia. *Eur J Nucl Med* 5:193, 1980.

239. Simpson IA, Sahn DJ: Quantification of valvular regurgitation by Doppler echocardiography. *Circulation* 84:suppl I-188, 1991.

Radionuclide Imaging in Nonischemic Cardiomyopathy

Daniel Edmundowicz
William P. Follansbee

The classification of heart muscle disease has evolved over decades. Wallace Brigden[1] first used the term "cardiomyopathy" in 1957 to describe "non coronary disease of the heart muscle of unknown etiology." Goodwin and his colleagues described cardiomyopathies in the 1960s as "primary heart muscle diseases" and attempted the first clinical classification of congestive, restrictive, and obstructive disorders.[2] Substantive modifications followed as epidemiologic, anatomic, and functional differences were identified.[3,4,5,6,7,8,9,10,11] The World Health Organization and the International Society and Federation of Cardiology (WHO/ISFC) proposed a classification of myocardial disease in 1980 based on clinical, hemodynamic, and structural features.[11] Myocardial disorders resulting from coronary artery disease, systemic or pulmonary hypertension, valvular heart disease, and congenital cardiac anomalies were purposefully excluded from these classifications. Recognizing that the difference between cardiomyopathy and specific heart muscle disease has become indistinct, the 1995 WHO/ISFC task force has reclassified heart muscle disease by the dominant pathophysiology or, if possible, by etiological and pathogenetic factors.[12] Under this scheme, cardiomyopathies are generally defined as diseases of the myocardium associated with cardiac dysfunction and are classified as dilated cardiomyopathy, hypertrophic cardiomyopathy, restrictive cardiomyopathy, and arrhythmogenic right ventricular cardiomyopathy. Previously described "specific heart muscle diseases" are now classified as "specific cardiomyopathies" and are used to describe heart muscle diseases that are associated with specific cardiac or systemic disorders (Table 25-1).

Nuclear imaging procedures, particularly those used to assess ventricular function, are useful in the diagnosis, clinical evaluation, and classification of myocardial disorders. The focus of this chapter will be to discuss the specific clinical findings and contributions of radionuclide ventriculography and myocardial perfusion imaging in hypertrophic, dilated, and restrictive cardiomyopathy. In addition, selected specific cardiomyopathies in which nuclear imaging techniques have had a demonstrated diagnostic or prognostic role, including viral myocarditis, AIDS, diabetes mellitus, rheumatoid arthritis, scleroderma, systemic lupus erythematosus, sarcoidosis, and myocardial toxicities including alcohol and cocaine, will be briefly discussed and are summarized in Table 25-2. Finally, the use of radionuclide imaging in the evaluation and follow-up of patients undergoing cardiac transplantation will be examined.

HYPERTROPHIC CARDIOMYOPATHY

Hypertrophic cardiomyopathy (HCM) is a primary myocardial disease of variable anatomy, physiology, clinical presentation, and prognosis. Common to all variations is abnormal left ventricular hypertrophy that is not secondary to chronic pressure overload. The pattern of hypertrophy typically involves substantial portions of the

Table 25-1 Classification of Cardiomyopathies

Dilated Cardiomyopathy

Hypertrophic Cardiomyopathy

Restrictive Cardiomyopathy

Arrhythmogenic Right Ventricular Cardiomyopathy

Unclassified Cardiomyopathies
  (eg, fibroelastosis)

Specific Cardiomyopathies
  Ischemic Cardiomyopathy
  Valvular Cardiomyopathy
  Hypertensive Cardiomyopathy
  Inflammatory Cardiomyopathy
    (eg, Chagas' disease, HIV, enterovirus, adenovirus, CMV)
  Metabolic Cardiomyopathy
    (eg, diabetes mellitus, thyroid disorders, familial storage diseases)
  General Systemic Disease
    (eg, connective tissue disorders and granulomatous diseases)
  Muscular Dystrophies
  Neuromuscular Disorders
  Sensitivity and Toxic Reactions
  Peripartal Cardiomyopathy

Source: Modified from WHO/IFSC Task Force[12]

septum and anterolateral left ventricular free wall, but is variable.[13] Anatomic and pathologic characteristics have been well delineated by two-dimensional and M-mode echocardiography. Features include abnormal septal hypertrophy, which is typically disproportionate to posterior wall hypertrophy; apical ventricular hypertrophy; systolic anterior motion of the mitral valve; narrow septal-mitral valve separation at end diastole; and mid-systolic closure of the aortic valve.[14,15,16,17]

The pathophysiologic characteristics of HCM are even more complex and variable than the anatomy. Early invasive hemodynamic investigations focused attention on dynamic left ventricular outflow tract obstruction, for which the term hypertrophic obstructive cardiomyopathy (HOCM) has been used.[18] Potential mechanisms for such an obstruction have been proposed by a multidisciplinary approach using angiographic, echocardiographic, and radionuclide techniques[19,20,21,22,23,24] and are summarized in Table 25-3. Outflow tract obstruction, however, is only one element of the pathology in this disease and probably occurs in only about 25 percent of afflicted patients.[25] Other important physiologic abnormalities include reduced left ventricular afterload with hyperdynamic systolic function,[26,27] and, more commonly, impaired left ventricular relaxation with or without increased end-diastolic pressure.[28] When impairment of ventricular distensibility causes increased diastolic filling pressures and restriction of diastolic filling volume, symptoms of both pulmonary venous hypertension and compromised forward stroke volume result.[29,30,31]

Nuclear imaging techniques such as radionuclide angiography[25,32,33,34,35,36,37] and thallium scintigraphy[38,39,40,41,42,43,44,45,46,47,48] have been shown to be useful in the evaluation of patients with HCM. Multiple gated

blood pool imaging has been used to demonstrate asymmetric septal hypertrophy in a fashion not unlike that of biventricular cineangiography in the catheterization laboratory.[49] Both techniques can be used to characterize patterns of myocardial hypertrophy, identify systolic cavity obliteration, and demonstrate narrowing of the left ventricular outflow tract.[50] Radionuclide angiography and thallium scintigraphy are helpful in detecting patterns of hypertrophy that are not well suited to echocardiographic analysis, particularly apical hypertrophy.[51]

Figure 25-1 is a study of a 41-year-old man who was referred for evaluation of chest pain. An exercise thallium study suggested marked left ventricular hypertrophy, particularly in the apical portion of the anterior wall and septum. An echocardiogram was performed but was nondiagnostic because of poor acoustic windows. A radionuclide ventriculography study revealed a hyperkinetic left ventricle with a dramatically increased silhouette and obliteration of the cavity in systole. The findings were interpreted as being indicative of hypertrophic cardiomyopathy. Subsequent cardiac catheterization revealed angiographically normal coronary arteries, a left ventricular end-diastolic pressure of 40 mmHg, and a provocable left ventricular outflow tract gradient.

Several investigators have demonstrated the utility of radionuclide angiography in identifying impaired left ventricular relaxation in HCM. Abnormal parameters include a decreased peak filling rate measured in end-diastolic volumes per second,[36] an increased time to peak filling rate,[32,36,37] a prolonged isovolumic relaxation time,[33] and an increased atrial contribution to ventricular filling.[35] It has been suggested that the reduced peak filling rate is a significant predictor of disease-related death in HCM.[35]

Myocardial perfusion abnormalities are common in HCM. Although there is no increased predisposition to atherosclerotic coronary artery disease, findings suggestive of ischemia are common, even in the absence of coronary blockage. These include the presence of abnormal lactate metabolism during atrial pacing, reduced coronary vasodilator reserve[52,53,54] and autopsy evidence of left ventricular necrosis, widespread fibrosis, and even transmural scarring.[55,56,57,58] Potential mechanisms for myocardial ischemia in the absence of epicardial coronary artery disease in HCM include 1) inadequate capillary density relative to the greatly increased left ventricular mass;[25] 2) systolic compression of large intramyocardial coronary arteries;[59] 3) excessive myocardial oxygen demand caused by increased wall tension in the face of resting LV outflow-tract obstruction;[25] 4) impaired ventricular relaxation decreasing the time available for coronary flow during diastole;[60] and 5) small-vessel disease characterized by thickening of the vessel wall and a decrease in luminal size contributing to limitation of coronary flow reserve.[56]

Table 25-2   Radionuclide Imaging in Cardiomyopathies

Cardiomyopathy	Applicable Radionuclide Study	Typical Pathology	Characteristic Findings	Comments	References
Hypertrophic	RNA	Ventricular hypertrophy	Asymmetric hypertrophy (apical)		49,51
			Systolic cavity obliteration		50
			LVOT narrowing		50
		Impaired LV relaxation	Decreased PFR		36
			Increased time to PFR		32,36,37
			Prolonged isovolumic relaxation		33
			Increased atrial contribution to ventricular filling		35
	Thallium Scintigraphy		Fixed or only partially reperfusing defects	Usually poor LV function	44
			Reversible defects	Preventable with verapamil therapy	46
Dilated	RNA	Globular, hypokinetic LV	Diffusely impaired wall motion with chamber dilatation	May be segmental	
	Thallium Scintigraphy		Small, patchy perfusion defects	Contrast to extensive segments in CAD	66,81,82
			Increased lung thallium activity		79
Restrictive	RNA	Restricted and/or prolonged LV filling	"Dip and plateau" contour of early diastolic filling pressure	PFR may be normal (See text)	12
			Generalized prolongation of diastolic filling	Typical of amyloid	86,87
		Reduced diastolic volume of either or both ventricles		Usually normal LV systolic function	
Myocarditis	Gallium 67	Active inflammation	Diffuse myocardial uptake		100,101,102
	Indium 111		Diffuse myocardial uptake		104,105
AIDS	RNA	Abnormal LV systolic function			110
		Infiltrating myocardial tumors	Restrictive LV diastolic filling		109
Diabetes	Exercise RNA	Impaired LV relaxation	Abnormal LVEF response to exercise Decreased PFR		127,128,135

Exercise-induced perfusion abnormalities have been described in patients with HCM, many of whom do not experience symptoms of angina pectoris.[44] Fixed or only partially reversible defects suggestive of myocardial scar or severe ischemia occur primarily in patients with impaired systolic performance.[44] Completely reversible perfusion abnormalities occur predominantly in patients with preserved systolic LV function. They correlate well with metabolic evidence of stress-induced ischemia,[46] and are prevented in the majority of these patients with verapamil therapy.[44,45] Finally, although it had been suggested that thallium perfusion abnormalities identify a subgroup of patients with HCM at increased risk of potentially lethal arrhythmias,[61] recent evidence suggests that sudden cardiac arrest or syncope in these patients may more frequently be related to myocardial ischemia.[62]

A relatively new radionuclide imaging technique might have utility in the assessment of patients with HCM. Nearly 60 percent of energy in normal myocardium is supplied by β-oxidation of fatty acids. The myocardial accumulation of β-methyliodophenylpentadecanoic acid (BMIPP) has been correlated with the intracellular concentration of adenosine triphosphate, suggesting that it may be an indicator of myocardial energy production associated with ventricular wall motion.[63] In patients with HCM, decreased BMIPP and

Table 25-2 (*Continued*)

Cardiomyopathy	Applicable Radionuclide Study	Typical Pathology	Characteristic Findings	Comments	References
Rheumatoid	RNA	Impaired LV relaxation	Decreased PFR		144
Scleroderma	Thallium Scintigraphy	Abnormal microvasculature Patchy myocardial fibrosis	Rest or exercise-induced perfusion abnormalities	Patients with large defects have low LVEF by RNA	151
Scleroderma	Thallium Scintigraphy	Abnormal microvasculature	Cold-induced perfusion defects		159
	RNA		Cold-induced abnormal LV function	Improved with vasodilators	160
SLE	RNA	Immune complex deposition	LV wall motion abnormalities	Worsened with exercise	166
	Thallium Scintigraphy		Both exercise induced and fixed defects		177
Sarcoidosis	Thallium Scintigraphy	Granuloma deposition	Abnormal distribution at rest		185
	Gallium 67		Increased myocardial uptake in areas of thallium defects	Improved with steroids (see text)	188,189,190
Alcohol	RNA	Direct toxic effect?	Decreased LV function		194
			Dilated LV with decreased wall thickness		199
			Normal LV size with increased wall thickness		199
Cocaine	RNA	Toxicity or myocarditis	Decreased LV function	Global and segmental abnormalities	206
	Thallium Scintigraphy	Vasospasm Coronary thrombosis	Regional perfusion defects		209

RNA: Radionuclide angiocardiogram PFR: Peak Filling Rate LV: Left Ventricle EF: Ejection Fraction LVOT: Left Ventricular Outflow Tract CAD: Coronary Artery Disease

thallium uptake has been observed, which suggests that ischemia may play a role in impaired fatty acid metabolism in this disease.[64,65]

DILATED CARDIOMYOPATHY

Dilated cardiomyopathy is a common disorder of multifactorial etiology.[4] This entity is characterized by dilation

Table 25-3 Factors Influencing the Presence of Left Ventricular Outflow Obstruction

Small LV cavity with hyperdynamic systolic function

Thickening of the basal ventricular septum with enchroachment on the LV outflow tract

Abnormal papillary muscle position drawing the mitral valve chordae anteriorly

"Venturi effect" of accelerated blood through the narrowed outflow tract drawing the anterior mitral leaflet toward the ventricular septum

Adapted from Louie and Edwards[27]

of the ventricles, which usually precedes the clinical signs and symptoms of heart failure. Affected patients have a globular, poorly contracting left ventricle, with variable right ventricular size and systolic function ranging from normal to severely abnormal.[10] The reason for the variability in right ventricular involvement is unclear, but it does not appear to be primarily related to the degree of pulmonary hypertension that is present.[66]

The true etiology of dilated cardiomyopathy remains obscure in most cases, and it may be difficult to distinguish this entity from other known processes that lead to a similar clinical presentation, such as advanced ischemic disease.[10] Angina pectoris and Q waves on the electrocardiogram are both more common in patients with coronary disease, whereas left bundle branch block is more common in those with dilated cardiomyopathy.[66]

Nuclear cardiology procedures can serve a useful function in the clinical diagnostic evaluation of patients with dilated cardiomyopathy.[67,68,69,70,71,72,73,74,75,76] In a general sense, radionuclide ventriculography permits the characterization of left ventricular size, global left ventricular function, and regional ventricular wall motion. Although reduced wall motion is typically diffuse in dilated cardiomyopathy, segmental wall motion abnor-

ANT   45 LAO   70 LAO

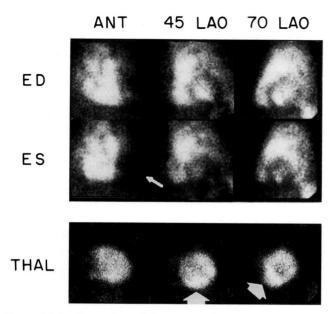

ED

ES

THAL

Figure 25-1 The radionuclide angiocardiograms and exercise thallium scintigrams are shown in the anterior (ANT), 45° left anterior oblique (LAO), and 70° LAO projections. The radionuclide ventriculograms show a prominent silhouette surrounding the left ventricle, particularly in the anterior wall and apex (ANT and 70° LAO view). There is end-systolic cavity obliteration on the anterior projection (small arrow). The thallium study suggests left ventricular hypertrophy, particularly in the apical regions (45° and 70° LAO views, large arrow). ED = end diastole; ES = end systole; THAL = thallium.

malities do occur. Greenberg et al suggested that wall motion analysis was helpful only at the extremes (prominently segmental or clearly diffuse) but had little predictive value in the middle range.[77] The presence of a ventricular aneurysm is the only abnormality that significantly increases the odds of ischemic etiology.[67,68]

In addition to wall motion analysis of patients with dilated cardiomyopathy, blood pool scintigraphy can also provide an assessment of pulmonary capillary wedge pressure by quantitating the regional radioactivity in the apex of the lung relative to the base.[78] In patients with mitral regurgitation and pulmonary vascular congestion, preserved ventricular function assessed by radionuclide ventriculography would suggest primary mitral valve disease in contrast to mitral regurgitation secondary to progressive left ventricular dysfunction and dilatation. The former patients might be candidates for mitral valve replacement; the latter are not.

Thallium imaging can be useful in distinguishing dilated cardiomyopathy from coronary artery disease with left ventricular dysfunction. Patients with dilated cardiomyopathy have increased lung thallium activity, reflecting elevated left ventricular filling pressure.[79] The majority of patients with dilated cardiomyopathy do not have perfusion defects.[70,73,75] When perfusion defects are present, they are typically small and patchy and usually

can be differentiated from those seen in patients with coronary artery disease, which are generally more extensive and segmental.[80] Thallium defects in patients with dilated cardiomyopathy are probably, at least in part, a result of geometric changes in the ventricle, which can create apparent but artifactual defects due to attenuation.[81] In other instances, thallium defects might also be a reflection of underlying myocardial fibrosis or of a diminution of coronary vasodilatory reserve.[66,82] Tauberg et al demonstrated that an absence of severe perfusion defects in dilated cardiomyopathy had a 94 percent predictive value for absence of coronary artery disease (CAD) as the etiology, whereas large perfusion defects had a 97 percent predictive value for presence of CAD.[75] When present in dilated cardiomyopathy, large perfusion defects are associated with a poor prognosis, but do not add to the predictive value of conventional parameters such as increased left ventricular end-diastolic pressure, increased cardiothoracic dimensions, and the presence of ventricular tachycardia.[70]

Figure 25-2 shows findings from 2 patients with dilated cardiomyopathy with similar radionuclide ventriculography studies. The thallium scan in the patient with dilated cardiomyopathy (2-A) reveals a dilated heart but essentially normal thallium distribution; the scan in the patient with coronary artery disease and left ventricular dysfunction (2-B) shows large perfusion defects.

RESTRICTIVE CARDIOMYOPATHY

Restrictive cardiomyopathy is probably the least common type of cardiomyopathy and is characterized by restrictive filling and reduced diastolic volume of either or both ventricles with normal or near normal systolic function.[12] Interstitial fibrosis may or may not be present and may be idiopathic or associated with other diseases such as amyloidosis. Eosinophilic endomyocardial disease is included in the task force's definition of restrictive cardiomyopathy and has served as the basis from which existing diagnostic criteria have been described.[10]

Patients with restrictive cardiomyopathy demonstrate rapid completion of ventricular filling in early diastole and little or no further filling in mid or late diastole, creating a characteristic "dip and plateau" contour of early diastolic pressure.[83,84,85] Patients with amyloidosis, however, may demonstrate a generalized prolongation of left ventricular diastolic filling.[86,87] Idiopathic restrictive cardiomyopathy, the occurrence of classic restrictive hemodynamics in the absence of specific histologic changes of the myocardium, is the purest form of this disease and was reported in 9 patients by Benotti and co-workers in 1980.[88] All patients studied demonstrated elevated right and left ventricular filling pressures, a dip and pla-

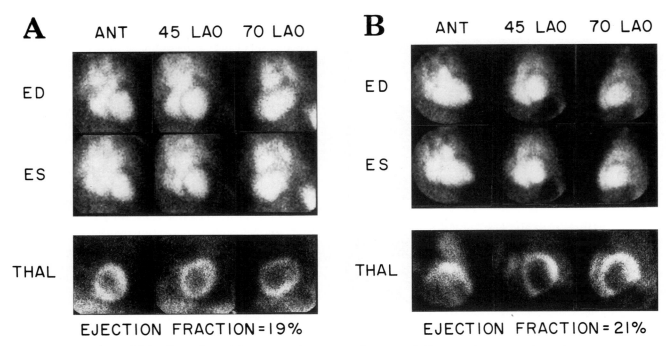

A ANT 45 LAO 70 LAO

ED

ES

THAL

EJECTION FRACTION = 19%

B ANT 45 LAO 70 LAO

ED

ES

THAL

EJECTION FRACTION = 21%

Figure 25-2 The radionuclide angiocardiograms and exercise thallium scintigrams are shown in a patient with idiopathic cardiomyopathy (**A**) and a patient with ischemic cardiomyopathy (**B**). In both cases the left ventricle is markedly dilated and diffusely hypokinetic with similar ejection fractions (19 percent and 21 percent, respectively). In patient **A** the thallium study shows somewhat diminished perfusion of the anteroseptal wall on the 70° left anterior oblique (LAO) projection, but otherwise is normal, with the exception of the dilated size of the ventricle. In contrast, the thallium study in patient **B** shows major perfusion abnormalities of the inferior wall (all three projections), septum (45° LAO), apex (anterior and 45° LAO), and of the right ventricular apex (45° LAO). At cardiac catheterization, patient **A** had a normal coronary angiogram. Patient **B** has severe triple-vessel coronary artery disease. ED = end diastole; ES = end systole; THAL = thallium.

teau diastolic pressure pattern, normal or near normal systolic function, and no evidence of pericardial constriction or other known cause for the abnormalities.

Radionuclide imaging techniques may have some utility in restrictive cardiomyopathy by identifying and characterizing abnormal diastolic filling parameters. Caution must be used when measuring peak filling rate with radionuclide ventriculography, however, since rapid early diastolic filling as described earlier may result in normal PFR in some patients despite the presence of relaxation abnormalities. Hence, the morphology of the entire ventricular filling curve needs to be examined. The percentage of total diastolic filling that is contributed by atrial systole may be a useful additional parameter in assessing diastolic function.

It is also important to recognize that diastolic filling abnormalities in certain restrictive disorders such as amyloidosis and endomyocardial fibrosis exist in a continuum and are sometimes not demonstrable despite provocative maneuvers including volume loading or exercise.[83,89] Patients with amyloidosis, for example, may initially show mild abnormal diastolic relaxation charac-

terized by a long isovolumic relaxation time, reduced rate of acceleration to a low early peak velocity, slow deceleration rate, and an increased contribution of atrial systole to total diastolic filling. It may not be until late in the disease process that a restrictive physiology is demonstrated, at which time prognosis is often poor.[90]

SPECIFIC CARDIOMYOPATHIES

Myocarditis

Myocarditis refers to a process characterized by inflammatory infiltrates of the myocardium with necrosis or degeneration of myocytes, not typical of the ischemic damage associated with coronary artery disease.[91] The clinical manifestations are quite variable and may include isolated left ventricular failure or biventricular failure, symptomatic dysrhythmias with or without congestive failure, and chest pain syndromes mimicking acute myocardial infarction.[92] Whereas diffuse ventricular hypokinesis is common, segmental wall motion abnormalities and left ventricular aneurysm formation have been frequently described.[93,94,95] The actual incidence and natural history of viral myocarditis are unknown, since it is likely that many cases are subclinical and never come to diagnosis.

Although the etiology of primary dilated cardiomyopathy is unknown, it is suspected that in many instances the cardiomyopathy is a result of recent or remote viral infection, particularly from Coxsackie B virus.[96] The development and clinical application of enterovirus group-specific hybridization probes and the polymerase chain reaction has allowed the detection of enteroviral RNA sequences in endomyocardial biopsy samples from patients in all stages of the disease.[94] However, because of the small sample size of the biopsy specimens and the patchy distribution of the inflammatory lesions, it is likely that endomyocardial biopsy might be limited in its ability to detect the infectious process, or to quantify the inflammatory component. Furthermore, because biopsy is an invasive procedure, it would be desirable to have a noninvasive method that is sensitive and specific in detecting active myocardial inflammation.

Gallium-67 citrate has been shown to accumulate in areas of active inflammation and has been used clinically for the detection of localized inflammation in nearly every organ system in the body. It has been demonstrated that ^{67}Ga binds to lymphocyte plasma membranes and has a high affinity for both transferrin and lactoferrin.[97,98] The accumulation of ^{67}Ga in microbial abscesses is explained partially by high lactoferrin levels in neutrophils. In addition, iron avid molecules, called siderophores, produced by bacteria, complex with gallium in a manner similar to iron. They are then taken up by a specific bacterial transport mechanism, explaining the observation that neutropenic animals with abscesses still accumulate ^{67}Ga.[99]

With the use of endomyocardial biopsy as a "gold standard," the reported sensitivity and specificity of ^{67}Ga citrate imaging for the detection of myocarditis have varied widely. Strain et al reported a sensitivity of 44 percent and a specificity of 100 percent,[100] whereas O'Connell et al, in a much larger study, reported a sensitivity of 87 percent and specificity of 86 percent.[101] In part, the differences between these two series might reflect differences in criteria for scan interpretation. Of importance, the predictive value of a positive result in this latter study was only 36 percent. Gallium-67 uptake by the heart has also been well demonstrated in acute transient myocarditis,[102] bacterial endocarditis,[99] pericarditis,[103] and other noninfectious diseases to be discussed later.

Yasuda and colleagues have used imaging with ^{111}In monoclonal antimyosin antibody to aid in the diagnosis of acute myocarditis.[104] This procedure was performed on 28 patients clinically suspected of having myocarditis, 25 of whom had a left ventricular ejection fraction of less than 45 percent. The results were compared with those of right ventricular endomyocardial biopsy performed within 48 h of the scan. Nine patients with a positive antimyosin scan had biopsy evidence of myocarditis, and all 11 patients with a negative antimyosin scan showed no evidence of myocarditis on right ventricular biopsy (overall sensitivity, 100 percent; specificity, 58 percent). However, in using endomyocardial biopsy as the gold standard, it must be recognized that it has significant limitations in accurately establishing the diagnosis of myocarditis. Hence, the actual specificity of the imaging technique is likely to be underestimated. Dec et al and Narula et al performed similar clinical evaluations of sensitivity and specificity of antimyosin imaging using endomyocardial biopsy as the gold standard."[105,106] Sensitivity ranged from 83 to 100 percent in biopsy-proven myocarditis; specificity ranged from 35 to 58 percent. The predictive value of a positive scan for the presence of myocarditis in these studies ranged from 33 to 43 percent and that of a negative scan for the absence of myocarditis from 92 to 100 percent. These promising results suggest a potential role for ^{111}In monoclonal antimyosin imaging as a screening tool and a guide for the use of endomyocardial biopsy in patients with objective evidence of left ventricular dysfunction and clinical suspicion of myocarditis. However, the radiation burden of ^{111}In antimyosin antibody is not insignificant, particularly in young patients, and the therapeutic implications of detected myocarditis require clarification.

AIDS

Active myocarditis is a common finding at autopsy in HIV-infected patients, with a prevalence ranging from 34 percent to 52 percent.[107,108] Anderson et al retrospectively evaluated 71 consecutive necropsy patients who died from AIDS and found focal myocarditis, unassociated with opportunistic pathogens or drugs, in 37 patients.[108] The histologic appearance was consistent with viral infection in most patients studied, and 28 of 37 patients had documented presence of CMV, suggesting its role as a possible causative agent. Interestingly, myocarditis was present in all cases of biventricular dilation in this series.

A wide range of clinical cardiac problems have been associated with HIV infections. Infiltrating tumors including lymphomas and Kaposi's sarcoma have been shown to result in restrictive left ventricular diastolic filling patterns. Pericardial effusion, infective endocarditis, and pulmonary hypertension with right heart failure have also been described in HIV patients.[109] The most clinically significant HIV-associated heart disease emerging over the past several years, however, has been left ventricular dysfunction. Cohen et al provided the first report of AIDS-related congestive cardiomyopathy in 3 patients who died with acute cardiac illnesses.[110] All three patients demonstrated abnormal left ventricular systolic function by either echocardiography or radionuclide angiography. Of the three patients, two were subjected to postmortem examination and showed marked four-chamber dilatation, myofibrillar loss, and focal myocarditis.

Since Cohen's initial description, there have been numerous additional case reports of AIDS-associated dilated cardiomyopathy in the adult[111,112,113,114] and pediatric[115] populations. Additionally, Herskowitz et al prospectively evaluated 69 HIV-infected patients without symptomatic heart disease by echocardiography and found a 14.5 percent prevalence of global left ventricular hypokinesia.[116] During 18 mo of follow-up, 4 patients (5.8 percent) developed symptoms of congestive heart failure. The authors concluded that this relatively high rate of ventricular dysfunction in the HIV-infected population studied suggested that early contractile abnormalities may involve a significant number of patients, a subgroup of whom appear to progress to symptomatic congestive heart failure.

The pathogenesis of HIV cardiomyopathy is not clearly established. Current hypotheses associate this disorder with postviral cardiac autoimmunity,[117] selenium deficiency,[118] and hypersensitivity to toxicity of agents used in the therapy of HIV such as nucleoside analogues and pentamidine.[119] A direct role for HIV-mediated myocyte injury has been difficult to characterize since the HIV genome has been isolated in postmortem cardiac tissue from patients both with and without cardiac dysfunction during life.[120,121]

Gallium-67 imaging has been shown to be beneficial in diagnosing myocarditis in the AIDS population in some studies. Cregler et al described two intravenous drug–abusing AIDS patients who were admitted with chest pain and dyspnea and found to have global left ventricular hypokinesis by echocardiography.[122] Both patients underwent ^{67}Ga scanning, which revealed diffuse intense uptake in the myocardium. The authors suggested that unexplained cardiovascular dysfunction in a patient with AIDS should raise the possibility of myocarditis, and ^{67}Ga scanning might be used to help confirm its presence. Similarly, focal cardiac gallium uptake has been described in the pediatric AIDS population[123] and in the presence of myocarditis from opportunistic infections.[124]

HIV-related cardiomyopathy may be easily overlooked because of the vagueness of associated symptoms. Breathlessness and abnormal lung fields on chest x-rays in AIDS patients are frequently attributed to pulmonary involvement by opportunistic infection. Fatigue may be mistakenly attributed to anemia commonly found in

AIDS, rather than being recognized as a manifestation of decreased cardiac output from myocardial dysfunction. Myocardial depression secondary to sepsis is an important diagnostic consideration in immunocompromised patients, particularly patients with AIDS, who have pulmonary congestion. Patients with septic shock may have significantly reduced ejection fraction with transient ventricular dilatation, while the cardiac index remains normal or even supranormal. Clearly, radionuclide ventriculography or echocardiography can have an important role in evaluation of AIDS patients with cardiovascular symptoms.

Given the recent advances in treatment of opportunistic infections and antiretroviral therapy, it is likely that the patients previously dying of noncardiac illnesses will survive to manifest symptoms of HIV cardiomyopathy. The noninvasive assessment of ventricular function will continue to have a crucial role in identifying those HIV-infected patients, both symptomatic and asymptomatic, with ventricular dysfunction and will aid in the ongoing search for pathogenic mechanisms for these conditions.

Endocrine and Metabolic Abnormalities

DIABETES MELLITUS

The Framingham study demonstrated that patients with diabetes mellitus, particularly those with insulin-dependent disease, have an increased morbidity and mortality due to all types of cardiovascular disease.[125] Abnormal myocardial function and perfusion in asymptomatic diabetics in the absence of coronary atherosclerosis or systemic hypertension has been suggested by multiple studies utilizing echocardiography[126,127,128,129] and radionuclide techniques.[130,131,132,133,134] Ventricular function abnormalities appear to be predominantly diastolic, at least initially, and are identified by prolonged indices of diastolic relaxation.[127,128,129,134] Most studies have agreed that there is an association between microvascular disease in other organs and evidence of diabetic cardiomyopathy. This finding, if true, suggests that the cardiac dysfunction is likewise a result of small-vessel disease.[127,129]

Nuclear cardiac procedures are well suited to the noninvasive evaluation of patients with diabetes mellitus who are at risk for myocardial complications. Typically these patients have normal left ventricular ejection fractions at rest, as measured by radionuclide ventriculography, but between 13 and 35 percent of them have an abnormal left ventricular ejection fraction response to exercise.[127,128] Follansbee and colleagues reported findings from a study of 128 type I (insulin-dependent) diabetics who had had diabetes mellitus for a mean duration of 20 y.[135] The population was separated into two groups, based on the presence or absence of microvascular disease in the retina or kidneys. Twenty-one percent of the patients with microvascular disease had an abnormal left ventricular ejection fraction response to exercise, whereas only 7 percent of the patients without microvascular disease were abnormal (p < 0.02).

Abnormal left ventricular function during exercise could be a manifestation of occult diabetic cardiomyopathy or, alternatively, could be a manifestation of occult underlying coronary artery disease. Exercise thallium scintigraphy has been used to differentiate these two possibilities.[130,131,133,135,136] If the exercise thallium study is normal, significant underlying coronary artery disease sufficient to account for the left ventricular dysfunction during exercise is improbable. If the thallium scan is abnormal, the findings may be less specific. It is conceivable that diabetic cardiomyopathy could cause false-positive thallium perfusion abnormalities, particularly if microvascular disease is present in the heart. Nevertheless, false-positive thallium scans in diabetic patients appear to be uncommon.[135] Accordingly, if a clear segmental perfusion abnormality is present on a thallium study of a diabetic patient, coronary artery disease should be assumed unless ruled out by coronary angiography.

As noted previously, studies using echocardiography have suggested that there is a high prevalence of abnormalities of diastolic function in patients with diabetes mellitus. However, in a recent study of 122 patients with diabetes mellitus, Follansbee and co-workers noted that abnormalities of diastolic function were infrequent and mild.[137] Since abnormalities in diastolic function determined by echocardiography and radionuclide ventriculography have been correlated,[132] it would follow that if clinically significant abnormalities in diastolic function are present in patients with diabetes, they might be detected by both techniques. Hence, the differences in findings between the echocardiographic and radionuclide studies might more likely be a reflection of the populations examined. It is of interest to note that indices of diastolic filling are dependent on changes in preload and sympathetic tone.[138] Kahn and co-workers, using radionuclide ventriculography, found abnormal diastolic filling indices in diabetic patients, but this finding was limited to patients who had autonomic neuropathy.[139] The index of autonomic function that correlated most strongly with impaired diastolic filling rates in the population studied by Kahn et al was the presence of orthostatic hypotension. Similarly, Erbas et al, using radionuclide ventriculography, found subclinical left ventricular diastolic dysfunction and sympathetic overactivity in patients with diabetes and autonomic cardiac neuropathy.[134] These findings raise the possibility that at least a portion of the abnormal diastolic filling rates observed in this population might be a result of neurologic rather than primary myocardial abnormalities.

Rheumatic Connective Tissue Disorders

RHEUMATOID ARTHRITIS

Cardiac involvement in rheumatoid arthritis (RA) occurs, but it is usually clinically silent. Necropsy studies suggest a prevalence of cardiac abnormalities in this disorder of 30 to 50 percent, whereas clinically detectable disease is apparent in only 2 to 10 percent of afflicted patients.[140] Recently, Corrao et al examined 35 RA patients without cardiac symptoms or extra-cardiac complaints with echocardiography, and compared the findings to a control group of 52 age-matched volunteers without RA or cardiac symptoms.[141] The RA patients were subdivided based on the stage and duration of their disease. Abnormalities found in asymptomatic patients included pericardial effusion (57 percent), dilated aortic root (34 percent), and valvular thickening (43 percent). There was no statistically significant difference between the groups of RA patients based on the stage or duration of their disease. There was no correlation between cardiac abnormalities, erythrocyte sedimentation rate, or drug therapy.

Increased cardiovascular mortality from cardiac failure has been documented in both male and female patients with RA.[142] Decreased mitral E-F slope, increased isovolumic relaxation time, and lower peak filling rate have been described in patients with RA and have been ascribed to either valvular stiffness from granulomata or abnormalities in left ventricular diastolic function.[143,144] Diastolic dysfunction can lead to impairment of left ventricular systolic function, but it remains to be seen if diastolic abnormalities lead to increased occurrence of cardiac failure or mortality in RA.

The role of nuclear imaging procedures in the cardiac evaluation of patients with RA has not been systematically examined but probably is limited. As noted, clinically significant myocardial involvement is relatively rare. In isolated cases, there could be a potential role for ^{67}Ga citrate imaging in the evaluation of pericardial disease.[103] Radionuclide ventriculography assessment of diastolic ventricular function could also be helpful in selected cases. Since significant coronary arteritis is rare, the role of thallium scintigraphy is likely to be limited. In RA patients with chest pain, pharmacologic stress testing with dobutamine, dipyridamole, or adenosine facilitates scintigraphic detection of coronary disease despite the presence of debilitating joint disease, which limits the patient's ability to perform exercise stress.

SYSTEMIC SCLEROSIS (SCLERODERMA)

Cardiac involvement in systemic sclerosis (progressive systemic sclerosis or scleroderma) was first recognized by Weiss et al in 1943.[145] The manifestations include pericardial disease, myocardial disease, conduction system disease, and dysrythmias.[146] Clinical cardiac involvement, particularly congestive heart failure, portends an unfavorable prognosis.[147] The ECG is normal in approximately half the patients with systemic sclerosis, but ventricular conduction abnormalities, septal infarction pattern, and atrial and ventricular dysrhythmias are not uncommon and may be used as potential indicators of myocardial involvement in the disease, which otherwise might be clinically inapparent.[148]

The prevalence of clinically recognized cardiac involvement in systemic sclerosis appears to be much less than that suggested by autopsy studies.[149,150] Radionuclide techniques have proven useful in detecting subclinical disease. Follansbee et al used exercise thallium scintigraphy and exercise radionuclide ventriculography to examine a series of 26 patients with diffuse scleroderma.[151] Whereas only 6 patients had clinical evidence of cardiac involvement, 20 had abnormal thallium scans, including 10 who had exercise-induced thallium perfusion abnormalities in the absence of coronary artery disease at angiography. These redistributing defects suggest the presence of impaired microvascular circulation. Moreover, thallium perfusion defect size was related to left ventricular function in this group of patients. Those with larger perfusion abnormalities, as a group, had a lower left ventricular ejection fraction by radionuclide ventriculography than did the patients with smaller defects. These findings demonstrate that clinically inapparent systemic sclerosis can be detected by thallium scintigraphy even before significant myocardial dysfunction has occurred.

In a similar study of patients with systemic sclerosis with the CREST (calcinosis, Raynaud's phenomenon, esophageal dysmotility, sclerodactyly, telangiectasia) syndrome, Follansbee and co-workers noted that thallium perfusion abnormalities in this subgroup are much smaller than those seen in patients with diffuse scleroderma.[152] Additionally, exercise-induced thallium defects were not seen in this subgroup, and the thallium perfusion abnormalities that were present were not associated with left ventricular dysfunction either at rest or during exercise. Therefore, radionuclide studies suggest that significant cardiac involvement in the CREST syndrome is unlikely.

Pathologic studies have indicated that the characteristic myocardial lesion of systemic sclerosis is diffuse, patchy myocardial fibrosis.[153] The coexistence of contraction band necrosis with the fibrosis led Bulkley et al to hypothesize that myocardial damage may be a result of coronary arteriolar vasospasm, a "myocardial Raynaud's phenomenon."[153] Alexander et al performed thallium imaging and echocardiography during cold pressor challenge in a small series of patients with systemic sclerosis.[154] In these patients, they noted a nearly universal prevalence of cold-induced thallium perfusion abnormalities with associated segmental wall motion abnormalities. They proposed that the defects were a result

of cold pressor–induced coronary vasospasm. Likewise, Gustafsson et al performed SPECT thallium imaging in 21 patients with systemic sclerosis and no other evidence of cardiac disease.[155] They used cooling of the trunk with ice bags for cold provocation and avoided a change in the heart rate/blood pressure product seen in response to the painful effects of cold pressor stress used in other studies. They demonstrated reversible perfusion defects of the myocardium in 12 out of the 21 patients and isolated nonreperfusing defects in 3 patients.

Because of the possible presence of vasospasm in the coronary microcirculation, several studies have investigated the potential role of coronary vasodilator therapy in systemic sclerosis.[156,157,158,159,160] Kahan and colleagues performed SPECT thallium scintigraphy before and after 20 mg of nifedipine in a population of patients with systemic sclerosis.[156] These investigators noted a high prevalence of segmental thallium perfusion abnormalities at rest, which appeared to improve after nifedipine therapy. In a subsequent study, the same group noted a similar response with the use of nicardipine.[158] Coronary vasodilators dipyridamole[157] and captopril[161] have also been shown to significantly improve resting myocardial perfusion in patients with scleroderma without significantly effecting heart rate or systolic blood pressure.

Follansbee and co-workers performed cold pressor thallium and radionuclide ventriculogram studies pre- and posttherapy with diltiazem in a population of patients with diffuse scleroderma; they compared their findings with those from a group of patients who had Raynaud's disease without systemic sclerosis.[159,160] It was noted that patients with systemic sclerosis had more cold-induced thallium perfusion abnormalities than did those with Raynaud's disease. There was no significant decrease in the thallium defects with diltiazem therapy, but the decrease in left ventricular ejection fraction during cold pressor challenge was lessened by diltiazem in the patients with systemic sclerosis. Likewise, Kahan et al studied 20 scleroderma patients using resting gated blood pool imaging.[162] They demonstrated an improvement in left ventricular ejection fraction (from 65.4 +/− 2.3 percent to 71.3 +/− 2.3 percent) and segmental wall motion 90 min after a 40-mg dose of oral nicardipine. Although a decrease in blood pressure and reflex increase in sympathetic tone may improve resting left ventricular function, no significant modulations in systolic blood pressure or heart rate were noted in their study.

Taken together, these radionuclide studies in patients with systemic sclerosis consistently show improved left ventricular perfusion and function as a result of the use of coronary vasodilators without associated significant changes in systemic blood pressure or heart rate. These findings are consistent with the hypothesis that there is abnormal intramyocardial blood flow in systemic sclerosis that is likely a result of a disordered microcirculation and, possibly, a superimposed vasospastic component.

SYSTEMIC LUPUS ERYTHEMATOSUS

The cardiac manifestations of systemic lupus erythematosus include pericarditis, myocarditis, endocarditis (Libman-Sacks), and coronary artery disease. Myocarditis is characterized by decreases in cardiac output, systolic ventricular function, ventricular diastolic compliance, and coronary vascular reserve.[163,164,165,166] Bidani et al demonstrated myocardial immune complex aggregates in 9 of 10 autopsy patients with lupus and suggested that immune complex deposition may lead to complement activation, inflammation, and myocardial damage.[167] Similar immunopathologic mechanisms may be responsible for coronary vasculitis in this disease.[168] Premature coronary artery disease may be due to arteritis or to atherosclerosis.[169] Arteritis typically involves the smaller vessels but can involve the large epicardial coronary arteries and cause myocardial infarction.[170,171] Accelerated coronary atherosclerosis is a well-documented complication of lupus and has also resulted in unexpected myocardial infarction.[172,173,174,175] Additionally, corticosteroid therapy might predispose to premature coronary atherosclerosis in this population.[176]

Bahl et al assessed left ventricular systolic function by means of both rest and exercise radionuclide ventriculography.[166] They studied 20 consecutive patients with systemic lupus and found normal resting left ventricular function in all. Four patients, despite overall normal LV function, had resting wall motion abnormalities. Eight of the 20 patients could exercise on a bicycle ergonometer and 3 had abnormal ventriculographic responses (new or worsening regional wall motion or significant decline in left ventricular ejection fraction). Hosenpud et al described exercise thallium studies of 26 patients with systemic lupus.[177] None of them had angina pectoris or myocardial infarction, although 9 had atypical chest pain and 19 had risk factors for coronary disease. Of these patients, 10 had abnormal thallium scans, including 5 with exercise-induced defects, 4 with fixed defects, and 1 with both. In view of these combined findings and the known risk of coronary artery disease in the lupus population, it is advisable to perform an exercise thallium study in any patient with lupus who has either multiple cardiac risk factors, chest pain, or resting wall motion abnormalities by radionuclide ventriculography or echocardiography. If the study is positive, coronary arteriography is then recommended to exlude the presence of obstructive atherosclerotic coronary artery disease.

Finally, Morguet et al used standard planar imaging after injection of 2 mCi of ^{111}In-antimyosin Fab to identify myocardial involvement in 2 patients with lupus myocarditis.[178] Indium-111-antimyosin Fab is a specific marker for myocellular injury that has been evaluated in various conditions associated with localized or disseminated myocardial injury. Both lupus patients in Morguet's study experienced chest pain and had abnormal ECGs and normal coronary anatomy at angiography. One patient had an abnormal thallium scan demonstrating both fixed and redistributing defects. Positive ^{111}In-antimyosin Fab scanning led to endomyocardial biopsy confirming lupus myocarditis in one patient and symptomatic improvement after aggressive immunosuppressive therapy in both patients. Indium-111-antimyosin Fab imaging may provide important diagnostic information and guide management in lupus patients with myocardial involvement. As the authors suggest, however, the sensitivity and specificity of this technique must be more fully studied before its broad clinical use can be recommended.

SARCOIDOSIS

Sarcoidosis is a multisystemic granulomatous disorder that occurs most commonly in the second and third decades of life. Autopsy studies suggest that myocardial involvement in sarcoidosis can occur in up to 27 percent of patients.[179] This might be an overestimation, since the overall mortality of the disease worldwide is about 5 percent,[180] and autopsy studies are likely to be biased toward more advanced disease. The clinical features of myocardial involvement are dysrhythmias (including ventricular tachycardia), conduction system disease (including complete heart block), sudden death, congestive heart failure, electrocardiographic infarction pattern, and papillary muscle dysfunction.[179,181,182]

Pathologically, any region of the heart may become the site of granuloma deposition, with the most common areas being the left ventricular free wall and interventricular septum.[183] Granulomata may frequently involve the papillary muscles with mitral or tricuspid regurgitation, but involvement of the valve tissue itself is rare.[181] The atria may be involved, but are relatively spared compared to the extent of involvement seen in the ventricles.[182] Granulomatous involvement with accompanying focal fibromuscular dysplasia can be found in the small coronary arteries.[182] This condition suggests that the pathologic damage that occurs in the myocardium may be a result of ischemic injury in addition to direct granulomatous infiltration. Ventricular aneurysms can occur and may be a source of ventricular tachycardia.[184]

Thallium scintigraphy has had demonstrated value in detecting cardiac involvement in sarcoidosis.[179,185,186,187,188,189,190,191] In a study of 44 consecutive patients with sarcoidosis but no clinical evidence of cardiac involvement, Kinney et al demonstrated that 14 (32 percent) had abnormal thallium distribution in the left ventricle at rest, and 4 (9 percent) had abnormal right ventricular uptake.[185] The presence of thallium defects appeared to correlate with abnormalities of left ventricular function as demonstrated by echocardiography, although the echocardiographic abnormalities described were rather nonspecific.

The combination of ^{201}Tl perfusion imaging with ^{67}Ga imaging appears to be useful in the diagnostic evaluation of sarcoid patients. Several investigators have demonstrated abnormal ^{67}Ga myocardial uptake in sarcoid patients that corresponds closely to areas of perfusion abnormalities on rest ^{201}Tl images.[189,188,190] After corticosteroid therapy, ^{67}Ga accumulation in the myocardium and other organs disappeared, and the ^{201}Tl uptake became more homogenous. Hirose et al studied 75 nonselected patients with sarcoidosis and found that left ventricular ejection fraction by radionuclide ventriculography was related to the severity of sarcoid involvement as demonstrated by thallium perfusion imaging and gallium myocardial scans.[191] They suggested that LV ejection fraction reflects the severity of sarcoid heart disease and may be a helpful prognostic indicator of disease status during follow-up. Although further investigation and validation is needed, dual isotope imaging with ^{201}Tl and ^{67}Ga may aid in characterizing myocardial sarcoid and prove beneficial in differentiating myocardial sarcoid from underlying coronary artery disease.

Myocardial Toxicities

ALCOHOL

Congestive cardiomyopathy with fulminant biventricular myocardial dysfunction has been associated with chronic alcohol abuse and seems to be particularly associated with binge drinking. It is estimated that 1 percent of chronic alcoholics develop cardiac failure[192] that is reversible with abstinence.[193] There are likely to be important underlying risk factors for the development of alcoholic cardiomyopathy. Acute alcohol ingestion can have more profound cardiac inhibitory effects on patients with prior underlying cardiac disease than it does in normal individuals.[194] There also appears to be a sex differential in cardiac risk, with female patients having a lesser incidence of cardiomyopathy than males even at equivalent levels of chronic alcohol ingestion.[195]

Alcohol-related ventricular dysfunction is frequently subclinical but can be detected by echocardiography combined with systolic time intervals.[196,197] Alcoholics with cirrhosis have appeared to be spared from cardiomyopathy, but echocardiographic studies have suggested that this might in part be an artifact of cardiac unloading resulting from the decreased peripheral vascular resistance associated with cirrhosis.[198] The manifestations of subclinical cardiomyopathy appear to fall into at least two categories. One category is characterized by normal diastolic ventricular dimensions with increased left ventricular wall thickness and left ventricular mass; the other is characterized by increased diastolic dimensions with normal or decreased relative wall thickness.[199] It has been suggested that an abnormality of diastolic compliance is an important pathophysiologic component of alcoholic cardiomyopathy.[200]

Although nuclear cardiac studies have not been applied in any systematic fashion to the evaluation of alcoholics, quantification of ventricular function may readily be performed by radionuclide ventriculography. Abnormalities of diastolic function might also be characterized by these techniques. Serial radionuclide examinations of individual patients could be useful as a guide to therapy and to confirm improvement in ventricular function with abstinence.[201]

There is also a potential role for thallium studies in the evaluation of alcoholic patients. The pathogenesis of myocardial injury from alcohol has not been clearly defined, but there is some evidence to suggest that the injury might, at least in part, be ischemically mediated.[202] Acute myocardial infarction in the presence of normal extramural coronary arteries has been documented in alcoholics.[203] Possibly it is a manifestaion of coronary artery vasospasm or coronary thrombosis with recanalization. However, histologic abnormalities of the small intramyocardial arteries have also been described in alcoholics.[202,203] One model of myocardial injury that has been proposed suggests that the initial damage occurs at the level of the endothelial cells in the small intramyocardial arteries. This causes transudation of fluid and proteins into the intramural and perivascular spaces, which in turn causes arterial fibrosis and a compromise in coronary vascular reserve, ultimately leading to ischemic myocardial damage.[202] If this model is correct, then exercise thallium scintigraphy might be helpful in identifying these abnormalities in a manner analagous to that already demonstrated in a possibly similar condition—that of cardiac scleroderma.[151] However, this model remains only speculative, particularly since evidence of small-vessel disease in other organs of alcoholic patients is lacking.

Overall, therefore, thallium imaging has at least theoretic potential utility in the evaluation of alcoholic cardiomyopathy. First, from an investigational standpoint it would provide objective evidence of the presence of an abnormality in myocardial perfusion, which thus far has only been presumed. Second, if these abnormalities are confirmed, then thallium scintigraphy could have the additional clinical potential of identifying patients with occult alcoholic cardiac disease in whom intervention might be beneficial in avoiding advanced toxicity. Third, and probably most useful clinically, thallium imaging has a role in ruling out coexisting coronary artery disease in alcoholic patients.

COCAINE

Cocaine blocks the synaptic reuptake of norepinephrine and dopamine, thereby potentiating sympathetic stimulation in a dose-dependent manner. Physiologic effects include increased heart rate, increased blood pressure, and systemic vasoconstriction of small arteries.[204] The cardiac complications of cocaine use have been well described and include sudden death, myocardial infarction, aortic dissection, dysrythmia, myocarditis and cardiomyopathy.[205,206] Myocardial infarction is the most frequent of these, with more than 100 cases reported in the literature since 1982.[207] Mechanisms that have been proposed for cocaine-induced myocardial ischemia include 1) coronary thrombosis, 2) increased myocardial oxygen demand in the setting of limited myocardial oxygen supply, 3) coronary artery vasoconstriction, and 4) accelerated atherosclerosis.[206]

Myocardial thallium imaging has been used to characterize the effect of cocaine on myocardial blood flow in the canine model. Oster et al demonstrated the appearance of regional perfusion defects of the septum and apex after the intravenous administration of cocaine to six mongrel dogs.[208] They postulated the effect was due to a summation of subepicardial and intramural vascular spasm. Yuen-Green et al used ^{99m}Tc sestamibi myocardial imaging to demonstrate the usefulness of imaging at rest and during chest pain for the diagnosis of cocaine-induced myocardial ischemia and infarction.[209] They imaged a 35-year-old woman with nonobstructive coronary artery disease who was admitted with acute myocardial infarction after intranasal cocaine use. On the seventh post-MI day, the patient had recurrent chest pain without new ECG abnormalities. She was given ^{99m}Tc sestamibi during a 2-h episode of chest pain and then underwent SPECT imaging. Repeat imaging was performed after she had been free of chest pain for 48 h. The images aquired during the chest pain episode revealed severely reduced perfusion of the anterior wall and septum from apex to mid-ventricle. Subsequent images after resolution of chest pain showed partially reversible defects in the anterior wall and septum indicative of previous MI and residual ischemia in the LAD territory. It was felt that the lingering effects of cocaine were inducing persistent symptomatic vasospasm in this patient's peri-infarct period.

Acute depression of myocardial function has been shown to occur after the use of cocaine, possibly as a direct toxic effect on cardiac muscle or myocarditis.[206] Several investigators have reported patients with dilated cardiomyopathy and normal coronary arteries following the long-term use of cocaine.[210,211,212] Radionuclide angiography has been used to follow left ventricular function in patients with myocardial dysfunction associated with long-term cocaine use and has revealed global and segmental abnormalities of wall motion.[206] Although specific nuclear imaging applications in cocaine heart disease have yet to enter clinical trials, standard myocardial perfusion imaging and radionuclide angiography have proven beneficial in confirming the presence or absence of underlying obstructive coronary disease or myocardial dysfunction in patients abusing cocaine who might otherwise be at low risk of such disease.

CARDIAC TRANSPLANTATION

Cardiac transplantation is an effective treatment in the terminal stage of chronic congestive heart failure. The success of cardiac transplantation has been bolstered by advances in immunosuppressive therapy, including the use of cyclosporine. Nevertheless, patient survival following cardiac transplantation is threatened by transplant rejection and coronary vasculopathy.

Transplant Rejection

Percutaneous endomyocardial biopsy is the standard method for diagnosis of cardiac transplant rejection. Histopathologic examination of the biopsy samples can reveal perivascular or interstitial cellular infiltrates and evidence of myocyte necrosis. Endomyocardial biopsy samples can often provide definitive evidence of allograft rejection and guide antirejection therapy before severe rejection or extensive myocyte necrosis occurs. The principal disadvantages of allograft surveillance by endomyocardial biopsy are the invasive nature of the procedure and dependence on clinical evidence of allograft rejection to guide the timing of the biopsy procedure.

Several noninvasive methods have been proposed to evaluate patients for evidence of cardiac transplant rejection. Reduction in QRS voltage by electrocardiography,[213] increases in left ventricular mass, or decreases in diastolic compliance by echocardiography[214,215] can be observed but are indicative of an advanced stage of rejection. Detection of allograft rejection at an earlier stage of resultant left ventricular diastolic dysfunction may be possible with Doppler echocardiography[216,217] or with radionuclide ventriculography,[218] but confirmatory studies are needed. Other approaches have examined tissue biochemical characteristics of the transplanted heart in an attempt to detect allograft rejection at an earlier stage. For example, magnetic resonance spectroscopy has demonstrated a reduced ratio of phosphocreatine to inorganic phosphate early in the course of transplant rejection.[219,220] Others have used spin echo magnetic resonance imaging in patients who are at least 25 d past allograft transplantation to demonstrate altered T_1 or T_2 proton relaxation times in the presence of transplant rejection.[221,222]

Nuclear medicine imaging methods have also been studied in the detection of acute transplant rejection. Technetium-99m pyrophosphate and ^{201}Tl imaging were found to lack sensitivity for detection of allograft rejection.[223,224] In an attempt to detect the inflammatory reaction associated with transplant rejection ^{67}Ga citrate has been evaluated in heart transplant patients. Meneguetti and co-workers examined 46 gallium studies and endomyocardial biopsies in 7 transplant recipients and found that gallium imaging was 83 percent sensitive for the detection of rejection.[225] However, the overall agreement with biopsy was only 52 percent. The usefulness of this technique is also limited by the time required to complete a study and by the radiation exposure, particularly when serial studies are used.

Since rejection is mediated by lymphocytic infiltration, administration of autologous lymphocytes labeled with ^{111}In might provide a scintigraphic marker of cardiac transplant rejection. Eisen and co-workers assessed the ability of ^{111}In-labeled lymphocytes to detect rejection in an orthotopic heart transplant model in dogs.[226] They used ^{99m}Tc to label the blood pool to develop a correction factor for lymphocytes that were in the blood pool rather than in the myocardium itself.[226,227] With this correction, the technique had very good sensitivity and specificity for detecting rejection, both when compared with serial biopsies and when compared with examination of the whole hearts at autopsy. Importantly, correlation of the scintigraphic and histologic findings was maintained in the presence of mild rejection. Rosenbloom and colleagues assessed the reliability of this technique in a canine model for assessing the treatment of transplant rejection; again they noted a good correlation between the scintigraphic findings and the histologic findings.[228] In a recent preliminary report, Rubin and associates studied 7 patients 5 ± 2 mo after cardiac transplantation and showed the feasibility of ^{111}In-labeled lymphocyte imaging for detection of histologic transplant rejection.[229]

Although the ^{111}In-labeled lymphocyte technique is therefore promising, it is not without some limitations. First, it is unlikely that the technique could differentiate between rejection and other processes, particularly infections, that might involve lymphocytic infiltration in the myocardium. The technique is also technically demanding. Finally, the direct radiation burden of the technique, particularly to the lymphocytes themselves, is of concern and requires further study.[227] Although the estimated risk of fatal malignancy over 30 y from a 0.9- to 4.8-MBq patient dose of ^{111}In-lymphocytes is low,[230] patients on chronic cyclosporine therapy have already shown evidence of an increased predisposition to lymphoma; it is unknown whether the radiation exposure to the lymphocytes from the ^{111}In studies would

have any potentiating effect on this malignancy potential.

A different imaging modality that has been evaluated with regard to its ability to detect cardiac transplant rejection involves ^{111}In attached to a monoclonal antimyosin antibody Fab fragment specific for cardiac myosin. Addonizio and co-workers investigated the utility of ^{111}In-labeled antimyosin fragments for detecting rejection in six dogs with heterotopic heart transplantations.[231] Using SPECT imaging, they found a good correlation between the ratio of indium activity in the heterotopic transplanted heart compared with the native heart and histologic rejection scores ($r = 0.97$). However, their experimental model involved severe rejection and did not necessarily indicate the reliability of the method for detecting lesser severities of rejection. Frist et al evaluated the technique in 20 studies performed on 18 patients with orthotopic heart transplantations.[232] In 16 of the 20 studies there was good agreement between the scintigraphic findings and the results of biopsy. In four instances, the results were discordant.

Indium-111 antimyosin activity in the myocardium varies over time following cardiac transplantation. During the first month after transplantation, cardiac ^{111}In antimyosin visualization appears to result directly from myocardial necrosis related to the transplant surgical procedure.[233,234] In the absence of rejection, antimyosin uptake then normalizes over a mean of 10 mo. Therefore, abnormal ^{111}In antimyosin studies between 1 mo and 1 y after cardiac transplantation may result from late normalization following transplant surgery or may reflect acute rejection. Ballester and colleagues observed that none of their 23 transplant patients who had a gradual decrease in ^{111}In antimyosin heart-to-lung ratio during the first 3 mo after surgery showed rejection-related complications. Persistent ^{111}In antimyosin uptake over the first 3 mo was associated with complications in 5 of 9 patients (56 percent).[235]

After 1 y following cardiac transplantation, a normal ^{111}In antimyosin scan places the patient at low risk. Ballester et al reported findings from 21 patients who were more than 1 y post-transplantation.[236] Indium-111 antimyosin antibody imaging was performed 22 ± 9 mo following transplantation. Subsequently, 102 endomyocardial biopsies were performed during a mean of 18 mo of follow-up. The mean number of rejection episodes was 0.11 ± 0.33 among 9 patients with a normal ^{111}In antimyosin scan (ie, heart-to-lung ratio less than 1.54) versus 1.41 ± 1.44 among 12 patients with an abnormal ^{111}In antimyosin scan at study entry (p<0.01). The authors suggested that beginning 1 y after cardiac transplantation, in patients with a normal ^{111}In antimyosin scan, quarterly endomyocardial biopsies can be avoided and surveillance for transplant rejection can be accomplished at longer intervals (e.g., yearly) by antimyosin imaging.[234,236]

Coronary Vasculopathy

Transplant coronary artery disease is the major factor limiting long-term survival after heart transplantation. Allograft vascular disease, which occurs both as a tubular segmental disease and as a diffuse concentric coronary narrowing with distal artery obliteration, appears to be a result of chronic vascular rejection.[237,238] Detection of coronary vasculopathy is made difficult by the frequent absence of angina pectoris in association with coronary artery narrowing in the denervated transplanted heart.[239]

Surveillance for coronary vasculopathy in the transplanted heart has been accomplished by periodic coronary arteriography. However, it is precisely because of the diffuse reduction in luminal caliber in transplant vasculopathy that coronary arteriography often severely underestimates the presence and severity of coronary disease.[240] Numerous patients have been described in whom greater than 80 percent diameter luminal narrowings were present in a coronary artery at the time of autopsy or retransplantation, but the lesions were undetected by a temporally proximate coronary arteriogram.[241] In a study of 360 patients who underwent annual coronary arteriography for cardiac transplant surveillance, Uretsky and associates identified 26 patients who developed myocardial infarction, heart failure from previous myocardial infarction, or sudden cardiac death. Only 33 percent of patients who developed a cardiac event had evidence of a greater than 50 percent coronary artery stenosis on the preceding annual surveillance coronary arteriogram.[242] A logical alternative to coronary arteriography would be a technique that can assess the entire coronary artery diameter including portions of the diameter that are obstructed by intimal hyperplasia or atherosclerotic plaque. Intracoronary ultrasound has proven useful in this assessment[243,244,245,246,247,248,249] and also provides prognostic information that may be used to guide revascularization or retransplantation strategies.[250] Limitations of intracoronary ultrasound in the detection of transplant vasculopathy include its invasive nature and the size of the probe, which limits detection of diffuse distal vessel disease.[251]

Accurate noninvasive detection of coronary vasculopathy would facilitate cardiac surveillance in transplant patients, but to date has not provided an acceptable alternative to invasive approaches. Derumeaux and colleagues studied 37 patients with dobutamine (up to 40 μg/kg/min) echocardiography at the time of annual coronary arteriography 40 $\pm$ 20 mo following cardiac transplantation.[252] Dobutamine stress echocardiography was normal in 21 of 23 patients with a normal coronary arteriogram. Dobutamine-induced hypokinesia was visualized in each of 7 patients with a greater than 50 percent angiographic stenosis and in 5 of 7 patients with

an angiographic stenosis less than 50 percent of the luminal diameter. Confirmation of these results in larger studies is needed.

Despite some inconclusive or unfavorable initial reports,[253,254] myocardial perfusion imaging has shown promise in recent studies for diagnostic and prognostic assessment of transplant vasculopathy. Ciliberto and associates reported results of exercise planar ^{201}Tl imaging in 50 heart transplant patients who were imaged within 48 h of scheduled annual coronary arteriography.[255] Thirty-five patients had normal coronary arteriograms and normal exercise thallium scans. Seven patients had a 50 percent or greater angiographic coronary stenosis and an abnormal exercise ^{201}Tl scan. Eight patients had a less than 50 percent angiographic coronary artery stenosis, and 3 of the 8 had an abnormal myocardial perfusion scan. During 13 $\pm$ 3 mo of follow-up, no patient with a normal exercise ^{201}Tl scintigram experienced a cardiac event, whereas 4 of 10 patients with an abnormal ^{201}Tl scintigram did develop a cardiac event. Perhaps more representative are the results reported by Rodney and co-authors.[256] Among 25 heart transplant recipients, exercise ^{201}Tl tomography was abnormal in 10 of 13 patients with a 50 percent or greater luminal diameter narrowing by angiography (sensitivity 77 percent) and was normal in 12 of 12 patients without significant narrowing (specificity 100 percent). Tomographic imaging with ^{99m}Tc sestamibi was also performed in 18 of the 25 study patients and provided no advantage compared with ^{201}Tl imaging. Nevertheless, the favorable prognostic information from ^{201}Tl imaging as described by Ciliberto et al[255] has recently been confirmed in a preliminary report by Verhoeven and associates.[257] In 47 cardiac transplant patients followed up for 40.1 $\pm$ 19.2 mo, stress myocardial perfusion imaging was the most significant predictor of survival (p < 0.001). The 5-y survival for patients with a normal ^{201}Tl perfusion scan was 96 percent compared with 26 percent for patients with an abnormal ^{201}Tl scan.

Future noninvasive assessment of cardiac transplant patients for evidence of coronary vasculopathy may include quantitative assessment of coronary blood flow reserve. Using ^{13}N ammonia and positron emission tomography, Zhao et al observed that myocardial blood flow decreased from 73 $\pm$ 21 to 56 $\pm$ 13, 51 $\pm$ 11, and 51 $\pm$ 27 mL/min/g of tissue in patients surviving 3 mo, 1, 2, and 3 y after transplantation.[258] The decrease in myocardial blood flow was more profound in 11 of the 43 study patients with angiographic evidence of diffuse concentric coronary artery narrowing.

SUMMARY

The list of disorders that can affect the myocardium, either primarily or secondarily, is an extensive one. Radionuclide studies, particularly ventricular function studies, can be useful in the evaluation of any of these, particularly in characterizing ventricular systolic and diastolic function. In certain of the disorders, however, radionuclide studies can also serve a specific role in detection, diagnosis, and guiding therapy. In addition, in specific entities they may have a role in the investigation of underlying pathophysiology and pathogenesis.

REFERENCES

1. Brigden W: Uncommon myocardial diseases: The noncoronary cardiomyopathies. *Lancet* 2:1179, 1957.

2. Goodwin JF, Gordon H, et al: Clinical aspects of cardiomyopathy. *Br Med J* 1:69, 1961.

3. Goodwin JF, Oakley CM: The cardiomyopathies. *Br Heart J* 34:545, 1972.

4. Roberts WC, Ferrans VJ: Pathologic anatomy of the cardiomyopathies. *Hum Pathol* 6:287, 1975.

5. Abelmann WH: The cardiomyopathies. *Hosp Pract* 6:101, 1971.

6. Goodwin JF: Prospects and predictions for the cardiomyopathies. *Circulation* 50:210, 1974.

7. Goodwin JF: Congestive and hypertrophic cardiomyopathies—a decade of study. *Lancet* II:731, 1970.

8. Ableman WH: Classification and natural history of primary myocardial disease. *Prog Myocard Dis* 27(2):73, 1984.

9. Boffa GM, Thiene G, Nava A, et al: Cardiomyopathy: A necessary revision of the WHO classification. *Int J Cardiol* 30:1, 1991.

10. Keren A, Popp RL: Assignment of patients into the classification of cardiomyopathies. *Circulation* 86:1622, 1992.

11. WHO/IFSC Task Force: Report of the WHO/ISFC task force on the definition and classification of cardiomyopathies. *Br Heart J* 44:672, 1980.

12. WHO/IFSC Task Force: Report of the 1995 World Health Organization/International Society and Federation of Cardiology task force on the definition and classification of cardiomyopathies. *Circulation* 93:841, 1996.

13. Maron BJ, Gottdiener JS, Epstein SE: Patterns and significance of distribution of left ventricular hypertrophy in hypertrophic cardiomyopathy: A wide angle, two-dimensional echocardiographic study of 125 patients. *Am J Cardiol* 48:418, 1981.

14. Chahine RA, Raizner AE, Ishimori T, et al: Echocardiographic, heamodynamic, and angiographic correlations in hypertrophic cardiomyopathy. *Br Heart J* 39:945, 1977.

15. Doi YL, McKenna WJ, Gehrke J, et al: M-mode echocardiography in hypertrophic cardiomyopathy: Diagnostic criteria and prediction of obstruction. *Am J Cardiol* 45:6, 1980.

16. Maron BJ, Epstein SE: Hypertrophic cardiomyopathy: Recent observations regarding the specificity of three hallmarks of the disease: asymmetric septal hypertrophy, septal disorganization and systolic anterior motion of the mitral leaflet. *Am J Cardiol* 45:141, 1980.

17. Shapiro LM, McKenna WJ: Distribution of left ventricular hypertrophy in hypertrophic cardiomyopathy: A two-dimensional echocardiographic study. *J Am Coll Cardiol* 2:437, 1983.

18. Braunwald E, Lambrew CT, et al: Idiopathic hypertrophic subaortic stenosis. I. A description of the disease based upon an analysis of 64 patients. *Circulation* 29–30:IV-3-IV-119, 1964 (suppl IV).

19. Henry WL, Clark CE, Griffith JM, Epstein SE: Mechanism of left ventricular outflow obstruction in patients with obstructive asymmetric septal hypertrophy (idiopathic hypertrophic subaortic stenosis). *Am J Cardiol* 35:337, 1975.

20. Spirito P, Maron BJ: Significance of left ventricular outflow tract cross-sectional area in hypertrophic cardiomyopathy: A two-dimensional echocardiographic assessment. *Circulation* 67:1100, 1983.

21. Wigle ED, Sasson Z, Henderson MA, et al: Hypertrophic cardiomyopathy: The importance of the site and extent of hypertrophy: A review. *Prog Card Dis* 28:1, 1985.

22. Yock PG, Hatle L, Popp RL: Patterns and timing of doppler-detected intracavitary and aortic flow in hypertrophic cardiomyopathy. *J Am Coll Card* 8:1047, 1986.

23. Wigle, ED: Hypertrophic cardiomyopathy: A 1987 viewpoint. *Circulation* 75:311, 1987.

24. Stewart WJ, Schiavone WA, Salcedo EE, et al: Intraoperative doppler echocardiography in hypertrophic cardiomyopathy: Correlations with the obstructive gradient. *J Am Coll Card* 10:327, 1987.

25. Maron BJ, Bonow RO, Cannon RO, et al: Hypertrophic cardiomyopathy, interrelations of clinical manifestations, pathophysiology, and therapy. *N Engl J Med* 316:789;844, 1987.

26. Pouleur H, Rousseau MF, van Eyll C, et al: Force-velocity-length relationships in hypertrophic cardiomyopathy: Evidence of normal or depressed myocardial contractility. *Am J Cardiol* 52:813, 1983.

27. Louie EK, Edwards LC: Hypertrophic cardiomyopathy. *Prog Card Dis* 36:275, 1994.

28. Bonow RO, Dilsizian V, Rosing DR, et al: Verapamil-induced improvement in left ventricular diastolic filling and increased exercise tolerance in patients with hypertrophic cardiomyopathy: Short and long term effects. *Circulation* 72:853, 1985.

29. Goodwin JF: The frontiers of cardiomyopathy. *Br Heart J* 48:1, 1982.

30. Sanderson JE, Gibson DG, Brown DJ, et al: Left ventricular filling in hypertrophic cardiomyopathy: An angiographic study. *Br Heart J* 39:661, 1977.

31. Sanderson JE, Traill TA, St. John Sutton MG, et al: Left ventricular relaxation and filling in hypertrophic cardiomyopathy: An echocardiographic study. *Br Heart J* 40:596, 1978.

32. Bryhn M, Persson S: Noninvasive findings in patients with hypertrophic and dilative cardiomyopathy: A combined echocardiographic and radionuclide angiographic study. *Clin Cardiol* 9:537, 1986.

33. Betocchi S, Bonow RO, Bacharach SL, et al: Isovolumic

relaxation period in hypertrophic cardiomyopathy: Assessment by radionuclide angiography. *J Am Coll Cardiol* 7:74, 1986.

34. Dilsizian V, Rocco TP, Bonow RO, et al: Cardiac blood-pool imaging II: Applications in noncoronary heart disease. *J Nucl Med* 31:10, 1990.

35. Chikamori T, Dickie S: Prognostic significance of radionuclide-assessed diastolic function in hypertrophic cardiomyopathy. *Am J Cardiol* 65:478, 1990.

36. Stewart RA, McKenna WJ: Assessment of diastolic filling indexes obtained by radionuclide ventriculography. *Am J Cardiol* 65:226, 1990.

37. Inoue T, Morooka S, Hayashi T, et al: Global and regional abnormalities of left ventricular diastolic filling in hypertrophic cardiomyopathy. *Clin Cardiol* 14:573, 1991.

38. Bulkley BH, Rouleau J, Strauss HW: Idiopathic hypertrophic subaortic stenosis: Detection by thallium-201 myocardial perfusion imaging. *N Engl J Med* 293:1113, 1975.

39. Rubin KA, Morrison J, Padnick MB, et al: Idiopathic hypertrophic subaortic stenosis: Evaluation of anginal symptoms with thallium-201 myocardial imaging. *Am J Cardiol* 44:1040, 1979.

40. Pitcher D, Wainwright R, Maisey M, et al: Assessment of chest pain in hypertrophic cardiomyopathy using exercise thallium-201 myocardial scintigraphy. *Br Heart J* 44:650, 1980.

41. Hanrath P, Mathey D, Muntz R, et al: Myocardial thallium-201 imaging in hypertrophic obstructive cardiomyopathy. *Eur Heart J* 2:177, 1981.

42. Suzuki Y, Kadota K, Nohara R, et al: Recognition of regional hypertrophy in hypertrophic cardiomyopathy using thallium-201 emission-computed tomography: Comparison with two-dimensional echocardiography. *Am J Cardiol* 53:1095, 1984.

43. Nagata S, Park YD, Minamikawa T, et al: Thallium perfusion and cardiac enzyme abnormalities in patients with familial hypertrophic cardiomyopathy. *Am Heart J* 109:1317, 1985.

44. O'Gara PT, Bonow RO, Maron BJ, et al: Myocardial perfusion abnormalities in patients with hypertrophic cardiomyopathy: Assessment with thallium-201 emission computed tomography. *Circulation* 76:1214, 1987.

45. Udelson JE, Bonow RO, O'Gara PT, et al: Verapamil prevents silent myocardial perfusion abnormalities during exercise in asymptomatic patients with hypertrophic cardiomyopathy. *Circulation* 79:1052, 1989.

46. Cannon RO, Dilsizian V, O'Gara PT, et al: Myocardial metabolic, hemodynamic, and electrocardiographic significance of reversible thallium-201 abnormalities in hypertrophic cardiomyopathy. *Circulation* 83:1660, 1991.

47. Takata J, Counihan PJ, Gane JN, et al: Regional thallium-201 washout and myocardial hypertrophy in hypertrophic cardiomyopathy and its relation to exertional chest pain. *Am J Cardiol* 72:211, 1993.

48. Cannon RO, Dilsizian V, O'Gara PT, et al: Impact of surgical relief of outflow obstruction on thallium perfusion abnormalities in hypertrophic cardiomyopathy. *Circulation* 85:1039, 1992.

49. Redwood DR, Scherer JL, Epstein SE: Biventricular cine-angiography in the evaluation of patients with asymmetric septal hypertrophy. *Circulation* 49:116, 1974.

50. Pohost GM, Vignola PA, McKusick KE, et al: Hypertrophic cardiomyopathy: Evaluation by gated cardiac blood pool scanning. *Circulation* 55:92, 1997.

51. Keren G, Belhassen B: Apical hypertrophic cardiomyopathy: Evaluation by noninvasive and invasive techniques in 23 patients. *Circulation* 71:45, 1985.

52. Thompson DS, Naqvi N, Juul SM, et al: Effects of propranolol on myocardial oxygen consumption, substrate extraction and hemodynamics in hypertrophic cardiomyopathy. *Br Heart J* 44:488, 1980.

53. Pasternac A, Noble J, Streulens Y, et al: Pathophysiology of chest pain in patients with cardiomyopathies and normal coronary arteries. *Circulation* 65:778, 1982.

54. Cannon RO, Rosing DR, Maron BJ, et al: Myocardial ischemia in patients with hypertrophic cardiomyopathy: Contribution of inadequate vasodilator reserve and elevated left ventricular filling pressures. *Circulation* 71:231, 1985.

55. St. John Sutton MG, Lie JT, Anderson KR, et al: Histopathological specificity of hypertrophic obstructive cardiomyopathy: Myocardial fibre disarray and myocardial fibrosis. *Br Heart J* 44:433, 1980.

56. Maron BJ, Wolfson JK, Epstein SE, et al: Intramural ("small vessel") coronary artery disease in hypertrophic cardiomyopathy. *J Am Coll Cardiol* 8:545, 1986.

57. Tanaka M, Fujiwara H, Onodera T, et al: Quantitative analysis of myocardial fibrosis in normals, hypertensive hearts, and hypertrophic cardiomyopathy. *Br Heart J* 55:575, 1986.

58. Maron BJ, Epstein SE, Roberts WC, et al: Hypertrophic cardiomyopathy and transmural myocardial infarction without significant atherosclerosis of the extramural coronary arteries. *Am J Cardiol* 43:1086, 1979.

59. Pichard AD, Meller J, Teicholz LE, et al: Septal perforator compression (narrowing) in idiopathic hypertrophic subaortic stenosis. *Am J Cardiol* 40:310, 1977.

60. St John Sutton MG, Tajik AJ, Gibson DG, et al: Echocardiographic assessment of left ventricular filling and septal and posterior wall dynamics in idiopathic hypertrophic subaortic stenosis. *Circulation* 57:512, 1978.

61. von Dahlin TO, Prisant LM, Frank MJ: Significance of positive or negative thallium 201 scintigraphy in hypertrophic cardiomyopathy. *Am J Cardiol* 64:498, 1989.

62. Dilsizian V, Bonow RO, Epstein SE, et al: Myocardial ischemia detected by thallium scintigraphy is frequently related to cardiac arrest and syncope in young patients with hypertrophic cardiomyopathy. *J Am Coll Cardiol* 22:796, 1993.

63. Fujibayashi Y, Yonekura Y, Takemura Y, et al: Myocardial accumulation of iodinated beta-methyl branched fatty acid analogue, iodine-123-15-p-iodophenyl-3-(R,S)-methylpentadexanoic acid (BMIPP), in relation to ATP concentration. *J Nucl Med* 31:1818, 1990.

64. Taki J, Nakajima K, Bunko H, et al: ^{123}I-labelled BMIPP fatty acid myocardial scintigraphy in patients with hypertrophic cardiomyopathy: SPECT comparison with stress [201]Tl. *Nucl Med Commun* 14:181, 1993.

65. Ohtsuki K, Sugihara H, Umamoto I, et al: Clinical evalua-

tion of hypertrophic cardiomyopathy by myocardial scintigraphy using ^{123}I-labelled 15-(p-iodophenyl)-3-R, S-methylpentadecanoic acid (^{123}I-BMIPP). *Nucl Med Commun* 15:441, 1994.

66. Johnson RA, Palacios I: Dilated cardiomyopathies of the adult. *N Engl J Med* 307:1051, 1119, 1982.

67. Wallis DE, O'Connell JB, Henkin RE, et al: Segmental wall motion abnormality in dilated cardiomyopathy: A common finding and good prognostic sign. *J Am Coll Cardiol* 4:674, 1984.

68. Yamaguchi S, Tsuiki K, Hayasaka M, et al: Segmental wall motion abnormalities in dilated cardiomyopathy: Hemodynamic characteristics and comparison with thallium-201 myocardial scintigraphy. *Am Heart J* 113:1123, 1987.

69. Eichhorn EJ, Kosinski EJ, Lewis SM, et al: Usefulness of dipyridamole-thallium-201 perfusion scanning for distinguishing ischemic from nonischemic cardiomyopathy. *Am J Cardiol* 62:945, 1988.

70. Doi YL, Chikamori T, Tukata J, et al: Prognostic value of thallium-201 perfusion defects in idiopathic dilated cardiomyopathy. *Am J Cardiol* 67:188, 1991.

71. Gaudio C, Tanzilli G, Mazzarotto P, et al: Comparison of left ventricular ejection fraction by magnetic resonance imaging and radionuclide ventriculography in idiopathic dilated cardiomyopathy. *Am J Cardiol* 67:411, 1991.

72. Glamann DB, Lange RA, Corbett JR, et al: Utility of various radionuclide techniques for distinguishing ischemic from nonischemic dilated cardiomyopathy. *Arch Intern Med* 152:769, 1992.

73. Chikamori T, Doi Y, Yonezawa Y, et al: Value of dipyridamole thallium-201 imaging in noninvasive differentiation of idiopathic dilated cardiomyopathy from coronary artery disease with left ventricular dysfunction. *Am J Cardiol* 69:650, 1992.

74. Tomai F, Ciavolella M, Crea F, et al: Left ventricular volumes during exercise in normal subjects and patients with dilated cardiomyopathy assessed by first-pass radionuclide angiography. *Am J Cardiol* 72:1167, 1993.

75. Tauberg SG, Orie JE, Bartlett BE, et al: Usefulness of thallium 201 for distinction of ischemic from idiopathic dilated cardiomyopathy. *Am J Cardiol* 71:674, 1993.

76. Juilliere Y, Marie PY, Danchin N, et al: Radionuclide assessment of regional differences in left ventricular wall motion and myocardial perfusion in idiopathic dilated cardiomyopathy. *Eur Heart J* 14:1163, 1993.

77. Greenberg JM, Murphy JH, Okada RD, et al: Value and limitations of radionuclide angiography in determining the cause of reduced left ventricular ejection fraction: Comparison of idiopathic dilated cardiomyopathy and coronary artery disease. *Am J Cardiol* 55:541, 1985.

78. Bateman TM, Gray RJ, Czer LS, et al: Regional distribution of pulmonary blood volume: An index of pulmonary capillary wedge pressure determined from blood pool scintigraphy. *Am J Cardiol* 51:1404, 1983.

79. Iskandrian AS, Hakki AH, Kane S: Resting thallium-201 myocardial perfusion patterns in patients with severe left ventricular dysfunction: Differences between patients with primary cardiomyopathy, chronic coronary artery disease, or acute myocardial infarction. *Am Heart J* 111:760, 1986.

80. Dunn RF, Uren RF, Sadick N, et al: Comparison of thallium-201 scanning in idiopathic dilated cardiomyopathy and severe coronary artery disease. *Circulation* 66:804, 1982.

81. Gewirtz H, Grotte GJ, Strauss HW, et al: The influence of left ventricular volume and wall motion on myocardial images. *Circulation* 59:1172, 1979.

82. Opherk D, Schwarz F, Mall G, et al: Coronary dilatory capacity in idiopathic dilated cardiomyopathy: Analysis of 16 patients. *Am J Cardiol* 51:1657, 1983.

83. Shabetai R: Pathophysiology and differential diagnosis of restrictive cardiomyopathy. *Cardiovasc Clin* 19:123, 1988.

84. Seward JB: Restrictive cardiomyopathy: Reassessment of definitions and diagnosis. *Curr Opin Cardiol* 3:391, 1988.

85. Johnson RA, Palacios I: Nondilated cardiomyopathies. *Adv Intern Med* 30:243, 1984.

86. Tyberg TI, Goodyer AVN, Hurst VW III, et al: Left ventricular filling in differentiating restrictive amyloid cardiomyopathy and constrictive pericarditis. *Am J Cardiol* 47:791, 1981.

87. Gerson MC, Colthar MS, Fowler NO: Differentiation of constrictive pericarditis and restrictive cardiomyopathy by radionuclide ventriculography. *Am Heart J* 118:114, 1989.

88. Benotti JR, Grossman W, Cohn PF: Clinical profile of restrictive cardiomyopathy. *Circulation* 61:1206, 1980.

89. Robbins MA, Pizzarello RA, Stechel PR, et al: Resting and exercise hemodynamics in constrictive pericarditis and a case of cardiac amyloidosis mimicking constriction. *Cathet Cardiovasc Diagn* 9:463, 1983.

90. Klein AL, Hatle LK, Taliercio CP, et al: Prognostic significance of Doppler measures of diastolic function in cardiac amyloidosis: A Doppler echocardiography study. *Circulation* 83:808, 1991.

91. Aretz HT: Diagnosis of myocarditis by endomyocardial biopsy. *Med Clin North Am* 70:1215, 1986.

92. Ramamurthy S, Talwar KK, Goswami KC, et al: Clinical profile of biopsy proven idiopathic myocarditis. *Int J Cardiol* 41:225, 1993.

93. Frustace A, Maseri A: Localized left ventricular aneurysms with normal global function caused by myocarditis. *Am J Cardiol* 70:1221, 1992.

94. Richardson PJ, Why HJ, Archard LC: Virus infection and dilated cardiomyopathy. *Postgrad Med J* 68:S17, 1992.

95. El-Khatib MR, Chason JL, Lerner AM: Ventricular aneurysms complicating Coxsackie virus group B, types 1 and 4 murine myocarditis. *Circulation* 59:412, 1979.

96. Cambridge G, Mac Arthur CG, Milder MS, et al: Antibodies to Coxsackie B viruses in congestive cardiomyopathy. *Br Heart J* 41:692, 1979.

97. Gelrud LG, Arseneau JS, et al: The kinetics of gallium-67 incorporation into inflammatory lesions: Experimental and clinical studies. *J Lab Clin Med* 83:489, 1974.

98. Merz T, Malmud L, McKusick K, et al: The mechanism of Ga-67 association with lymphocytes. *Cancer Res* 34:2495, 1974.

99. Desai SP, Yuille DL: The unsuspected complications of bacterial endocarditis imaged by gallium-67 scanning. *J Nuc Med* 34:955, 1993.

100. Strain JE, Fine EJ, et al: Comparison of myocardial biopsy and gallium-67 imaging for diagnosing myocarditis. *Circulation* 68:III-203, 1983 (abstr).
101. O'Connell JB, Henkin RE, Robinson JA, et al: Gallium-67 imaging in patients with dilated cardiomyopathy and biopsy-proven myocarditis. *Circulation* 70:58, 1984.
102. Veluvolu P, Kamrani F, Horton DP, et al: Acute transient myocarditis: Evaluation by gallium imaging. *Clin Nuc Med* 17:412, 1992.
103. O'Connell J, Robinson JA, Henkin RE, et al: Gallium citrate scanning for noninvasive detection of inflammation in pericardial diseases. *Am J Cardiol* 46:879, 1980.
104. Yasuda T, Palacios IF, Dec GW, et al: Indium 111-monoclonal antimyosin antibody imaging in the diagnosis of acute myocarditis. *Circulation* 76:306, 1987.
105. Dec GW, Palacios IF, Yasuda T, et al: Antimyosin antibody cardiac imaging: Its role in the diagnosis of myocarditis. *J Am Coll Cardiol* 16:97, 1990.
106. Narula J, Yasuda T, et al: Antimyosin scintigraphic detection of myocarditis: Sensitivity, specificity, heart/lung ratio, clinical outcome and intra/inter-observer variations. *J Nuc Med* 32:1019, 1991 (abstr).
107. Baroldi G, Corallo S, Moroni M, et al: Focal lymphocytic myocarditis in acquired immunodeficiency syndrome (AIDS): A correlative morphologic and clinical study in 26 consecutive fatal cases. *J Am Coll Cardiol* 12:463, 1988.
108. Anderson DW, Virmani R, Reilly JM, et al: Prevalent myocarditis at necropsy in the acquired immunodeficiency syndrome. *J Am Coll Cardiol* 11:792, 1988.
109. Anderson DW, Virmani R: Emerging patterns of heart disease in human immunodeficiency virus infection. *Hum Path* 21:253, 1990.
110. Cohen IS, Anderson DW, Virmani R, et al: Congestive cardiomyopathy in association with the acquired immunodeficiency syndrome. *N Engl J Med* 315:628, 1986.
111. Corboy JR, Fink L, Miller WT: Congestive cardiomyopathy in association with AIDS. *Radiology* 165:139, 1987.
112. Kaminski HJ, Katzman M, Wiest PM, et al: Cardiomyopathy associated with the acquired immune deficiency syndrome. *J Acquired Immune Defic Syndr* 1:105, 1988.
113. Miller RF, Gilson R, Hage C, et al: HIV-associated dilated cardiomyopathy. *Genitourin Med* 67:453, 1991.
114. Noreuil TO, Dinh HA: Dilated cardiomyopathy as an early and rapidly progressive presentation in a woman with acquired immunodeficiency syndrome. *South Med J* 86:465, 1993.
115. Joshi VV, Gadol C, Connor E, et al: Dilated cardiomyopathy in children with acquired immunodeficiency syndrome. *Hum Pathol* 19:69, 1988.
116. Herskowitz A, Vlahov D, Willoughby S, et al: Prevalence and incidence of left ventricular dysfunction in patients with human immunodeficiency virus infection. *Am J Cardiol* 71:955, 1993.
117. Herskowitz A, Willoughby S, Wu TC, et al: Immunopathogenesis of HIV-1-associated cardiomyopathy. *Clin Immunol Imunopathol* 68:234, 1993.
118. Kavanaugh-McHugh AL, Ruff A, Perlman E, et al: Selenium deficiency and cardiomyopathy in acquired immunodeficiency syndrome. *J Parent Ent Nutr* 15:347, 1991.
119. Herskowitz A, Willoughby S, Baughman KL, et al: Cardiomyopathy associated with anti-retroviral therapy in patients with human immunodeficiency virus infection: A report of six cases. *Ann Intern Med* 116:311, 1992.
120. Grody WW, Cheng L, Lewis W: Infection of the heart by the human immunodeficiency virus. *Am J Cardiol* 66:203, 1990.
121. Calabrese LH, Proffitt MR, Yen-Lieberman B, et al: Congestive cardiomyopathy and illness related to the acquired immunodeficiency syndrome (AIDS) associated with isolation of retrovirus from myocardium. *Ann Intern Med* 107:691, 1987.
122. Cregler LL, Sosa I, Ducey S, et al: Myopericarditis in acquired immunodeficiency syndrome diagnosed by gallium scintigraphy. *J Nat Med Assoc* 82:511, 1990.
123. Auringer ST, Sumner TE, Cowan RJ: Pediatric AIDS-related myocarditis: Focal cardiac gallium uptake. *Clin Nuc Med* 18:999, 1993.
124. Memel DS, DeRogatis AJ, Williams DC: Ga-67 citrate myocardial uptake in a patient with AIDS, toxoplasmosis, and myocarditis. *Clin Nuc Med* 16:315, 1991.
125. Garcia MJ, McNamara PM, Gordon T, et al: Morbidity and mortality in diabetics in the Framingham population: Sixteen year follow-up study. *Diabetes* 23:105, 1974.
126. Sanderson JE, Brown DJ, Rivellese A, et al: Diabetic cardiomyopathy? An echocardiographic study of young diabetics. *Br Med J* 1:404, 1978.
127. Shapiro LM: Echocardiographic features of impaired ventricular function in diabetes mellitus. *Br Heart J* 47:439, 1982.
128. Zarich SW, Arbuckle BE, Cohen LR, et al: Diastolic abnormalities in young asymptomatic diabetic patients assessed by pulsed Doppler echocardiography. *J Am Coll Cardiol* 12:1, 114, 1988.
129. Takenaka K, Sakamoto T, Amano K, et al: Left ventricular filling determined by Doppler echocardiography in diabetes mellitus. *Am J Cardiol* 61:1140, 1988.
130. Abenavoli T, Rubler S, Fisher VJ, et al: Exercise testing with myocardial scintigraphy in asymptomatic diabetic males. *Circulation* 63:54, 1981.
131. Vered A, Battler A, Segal P, et al: Exercise-induced left ventricular dysfunction in young men with asymptomatic diabetes mellitus (diabetic cardiomyopathy). *Am J Cardiol* 54:633, 1984.
132. Spirito P, Maron BJ, Bonow RO: Noninvasive assessment of left ventricular diastolic function: Comparative analysis of Doppler echocardiographic and radionuclide angiographic techniques. *J Am Coll Cardiol* 7:518, 1986.
133. Amano K, Sakamoto T, Oku J, et al: Diabetic cardiomyopathy: The relationship between 201 thallium myocardial scintigraphic perfusion defect and left ventricular function in asymptomatic diabetics. *Acto Cardiologica* 2:75, 1988.
134. Erbas T, Erbas B, Gedik O, et al: Scintigraphic evaluation of left ventricular function and correlation with autonomic cardiac neuropathy in diabetic patients. *Cardiology* 81:14, 1992.
135. Follansbee WP, Curtiss EI, et al: Diabetic cardiomyopathy: Final results from the epidemiology of diabetes complications study. *Circulation* 80(suppl II):II-206, 1989.

136. Mildenberger RR, Barsshlomo B, Druck MN, et al: Clinically unrecognized ventricular dysfunction in young diabetic patients. *J Am Coll Cardiol* 4:234, 1984.

137. Follansbee WP, Schulman DS, et al: Diastolic function in diabetes: Results from the Epidemiology of Diabetic Complications Study. *Circulation* 80(suppl II):II-76, 1989 (abstr).

138. Plotnick GD, Kahn B, Rogers WJ, et al: Effect of postural changes, nitroglycerin and verapamil on diastolic ventricular function as determined by radionuclide angiography in normal subjects. *J Am Coll Cardiol* 12:121, 1988.

139. Kahn JK, Zola B, Juni JE, et al: Radionuclide assessment of left ventricular diastolic filling in diabetes mellitus with and without cardiac autonomic neuropathy. *J Am Coll Cardiol* 7:1303, 1986.

140. Pizzarello RA, Goldberg J: The heart in rheumatoid arthritis, in Utsinger PD, Svaifler NJ, Ehrlich GE (eds): *Rheumatoid Arthritis: Aetiology, Diagnosis and Management.* Philadelphia, JB Lippincott, 1985, pp 41–440.

141. Corrao S, Salli L, Arnone S, et al: Cardiac involvement in rheumatoid arthritis: Evidence of silent heart disease. *Eur Heart J* 16:253, 1995.

142. Mutru O, Laakso M, Isomake H, et al: Cardiovascular mortality in patients with rheumatoid arthritis. *Cardiology* 76:71, 1989.

143. Prakash R, Atassi A, Poske R, et al: Prevalence of pericardial effusion and mitral-valve involvement in patients with rheumatoid arthritis without cardiac symptoms: An echocardiographic evaluation. *N Eng J Med* 289:597, 1973.

144. Mustonen J, Laakso M, Hirvonen T, et al: Abnormalities in left ventricular diastolic function in male patients with rheumatoid arthritis without clinically evident cardiovascular disease. *Eur J Clin Inves* 23:246, 1993.

145. Weirs S, Stead EA Jr, et al: Scleroderma heart disease: With a consideration of certain other visceral manifestations of scleroderma. *Arch Intern Med* 71:749, 1943.

146. Follansbee WP: The cardiovascular manifestations of systemic sclerosis (scleroderma). *Curr Probl Cardiol* 11:242, 1986.

147. Medsger TA Jr, Masi AT, Rodnan GP, et al: Survival with systemic sclerosis (scleroderma): A life-table analysis of clinical and demographic factors in 309 patients. *Ann Intern Med* 75:369, 1971.

148. Follansbee WP, Curtiss EI, Rahko PS, et al: The electrocardiogram in systemic sclerosis (scleroderma): A study of 102 consecutive cases with functional correlations and a review of the literature. *Am J Med* 79:183, 1985.

149. D'Angelo WA, Fries JF, Masi AT, et al: Pathologic observations in systemic sclerosis (scleroderma): A study of fifty-eight autopsy cases and fifty-eight matched controls. *Am J Med* 46:428, 1969.

150. Medsger TA Jr, Massi AT: Survival with scleroderma-II: A life-table analysis of clinical and demographic factors in 358 male U.S. veteran patients. *J Chronic Dis* 26:647, 1973.

151. Follansbee WP, Curtiss EI, Medsger TA Jr, et al: Physiologic abnormalities of cardiac function in progressive systemic sclerosis with diffuse scleroderma. *N Engl J Med* 10:142, 1984.

152. Follansbee WP, Curtiss EI, Medsger TA Jr, et al: Myocar-

153. Bulkley BH, Ridolfi RL, Salyer WR, et al: Myocardial lesions of progressive systemic sclerosis: A cause of cardiac dysfunction. *Circulation* 53:483, 1976.

154. Alexander EL, Firestein GS, Weiss JL, et al: Reversible cold-induced abnormalities in myocardial perfusion and function in systemic sclerosis. *Ann Int Med* 105:661, 1986.

155. Gustafsson R, Mannting F, Kazzam E, et al: Cold-induced reversible myocardial ischaemia in systemic sclerosis. *Lancet* 2:475, 1989.

156. Kahan A, Devaux JY, Amor B, et al: Nifedipine and thallium-201 myocardial perfusion in progressive systemic sclerosis. *N Engl J Med* 314:1397, 1986.

157. Kahan A, Devaux JY, Amor B, et al: Pharmacodynamic effect of dipyridamole on thallium-201 myocardial perfusion in progressive systemic sclerosis with diffuse scleroderma. *Ann Rheum Dis* 45:718, 1986.

158. Kahan A, Devaux JY, Amor B, et al: Nicardipine improves myocardial perfusion in systemic sclerosis. *J Rheumatol* 15:1395, 1988.

159. Follansbee WP, Kiernan JM, et al: Cold-induced thallium perfusion abnormalities in diffuse scleroderma and Raynaud's disease: Response to diltiazem therapy. *Arthritis Rheum* 29:S52, 1987.

160. Follansbee WP, Kiernan JM, et al: Left ventricular function during cold pressor stimulation in diffuse scleroderma, Raynaud's disease, and normals: Response to diltiazem therapy. *Arthritis Rheum* 29:S52, 1987.

161. Kahan A, Devaux JY, Amor B, et al: The effect of captopril on thallium-201 myocardial perfusion in systemic sclerosis. *Clin Pharmacol Ther* 47:483, 1990.

162. Kahan A, Devaux JY, Amor B, et al: Pharmacodynamic effect of nicardipine on left ventricular function in systemic sclerosis. *J Cardiovasc Pharmacol* 15:249, 1990.

163. Strauer BE, Brune I, Schenk H, et al: Lupus cardiomyopathy: Cardiac mechanics, hemodynamics, and coronary blood flow in uncomplicated systemic lupus erythematosus. *Am Heart J* 92:715, 1976.

164. Klinkhoff AV, Thompson CR, Reid GO, et al: M-mode and two-dimensional echocardiographic abnormalities in systemic lupus erythematosus. *J Am Med Assoc* 253:3273, 1985.

165. Leung WH, Wong KL, Lau CP, et al: Doppler echocardiographic evaluation of left ventricular diastolic function in patients with systemic lupus erythematosus. *Am Heart J* 120:82, 1990.

166. Bahl VK, Aradhye S, Vasan RS, et al: Myocardial systolic function in systemic lupus erythematosus: A study based on radionuclide ventriculography. *Clin Cardiol* 15:433, 1992.

167. Bidani AK, Roberts JL, Schwartz JL, et al: Immunopathology of cardiac lesions in fatal SLE. *Am J Med* 69:849, 1980.

168. Korbet SM, Schwartz MM, Lewis EJ: Immune complex deposition and coronary vasculitis in systemic lupus erythematosus. *Am J Med* 77:141, 1984.

169. Homcy CJ, Liberthson RR, Fallon JT, et al: Ischemic

heart disease in systemic lupus erythematosus in the young patient: Report of six cases. *Am J Cardiol* 49:478, 1982.

170. Bonfiglio TA, Botti RE, Hagstrom JW: Coronary arteritis, occlusion, and myocardial infarction due to lupus erythematosus. *Am Heart J* 83:153, 1972.

171. Heibel RH, O'Toole JD, Curtiss EI, et al: Coronary arteritis in systemic lupus erythematosus. *Chest* 69:700, 1976.

172. Tsakraklides VG, Blieden LC, Edwards JE: Coronary atherosclerosis and myocardial infarction associated with systemic lupus erythematosus. *Am Heart J* 87:637, 1974.

173. Meller J, Conde CA, Deppisch LM, et al: Myocardial infarction due to coronary atherosclerosis in three young adults with systemic lupus erythematosus. *Am J Cardiol* 35:309, 1975.

174. Haider YS, Roberts WC: Coronary arterial disease in systemic lupus erythematosus: Quantification of degrees of narrowing in 22 necropsy patients (21 women) aged 16 to 37 years. *Am J Med* 7:775, 1981.

175. Spiera H, Rothenberg RR: Myocardial infarction in four young patients with SLE. *J Rheumatol* 10:464, 1983.

176. Bulkley BH, Roberts WC: The heart in systemic lupus erythematosus and the changes induced in it by corticosteroid therapy. *Am J Med* 58:243, 1975.

177. Hosenpud JD, Montanaro A, Hart MV, et al: Myocardial perfusion abnormalities in asymptomatic patients with systemic lupus erythematosus. *Am J Med* 77:286, 1984.

178. Morguet AJ, Sandrock D, Stille-Siegener M, et al: Indium-111-antimyosin Fab imaging to demonstrate myocardial involvement in systemic lupus erythematosus. *J Nucl Med* 36:1432, 1995.

179. Silverman KJ, Hutchins GM, Bulkley BH: Cardiac sarcoid: A clinicopathologic study of 84 unselected patients with systemic sarcoidosis. *Circulation* 58:1204, 1978.

180. Silztbach LE, James DG, Neville E, et al: Course and prognosis of sarcoidosis around the world. *Am J Med* 57:947, 1974.

181. Ghosh P, Fleming HA, Greshham GA, et al: Myocardial sarcoidosis. *Br Heart J* 34:769, 1972.

182. James TN: Clinicopathologic correlations: De subitaneis mortibus. XXV. Sarcoid heart disease. *Circulation* 56:320, 1977.

183. Swanton RH: Sarcoidosis of the heart. *Eur Heart J* 9(Suppl G):169, 1988.

184. Lull RJ, Dunn BE, Gregoratos G, et al: Ventricular aneurysm due to cardiac sarcoidosis with surgical cure of refractory ventricular tachycardia. *Am J Cardiol* 30:282, 1972.

185. Kinney EL, Jackson GL, Reeves WC, et al: Thallium scan myocardial defects and echocardiographic abnormalities in patients with sarcoidosis without clinical cardiac dysfunction: An analysis of 44 patients. *Am J Med* 68:497, 1980.

186. Bulkley BH, Rouleau JR, Whitaker JQ, et al: The use of thallium 201 for myocardial perfusion imaging in sarcoid heart disease. *Chest* 72:27, 1977.

187. Makler PT, Lavine SJ, Denenberg BS, et al: Redistribution on the thallium scan in myocardial sarcoidosis: Concise communication. *J Nucl Med* 22:428, 1981.

188. Kurata C, Sakath K, Taguchi T, et al: SPECT imaging with Tl-201 and Ga-67 in myocardial sarcoidosis. *Clin Nucl Med* 15:408, 1990.

189. Taki J, Nakajima K, Bunko H, et al: Cardiac sarcoidosis demonstrated by Tl-201 and Ga-67 SPECT imaging. *Clin Nucl Med* 15:636, 1990.

190. Tawarahara K, Kurata C, Okayama K, et al: Thallium-201 and gallium-67 single photon emission computed tomographic imaging in cardiac sarcoidosis. *Am Heart J* 124:1383, 1992.

191. Hirose Y, Ishida Y, Hayashida K, et al: Myocardial involvement in patients with sarcoidosis: An analysis of 75 patients. *Clin Nucl Med* 19:522, 1994.

192. Fink R, Marjot DH, Rosalki SB: Detection of alcoholic cardiomyopathy by serum enzyme and isoenzyme determination. *Ann Clin Biochem* 16;165, 1979.

193. Jacob AJ, McLaren KM, Boon NA: Effects of abstinence on alcoholic heart muscle disease. *Am J Cardiol* 68:805, 1991.

194. Gould L, Zahir M, DeMartino A, et al: Cardiac effects of a cocktail. *JAMA* 218:1799, 1971.

195. Wu CF, Sudhakar M, Ghazanfar J, et al: Preclinical cardiomyopathy in chronic alcoholics: A sex difference. *Am Heart J* 91:281, 1976.

196. Cregler LL, Worner TM, Mark H: Echocardiographic abnormalities in chronic asymptomatic alcoholics. *Clin Cardiol* 12:122, 1989.

197. Zambrano SS, Mazzotta JF, Sherman D, et al: Cardiac dysfunction in unselected chronic alcoholic patients: Noninvasive screening by systolic time intervals. *Am Heart J* 87:318, 1974.

198. Ahmed SS, Howard M, ten Hove M, et al: Cardiac function in alcoholics with cirrhosis: Absence of overt cardiomyopathy—myth or fact? *J Am Coll Cardiol* 3:696, 1984.

199. Mathews EC Jr, Gardin JM, Henry WL, et al: Echocardiographic abnormalities in chronic alcoholics with and without overt congestive heart failure. *Am J Cardiol* 47:570, 1981.

200. Askanas A, Udoshi M, Sadjaki SA: The heart in chronic alcoholism: A noninvasive study. *Am Heart J* 99:9, 1980.

201. Hung J, Harris PJ, Kelly DT, et al: Improvement of left ventricular function in alcoholic cardiomyopathy documented by serial gated cardiac pool scanning. *Aust Nz J Med* 9:420, 1979.

202. Factor SM: Intramyocardial small-vessel disease in chronic alcoholism. *Am Heart J* 92:561, 1976.

203. Regan TJ, Wu CF, Weisse AB, et al: Acute myocardial infarction in toxic cardiomyopathy without coronary obstruction. *Circulation* 51;453, 1975.

204. Morris DC: Cocaine heart disease. *Hosp Pract* 26:83, 1991.

205. Isner JM, Estes NA 3d, Thompson PD, et al: Acute cardiac events temporally related to cocaine abuse. *N Engl J Med* 315:1438, 1986.

206. Mouhaffel AH, Madu EC, Satmary WA, et al: Cardiovascular complications of cocaine. *Chest* 107:1426, 1995.

207. Minor RL Jr, Scott BD, Brown DD, et al: Cocaine-induced myocardial infarction in patients with normal coronary arteries. *Ann Intern Med* 115:797, 1991.

208. Oster ZH, Som P, Wang GJ, et al: Imaging of cocaine-induced global and regional myocardial ischemia. *J Nucl Med* 32:1569, 1991.

209. Yuen-Green MS, Yen CK, Lim AD, et al: Tc-99m sestamibi myocardial imaging at rest for evaluation of cocaine-induced myocardial ischemia and infarction. *Clin Nuc Med* 17:923, 1992.

210. Wiener RS, Lockhart JT, Schwartz RG: Dilated cardiomyopathy and cocaine abuse: Report of two cases. *Am J Med* 81:699, 1986.

211. Duell PB: Chronic cocaine abuse and dilated cardiomyopathy. *Am J Med* 83:601, 1987.

212. Chokshi SK, Moore R, Pandian NG, et al: Reversible cardiomyopathy associated with cocaine intoxication. *Ann Intern Med* 111:1039, 1989.

213. Haberl R, Weber M, Reichenspurner H, et al: Frequency analysis of the surface electrocardiogram for recognition of acute rejection after orthotopic cardiac transplantation in man. *Circulation* 76:101, 1987.

214. Dubroff JM, Clark MB, Wong CYH, et al: Changes in left ventricular mass associated with the onset of acute rejection after cardiac transplantation. *J Heart Transplant* 3:105, 1984.

215. Dawkins KD, Oldershaw PJ, Billingham ME, et al: Changes in diastolic function as a noninvasive marker of cardiac allograft rejection. *J Heart Transplant* 3:286, 1984.

216. Valantine HA, Fowler MB, Hunt SA, et al: Changes in Doppler echocardiographic indexes of left ventricular function as potential markers of acute cardiac rejection. *Circulation* 76(suppl V):V-86, 1987.

217. Derumeaux G, Mouton D, Cochonneau O, et al: Accuracy of doppler tissue imaging to detect cardiac allograft acute rejection. *Circulation* 92(suppl I):I-735, 1995 (abstr).

218. Latre JM, Arizon JM, Jimenez-Heffernan A, et al: Noninvasive radioisotopic diagnosis of acute heart rejection. *J Heart Lung Transplant* 11:453, 1992.

219. Canby RC, Evanochko WT, Barrett LV, et al: Monitoring the bioenergetics of cardiac allograft rejection using in vivo P-31 nuclear magnetic resonance specroscopy. *J Am Coll Cardiol* 9:1067, 1987.

220. Fraser CD Jr, Chacko VP, Jacobus WE, et al: Evidence of 31p nuclear magnetic resonance studies of cardiac allografts that early rejection is characterized by reversible biochemical changes. *Transplantation* 48:1068, 1989.

221. Wisenberg G, Pflugfelder PW, Kostuk WJ, et al: Diagnostic applicability of magnetic resonance imaging in assessing human cardiac allograft rejection. *Am J Cardiol* 60:130, 1987.

222. Smart FW, Young JB, Weilbaecher D, et al: Magnetic resonance imaging for assessment of tissue rejection after heterotopic heart transplantation. *J Heart Lung Transplant* 12:403, 1993.

223. Yamamoto S, Bergsland J, Michalek SM, et al: Uptake of myocardial imaging agents by rejecting and nonrejecting cardiac transplants: A comparative clinical study of thallium 201, technetium 99m, and gallium 67. *J Nucl Med* 30:1464, 1989.

224. Barak JH, LaRaia PJ, Boucher CA, et al: Thallium kinetics in rat cardiac transplant rejection. *Transplantation* 45:687, 1988.

225. Meneguetti JC, Camargo EE, Soares J Jr, et al: Gallium-67 imaging in human heart transplantation: Correlation with endomyocardial biopsy. *J Heart Transplant* 6:171, 1987.

226. Eisen HJ, Rosenbloom M, Laschinger JC, et al: Detection of rejection of canine orthotopic cardiac allografts with indium-111 lymphocytes and gamma scintigraphy. *J Nucl Med* 29:1223, 1988.

227. Eisen HJ, Eisenberg SB, Saffitz JE, et al: Noninvasive detection of rejection of transplanted hearts with indium-111-labeled lymphocytes. *Circulation* 75:868, 1987.

228. Rosenbloom M, Eisen HJ, Laschinger J, et al: Noninvasive assessment of treatment of cardiac allograft rejection with indium-111-labeled lymphocytes. *Transplantation* 46:341, 1988.

229. Rubin PJ, Hartman JJ, Bakke JE, Bergmann SR: Imaging of cardiac transplant rejection with indium-111-labeled lymphocytes. *Circulation* 92(Suppl I):I-577, 1995 (abstr).

230. Thakur MI, McAfee JG: The significance of chromosomal aberrations in indium-111-labeled lymphocytes. *J Nucl Med* 25:922, 1984.

231. Addonizio LJ, Michler RE, Marboe C, et al: Imaging of cardiac allograft rejection in dogs using indium-111 monoclonal antimyosin Fab. *J Am Coll Cardiol* 9:55, 1987.

232. Frist W, Yasuda T, Segall G, et al: Noninvasive detection of human cardiac transplant rejection with indium-111 antimyosin (Fab) imaging. *Circulation* 76(Suppl V):V-81, 1987.

233. Carrio I, Berna L, Ballester M, et al: Indium-111 antimyosin scintigraphy to assess myocardial damage in patients with suspected myocarditis and cardiac rejection. *J Nucl Med* 29:1893, 1988.

234. Khaw B-A, Narula J: Antibody imaging in the evaluation of cardiovascular diseases. *J Nucl Cardiol* 1:457, 1994.

235. Ballester M, Obrador D, Carrio I, et al: Early postoperative reduction of monoclonal antimyosin antibody uptake is associated with absent rejection-related complications after heart transplantation. *Circulation* 85:61, 1992.

236. Ballester M, Obrador D, Carrio I, et al: Indium-111-monoclonal antimyosin antibody studies after the first year of heart transplantation: Identification of risk groups for developing rejection during long-term follow-up and clinical implications. *Circulation* 82:2100, 1990.

237. Billingham ME: Cardiac transplant atherosclerosis. *Transplantation Proc* 19(Suppl 5):19, 1987.

238. Gao S-Z, Alderman EL, Schroeder JS, et al: Accelerated coronary vascular disease in the heart transplant patient: Coronary arteriographic findings. *J Am Coll Cardiol* 12:334, 1988.

239. Stark RP, McGinn AL, Wilson RF: Chest pain in cardiac-transplant recipients: Evidence of sensory reinnervation after cardiac transplantation. *N Eng J Med* 324:1791, 1991.

240. O'Neill BJ, Pflugfelder PW, Singh NR, et al: Frequency of angiographic detection and quantitative assessment of

coronary arterial disease one and three years after cardiac transplantation. *Am J Cardiol* 63:1221, 1989.

241. Russell ME, Fujita M, Masek MA, et al: Cardiac graft vascular disease, nonselective involvement of large and small vessels. *Transplantation* 56:762, 1993.

242. Uretsky BF, Kormos RL, Zerbe TR, et al: Cardiac events after heart transplantation: Incidence and predictive value of coronary arteriography. *J Heart Lung Transplant* 11:S45, 1992.

243. St Goar FG, Pinto FJ, Alderman EL, et al: Intracoronary ultrasound in cardiac transplant recipients: In vivo evidence of "angiographically silent" intimal thickening. *Circulation* 85:979, 1992.

244. Ventura HO, White CJ, Jain SP, et al: Assessment of intracoronary morphology in cardiac transplant recipients by angioscopy and intravascular ultrasound. *Am J Cardiol* 72:805, 1993.

245. Heroux AL, Silverman P, Costanzo MR, et al: Intracoronary ultrasound assessment of morphological and functional abnormalities associated with cardiac allograft vasculopathy. *Circulation* 89:272, 1994.

246. Caracciolo EA, Wolford TL, Underwood RD, et al: Influence of intimal thickening on coronary blood flow responses in orthotopic heart transplant recipients: A combined intravascular Doppler and ultrasound imaging study. *Circulation* 92(Suppl II):II-182, 1995.

247. Tuzcu EM, Hobbs RE, Rincon G, et al: Occult and frequent transmission of atherosclerotic coronary disease with cardiac transplantation: Insights from intravascular ultrasound. *Circulation* 91:1706, 1995.

248. Clausell N, Butany J, Molossi S, et al: Abnormalities in intramyocardial arteries detected in cardiac transplant biopsy specimens and lack of correlation with abnormal intracoronary ultrasound or endothelial dysfunction in large epicardial coronary arteries. *J Am Coll Cardiol* 26:110, 1995.

249. Rickenbacher PR, Pinto FJ, Chenzbraun A, et al: Incidence and severity of transplant coronary artery disease early and up to 15 years after transplantation as detected by intravascular ultrasound. *J Am Coll Cardiol* 25:171, 1995.

250. Rickenbacher PR, Pinto FJ, Lewis NP, et al: Prognostic importance of intimal thickness as measured by intracoronary ultrasound after cardiac transplantation. *Circulation* 92:3445, 1995.

251. Jamieson SW: Investigation of heart transplant coronary atherosclerosis. *Circulation* 85:1211, 1992.

252. Derumeaux G, Redonnet M, Mouton-Schleifer D, et al: Dobutamine stress echocardiography in orthotopic heart transplant recipients. *J Am Coll Cardiol* 25:1665, 1995.

253. McKillop JH, Goris ML: Thallium-201 myocardial imaging in patients with previous cardiac transplantation. *Clin Radiol* 32:447, 1981.

254. Smart FW, Ballantyne CM, Cocanougher B, et al: Insensitivity of noninvasive tests to detect coronary artery vasculopathy after heart transplant. *Am J Cardiol* 67:243, 1991.

255. Ciliberto GR, Mangiavacchi M, Banfi F, et al: Coronary artery disease after heart transplantation: Non-invasive evaluation with exercise thallium scintigraphy. *Eur Heart J* 14:226, 1993.

256. Rodney RA, Johnson LL, Blood DK, Barr ML: Myocardial perfusion scintigraphy in heart transplant recipients with and without allograft atherosclerosis: A comparison of thallium 201 and technetium 99m sestamibi. *J Heart Lung Transplant* 13:173, 1994.

257. Verhoeven PPAM, Lee FA, Ramahi TM, Wackers FJTh: Prognostic value of normal thallium-201 stress myocardial perfusion imaging at one year after heart transplantation. *Circulation* 92(Suppl I):I-578, 1995 (abstr).

258. Zhao X-M, Delbeke D, Sandler MP, et al: Nitrogen-13-ammonia and PET to detect allograft coronary artery disease after heart transplantation. Comparison with coronary angiography. *J Nucl Med* 36:982, 1995.

Cardiac Trauma

James M. Hurst
Jay A. Johannigman

NONPENETRATING CHEST TRAUMA

One is accustomed to look upon the heart as an organ which almost always escapes any of the ordinary injuries to which the rest of the body is subjected. The thoracic cage affords what is usually considered to be practically a perfect protection to the heart. No such immunity to injury from contusive or compressive forces is extended to the liver, spleen, kidneys, brain or other organs of the body. It is remarkable that this belief developed, because the heart, lying against the sternum, is vulnerable to any such impact over the sternum and, buttressed against the bodies of the thoracic vertebrae posteriorly, is vulnerable to compressive forces applied to the chest. There can be little doubt that the heart is the recipient of many injuries. Most of those probably produce no functional disturbances and are not recognized. Some of them *do* produce functional disturbances and usually these are not recognized.[1]

The capricious nature of these injuries was documented by Bright and Beck in 1935 as they reported 23 patients evaluated for blunt cardiac injury without cardiac rupture.[1] On the basis of their analysis, they outlined five various ways in which nonpenetrating wounds of the heart were produced:

1. Direct blow to the precordium, producing fracture of the sternum or ribs and broken ends that were driven into the heart.

2. Contusion or compression of the heart between the sternum anteriorly and the vertebrae posteriorly.
3. The application of indirect forces such as sudden compression of the legs or abdomen.
4. Laceration of the thoracic viscera, as in a fall sustained from a height.
5. Concussion of the heart.

Other than clinical evaluation, electrocardiography provided the only indirect means for the evaluation of cardiac function in those years. The authors noted the limited usefulness in obtaining radiographic examinations for cardiac contusion. Although the severity of these injuries was noted and discussed, the authors indicated that "it is unlikely that death always follows a nonpenetrating wound." They concluded that the vast majority of nonpenetrating wounds of the heart were not clinically recognizable.

Bright and Beck noted that patients with cardiac contusion followed one of the following clinical courses:

1. The symptoms disappear hours or days after the accident and the patient remains clinically well.
2. The symptoms persist for years and are accentuated by exercise.
3. The heart fails hours to days after the accident.
4. Contusion softens and rupture ensues.

Pathologic Findings

An elegant pathologic study of cardiac contusion was provided in 1938 by Moritz and Atkins, who employed a canine model and induced cardiac trauma by the external application of force.[2] When dogs succumbed to electrical conduction abnormalities, ventricular fibrillation was evident more consistently in those with the most severe cardiac damage. Immediate asystole following contusion was noted in several of the dogs exhibiting complete laceration of the right ventricle. From a pathologic standpoint, the most outstanding macroscopic characteristic of the myocardial lesions within 24 h of injury was hemorrhage with or without identifiable laceration. Both large and small lacerations were obvious but, at times, massive interstitial hemorrhage seemed to mask many smaller lesions. Within 24 h of the production of the lesion, the contused segment became infiltrated with polymorphonuclear leukocytes and, at the end of 3 days, the leukocytic infiltration became dense and diffuse. There was marked interstitial edema in addition to the hemorrhage and leukocytes. The infiltrate progressed over a number of days to a predominantly lymphocytic infiltration. Hearts examined 30 to 60 days after contusion revealed advanced organization and lesions with scar formations that were microscopically indistinguishable from those due to myocardial infarction. Pericardial adhesions were not a prominent finding of early investigations unless the pericardium had been lacerated by the application of external force.

Experimental Studies

Early experiments by Bright and Beck employed a canine model of cardiac contusion. Direct myocardial impact was performed by striking the myocardium with a metal dilator weighing 40 g. Their observations documented the most immediate response to cardiac injury to be tachycardia, often to rates of 160 to 180 beats/min, followed by wide fluctuations of arterial pressure. Early measurements of venous pressure in the laboratory documented immediate rises in central venous pressure to 10 to 15 cmH$_2$O, but with rapid return to normal. Various electrocardiogram (ECG) abnormalities were noted in the animal model. They ranged from clinically insignificant ST-segment elevation to alterations in Q-wave morphology and lethal arrhythmias including ventricular fibrillation and asystole.[2,3] It was noted that blood injected into the interventricular septum produced similar findings on the ECG.

Leidtke et al used radioactive microspheres in a swine model to assess the effects of blunt injury on coronary vasomotion and global myocardial performance.[4] In the absence of large-vessel spasm following impact, they reported a transmural redistribution of small-vessel perfusion. This was observed with a concomitant decrease in coronary vascular resistance in tissue perfused by the experimentally injured vessels. This is a condition similar to the change in the epicardial-to-endocardial blood-flow ratio important in myocardial ischemia. These studies essentially eliminated the school of thought that held a major etiology of myocardial contusion to be large-vessel coronary artery spasm and/or thrombosis.

Subsequent studies focused on the biomechanical response of the heart and great vessels to blunt chest trauma in order to explain the constellation of injuries often remote from the impact site.[5,6] Stein et al employed a canine model to evaluate responses to impact velocities corresponding to automobile injuries at 27 mph (12 m/s) and 40 mph (18 m/s). Intracavitary and aortic pressures rose rapidly to levels many times greater than those in control animals following blunt chest injury. Aortic pressure reached 450 mmHg (following impact delivered at 12 m/s) to 710 mmHg (at 18 m/s). Left ventricular pressure reached 1030 ± 200 mmHg with impact delivered at 18 m/s. Right ventricular pressure reached 550 mmHg at 18 m/s. While this is much lower than the corresponding left ventricular pressure, the thin-walled right ventricle is less well equipped to deal with pressures of this magnitude. Transient "overpressure" situations probably explain areas of hemorrhage or valvular damage at sites remote from the impact.

Global disruption of myocardial performance was readily observed. Myocardial contractility (dp/dt) decreased by as much as 35 percent after an impact at 18 m/s. Interstitial hemorrhage, the most common pathologic lesion in myocardial contusion, produced decreased ventricular compliance which at times was dramatic. This is readily appreciated by the abnormal pressure–volume relationships that exist after myocardial contusion.[7]

Cooper et al studied biomechanical stress to the anterior chest and the specific cardiac lesions that resulted.[6] This experimental design employed a porcine model subjected to impact with a cylinder moving at 12 m/s. This closely resembles the characteristics of an automobile steering-column impact. Thirteen radiopaque markers were attached to the left ventricular epicardium and the adventitia of the aorta. High-speed cineradiography was taken during impact. Injury severity was positively correlated with the maximal chest wall displacement (P_{max}) versus anteroposterior chest diameter (AP). Myocardial contusion was evident at postmortem examination if the P_{max}/AP reached 0.2. Cardiac rupture occurred if P_{max}/AP reached 0.27. Maximum ventricular compression occurred 5 ms after impact. During impact, there was substantial displacement of the heart not only toward the vertebral bodies but also significantly into the right chest. Marked elongation of great vessels occurred as a result of this displacement. Undoubtedly this distortion of vascular structures combined with sudden marked elevation in intravascular pressures leads to severe injuries observed at points removed from the impact.

Diagnosis

Many types of cardiac injury may result from blunt chest trauma[8] (see Table 26-1). Prior to the availability of creatine kinase isoenzymes, the diagnosis of nonpenetrating cardiac trauma was based almost entirely on (1) the clinical history, (2) physical examination, and (3) ECG. In the recent past, the techniques of cardiac isoenzyme assay and radionuclide-imaging studies have been added to the clinicians armamentarium. The most common symptom of cardiac contusion is chest pain, but this symptom is difficult to interpret in the presence of pain related to chest wall trauma. A new murmur or rub or evidence of pericardial tamponade may suggest cardiac injury but is usually absent in cardiac contusion. Severe cardiac injury may occur in the absence of external evidence of thoracic injury or may be overshadowed by other more visible injuries. In some cases, cardiac damage may result from injuries in which the abdomen or lower extremities are compressed, producing a *hydraulic ram effect* in the absence of direct thoracic trauma.

The ECG may be very helpful if changes diagnostic of myocardial necrosis appear. The appearance of new pathologic Q waves in cardiac contusion, however, seems to be uncommon.[9–11] Sutherland et al[10] noted new pathologic Q waves in two of 42 patients with radionuclide angiographic evidence of myocardial contusion. Potkin et al[9] observed intraventricular conduction abnormalities, mostly right bundle branch block, in 18 of 100 patients with severe chest wall injury. This included one of five patients with autopsy confirmation of myo-

Table 26-1 Types of Cardiac Injury from Blunt Trauma

I. Myocardium
  A. Contusion
  B. Laceration
  C. Rupture
  D. Septal perforation
  E. Aneurysm, pseudoaneurysm
  F. Thrombosis, systemic embolism

II. Pericardium
  A. Pericarditis
  B. Postpericardiotomy syndrome
  C. Constrictive pericarditis
  D. Pericardial laceration
  E. Hemorrhage
  F. Cardiac herniation

III. Endocardial structures
  A. Rupture of papillary muscle
  B. Rupture of chordae tendineae
  C. Rupture of atrioventricular and semilunar valves

IV. Coronary artery
  A. Thrombosis
  B. Laceration
  C. Fistula

From Jackson and Murphy,[8] reproduced by permission of the American Heart Association, Inc.

cardial contusion. Most often, the ECG findings in cardiac contusion consist of nonspecific ST-segment and T-wave abnormalities. Similar nonspecific ECG findings were prevalent in patients with chest injury but no autopsy evidence of myocardial contusion.[9] A totally normal ECG may provide useful evidence that cardiac contusion is either absent or, if present, poses only a minimal risk to the patient. Only three of 41 patients with documented cardiac contusion had a normal admission ECG in the study by Snow et al.[12] Similarly, in the series of Sutherland et al,[10] few patients with radionuclide evidence of cardiac contusion had a normal ECG. Four of five patients with autopsy evidence of cardiac contusion had an abnormal ECG during the hospital course in the study by Potkin et al.[9] Importantly, three patients who died from sudden cardiac death in the study by Sutherland et al[10] had an abnormal ECG during the hospital course. Blair described three patients who had autopsy-proven myocardial contusion with a normal admission ECG.[11] However, ECG abnormalities developed within 24 to 36 h following admission. In a recent series by Biffl et al, the majority of ECG abnormalities (14 of 17) were present at the time of admission and all rhythm disturbances were manifested within 24 h. The majority of authors currently advocate telemetry monitoring for a 24-h period for those patients whose sole presentation criteria is an abnormal ECG.[13]

Serum enzyme levels are often elevated in trauma victims in the absence of cardiac damage. The availability of creatine kinase muscle–brain (MB) fraction measurement provides a tool that is more specific for cardiac necrosis but may still have limited specificity in trauma patients for myocardial contusion.[14] Of 15 patients studied by Potkin et al[8] following chest trauma, only one of five patients with pathologic evidence of myocardial contusion had a creatine kinase MB fraction greater than or equal to 2 percent of the total serum creatine kinase. Six of the remaining 10 patients with no pathologic evidence of cardiac contusion did have a 2 percent or greater level of creatine kinase MB fraction. The Denver General Trauma Group has adopted a more aggressive interpretation of the utility of cardiac enzymes based on a 4-year review of their experience.[13] In this series of 359 patients at risk for myocardial contusion, 107 were felt to meet diagnostic criteria. The addition of cardiac enzyme analysis failed to identify independently any patient at risk for development of cardiac complications. Based on this experience, the Denver Group advocates the elimination of cardiac enzymes from the practice guidelines for the management of the patient with suspected myocardial contusion.

Soliman and Waxman[15] reviewed 104 consecutive patients admitted for blunt chest trauma. Substantial chest injury was the sole admission criterion. An overwhelming number of these patients' injuries were the result of motor vehicle accidents with speeds exceeding

35 mph. The purpose of this study was to evaluate a conventional approach for the diagnosis of myocardial contusion after blunt chest injury. Although many patients had significant clinical findings, no single clinical finding (cardiac enzyme level, chest x-ray, or ECG) by multivariate analysis correctly predicted the high-risk group of patients who would subsequently develop complications related to myocardial contusion. Of the 104, 24 (23 percent) developed what the authors described as serious complications (none described as fatal). The investigators' conclusion was that a conventional diagnostic approach failed to identify patients who were likely to develop complications as a result of myocardial contusion. Therefore they suggested a more sophisticated approach, including two-dimensional echocardiography or radionuclide imaging for more precise definition of these lesions.

Radionuclide imaging with the infarct-avid tracer ^{99m}Tc pyrophosphate has been proposed for detection of myocardial contusion.[16-18] Brantigan et al[19] studied 29 patients with chest injury and ECG changes suggestive of myocardial contusion and found a positive pyrophosphate scan in only two patients. In each of five patients with autopsy documentation of cardiac contusion, Potkin et al[9] found a normal ^{99m}Tc-pyrophosphate scan. It has been suggested that ECG gating or tomographic approaches to ^{99m}Tc-pyrophosphate imaging may improve the utility of this procedure in cardiac contusion. This hypothesis remains unproven. Certainly, many patients who require diagnosis of cardiac contusion cannot easily be moved to a tomographic imaging facility at the time when a correct diagnosis is needed most. Currently, the role of ^{99m}Tc-pyrophosphate imaging in myocardial contusion remains to be established.

A potentially important role of radionuclide ventriculography in the detection of cardiac contusion (Fig. 26-1) is suggested by several studies.[10,11,16-24] Sutherland and associates[10] studied 77 patients with multisystem trauma, including severe blunt chest injury. The severity of injury was underlined by a requirement for mechanical ventilation in 70 of the 77 patients in order to maintain the arterial oxygen tension greater than 70 mmHg and the arterial carbon dioxide tension at 37 to 42 mmHg. The low mean age of 31 years suggests that preexisting heart disease prior to trauma was uncommon or absent. Of these patients, 42 (55 percent) had one or more focal abnormalities of right or left ventricular wall motion. This included involvement of the right ventricle only in 27 patients, left ventricle only in seven patients, biventricular involvement in seven patients, and septal involvement only in one patient. Right and left ventricular ejection fractions were significantly ($p < 0.01$) lower (31 ± 11 percent and 47 ± 14 percent, respectively) compared with the 35 chest trauma patients with no scintigraphic wall-motion abnormality. Among 42 patients with scintigraphic wall-motion abnormalities, only 11 (26 per-

cent) had ECG findings described as typical for acute myocardial injury (consisting of "a combination of sinus tachycardia, right bundle branch block, ST-segment elevation, and peaked T waves"). Only six of these patients had evidence of right bundle branch block and none had new infarction Q waves. The mean serum creatine kinase levels were not different in patients with, compared to patients without, scintigraphic regional wall-motion abnormality. Three of the 77 patients studied experienced sudden cardiac death. Each patient had ECG changes described as typical for myocardial contusion as well as scintigraphic regional wall-motion abnormality and pathologic evidence of myocardial contusion.

Similar findings have been reported by Harley and associates[20] using first-pass radionuclide angiography. In 74 consecutive patients with blunt chest trauma, biventricular radionuclide angiography was performed 24 to 48 h following admission to the hospital. Chest pain of musculoskeletal origin was the most common symptom, whereas no patient had pain suggestive of angina pectoris. ECG abnormalities were present at the time of admission in 21 (28 percent) of 74 patients, including right bundle branch block in three patients and infarction Q waves in four patients. The creatine kinase MB isoenzyme level was elevated in just six of 74 patients and was accompanied by ECG changes in only two patients. Radionuclide angiography demonstrated an abnormal right ventricular ejection fraction (defined in this study as <40 percent) in 36 patients, an abnormal left ventricular ejection fraction (<50 percent) in 32 patients, and abnormal left ventricular regional wall motion in 42 patients. Only 19 of 74 patients had a normal radionuclide study.

Most recently, Hendel's group[25] has reported on the use of ^{111}In-labeled antimyosin scanning as a sensitive means of diagnosing cardiac injury. This group studied 17 patients with severe multisystem trauma and thoracic injury. Blinded interpretation of the antimyosin scans revealed only one scan with positive focal myocardial uptake; this same patient had the only discrete wall-motion abnormality on the echocardiogram. This same patient had ST depression and ectopy by ECG but normal creatine kinase MB. This technique may offer promise since it identifies the subset of patients with discrete myocardial damage who are at greatest risk for development of complications. In the study by Hendel and associates, ^{111}In-labeled antimyosin was injected 65 ± 21 h following chest injury. It is not currently known whether antimyosin injection and imaging can be performed successfully earlier following blunt chest trauma, at a time when the imaging results are more likely to aid in patient management.

Thallium-201 myocardial scintigraphy has also been evaluated for use in establishing the diagnosis of myocardial contusion. Preliminary evidence by Waxman et al[26] suggested that ^{201}Tl scanning may successfully detect patients who are at high risk for developing dysrhythmias

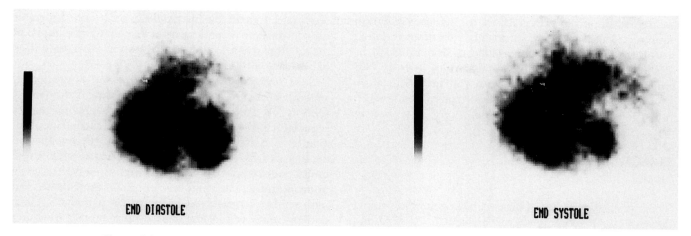

Figure 26-1 Rest radionuclide ventriculogram in the left anterior oblique projection from a 25-year-old woman with chest trauma and electrocardiographic evidence of myocardial contusion. The right ventricle is dilated with right ventricular ejection fraction of 31 percent. Left ventricular global and regional function is normal.

as a result of blunt chest trauma. Bodin et al[27] performed planar ^{201}Tl scans in 55 critically ill patients a mean of 8 days after blunt chest trauma. A resting thallium perfusion defect was detected in 38 of the 55 patients and a corresponding two-dimensional echocardiographic finding of segmental hypokinesis or pericardial effusion was present in 17 of these patients. No patient with a normal thallium scan had an echocardiographic abnormality. An abnormal ECG was described in 51 of 55 study patients but consisted of ST-T-wave changes in the vast majority of cases. Further confirmation of the diagnostic and prognostic utility of ^{201}Tl imaging in myocardial contusion is needed.

Echocardiography

In seven patients with chest trauma, Miller and associates[28] showed that transthoracic two-dimensional echocardiography can demonstrate right ventricular dilatation, right ventricular wall-motion abnormality, right ventricular wall thinning, and right ventricular mural thrombi. Hiatt and associates[29] found two-dimensional echocardiography helpful to triage patients with blunt chest trauma, but they emphasized the importance of clinical and ECG correlation to separate acute from chronic cardiac disease. Several examples of traumatic tricuspid regurgitation have been demonstrated by two-dimensional echocardiography.[28–31] The echocardiogram is a highly effective tool for demonstrating pericardial effusion.[32–34] Transthoracic two-dimensional echocardiography may be technically unsatisfactory in 10 to 20 percent of chest trauma patients.[32]

With the recent introduction of transesophageal echocardiography (TEE), yet another tool has been added to the clinician's potential armamentarium for evaluating the presence of myocardial contusion. The TEE probe consists of a 3- or 5-MHz transducer mounted at the tip of a standard adult gastroscope and interfaced with a standard ultrasonograph. In the conscious patient, the instrument is introduced under topical anesthesia in a fashion similar to endoscopy. In the operating room, the probe is introduced manually and advanced under ultrasound guidance. Much of the expertise with this technique has been generated from the operative setting, where the probe is placed and subsequently left in position for continuous dynamic monitoring of ventricular performance and cardiac output during cardiac surgery.

The value of traditional transthoracic echocardiography in the evaluation of myocardial contusion is often limited by interposed fat, air, subcutaneous emphysema, edema, or thoracic/sternal fractures. TEE largely eliminates these problems and provides an image of enhanced clarity due to the direct anatomical proximity of the esophagus to the heart.[35] A significant additional advantage of TEE is its ability to detect thoracic aortic trauma. Patients at risk for myocardial contusion also are at risk for thoracic aortic transection. Prompt recognition and intervention for aortic transection is of paramount importance since mortality may be as high as 50 percent per day with this lesion. In some centers with extensive experience with TEE, this procedure has replaced computed-tomographic scanning and aortography in diagnosing aortic dissection.[36] Taams et al evaluated TEE for accuracy in diagnosing aortic transection and found that TEE yielded a correct diagnosis in all 15 patients and was in fact more accurate than angiography.[37] In the setting of thoracic trauma, it is important to establish the presence of myocardial contusion because of the implications of altered cardiac performance.[38] In the acutely traumatized patient at risk for myocardial contusion, emergent operative intervention is often required before the presence of myocardial dysfunction can be documented adequately. Intraoperative or bedside TEE appears to provide a reliable route for the visualization of cardiac function in this subset of trauma patients.

CLINICAL APPLICATIONS

The reported incidence of blunt cardiac injury in trauma patients is approximately 6 to 7 percent.[18,39–41] Although this may represent the most common unsuspected visceral injury resulting in fatality,[42] the true incidence has remained largely unknown. As has been discussed, this is primarily because it is not possible to make an accurate diagnosis with the currently available diagnostic methods. Several important questions have been raised.

What is the best way to screen for myocardial contusion? Historical aspects of the accident, as listed here, are important in determining the need for initial screening:

1. History compatible with injury that may result in myocardial contusion
   a. High-speed/head-on collision
   b. Significant deformity of steering column
2. Multiple rib fractures
3. Spinal fracture
4. Pulmonary contusion
5. Flail chest
6. Significant precordial contusion

Should any of these conditions be met, the following methods for evaluation are available: (1) ECG, (2) chest x-ray, (3) creatine kinase isoenzymes, (4) ^{99m}Tc-pyrophosphate myocardial scintigraphy, (5) TEE or transthoracic two-dimensional echocardiography, and (6) radionuclide ventriculography. Although the ECG may be nonspecific for the diagnosis of cardiac contusion in many cases, the presence of new infarction Q waves, right bundle branch block, or an injury pattern is diagnostically helpful and may have important prognostic implications. The presence of substantial creatine kinase MB fraction (e.g., ≥5 percent of total creatine kinase) can also identify a patient at risk for cardiac complications.[12] The clinical usefulness of ^{99m}Tc-pyrophosphate scintigraphy is doubtful. Two-dimensional echocardiography is a valuable noninvasive tool for the investigation of cardiac contusion, in part because of the potential for examination at the bedside. However, the sensitivity and specificity of echocardiography for detection of myocardial contusion are not clearly established.[28,29,32–34,43] At present, radionuclide ventriculography appears to be a sensitive noninvasive tool for the detection of myocardial

contusion. In many hospitals, the availability of portable echocardiographic and radionuclide-imaging equipment may dictate test selection for the noninvasive evaluation of patients with chest trauma.

Are the complications of myocardial contusion of significant severity to warrant widespread screening? Only a few studies contain an in-depth review of the sequelae of well-documented myocardial contusion.[10,12,29] Sutherland et al reported three unexpected cardiac deaths in a series of 77 patients with severe multisystem trauma.[10] Snow et al reported 300 cases of nonpenetrating chest injuries with only three deaths but with serious cardiac morbidity in 28 patients.[12] Three patients required placement of a transvenous pacemaker while three others required intraaortic balloon counterpulsation for the treatment of cardiogenic shock. The low incidence of cardiac death in these and other series[44] suggests that routine screening of all chest trauma patients with costly tests such as radionuclide ventriculography or two-dimensional echocardiography will be an inefficient and expensive approach to the reduction of mortality from cardiac contusion.[45] Patients with an abnormal ECG on hospital admission are those most likely to benefit from further screening for cardiac contusion. At this time, radionuclide ventriculography and TEE are the noninvasive tests most likely to provide clinically useful data on further testing (Fig. 26-2).

A recent editorial addressed the management of patients with significant thoracic trauma who are at risk for myocardial injury. In this editorial, Mattox and associates called for a reevaluation of the diagnostic criteria of "myocardial contusion." These authors cited the disparate diagnostic approach to the clinical entity of myocardial contusion and made the following conclusions:

1. Asymptomatic patients with anterior chest wall concussion should not be housed in an intensive care unit for continuous ECG monitoring, serial determination of creatine kinase-MB enzyme levels or cardiac imaging unless less intensive facilities are not available. Asymptomatic patients should be admitted to an intermediate care unit or a general ward nursing unit for telemetered monitoring or ECG monitoring.
2. When traumatic cardiac diagnoses are used for admission, injury severity scoring, discharge summary, billing, or reimbursement purposes, specific descriptions should be used such as:
   a. Blunt cardiac injury with septal rupture
   b. Blunt cardiac injury with free wall rupture
   c. Blunt cardiac injury with coronary artery thrombosis
   d. Blunt cardiac injury with cardiac failure
   e. Blunt cardiac injury with minor ECG or enzyme abnormality
   f. Blunt cardiac injury with complex arrhythmia.[46]

Algorithm for Evaluation of Patients with Myocardial Contusion

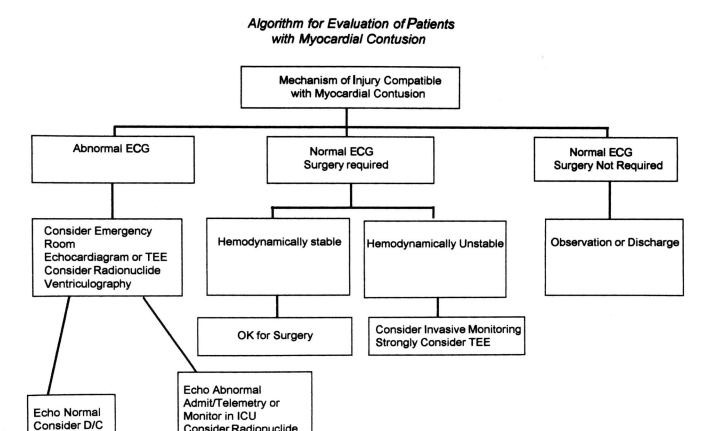

Figure 26-2 Possible algorithm for evaluation of patients with myocardial contusion. TEE, transesophageal echocardiography; D/C, discharge; ICU, intensive care unit.

What is the management plan for patients with myocardial contusions who require emergency surgery? In only one series has this topic been discussed in detail. Snow et al reported that 27 of their 300 patients with nonpenetrating chest injuries required emergency thoracic and/or abdominal surgery.[12] There was "little morbidity" and there were no deaths. In seven patients studied by Harley et al,[20] the timing of surgical intervention was influenced by normal or abnormal radionuclide angiographic studies. Based on abnormal findings from radionuclide angiography, three patients with potentially operable injuries were treated conservatively. This included a patient with a documented splenic rupture, a patient with a hip fracture, and a patient with a fractured femoral shaft. There were no untoward effects resulting from this approach. Conversely, three patients with ECG abnormalities but a normal radionuclide angiogram were sent to surgery, and no cardiac complications were reported. Patients in whom myocardial contusion is suspected prior to emergency surgery are often not candidates for the delay necessary to obtain radionuclide angiography. Appropriate invasive hemodynamic monitoring and pharmacologic support may be necessary in patients exhibiting one or more of the following: (1) unexplained hypotension after correction of volume deficit, (2) unexplained hypoxia, (3) significant dysrhythmia, or (4) inappropriate response to volume challenge. TEE provides a particularly effective means of evaluating the patient with significant thoracic trauma who must undergo emergency surgery. The technique of TEE enables dynamic cardiac imaging that provides information regarding cardiac performance. Equally valuable in this group of patients with thoracic injuries is the ability of TEE to survey for other significant thoracic injuries. Patients who are at risk for blunt cardiac injury have usually experienced a significant deceleration force. These patients are therefore also at risk for thoracic aortic transection. Review work by Kearney et al[47] and Shapiro et al[48] has demonstrated that TEE may be equivalent, or even superior to, aortography in the detection of thoracic aorta transection. Thus, TEE allows the patient with thoracic trauma to have a thorough and dynamic evaluation of cardiac performance and aortic anatomy without delaying emergency surgery.

What is the usual course of myocardial contusion? Sutherland et al reported improvement or resolution of radionuclide abnormalities in 84 percent of patients at 8 to 16 days.[10] In his own series of patients, the author has seen only two abnormal repeat radionuclide studies 72 h after the initial screen. Regardless of the study interval, patients in whom rescanning reveals normal ventricular function may be assumed to have clinically important resolution of their cardiac injury.

Is radionuclide screening cost-effective? No study has formally addressed the question of the cost effectiveness of the radionuclide ventriculogram in the patient with chest trauma. If the test is to be cost-effective, patients must be appropriately selected and the test results must contribute to patient care by improving the clinical outcome and/or reducing costs. It has been suggested that patients with nonpenetrating chest trauma require monitoring in an intensive care setting for 72 h with serial ECG and cardiac enzyme studies. Considering the low mortality associated with cardiac contusion, this is a very costly approach. In some[12] but not all[11] series, chest trauma patients with a completely normal admission ECG were found to have a very low likelihood of cardiac contusion and were unlikely to develop cardiac complications. If the ECG remains normal for 24 to 36 h following admission, cardiac contusion is unlikely to be present.[11] Such patients may not require observation beyond 36 h in a monitored environment. In patients with an ECG abnormality, a normal radionuclide ventriculogram may permit early transfer from the monitored unit, resulting in elimination of costly intensive care (Fig. 26-2).

PENETRATING WOUNDS

Immediate Diagnosis and Management

Penetrating cardiac wounds are among the most urgent challenges facing the trauma surgeon. The patient with wounds between lines drawn vertically through the nipples, from the epigastrium to the clavicles, anteriorly and posteriorly, should be evaluated promptly for the possibility of cardiac tamponade. Immediate operation is usually required in hemodynamically unstable patients and in stable patients with evidence of pericardial tamponade following penetrating cardiac injury.[49,50] Initially, noninvasive evaluation is usually limited to stable patients without urgent signs of tamponade. M-mode and two-dimensional echocardiography are logically employed in this setting to exclude the presence of hemopericardium.

Sequelae

Unless a lesion that may preclude survival is found, repair of intracardiac lesions is best deferred until a later date. A variety of intracardiac lesions are possible after penetrating trauma, including septal defects, valvular lesions, damage to conduction bundles, coronary arteriovenous fistulas, ventricular aneurysms, aortopulmonary fistulas, aorto–right ventricular fistulas, and hemopericardium.[51-58] An extensive review of penetrating cardiac wounds reveals that the right and left ventricules are, respectively, involved approximately 43 percent and 33 percent of the time.[59]

In addition to electrocardiography, two-dimensional echocardiography,[57] Doppler echocardiography, and radionuclide angiography are currently available diagnostic techniques for characterizing sequelae of penetrating chest wounds. Radionuclide ventriculography may potentially contribute in a number of ways:

1. Detection of abnormal bleeding in the pericardial space.
2. Detection of shunts by first-pass radionuclide angiography.
3. Detection of thrombus within the cardiac chambers.
4. Quantitation of the volume of the cardiac chambers.
5. Accurate reproducible measurement of right and left ventricular ejection fractions.

Segmental wall-motion abnormalities may suggest the possibility of ischemic or direct myocardial injury.[22,23] The presence of left ventricular pseudoaneurysm may be suggested by echocardiography or radionuclide ventriculography. Cardiac catheterization remains the "gold standard" for the definition of intracardiac lesions and the quantitation of shunts prior to definitive surgical correction.

REFERENCES

1. Bright EF, Beck CS: Non-penetrating wounds of the heart: An experimental and clinical study. *Am Heart J* 10:293, 1935.
2. Moritz AR, Atkins JP: Cardiac contusion: An experimental and pathologic study. *Arch Pathol* 25:445, 1938.
3. Doty DB, Anderson AE, Rose EF, et al: Cardiac trauma: Clinical and experimental correlations of myocardial contusion. *Ann Surg* 180:452, 1974.
4. Liedtke AJ, Allen RP, Nellis SH: Effects of blunt cardiac trauma on coronary vasomotion, perfusion, myocardial mechanics, and metabolism. *J Trauma* 20:777, 1980.
5. Stein PD, Sabbah HN, Viano DC, et al: Response of the heart to non-penetrating cardiac trauma. *J Trauma* 22:364, 1982.

6. Cooper GJ, Maynard RL, Pearce BP, et al: Cardiovascular distortion in experimental non-penetrating chest impact. *J Trauma* 24:188, 1984.

7. Sabbah HN, Stein PD, Hawkins ET, et al: Right ventricular outflow obstruction secondary to non-penetrating blunt trauma to the canine myocardium. *J Trauma* 22:1009, 1982.

8. Jackson DH, Murphy GW: Nonpenetrating cardiac trauma. *Mod Concepts Cardiovasc Dis* 45:123, 1976.

9. Potkin RT, Werner JA, Trobaugh GB, et al: Evaluation of non-invasive tests of cardiac damage in suspected cardiac contusion. *Circulation* 66:627, 1982.

10. Sutherland GR, Driedger AA, Holliday RL, et al: Frequency of myocardial injury after blunt chest trauma as evaluated by radionuclide angiography. *Am J Cardiol* 52:1099, 1983.

11. Blair E, Topuzlu C, Davis JH: Delayed or missed diagnosis in blunt chest trauma. *J Trauma* 11:129, 1971.

12. Snow N, Richardson JD, Flint LM: Myocardial contusion: Implications for patient with multiple traumatic injuries. *Surgery* 92:744, 1982.

13. Biffl WL, Moore FA, Moore EE, et al: Cardiac enzymes are irrelevant in the patient with suspected myocardial contusion. *Am J Surg* 169:523, 1994.

14. Keller KD, Shatney CH: Creatine phosphokinase-MB assays in patients with suspected myocardial contusion: Diagnostic test or test of diagnosis? *J Trauma* 28:58, 1988.

15. Soliman MH, Waxman K: Value of a conventional approach to the diagnosis of traumatic cardiac contusion after chest injury. *Crit Care Med* 15:218, 1987.

16. Go RT, Doty DB, Chiu CL, et al: A new method of diagnosing myocardial contusion in man by radionuclide imaging. *Radiology* 116:107, 1975.

17. Coleman J, Gonzalez A, Harlaftis N, et al: Myocardial contusion: Diagnostic value of cardiac scanning and echocardiography. *Surg Forum* 27:293, 1976.

18. Downey J, Chagrasulis R, Fore D, et al: Accumulation of technetium-99m stannous pyrophosphate in contused myocardium. *J Nucl Med* 18:1171, 1977.

19. Brantigan CO, Burdick D, Hopeman AR, et al: Evaluation of technetium scanning for myocardial contusion. *J Trauma* 18:460, 1978.

20. Harley DP, Mena I, Narahara KA, et al: Traumatic myocardial dysfunction. *J Thorac Cardiovasc Surg* 87:386, 1984.

21. Rosenbaum RC, Johnston GS: Posttraumatic cardiac dysfunction: Assessment with radionuclide ventriculography. *Radiology* 160:91, 1986.

22. Datz FL, Lewis SE, Parkey RW, et al: Radionuclide evaluation of cardiac trauma. *Semin Nucl Med* 10:187, 1980.

23. Simon TR, Parkey RW, Lewis SE: Role of cardiovascular nuclear medicine in evaluating trauma and the postoperative patient. *Semin Nucl Med* 13:123, 1983.

24. Lee VW, Allard JC, Berger P, et al: Right ventricular tardokinesis in cardiac contusion: A new observation on phase images. *Radiology* 167:737, 1988.

25. Hendel RC, Cohn S, Aurigemma G, et al: Focal myocardial injury following blunt chest trauma: A comparison of indium-111 antimyosin scintigraphy with other noninvasive methods. *Am Heart J* 123:1208, 1992.

26. Waxman K, Soliman MH, Braunstein P, et al: Diagnosis of traumatic cardiac contusion. *Arch Surg* 121:689, 1986.

27. Bodin L, Roube JJ, Viars P: Myocardial contusion in patients with blunt chest trauma as evaluated by thallium 201 myocardial scintigraphy. *Chest* 94:72, 1988.

28. Miller FA, Seward JB, Gersh BJ, et al: Two-dimensional echocardiographic findings in cardiac trauma. *Am J Cardiol* 50:1022, 1982.

29. Hiatt JR, Yeatman LA Jr, Child JS: The value of echocardiography in blunt chest trauma. *J Trauma* 28:914, 1988.

30. Bardy GH, Talano JV, Meyers S, et al: Acquired cyanotic heart disease secondary to traumatic tricuspid regurgitation: Case report with a review of the literature. *Am J Cardiol* 44:1401, 1979.

31. Sheikhzadeh A, Langbehn AF, Ghabusi P, et al: Chronic traumatic tricuspid insufficiency. *Clin Cardiol* 7:299, 1984.

32. Reid CL, Kawanishi DT, Rahimtoola SH, et al: Chest trauma: Evaluation by two-dimensional echocardiography. *Am Heart J* 113:971, 1987.

33. Beggs CW, Helling TS, Evans LL, et al: Early evaluation of cardiac injury by two-dimensional echocardiography in patients suffering blunt chest trauma. *Ann Emerg Med* 16:542, 1987.

34. Hossack KF, Moreno CA, Vanway CW, Burdick DC: Frequency of cardiac contusion in nonpenetrating chest injury. *Am J Cardiol* 61:391, 1988.

35. Seward JB, Khandheria BH, Oh JK, et al: Transesophageal echocardiography: Technique, anatomic correlations, implementation, and clinical applications. *Mayo Clin Proc* 63:649, 1988.

36. Cujec B, Sullivan H, Wilansky S, et al: Transesophageal echocardiography: Experience of a Canadian center. *Can J Cardiol* 5:255, 1989.

37. Taams MA, Gussenhoven WJ, Schippers LA, et al: The value of transesophageal echocardiography for diagnosis of thoracic aorta pathology. *Eur Heart J* 9:1308, 1988.

38. Kram HB, Appel PL, Shoemaker WC: Increased incidence of cardiac contusion in patients with traumatic thoracic aortic rupture. *Ann Surg* 208:615, 1988.

39. Symbas PN: Traumatic heart disease. *Curr Probl Cardiol* 7:3, 1982.

40. Harley DP, Mena I, Miranda R, et al: Myocardial dysfunction following blunt chest trauma. *Arch Surg* 118:1384, 1983.

41. Michelson WB: CPK-MB isoenzyme determinations: Diagnostic and prognostic value in evaluation of blunt chest trauma. *Ann Emerg Med* 9:562, 1980.

42. Liedtke AJ, DeMuth WE: Nonpenetrating cardiac injuries: A collective review. *Am Heart J* 86:687, 1973.

43. Fabian TC, Mangiante EC, Patterson CR, et al: Myocardial contusion in blunt trauma: Clinical characteristics, means of diagnosis, and implications for patient management. *J Trauma* 28:50, 1988.

44. Beresky R, Klingler R, Peake J: Myocardial contusion: When does it have clinical significance? *J Trauma* 28:64, 1988.

45. Schamp DJ, Plotnick GD, Croteau D, et al: Clinical significance of radionuclide angiographically determined abnormalities following acute blunt chest trauma. *Am Heart J* 116:500, 1988.

46. Mattox KL, Flint LM, Carrico CJ, et al: Blunt cardiac injury. *J Trauma* 33:649, 1992.

47. Smith MD, Cassidy JM, Souther S, et al: Transeophageal echocardiography in the diagnosis of traumatic rupture of the aorta. *N Engl J Med* 332:356, 1995.

48. Shapiro MJ, Yanofsky SD, Trapp J, et al: Cardiovascular evaluation in blunt thoracic trauma using transesophageal echocardiography (TEE). *J Trauma* 31:835, 1991.

49. Marshall WG, Bell JL, Kouchoukos NT: Penetrating cardiac trauma. *J Trauma* 24:147, 1984.

50. Borja AR, Lansing AM, Ransdell HT: Immediate operative treatment for stab wounds of the heart: Experience with 54 consecutive cases. *J Thorac Cardiovasc Surg* 59:662, 1970.

51. Fallahnejad M, Kutty ACK, Wallace HW: Secondary lesions of penetrating cardiac injuries. *Ann Surg* 191:228, 1980.

52. Whisennand HH, Van Pelt SA, Beall AC, et al: Surgical management of traumatic intracardiac injuries. *Ann Thorac Surg* 28:530, 1979.

53. O'Connor F, Miranda AL, Tellez G, et al: Traumatic ventricular septal defect: A case of early repair and review of the literature. *Intern Surg* 64:31, 1979.

54. Morgan S. Maturana G, Urzua J, et al: Elective correction of intracardiac lesions resulting from penetrating wounds of the heart. *Thorax* 34:459, 1979.

55. Thandroyen FT, Matisonn RE: Penetrating thoracic trauma producing cardiac shunts. *J Thorac Cardiovasc Surg* 81:569, 1981.

56. Goddard P. Jones AG, Wisheart JD: Self-inflicted stab wounds causing aorta-right ventricular fistula. *Br Heart J* 46:101, 1981.

57. Sklar J, Clarke D, Campbell D, et al: Traumatic ventricular septal defect and lacerated mitral leaflet. *Chest* 81:247, 1982.

58. Phillips TF, Rodriguez A, Cowley RA: Right ventricular outflow obstruction secondary to right sided tamponade following myocardial trauma. *Ann Thorac Surg* 36:353, 1983.

59. Karrel R, Schaffer MA, Franaszek JB: Emergency diagnosis, resuscitation and treatment of acute penetrating cardiac trauma. *Ann Emerg Med* 11:504, 1982.

Pediatric Nuclear Cardiology

Michael J. Gelfand
David W. Hannon

Nuclear cardiology methods have had less impact on pediatric cardiology than on adult cardiology. Most pediatric heart disease results from congenital malformations of the heart and great vessels. Unfortunately, nuclear medicine techniques are limited in their spatial resolution—structures that overlie each other are separated with difficulty. As a result, nuclear cardiology is usually of limited value in the anatomic characterization of the congenital heart abnormalities. Nevertheless, it has been useful in the detection and quantification of the pathophysiologic consequences of many congenital cardiac malformations. We will review applications of nuclear medicine in pediatric cardiology and attempt to assess each in terms of its clinical utility.

FIRST-PASS RADIONUCLIDE ANGIOGRAPHY

Identification and Quantitation of Left-to-Right Shunts

Identification of left-to-right shunts by analysis of pulmonary dilution curves was first suggested by Folse and Braunwald in 1962.[1] As a bolus of radionuclide passed through the lungs under a single-crystal scintillation probe, identification of an early recirculation peak allowed separation of patients without left-to-right shunts from those with left-to-right shunts due to patent ductus arteriosus, ventricular septal defect, or atrial septal defect. Other anatomic lesions with left-to-right shunts,

such as anomalous pulmonary venous return, aortico-pulmonary window, ruptured sinus of Valsalva aneurysm, and surgical systemic-to-pulmonary shunts, could also be evaluated.[1,2]

In the original studies, a single-crystal scintillation probe was used, but now the gamma camera and dedicated computer are used to record the first-pass radionuclide angiogram. Using the computer, an area of interest is located over a part of lung that is free of counts originating from the heart chambers and great vessels (Fig. 27-1). The pulmonary dilution time-activity curve is then derived from the counts integrated over this area of interest over successive equal time intervals (usually 0.5 s). With the gamma camera and computer, the area of interest defines the volume of tissue used in creation of the pulmonary time-activity curve much more accurately than with a single-probe system, especially in infants and small children. Unfortunately, the sensitivity of the gamma camera-computer system is considerably less than that of the single-probe system, necessitating the use of considerably larger administered activities. Gould et al showed excellent agreement between single-crystal nuclear probe shunt quantitation and gamma camera-derived shunt measurements in 29 patients.[3]

Early Methods: The C_2/C_1 and Area Ratio Methods

Three methods of analysis of these curves have been developed. The C_2/C_1 method illustrated in Fig. 27-2A

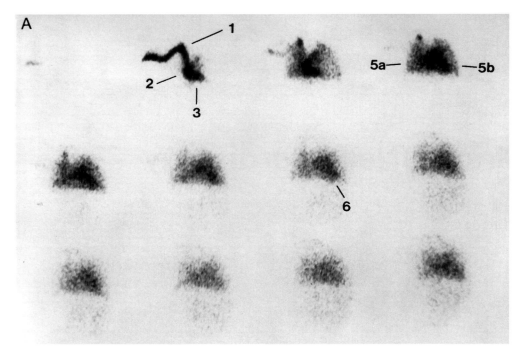

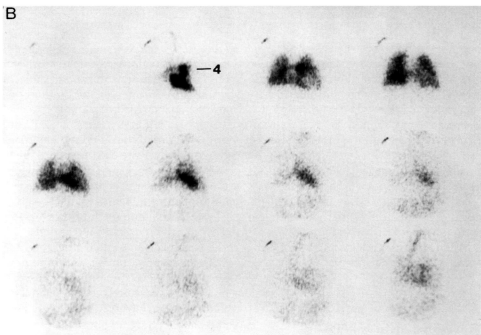

Figure 27-1 A 1-year-old boy with a large ventricular septal defect. Frames are 1.5 s in duration in an anterior projection. **A:** The first-pass transit of a bolus of radionuclide through the heart and great vessels is shown. Activity passes sequentially through the superior vena cava (1), right atrium (2), right ventricle (3), right (5a) and left (5b) lungs, and left ventricle (6). Persistent activity in the lungs is due to the large left-to-right shunt. **B:** The same infant 2 h after cardiopulmonary bypass and closure of the ventricular septal defect. The main pulmonary artery (4) is better seen on this study. The lungs clear rapidly of activity after the initial transit of the bolus. **C:** An area of interest has been created for the right lung that will later be used to create a time-activity curve for the lung. The medial portion of the lung was excluded from the area of interest in this patient, because of overlap, in this projection, of superior vena cava and right atrium with right lung.

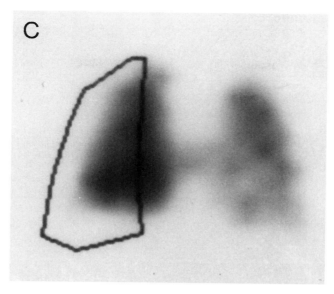

Figure 27-1 *(Continued)*

was first described by Folse and Braunwald and later applied by others.[1-11] C_2/C_1, calculated as in Fig. 27-2**A**, was less than 0.42 for 16 patients without left-to-right shunts and greater than 0.45 for 17 patients with left-to-right shunts.[1] However, not all authors were able to separate patients with left-to-right shunts from those without shunts.[4,6,10,11] As indicated in Table 27-1, there was some correlation between C_2/C_1 and Q_p/Q_s, the pulmonary to systemic flow ratio, but not a close enough relationship to allow shunt quantitation.[7,9,11]

The area-ratio method was developed by Flaherty et al and allowed quantitation of left-to-right shunts.[12]

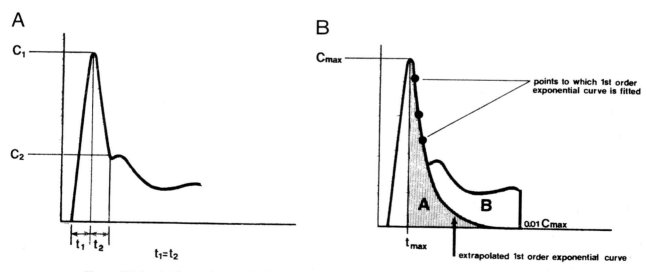

Figure 27-2 **A:** The C_2/C_1 method. The time t_1 from the arrival of the bolus to the peak of the pulmonary dilution curve is measured. A time interval t_2, equal to t_1, is measured beginning at the peak of the curve. The ratio of counts C_2/C_1 at t_2 and t_1, respectively, is computed. **B:** The area-ratio method. A single-component exponential curve is fitted to the downslope of the pulmonary dilution curve to a point where it has a magnitude of 1 percent of the peak count level C_{max} of the pulmonary dilution curve. Area A is the area below the extrapolated curve from the time of occurrence of C_{max} until the time at which the extrapolated curve falls to $0.01 \cdot C_{max}$. Area B is the area below the original curve and above the extrapolated curve between the same time limits. The ratio B/A is calculated.

Table 27-1   Left-to-Right Shunt Quantitation

Author	Number Normal and/or without Shunts	Number with Shunts	Correlation Coefficient, r
C_2/C_1 Method			
Alazraki[7]	8	40	0.81
Maltz[9]	13	22	0.71
Alderson[11]	20	30	0.84
Area-Ratio Method			
Flaherty[12]	30	80	0.94
Anderson[13]	6	20	0.95
Alderson[11]	20	30	0.86
Gelfand[14]	0	16	0.85
Gamma-Variate Method			
Maltz[9]	13	22	0.91
Seward[15]	8	23	0.94
Askenazi[16]	21	84	0.94
(includes Maltz[9])			
Johnson[17]	5	18	0.93
Gelfand[14]	0	16	0.93
Baker[19]			
All subjects	16	84	0.83
ASD	0	32	0.64
VSD	0	52	0.86
Inhalation Method			
Boucher[175]	21	20	0.83
Watson[177]	37	40	0.9

Note: ASD = atrial septal defect; VSD = ventricular septal defect.

Observers using both single-probe and gamma camera-computer systems generally reported a close correlation between B/A, the calculated ratio of two areas defined as in Fig. 27-2B, and Q_p/Q_s.[11-14] Since the normal range of values varied from institution to institution before use of this method, a small series of patient results must be accumulated and a regression equation must be calculated with Q_p/Q_s by the Fick method or another method before routine clinical application is possible.

Gamma-Variate Method

The gamma-variate method, first reported by Maltz and Treves, also utilizes curve fitting.[9] The gamma-variate function describes a curve with rapid upslope and exponential decay and resembles the pulmonary dilution curve of a normal subject after an intravenous bolus injection. The pulmonary dilution time-activity curve before recirculation is fitted to the gamma-variate func-

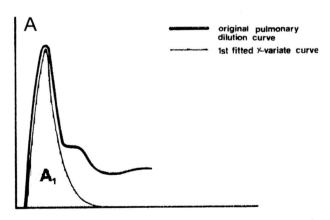

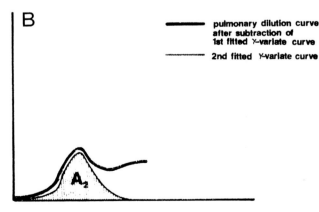

Figure 27-3   **A:** A gamma-variate curve is fitted to the pulmonary dilution curve. The area under this curve A_1 is calculated, representing Q_p, the quantity of blood flowing through the lungs. **B:** Each point on the gamma-variate curve in A is subtracted from the corresponding point in the original pulmonary dilution curve. The resultant curve is illustrated, representing recirculation of activity through the lungs. Using the portion of this resultant curve from beginning of its upslope until immediately after its peak, a second gamma-variate curve is fitted. The area under this second gamma-variate curve A_2 represents pulmonary flow less systemic flow ($Q_p - Q_s$). The ratio $A_1/(A_1 - A_2)$ is equal to Q_p/Q_s.

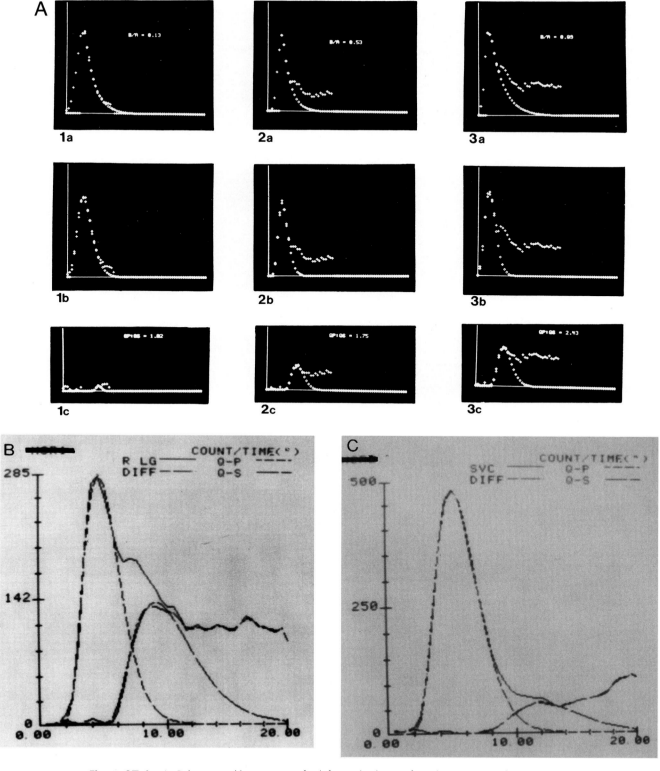

Figure 27-4   **A:** Pulmonary dilution curves for left-to-right shunts of Q_p/Q_s = 1.0 (column 1), 1.6 (column 2), and 2.5 (column 3), as measured by Fick oximetry. Calculated values of B/A by the area-ratio method (row a) are 0.13, 0.53, and 0.89, respectively. Calculated values of Q_p/Q_s by the gamma-variate method are 1.02, 1.75, and 2.43, respectively. **B:** The gamma-variate method is used to calculate Q_p/Q_s for the patient depicted in Fig. 27-1. On the preoperative study, Q_p/Q_s was equal to or greater than 3.0. **C:** On the postoperative study, Q_p/Q_s = 1.3.

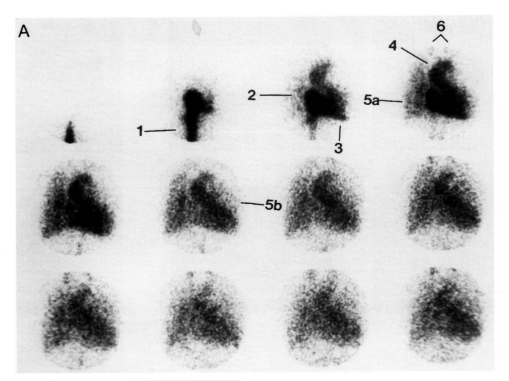

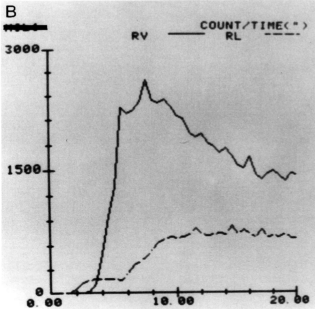

Figure 27-5   **A:** A 13-year-old girl with a severe tetralogy of Fallot (pulmonary atresia with ventricular septal defect) and a Waterston shunt (surgical ascending aorta to right pulmonary artery side-to-side anastomosis). After lower extremity injection, activity travels from the inferior vena cava (1) through the right atrium (2) and right ventricle (3) and into the aorta (4), which overrides the ventricular septal defect. The blood that reaches the lungs arrives via bronchial arteries and the Waterston shunt. More activity reaches the right lung (5a) than the left lung (5b). The right-to-left shunt is apparent with activity in the aorta and carotid arteries (6) simultaneously with arrival of activity in the lungs. **B:** Time-activity curves derived from areas of interest over the right ventricle (RV) and right lung (RL). There is no well-defined peak on the right lung time-activity curve. **C:** Shortly after surgical correction of the tetralogy of Fallot by closure of VSD and placement of a right ventricle to pulmonary artery conduit (7). Persistent lung activity is, in large part, due to persistent bronchial artery flow, especially to the right lower lung (arrow).

tion as shown in Fig. 27-3A. This fitted curve is subtracted from the pulmonary dilution curve; the resultant curve represents recirculation. If an early recirculation peak can be identified (before the normal recirculation that occurs after transit through the systemic capillary bed), a second gamma-variate function is fitted to the resultant curve, as in Fig. 27-3B. The points that are used in fitting the second gamma-variate curve should include no more than one or two data points after the peak of the early recirculation curve. The area under the first fitted curve (A_1) represents the quantity of blood

flowing through the lungs (Q_p). The area under the second fitted curve (A_2) represents recirculation and is equal to pulmonary flow (Q_p) less systemic flow (Q_s), that is, $Q_p - Q_s$. Thus, the ratio of $A_1/(A_1 - A_2)$ represents the ratio Q_p/Q_s in the manner in which it is most often expressed.

Several observers have reported excellent correlation between Q_p/Q_s calculated by the gamma-variate method and Q_p/Q_s determined by Fick oximetry.[9,11,15–17] However, several limitations exist. Care must be taken in determining the portion of this curve to which the

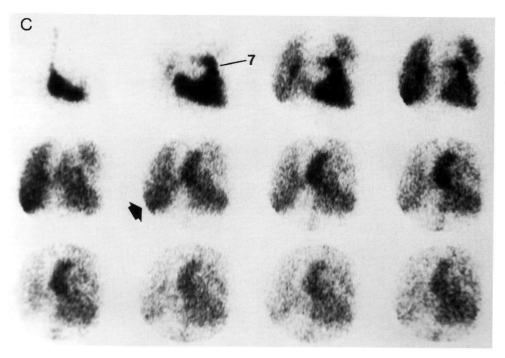

Figure 27-5 *(Continued)*

gamma-variate function is fitted. Also, as the size of the left-to-right shunt increases, the area under the second fitted curve (A_2) increases, making the calculation $Q_p/Q_s = A_1/(A_1 - A_2)$ unreliable. Published series do not attempt to quantitate shunts larger than $Q_p/Q_s = 3.0$. Despite these problems, the gamma-variate function is the preferred radionuclide method for quantitation of left-to-right shunts.

Alderson et al, using implantable flow meters in dogs and surgically created atrial septal defects, found that the gamma-variate radionuclide method correlated better with flow meter readings than did Fick oximetry.[18] Presumably this was due to difficulty, when an atrial septal defect is present, in obtaining the true mixed venous oxygen concentration required by the Fick method. Therefore, it appears that the radionuclide method is more accurate for shunt quantitation in the presence of an atrial septal defect than the Fick method to which it is usually compared. A clinical study by Baker et al seems to confirm this observation in humans. In 100 children with left-to-right shunts, the correlation between shunt size calculated by Fick oximetry and first-pass radionuclide angiography was much better in those with ventricular septal defects than in those with atrial septal defects. This was interpreted as demonstrating the superiority of radionuclide over oximetric shunt measurement in atrial septal defects.[19]

Figure 27-4 illustrates application of the area-ratio method (1a, 2a, 3a) and sequential fitting of gamma-variate curves to the first pulmonary transit (1b, 2b, 3b) and to the early recirculation peak (1c, 2c, 3c). The pulmonary dilution curves demonstrate no shunt (1a, 1b, 1c), a small left-to-right shunt with a Q_p/Q_s of 1.6 by the Fick method (2a, 2b, 2c), and a moderate left-to-right shunt with a Q_p/Q_s of 2.5 by the Fick method (3a, 3b, 3c), respectively.

Pitfalls

A compact bolus injection is necessary for accurate quantitation by any of these methods. The time-activity curve over the vena cava or right heart should be checked for bipartite or double-peaked bolus injections that may create an artifact in the pulmonary dilution curves suggestive of left-to-right shunts when, in reality, no shunt is present.[20] A widened bolus due to slow injection may also give an inaccurate quantitative result. Effective methods for bolus injection have been described that use a special unidirectional dual-port stopcock or a standard stopcock and an intravenous extension tube, both in conjunction with a saline-filled syringe for flushing the bolus of radionuclide.[21,22] In adults and older children, injections using a central venous catheter or a short Teflon catheter in an external jugular vein are most often successful. In infants and small children, bolus injection is usually successful when a short Teflon catheter is used in a peripheral vein of the upper extremity. Injection should be made when the child is not crying and should not be made during a Valsalva maneuver; either may disrupt the continuity of the bolus of activity before it

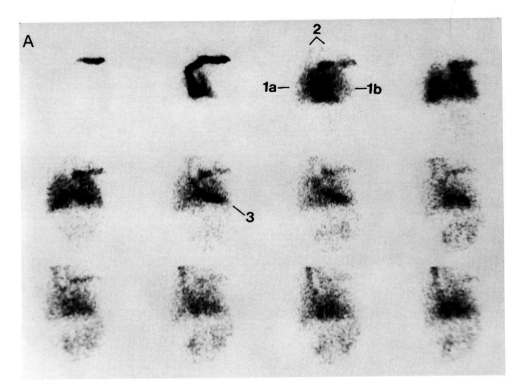

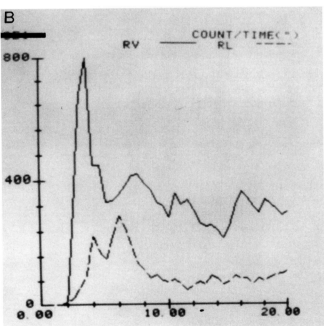

Figure 27-6 A 2-year-old with tetralogy of Fallot and bidirectional shunting, including only a small right-to-left shunt. **A:** Activity reaches the lungs (1a, 1b) simultaneously with the arrival of small amounts of activity in the systemic circulation (carotid arteries, 2). The left ventricle (3) is seen after peak lung activity and after activity returns from the lungs via the pulmonary veins. Activity in the right ventricle preferentially enters the aorta overriding the VSD rather than crossing the VSD into the left ventricle. **B:** Time-activity curves derived from areas of interest over the right ventricle and right lung. There are two peaks on the pulmonary dilution curve (RL). It is difficult to be certain if the second peak represents a left-to-right shunt, bronchial blood flow (less likely in this patient), or "noise" due to limited count statistics. The second peak on the right ventricular time-activity curve is due to activity in the left ventricle falling within the right ventricular area of interest. **C:** Two hours after surgical correction (pulmonary valvotomy and closure of the VSD), the right-to-left shunt is no longer present.

reaches the right heart and cause an error in the estimation of Q_p/Q_s. Technical problems with adequate bolus injections would be expected in premature infants (where shunt quantitation for determining the significance of the patent ductus arteriosus may be useful). However, Treves et al have reported successful application of this technique in these infants using a portable scintillation camera and computer in the intensive care nursery.[23]

Attempts to further improve quantitation, using deconvolution analysis to remove the effect of inadequate bolus injection, have met with varied success.[24] Removal of the primary systemic recirculation peak to facilitate fitting of the early abnormal recirculation curve has also been attempted.[25]

Investigators have reported or postulated inaccurate results using the various shunt determination methods

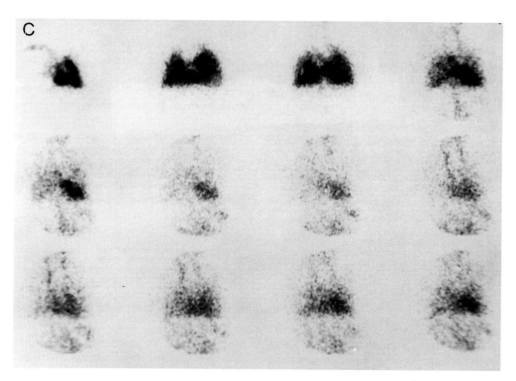

Figure 27-6   (Continued)

in the presence of right-sided valvular incompetence, bidirectional shunts, Valsalva maneuver or crying at the time of injection, severe congestive heart failure, severe aortic or mitral valve disease, or severe pulmonic stenosis.[1,4,11–14,20] Alderson et al also found that in patients with severe valvular disease (mitral insufficiency, mitral stenosis, and pulmonary stenosis) without shunts, abnormal C_2/C_1 values were obtained. This finding was less frequent with the area-ratio and gamma-variate methods.[11] When pulmonic stenosis was created surgically by banding in experimental animals with left-to-right shunts, measurement of Q_p/Q_s by the gamma-variate method remained accurate.[18]

Bronchial arterial circulation may persist after correction of cyanotic congenital heart defects (Fig. 27-5). Peak flow to the lungs via the pulmonary artery will occur before bronchial flow reaches the lungs, creating a pulmonary dilution curve indistinguishable from a left-to-right shunt.

Surgical Systemic-to-Pulmonary Shunts

Several surgical systemic-to-pulmonary shunts have been used to improve pulmonary blood flow in cyanotic heart disease. These include the Blalock-Taussig anastomosis (subclavian artery to pulmonary artery on either side), a modification of this procedure using synthetic graft material to create a subclavian artery to pulmonary artery shunt, the Waterston anastomosis (ascending aorta to right pulmonary artery), and the Potts anastomosis (descending aorta to left pulmonary artery). Examples have been published of increased recirculation to the lung on the side of the shunt after systemic-to-pulmonary anastomosis, demonstrated by analysis of pulmonary dilution curves.[1,7] However, this method is often of limited utility. The method is only successful when there is a well-defined peak on the pulmonary dilution curve, representing flow through the lungs from the right ventricle and pulmonary artery, on which the recirculation peak may be superimposed.

Unfortunately, in patients in whom the question arises of the patency of a surgical systemic-to-pulmonary shunt, there is usually very little or no blood entering the lungs via the right ventricle and pulmonary artery. Therefore, an initial peak on the pulmonary dilution curve distinct from the recirculation peak cannot be identified (Figs. 27-5 and 27-6). In many cardiac conditions such as single ventricle, critical pulmonary stenosis, pulmonary atresia, tricuspid atresia, and truncus arteriosus, all tracer from an intravenous bolus reaches the lungs at about the same time, whether through preexisting or surgically created routes (Fig. 27-5). Thus, although the first-pass angiogram provides useful information on the relative perfusion of each lung in such patients (see section on cyanotic heart disease), further analysis of the pulmonary dilution curves is usually of little value.

First-Pass Ejection-Fraction Determination

First-pass right and left ventricular ejection fractions have been calculated in children by the same methods used in adults. Hurwitz et al have established normal first-pass right and left ejection-fraction values in children using a single-crystal camera. In their patients, a value of less than 41 percent was considered abnormal for right ventricular ejection fraction and a value of less than 50 percent abnormal for left ventricular ejection fraction.[26] Brenner et al have used a multicrystal scintillation camera to determine left ventricular ejection fraction in children with cardiomyopathy and myocarditis.[27]

Cardiac Output Determination

With the use of the Stewart-Hamilton principle, cardiac output may be measured in children in the same way that it is measured in adults, using the area under the first-pass curve from the right and left ventricles along with an equilibrium measurement of counts within the heart and a measured or estimated total blood volume. Cardiac output (CO) is then calculated as follows:

$$CO = \frac{\text{blood volume} \times \text{equilibrium blood counts}}{\text{area under first-pass ventricular curve}}$$

Rabinovitch et al first reported the use of this technique in pediatric patients with good agreement between radionuclide and Fick cardiac output measurements when measured blood volumes were used ($r = 0.88$).[28] A tendency to overestimate cardiac output by the first-pass radionuclide method in children was noted. Covitz and Eubig found a similar correlation ($r = 0.74$) with Fick when an estimated blood volume was used in 9 children.[29]

First-Pass Transit Times

Jones et al demonstrated that normal pulmonary transit times are shorter in children than in adults.[30] In their laboratory the normal adult pulmonary transit time is 6.3 ± 1.5 s. In children 6 to 15 years old, the normal value is approximately 4.5 s, with 2.5 s the normal value for ages 1 to 5 years. Appreciation of these differences is important when using transit times to estimate cardiac function in children.

Quantitation of Right-to-Left Shunts

Quantitation of right-to-left shunting in children with cyanotic congenital heart disease has been performed by

analyzing the area under an "early peak" in the left ventricular time-activity curve.[31] However, in many cyanotic lesions (eg, tetralogy of Fallot), the degree of shunting is apparent only at the level of the aorta, so this method may not be consistently useful. Peter et al obviated this problem by analyzing the carotid artery time-activity curve on first-pass studies acquired with a multicrystal camera.[32] However, because of the reduced count rate obtained from a single-crystal gamma camera with conventional collimation, right-to-left shunt quantitation using carotid artery time-activity curves has not been widely applied in small children.

Anatomic Characterization

The advent of the Anger scintillation camera and the availability of radiopharmaceuticals labeled with ^{99m}Tc led to many publications describing the application of first-pass radionuclide angiography in congenital heart disease.[4,21,33–50] A normal first-pass radionuclide angiogram in a small child is illustrated in Fig. 27-1B. Although this technique failed to gain wide application in the diagnosis of congenital heart disease, the first transit of radionuclide through the chest always provides some information about anatomy and flow patterns.

The first-pass angiogram may define abnormalities of the superior and inferior vena cava. Depending on the site of the injection, diagnosis may be made of persistence of the left superior vena cava (emptying into the coronary sinus or left atrium), absence of the normal right superior vena cava, abnormal right atrial situs, and bilateral or left inferior vena cava (at times changing sides in the liver, possibly with azygos or hemiazygos continuation).[4,35,41–43,47,48] Also, polysplenia may be inferred when there is interruption of the inferior vena cava with azygos continuation.[50]

Cyanotic Heart Disease

First-pass radionuclide angiography may identify a number of congenital cyanotic cardiac anomalies. However, as the abnormal morphology of many of these conditions is usually identified by pediatric echocardiography, the demand for and utility of these studies may be limited. Importantly, in cyanotic children particular care should be taken not to introduce air bubbles during intravenous injection, as they may embolize into the systemic circulation.

The total amount of pulmonic blood flow and the amount of blood flow to each lung is variable in tetralogy of Fallot, depending on the severity of the patient's pulmonic stenosis and the presence of stenoses of the branch pulmonary arteries. An approximation of the relative

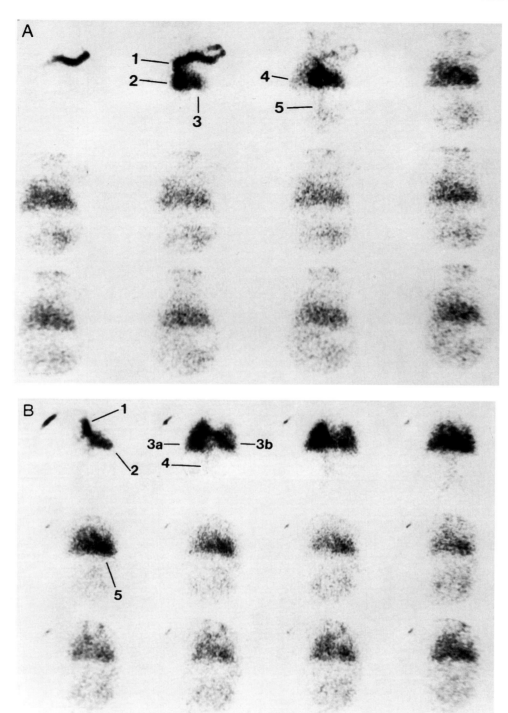

Figure 27-7 D-transposition of the great vessels in a 7-month-old. Shortly after birth, an atrial septal defect was enlarged by balloon septostomy. **A:** Activity moves through the superior vena cava (1) to the right atrium (2). A small amount of activity crosses the atrial septum and reaches the right (4) and left lungs via the left atrium and ventricle. Most of injected activity continues its transit from the right atrium to the right ventricle (3) and aorta (5). **B:** Senning correction in the same patient, by plication of atrial wall creating an intraatrial baffle that directs blood from the systemic veins to the left ventricle and pulmonary artery, and from the pulmonary veins to the right ventricle and aorta. Activity is noted to move rapidly from the superior vena cava (1) through the atrium on one side of the atrial baffle to the left ventricle (2) and right (3a) and left (3b) lungs. Reflux down the inferior vena cava (4) may be normally seen. Activity returns from the lungs through the atrium on the other side of the atrial baffle to the right ventricle (5) and into the systemic circulation.

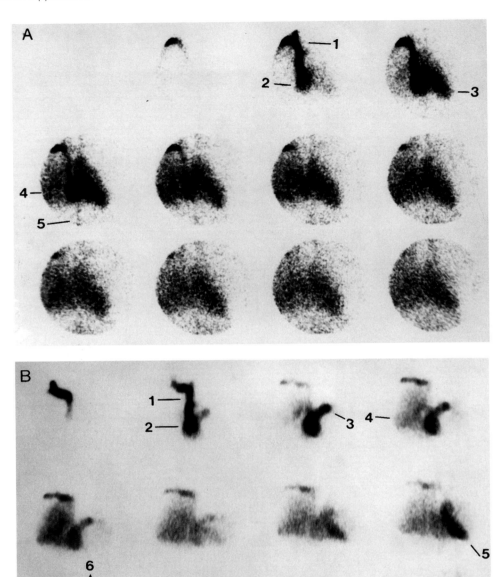

Figure 27-8   A 12-year-old with tricuspid atresia with Waterston (side-to-side ascending aorta to right pulmonary artery) and left Blalock-Taussig (subclavian artery-to-pulmonary artery) shunts. **A:** Activity appears sequentially in the superior vena cava (1), right atrium (2), and left ventricle (3). The right lung (4) and the systemic circulation (5) are visualized simultaneously. Left lung flow is markedly reduced, in this case, owing to increased vascular resistance on that side rather than to a stenotic vessel. **B:** After the Fontan procedure (closure of septal defects and placement of a conduit from the right atrium to the pulmonary artery), activity moves from superior vena cava (1) to right atrium (2), conduit (3), right lung (4), left ventricle (5), and systemic circulation (6). **C:** On gated equilibrium images, a right ventricle is not identified. The right atrium (1) fills as the left ventricle contracts (2). LAO = left anterior oblique; ANT = anterior; ED = end diastole; ES = end systole.

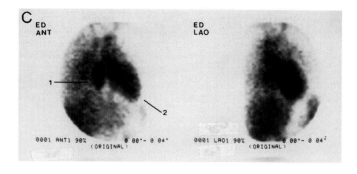

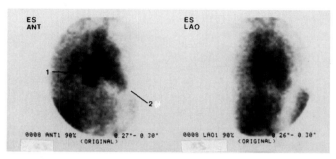

Figure 27-8 (Continued)

flow to each lung may be determined from the first-pass angiogram (Fig. 27-5). In tetralogy of Fallot, the normally situated right ventricle fills with radionuclide followed by near simultaneous filling of the lungs and aorta. Usually, the left ventricle is seen after the lungs are visualized (Fig. 27-6).[41,42,46]

In transposition of the great vessels with intact ventricular septum, there is often little radioactivity in the lungs.[46] The right ventricle fills before the aorta. Some activity enters the left atrium across the atrial or ventricular septum, allowing a variable, though usually decreased, amount of activity to reach the lungs (Fig. 27-7). If a lateral first-pass study is performed, the origin of the aorta may be identified anterior to the superior vena cava, filling from the right ventricle.[39,41]

In pulmonary atresia, the anterior pulmonary artery is not visualized,[41] and the left atrium is seen before the lungs.[46] In tricuspid atresia and Ebstein's anomaly, the left atrium may be visualized before the lungs.[46] In Ebstein's anomaly, the right atrium is noted to be very large.[35,41] Cases of right superior vena cava drainage into the left atrium have been identified.[44] However, early appearance of radionuclide in the left heart may occur in pulmonary disorders, including persistent fetal circulation of the neonate, due to pulmonary hypertension with shunting through the foramen ovale from the right to the left atrium.[41,49] The similar findings in pulmonary atresia with intact ventricular septum, tricuspid atresia, and some cases of right-to-left shunting through the foramen ovale limit the diagnostic specificity of the study. There is no clear published evidence that the many defects with single ventricle or single-

ventricle physiology can be identified by characteristic sequences of images. Total anomalous pulmonary venous return below the diaphragm gives characteristic images. In this anomaly, flow is noted below the diaphragm after visualization of the lungs and before filling of the left heart.[4,40] Total anomalous pulmonary venous return above the diaphragm will show marked persistence of lung activity and a small right-to-left shunt.

Acyanotic Heart Disease

In acyanotic congenital heart disease with left-to-right shunting, the level of the shunt may be identified in some cases. In atrial septal defect, early recirculation to the right atrium and ventricle will occur after the initial pulmonary transit, and may, at times, be noted on the sequence of first-pass images.[21,38,42,49] Similar early identification of radionuclide in the right ventricle may be possible after the first pulmonary transit in ventricular septal defect.[21,38,42,49,51] Gates found that appropriately timed functional images aided in the visual identification of these abnormal flow patterns.[52] In patent ductus arteriosus, evidence of early recirculation on time-activity curves is seen only in the lungs.[21,49] In partial anomalous venous return to the superior vena cava, early recirculation to the superior vena cava and right heart may be visualized.[49] In all these cases, time-activity curves for individual chambers and pulmonary dilution curves may all be of value when the individual structures can be

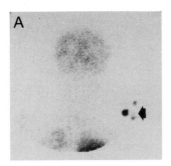

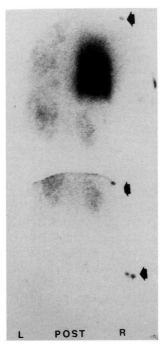

Figure 27-9   The ^{99m}Tc-macroaggregated albumin study in the patient in Fig. 27-8 is shown. Activity injected into a peripheral systemic vein reaches the lungs but also the systemic circulation via the right-to-left shunt. **A:** Activity is noted in the brain and kidneys. The left lung has markedly decreased perfusion. (Arrows indicate radioactive markers placed for orientation.) **B:** Areas of interest are placed over each lung and over all of the rest of the body. In this patient 29 percent of pulmonary venous return went to the body and 71 percent went to the lungs. Left lung circulation was only 11 percent of total lung blood flow. R = right; L = left; POST = posterior.

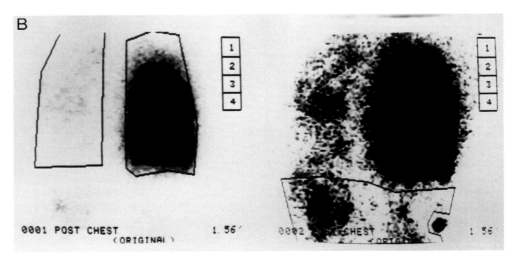

identified, and when regions of interest free of "cross-talk" can be placed over the structures. Any large shunt will result in persistent lung activity, the so-called smudge sign described by Kriss et al (Fig. 27-1A).[42]

Surgical Shunts and Postsurgical Changes

The patency of a superior vena cava to right pulmonary artery shunt (Glenn shunt) may be demonstrated by radionuclide angiography after tracer injection in an upper extremity or external jugular vein. In the presence of a patent shunt, the superior vena cava is visualized followed by the right lung and left heart.[35,36,42,45] Injection in a lower extremity will fill the right atrium followed by the left lung. However, after several years, late perfusion of both lungs via collaterals may be prominent. Moreover, Cloutier et al have demonstrated by radionuclide technique the late occurrence of intrapulmonary right-to-left shunting in such patients, presumably through arteriovenous fistulas.[53]

With a subclavian artery-to-pulmonary artery (Blalock-Taussig) anastomosis, there may be increased flow to the lung on the side of the shunt. Also, an ascending aorta to right pulmonary artery shunt (Waterston) may show increased flow to the right lung (Figs. 27-5A and 27-8).[49] Complete obstruction of a pulmonary artery after a shunt procedure will result in no flow to the involved lung.[47] After any of these surgical shunt procedures, flow to the side opposite the site of the shunt may be predominant owing to streaming effects, stenosis, or differences in vascular resistance of the pulmonary arteries.

After the Mustard or Senning procedures for total correction of transposition of the great vessels, baffle obstruction may be indicated by interruption of the normal pattern of flow in the superior vena cava and by collateral circulation.[49] After either correction, initial atrial visualization is followed sequentially by visualization of the left ventricle, lung, right ventricle, and systemic circulation (Fig. 27-7B). A residual right-to-left intraatrial shunt or "baffle leak" can also be

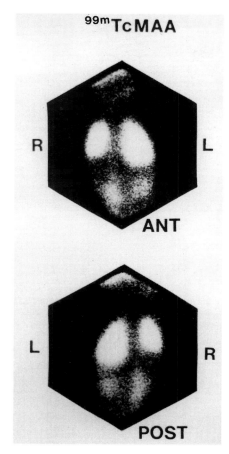

Figure 27-10 A right-sided systemic-to-pulmonary artery shunt has resulted in decreased activity and an apparent decrease in flow to the base of the right lung. Blood flow reaching this area is composed of pulmonary venous return (devoid of ^{99m}Tc- labeled macroaggregated albumin) and activity that has reached the left heart via the right-to-left shunt. The concentration of activity moving through the surgical shunt is lower than in the blood reaching the lungs via the pulmonary artery from the right ventricle. Therefore, areas of the lung fed by the surgical shunt have less activity than those fed by the pulmonary artery from the right ventricle. R = right; L = left; ANT = anterior; POST = posterior.

seen on the first-pass angiogram. Recently radionuclide angiography has been used in children with transposition of the great vessels who have undergone the arterial switch or physiologic repair. Postsurgical anatomy and function and the presence of residual shunts were assessed.[54]

The Fontan repair for tricuspid atresia and other lesions with a single functional ventricle uses the right atrium as the pulmonary "ventricle" via a right atrial-pulmonary artery anastomosis or conduit. On first-pass angiography, the conduit from the right atrium to the lungs is easily seen (Fig. 27-8B). Postoperative leaks from right to left through the atrial septum repair also may be seen.[55] Evaluation of right atrial function, contrary to initial evidence, has not been of value in prediction of outcome after the Fontan repair.

Radioactive Noble Gases for Detection of Right-to-Left Shunts

Xenon 133, after intravenous injection in saline, will reach the left ventricle and systemic circulation only in the presence of a right-to-left shunt.[20,51,56] Similarly, a continuous intravenous infusion of ^{81m}Kr in saline also will reach the left heart only when there is a right-to-left shunt.

TECHNETIUM-99m-LABELED MACROAGGREGATED ALBUMIN FOR DETECTION AND QUANTITATION OF RIGHT-TO-LEFT SHUNTS

Technetium-99m-labeled macroaggregated albumin is a standard lung imaging agent. Its use in the quantitation of relative blood flow to the lungs after intravenous injection and of flow to various portions of the systemic circulation after intraarterial injection has been validated experimentally.[57-60] In patients with right-to-left shunts, particles of macroaggregated albumin will be distributed both to the lungs and via the right-to-left shunt to the systemic circulation (Fig. 27-9). Intravenous injection of this radiopharmaceutical has been used to determine the amount of right-to-left shunting, allowing quantitation of the relative proportions of systemic venous return that are distributed to the pulmonary circulation and to the systemic circulation.[57-60]

Technique

After placement of an intravenous line and after the patient has become quiet, ^{99m}Tc-macroaggregated human serum albumin is injected intravenously. The number and size of particles must be carefully controlled. Images of the entire body are taken for equal intervals of time all in an anterior or all in a posterior projection. With the use of the computer, nonoverlapping areas of interest are defined over the lungs and then over the rest of the body, excluding any extravasated activity at the injection site. The percentage of right-to-left shunt is calculated as

$$\frac{\text{Total body counts} - \text{total lung counts}}{\text{Total body counts}} \times 100$$

Gates compared measurement of right-to-left shunting by the macroaggregated albumin method with measurement of the same parameter by the Fick oximetry method done at cardiac catheterization. Studies were excluded if the patient was crying at the time of injection or where

A

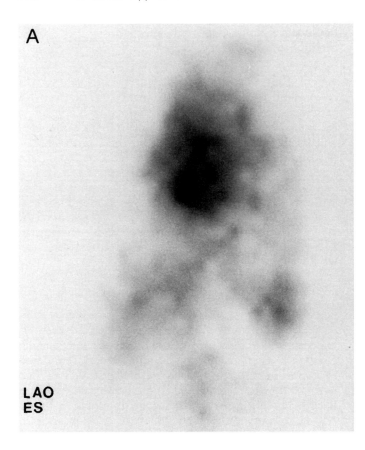

LAO
ES

Figure 27-11 A 1-year-old with ventricular septal defect. **A:** End-systolic image (ES) from an equilibrium gated ventriculogram obtained in the left anterior oblique (LAO) projection with a low energy all-purpose collimator. The image is small and the margins of the left and right ventricles are difficult to identify on a static frame from the cine study. **B:** An end-systolic image from the same equilibrium gated study in the same patient using a pinhole collimator. Image processing has included temporal smoothing and addition of adjacent frames. Image size is adequate and the margins of both ventricles are well defined. (From Hannon et al,[90] reproduced with permission.)

there was evidence of free pertechnetate on images. For 18 patients the two methods correlated with $r = 0.82$.[59]

Injection should not be made in a crying patient because the increased pulmonary resistance during crying will increase both the visible cyanosis and the measured shunt.[61] Also, if the bladder is visualized, excessive free pertechnetate is present. The free pertechnetate outside the lungs will increase the counts over the body, resulting in an overestimation of the right-to-left shunt and invalidating the study.[62] In addition, the percentage of total pulmonary counts is determined for each lung. Ideally, images are taken in both anterior and posterior projections, and errors due to absorption of counts by overlying tissues are removed by calculation of the geometric mean of the conjugate views. In practice, this is rarely done, as increasing breakdown of the radiopharmaceutical over time may create additional errors.

On images of a child with cyanotic congenital heart disease, there will be visualization of the lungs, brain, and kidneys. Liver, spleen, and myocardial uptake may also be noted at times (Figs. 27-9 and 27-10). Although the quantitation of total right-to-left shunt is useful, the use of macroaggregated albumin to diagnose cyanotic congenital heart disease may give misleading results. Total anomalous pulmonary venous return implies an obligate right-to-left shunt, usually through the foramen ovale. However, this diagnosis may be falsely excluded

B

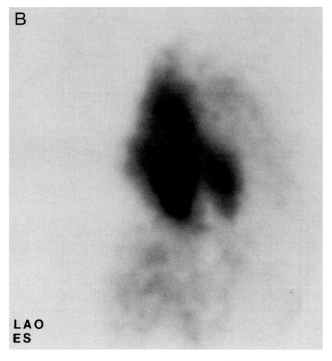

LAO
ES

Figure 27-11 *(Continued)*

by the macroaggregated albumin technique, since the high pulmonary-to-systemic flow ratio causes almost all particles to impact in the lungs and gives the appearance of no significant right-to-left shunt. Conversely, patients with pulmonary hypertension, a patent foramen ovale, and no structural congenital heart disease (eg, infants with persistent fetal circulation) may demonstrate a significant right-to-left shunt.[63,64]

Safety

Gates recommends injection of 0.2 mg of albumin with particles all within a size range of 10 to 50 μm.[65] In other institutions where the procedure is carried out, particle number rather than milligrams of albumin is used as a criterion, with number of particles per injection ranging from 30,000 to 150,000. At the Cincinnati Children's Hospital, between 20,000 and 50,000 particles have been used, depending on the size of the patient, without adverse effect. However, this small number of particles often gives a nonuniform appearance to the lung images. Particle size must be determined before injection by inspection with a microscope and hemocytometer and, when particle number is used as a safety criterion, the number of particles must also be determined. Evidence for safety of the procedure, in which particles of macroaggregated albumin will reach the cerebral circulation, comes from experimental[66–68] and clinical experience[61,68–72] in the use of the radiopharmaceutical in brain imaging after intracarotid injection. In human studies, when 5- to 30-μm particles were injected by direct carotid puncture, morbidity was no different from that experienced in a similar group that underwent cerebral arteriography alone.[68–71] After intravenous injection using the 0.2-mg dose of albumin, Gates et al estimated a 6000-fold safety margin with the dose they employed and reported no complications.[61,72]

Surgical Systemic-to-Pulmonary Shunts

Besides quantification of right-to-left shunting in cyanotic heart disease, ^{99m}Tc-labeled macroaggregated albumin may be used to evaluate the adequacy of surgical systemic-to-pulmonary shunts. If there is blood flow into the lungs via the right heart and pulmonary artery, the portion of the lungs perfused by that route will receive blood with a high concentration of macroaggregates. If there is also blood flow from a surgical systemic-to-pulmonary shunt, the portion of the lungs receiving blood from the shunt will receive additional blood that has a relatively low concentration of macroaggregates—the blood in the left heart having been diluted by pulmonary venous return devoid of particles. Therefore, creation of a functioning surgical systemic-to-pulmonary shunt will cause an increase in the percentage of particles distributed in the lungs, but the increase in lung uptake will not reflect the full increase in pulmonary blood flow due to the shunt. Figure 27-10 illustrates uptake in the lungs, liver, and kidneys in a patient with a right-to-left shunt. The region of decreased flow at the base of the right lung is due to perfusion by blood with a lower concentration of albumin macroaggregates from a right-sided systemic-to-pulmonary shunt. In contrast, when all blood enters the lungs from a single ventricle or when single-ventricle physiology is present, the increase in blood flow will be accurately reflected by a similar increase in the percentage of lung uptake. In this latter case, all blood delivered to the lung has the same concentration of macroaggregates.

Experimental work in dogs indicated that 75 percent of blood flow from an end-to-side subclavian-to-pulmonary artery shunt went to the lung on the side of the shunt, whereas most blood from the right ventricle went to the lung opposite the shunt.[73]

Another experiment in dogs with surgically created atrial septal defects, pulmonic stenosis, and shunts from the ascending aorta to the right pulmonary artery showed predominant flow of blood from the left ventricle to the right lung and from the right ventricle to the left lung.[74] Therefore, one would expect a high concentration of activity in the lung opposite the shunt from venous blood with a high concentration of macroaggregates and a low concentration of activity in the lung ipsilateral to the shunt from systemic blood with a low concentration of macroaggregates.

In clinical practice, results have been less straightforward. Several series found the expected distribution of pulmonary activity, that is, less than half of total lung activity on the side of the shunt.[75–77] However, in other series results have been confusing, with the greatest activity on the side either ipsilateral to or contralateral to the surgical systemic-to-pulmonary shunt.[78–80] The matter is further confused by a high frequency of preexisting branch pulmonary artery stenoses, especially in tetralogy of Fallot.[72,80] Similarly, in tetralogy of Fallot and in transposition of the great vessels, there may be a preexisting predominance of flow to the right lung.[72,81–83] It appears that, in the presence of a functioning systemic-to-pulmonary shunt, either the ipsilateral or contralateral lung may receive the greatest number of particles, with the distribution again being dependent on factors such as the individual surgical anastomosis, the resistance in the right and left pulmonary arteries, and streaming effects.[72,81,84] Gates stated that evaluation of perfusion images alone is inadequate; the best indication of a functioning shunt is a decrease in the calculated size of the right-to-left shunt after surgery.[84] The situation is relatively straightforward only if there is complete mixing of systemic and pulmonary venous blood, as in tricuspid atresia, pulmonary atresia, or single-ventricle physiology. Tamir et al found that lung perfusion imaging was more sensitive in detecting abnormal lung perfusion than was chest radiography. They found lung perfusion scans valuable in identifying those children who needed a special intervention at time of complete repair and in the evaluation of the results of transcatheter interventions.[85]

Function of an anastomosis from the superior vena cava to the right pulmonary artery (Glenn shunt) also may be studied by injection of labeled macroaggregates. In this case the right lung is imaged after injection in an upper-extremity vein and the left lung is imaged after lower-extremity injection.[75,79] Baker et al modified this technique, using injections at multiple sites during cardiac catheterization together with digital image subtraction to define dual blood supplies to portions of the lungs in patients with pulmonary atresia and ventricular septal defect.[86] This allowed surgical ligation of large collaterals without compromising pulmonary blood supply.

After repair of congenital cyanotic heart disease, lung perfusion is often asymmetric. After total correction of tetralogy of Fallot, pulmonary flow is most often decreased on the side of the shunt.[79,81] After the Mustard procedure for correction of transposition of the great vessels, a predominance of flow to the right lung may remain.[82] Absent perfusion of the lung may be due to thrombosis of a pulmonary artery after a surgical systemic-to-pulmonary artery shunt.[75]

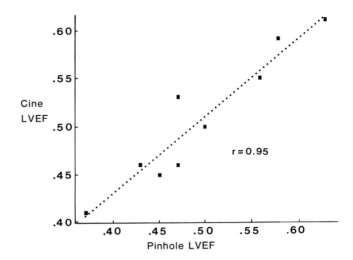

Figure 27-12   Left ventricular ejection fraction (LVEF) obtained by pinhole collimated gated equilibrium ventriculography correlated well (r = 0.95) with LVEF calculated from contrast cine ventriculography at cardiac catheterization. (From Hannon et al,[90] reproduced with permission.)

GATED STUDIES FOR VENTRICULAR FUNCTION

Choice of Radiopharmaceutical

Technetium-99m human serum albumin (HSA) or, more commonly, ^{99m}Tc red blood cells, labeled by various methods, may be used for gated equilibrium blood pool imaging. Technetium-99m HSA is prepared using a commercial kit and ^{99m}Tc pertechnetate eluted from a generator. Some investigators prefer ^{99m}Tc HSA because it requires only a single injection in children who are often apprehensive and who may have limited venous access.[87] However, in adults it has been shown that the ratio of heart counts to background counts is significantly lower for ^{99m}Tc HSA than for the various forms of ^{99m}Tc-labeled red blood cells, and clinical experience suggests that this is also true in children. Red blood cells may be labeled by in vivo, semi–in vivo, and kit methods. To avoid multiple venipunctures and to facilitate a bolus injection, a short intravenous Teflon catheter may be placed in the hand in infants or the antecubital fossa in older children. Millar et al indicated that Teflon may interfere with the in vivo red blood cell labeling; however, this effect has not been observed in our experience.[88] If all stopcocks

and intravenous tubing attached to the intravenous catheter are replaced after the initial injection of stannous pyrophosphate and the catheter is flushed with at least 5 mL of normal saline, excellent labeling of red blood cells is achieved despite use of a Teflon catheter and a single injection site.

Radiation Dosimetry

With an administered activity of 200 μCi/kg, the absorbed radiation dose for ^{99m}Tc HSA is 0.21 rad to the bone marrow with an average whole body dose of 0.20 rad.[89] For ^{99m}Tc red blood cells, the bone marrow absorbed dose is 0.31 rad, and the whole body dose is 0.22 rad.[90] At this time, for purposes of radiation dosimetry, one must assume that pediatric biodistribution and pharmacokinetics are identical to those of adults. This results in an absorbed radiation dose that varies little with age as long as the administered activity per kilogram is kept constant. Many investigators use a somewhat larger administered activity per kilogram in children, particularly in smaller infants, resulting in a proportionate increase in absorbed radiation dose. Although others have recommended 2 to 3 mCi as a minimum ^{99m}Tc dose, we have had good results with 1 to 1.5 mCi as a minimum activity.

Choice of Collimation

In children weighing over 12 kg, the gated radionuclide ventriculogram is performed using a parallel-hole general-purpose low-energy collimator—the same collimator that would be used in adults. In infants weighing under 12 kg, the cardiac ventricles are small and their margins are difficult to define on individual cine images, even though there is obvious evidence of ventricular contraction on the cine images. In these small infants, pinhole collimation has been used to acquire magnified gated equilibrium studies in the LAO view (Fig. 27-11).[91] The pinhole collimator has been used extensively in adults for imaging of small thyroid nodules, in children for imaging of the hips and scrotum,[91–93] and for cardiac imaging in small laboratory animals.[95] Pinhole collimation has the disadvantage that it is insensitive, with a very low proportion of photons reaching the crystal detector. This has been overcome by increasing the study acquisition time to 15 min and by image-processing methods that compensate for the poor count statistics. The spatial distortion near the edges of the field of view with pinhole collimation is minimized by proper positioning of the collimator so that the heart is centered away from the edges of the field of view.

In our laboratory, processing involves adding pairs of temporally adjacent image frames together, which effectively doubles the time per frame. A three-point temporal smoothing filter is applied, resulting in an eight-frame cine format that can be displayed in a flicker-free manner. Definition of the ventricular margins on the processed images is adequate for delineation of end-diastolic and end-systolic areas of interest. Areas of interest are applied to the original unprocessed images for calculation of ejection fraction by standard methods. The left ventricular ejection fraction from the pinhole technique was correlated with the left ventricular cine angiographic ejection fraction obtained at the same time as cardiac catheterization. A satisfactory correlation coefficient of $r = 0.95$ was obtained (Fig. 27-12).[91] Delineation of the right ventricular margins was also possible in many cases where it was impossible on the conventionally collimated gated study.[91] This is of particular value for calculation of right ventricular ejection fraction in patients with transposition of the great vessels where the right ventricle is the systemic pump. The improved spatial resolution of pinhole collimation gated studies is useful for detecting septal and apical wall motion abnormalities in children. These have been found frequently in the postoperative period and are usually due to transient myocardial dysfunction after open heart surgery and cardioplegic arrest. In the past, the apical left ventricular venting technique often produced readily apparent apical dyskinesia.[96] Wall motion abnormalities may also be seen in children after myocardial infarction from anomalous origin of the left coronary artery and from Kawasaki disease (Fig. 27-13).

Absolute ventricular volume calculation from gated equilibrium studies is not possible using pinhole collimation owing to variation in sensitivity and magnification dependent on the distance between the collimator aperture and the left ventricle.

Parametric Images

Parametric image processing methods may be applied to the series of gated cine images in the same manner as in adult studies. Using Fourier analysis, amplitude and phase images are easily obtained. As in adult studies, left ventricular wall motion abnormalities are clearly demonstrated, but these findings are relatively uncommon. Often, however, a change in contractility (eg, after cardiopulmonary bypass) not only results in a decrease in ejection fraction but also in a striking change in the Fourier amplitude image (Fig. 27-14).[97]

A parametric image that is composed of amplitudes of the fundamental frequency for pixels that are in phase with ventricular contraction, that is, a ventricular amplitude image, is useful in definition of the margins of the right ventricle. This facilitates separation of the right ventricle from the right atrium.[91] This is particularly useful for delineation of areas of interest before calculation of right ventricular ejection fraction. In addition, these parametric images may be used for calculation of regurgitant ratios, as has been demonstrated in adult patients. As in adults, changes in contractility, whether global or focal, are reflected on these images.

Measurement of Ventricular Volume

Nongeometric, counts-based absolute right and left ventricular volumes in children were first assessed by Parrish et al using a variation of previously described adult methods.[97] They defined a regression equation based on patient size for cardiac-to-camera distance determination [distance d (in cm) $= 3.7 \times$ body surface area (m^2) $+$ 3.6] and an assumed attenuation coefficient (μ) of 0.1 cm^{-1} to calculate volume:

$$\text{Volume} = \frac{\substack{\text{(background corrected} \\ \text{ventricular counts)} \times e^{\mu d}}}{\substack{\text{(frame duration} \times \text{collected cycles} \\ \times \text{count rate/mL blood sample)}}}$$

The correlation for right and left ventricular end-diastolic volumes by cineangiography and radionuclide angiography was greater than 0.90. Guiteras et al used a cardiac phantom to determine that an attentuation coefficient of 0.11 cm^{-1} was appropriate for cardiac volumes in the pediatric age range.[99]

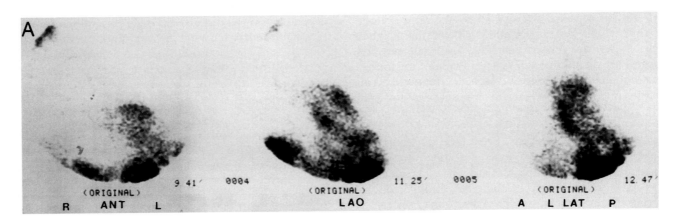

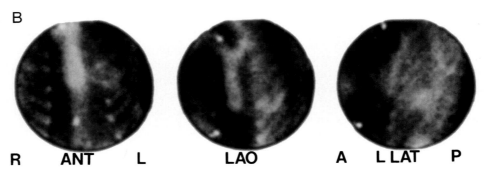

Figure 27-13 Acute myocardial infarction in a 16-year-old with coronary artery aneurysms after Kawasaki syndrome. **A:** Rest ^{201}Tl images show hypoperfusion of the apical half of the left ventricle and more extensive hypoperfusion in the inferior and posterior walls. **B:** Extensive uptake of ^{99m}Tc-pyrophosphate is present. **C:** A gated equilibrium study performed 3 mo after the myocardial infarction shows severe apical hypokinesia (arrows). **D:** On a ^{201}Tl study 3 mo later, perfusion is considerably improved. R = right; L = left; ANT = anterior; LAO = left anterior oblique; L LAT = left lateral; A = anterior; P = posterior; ED = end diastole; ES = end systole.

Regurgitant Ratios

As in adults, the ratio of left ventricular to right ventricular stroke counts has been used to estimate the severity of valvular regurgitation. In 60 children, Parrish et al determined a normal range of 0.70 to 1.38 for the stroke-count ratio and demonstrated a good correlation ($r = 0.88$) with cineangiographic stroke-volume ratios.[100] Hurwitz and associates have considered 0.9 to 1.5 to be normal in children and used stroke-count ratios below this level to detect patients with tricuspid regurgitation after Mustard operation for transposition of the great arteries.[101]

Evaluation of Patients After Surgical Repair of Congenital Heart Disease

Early and late postoperative evaluation of children undergoing cardiac surgery has been described using gated equilibrium studies. Depressed left ventricular ejection fractions, residual shunts, and wall motion abnormalities in children may be assessed in the postoperative intensive care unit.[96] A few patients with bleeding severe enough to require reoperation have shown evidence on gated images of active bleeding, with accumulation of activity around the heart (Fig. 27-15). In another study of children during the immediate postoperative period, Covitz et al found a transient decline in left ventricular ejection fraction that was related to aortic cross clamp time.[102] More recently, Hammon et al showed that in 15 children an abnormal left ventricular ejection fraction 72 to 96 h after cardiac surgery correlated with low myocardial ATP levels measured at the conclusion of aortic cross-clamping.[103] At our institution, radionuclide angiography has been particularly valuable in those with complex intracardiac repairs and in those who require inotropic support postoperatively.[96] On the postoperative study, the presence of significant left ventricular dysfunction (left ventricular ejection fraction < 30 percent) correlates with a more complicated postoperative course and the need for inotropic support. A persistent postoperative depression in ejection fraction has been associated

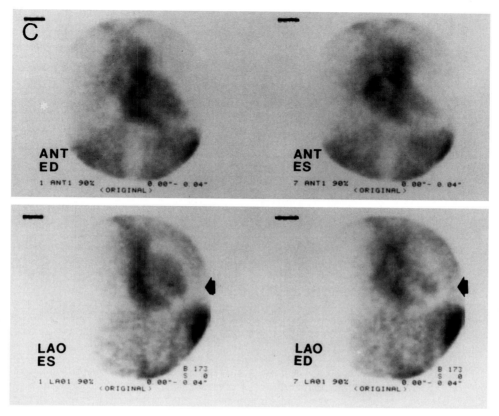

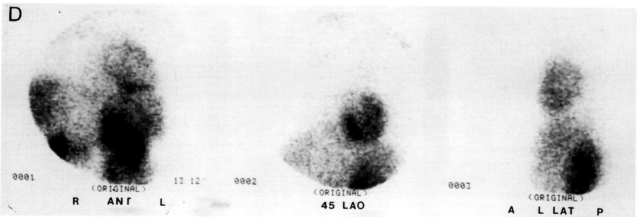

Figure 27-13 *(Continued)*

with a complicated postoperative course and a poor long-term prognosis.[104]

Gated equilibrium studies have also been used in the delayed postoperative assessment of patients after surgery for congenital heart disease. After repair of transposition of the great vessels or tricuspid atresia, occult resting ventricular dysfunction has been found in patients despite an asymptomatic clinical status.[55,105,106] Bove et al have shown that residual pulmonic valve incompetence after repair of tetralogy of Fallot results in lower right and left ventricular ejection fractions than when the pulmonary valve is competent.[107] In a follow-up study, they demonstrated recovery of right ventricular ejection fraction after pulmonary valve replacement.[108] With a modified surgical technique, the radionuclide right ventricular ejection fraction was preserved even in patients with residual pulmonic incompetence.[109] Also of interest is the observation by Burns et al that late ventricular arrhythmias in adults 5 to 27 y after tetralogy repair correlate with abnormal radionuclide left ventricular ejection fraction.[110] Kavey et al have since published similar findings.[111] In children with transposition of the great vessels who underwent the arterial switch procedure, Treves et al used first-pass ventriculography to

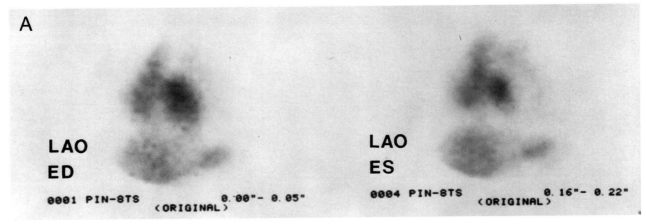

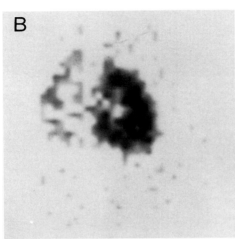

Figure 27-14 A 2-month-old with a large ventricular septal defect. **A:** The pinhole collimated gated equilibrium ventriculogram obtained before surgery shows good contractility with left ventricular ejection fraction (LVEF) of 60 percent. **B:** The amplitude functional image obtained by Fourier analysis shows excellent left ventricular wall motion. LAO = left anterior oblique; ED = end diastole; ES = end systole. **C:** Two h after repair of the ventricular septal defect, the pinhole gated equilibrium study shows a marked decrease in contractility with a fall in LVEF to 34 percent. The patient had a complicated course after surgery and required prolonged inotropic and ventilatory support. **D:** The Fourier amplitude functional image shows loss of contractility of the apical portions of the left ventricle (arrowhead). LAO = left anterior oblique; ED = end diastole; ES = end systole.

evaluate the left and right ventricles for global dysfunction and evidence of ischemia and infarction.[54] In recent studies, patients with cyanotic heart disease had no change in resting left ventricular ejection fraction after external conduit surgery for tetralogy of Fallot and after atriopulmonary connection (Fontan procedure) for single-ventricle physiology.[112,113]

Evaluation of Patients Undergoing Cancer Chemotherapy

Doxorubicin hydrochloride (Adriamycin) is an antineoplastic anthracycline drug widely used in pediatric cancer chemotherapy. Cardiotoxicity has been reported in a significant number of patients receiving more than 550 mg/m² total dose, but it is apparent that a wide variability in drug tolerance exists. In children treated with doxorubicin, Hutter et al used radionuclide angiography to detect left ventricular dysfunction but recommended serial echocardiography for screening and follow-up.[114] In clinical practice, either serial echocardiography, when performed by skilled personnel, or radionuclide angiography may be used to monitor for doxorubicin cardiotoxicity. There is evidence in adults that abnormal exercise radionuclide ejection fraction may correlate with endomyocardial biopsy findings, but experience in children is lacking.[115]

Exercise Studies

Radionuclide ventriculography has been performed in children undergoing supine or upright bicycle exercise and isometric exercise in several clinical settings. Parrish et al have performed exercise gated ventriculography in 32 children, aged 5 to 19 years, without heart disease, and from their results defined a decrease in ejection fraction of more than five absolute percentage points as abnormal.[116] Abnormal ventricular ejection fraction responses to exercise have been found in children and young adults with tricuspid atresia,[117,118] tetralogy of Fallot,[112,119] Mustard's repair of transposition,[120–122] sickle cell anemia,[123] thalassemia,[124] Ebstein's anomaly,[125] cystic

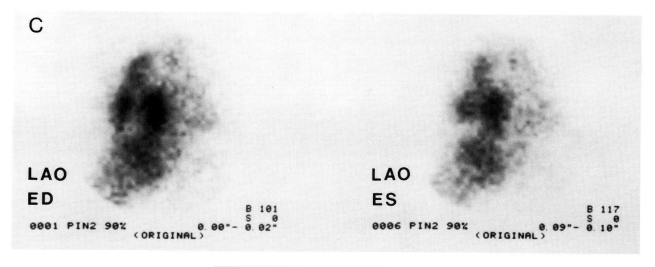

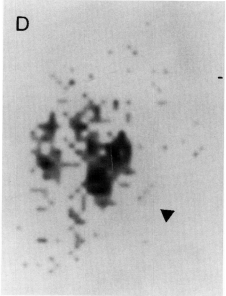

Figure 27-14 *(Continued)*

fibrosis,[126] and Duchenne's muscular dystrophy,[127] and after external conduit for cyanotic heart disease.[112] In patients with single-ventricle physiology, Akagi et al found that abnormal exercise ejection fraction responses were correlated with the interval of time after Fontan procedure. This suggests that this group of patients may need continued follow-up of exercise cardiac performance.[112] Also, exercise ejection-fraction response may be measured in children with significant aortic valve regurgitation, as is frequently done in adults. Hurwitz et al demonstrated that left ventricular function can be studied before and during dobutamine infusion, in lieu of evaluation during exercise.[128]

In the study by Parrish et al, abnormal right (systemic) and left ventricular ejection-fraction responses to exercise were found in most patients after the Mustard operation, despite normal exercise capacity and blood pressure responses.[120] Likewise, Benson et al found no difference in peak exercise work load, heart rate, or blood pressure response between postoperative transposition patients with normal versus abnormal exercise ejection-fraction responses.[122] Murphy et al did find that the maximal work load obtainable during exercise was predictive of ejection-fraction response to exercise in patients a mean of 9 y after Mustard operation.[121] However, right ventricular ejection-fraction measurements may be difficult to reproduce in children. When Schaffer et al measured equilibrium right ventricular ejection fractions in 13 children with hypercholesterolemia, interobserver and intraobserver variability was high.[129] Such studies illustrate that the prognostic significance of an abnormal exercise ejec-

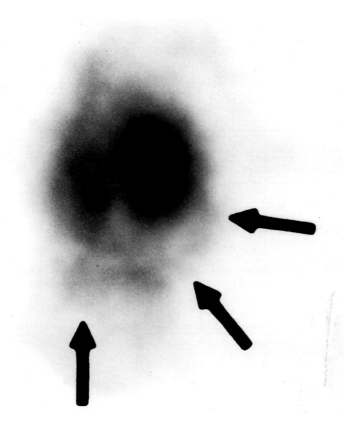

Figure 27-15 A 1-year-old 2 h after closure of a ventricular septal defect and removal of a pulmonary artery band that had been placed earlier to limit pulmonary arterial flow. The pinhole collimated image in end diastole shows blood in the pericardium. (From Hannon et al,[90] reproduced with permission.)

tion-fraction response after open heart repair of congenital heart diseases is not established.

Diastolic Function

The techniques of diastolic functional assessment are treated in detail in Chap. 15. In pediatrics, few studies of diastolic function have been done. Shaffer et al noted an improved peak filling rate and reduced time to peak filling after verapamil treatment in 10 children with hypertrophic cardiomyopathy. These findings are similar to those described previously in adults.[130] Akagi et al measured peak filling rate and time to peak filling in 20 normal children and demonstrated abnormal values for these diastolic function parameters in patients after Fontan procedure for single ventricle.[131]

MYOCARDIAL PERFUSION STUDIES

Myocardial perfusion scintigraphy with ^{201}Tl or the ^{99m}Tc myocardial perfusion agents has a limited role in pediatric cardiology. Except in populations where homozygous hypercholesterolemia is common, coronary artery disease is largely limited to congenital coronary lesions and Kawasaki disease. An important congenital lesion of the coronary arteries is an anomalous origin of the left coronary artery from the pulmonary artery. Myocardial perfusion images will demonstrate perfusion defects, usually extensive, with left ventricular enlargement, in patients who already have undergone myocardial infarction. After reanastomosis of the left coronary artery to the aorta, the patient may be evaluated for residual ischemia.[132,133,134] Patients with coronary artery to coronary sinus fistulas also may be evaluated in the same manner.[135]

After Kawasaki syndrome, approximately 15 percent of children develop aneurysms of the coronary arteries (Figs. 27-13 and 27-16). Treves et al first reported a case of decreased myocardial ^{201}Tl uptake in an infant with Kawasaki syndrome who later died. In this case planar ^{201}Tl scintigraphy was normal, but single photon emission computed tomography revealed diminished anterolateral left ventricular uptake.[136] Ueda et al reported a child with Kawasaki disease and myocardial infarction in whom decreased myocardial ^{201}Tl uptake was present by conventional planar scintigraphy.[137] Kato et al used resting ^{201}Tl myocardial perfusion scintigrams to study 34 patients with Kawasaki syndrome who had follow-up coronary arteriograms a mean of 4 y following presentation with symptoms. All 15 children with angiographic regression of their coronary artery aneurysms

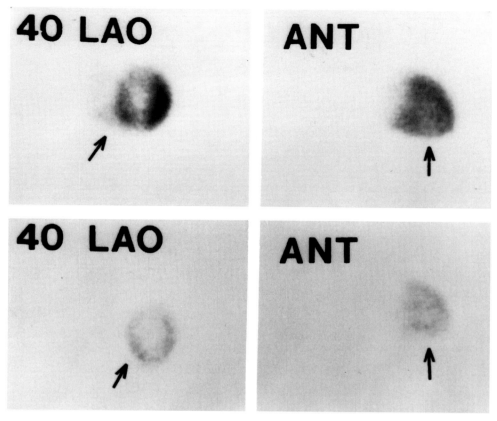

Figure 27-16 An 11-year-old with aneurysms of the right and left coronary arteries and posterior descending artery thrombosis after Kawasaki syndrome. On ^{201}Tl images, there is septal and probable inferior wall hypoperfusion (arrows) immediately after treadmill exercise. Delayed images show redistribution into the septum and possibly also into the inferior wall (arrows). When coronary artery bypass surgery was performed, a small inferior wall infarct was found. ANT = anterior; 40 LAO = 40° left anterior oblique.

had a normal follow-up ^{201}Tl scintigram. Of 19 children with an abnormal follow-up coronary arteriogram, 31 percent had abnormal myocardial perfusion scintigrams at rest.[138] Thallium 201 may be useful in detecting the presence of stress-induced myocardial ischemia in these patients (Figs. 27-16 and 27-17). Miyagawa et al performed stress ^{201}Tl imaging with exercise or intravenous dipyridamole in 112 children with coronary artery lesions from Kawasaki syndrome. SPECT ^{201}Tl images were much more sensitive than planar images and compared favorably with coronary angiograms in detecting coronary arterial lesions.[139] Similar results were obtained by Ono et al and Kondo et al.[140,141]

A rest-stress study by Paridon et al raises concern about post–Kawasaki syndrome patients with angiographically normal coronary arteries. Of 27 patients who never had angiographic abnormalities after Kawasaki syndrome, 37 percent had reversible poststress perfusion defects, and 63 percent of 8 patients with resolved coronary artery aneurysms had similar reversible perfusion defects. Myocardial perfusion defects, mostly reversible, were present in all patients with coronary artery aneu-

rysms.[142] Collateral circulation appears to occur only when total occlusion of a coronary artery is present; and these patients have myocardial perfusion abnormalities similar to those with severe stenosis of a coronary artery.[143] Long-term follow-up of Kawasaki syndrome patients may become increasingly important because of the discovery of early-onset adult-type coronary artery disease in some of these patients.[143,144]

Gallium 67, ^{111}In white blood cell imaging, and ^{99m}Tc-HMPAO-white blood cell imaging all show myocardial uptake in some patients during the acute phase of Kawasaki syndrome, but prediction of later aneurysm formation has not been reported with this technique.[145,146,147]

Thallium-201 imaging at rest has also been used in identification of asymmetric septal hypertrophy[148] and for detection of the presence of a ventricular septum in children with single-ventricle physiology.[149] However, in both cases, there is no evidence to suggest that it is superior to echocardiography in these applications.

In asphyxiated newborns, transient myocardial ischemia was demonstrated by Finley et al. In these patients the pattern of ^{201}Tl uptake resembles that seen in some

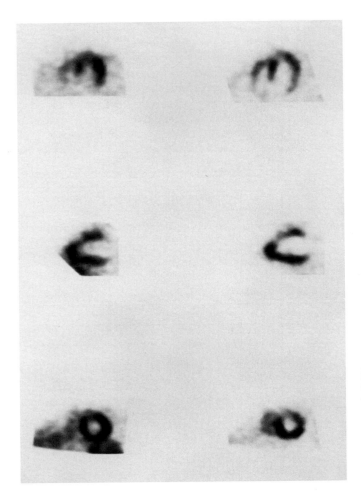

Figure 27-17 A 13-year-old with Kawasaki syndrome. Rest ^{201}Tl (left column) and poststress ^{99m}Tc-sestamibi studies (right column) with representative matching horizontal long axis (top), vertical long axis (middle) and short axis sections (bottom). There is a moderately large area of anterior hypoperfusion on the poststress images that is better perfused on rest images. Angiography demonstrated left main and right coronary aneurysms, with complete occlusion of the left main coronary artery, and retrograde filling from the right coronary and left circumflex arteries.

older patients with severe heart failure and pulmonary edema in whom the lung uptake exceeds myocardial uptake. Thus, it is not clear if the poor myocardial uptake in these infants is absolute and related to myocardial injury or ischemia, or represents a relative decrease in the presence of increased lung uptake. On repeat studies, normal myocardial perfusion was noted in these infants.[150] Children with congestive cardiomyopathy and heart failure may show this nonspecific pattern as well, but in a few patients local defects have been observed in the myocardial wall.[148]

Saji et al found localized resting ^{201}Tl perfusion defects in 9 of 12 children with the diagnosis of myocarditis. These patients had normal coronary arteriography but abnormal endomyocardial biopsies. They concluded that ^{201}Tl uptake was not only dependent on regional coronary flow, but also on the degree of pathologic change in the myocardial cells in these patients.[151] Perfusion defects with ^{201}Tl have also been described in thalassemia and in Duchenne's and other forms of muscular dystrophy.[152,153,154,155,156]

Flynn and associates compared myocardial perfusion scintigrams performed with ^{201}Tl and ^{99m}Tc 2-methoxy-

isobutylisonitrile (sestamibi) in 11 infants who had undergone the arterial switch procedure for transposition of the great arteries. Uniform myocardial perfusion was documented in each infant with both tracers.[157] Images obtained with ^{99m}Tc sestamibi required a shorter acquisition time, involved less radiation exposure to the infant, and were qualitatively comparable or superior to those obtained with ^{201}Tl. In other studies, a moderate number of patients who had undergone the arterial switch procedure had perfusion defects at rest and under stress.[158,159,160] In general, rest studies were more likely to demonstrate perfusion abnormalities than poststress studies, suggesting that most of the perfusion abnormalities were fixed.

Right Ventricular and Pulmonary Hypertension

Increased ^{201}Tl uptake has been demonstrated in patients with right ventricular hypertension. Rabinovitch et al were able to approximately quantitate the right ventricular pressure in 24 patients with congenital heart disease from the ratio of right ventricular to left ventricular myocardial counts in the left anterior oblique projection.[161] A close relationship between the right ventricular to left ventricular systolic pressure ratio and ratio of right ventricular to left ventricular counts was shown by Nakajima, Ishii, and their collaborators.[162,163] Another approach to the detection of right-sided pressure overload was taken by Takeda, who found that the difference in the blood pool phase angles between the right and left ventricles was increased in children with left-to-right shunts and pulmonary hypertension.[164]

In adults with pulmonary hypertension, Friedman and Holman measured right ventricular ejection fraction in the right ventricular free wall in late systole and found it to be abnormally low compared with that of adults with normal pulmonary artery pressures.[165] Subsequently this method was applied to 17 infants with ventricular septal defects.[166] Pinhole collimation was used to delineate the right ventricular free wall from a parametric ejection-fraction image. In these infants, as in Friedman and Holman's adult patients, right ventricular and pulmonary hypertension was accurately detected by low second-half systolic ejection fraction in the right ventricular free wall. In children with septal defects and pulmonary hypertension, the reactivity of the pulmonary vascular bed has been assessed by radionuclide first-pass measurement of left-to-right shunting before and during oxygen inhalation.[167] Patients with nonreactive pulmonary vasculature had Q_p/Q_s ratios of 2.3 or less, which also did not increase with oxygen inhalation.

POSITRON EMISSION TOMOGRAPHY AND SHORT-HALF-LIFE GENERATOR-PRODUCED RADIONUCLIDES

An interesting new development with great potential for pediatric application has been the experimental use of short-half-life radionuclides. Reduction of absorbed radiation dose is of greater importance in children than adults. The new short-lived radionuclides include ^{178}Ta, ^{191m}Ir, ^{195m}Au, and ^{81m}Kr. Tantalum 178 ($t_{1/2} = 9.3$ min), produced from a ^{178}W generator ($t_{1/2} = 21$ d), has a gamma energy too low for optimal use with conventional sodium iodide crystal cameras. Lacy has developed an investigational multiwire scintillation camera that uses multiple conducting wires to register the electron discharge from a xenon gas detector. The camera is able to provide high-resolution images with this radionuclide.[168,169] Because of its short half-life, ^{178}Ta is suitable for gated equilibrium studies, but at a significantly lower radiation dose than ^{99m}Tc. Gold 195m ($t_{1/2} = 30.6$ s), produced from a ^{195m}Hg generator ($t_{1/2} = 41$ h), is suitable for first-pass studies with a conventional gamma camera, again at a reduced absorbed radiation dose.[170,171] Iridium 191m ($t_{1/2} =$

5.0 s), produced by an ^{191}Os generator ($t_{1/2} = 15.4$ d), may be used for first-pass radionuclide angiograms, including first-pass studies of the left ventricle.[172,173] Krypton 81m ($t_{1/2} = 13$ s), produced from a ^{81}Rb generator ($t_{1/2} = 4.6$ h) and administered in saline, has also been given by continuous infusion to study right heart function by the gated technique.[174] The cyclotron-produced positron emitter, ^{15}O ($t_{1/2} = 2$ min), in the form of labeled carbon dioxide, has been used to quantitate left-to-right shunts (see Table 27-1).[175-177] As in adults, the positron emitter ^{82}Rb ($t_{1/2} = 76.4$ s), produced by a ^{82}Sr generator ($t_{1/2} = 25.6$ d), may be substituted for ^{201}Tl for myocardial perfusion imaging.[178,179]

REFERENCES

1. Folse R, Braunwald E: Pulmonary vascular dilution curves recorded by external detection in the diagnosis of left-to-right shunts. *Br Heart J* 24:166, 1962.
2. Rosenthall L: Nucleographic screening of patients for left-to-right cardiac shunts. *Radiology* 99:601, 1971.
3. Gould BA, Turner J, Keeling DH, et al: Bedside nuclear probe for detection and quantification of left to right intracardiac shunts. *Br Heart J* 59:463, 1988.
4. Hagan AD, Friedman WF, Ashburn WL, et al: Further application of scintillation scanning technics to the diagnosis and management of infants and children with congenital heart disease. *Circulation* 45:858, 1972.
5. Clarke JM, Deegan T, McKendrick CS, et al: Technetium-99m in the diagnosis of left-to-right shunts. *Thorax* 21:79, 1966.
6. Kinoshita M, Nakao K, Nohara Y, et al: Detection of circulatory shunts by means of external counting method: Differentiation between ASD and VSD, semiquantitative estimation of left-to-right shunt, and the detection of right-to-left shunt. *Jpn Circ J* 33:815, 1969.
7. Alazraki NP, Ashburn WL, Hagan A, et al: Detection of left-to-right cardiac shunts with the scintillation camera pulmonary dilution curve. *J Nucl Med* 13:142, 1972.
8. Rosenthall L, Mercer EN: Intravenous radionuclide cardiography for the detection of cardiovascular shunts. *Radiology* 106:601, 1973.
9. Maltz DL, Treves S: Quantitative radionuclide angiocardiography: Determination of $Q_p:Q_s$ in children. *Circulation* 47:1049, 1973.
10. Van Aswegen A, Lotter MG, Minnaar PC, et al: Die vasstelling van linker-na-regte kardiale aftakkings met behulp van gamma-kamera-flikkergrafie. *S Afr Med J* 47:1700, 1973.
11. Alderson PO, Jost RG, Strauss AW, et al: Radionuclide angiocardiography: Improved diagnosis and quantitation of left-to-right shunts using area ratio techniques in children. *Circulation* 51:1136, 1975.
12. Flaherty JT, Canent RV Jr, Boineau JP, et al: Use of externally recorded radioisotope-dilution curves for

quantitation of left to right shunts. *Am J Cardiol* 20:341, 1967.

13. Anderson PAW, Jones RH, Sabiston DC Jr: Quantitation of left-to-right cardiac shunts with radionuclide angiography. *Circulation* 49:512, 1974.

14. Gelfand MJ, Breitweser J, Dillon T, et al: Comparison of scintigraphic and echocardiographic methods for estimation of left-to-right shunts. *J Nucl Med* 18:597, 1977 (abstr).

15. Seward JB, Nolan NG, Tancredi RG: Rapid quantitation of left-to-right intracardiac shunts by use of a computer-interfaced gamma camera. *Proceedings of Fifth Symposium on Sharing of Computer Programs and Technology in Nuclear Medicine, Salt Lake City, Utah,* Jan 15–16, 1975 (Conf-750124), pp 66–76.

16. Askenazi J, Ahnberg DS, Korngold E, et al: Quantitative radionuclide angiography: Detection and quantitation of left to right shunts. *Am J Cardiol* 37:382, 1976.

17. Johnson PM, Boxer RA, Esser PD, et al: Quantitative pulmonary radioangiography: A reliable method for measuring left-to-right shunts. *J Nucl Med* 19:745, 1978 (abstr).

18. Alderson PO, Gaudiani VA, Watson DC, et al: Quantitative radionuclide angiocardiography in animals with experimental atrial septal defects. *J Nucl Med* 19:364, 1978.

19. Baker EJ, Ellam SV, Lorber A, et al: Superiority of radionuclide over oximetric measurement of left to right shunts. *Br Heart J* 53:535, 1985.

20. Greenfield LD, Bennett LR: Comparison of heart chamber and pulmonary dilution curves for the diagnosis of cardiac shunts. *Radiology* 111:359, 1974.

21. Treves S, Maltz DL, Adelstein SJ: Intracardiac shunts, in James AE Jr, Wagner HN Jr, Cooke RE (eds): *Pediatric Nuclear Medicine.* Philadelphia, Saunders, 1974, pp 231–246.

22. Lane SD, Patton DD, Staab EV, et al: Simple technique for rapid bolus injection. *J Nucl Med* 13:118, 1972.

23. Treves S, Collins-Nakai R, Ahnberg DS, et al: Quantitative radionuclide angiocardiology (RAC) in premature infants with patent ductus arteriosus (PDA) and respiratory distress syndrome (RDS). *J Nucl Med* 17:554, 1976 (abstr).

24. Alderson PO, Douglass KH, Mendenhall KG, et al: Quantitation of left-to-right cardiac shunts after deconvolution analysis of pulmonary time-activity curves. *J Nucl Med* 19:697, 1978 (abstr).

25. Esser PD: Improved precision in the quantitation of Q_p/Q_s in left-to-right shunts. *J Nucl Med* 19:740, 1978 (abstr).

26. Hurwitz RA, Treves S, Kuruc A: Right ventricular and left ventricular ejection fraction in pediatric patients with normal hearts: First-pass radionuclide angiocardiography. *Am Heart J* 107:726, 1984.

27. Brenner JI, Moschler R, Baker K, et al: Evaluation of left ventricular performance in infants and children using radionuclide angiography. *Pediatr Cardiol* 2:115, 1982.

28. Rabinovitch M, Rosenthal A, Ahnberg DS, et al: Cardiac output determination by radionuclide angiography in patients with congenital heart disease. *Am J Cardiol* 39:309, 1977 (abstr).

29. Covitz W, Eubig C: Modifying nuclear cardiac studies for children. *Clin Res* 27:796A, 1979 (abstr).

30. Jones RH, Scholz PM, Anderson PAW: Radionuclide studies in patients with congenital heart disease. *Cardiovasc Clin* 10:225, 1979.

31. Hurley PJ, Poulose KP, Wagner HN Jr: Radionuclide angiocardiography for detecting right-to-left intracardiac shunts. *J Nucl Med* 10:344, 1969 (abstr).

32. Peter CA, Armstrong BE, Jones RH: Radionuclide quantitation of right-to-left intracardiac shunts in children. *Circulation* 64:572, 1981.

33. Kriss JP, Yeh SH, Farrer PA, et al: Radioisotope angiocardiography. *J Nucl Med* 7:367, 1966 (abstr).

34. Burke G, Halko A, Goldberg D: Dynamic clinical studies with radioisotopes and the scintillation camera. IV. ^{99m}Tc-sodium pertechnetate cardiac blood-flow studies. *J Nucl Med* 10:270, 1969.

35. Graham TP Jr, Goodrich JK, Robinson AE, et al: Scinti-angiocardiography in children: Rapid sequence visualization of the heart and great vessels after intravenous injection of radionuclide. *Am J Cardiol* 25:387, 1970.

36. Hurley PJ, Strauss HW, Wagner HN Jr: Radionuclide angiocardiography in cyanotic congenital heart disease. *Johns Hopkins Med J* 127:46, 1970.

37. Hurley PJ, Strauss HW, Wagner HN Jr: Radionuclide angiography and cine-angiography in screening patients for cardiac disease. *J Nucl Med* 11:633, 1970 (abstr).

38. Kriss JP, Freedman GS, Enright LP, et al: Radioisotopic angiocardiography: Preoperative and postoperative evaluation of patients with diseases of the heart and aorta. *Radiol Clin N Am* 9:369, 1971.

39. Wesselhoeft H, Hurley PJ, Wagner HN Jr: Nuclear angiocardiography in the differential diagnosis of congenital heart disease in infants. *J Nucl Med* 12:406, 1971 (abstr).

40. Alazraki NP, Ashburn WL: Radionuclide imaging in the evaluation of cardiac disease: The role of myocardial perfusion imaging and radionuclide angiography. *J Nucl Biol Med* 16:224, 1972.

41. Hurley PJ, Wesselhoeft H, James AE, Jr: Use of nuclear imaging in the evaluation of pediatric cardiac disease. *Semin Nucl Med* 2:353, 1972.

42. Kriss JP, Enright LP, Hayden WG, et al: Radioisotopic angiocardiography: Findings in congenital heart disease. *J Nucl Med* 13:31, 1972.

43. Freedom RM, Treves S: Splenic scintigraphy and radionuclide venography in the heterotaxy syndrome. *Radiology* 107:381, 1973.

44. Park HM, Smith ET, Silberstein EB: Isolated right superior vena cava draining into left atrium diagnosed by radionuclide angiocardiography. *J Nucl Med* 14:240, 1973.

45. Stocker FP, Kinser J, Weber JW, et al: Pediatric radiocardioangiography. Shunt diagnosis. *Circulation* 47:819, 1973.

46. Treves S, Maltz DL: Radionuclide angiocardiography. *Postgrad Med* 56:99, 1974.

47. Ferrer PL, Gottlieb S. Kallos N, et al: Applications of diagnostic ultrasound and radionuclides to cardiovascular diagnosis. Part II. Cardiovascular disease in the young. *Semin Nucl Med* 5:387, 1975.

48. Stevens JS, Mishkin FS: Persistent left superior vena cava

demonstrated by radionuclide angiography: Case report. *J Nucl Med* 16:469, 1975.

49. Treves S, Collins-Nakai RL: Radioactive tracers in congenital heart disease. *Am J Cardiol* 38:711, 1976.

50. Roguin N, Lam M, Frenkel A, Front D: Radionuclide angiography of azygos continuation of inferior vena cava in left atrial isomerism (polysplenia syndrome). *Clin Nucl Med* 12:708, 1987.

51. Uhrenholdt A: Detection of cardiac right-to-left shunts by external counting of ^{133}Xe. *Scand J Clin Lab Invest* 28:395, 1971.

52. Gates GF: Assessment of radionuclide angiocardiograms using color/time images. *Radiology* 129:483, 1978.

53. Cloutier A, Ash JM, Smallhorn JF, et al: Abnormal distribution of pulmonary blood flow after the Glenn shunt or Fontan procedure: Risk of development of arteriovenous fistulae. *Circulation* 72:471, 1985.

54. Treves ST, Newberger J, Hurwitz R: Radionuclide angiocardiography in children. *J Am Coll Cardiol* 5:120S, 1985.

55. Janos GG, Gelfand MJ, Schwartz DC, et al: Postoperative evaluation of the Fontan procedure by radionuclide angiography. *Am Heart J* 104:785, 1982.

56. Bosnjakovic VB, Bennett LR, Greenfield LD, et al: Dual-isotope method for diagnosis of intracardiac shunts. *J Nucl Med* 14:514, 1973.

57. Tow DE, Wagner HN Jr, Lopez-Majano V, et al: Validity of measuring regional pulmonary arterial blood flow with macroaggregates of human serum albumin. *Am J Roentgenol Radium Ther Nucl Med* 96:664, 1966.

58. Gates GF, Orme HW, Dore EK: Measurement of cardiac shunting with technetium labeled albumin aggregates. *J Nucl Med* 12:746, 1971.

59. Gates GF, Orme HW, Dore EK: Cardiac shunt assessment in children with macroaggregated albumin technetium-99m. *Radiology* 112:649, 1974.

60. Gates GF: *Radionuclide Scanning in Cyanotic Heart Disease.* Springfield, Ill, Thomas, 1974.

61. Gates GF: *Radionuclide Scanning in Cyanotic Heart Disease.* Springfield, Ill, Thomas, 1974, p 35.

62. Gates GF, Goris ML: Suitability of radiopharmaceuticals for determining right-to-left shunting: Concise communication. *J Nucl Med* 18:255, 1977.

63. Hurley PJ: Patent foramen ovale demonstrated by lung scanning. *J Nucl Med* 13:177, 1972.

64. Gates GF: *Radionuclide Scanning in Congenital Heart Disease.* Springfield, Ill, Thomas, 1974, p 28.

65. Gates GF: *Radionuclide Scanning in Congenital Heart Disease.* Springfield, Ill, Thomas, 1974, pp 9–11.

66. Kennady JC, Taplin GV: Albumin macroaggregates for brain scanning: Experimental basis and safety in primates. *J Nucl Med* 6:566, 1965.

67. Murphy E, Cervantes C, Maass R: Radioalbumin macroaggregate brain scanning: A histopathologic investigation. *Am J Roentgenol Radium Ther Nucl Med* 102:88, 1968.

68. King EG, Wood DE, Morley TP: The use of macroaggregates of radioiodinated human serum albumin in brain scanning. *Can Med Assoc J* 95:381, 1966.

69. Rosenthall L: Human brain scanning with radioiodinated

70. Kanafani SB, Constantino GL: Perfusion I-131 macroaggregate brain scanning: A clinical evaluation of its diagnostic efficiency. *Am J Roentgenol Radium Ther Nucl Med* 106:333, 1969.

71. Verhas M, Schoutens A, Demol O, et al: Use of ^{99m}Tc-labeled albumin microspheres in cerebral vascular disease. *J Nucl Med* 17:170, 1976.

72. Gates GF, Orme HW, Dore EK: The hyperperfused lung: Detection in congenital heart disease. *JAMA* 233:782, 1975.

73. Fort L III, Morrow AG, Pierce GE, et al: The distribution of pulmonary blood flow after subclavian-pulmonary anastomosis: An experimental study. *J Thorac Cardiovasc Surg* 50:671, 1965.

74. Oldham HN Jr, Simpson L, Jones RH, et al: Differential distribution of pulmonary blood flow following aorto-pulmonary anastomosis. *Surg Forum* 21:201, 1970.

75. Friedman WF, Braunwald E, Morrow AG: Alterations in regional pulmonary blood flow in patients with congenital heart disease studied by radioisotope scanning. *Circulation* 37:747, 1968.

76. Haroutunian LM, Neill CA, Wagner HN Jr: Radioisotope scanning of the lung in cyanotic congenital heart disease. *Am J Cardiol* 23:387, 1969.

77. Tong ECK, Liu L, Potter RT, et al: Macroaggregated RISA lung scan in congenital heart disease. *Radiology* 106:585, 1973.

78. Mishkin F, Knote J: Radioisotope scanning of the lungs in patients with systemic-pulmonary anastomoses. *Am J Roentgenol Radium Ther Nucl Med* 102:267, 1968.

79. Draulans-Noe HA, Evenblij H: The value of radioisotope scanning in the study of pulmonary circulation in patients with tetralogy of Fallot and systemic pulmonary anastomosis. *J Nucl Med Biol* 16:145, 1972.

80. Puyau FA, Meckstroth GR: Evaluation of pulmonary perfusion patterns in children with tetralogy of Fallot. *Am J Roentgenol* 122:119, 1974.

81. Alderson PO, Boonvisut S, McKnight RC, et al: Pulmonary perfusion abnormalities and ventilation perfusion imbalance in children after total repair of tetralogy of Fallot. *Circulation* 53:332, 1976.

82. Vidne B, Duszynski D, Subramanian S: Pulmonary flow distribution in transposition of the great arteries. *Am J Cardiol* 37:178, 1976 (abstr).

83. Lin C-Y: Lung scan in cardiopulmonary disease. I. Tetralogy of Fallot. *J Thorac Cardiovasc Surg* 61:370, 1971.

84. Gates GF, Orme HW, Dore EK: Surgery of congenital heart disease assessed by radionuclide scintigraphy. *J Thorac Cardiovasc Surg* 69:767, 1975.

85. Tamir A, Melloul M, Berant M, et al: Lung perfusion scans in patients with congenital heart defects. *J Am Coll Cardiol* 19:383, 1992.

86. Baker EJ, Malamitsi J, Jones ODH, et al: Use of radionuclide labeled microspheres to show the distribution of the pulmonary perfusion with multifocal pulmonary blood supply. *Br Heart J* 52:72, 1984.

87. Covitz W, Eubig C: Radionuclide studies of the circulation, special technical considerations in children, in Fried-

man WF, Higgins CB (eds): *Pediatric Cardiac Imaging.* Philadelphia, Saunders, 1984, p 92.

88. Millar AM, Wathen CG, Muir AL: Failure of labelling of red blood cells with ^{99m}Tc: Interaction between intravenous cannulae and stannous pyrophosphate. *Eur J Nucl Med* 8:502, 1983.

89. Package insert. Technetium-99m-HSA unit dose. Emeryville, California, Medi-Physics, Inc., 1981.

90. Package insert. Technescan PYP. St Louis, Mallinckrodt, 1984.

91. Hannon DW, Gelfand MJ, Bailey WW, et al: Pinhole radionuclide ventriculography in small infants. *Am Heart J* 111:316, 1986.

92. Gelfand MJ, Williams PJ, Rosenkrantz JG: Pinhole imaging: Utility in testicular imaging in children. *Clin Nucl Med* 5:237, 1980.

93. Hurley PJ, Strauss HW, Pavoni P, et al: The scintillation camera with pinhole collimator in thyroid imaging. *Radiology* 101:133, 1971.

94. Danigelis JA, Fisher RL, Ozonoff MB, et al: ^{99m}Tc-polyphosphate bone imaging in Legg-Perthes disease. *Radiology* 115:407, 1975.

95. Green MV, Cannon RO, Findley SL, et al: A method for in vivo assessment of cardiac function in small animals. *J Am Coll Cardiol* 1:710, 1983 (abstr).

96. Janos GG, Gelfand MJ, Benzing G, et al: Radionuclide angiography and ventriculography after open heart surgery. *J Nucl Med* 22:P37, 1981 (abstr).

97. Schaffer MS, deSouza M, Olley PM, et al: Qualitative phase analysis in pediatric nuclear cardiology: Isolation of cardiac chambers and identification of asynchronous contraction patterns. *Pediatr Cardiol* 5:179, 1984.

98. Parrish MD, Graham TP Jr, Born ML, et al: Radionuclide ventriculography for assessment of absolute right and left ventricular volumes in children. *Circulation* 66:811, 1982.

99. Guiteras P, Green M, DeSouza M, et al: Count based scintigraphic method to calculate ventricular volumes in children: In vitro and clinical validation. *J Am Coll Cardiol* 5:963, 1985.

100. Parrish MD, Grahm TP Jr, Born ML, et al: Radionuclide stroke count ratios for assessment of right and left ventricular volume overload in children. *Am J Cardiol* 51:261, 1983.

101. Hurwitz RA, Treves S, Freed M, et al: Quantitation of aortic and mitral regurgitation in the pediatric population: Evaluation by radionuclide angiocardiography. *Am J Cardiol* 51:252, 1983.

102. Covitz W, Eubig C, Moore HV, et al: Assessment of cardiac and renal function in children immediately after open-heart surgery: The significance of a reduced radionuclide ejection fraction (postoperative ejection fraction). *Pediatr Cardiol* 5:167, 1984.

103. Hammon JW Jr, Graham TP Jr, Boucek RJ Jr, et al: Myocardial adenosine triphosphate content as a measure of metabolic and functional myocardial protection in children undergoing cardiac operation. *Ann Thorac Surg* 44:467, 1987.

104. Hannon DW, Gelfand MJ: Unpublished data.

105. Hurwitz RA, Papanicolaou N, Treves S, et al: Radionuclide angiocardiography in evaluation of patients after repair of transposition of the great arteries. *Am J Cardiol* 49:761, 1982.

106. Hurwitz RA, Caldwell RL, Girod DA, et al: Ventricular function in transposition of the great arteries: Evaluation by radionuclide angiocardiography. *Am Heart J* 110:600, 1985.

107. Bove EL, Byrum CJ, Thomas FD, et al: The influence of pulmonary insufficiency on ventricular function following repair of tetralogy of Fallot: Evaluation using radionuclide ventriculography. *J Thorac Cardiovasc Surg* 85:691, 1983.

108. Bove EL, Kavey RE, Byrum CJ, et al: Improved right ventricular function following late pulmonary valve replacement for residual pulmonary insufficiency or stenosis. *J Thorac Cardiovasc Surg* 90:50, 1985.

109. Kavey RE, Bove EL, Byrum CJ, et al: Postoperative functional assessment of a modified surgical approach to repair of tetralogy of Fallot. *J Thorac Cardiovasc Surg* 93:533, 1987.

110. Burns RJ, Liu PP, Druck MN, et al: Analysis of adults with and without complex ventricular arrhythmias after repair of tetralogy of Fallot. *J Am Coll Cardiol* 4:226, 1984.

111. Kavey E, Thomas FD, Byrum CJ, et al: Ventricular arrhythmias and biventricular dysfunction after repair of tetralogy of Fallot. *J Am Coll Cardiol* 4:126, 1984.

112. Suda K, Iwatani H, Mori C, et al: Radionuclide assessment of left ventricular performance on exercise after external conduit operation. *Acta Paediat Jap* 35:283, 1993.

113. Akagi T, Benson LN, Green M, et al: Ventricular performance before and after Fontan repair for univentricular atrioventricular connection: Angiographic and radionuclide assessment. *J Am Coll Cardiol* 20:920, 1992.

114. Hutter JJ Jr, Sahn DJ, Woolfenden JM, et al: Evaluation of the cardiac effects of doxorubicin by serial echocardiography. *Am J Dis Child* 135:653, 1981.

115. Druck MN, Gulenchyn KY, Evans WK, et al: Radionuclide angiography and endomyocardial biopsy in the assessment of doxorubicin cardiotoxicity. *Cancer* 53:1667, 1984.

116. Parrish MD, Boucek RJ Jr, Burger J, et al: Exercise radionuclide ventriculography in children: Normal values for exercise variables and right and left ventricular function. *Br Heart J* 54:509, 1985.

117. Baker EJ, Jones ODH, Joseph MC, et al: Radionuclide measurement of left ventricular ejection fraction in tricuspid atresia. *Br Heart J* 52:572, 1984.

118. Harder JR, Gilday DL, de Souza M, et al: Radionuclide assessment of left ventricular function in patients with tricuspid atresia. *Am J Cardiol* 47:431, 1981 (abstr).

119. Reduto LA, Berger HJ, Johnstone DE, et al: Radionuclide assessment of right and left ventricular exercise reserve after total correction of tetralogy of Fallot. *Am J Cardiol* 45:1013, 1980.

120. Parrish MD, Graham TP Jr, Bender HW, et al: Radionuclide angiographic evaluation of right and left ventricular function during exercise after repair of transposition of the great arteries: Comparison with normal subjects and patients with congenitally corrected transposition. *Circulation* 67:178, 1983.

121. Murphy JH, Barlai-Kovach MM, Mathews RA, et al: Rest and exercise right and left ventricular function late after the Mustard operation: Assessment by radionuclide ventriculography. *Am J Cardiol* 51:1520, 1983.

122. Benson LN, Bonet J, McLaughlin P, et al: Assessment of right ventricular function during supine bicycle exercise after Mustard's operation. *Circulation* 65:1052, 1982.

123. Covitz W, Eubig C, Balfour IC, et al: Exercise-induced cardiac dysfunction in sickle cell anemia: A radionuclide study. *Am J Cardiol* 51:570, 1983.

124. Leon MB, Borer JS, Bacharach SL, et al: Detection of early cardiac dysfunction in patients with severe beta-thalassemia and chronic iron overload. *N Engl J Med* 301:1143, 1979.

125. Benson LN, Child JS, Schwaiger M, et al: Left ventricular geometry and function in adults with Ebstein's anomaly of the tricuspid valve. *Circulation* 75:353, 1987.

126. Chipps BE, Alderson PO, Roland JMA, et al: Noninvasive evaluation of ventricular function in cystic fibrosis. *J Pediatr* 95:379, 1979.

127. Iorio F, Ferro-Luzzi M, Genuini I, et al: Equilibrium radionuclide ventriculography in Duchenne's cardiomyopathy. *Nucl Med Commun* 9:357, 1988.

128. Hurwitz RA, Siddique A, Caldwell RL, et al: Assessment of ventricular function in infants and children: Response to dobutamine infusion. *Clin Nucl Med* 15:556, 1990.

129. Schaffer MS, de Souza M, Gilday DL, et al: Exercise radionuclide right ventriculography in children. *Pediatr Cardiol* 8:235, 1987.

130. Shaffer EM, Rocchini AP, Spicer RL, et al: Effects of verapamil on left ventricular diastolic filling in children with hypertrophic cardiomyopathy. *Am J Cardiol* 61:413, 1988.

131. Akagi T, Benson LN, Gilday DL, et al: Influence of ventricular morphology on diastolic filling performance in double-inlet ventricle after the Fontan procedure. *J Am Coll Cardiol* 22:1948, 1993.

132. Finley JP, Howman-Giles R, Gilday DL, et al: Thallium-201 myocardial imaging in anomalous left coronary artery arising from the pulmonary artery: Application before and after medical and surgical treatment. *Am J Cardiol* 42:675, 1978.

133. Rabinovitch M, Rowland TW, Castaneda AR, et al: Thallium-201 scintigraphy in patients with anomalous origin of the left coronary artery from the main pulmonary artery. *J Pediatr* 94:244, 1979.

134. Seguchi M, Nakanishi T, Nakazawa M, et al: Myocardial perfusion after aortic implantation for anomalous origin of the left coronary artery from the pulmonary artery. *Eur Heart J* 11:213, 1990.

135. Raifer SI, Oetgen WJ, Weeks KD Jr, et al: Thallium-201 scintigraphy after surgical repair of hemodynamically significant primary coronary artery anomalies. *Chest* 81:687, 1982.

136. Treves S, Hill TC, Van Praagh R, et al: Computed tomography of the heart using thallium 201 in children. *Radiology* 132:707, 1979.

137. Ueda K, Saito A, Nakano H, et al: Thallium-201 scintigraphy in an infant with myocardial infarction following mucocutaneous lymph node syndrome. *Pediatr Radiol* 9:183, 1980.

138. Kato H, Ichinose E, Yoshioka F, et al: Fate of coronary aneurysms in Kawasaki disease: Serial coronary angiography and long-term follow-up study. *Am J Cardiol* 49:1758, 1982.

139. Miyagawa M, Murase K, Mochizaki T, et al: Assessment of stress thallium-201 myocardial emission tomography in Kawasaki disease. *J Nucl Med* 29:791, 1988 (abstr).

140. Kondo C, Hiroe M, Nakanishi T, Takao A: Detection of coronary artery stenosis in children with Kawasaki disease: Usefulness of pharmacologic stress ^{201}Tl myocardial tomography. *Circulation* 80:615, 1989.

141. Ono Y, Kohata T, Iwatani H, et al: Usefulness and limitations of stress 201-thallium myocardial imaging in patients with Kawasaki disease. *J Cardiol* 21:437, 1991.

142. Paridon SM, Gallioto FM, Vincent JM, et al: Exercise capacity and incidence of myocardial perfusion defects after Kawasaki disease in children and adolescents. *J Am Coll Cardiol* 25:1420, 1995.

143. Tatara L, Kusakawa S, Itoh K, et al: Collateral circulation in Kawasaki disease with coronary occlusion or severe stenosis. *Am Heart J* 121:797, 1991.

144. Bertrand A: Kawasaki disease: Unsafe at any age? *J Am Coll Cardiol* 25:1425, 1995.

145. Sty JR, Chusid MJ, Dorrington A: Ga-67 imaging: Kawasaki disease. *Clin Nucl Med* 6:112, 1981.

146. Williamson MR, Williamson SL, Seibert JJ: Indium-111 leukocyte scanning localization for detecting early myocarditis in Kawasaki disease. *AJR* 146:255, 1986.

147. Kao CH, Hsieh KS, Chen YC, et al: Labeled WBC cardiac imaging and two-dimensional echocardiography to evaluate high-dose gamma globulin treatment in Kawasaki disease. *Clin Nucl Med* 20:813, 1995.

148. Gilday DL, de Souza M: Pediatric nuclear cardiology, in Come PC (ed): *Diagnostic Cardiology Noninvasive Imaging Technique.* New York, Lippincott, 1985, p 168.

149. Neill C, Kelly D, Bailey I, et al: Thallium-201 myocardial scintigraphy in single ventricle. *Circulation* 53–54 (suppl II):II-46, 1976 (abstr).

150. Finley JP, Howman-Giles RB, Gilday DL, et al: Transient myocardial ischemia of the newborn infant demonstrated by thallium myocardial imaging. *J Pediatr* 94:263, 1979.

151. Saji T, Matsuo N, Hashiguchi R, et al: Radionuclide imaging for assessment of myocarditis and postmyocarditic state in infants and children: Thallium-201 myocardial imaging and technetium-99m-HSA gated equilibrium ventriculography. *Jpn Heart J* 26:413, 1985.

152. Perloff JK, Henze E, Schelbert HR: Alterations in regional myocardial metabolism, perfusion, and wall motion in Duchenne muscular dystrophy studied by radionuclide imaging. *Circulation* 69:33, 1984.

153. Hellenbrand WE, Berger HJ, O'Brien RT, et al: Left ventricular performance in thalassemia: Combined noninvasive radionuclide and echocardiographic assessment. *Circulation* 55-56 (suppl III):III-49, 1977 (abstr).

154. Nagamachi S, Jinnouchi S, Hoshi H, et al: Serial changes of the myocardium in patients with Duchenne's muscular dystrophy followed by cardiac nuclear imaging: 5 years' observation. *Nippon Acta Radiologica* 50:1415, 1990.

155. Tamura T, Shibuya N, Hashiba K, et al: Evaluation of myocardial damage in Duchenne's muscular dystrophy

with thallium-201 myocardial SPECT. *Jpn Heart J* 34:51, 1993.

156. Nagamachi S, Inoue K, Jinnouchi S, et al: Cardiac involvement of progressive muscular dystrophy (Becker type, limb-girdle type and Fukuyama type) evaluated by radionuclide method. *Ann Nucl Med* 8:71, 1994

157. Flynn B, Wernovsky G, Summerville DA, et al: Comparison of technetium-99m MIBI and thallium-201 chloride myocardial scintigraphy in infants. *J Nucl Med* 30:1176, 1989.

158. Vogel M, Smallhorn JF, Gilday D, et al: Assessment of myocardial perfusion in patients after the arterial switch operation. *J Nucl Med* 32:237, 1991.

159. Weindling SN, Wernovsky G, Colan SD, et al: Myocardial perfusion, function and exercise tolerance after the arterial switch operation. *J Am Coll Cardiol* 23:424, 1994.

160. Hayes AM, Baker EJ, Kakadeker A, et al: Influence of anatomic correction for transposition of the great arteries on myocardial perfusion: Radionuclide imaging with technetium-99m 2-methoxyisobutyl isonitrile. *J Am Coll Cardiol* 24:769, 1994.

161. Rabinovitch M, Fischer KC, Treves S: Quantitative thallium-201 myocardial imaging in assessing right ventricular pressure in patients with congenital heart defects. *Br Heart J* 45:198, 1981.

162. Nakajima K, Taki J, Ohno T, et al: Assessment of right ventricular overload by a thallium-201 SPECT study in children with congenital heart disease. *J Nucl Med* 32:2215, 1991.

163. Ishii I, Nakajima K, Taki J, et al: Assessment of congenital heart disease by a thallium-201 SPECT study in children: Accuracy of estimated right to left ventricular pressure ratio. *Jpn J Nucl Med* 30:41, 1993.

164. Takeda K: Ventricular performance in congenital left-to-right shunt: Temporal Fourier analysis of gated blood-pool data. *J Nucl Med* 24:829, 1983.

165. Friedman BJ, Holman BL: Scintigraphic prediction of pulmonary arterial systolic pressure by regional right ventricular ejection fraction during the second half of systole. *Am J Cardiol* 50:1114, 1982.

166. Hannon DW, Gelfand MJ, Kaplan S: Radionuclide regional RV ejection fraction detects pulmonary hypertension in infants with VSD. *Circulation* 72 (suppl III):III-30, 1985 (abstr).

167. Fujii AM, Rabinovitch M, Keane JF, et al: Radionuclide angiocardiographic assessment of pulmonary vascular reactivity in patients with left to right shunt and pulmonary hypertension. *Am J Cardiol* 49:356, 1982.

168. LeBlanc AD, Lacy JL, Johnson PC, et al: Ta-178 as an imaging agent for Anger and multicrystal cameras. *J Nucl Med* 22:P75, 1981 (abstr).

169. Babich JW, LeBlanc AD, Lacy J, et al: Biological fate of tungsten-178 and tantalum-178. *J Nucl Med* 24: P122, 1983 (abstr).

170. Brihaye C, Guillaume M, Lavi N, et al: Development of a reliable Hg-195m-Au-195m generator for the production of Au-195m, a short-lived nuclide for vascular imaging. *J Nucl Med* 23:1114, 1982.

171. Mena I, Narahara KA, deJong R, et al: Gold-195m, an ultra short-lived generator produced radionuclide: Clinical application in sequential first pass ventriculography. *J Nucl Med* 24:139, 1983.

172. Treves S, Kulprathipanja S, Hnatowich DJ: Angiocardiography with iridium-191m: An ultrashort-lived radionuclide (T 4.9 sec). *Circulation* 54:275, 1976.

173. Cheng C, Treves S, Samuel A, et al: A new osmium-191-iridium-191m generator. *J Nucl Med* 21:1169, 1980.

174. Knapp WH, Helus F, Lambrecht RM, et al: Kr-81m for determination of right ventricular ejection fraction (RVEF). *Eur J Nucl Med* 5:487, 1980.

175. Boucher CA, Beller GA, Ahluwalia B, et al: Inhalation imaging for detection and quantitation of left-to-right shunts. *Circulation* 53–54(suppl II):II-145, 1976 (abstr).

176. Watson D, Janowitz W, Kenny P, et al: Detection of left-to-right shunts by inhalation of oxygen-15 labelled carbon dioxide. *Circulation* 53–54(suppl II):II-145, 1976 (abstr).

177. Watson DD, Kenay PJ, Janowitz WR, et al: Detection of left-to-right shunts by inhalation of oxygen-15 labelled carbon dioxide, in Serafini AN, Gilson AJ, Smoak Wm (eds): *Nuclear Cardiology: Principles and Methods.* New York, Plenum, 1977, pp 49–63.

178. Neirinckx RD, Kronauge JF, Gennaro GP, et al: Evaluation of inorganic absorbents for the rubidium-82 generator: I. Hydrous SnO_2. *J Nucl Med* 23:245, 1982.

179. Goldstein RA, Mullani NA, Marani SK, et al: Myocardial perfusion with rubidium-82. II. Effects of metabolic and pharmacologic interventions. *J Nucl Med* 24:907, 1983.

Imaging Intracardiac Thrombi with Nuclear Medicine Techniques

John R. Stratton

Intracardiac thrombi include those in the coronary arteries, in the cardiac chambers (left ventricular, left atrial, or right heart), and those attached to valves (valve thrombi and valvular vegetations). The clinical importance of the thrombus depends on its location. Coronary artery thrombi cause most acute myocardial infarctions and sudden cardiac deaths as well as some episodes of unstable angina. Thrombi in the right heart can cause pulmonary emboli, and thrombi in the left atrium or ventricle or on left-sided valves can embolize and cause stroke or organ ischemia. Overall, it is estimated that approximately 15 percent of all strokes are due to cardiac emboli, most commonly from the left atrium or left ventricle.[1,2] Thus, intracardiac thrombi are of great importance in clinical medicine.

Given the central role of intracardiac thrombi in causing disease, the development of noninvasive, or minimally invasive, methods capable of diagnosing the presence of intracardiac thrombi and their response to therapy would have great clinical benefit. Thrombosis imaging using nuclear medicine techniques involves the injection of a radioactive tracer that preferentially accumulates in thrombi. To date, no widely available and accurate nuclear imaging method of detecting the majority of intracardiac thrombi has been developed, but significant progress has been made.

The main focus of this chapter is to review the use of nuclear medicine techniques to detect intracardiac thrombi in humans. Where possible, nuclear medicine techniques are compared with other more conventional and widely available methods. Multiple new approaches to thrombus detection using nuclear medicine techniques are being explored in animal models, including the labeling of monoclonal antibodies directed against platelets, fibrin, or other thrombus components, or the labeling of other compounds such as tissue plasminogen activator (t-PA) or annexin V that localize in thrombi. To this point, however, nearly all nuclear medicine imaging of intracardiac thrombi in humans has utilized indium-111 (^{111}In)-labeled platelets. Thus, the majority of information presented in this chapter relates to ^{111}In platelet imaging.

PLATELET-LABELING AND IMAGING TECHNIQUES

By far, the most technically challenging part of platelet imaging is the preparation of a viable population of labeled platelets, since platelets can be relatively easily damaged during the labeling process by improper centrifugation, the use of normal saline, or the use of improper anticoagulant or pH. Damaged platelets may have reduced survival or aggregability and may not participate in thrombosis.[3] Despite the traumas of labeling, several studies have demonstrated near-normal aggregation patterns of labeled platelets by using several labeling techniques,[4-13] and Thakur and associates reported no marked change in the ultrastructure of labeled platelets when using their labeling methods.[12,14] Moreover, platelet recovery[4,5,7,15-17] and survival[18-22] with ^{111}In platelets have been comparable to those achieved with chromium-51 labeling. Additional evidence that labeled platelets retain viability is the demonstration of labeled platelet uptake in areas of active thrombosis.

Thakur and associates[11] originally described the preparation of ^{111}In–oxine-labeled platelets in 1976. Subsequently, several other methods have been described.[2-25] Several steps are common to all labeling approaches. Initially, platelets are separated from other blood cells and plasma. Whole blood is drawn into an anticoagulant mixture, and platelet-rich plasma is separated by a "soft" centrifugation (640 to 2000 g). A platelet pellet is then formed, washed, and resuspended in plasma, Ringer citrate dextrose, modified Tyrode solution, or another physiologic solution. Indium alone will not penetrate the platelet membrane because it is not lipid soluble, so indium is complexed to oxine or another chelate. The platelets are incubated with the indium chelate mixture for up to 30 min. The labeled platelets are then typically recentrifuged, washed, and resuspended in autologous platelet-poor plasma. The injected dose ranges between 100 and 500 μCi in human studies. Depending on the technique, labeling requires 30 min to $3\frac{1}{2}$ h. Contamination with other cells (leukocytes and erythrocytes) has been estimated to be less than 5 percent.[18] Different labeling methods vary with regard to the blood volume utilized, the chelate (oxine, tropolone, acetylacetone, or mercaptopyridine-N-oxide), the centrifugal forces, the medium in which platelets are labeled (acid citrate dextrose, saline, plasma, or Tyrode buffer), the labeling efficiency, and the duration of the procedure. Techniques also vary as to whether the platelets are labeled in an open test tube, using a laminar flow hood to minimize airborne contamination, or in a closed blood-bag system, which effectively eliminates the possibility of airborne contamination.

Once the ^{111}In complex is inside the cell, the oxine or other ligand is probably displaced, with subsequent binding of the ^{111}In to intracellular components (cytoplasmic proteins, organelles, and the cell membrane) almost irreversibly. Over 70 percent of the ^{111}In is located in the platelet cytosol,[6,23] and the remainder is distributed between the α and dense granules and the platelet membrane. Our studies and others have noted that less than 5 to 10 percent of the ^{111}In is "free" unattached indium following intravenous injection, and that there is minimal elution of ^{111}In over time.[24,25]

Several authors have described preliminary studies using a technetium-99m (^{99m}Tc)-based label, the lipophilic ^{99m}Tc–HMPAO complex.[26-33] With these methods, the label is continuously lost from the platelets, which leads to renal excretion of the label and to significant kidney and bladder activity.

Radiation dosimetry in humans for ^{111}In-labeled platelets based on Medical Internal Radiation Dose estimates has been reported. For each 1 mCi injected, the estimated spleen dose is 30 rad, the red marrow dose is 1.1 rad, the liver dose is 2.1 rad, the male gonad dose is 0.25 rad, the ovarian dose is 0.46 rad, the blood dose is 0.52 rad, and the remainder of the body dose is 0.58 rad.[34] Because of the splenic dose, although it is within acceptable limits, we limit the total injected dose to 0.33 mCi per study and the total injected dose to 1 mCi per year. We do not study women of childbearing potential.

Imaging Techniques

Indium-111 releases two gamma rays at 171 and 245 keV that are responsible for 87 percent of the energy released. The 4-day half-life of normal circulating platelets corresponds reasonably well to the 2.8-day half-life of ^{111}In, thus allowing the assessment of the dynamics of platelet deposition over most of the platelet life span.

The key points in imaging ^{111}In platelets are to image long enough at each imaging time to get adequate counts and to image late enough following platelet injection to achieve the optimal thrombus-to-background ratio. Simultaneous collection of both 171- and 245-keV photopeaks of ^{111}In is desirable. We use a medium-energy parallel-hole collimator and 15 to 20 percent energy windows. The low count rates obtained from cardiac structures necessitates relatively long imaging times. For planar images of the thorax and heart, we typically obtain 300,000 counts per view. Due to the long platelet life span, there is substantial blood-pool background for several days following injection. Therefore, serial imaging over a period of 4 to 5 days is usually necessary to distinguish areas of thrombosis from circulating blood-pool activity. Thrombi typically become progressively more apparent on later images because of continued accumulation of labeled platelets over time, as well as a reduction in the circulating background blood pool as senescent platelets are removed from the circulation.

Extended imaging clearly improves lesion detection; in one study of patients with left ventricular thrombi, only half of the images were positive at 24 h after injection compared with images obtained at 48 or 72 h.[35] Despite the low count rates, we have found tomographic imaging of labeled platelets to be feasible; tomographic imaging probably improves thrombus detection as well as enabling improved quantification of platelet uptake.[36,37]

Image Quantitation Techniques

There are no standardized approaches for quantification of ^{111}In-labeled platelet images in humans.[38] Experimental studies have demonstrated that small areas of deposition, or relatively large changes induced by drugs, cannot be adequately assessed by simple visual analysis of the images,[39] emphasizing the need for accurate quantitative techniques. To quantify thrombus activity, localized platelet activity in a region has been compared with a noninvolved area in the same image, with simultaneously collected whole blood activity, with injected ^{111}In dose, or with whole body activity. Although no quantitative methods have been validated in human studies, several techniques have been assessed in animal models. Blood-pool subtraction techniques have been attempted in order to subtract the circulating blood-pool activity.[40–42] Blood-pool subtraction has offered no clear-cut improvement compared with other methods either for thrombus detection or for quantification.[43–45] The superiority of blood-pool subtraction techniques to simpler methods has not been established, and it is quite possible to generate artifacts by using blood-pool subtraction that can be misinterpreted as thrombi.

LEFT VENTRICULAR THROMBI

Background

Left ventricular thrombi are important because they cause embolic stroke and systemic emboli. Overall, it is estimated that approximately 25 percent of all cardiogenic emboli are due to left ventricular thrombi.[46] Nearly all left ventricular thrombi occur in one of two settings: prior anterior myocardial infarction or dilated cardiomyopathy.

The majority of left ventricular thrombi form at the time of an acute anterior myocardial infarction. Left ventricular thrombi form in approximately 30 percent of patients with acute anterior infarction not treated with thrombolytics or early full-dose heparin, but almost never (less than 1 percent) in other types of infarction such as nontransmural, lateral, or inferior infarction.[46] In the setting of acute infarction, if a left ventricular thrombus forms, the risk of an embolic event is quite high at approximately 15 percent within the first 4 weeks in the absence of anticoagulation.[46,47] Although early heparin therapy reduces the development of left ventricular thrombi in acute anterior myocardial infarction, 11 to 18 percent of patients with anterior infarction treated with full-dose heparin still develop left ventricular thrombi, compared with 32 to 37 percent of untreated patients.[48,49] In addition, in a GISSI-II (Gruppo Italizao per lo Studio della Sopravvivenza sell'Infarto) substudy, even patients with acute anterior infarction treated with thrombolytic agents (t-PA or streptokinase) plus high-dose subcutaneous heparin (12,500 b.i.d.) still had a 27 percent incidence of left ventricular thrombi.[50] Thus, even with contemporary management of acute anterior infarction, a relatively high percentage will develop ventricular thrombi that can serve as a significant risk for emboli.

Although some of the left ventricular thrombi that form with acute infarction resolve spontaneously or with anticoagulant therapy, a significant proportion remain and become chronic left ventricular thrombi.[46] In the largest available study, 13 percent of patients (137 of 1071) with remote (less than 1 month) anterior infarction had left ventricular thrombi.[51] Thus, a substantial proportion of patients with acute anterior infarction will go on to have chronic left ventricular thrombi. The embolic risk of a chronic left ventricular thrombus is clearly less than that of an acute thrombus, but still significant. In retrospective studies of patients with chronic left ventricular thrombi, Kneissl et al[51] noted that 8 percent of patients with chronic thrombus had a prior history of an embolic event compared with only 1 percent of patients without a left ventricular thrombus. Similarly, we found that 19 percent of patients with left ventricular thrombus had a prior embolic event compared with 5 percent of controls.[52] In a prospective study of patients with chronic thrombi, almost all due to prior anterior infarction, we noted an embolic rate of 7 percent per year.[52] Thus, chronic left ventricular thrombi represent an embolic risk similar to that seen with chronic atrial fibrillation of approximately 5 to 7 percent per year.

The second setting in which left ventricular thrombi occur is with idiopathic dilated congestive cardiomyopathy. The prevalence of left ventricular thrombi in patients with nonischemic cardiomyopathies has been very variably reported, ranging from 11 to 60 percent.[53–56] There are many fewer data regarding the embolic risk in these subjects, but it is reasonable to expect based on limited data that the embolic risk is similar to that seen with left ventricular thrombi due to myocardial infarction.[53,56] For example, Falk and colleagues found an embolic rate of 27 percent over a mean follow-up of 22 months in 25 patients with nonischemic cardiomyopathy with left ventricular thrombi.[53]

Diagnosis of Left Ventricular Thrombi by Indium-111 Platelet Imaging

Indium-111 platelet imaging can detect left ventricular thrombi in humans (Figs. 28-1 and 28-2).[35,45–47,52,57–77] Delayed imaging in multiple views is essential for accurate thrombus detection.[62,78] Of the first 10 patients with left ventricular thrombi studied in our laboratory, none were positive at 2 h following platelet injection and half were positive at 24 h, while all were positive at 48 to 72 h following injection.[78] Similarly, Ezekowitz et al noted that the sensitivity of platelet imaging increased two to three fold at 3 to 4 days compared with earlier imaging at 1 to 2 days after platelet injection.[62] Early imaging, however, is useful because it defines the area

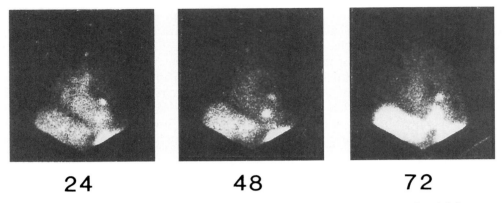

Figure 28-1 Anterior, 300,000-count images are shown obtained at 24, 48, and 72 h following injection of ^{111}In platelets in a patient with a large left ventricular thrombus. In the 24-h image, there is relatively marked blood-pool activity present in the region of the heart, with a possible hot spot on the superior portion of the cardiac silhouette. The liver is in the *lower left* portion of the image and the spleen is in the *lower right* portion of the image. On the 48-h image, the area of increased uptake is more pronounced relative to the circulating blood-pool activity in the remainder of the heart. On the 72-h image, the uptake is even more apparent. This series of images demonstrates that late imaging of left ventricular thrombi is typically necessary.

of the blood pool with the greatest activity. Hot spots appearing later can be assumed to be due to thrombi. For example, by using both the early and late images, Ezekowitz et al noted an 11 percent increase in sensitivity for left ventricular thrombi from 54 percent using only the late images to 65 percent when using both the early

and late images.[62] Thus, imaging on day 0 and again on days 3 to 4 in multiple views maximizes the diagnostic accuracy. For positive diagnosis, it is important to note an increase in localized activity over time, which is clearly distinguishable from the background circulating blood-pool activity.

INDIUM-111 PLATELET TOMOGRAPHY-LV THROMBUS

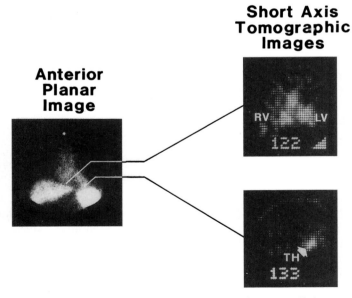

Figure 28-2 Planar and tomographic images from a patient with an apical left ventricular thrombus are displayed. These images were obtained 48 h after labeled platelet injection. The planar image showed localized uptake at the left ventricular apex. Single photon emission computed tomographic imaging was also obtained, and the cardiac short-axis slices are displayed. The *top right* image is a slice obtained near the base of the heart and shows activity in the right ventricle (RV) and left ventricle (LV). On the *bottom right* image, highly localized uptake in the apical left ventricular thrombus is demonstrated.

Sensitivity and Specificity of Indium-111 Platelet Imaging for Detection of Left Ventricular Thrombi

In an animal model, Seabold and colleagues assessed the diagnostic accuracy of ^{111}In platelet imaging for detection of left ventricular thrombi. The apparent sensitivity of platelet imaging for thrombus detection decreased over time following thrombus formation. Among recently formed thrombi, 75 percent (nine of 12) were detected by platelet imaging.[79] In contrast, among 1-week-old thrombi, only 57 percent (four of seven) were detected. In humans, Belotti et al demonstrated that the uptake of platelets on the surface of recently formed left ventricular thrombi is greater than on older thrombi, similar to the findings in animal models.[57]

In a study in humans, Ezekowitz and colleagues found an overall sensitivity of 65 percent and a specificity of 99 percent when platelet-imaging findings were compared with surgical or autopsy findings.[62] Similar but smaller studies have had similar findings. Thus, only about two-thirds of left ventricular thrombi have externally detectable platelet uptake by platelet imaging. However, the specificity is quite high; that is, the risk of a false-positive result with labeled platelet imaging is extremely low. The failure to detect some thrombi probably relates to decreased uptake of ^{111}In platelets by thrombus over time, small thrombus size, and possibly the effects of antithrombotic drugs.

Stratification of Embolic Risk with Platelet Imaging

Platelet imaging of left ventricular thrombi can be used to predict the subsequent risk of embolization. We compared the embolic rate in 33 patients with positive ^{111}In platelet images for left ventricular thrombi with the rate in 65 patients with negative images during a mean follow-up of 31 ± 24 months (Fig. 28-3).[67] The groups were similar with respect to all clinical features, including the prevalence of anterior infarction, antithrombotic therapy, the prevalence of aneurysm formation, and the time after infarction. During follow-up, embolic events occurred in 12 percent of patients (four of 33) with positive platelet images for left ventricular thrombi, compared with only 2 percent of patients (one of 65) with negative images ($p = 0.02$). By actuarial methods, at 5 years of follow-up, only 71 percent of patients with initially positive images were embolus free, compared with 98 percent of patients with negative images.

Next, we examined just a subset of patients who had a left ventricular thrombus already documented by echocardiography, and asked whether platelet imagng findings in patients who already had a positive echocardiogram would help to stratify embolic risk. We identified 53 patients with a left ventricular thrombus by echocar-

diography, 29 of whom had a positive platelet image while the remaining 24 patients had a negative platelet image. Among patients with a positive echocardiogram and a positive platelet image, embolic events occurred in 23 percent versus 4 percent in patients with just a positive echocardiogram but a negative platelet image ($p = 0.03$).[67] Thus, platelet imaging can help to stratify embolic risk in patients with left ventricular thrombi already identified by echocardiography. If the echocardiogram is positive but the platelet scan is negative, indicating hematologic inactivity, the embolic risk is low.

These data have been confirmed by Benichou and colleagues. Among 30 patients with a positive two-dimensional echocardiogram, the embolic incidence was 21 percent (four of 19) among patients with positive ^{111}In platelet exams compared with 0 percent (0 of 11) among patients with negative platelet exams ($p < 0.01$).[80]

In addition, Benichou et al[80] noted that, among patients with left ventricular thrombi documented by two-dimensional echocardiography, those who also had positive platelet images were significantly less likely to have thrombus resolution compared with patients who had negative platelet images. At 1½ months of follow-up, among patients with a positive ^{111}In platelet study, only 13 percent (two of 16), had thrombus resolution, compared with 80 percent resolution if the platelet scan was negative ($p < 0.01$). These findings strongly suggest that platelet-imaging findings may be used to predict whether a thrombus will resolve.

Effects of Antithrombotic Drugs on Platelet Imaging of Left Ventricular Thrombi

Antithrombotic drug effects have been assessed in several studies. Benichou et al,[80] Yamada et al,[81] and our group[66] have found that therapy with warfarin or similar agents reduces labeled platelet uptake in most patients (Fig. 28-4). In the largest study, by Yamada and colleagues, platelet imaging in 10 of 11 patients with left ventricular thrombi treated with vitamin-K antagonists became negative, while only one of nine control subjects who was not treated became negative.[81]

The effects of platelet inhibitory agents have been less impressive. In a randomized trial of patients with acute myocardial infarction, Funke-Kupper and colleagues found no effect of aspirin in a dose of 100 mg/day in preventing the development of left ventricular thrombi or in reducing the activity of established thrombi as studied by platelet imaging.[73] Similarly, in uncontrolled studies, neither aspirin in variable doses (300 to 2400 mg daily):[70] nor low-dose subcutaneous heparin[65,71] prevented detection by platelet imaging of established left ventricular thrombi.

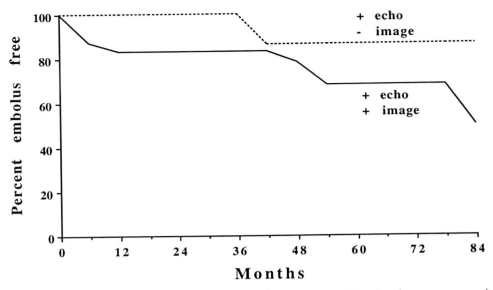

Figure 28-3 The graph depicts the probability of remaining embolus free for two groups of patients, one who had a positive echocardiogram as well as a positive ^{111}In image (*bottom curve*), and the second group who had a positive echocardiogram but a negative platelet image (*top curve*) indicating a hematologically inactive thrombus. In patients with a positive echocardiogram and a positive ^{111}In platelet study, embolic events occurred in 23 percent compared with 4 percent in patients with a positive echocardiogram but a negative platelet image ($p < 0.05$).

Among 32 patients with initially positive platelet images for left ventricular thrombi, the effects of the platelet inhibitory agents ticlopidine and indobufen were compared. On follow-up platelet imaging, reduced deposition was seen in only 11 percent of controls, compared with 42 percent of those treated with indobufen and 63 percent of those treated with ticlopidine.[58]

In patients with chronic left ventriculaar thrombi, we prospectively assessed the effects of sulfinpyrazone (200 mg q.i.d.), aspirin (325 mg t.i.d.) plus dipyridamole (75 mg t.i.d.), or high-dose warfarin therapy.[66] We initially established the reproducibility of the platelet-imaging findings by repeating studies on five subjects with thrombi who were restudied on no medications; the findings in all studies remained positive. Among seven patients treated with sulfinpyrazone, five had decreased platelet deposition (three became negative and two equivocal). Among six patients treated with aspirin plus dipyridamole, three had decreased deposition (one became negative and three equivocal). In contrast, among four warfarin-treated patients, three became negative and one was unchanged.[66]

BASELINE

WARFARIN

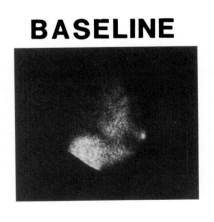

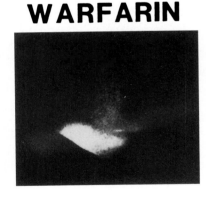

Figure 28-4 Indium-111 platelet images at 48 h are displayed in a patient who had relatively marked uptake in an apical left ventricular thrombus at baseline. After 2 weeks of warfarin therapy, active uptake was no longer detected by platelet imaging, and the thrombus had resolved by two-dimensional echocardioraphy.

A very interesting finding to emerge from these prior studies[58,66] is that despite a reduction in thrombus activity demonstrated by platelet imaging, a change in thrombus size by echocardiography was extremely rare in patients treated with platelet-inhibitory agents. In our study, echocardiography demonstrated only no change or a miimal reduction in estimated thrombus size. Similarly, in the study by Bellotti et al, none of the 32 subjects had complete thrombus resolution by echocardiography and only one subject had an apparent reduction in thrombus size. These results strongly suggest that platelet-active agents can diminish left ventricular thrombus activity as assessed by platelet imaging without necessarily grossly altering thrombus size, at least during short-term therapy. Thus, platelet imaging may be superior to echocardiography as an early indicator of antithrombotic drug effect in patients with left ventricular thrombi. Based on the data just presented,[67,80] it is reasonable to postulate that converting a positive platelet image to a negative platelet image with antithrombotic therapy would be associated with a reduction in the embolic risk.

COMPARISON TO OTHER TECHNIQUES

Two-dimensional echocardiography is clearly the diagnostic procedure of choice for left ventricular thrombi. It is relatively quick, involves no radiation exposure, is very widely available, and has an acceptably high sensitivity ranging from 77 to 95 percent, with a similarly high specificity of 88 to 100 percent.[61,82–85] Thus, not only is echocardiography more widely available than platelet scintigraphy, it is more accurate. In addition to providing diagnostic information about left ventricular thrombi, two-dimensional echocardiography also often provides important information about the presence and extent of left ventricular dysfunction and the presence and severity of valvular lesions. This additional information may be clinically important in many patients, both prognostically and in making management decisions.

Several studies have assessed platelet-imaging findings in patients with two-dimensional echocardiographically documented left ventricular thrombi. As shown in Table 28-1, among patients with left ventricular thrombi documented by echocardiography, only approximately 50 to 60 percent have positive ^{111}In platelet images. The reason for this discrepancy is multifactorial. Platelet imaging can detect only those thrombi that are hematologically active, with ongoing platelet incorporation. Thrombi with either no incorporation of platelets, or low levels of platelet uptake, will not be externally detectable. Among left ventricular thrombi that were detected by platelet imaging, the thrombus-to-blood ratio in surgically resected specimens in patients with positive images

Table 28-1   Indium-111 Platelet-Imaging Findings in Patients with Two-Dimensional Echocardiograms Positive for Left Ventricular Thrombi

Author	Reference	Number of Left Ventricular Thrombi by Echo	Percent with Positive [111]In Images
Stratton 1	35	15	60
Stratton 2	67	65	45
Benichou 1	69	18	89
Benichou 2	80	30	63
Funke-Kupper	73	17	53
Tsuda	77	15	60
Total		160	56

was between 10 : 1 to 355 : 1 compared with a thrombus-to-blood ratio in patients with negative images of only 0.03 : 1 to 16 : 1.[35,61] Additionally, as noted above, older thrombi tend to have less up..ke. Moreover, some thrombi may be too small to detect by platelet imaging, and other thrombi may have platelet uptake inhibited by antithrombotic drugs.

Echocardiography, however, does have several limitations for the diagnosis of left ventricular thrombus. About 5 to 10 percent of studies are technically poor and cannot adequately exclude the presence of a thrombus. Anatomic structures such as trabeculations, aberrant bands, papillary muscles, and tumors are occasionally mistaken for thrombi and cause falsely abnormal (false-positive) studies.[83,86,87] In addition, echocardiographic artifacts due to noise or resolution problems can cause false-positive studies. In cases where the echocardiogram is equivocal or of poor technical quality, platelet imaging may be of use. Also, it is possible that platelet-imaging findings may be superior to echocardiography for stratification of embolic risk.

Embolic risk can also be stratified using two-dimensional echocardiography.[46,47] Multiple studies have demonstrated that both thrombus mobility and thrombus protrusion are associated with a higher embolic rate.[46,52,88–92] From pooled data, mobile thrombi have been associated with a very high 63 percent embolic prevalence (59 of 93) compared with an embolic prevalence of only 11 percent (31 of 294) for immobile thrombi.[47] Similarly, for protruding thrombi, the embolic prevalence of 51 percent (70 of 138) has been much higher than the embolic prevalence of 8 percent (20 of 249) with flat thrombi.

Whether ^{111}In platelet imaging is superior to simple echocardiographic features in predicting embolic risk has not been determined with certainty. In our study of 58 patients with positive echocardiograms, eight of whom had embolic events, only platelet imaging findings were significantly different between the groups with and without embolic events, while the prevalence of mobile or protruding thrombi was not significantly different.[67]

These findings suggest that platelet-imaging findings may be of more use for determining embolic risk than are echocardiographic features. However, these findings need confirmation in a larger study.

There has been limited experience with other nuclear imaging techniques for detecting left ventricular thrombi in humans. In two patients with chronic left ventricular thrombi who had positive ^{111}In platelet images, antifibrin antibody imaging using ^{99m}Tc-labeled T2G1s monoclonal antifibrin antibody fragment was negative in both subjects.[93] In contrast, two relatively small studies have noted encouraging results when using gallium-67 (^{67}Ga) fibrinogen[94,95] In one study, ^{67}Ga–DFO–DAS–fibrinogen imaging detected left ventricular thrombi in 11 subjects after acute myocardial infarction; however, only five of these 11 subjects had a positive two-dimensional echocardiogram.[94] Due to the relatively high sensitivity of two-dimensional echocardiography, it would seem quite possible that many of the positive studies noted with gallium–fibrinogen imaging were falsely positive.

Another technique that has been described for detecting left ventricular thrombi has been radionuclide angiography.[85,96,97] The findings compatible with a left ventricular thrombus by radionuclide angiography are a discrete filling defect or a squared or cut-off ventricular apex in an area of abnormal wall motion. However, the sensitivity is relatively low. We studied a total of 70 patients who had left ventricular thrombi proven or disproven by other methods: 22 patients had thrombi while 48 did not. If equivocal readings were considered negative, the sensitivity of radionuclide angiography was only 55 percent while the specificity was 94 percent. At best, this technique should be considered only as suggestive of left ventricular thrombi. For definitive diagnosis, however, these findings should be confirmed by another noninvasive study, typically two-dimensional echocardiography.

Other imaging techniques that can detect left ventricular thrombi include x-ray computed tomographic imaging[98-102] and magnetic resonance imaging.[103-107] For both of these methodologies, however, there have been no large studies to document sensitivity or specificity. Moreover, relative to echocardiography, they are less available and costlier.

Thus, a number of imaging techniques are available for the identification of left ventricular thrombi. Echocardiography is clearly the method of choice. However, technically inadequate studies may occur in up to one-quarter of patients, and the rate of false-positive studies may also be as high as 20 percent. The accuracy of the echocardiographic information depends critically upon the skill and thoroughness of the technician. Radionuclide angiography has a relatively poor sensitivity. X-ray computed tomography and magnetic resonance imaging may be potentially helpful, but their accuracy has not been well defined, and they are costlier than echocardiography. Indium-111 platelet imaging has not been widely utilized. However, it may well be complimentary to echo-

cardiography, especially in patients who have technically inadequate echocardiograms. Moreover, it is quite possible that even among patients with left ventricular thrombi diagnosed by two-dimensional echocardiography, platelet imaging may further stratify embolic risk and therefore help in making important decisions regarding anticoagulant therapy.

LEFT ATRIAL THROMBI

Left atrial thrombi occur in approximately 10 to 15 percent of patients with atrial fibrillation and are associated with an increased risk of embolic stroke and peripheral emboli. In animal models, Vandenberg et al assessed the utility of ^{111}In platelet imaging for the detection of left atrial appendage thrombi.[108] Among animals with acute thrombi, platelet imaging detected 100 percent of left atrial thrombi (17 of 17). Among animals with chronic thrombi (4 to 8 days old), however, platelet imaging detected only 20 percent (two of 10). Thus, although acute atrial thrombi could be detected in this model, the sensitivity for detection of chronic thrombi was poor because of diminished incorporation of labeled platelets onto older thrombi.

There are only limited data regarding the ability of ^{111}In platelet imaging to detect left atrial thrombi in humans.[64,68,109-113] In the largest study, of 28 patients with mitral valve disease, findings compatible with a left atrial thrombus were seen in seven.[110] Among 12 patients who had operative or autopsy confirmation, platelet imaging detected four of five proven thrombi and was negative in all seven patients without thrombi.

Alternative diagnostic methods for the detection of left atrial thrombi are transesophageal echocardiography, x-ray computed tomography, and magnetic resonance imaging. Unlike the situation with left ventricular thrombi where the accuracy of transthoracic echocardiography is quite high, transthoracic echocardiography has a very low sensitivity of less than 50 percent for the detection of left atrial thrombi.[114,115] In contrast, transesophageal echocardiography, which is able to visualize the left atrial appendage where most left atrial thrombi occur, has a much higher sensitivity of at least 83 percent.[115-120] Currently, transesophageal echocardiography is the diagnostic procedure of choice for the detection of left atrial thrombi.

RIGHT ATRIAL AND RIGHT VENTRICULAR THROMBI

Thrombus formation in the right heart chambers is an unusual event, but can occur in the presence of atrial fibrillation, right ventricular infarction, dilated cardio-myopathy, or with thromboemboli from the periphery. Minimal data are available regarding the ability of nuclear imaging techniques to detect thrombi located in the right heart. There has been a single report of the detection of a right ventricular thrombus by ^{111}In platelet imaging.[71] In addition, the detection of right atrial thrombi by ^{111}In platelet imaging has been described.[112,113] In addition, platelet deposition has been detected in right-sided extracardiac conduits in humans.[121,122]

Other techniques that have been used to detect right heart thrombi in small numbers of patients include transthoracic or transesophageal echocardiography,[84,102,104,113,118,120,123–129] x-ray computed tomographic scanning,[102,112,113] and gated nuclear magnetic resonance imaging.[103,104,125,127] Transesophageal echocardiography appeared superior to transthoracic echocardiography for the detection of right heart thrombi.[118,130,131] Studies using two-dimensional echocardiography in patients with documented pulmonary emboli have noted the finding of right atrial or right ventricular thrombi in 4 to 17 percent of patients.[132–135]

At the present, transthoracic and transesophageal echocardiography are the diagnostic modalities of choice for the detection of right heart thrombi, but definitive studies delineating the sensitivity and specificity of either technique have not yet been reported.

VEGETATIONS AND VALVULAR THROMBI

The detection of vegetations due to infective endocarditis, which are composed primarily of platelets and fibrin, was demonstrated in an animal model by Riba and colleagues using ^{111}In platelets.[136] Indium-111 platelet uptake in vegetations averaged 100-fold greater than in blood. Despite these experimental results, however, detection of vegetations in humans with endocarditis has not been possible.[137]

Also in animal models, platelet deposition has been demonstrated in the region of prosthetic valves.[137–141] Acar and colleagues extended these findings into humans[142] by studying 41 patients with 45 valve prostheses (mechanical, 37; and biological, 8). All patients had suspected valve thrombi on the basis of prior thromboembolic events. Platelet imaging was abnormal in 51 percent (24 of 41). Among 10 cases in which there was proof of prosthetic thrombus at surgery or autopsy, platelet imaging was positive in eight. These authors concluded that platelet imaging is a useful means for detecting prosthetic valve thrombi. Among the patients who did not have surgery or autopsy validation, platelet imaging was positive in 16 of 31. These exciting findings have not yet been confirmed in another study. A single case of

prosthetic valve thrombosis detected by ^{111}In platelet imaging was reported by Otaki et al.[143]

Transthoracic and transesophageal echocardiography remain the procedures of choice for diagnosing valvular vegetations or valve thrombi.

CORONARY ARTERY THROMBI

The formation of a coronary artery thrombus is the final common pathway leading to the majority of episodes of acute myocardial infarction and sudden cardiac death. The noninvasive detection of coronary thrombi is the holy grail of noninvasive cardiovascular imaging. In animal models, labeled platelets have detected coronary artery thrombi when blood-pool subtraction techniques[144] or unprocessed images were used.[145] However, thrombi over 24 h old or those that were small (11 to 17.5 mg) were not externally detectable.

There are no convincing data that coronary artery thrombi can be externally imaged by using labeled platelets or other thrombosis tracers as yet in humans. Fox and colleagues described the possible detection of coronary thrombi in nine patients by using a blood-pool subtraction technique,[146] but they offered no independent confirmation of the presence or absence of thrombus, and only one thrombus was detected on an unprocessed image. It is possible that their early encouraging findings were due either to platelet uptake on left ventricular thrombi or to platelet accumulation in the infarct zone, which has been documented,[147,148] or simply due to the artifacts of blood-pool subtraction. Similarly, although platelet accumulation has been demonstrated at coronary angioplasty sites in many animal models, preliminary reports on studies in humans have noted no detectable platelet deposition within coronary arteries.[3,149] In addition, platelet uptake in 10 patients with recently implanted saphenous vein bypass grafts was not detectable.[137]

Overall, there have been no convincing displays of platelet deposition detected within the coronary arteries or in vein bypass grafts in humans. There are many reasons why these negative results might be expected, including the small size of coronary thrombi, the poor intrinsic spatial resolution of gamma imaging systems, the relatively low injected isotope doses, the surrounding background activity, cardiac motion, and attenuation effects. The net result has been an inability to image coronary artery thrombi to date.

PULMONARY EMBOLI AND DEEP VENOUS THROMBOSIS

In animal models, acute pulmonary emboli have been detected by ^{111}In platelet imaging, but thrombi more than

24 h old could not be detected. In addition to age, heparin blocked the ability to image platelet uptake on pulmonary emboli.[150] In humans, there are only isolated case reports[151-154] describing the detection of pulmonary emboli with labeled platelets. In one study, platelet imaging failed to detect pulmonary emboli in 11 of 12 heparinized patients.[155] Among 146 patients studied following abdominal or pelvic surgery, Clarke-Pearson and colleagues detected five asymptomatic pulmonary emboli.[156] Thus, platelet imaging appears to offer little for the diagnosis of pulmonary emboli.

In contrast, labeled platelets have shown much greater promise for the detection of deep venous thrombosis. Labeled platelets have successfully imaged both calf and proximal leg thrombi.[157-159] Thrombus age seems to be an important determinant of whether platelet imaging will detect a thrombus;[157-162] older thrombi have either taken longer to visualize or have been undetectable. Both heparin at high doses and prostacyclin have been shown to block platelet incorporation.[157,158] The diagnostic accuracy of ^{111}In platelet imaging for the detection of deep venous thrombosis has not been conclusively established. Existing studies have reported a wide range in sensitivities from 38 to 100 percent.[156,163-167] Specificity has ranged from 67 to 100 percent. In a study by Seabold and colleagues of 31 patients, only two of whom were receiving heparin, the sensitivity was 100 percent and the specificity 89 percent. However, the sensitivity of platelet imaging may drop substantially if patients are receiving heparin.[166] In a study by Ezekowitz and colleagues, platelet imaging was positive in 80 percent (four of five) of patients not receiving heparin, but in only 33 percent (five of 15) of patients who were receiving heparin;[163,168] deep venous thrombi in this study were documented by contrast venography. As in platelet imaging of other conditions, late imaging to at least 24 h after labeled platelet injection is crucial. In one study that imaged nonheparinized subjects at only 2 h after injection, the sensitivity was less than 50 percent,[167] while, in a study that imaged patients to 24 h after platelet injection, the sensitivity improved from 69 percent at 4 h to 100 percent at 24 h.[166]

Platelet imaging has also been used to monitor patients who are at high risk for developing deep venous thrombi.[169-173] Positive images have been seen in 30 percent of patients following abdominal or pelvic surgery,[156] in 64 percent of patients with femur fractures,[172] and in 45 percent of patients with respiratory failure.[173]

To summarize, the strength of platelet imaging for detecting venous thrombosis has been that it can detect thrombi in multiple locations, including the calf, thigh, and pelvic thrombi, unlike some techniques. The sensitivity of platelet imaging for the detection of deep venous thrombosis appears to decline if there is concomitant heparin therapy, if imaging is not delayed sufficiently following platelet injection, or with advanced thrombus age. In addition, currently many other noninvasive methods are capable of detecting deep venous thrombi in many settings. Thus, clinically, platelet imaging has not assumed a role as an important diagnostic method for deep venous thrombosis. Several new alternative nuclear medicine approaches to the noninvasive detection of deep venous thrombi are reviewed in the next section.

EMERGING NUCLEAR MEDICINE THROMBOSIS-IMAGING AGENTS

Thrombi are formed of varying proportions of platelets, fibrin, and other blood elements. Thus, it is rational to attempt to image thrombi by using agents that have a high specificity for one or more of these elements. Several radiolabeled tracers have been tested in animal models, including labeled fibrinogen, t-PA, fibrin fragment E1, thrombospondin, annexin V, radiolabeled peptides, small proteins that bind with certain receptors, and monoclonal antibodies directed against platelets, fibrinogen, or fibrin.[174-178]

The most studied new agent has been antifibrin antibodies labeled with ^{111}In or [99m]Tc. Antifibrin antibodies bind specifically to fibrin, but not to circulating fibrinogen. Since fibrin is present only in areas of active thrombosis, and venous thrombi are throught to be composed primarily of fibrin, the rationale for antifibrin antibody imaging of venous thrombi is convincing.

In reported human studies, labeled antifibrin antibodies have appeared promising for the early diagnosis of deep venous thrombosis in humans, with sensitivities in the range of 81 to 97 percent and specificities of 73 to 100 percent compared with contrast venography.[179-185] Moreover, sensitivity appears to remain high even in patients receiving heparin. In addition, antifibrin antibody imaging does not need to be delayed as long as ^{111}In platelet imaging.[179-184] Vorne and colleagues compared ^{111}In labeled monoclonal antifibrin antibodies with ^{99m}Tc–HMPAO-labeled platelets in 18 patients who had venography as the gold-standard test.[26] Heparin significantly inhibited the uptake of technetium-labeled platelets, but not of indium-labeled monoclonal antibodies. Neither of the noninvasive nuclear techniques had a 100 percent sensitivity for detection of deep venous thrombosis.[26] Although the detection of deep venous thrombi by using a variety of monoclonal antibodies or antibody fragments labels in humans has been encouraging,[179-185] no antifibrin imaging agents have yet been approved by the United States Food and Drug Administration for clinical use.

For imaging of arterial thrombi, antifibrin antibody imaging has been disappointing. In an animal model in our laboratory,[186] antifibrin imaging detected all acute arterial thrombi within 2 h of labeled antibody injection, but subsequent findings in human studies were quite discouraging.[93] Using [99mTc]-labeled T2G1s monoclonal antifibrin antibody fragment (Fab'), we studied 18 patients with arterial thrombi. Antifibrin antibody imaging was positive in only 61 percent of 18 patients with large-vessel chronic arterial thrombi compared with a 100 percent positive rate using [111In]-labeled platelets.[93] In addition, target-to-background ratios for the antifibrin antibody imaging from tomographic images were less than with labeled platelets. Thus, antifibrin imaging has not been successful in imaging arterial thrombi in humans, possibly because arterial thrombi have a preponderance of platelets rather than fibrin.

In another labeled antibody approach, Tromholt et al described the use of an [111In]-labeled monoclonal antibody against t-PA in eight patients with venographically verified deep venous thrombosis.[187] This technique detected the site of thrombus in all patients at 24 h after injection. Peters, Lavender, and colleagues have described the use of an [111In]-labeled platelet-specific monoclonal antibody, P256, for the detection and monitoring of deep venous thrombosis.[188–191]

Labeled fragment E1, which is a 60-kD fragment of human fibrin that binds to fibrin dimers and polymers but not to fibrinogen or fibrin monomer, has also been studied.[174,192–195] Very little human data are available, but preliminary studies suggest it has promise for detecting venous thrombi.[193] Since it binds to fibrin, however, it may have limited value in the detection of arterial thrombi.

The synthetic peptide P280 is a 26-amino-acid dimer that binds with high affinity to the glycoprotein IIb/IIIa receptor expressed on activated platelets. In preliminary canine studies of venous thrombi, [99mTc]-labeled P280 accumulated in fresh thrombi with thrombus-to-background ratios when using region-of-interest analysis of 2.3 at 4 h after injection.[178,196] In preliminary human studies in nine subjects, [99mTc]-labeled P280 detected deep venous thrombi in eight of nine cases within 1 h after injection.[197] In addition, uptake compatible with pulmonary emboli was detectable in two subjects. Blood clearance was rapid, with less than 5 percent of the injected dose circulating 1 h after injection. The in vivo thrombus-to-background ratios obtained from region-of-interest analysis averaged 1.6 to 1.8 at 1 to 4 h after injection, and dropped to 1.4 at 24 h. These very encouraging early findings need to be extended.

Other approaches that have been tested in animal models but not in humans to our knowledge have been the use of antibodies to an antigen expresssed only on activated platelets, which is the α-granule protein GMP-140 also known as the PADGEM protein.[198,199] An inactive labeled t-PA has also been assessed in animal models.[200] In addition, peptide sequences that bind to platelets

have been tested in animal models.[178] However, none of these has yet been reported in human trials.

Another approach that has shown promise in animal studies and is soon to be tested in humans is labeled annexin V.[175,176] Annexin V is a human phospholipid-binding protein that binds to the phosphatidylserine residues that become exposed on the extracellular face of activated platelets. In pigs with left atrial thrombi, we found that [99mTc]-labeled annexin V offered a mean thrombus-to-whole blood ratio of 14.2 ± 10.6 for the entire thrombus and detected most left atrial thrombi when tomographic imaging techniques were used within 2 h after intravenous injection. Annexin V has a higher affinity for the thrombus relative to thrombin-targeted or t-PA-targeted approaches, and it has selective binding to activated but not quiescent platelets.

SUMMARY AND CONCLUSIONS

Thrombosis imaging with [111In]-labeled platelets has allowed the noninvasive detection of some intracardiac thrombi in humans and has also served as a useful research tool in experimental animal studies. However, it has several significant constraints that have limited its clinical utility in the diagnosis of intracardiac thrombi. These include the time-consuming and costly labeling and imaging methods. Rapid diagnosis is not possible since delayed imaging is always necessary. In addition, the resolution of platelet imaging has been limited by the relatively high circulating blood-pool activity that occurs and in part by the inherent limitations of all gamma imaging techniques.[110] Some of the most important but small intracardiac thrombi, such as coronary artery thrombi, cannot be detected with current platelet-imaging methods.

For the present, echocardiography, either transthoracic or transesophageal, remains the method of choice for the diagnosis of nearly all right or left heart thrombi. Alternative, but more expensive and less well documented, approaches include x-ray computed tomographic scanning and gated nuclear magnetic resonance imaging. The diagnosis of intracoronary thrombi has not yet been possible by any noninvasive methodology.

For nuclear thrombosis imaging to achieve an important role in clinical medicine, improvements in imaging techniques as well as improved thrombosis tracers are needed. Improved thrombosis imaging may be possible with labeling of compounds such as the small peptide P280, annexin V, t-PA, or a variety of monoclonal antibodies that are incorporated into thrombi. These new approaches, to be successful, must offer thrombus-to-background ratios that exceed those achieved with [111In]-

labeled platelets at earlier times following intravenous injection.

ACKNOWLEDGEMENT

This work was supported by the Medical Research Service of the Department of Veterans Affairs.

REFERENCES

1. Sherman D, Hart R: Thromboembolism and antithrombotic therapy in cerebrovascular disease. *J Am Coll Cardiol* 8:88B, 1986.
2. Sherman DG, Dyken ML, Fisher M, et al: Antithrombotic therapy for cerebrovascular disorders. *Chest* 102(Supplement):529S, 1992.
3. Thakur ML: A look at radiolabeled blood cells. *Int J Rad Appl Instrum* [B] 13:147, 1986.
4. Heaton WA, Davis HH, Welch MJ, et al: Indium-111: A new radionuclide label for studying human platelet kinetics. *Br J Haematol* 42:613, 1979.
5. Hawker RJ, Hawker LM, Wilkinson AR: Indium (^{111}In)-labelled human platelets: Optimal method. *Clin Sci* 58:243, 1980.
6. Hudson EM, Ramsey RB, Evatt BL: Subcellular localization of indium-111 in indium-111-labeled platelets. *J Lab Clin Med* 97:577, 1981.
7. Heyns AD, Lotter MG, Badenhorst PN, et al: Kinetics, distribution and sites of destruction of ^{111}indium-labelled human platelets. *Br J Haematol* 44:269, 1980.
8. Mathias CJ, Welch MJ: Radiolabeling of platelets. *Semin Nucl Med* 14:118, 1984.
9. Schmidt KG, Rasmussen JW, Arendrup H: Function ex vivo of ^{111}In-labelled human platelets: Simultaneous aggregation of labelled and unlabelled platelets induced by collagen. *Scand H Haematol* 29:51, 1982.
10. Schmidt KG, Rasmussen JW, Lorentzen M: Function and morphology of 111-In-labelled platelets: In vitro, in vivo and ex vivo studies. *Haemostasis* 11:193, 1982.
11. Thakur ML, Welch MJ, Joist JH, Coleman RE: Indium-111 labeled platelets: Studies on preparation and evaluation of in vitro and in vivo functions. *Thromb Res* 9:345, 1976.
12. Thakur ML, Walsh L, Malech HL, Gottschalk A: Indium-111-labeled human platelets: improved method, efficacy, and evaluation. *J Nucl Med* 22:381, 1981.
13. Isaka Y, Kimura K, Matsumoto M, et al: Functional alterations of human platelets following indium-111 labelling using diferent incubation media and labelling agents. *Eur J Nucl Med* 18:326, 1991.
14. Thakur ML, Sedar AW: Ultrastructure of human platelets following indium-111 labeling in plasma. *Nucl Med Commun* 8:69, 1987.
15. Goodwin DA, Bushberg JT, Doherty PW, et al: Indium-111-labeled autologous platelets for location of vascular thrombi in humans. *J Nucl Med* 19:626, 1978.
16. Klonizakis I, Peters AM, Fitzpatrick ML, et al: Radionuclide distribution following injection of ^{111}indium-labelled platelets. *Br J Haematol* 46:595, 1980.
17. Stratton JR, Ballem PJ, Gernsheimer T, et al: Platelet destruction in autoimmune thrombocytopenic purpura: Kinetics and clearance of indium-111-labeled autologous platelts. *J Nucl Med* 30:629, 1989.
18. Dewanjee MK, Wahner HW, Dunn WL, et al: Comparison of three platelet markers for measurement of platelet suvival time in healthy volunteers. *Mayo Clin Proc* 61:327, 1986.
19. Heaton WAL: Indium-111 (^{111}In) and chromium-51 (^{51}CR) labeling of platelets: Are they comparable? *Transfusion* 26:16, 1986.
20. Peters AM, Lavender JP: Platelet kinetics with indium-111 platelets: Comparison with chromium-51 platelets. *Semin Thromb Hemost* 9:100, 1983.
21. Schmidt KG, Rasmussen JW, Rasmusen AD, Arendrup H: Comparative studies of the in vivo kinetics of simultaneously injected ^{111}In and ^{51}CR-labeled human platelets. *Scand J Haematol* 30:465, 1983.
22. Wadenvik H, Kutti J: The in vivo kinetics of ^{111}In- and ^{51}Cr-labelled platelets: A comparative study using both stored and fresh platelets. *Br J Haematol* 78:523, 1991.
23. Joist JH, Baker RK, Welch MJ: Methodologic and basic aspects of indium-111 platelets. *Semin Thromb Hemost* 9:86, 1983.
24. Peters AM, Klonizakis I, Lavender JP, Lewis SM: Elution of ^{111}indium from retriculoendothelial cells. *J Clin Pathol* 35:507, 1982.
25. Kotze HF, Lotter MG, Heyns AD, et al: ^{111}In-labelled baboon platelets: The influence of in vivo redistribution and contaminating ^{114m}In on the radiation dose. *Int J Rad Appl Instrum* [B] 14:593, 1987.
26. Vorne MS, Honkanen TT, Lantto TJ, et al: Thrombus imaging with ^{99m}Tc–HMPAO-labeled platelets and ^{111}In-labeled monoclonal antifibrin antibodies. *Acta Radiol* 34:59, 1993.
27. Dewanjee MK, Robinson RP, Hellman RL, et al: Technetium-99m-labeled platelets: comparison of labeling with a new lipid-soluble Sn(II)-mercaptopyridine-N-oxide and ^{99m}Tc–HMPAO. *Int J Rad Appl Instrum* [B] 18:461, 1991.
28. Sundrehagen E, Urdal P, Heggli DE, et al: Radiolabelling of platelets with technetium-99m. *Thromb Res* 57:737, 1990.
29. Hardeman MR: Thrombocytes labelled with ^{99m}Tc–HMPAO: In vitro studies and preliminary clinical experience. *Prog Clin Biol Res* 355:49, 1990.
30. Becker W, Borst U, Krahe T, Borner W: Tc-99m–HMPAO labelled human platelets: In vitro and in vivo results. *Eur J Nucl Med* 15:296, 1989.
31. Vorne M, Honkanen T, Karppinen K, et al: Radiolabelling of human platelets with ^{99m}Tc–HMPAO. *Eur J Haematol* 42:487, 1989.
32. Becker W, Borner W, Borst U: ^{99m}Tc hexamethylpropyleneamineoxime (HMPAO) as a platelet label: Evaluation

of labelling parameters and first in vivo results. *Nucl Med Commun* 9:831, 1988.

33. Honkanen T, Jauhola S, Karppinen K, er al: Venous thrombosis: A controlled study on the performance of scintigraphy with ^{99m}Tc–HMPAO-labelled platelets versus venography. *Nucl Med Commun* 13:88, 1992.

34. Robertson JS, Ezekowitz MD, Dewanjee MK, et al: MIRD dose estimate no. 15: Radiation absorbed dose estimates for radioindium-labeled autologous platelets. *J Nucl Med* 33:777, 1992.

35. Stratton JR, Ritchie JL, Hamilton GW, et al: Left ventricular thrombi: In vivo detection by indium-111 platelet imaging and two dimensional echocardiography. *Am J Cardiol* 47:874, 1981.

36. Stratton JR, Ritchie JL: Effect of suloctidil on tomographically quantitated platelet accumulation in Dacron aortic gratfs. *Am J Cardiol* 58:152, 1986.

37. Stratton JR, Ritchie JL: Reduction of indium-111 platelet deposition on Dacron vascular grafts in humans by aspirin plus dipyridamole. *Circulation* 73:325, 1986.

38. Stratton JR: Thrombosis imaging using indium-111 labeled platelets, in Schelbert HR, Skorton DJ, Wolf DJ (eds): *Cardiac Imaging: Principles and Practice,* 2nd ed. New York, WB Saunders, 1996 (in press).

39. Wu KK, Chen YC, Fordham E, et al: Differential effects of two doses of aspirin on platelet–vessel wall interaction in vivo. *J Clin Invest* 68:382, 1981.

40. Allen BT, Mathias CJ, Sicard GA, et al: Platelet deposition on vascular grafts: The accuracy of in vivo quantification and the significance of in vivo platelet reactivity. *Ann Surg* 203:318, 1986.

41. Mathias CJ, Welch MJ: Dual isotope scintigraphy for the detection of platelet deposition in Heyns A, Badenhorst PN, Lötter MG (eds): *Platelet Kinetics and Imaging,* vol 1. Boca Raton, FL: CRC, 1985, pp 89–106.

42. Powers WJ, Hopkins KT, Welch MJ: Validation of the dual radiotracer method for quantitative In-111 platelet scintigraphy. *Thomb Res* 34:135, 1984.

43. Wakefield TW, Lindblad B, Graham LM, et al: Nuclide imaging of vascular graft–platelet interactions: Comparison of indium excess and technetium subtraction techniques. *J Surg Res* 40:388, 1986.

44. Powers WJ: In-111 platelet scintigraphy: Carotid atherosclerosis and stroke. *J Nucl Med* 25:626, 1984.

45. Machac J, Vallabhajosula S, Goldman ME, et al: Value of blood-pool subtraction in cardiac indium-111-labeled platelet imaging. *J Nucl Med* 30:1445, 1989.

46. Stratton JR: Common causes of cardiac emboli: Left ventricular thrombi and atrial fibrillation. *West J Med* 151:172, 1989.

47. Stratton JR: Chronic left ventricular thrombi: embolic potential and therapy. *G Ital Cardiol* 24:269, 1994.

48. Turpie AG, Robinson JG, Doyle DJ, et al: Comparison of high-dose with low-dose subcutaneous heparin to prevent left ventricular mural thrombosis in patients with acute transmural anterior myocardial infarction. *N Engl J Med* 320:352, 1989.

49. SCATI: Randomised controlled trial of subcutaneous calcium–heparin in acute myocardial infarction: The SCATI (Studio sulla Calciparina nell'Angina e nella Trombosi Ventricolare nell'Infarto) Group. *Lancet* 2:182, 1989.

50. Vecchio C, Chiarella F, Lupi G, et al: Left ventricular thrombus in anterior acute myocardial infarction after thrombolysis: A GISSI-2 connected study. *Circulation* 84:512, 1991.

51. Kneissl D, Bubenheimer P, Roskamm H: Ventricular thrombi in the chronic infarct stage: Echocardiographic findings, clinical apsects, relations to anticoagulation. *Z Kardiol* 74:639, 1985.

52. Stratton JR, Resnick AD: Increased embolic risk in patients with left ventricular thrombi. *Circulation* 75:1004, 1987.

53. Falk RH, Foster E, Coats MH: Ventricular thrombi and thromboembolism in dilated cardiomyopathy: A prospective follow-up study. *Am Heart J* 123:136, 1992.

54. Yokota Y, Kawanishi H, Hayakawa M, et al: Cardiac thrombus in dilated cardiomyopathy: Relationship between left ventricular pathophysiology and left ventricular thrombus. *Jpn Heart J* 30:1, 1989.

55. Ciaccheri M, Castelli G, Cecchi F, et al: Lack of correlation between intracavitary thrombosis detected by cross sectional echocardiography and systemic emboli in patients with dilated cardiomyopathy. *Br Heart J* 62:26, 1989.

56. Katz SD, Marantz PR, Biasucci L, et al: Low incidence of stroke in ambulatory patients with heart failure: A prospective study. *Am Heart J* 126:141, 1993.

57. Bellotti P, Claudiani F, Chiarella F, et al: Activity of left ventricular thrombi of different ages: Assessment with indium-oxine platelet imaging and cross-sectional echocardiography. *Eur Heart J* 8:855, 1987.

58. Bellotti P, Claudiani F, Chiarella F, et al: Left ventricular thrombi: Changes in size and in platelet deposition during treatment with indobufen and ticlopidine. *Cardiology* 77:272, 1990.

59. Claudiani F, Bellotti P, Strada P, et al: Semiquantitative imaging of left ventricular thrombi with ^{111}In–oxine labelled platelets. *J Nucl Med Allied Sci* 31:287, 1987.

60. Ezekowitz MD, Leonard JC, Smith EO, et al: Identification of left ventricular thrombi in man using indium-111-labeled autologous platelets: A preliminary report. *Circulation* 63:803, 1981.

61. Ezekowitz MD, Wilson DA, Smith EO, et al: Comparison of indium-111 platelet scintigraphy and two-dimensional echocardiography in the diagnosis of left ventricular thrombi. *N Engl J Med* 306:1509, 1982.

62. Ezekowitz MD, Burrow RD, Heath PW, et al: Diagnostic accuracy of indium-111 platelet scintigraphy in identifying left ventricular thrombi. *Am J Cardiol* 51:1712, 1983.

63. Ezekowitz MD: Imaging techniques for identifying left ventricular thrombi. *Am J Cardiac Imaging* 8:81, 1994.

64. Kimura M, Ojima K, Tsuda T, et al: Indium-111–oxine labeled platelet scintigraphy for detection of intracardiac and intravascular thrombi. *J Cardiogr* 13:499, 1983.

65. Salehi NF, Chan WC, McHutchinson J, et al: Early detection of left ventricular mural thrombi after acute Q wave myocardial infarction using ^{111}In oxine-labelled autologous platelets. *Nucl Med Commun* 111:857, 1990.

66. Stratton JR, Ritchie JL: The effects of antithrombotic drugs in patients with left ventricular thrombi: Assess-

ment with indium-111 platelet imaging and two-dimensional echocardiography. *Circulation* 69:561, 1984.

67. Stratton JR, Ritchie JL: Indium-111 platelet imaging of left ventricular thrombi: Predictive value for systemic emboli. *Circulation* 81:1182, 1990.

68. Benichou M, Camilleri JF, Bernard PJ, et al: Comparison of two-dimensional echocardiography with scanography and indium-111 platelet scintigraphy in detection of intracardiac thrombi. *Acta Cardiol* 43:93, 1988.

69. Benichou M, Bernard PJ, Sarrat P, et al: Detection of intracardiac thrombi by scintigraphy with indium-111-labeled platelets: Correlation with 2-dimensional echography and cardiac scanning. *Arch Mal Coeur* 77:1054, 1984.

70. Ezekowitz MD, Cox AC, Smith EO, Taylor FB: Failure of aspirin to prevent incorporation of indium-111 labelled platelets into cardiac thrombi in man. *Lancet* 2:440, 1981.

71. Ezekowitz MD, Kellerman DJ, Smith EO, Streitz TM: Detection of active left ventricular thrombosis during acute myocardial infarction using indium-111 platelet scintigraphy. *Chest* 86:35, 1984.

72. Funke-Kupper AJ, Verheugt FW, Jaarsma W, et al: Detection of ventricular thrombosis in acute myocardial infarction: Value of indium-111 platelet scintigraphy in relation to two-dimensional echocardiography and clinical course. *Eur J Nucl Med* 12:337, 1986.

73. Funke-Kupper AJ, Verheugt FW, Peels CH, et al: Effect of low dose acetylsalicylic acid on the frequency and hematoloic activity of left ventricular thrombus in anterior wall acute myocardial infarction. *Am J Cardiol* 63:917, 1989.

74. Kessler C, Henningsen H, Reuther R, et al: Identification of intracardiac thrombi in stroke patients with indium-111 platelet scintigraphy. *Stroke* 18:63, 1987.

75. Verheugt FW, Lindenfeld J, Kirch DL, Steele PP: Left ventricular platelet deposition after acute myocardial infarction: An attempt at quantification using blood pool subtracted indium-111 platelet scintigraphy. *Br Heart J* 52:490, 1984.

76. Ikeoka K, Todo Y, Konishiike A, et al: Scintigraphic detection of thrombi using indium-111-labeled autologous platelets. *J Cardiogr* 15:67, 1985.

77. Tsuda T, Kubota M, Iwakubo A, et al: Availability of ^{111}In-labeled platelet scintigraphy in patients with postinfarction left ventricular aneurysm. *Ann Nucl Med* 3:15, 1989.

78. Stratton JR, Ritchie JL, Werner JA: Indium-111 platelet imaging from the detection of intracardiac thrombi in survivors of sudden cardiac death. *Clin Res* 28:68A, 1980 (abst).

79. Seabold JE, Schroder E, Conrad GR, et al: Indium-111 platelet scintigraphy and two-dimensional echocardiography for detection of left ventricular thrombus: Influence of clot size and age. *J Am Coll Cardiol* 9:1057, 1987.

80. Benichou M, Camilleri JR, Bernard PJ, et al: Development of left intraventricular thrombi: Monitoring by two-dimensional echocardiography and scintigraphy with indium-111-labelled platelets. *Arch Mal Coeur* 81:1317, 1988.

81. Yamada M, Onishi K, Fukunami M, et al: Assessment

of warfarin therapy under full dose using indium-111 platelet scintigraphy in patiens with intracardiac thrombi. *Jpn Circ J* 52:1357, 1988.

82. Visser CA, Kan G, David GK, et al: Two-dimensional echocardiography in the diagnosis of left ventricular thrombus: A prospective study of 67 patients with anatomic validation. *Chest* 83:228, 1983.

83. Stratton JR, Lighty GJ, Pearlman AS, Ritchie JL: Detection of left ventricular thrombus by two-dimensional echocardiography: Sensitivity, specificity, and causes of uncertainty. *Circulation* 66:156, 1982.

84. Sheiban I, Casarotto D, Trevi G, et al: Two-dimensional echocardiography in the diagnosis of intracardiac masses: A prospective study with anatomic validation. *Cardiovasc Intervent Radiol* 10:157, 1987.

85. Starling MR, Crawford MH, Sorensen SG, Grover FL: Comparative value of invasive and noninvasive techniques for identifying left ventricular mural thrombi. *Am Heart J* 106:1143, 1983.

86. Keren A, Billingham ME, Popp RL: Echocardiographic recognition and implications of ventricular hypertrophic trabeculations and aberrant bands. *Circulation* 70:836, 1984.

87. Boyd MT, Seward JB, Tajik AJ, Edwards WD: Frequency and location of prominent left ventricular trabeculations at autopsy in 474 normal human hearts: Implications for evaluation of mural thrombi by two-dimensional echocardiography. *J Am Coll Cardiol* 9:323, 1987.

88. Visser CA, Kan G, Meltzer RS, et al: Embolic potential of left ventricular thrombus after myocardial infarction: A two-dimensional echocardiographic study of 119 patients. *J Am Coll Cardiol* 5:1276, 1985.

89. Haugland JM, Asinger RW, Mikell FL, et al: Embolic potential of left ventricular thrombi detected by two-dimensional echocardiography. *Circulation* 70:588, 1984.

90. Jugdutt BI, Sivaram CA: Prospective two-dimensional echocardiographic evaluation of left ventricular thrombus and embolism after acute myocardial infarction. *J Am Coll Cardiol* 13:554, 1989.

91. Johannessen KA, Nordrehaug JE, von-der-Lippe G, Vollset SE: Risk factors for embolisation in patients with left ventricular thrombi and acute myocardial infarction. *Br Heart J* 60:104, 1988.

92. Keren A, Goldberg S, Gottlieb S, et al: Natural history of left ventricular thrombi: their appearance and resolution in the posthospitalization period of acute myocardial infarction. *J Am Coll Cardiol* 15:790, 1990.

93. Stratton JR, Cerqueira MD, Dewhurst TA, Kohler TR: Imaging arterial thrombosis: Comparison of technetium-99m-labeled monoclonal antifibrin antibodies and indium-111 platelets. *J Nucl Med* 35:1731, 1994.

94. Sakoda S, Kinoshita M, Suzuki T: Left ventricular thrombi detected by Ga-67–DFO–DAS–fibrinogen imaging and two-dimensional echocardiography. *J Cardiol* 19:87, 1989.

95. Itagane H, Hirota K, Teragaki M, et al: Detection of left ventricular thrombi after acute myocardial infarction using Ga-67–DFO–DAS–fibrinogen. *J Cardiol* 18:949, 1988.

96. Stratton JR, Ritchie JL, Hammermeister KE, Kennedy

JW, Hamilton GW: Detection of left ventricular thrombi with radionuclide angiography. *Am J Cardiol* 48:565, 1981.

97. Stratton J: Left ventricular thrombi: Identification by radionuclide angiography. *Prim Cardiol* 10:133, 1984.

98. Yoshida H, Tsunoda K, Yamada Z, et al: Assessment of an intracardiac mural thrombus by contrast enhanced computed tomography. *J Cardiogr* 12:645, 1982.

99. Nair CK, Sketch MH, Mahoney PD, et al: Detection of left ventricular thrombi by computerised tomography: A preliminary report. *Br Heart J* 45:535, 1981.

100. Kanemitsu H, Hirata S, Inagaki T, Ishikawa K: Detection of left ventricular thrombi by echotomography and computed tomography. *J Cardiogr* 11:945, 1981.

101. Goldstein JA, Schiller NB, Lipton MJ, et al: Evaluation of left ventricular thrombi by contrast-enhanced computed tomography and two-dimensional echocardiography. *Am J Cardiol* 57:757, 1986.

102. Foster CJ, Sekiya T, Love HG, et al: Identification of intracardiac thrombus: Comparison of computed tomography and cross-sectional echocardiography. *Br J Radiol* 60:327, 1987.

103. Dooms GC, Higgins CB: MR imaging of cardiac thrombi. *J Comput Assist Tomogr* 10:415, 1986.

104. Johnson DE, Vacek J, Gollub SB, et al: Comparison of gated cardiac magnetic resonance imaging and two-dimensional echocardiography for the evaluation of right ventricular thrombi: A case report with autopsy correlation. *Cathet Cardiovasc Diagn* 14:266, 1988.

105. Sechtem U, Theissen P, Heindel W, et al: Diagnosis of left ventricular thrombi by magnetic resonance imaging and comparison with angiocardiography, computed tomography and echocardiography. *Am J Cardiol* 64:1195, 1989.

106. Zeitler E, Kaiser W, Schuierer G, et al: Magnetic resonance imaging of aneurysms and thrombi. *Cardiovasc Intervent Radiol* 8:321, 1986.

107. Zeitler E, Kaiser W, Schuierer G, et al: Magnetic resonance imaging of clots in the heart and vascular system. *Ann Radiol (Paris)* 28:105, 1985.

108. Vandenberg BF, Seabold JE, Conrad GR, et al: Indium-111 platelet scintigraphy and two-dimensional echocardiography for the detection of left atrial appendage thrombi: Studies in a new canine model. *Circulation* 78:1040, 1988.

109. Kessler C, Henningsen H, Reuther R: Der Nachweis intrakardialer Thromben mit der ^{111}In-Plattchenszintigraphie. *Nervenarzt* 56:311, 1985.

110. Yamada M, Hoki N, Ishikawa K, et al: Detection of left atrial thrombi in man using indium-111 labelled autologous platelets. *Br Heart J* 51:298, 1984.

111. Ezekowitz MD, Kellerman DJ, Smith EO, Streitz TM: Left atrial mass: Diagnostic value of transesophageal 2-dimensional echocardiography and indium-111 platelet scintigraphy. *Am J Cardiol* 51:1563, 1983.

112. Takeda T, Ishikawa N, Sakakibara Y, et al: A giant tumor thrombus in the right atrium clearly detected by [111]In−oxine labeled platelet scintigraphy. *Eur J Nucl Med* 11:49, 1985.

113. Nishimura T, Misawa T, Park YD, et al: Visualization of right atrial thrombus associated with constrictive peri-carditis by indium-111 oxine platelet imaging. *J Nucl Med* 28:1344, 1987.

114. Shrestha N, Moreno F, Marciso F, et al: Two dimensional echocardiographic diagnosis of left atrial thrombus in rheumatic heart disease: A clinicopathological study. *Circulation* 67:341, 1983.

115. Acar J, Cormier B, Grimberg D, et al: Diagnosis of left atrial thrombi in mitral stenosis: Usefulness of ultrasound techniques compared with other methods. *Eur Heart J* 12:70, 1991.

116. Aschenberg W, Schluter M, Kremer P, et al: Transesophageal two-dimensional echocardiography for the detection of left atrial thrombus. *J Am Coll Cardiol* 7:163, 1986.

117. Tsai LM, Chen JH, Lin LJ, Yang YJ: Role of transesophageal echocardiography in detecting left atrial thrombus and spontaneous echo contrast in patients with mitral valve disease or non-rheumatic atrial fibrillation. *Taiwan I Hsueh Hui Tsa Chih* 89:270, 1990.

118. Mugge A, Daniel WG, Haverich A, Lichtlen PR: Diagnosis of noninfective cardiac mass lesions by two-dimensional echocardiography: Comparison of the transthoracic and transesophageal approaches. *Circulation* 83:70, 1991.

119. Pearson AC, Labovitz AJ, Tatineni S, Gomez CR: Superiority of transesophageal echocardiography in detecting cardiac source of embolism in patients with cerebral ischemia of uncertain etiology. *J Am Coll Cardiol* 17:66, 1991.

120. Olson JD, Goldenberg IF, Pedersen W, et al: Exclusion of atrial thrombus by transesophageal echocardiography. *J Am Soc Echocardiogr* 5:52, 1992.

121. Kawata H, Matsuda H, Isaka Y, et al: Imaging analysis of platelet deposition on the extracardiac valved conduit in humans. *ASAIO Trans* 35:190, 1989.

122. Agarwal KC, Wahner HW, Dewanjee MK, et al: Imaging of platelets in right-sided extracardiac conduits in humans. *J Nucl Med* 23:342, 1982.

123. Boulay F, Danchin N, Neimann JL, et al: Echocardiographic features of right atrial thrombi. *J Clin Ultrasound* 14:601, 1986.

124. K'Ad'ar K, Harty'anszky I, Kir'aly L, Bendig L: Right heart thrombus in infants and children. *Pediatr Cardiol* 12:24, 1991.

125. Coto V, Cocozza M, Oliviero U, et al: Restrictive cardiomyopathy in eosinophilic leukemia: Echocardiographic and nuclear magnetic resonance aspects. *Cardiologia* 35:341, 1990.

126. Eskilsson J, Tallroth G: Spontaneous disappearance of right atrial thromboembolus without pulmonary embolism. *Acta Cardiol* 41:301, 1986.

127. Galanti G, Poggesi L, Comeglio M, et al: Right ventricular thrombosis in association with dilated cardiomyopathy: Diagnosis by echocardiography and nuclear magnetic resonance. *Cardiologia* 34:889, 1989.

128. Paul V, Foster CJ, Brownlee WC: Cross-sectional echocardiographic demonstration of biventricular thrombus. *Int J Cardiol* 18:266, 1988.

129. Corman C, Roudaut R, Gosse P, et al: Thromboses of the right atrium: Echocardiographic aspects, practical management—Apropos of 8 cases. *Arch Mal Coeur* 79:464, 1986.

130. Feltes TF, Friedman RA: Transesophageal echocardiographic detection of atrial thrombi in patients with non-fibrillation atrial tachyarrhythmias and congenital heart disease. *J Am Coll Cardiol* 24:1365, 1994.

131. Alam M, Sun I, Smith S: Transesophageal echocardiographic evaluation of right atrial mass lesions. *J Am Soc Echocardiogr* 4:331, 1991.

132. Kasper W, Meinertz T, Henkel B, et al: Echocardiographic findings in patients with proved pulmonary embolism. *Am Heart J* 112:1284, 1986.

133. Chapoutot L, Metz D, Canivet E, et al: Mobile thrombus of the right heart and pulmonary embolism: Diagnostic and therapeutic problems—Apropos of 12 cases. *Arch Mal Coeur* 86:1039, 1993.

134. Franzoni P, Cuccia C, Zappa C, et al: Thromboembolus migrating into the right heart in pulmonary embolism: Echocardiographic and clinico-therapeutic aspects in 7 cases and review of the literature. *G Ital Cardiol* 19:7, 1989.

135. Mancuso L, Marchi S, Mizio G, et al: Echocardiographic detection of right-sided cardiac thrombi in pulmonary embolism. *Chest* 92:23, 1987.

136. Riba AL, Thakur ML, Gottschalk A, et al: Imaging experimental infective endocarditis with indium-111-labeled blood cellular components. *Circulation* 59:336, 1979.

137. Dewanjee MK: Cardiac and vascular imaging with labeled platelets and leukocytes. *Semin Nucl Med* 14:154, 1984.

138. Dewanjee MK, Didisheim P, Kaye MP, et al: Platelet deposition on and calcification of bovine pericardial valve. *Eur Heart J* 5(suppl D):1, 1984.

139. Dewanjee MK, Trastek VF, Tago M, et al: Noninvasive radioisotopic technique for detection of platelet deposition on bovine pericardial mitral-valve prosthesis and in vitro quantification of visceral microembolism in dogs. *Trans Am Soc Artif Intern Organs* 29:188, 1983.

140. Dewanjee MK, Kaye MP, Fuster V, Rao SA: Noninvasive radioisotopic technique for detection of platelet deposition in mitral valve prosthesis and renal microembolism in dogs. *Trans Am Soc Artif Intern Organs* 26:475, 1980.

141. Dewanjee MK, Trastek VF, Tago M, Kaye MP: Radioisotopic techniques for noninvasive detection of platelet deposition in bovine-tissue mitral-valve prostheses and in vitro quantification of visceral microembolism in dogs. *Invest Radiol* 19:535, 1984.

142. Acar J, Vahanian A, Dorent R, et al: Detection of prosthetic valve thrombosis using [111]indium platelet imaging. *Eur Heart J* 11:389, 1990.

143. Otaki M, Kawashima M, Yamaguchi A, Kitamura N: A case report of a thrombosed mitral prosthesis diagnosed by [111]In—oxine platelet scintigraphy. *Kokyu To Junkan* 39:501, 1991.

144. Bergmann SR, Lerch RA, Mathias CJ, et al: Noninvasive detection of coronary thrombi with In-111 platelets: Concise communication. *J Nucl Med* 24:130, 1983.

145. Riba AL, Thakur ML, Gottschalk A, Zaret BL: Imaging experimental coronary artery thrombosis with indium-111 platelets. *Circulation* 60:767, 1979.

146. Fox KA, Bergmann SR, Mathias CJ, et al: Scintigraphic detection of coronary artery thrombi in patients with acute myocardial infarction. *J Am Coll Cardiol* 4:975, 1984.

147. Laws KH, Clanton JA, Starnes VA: Kinetics and imaging of indium-111-labelled autologous platelets in experimental myocardial infarction. *Circulation* 67:110, 1983.

148. Romson JL, Hook BG, Rigot VH, et al: The effect of ibuprofen on accumulation of indium-111-labeled platelets and leukocytes in experimental myocardial infarction. *Circulation* 66:1002, 1982.

149. Callahan RJ, Bunting RW, Block PC: Evaluation of platelet deposition at the site of coronary angioplasty using indium-111 labeled platelets. *J Nucl Med* 24:P60, 1983 (abst).

150. Sinzinger H, Virgolini I: Nuclear medicine and atherosclerosis. *Eur J Nucl Med* 17:160, 1990.

151. Ezekowitz MD, Eichner ER, Scatterday R, Elkins RC: Diagnosis of a persistent pulmonary embolus by indium-111 platelet scintigraphy with angiographic and tissue confirmation. *Am J Med* 72:839, 1982.

152. Sostman HD, Neumann RD, Loke J, et al: Detection of pulmonary embolism in man with ^{111}In-labeled autologous platelets. *Am J Roentgenol* 138:945, 1982.

153. Poskitt KR, Payne MN, Lane IF, McCollum CN: Radiolabeled platelets in detecting the souce of recurrent pulmonary emboli: A case report. *Angiology* 38:62, 1987.

154. Uchida Y, Minoshima S, Anzai Y, Okada J, et al: A case of pulmonary embolism diagnosed by ^{111}In labeled platelet scintigraphy. *Kaku Igaku* 27:869, 1990.

155. Davis HH, Siegel BA, Sherman LA, et al: Scintigraphy with ^{111}In-labeled autologous platelets in venous thromboembolism. *Radiology* 136:203, 1980.

156. Clarke-Pearson DL, Coleman RE, Siegel R, et al: Indium 111 platelet imaging for the detection of deep venous thrombosis and pulmonary embolism in patients without symptoms after surgery. *Surgery* 98:98, 1985.

157. Moser KM, Fedullo PF: Imaging of venous thromboemboli with labeled platelets. *Semin Nucl Med* 14:188, 1984.

158. Moser KM, Fedullo PF: Imaging of venous thromboemboli with 111-In labeled platelets, in Heyns AD, Badenhorst PN, Lotter MG (eds): *Platelet Kinetics and Imaging*, vol 2. Boca Raton, FL: CRC, 1985, pp. 57–70.

159. Knight LC, Primeau JL, Siegel BA, Welch MJ: Comparison of In-111-labeled platelets and iodinated fibrinogen for the detection of deep vein thrombosis. *J Nucl Med* 19:891, 1978.

160. Dormehl IC, Jacobs DJ, du Plessis M, et al: Evaluation of the diagnostic efficacy of autologous ^{111}In-labelled platelets as a scanning agent for deep vein thrombosis in the chacma baboon. *Eur J Nucl Med* 10:432, 1985.

161. Dormehl IC, Jacobs DJ, Pretorius JP, et al: Baboon (*Papio ursinus*) model to study deep vein thrombosis using 111-indium-labeled autologous platelets. *J Med Primatol* 16:27, 1987.

162. Grossman ZD, Rosebrough SF, McAfee JG, et al: Imaging fresh venous thrombi in the dog with I-131 and In-111 labeled fibrin-specific monoclonal antibody and F(ab')₂ fragments. *Radiographics* 7:913, 1987.

163. Ezekowitz MD, Pope CF, Sostman HD, et al: Indium-111

platelet scintigraphy for the diagnosis of acute venous thrombosis. *Circulation* 73:668, 1986.

164. Fenech A, Hussey JK, Smith FW, et al: Diagnosis of deep vein thrombosis using autologous indium-III-labelled platelets. *BMJ* 282:1020, 1981.

165. Grimley RP, Rafiqi E, Hawker RJ, Drolc Z: Imaging of ^{111}In-labelled platelets: A new method for the diagnosis of deep vein thrombosis. *Br J Surg* 68:714, 1981.

166. Seabold JE, Conrad GR, Ponto JA, et al: Deep venous thrombophlebitis: Detection with 4-hour versus 24-hour platelet scintigraphy. *Radiology* 165:355, 1987.

167. Farlow DC, Ezekowitz MD, Rao SR, et al: Early image acquisition after administration of indium-111 platelets in clinically suspected deep venous thrombosis. *Am J Cardiol* 64:363, 1989.

168. Ezekowitz MD, Migliaccio F, Farlow D, et al: Comparison of platelet scintigraphy, impedance plethysmography gray scale and color flow duplex ultrasound and venography for the diagnosis of venous thrombosis. *Prog Clin Biol Res* 355:23, 1990.

169. Hansberry KL, Thompson IJ, Bauman J, et al: A prospective comparison of thromboembolic stockings, external sequential pneumatic compression stockings and heparin sodium/dihydroergotamine mesylate for the prevention of thromboembolic complications in urological surgery. *J Urol* 145:1205, 1991.

170. Siegel RS, Rae JL, Ryan NL, et al: The use of indium-111 labeled platelet scanning for the detection of asymptomatic deep venous thrombosis in a high risk population. *Orthopedics* 12:1439, 1989.

171. Depace NL, Elguezabal A, Kotler MN, Wagner B: Giant left atrium with massive mural thrombus in a patient with mitral stenosis. *J Med Soc NJ* 78:754, 1981.

172. Winter JH, Fenech A, Bennett B, Douglas AS: Preoperative antithrombin III activities and lipoprotein concentrations as predictors of venous thrombosis in patients with fracture of neck of femur. *J Clin Pathol* 36:570, 1983.

173. Winter JH, Buckler PW, Bautista AP, et al: Frequency of venous thrombosis in patients with an exacerbation of chronic obstructive lung disease. *Thorax* 38:605, 1983.

174. Knight LC: Scintigraphic methods for detecting vascular thrombus. *J Nucl Med* 34:554, 1993.

175. Tait JF, Cerqueira MD, Dewhurst TA, et al: Evaluation of annexin V as a platelet-directed thrombus targeting agent. *Thromb Res* 75:491, 1994.

176. Stratton JR, Dewhurst TA, Kasina S, et al: Selective uptake of radiolabeled annexin V on acute porcine left atrial thrombi. *Circulation* 92:3113, 1995.

177. Seabold JE, Rosebrough SF: Will a radiolabeled antibody replace indium-111-platelets to detect active thrombus? [Editorial; comment]. *J Nucl Med* 35:1738, 1994.

178. Knight LC, Radcliffe R, Maurer AH, et al: Thrombus imaging with technetium-99m synthetic peptides based upon the binding domain of a monoclonal antibody to activated platelets. *J Nucl Med* 35:282, 1994.

179. Lusiani L, Zanco P, Visona A, et al: Immunoscintigraphic detection of venous thrombosis of the lower extremities by means of human antifibrin monoclonal antibodies labeled with In-111. *Angiology* 40:671, 1989.

180. Jung M, Kletter K, Dudczak R, et al: Deep vein thrombosis: Scintigraphic diagnosis with In-111-labeled monoclonal antifibrin antibodies. *Radiology* 173:469, 1989.

181. Aronen H: Diagnosis of deep venous thrombosis of the leg using immunoscintigraphy with In-111-labelled monoclonal antifibrin antibody fragments. *Acta Radiol* 30:159, 1989.

182. Alavi A, Palevsky HI, Gupta N, et al: Radiolabeled antifibrin antibody in the detection of venous thrombosis: Preliminary results. *Radiology* 175:79, 1990.

183. Alavi A, Gupta N, Palevsky HI, et al: Detection of thrombophlebitis with ^{111}In-labeled anti-fibrin antibody: Preliminary results. *Cancer Res* 50:958s, 1990.

184. DeFaucal P, Peltier P, Planchon B, et al: Evaluation of indium-111-labeled antifibrin monoclonal antibody for the diagnosis of venous thrombotic disease. *J Nucl Med* 32:785, 1991.

185. El Kouri D, Dupas B, Peltier P, et al: Diagnosis of venous thrombosis: Evaluation of immunoscintigraphy with 99m technetium labelled antifibrin. *Presse Med* 23:931, 1994.

186. Cerqueira MD, Stratton JR, Vracko R, et al: Noninvasive arterial thrombus imaging with 99mTc monoclonal antifibrin antibody. *Circulation* 85:298, 1992.

187. Tromholt N, Hesse B, Folkenborg O, et al: Detection of deep venous thrombosis with indium 111-labelled monoclonal antibody against tissue plasminogen activator. *Eur J Nucl Med* 18:321, 1991.

188. Kingg AD, Bell SD, Stuttle AWJ, et al: Platelet imaging of thromboembolism: Natural history of postoperative deep venous thrombosis and pulmonary embolism illustrated using the indium-111 labelled platelet-specific monoclonal antibody, P-256. *Chest* 101:1597, 1992.

189. Stuttle AW, Klosok J, Peters AM, Lavender JP: Sequential imaging of post-operative thrombus using the In-111-labelled platelet-specific monoclonal antibody P256. *Br J Radiol* 62:963, 1989.

190. Stuttle AW, Peters AM, Loutfi I, et al: Use of an antiplatelet monoclonal antibody F(ab')₂ fragment for imaging thrombus. *Nucl Med Commun* 9:647, 1988.

191. Peters AM, Lavender JP, Needham SG, et al: Imaging thrombus with radiolabelled monoclonal antibody to platelets. *BMJ* 293:1525, 1986.

192. Knight LC: Imaging thrombi with radiolabelled fragment E1. *Nucl Med Commun* 9:849, 1988.

193. Knight LC, Maurer AH, Robbins PS, et al: Fragment E1 labeled with I-123 in the detection of venous thrombosis. *Radiology* 156:509, 1985.

194. Knight LC, Abrams MJ, Schwartz DA, et al: Preparation and preliminary evaluation of technetium-99m-labeled fragment E1 for thrombus imaging. *J Nucl Med* 33:710, 1992.

195. Knight L, Olexa S, Malmud L, Budzynski A: Specific uptake of radioiodinated fragment E1 by venous thrombi in pigs. *J Clin Invest* 72:2007, 1983.

196. Knight L, Lister-James J, Dean RT, Maurer A: Evaluation of Tc-99m labeled cyclic peptides for thrombus imaging. *J Nucl Med* 34(suppl):17P, 1993 (abst).

197. Muto P, Lastoria S, Varrella P, et al: Detecting deep venous thrombosis with technetium-99m-labeled synthetic peptide P280. *J Nucl Med* 36:1384, 1995.

198. Miller DD, Boulet AJ, Tio FO, et al: In vivo technetium-99m S12 antibody imaging of platelet alpha-granules in rabbit endothelial neointimal proliferation after angioplasty. *Circulation* 83:224, 1991.

199. Palabrica TM, Furie BC, Konsam MA, et al: Thrombus imaging in a primate model with antibodies specific for an exteral membrane protein of activated platelets. *Proc Natl Acad Sci USA* 86:1036, 1989.

200. Ord JM, Hasapes J, Daugherty A, et al: Imaging of thrombi with tissue-type plasminogen activator rendered enzymatically inactive and conjugated to a residualizing label. *Circulation* 85:288, 1992.

MIBG Scintigraphy of Myocardial Innervation

Michael W. Dae

The sympathetic nervous system has profound influences on myocardial function and pathophysiology. The heart is densely innervated with sympathetic nerves, which are distributed on a regional basis. Heterogeneity of myocardial sympathetic innervation, or autonomic imbalance, has long been hypothesized as a major mechanism underlying sudden cardiac death. Only in the past few years has it been possible to evaluate abnormalities in heart innervation in the intact animal. Recent developments in cardiac imaging have lead to the ability to map the distribution of the sympathetic nerves in vivo, using radiolabelled metaiodobenzylguanidine (MIBG). As a result, the pathophysiologic mechanisms relating alterations in sympathetic nerve activity to disease processes are now being explored.

MYOCARDIAL UPTAKE OF MIBG

Myocardial sympathetic nerves have been shown to take up exogenously administered catecholamines. Early studies in rat hearts showed rapid accumulation of tritiated norepinephrine[1] into sympathetic nerve endings by a high-affinity uptake process (uptake 1). Subsequently, a low-affinity, high-capacity nonneuronal uptake process was also found (uptake 2).[2] Further studies showed that the neuronally bound catecholamine was retained in storage vesicles for long periods of time, whereas the nonneuronally bound compound was rapidly metabo-

lized and subsequently washed out of the heart at a fairly rapid rate.[3] Numerous other substances with chemical structures similar to norepinephrine have also been shown to enter sympathetic nerves (false adrenergic transmitters).[4] Several years ago, MIBG, an analog of the false adrenergic transmitter, guanethidine, was developed.[5] Radioiodinated MIBG was shown to localize to the heart and other organs in several animal species and in humans.[6]

MIBG is thought to share similar uptake and storage mechanisms as norepinephrine,[7,8] but is not metabolized by monoamine oxidase or catechol-o-methyltransferase. Hence, MIBG localizes to myocardial sympathetic nerve endings (Fig. 29-1). Numerous studies have evaluated the characteristics of MIBG uptake and distribution in experimental models designed to alter global and regional function of myocardial sympathetic nerves.

Sisson et al assessed the myocardial uptake of iodine-125 (^{125}I) MIBG in rats treated with either 6-hydroxydopamine, which causes a chemical degeneration of sympathetic nerves, or desmethylimipramine, an uptake-1 inhibitor.[9] Significant reductions in MIBG uptake occurred with both treatments. The responses of MIBG to perturbations of sympathetic nerves were qualitatively similar to the responses of ^{3}H norepinephrine.

Dae et al examined the early and late distributions of ^{123}I-labeled MIBG in normal and globally denervated canine and human hearts.[10] Canine hearts were denervated by intravenous injections of 6-hydroxydopamine, while patients were studied a mean of 4.3 months following cardiac transplantation. Results in denervated hearts

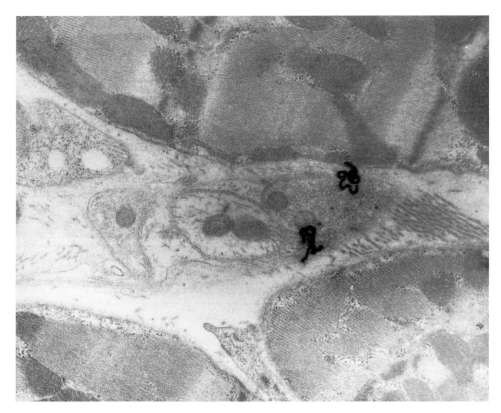

Figure 29-1   An electron microscopic autoradiograph of a rat heart. The two silver grains, formed by iodine-125 MIBG, are localized over a sympathetic nerve terminal.

were compared with normal controls. Normal hearts showed prominent uptake of MIBG on initial 5-min and 3-h delayed images (Figs. 29-2 and 29-3). Globally denervated canine hearts showed prominent uptake on initial images and absence of localization on delayed images, indicating complete washout of nonneuronally bound radionuclide (Fig. 29-2). The transplanted human heart showed no localization of MIBG on either the early or delayed images (Fig. 29-3). These studies suggest that the nonneuronal uptake mechanism (uptake 2) is not significant in human myocardium. This finding has significant implications for interpreting the myocardial behavior of MIBG in various pathologic situations such as dilated cardiomyopathy. Subsequent studies in transplanted human hearts showed evidence of reinnervation in about 50 percent of patients within 1 year of transplantation[11] (Fig. 29-4).

ASSESSMENT OF REGIONAL MYOCARDIAL INNERVATION

Validation Studies

To assess the feasibility of imaging noninvasively the distribution of myocardial sympathetic innervation in

dogs with regional denervation, Dae and colleagues evaluated the distribution of sympathetic nerve endings, using ^{123}I MIBG, and compared this with the distribution of myocardial perfusion, using thallium 201.[12] Regional denervation was induced by left stellate ganglion removal, right stellate ganglion removal, or application of phenol to the epicardial surface. Control dogs showed homogeneous and parallel distributions of MIBG and thallium in the major left ventricular mass. In the left stellectomized hearts, MIBG was reduced relative to thallium in the posterior left ventricle; whereas, in right stellectomized hearts, MIBG uptake was reduced in the anterior left ventricle (Plate 21). Phenol-painted hearts showed a broad area of decreased MIBG activity extending beyond the area of phenol application. The thallium distribution was homogeneous in all hearts. Norepinephrine content was greater in regions showing normal MIBG activity (550 ± 223 ng/g) compared with regions showing reduced MIBG activity (39 ± 44 ng/g) ($p <$ 0.001), confirming regional denervation. Others have also shown reduced MIBG uptake in regionally denervated dog hearts.[13]

In another series of experiments, Mori et al evaluated the contractile responses of hearts showing regional denervation by MIBG imaging.[14] Regional denervation was produced by the application of phenol to the midbasal epicardium. Ultrasonic crystals were placed to measure

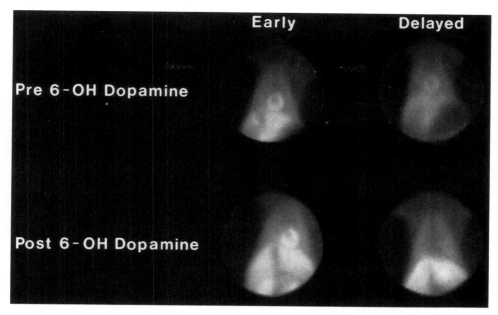

Figure 29-2 Early and delayed MIBG images in a dog studied at baseline (*top*) and 1 week after 6-hydroxydopamine treatment (*bottom*). There is prominent myocardial localization on both the early and delayed images at baseline. The post-6-hydroxydopamine images show prominent myocardial localization on the early images, whereas the delayed images show absence of myocardial localization. (From Dae et al,[10] Scintigraphic assessment of MIBG uptake in globally denervated human and canine hearts: Implications for clinical studies, *J Nucl Med* 33:1444, 1992, reproduced with permission.)

segmental shortening in response to left and right stellate stimulation, isoproterenol infusion, and tyramine infusion. Animals were studied acutely (1 to 2 h), after application of phenol, and chronically (3 to 14 days) after phenol application. At baseline, the area subsequently treated with phenol showed increased shortening in response to sympathetic nerve stimulation and isoproterenol infusion. One hour after the application of phenol (acute study), the contractile response of the midphenol region was reduced following nerve stimulation, consistent with interruption of nerve impulses by phenol treatment. MIBG uptake in the acutely denervated hearts was normal, however, consistent with preservation of neuronal function at the sympathetic nerve terminals. In the hearts studied 3 to 14 days after phenol treatment, the contractile responses were reduced after nerve stimulation, MIBG uptake was reduced, and there was no response to tyramine infusion. These results indicate that although phenol acutely interrupts conduction in axons crossing the phenol line, causing a *functional* denervation, the nerve endings remain viable for at least several hours. Within 3 to 14 days after the phenol application, the terminals of the transected efferent fibers degenerate, causing a *structural* denervation, as evidenced by the reduction in MIBG uptake. There was an increased contractile response to isoproterenol infusion acutely and chronically, indicating intact postsynaptic responses to beta-receptor stimulation.

Experimental Myocardial Ischemia and Infarction

The sympathetic nerves are acutely affected in regions of myocardial ischemia, as detected by enhanced washout of MIBG from the ischemic territory[15] (Fig. 29-5). The release of MIBG is not due to reflex neural increases in sympathetic tone during myocardial ischemia, but to local release from sympathetic nerve endings in the ischemic bed.[15] Transmural myocardial infarction can lead to a partially denervated ventricle,[16] which may predispose the heart to arrhythmia.[17] Dae and colleagues assessed MIBG uptake in dogs with transmural and nontransmural myocardial infarction.[18] Transmural myocardial infarction was produced by the injection of vinyl latex into the left anterior descending coronary artery, and nontransmural myocardial infarction was produced by ligation of the left anterior descending coronary artery. Hearts with transmural infarction showed zones of absent MIBG and thallium, indicating scar. Adjacent and distal regions showed reduced MIBG but normal thallium uptake, indicating viable but denervated myocardium (Plate 22). Denervation distal to the infarcted area was confirmed by reduced norepinephrine content and absence of nerve fluorescence. Nontransmural myocardial infarction also showed regional denervation. These findings demonstrate that in experimental myocardial infarction, the relative uptake of MIBG shows a spectrum: no uptake in the center of an infarct

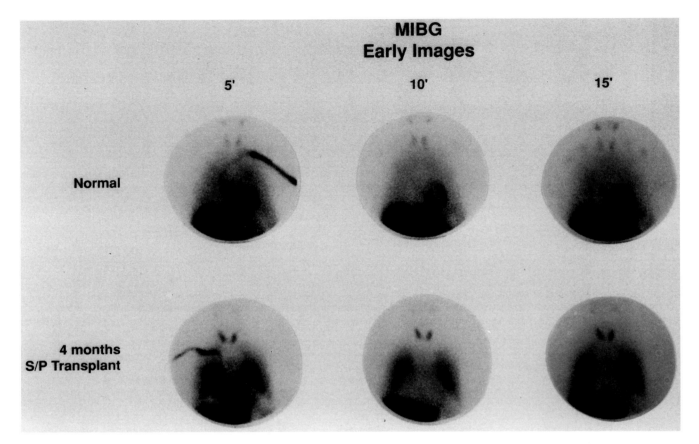

Figure 29-3 Five-minute static images taken at 5, 10, and 15 min after injection in a normal control (*top*) and in a patient studied 4 months after cardiac transplantation. After blood-pool clearance, there is absence of myocardial localization in the transplanted heart. (From Dae et al,[10] Scintigraphic assessment of MIBG uptake in globally denervated human and canine hearts: Implications for clinical studies, *J Nucl Med* 33:1444, 1992, reproduced with permission.)

with no flow, and relative decreased MIBG uptake in the perfused border zone of an infarct. This border zone may be transmural or nontransmural.

The mechanisms leading to denervation in transmural and nontransmural infarction may be different. Transmural myocardial infarction has been hypothesized to produce denervation secondary to necrosis of proximal sympathetic nerve trunks that travel in the subepicardium.[16] Viable myocardium distal to the infarction becomes denervated as a result of loss of proximal nerve input. As opposed to the distal denervation produced by transmural myocardial infarction, nontransmural infarction may lead to local ischemic damage of sympathetic nerve endings that are present within the ischemic zone. Studies of nontransmural infarction produced by intracoronary balloon occlusion (to avoid denervation due to injury of perivascular sympathetic nerves) confirmed that nontransmural myocardial infarction can produce regional denervation (Plate 23). These studies suggested that ischemia sufficient to cause myocardial necrosis is necessary before regional denervation develops.[15]

Partial denervation has been shown to occur in humans after myocardial infarction.[19–22] Stanton et al found a relationship between the presence of sympathetic denervation and the occurrence of spontaneous ventricular tachyarrhythmias, but not to sustained ventricular tachycardia induced at electrophysiologic testing.[20]

Diabetic Neuropathy

Recent studies have shown regional MIBG uptake abnormalities in the hearts of patients with diabetic neuropathy.[23] The functional significance of regional denervation in these patients is unknown.[24]

SCINTIGRAPHIC AND ELECTROPHYSIOLOGIC CORRELATIONS IN EXPERIMENTAL MYOCARDIAL INFARCTION

Schwartz et al demonstrated that stimulation of the left stellate ganglion or removal of the right stellate ganglion

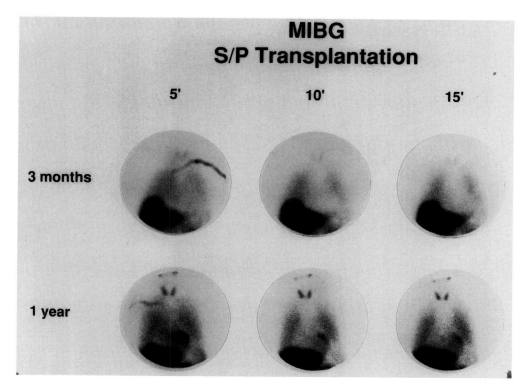

Figure 29-4 MIBG images from a patient studied at 3 months and 1 year after transplantation. MIBG myocardial localization is absent at 3 months but present at 1 year after transplantation. S/P, status post. (From De Marco et al,[11] J Am Coll Cardiol 25:927, 1995, reproduced with permission of the American College of Cardiology.)

lowered the ventricular fibrillation threshold.[25] In contrast, stimulation of the right stellate ganglion or removal of the left stellate ganglion raised the ventricular fibrillation threshold.[25,26] Randall et al have demonstrated an increased incidence of spontaneous junctional and ventricular arrhythmias particularly during exercise following denervation of the heart sparing the ventrolateral cardiac nerve.[27] These early studies led to the concept that heterogeneity of sympathetic innervation, or "sympathetic imbalance," could adversely affect the electrical stability of the heart.[28]

Minardo et al correlated MIBG scintigraphy with electrophysiologic responses to sympathetic stimulation in dogs with myocardial infarction.[29] During sympathetic stimulation, areas of viable myocardium with diminished MIBG uptake showed reduced shortening of the effective refractory period compared with normal basal myocardium. However, enhanced shortening of effective refractory period was found in the regions showing reduced MIBG uptake during norepinephrine infusion, indicating supersensitivity of the denervated regions. MIBG images returned to normal a mean of 14 weeks after infarction, consistent with reinnervation. Other studies have shown increased susceptibility to induced ventricular fibrillation or ventricular tachycardia in dogs with myocardial infarction and denervation.[17,30]

Newman and associates studied the effects of left stellate ganglion stimulation on regional epicardial monophasic action potential duration in dogs with chronic myocardial infarction.[31] These effects were correlated with MIBG and thallium imaging to identify areas of viable but denervated myocardium. During constant ventricular pacing, stellate stimulation shortened the action potential duration only in the innervated areas, whereas there was no change in action potential duration in the denervated areas (Fig. 29-6). This dispersion of refractoriness, which was accentuated during increased sympathetic tone, is thought to be a major underlying mechanism for ventricular arrhythmias. These results provide further confirmation of the electrophysiologic significance of scintigraphic denervation.

Several recent clinical studies have shown regional heterogeneity of MIBG uptake in patients with ventricular tachycardia and a "clinically normal heart."[32,33] In the report by Gill et al, patients with ventricular tachycardia had a higher proportion of asymmetric MIBG scans (47 percent) than subjects in the control group (0 percent).[33] Of patients with exercise-induced ventricular tachycardia and clinically normal hearts, 62 percent had asymmetric MIBG scans with a tendency toward reduced MIBG uptake in the septum. Dae and colleagues recently observed heterogeneous sympathetic innervation in a

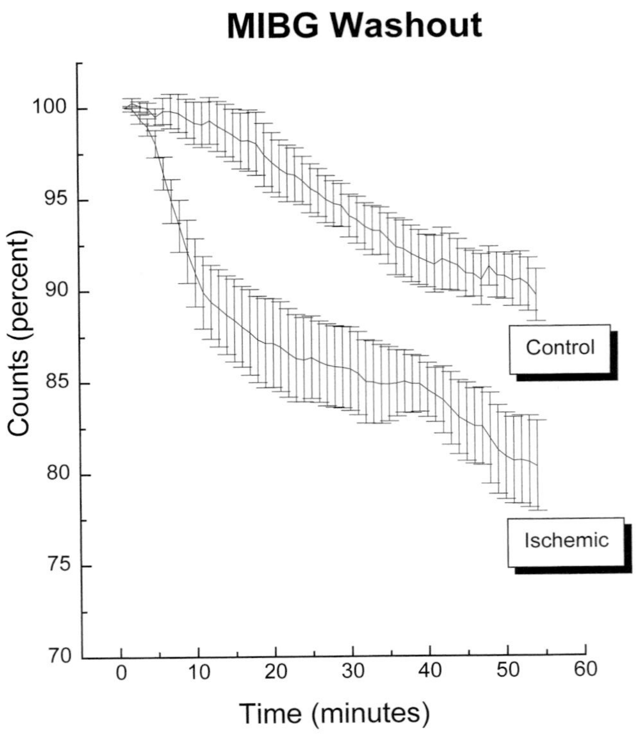

MIBG Washout

Figure 29-5 Composite time versus radioactivity curves (mean and standard error) from ischemic myocardium, showing enhanced MIBG washout during coronary occlusion and reperfusion, compared with nonischemic regions. The curves represent combined results from nine animals. (From Dae et al,[15] reproduced with permission.)

population of German shepherd dogs with inherited spontaneous ventricular arrhythmias and sudden death.[34] In a study of patients with arrhythmogenic right ventricular cardiomyopathy, 40 of 48 patients showed regional reductions in MIBG uptake located primarily in the basal posteroseptal left ventricle[35] (Plate 24). All of the patients in the control group showed homogeneous innervation. Abnormalities in MIBG scintigraphy in patients with arrhythmogenic right ventricular cardiomyopathy correlated with the site of origin of ventricular tachycardia, demonstrating regionally reduced uptake in 36 of 38 patients with right ventricular outflow tract tachycardia. The authors speculated that regional sympathetic denervation-related supersensitivity may be the underlying mechanism to explain the frequent provocation of ventricular arrhythmias by exercise or catecholamine infusion. The long QT syndrome is another condition associated with ventricular arrhythmias where abnormalities in regional MIBG uptake have been reported.[36] Dispersion of regional innervation[37] and repolarization[38] have also been identified in patients with dilated cardiomyopathy.

ASSESSMENT OF SYMPATHETIC NERVOUS SYSTEM ACTIVATION

One of the early physiologic responses to counteract depressed myocardial function is activation of a number of neurohumoral systems, such as the renin–angiotensin system, sympathetic nervous system, and the arginine–vasopressin system.[39] It is now widely accepted that excessive stimulation of these compensatory systems eventually leads to deterioration of ventricular function and may contribute to sudden cardiac death.[40] Sustained activation of the sympathetic nervous system is thought to play a major role in the etiology of sudden cardiac death.[41] More than 300,000 sudden cardiac deaths occur each year in the United States, accounting for 50 percent of all cardiac-related mortality.[42] The majority of these deaths occur among patients with prior healed myocardial infarctions and left ventricular dysfunction.[43] These deaths are thought to originate as ventricular tachycardia, which may degenerate into ventricular fibrillation. In most instances, there is no associated evidence for either acute infarction or significant ischemia.[43] Arrhythmia and sudden death are also important features of noncoronary cardiomyopathy and heart failure. Approximately 40 percent of patients with severe heart failure die suddenly, presumably of arrhythmia.[44]

The incidence of sudden death has been shown to correlate directly with both the extent of myocardial damage after infarction and the presence of complex spontaneous ventricular ectopy.[45,46] In addition, compelling evidence has emerged that implicates the sympathetic nervous system in the genesis of ventricular arrhythmias and sudden death. Beta-blocker therapy has been shown to reduce the incidence of total and sudden death in patients with myocardial infarction.[47] Beta blockers have been found to be particularly useful in decreasing the incidence of sudden death in patients with myocardial infarction and left ventricular dysfunction.[48] Elevated plasma catecholamines have been shown to identify patients with heart failure who are also at risk for sudden death.[49] Recent data showed significantly greater activation of myocardial sympathetic nerves in patients with left ventricular dysfunction and life-threatening ventricular arrhythmias compared with age-matched controls without a history of arrhythmia.[41]

Myocardial MIBG imaging may play a role in detecting sympathetic nervous system activation. In experimental studies, acute changes in adrenergic nerve activity of the heart have been assessed by measuring the rates of loss of neuronally bound MIBG. Sisson et al compared rates of loss of norepinephrine and MIBG in rat and dog hearts.[50] They used yohimbine, an α_2-adrenergic receptor antagonist, to increase the function of the sympathetic nerves, and clonidine, an α_2 agonist, to decrease the activity of the sympathetic nerves. In rat hearts, yohim-

Dog 116
Slice 2/6
VENTRICULAR PACING AT CL 300msec

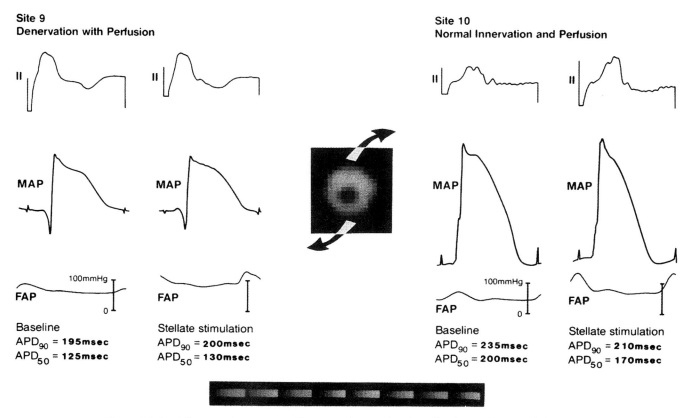

Site 9
Denervation with Perfusion

II

MAP

100mmHg

FAP   FAP

Baseline   Stellate stimulation
APD_{90} = **195msec** APD_{90} = **200msec**
APD_{50} = **125msec** APD_{50} = **130msec**

Site 10
Normal Innervation and Perfusion

II

MAP

100mmHg

FAP   FAP

Baseline   Stellate stimulation
APD_{90} = **235msec** APD_{90} = **210msec**
APD_{50} = **200msec** APD_{50} = **170msec**

Figure 29-6 A functional map (center) from a midventricular slice of a dog with regional denervation after myocardial infarction. The denervated area is *gray*, and the normally innervated area is *white*. Monophasic action potentials from the corresponding epicardial surfaces are also shown. There is a significant shortening of monophasic action potential duration in the normally innervated area, but no change in action potential duration in the denervated area, in response to stellate stimulation. Note that blood pressure (FAP, femoral arterial pressure) rose during stellate stimulation and that the electrocardiographic result (lead II) did not change. (From Newman et al,[31] reproduced with permission.)

bine induced similar increases in rates of loss of ^{3}H norepinephrine and ^{125}I MIBG, while clonidine induced similar decreases in rates of loss of ^{3}H norepinephrine and ^{125}I MIBG. Preliminary imaging studies in dog hearts with ^{123}I MIBG showed similar responses to yohimbine and clonidine. These results suggest that it may be possible to assess acute changes in efferent sympathetic activity to the heart, noninvasively. Although no studies have been reported to date in human hearts that compare MIBG washout kinetics with generally accepted standards for increased sympathetic tone such as norepinephrine spillover,[51] a number of clinical conditions thought associated with increased sympathetic tone have demonstrated enhanced washout of MIBG (Fig. 29-7). Henderson et al studied the myocardial distribution and kinetics of MIBG in images obtained from patients with conges-

tive cardiomyopathy compared with normal controls.[37] Patients with congestive cardiomyopathy had a 28 percent washout rate of MIBG from the heart over a period of 15 to 85 min following intravenous injection, as compared with a washout rate of 6 percent in the controls. The differences were highly significant ($p < 0.001$). In a recent study by Nakajima et al, patients with various cardiac disorders underwent planar MIBG imaging at 20 min and 3 h after injection.[52] A very high washout rate of more than 25 percent was seen in a number of cases of dilated cardiomyopathy (5 of 11), hypertrophic cardiomyopathy (11 of 24), ischemic heart disease (23 of 34), essential hypertension (five of 13), and hypothyroidism (six of 13). Mean washout rate in control patients was 9.6 percent. As demonstrated, enhanced MIBG washout can be seen in a number of different

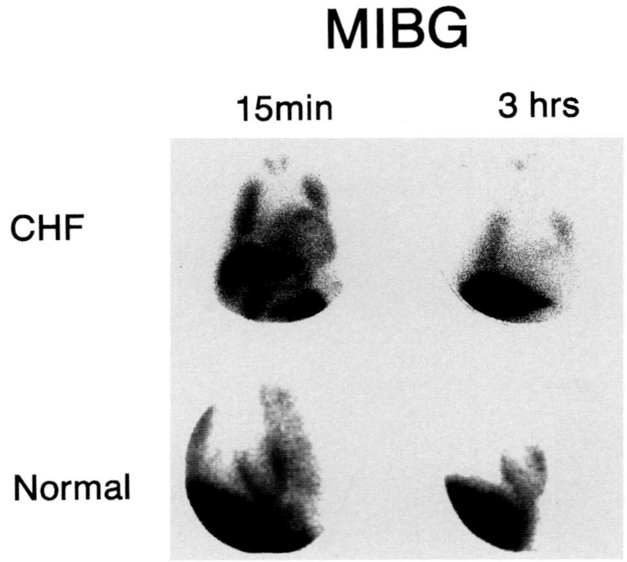

MIBG

15min   **3 hrs**

CHF

Normal

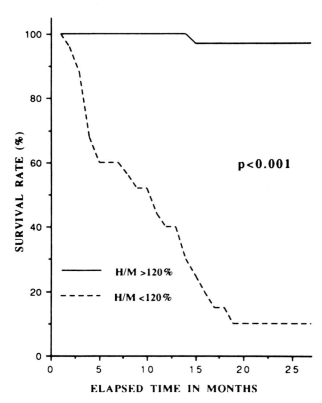

Figure 29-7 Planar iodine-123 MIBG images from the anterior projection at 15 min (*left*) and 3 h (*right*) from a patient with congestive heart failure due to dilated cardiomyopathy (*top*), compared with a control patient (*bottom*). Note the significant washout of MIBG at 3 h in the patient with congestive heart failure, whereas the control patient shows retention of MIBG. This washout of MIBG likely reflects enhanced activation of myocardial sympathetic nerves.

diseases. The mechanism in common is most likely activation of the sympathetic nervous system. It can also be seen that not all patients have the same degree of enhanced washout.

There are no reports to date to evaluate the prognostic utility of MIBG washout. In one study, however, Merlet et al reported the results of a prospective study of a group of 90 patients with congestive heart failure related to idiopathic dilated cardiomyopathy.[53] They assessed MIBG uptake, ejection fraction, cardiothoracic ratio on x-ray, and M-mode echocardiographic data, and followed the cases for up to 27 months. Multivariate life-table analysis showed that MIBG uptake, as assessed by the myocardial-to-mediastinal count ratio on anterior planar MIBG scans at 4 h after injection, was the best predictor for survival (Fig. 29-8). Myocardial-to-mediastinal ratio on delayed MIBG images has been shown to correlate inversely with MIBG washout.[52] Imamura et al recently demonstrated that the level of myocardial MIBG washout was related to the severity of heart failure, as measured by New York Heart Association classification[54] (Fig. 29-9). These interesting results suggest that there may be a significant role for MIBG imaging in the assessment of prognosis in patients with heart failure. Further studies involving larger numbers of patients are needed to evaluate the prognostic utility of MIBG uptake and washout kinetics.

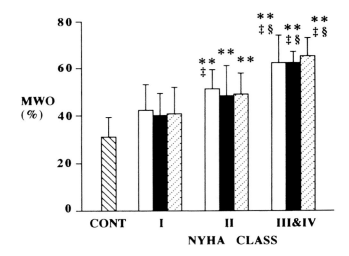

Figure 29-8 Survival curve, using life-table analysis, with a threshold value of 120 percent for heart-to-mediastinal MIBG ratio (H/M). A striking difference is seen for survival between patients with H/M less (*dotted line*) or greater (*unbroken line*) than 120 percent ($p < 0.001$). (From Merlet et al,[53] Prognostic valve of cardiac metaiodobenzylguanidine imaging in patients with heart failure, *J Nucl Med* 33:471, 1992, reproduced with permission.)

Figure 29-9 Functional cardiac status [New York Heart Association (NYHA) classification] versus myocardial washout (MWO) of MIBG in each heart failure group: *open bars*, dilated cardiomyopathy; *solid bars*, ischemic cardiomyopathy; *dotted bars*, valvular disease; **$p < 0.01$ versus control group (CONT); ‡$p < 0.01$ versus functional class I; §$p < 0.01$ versus functional class II. (From Imamura et al,[54] *J Am Coll Cardiol* 26:1594, 1995, reproduced with permission of the American College of Cardiology.)

CONCLUSION

There is an increasing body of literature confirming the feasibility of imaging the sympathetic innervation of the intact heart. These early studies suggest that the numerous hypotheses relating enhanced autonomic tone and autonomic imbalance to increased risk of arrhythmia and sudden death can be successfully tested. Future studies to compare functional abnormalities of the sympathetic nerves with myocardial perfusion, metabolism, and adrenergic receptor density may provide a more comprehensive understanding of the action of the autonomic nervous system in disease states. The ability to detect the distribution of innervation scintigraphically and to correlate these imaging findings with electrophysiologic assessment of vulnerability may provide important new understanding of the interaction of the sympathetic nerves and cardiac pathophysiology. In addition, a noninvasive means may be found to detect patients at risk for sudden death and possibly provide a basis for more rational approaches to therapy.

REFERENCES

1. Whitby LG, Axelrod J, Weil-Malherbe H: The fate of ^{3}H-norepinephrine in animals. *J Pharmacol Exp Ther* 132:193, 1961.
2. Iversen LL: Role of transmitter uptake mechanisms in synaptic neurotransmission. *Br J Pharmacol* 41:571, 1971.
3. Lightman SL, Iversen LL: The role of uptake in the extra-neuronal metabolism of catecholamines in the isolated rat heart. *Br J Pharmacol* 37:638, 1969.
4. Kopin I: False adrenergic transmitters. *Annu Rev Pharmacol* 8:377, 1968.
5. Wieland DM, Wu JL, Brown LE, et al: Radiolabeled adrenergic neuron-blocking agents: Adrenomedullary imaging with (131-I) iodobenzylguanidine. *J Nucl Med* 21:349, 1980.
6. Kline RC, Swanson DP, Wieland DM, et al: Myocardial imaging in man with I-123 metaiodobenzylguanidine. *J Nucl Med* 22:129, 1981.
7. Manger WM, Hoffman BB: Heart imaging in the diagnosis of pheochromocytoma and assessment of catecholamine uptake: Teaching editorial. *J Nucl Med* 24:1194, 1983.
8. Wieland DM, Brown LE, Rogers WL, et al: Myocardial imaging with a radioiodinated norepinephrine storage analog. *J Nucl Med* 22:22, 1981.
9. Sisson JC, Wieland DM, Sherman P, et al: Metaiodobenzylguanidine as an index of the adrenergic nervous system integrity and function. *J Nucl Med* 28:1620, 1987.
10. Dae M, De Marco T, Botvinick E, et al: Scintigraphic assessment of MIBG uptake in globally denervated human and canine hearts: Implications for clinical studies. *J Nucl Med* 33:1444, 1992.
11. De Marco T, Dae M, Yuen-Green M, et al: Iodine-123 metaiodobenzylguanidine scintigraphic assessment of the transplanted human heart: Evidence for late reinnervation. *J Am Coll Cardiol* 25:927, 1995.
12. Dae MW, O'Connell JW, Botvinick EH, et al: Scintigraphic assessment of regional cardiac adrenergic innervation. *Circulation* 79:634, 1989.
13. Sisson JC, Lynch JJ, Johnson J, et al: Scintigraphic detection of regional disruption of adrenergic neurons in the heart. *Am Heart J* 116:67, 1988.
14. Mori H, Pisarri T, Aldea G, et al: Usefulness and limitations of regional cardiac sympathectomy by phenol. *Am J Physiol* 257:HI523, 1989.
15. Dae M, O'Connell J, Botvinick E, Chin M: Acute and chronic effects of transient myocardial ischemia on sympathetic nerve activity, density, and norepinephrine content. *Cardiovasc Res* 30:270, 1995.
16. Barber MJ, Mueller TM, Henry DP, et al: Transmural myocardial infarction in the dog produces sympathectomy in noninfarcted myocardium. *Circulation* 67:787, 1983.
17. Herre J, Wetstein L, Lin YL, et al: Effect of transmural versus nontransmural myocardial infarction on inducibility of ventricular arrhythmias during sympathetic stimulation. *J Am Coll Cardiol* 11:414, 1988.
18. Dae M, Herre J, O'Connell J, et al: Scintigraphic assessment of sympathetic innervation after transmural versus nontransmural myocardial infarction. *J Am Coll Cardiol* 17:1416, 1991.
19. Dae M, Herre J, Botvinick E, et al: Scintigraphic assessment of adrenergic innervation after myocardial infarction. *Circulation* 74(suppl II):II-297, 1986.
20. Stanton MS, Tuli MM, Radtke NL, et al: Regional sympathetic denervation after myocardial infarction in humans detected noninvasively using I-123-metaiodobenzylguanidine. *J Am Coll Cardiol* 14:1519, 1989.
21. McGhie A, Corbett J, Akers M, et al: Regional cardiac adrenergic function using I-123 meta-iodobenzylguanidine tomographic imaging after acute myocardial infarction. *Am J Cardiol* 67:236, 1991.
22. Tomoda J, Yoshioka K, Shiina Y, et al: Regional sympathetic denervation detected by iodine 123 metaiodobenzylguanidine in non-W-wave myocardial infarction and unstable angina. *Am Heart J* 128:452, 1994.
23. Langer A, Freeman M, Josse R, Armstrong P: Metaiodobenzylguanidine imaging in diabetes mellitus: Assessment of cardiac sympathetic denervation and its relation to autonomic dysfunction and silent myocardial ischemia. *J Am Coll Cardiol* 25:610, 1995.
24. Wei K, Dorian P, Newman D, Langer A: Association between QT dispersion and autonomic dysfunction in patients with diabetes mellitus. *J Am Coll Cardiol* 26:859, 1995.
25. Schwartz PJ, Snebold NG, Brown AM: Effects of unilateral cardiac sympathetic denervation on the ventricular fibrillation threshold. *Am J Cardiol* 37:1034, 1976.
26. Schwartz PJ, Stone HL, Brown AM: Effects of unilateral stellate ganglion blockade on the arrhythmias associated with coronary occlusion. *Am Heart J* 92:589, 1976.
27. Randall WC, Kaye MP, Hageman GR, et al: Cardiac ar-

rhythmias in the conscious dog following surgically induced autonomic imbalance. *Am J Cardiol* 38:178, 1976.

28. Schwartz PJ: Sympathetic imbalance and cardiac arrhythmias, in Randall WC (ed): *Nervous Control of Cardiovascular Function.* New York, Oxford University Press, 1984, pp 225–252.

29. Minardo JD, Tuli MM, Mock BH, et al: Scintigraphic and electrophysiologic evidence of canine myocardial sympathetic denervation and reinnervation produced by myocardial infarction or phenol application. *Circulation* 78:1008, 1988.

30. Inoue H, Zipes D: Results of sympathetic denervation in the canine heart: Supersensitivity that may be arrhythmogenic. *Circulation* 75:877, 1987.

31. Newman D, Munoz L, Chin M, et al: Effects of canine myocardial infarction on sympathetic efferent neuronal function: Scintigraphic and electrophysiologic correlates. *Am Heart J* 126:1106, 1993.

32. Mitrani R, Klein L, Miles W, et al: Regional cardiac sympathetic denervation in patients with ventricular tachycardia in the absence of coronary artery disease. *J Am Coll Cardiol* 22:1344, 1993.

33. Gill J, Hunter G, Gane J, et al: Asymmetry of cardiac ^{123}I meta-iodobenzylguanidine scans in patients with ventricular tachycardia and a "clinically normal" heart. *Br Heart J* 69:6, 1993.

34. Dae M, Ursell P, Lee R, et al: Heterogeneous sympathetic innervation in German shepherd dogs with inherited ventricular arrhythmia and sudden death. *J Am Coll Cardiol* 25:20A, 1995 (abstr).

35. Wichter T, Hindricks G, Lerch H, et al: Regional myocardial sympathetic dysinnervation in arrhythmogenic right ventricular cardiomyopathy: An analysis using ^{123}I-metaiodobenzylguanidine scintigraphy. *Circulation* 89:667, 1994.

36. Muller K, Jakob H, Neuzner J, et al: ^{123}I-metaiodobenzylguanidine scintigraphy in the detection of irregular regional sympathetic innervation in long QT syndrome. *Eur Heart J* 14:316, 1993.

37. Henderson EB, Kahn JK, Corbett J, et al: Abnormal I-123 metaidobenzylguanidine myocardial washout and distribution may reflect myocardial adrenergic derangement in patients with congestive cardiomyopathy. *Circulation* 78:1192, 1988.

38. Tomaselli G, Beuckelmann D, Calkins H, et al: Sudden cardiac death in heart failure: The role of abnormal repolarization. *Circulation* 90:2534, 1994.

39. Consensus Trial Study Group: Effects of enalapril on mortality in severe congestive heart failure. *N Engl J Med* 316:1429, 1986.

40. Eichhorn E, Hjalmarson A: Beta-blocker treatment for chronic heart failure. *Circulation* 90:2153, 1994.

41. Meredith I, Broughton A, Jennings G, Esler M: Evidence of a selective increase in cardiac sympathetic activity in patients with sustained ventricular arrhythmias. *N Engl J Med* 325:618, 1991.

42. Myerburg R, Kessler K, Castellanos A: Sudden cardiac death: Structure, function, and time-dependence of risk. *Circulation* 85(suppl I):I-2, 1992.

43. Hurwitz J, Josephson M: Sudden cardiac death in patients with chronic coronary heart disease. *Circulation* 85(suppl I):I-43, 1992.

44. Francis G: Development of arrhythmias in the patient with congestive heart failure: Pathophysiology, prevalence, and prognosis. *Am J Cardiol* 57:3B, 1986.

45. Follansbee W, Michelson E, Morganroth J: Nonsustained ventricular tachycardia in ambulatory patients: Characteristics and association with sudden cardiac death. *Ann Intern Med* 92:741, 1980.

46. Gang E, Bigger J, Livell F: A model of chronic arrhythmias: The relationship between electrically inducible ventricular tachycardia, ventricular fibrillation threshold, and myocardial infarct size. *Am J Cardiol* 50:469, 1982.

47. Yusuf S, Peto R, Lewis J, et al: Beta-blockade during and after myocardial infarction: An overview of the randomized trials. *Prog Cardiovasc Dis* 25:335, 1985.

48. Chadda K, Goldstein S, Byington R, Curb J: Effect of propranalol after acute myocardial infarction in patients with congestive heart failure. *Circulation* 73:503, 1986.

49. Cohn J, Levine T, Olivari M, et al: Plasma norepinephrine as a guide to prognosis in patients with chronic congestive heart failure. *N Engl J Med* 311:819, 1984.

50. Sisson J, Bolgas G, Johnson J: Measuring acute changes in adrenergic nerve activity of the heart in the living animal. *Am Heart J* 121:1119, 1991.

51. Kingwell B, Thompson J, Kaye D, et al: Heart rate spectral analysis, cardiac norepinephrine spillover, and muscle sympathetic nerve activity during human sympathetic nervous activation and failure. *Circulation* 90:234, 1994.

52. Nakajima K, Taki J, Tonami N, Hisada K: Decreased 123-I MIBG uptake and increased clearance in various cardiac diseases. *Nucl Med Commun* 15:317, 1994.

53. Merlet P, Valette H, Dubois R, et al: Prognostic valve of cardiac metaiodobenzylguanidine imaging in patients with heart failure. *J Nucl Med* 33:471, 1992.

54. Imamura Y, Ando H, Mitsuoka W, et al: Iodine-123 metaiodobenzylguanidine images reflect intense myocardial adrenergic nervous activity in congestive heart failure independent of underlying cause. *J Am Coll Cardiol* 26:1594, 1995.

INDEX

Page numbers followed by f and t indicate figures and tables, respectively.

ISBN 0-07-032848-X